Textbook of
VETERINARY
DIAGNOSTIC
RADIOLOGY

Textbook of
VETERINARY DIAGNOSTIC RADIOLOGY

THIRD EDITION

DONALD E. THRALL, DVM, PhD

Professor of Radiology
College of Veterinary Medicine
North Carolina State University
Raleigh, North Carolina

W.B. SAUNDERS COMPANY

A Division of Harcourt Brace & Company
Philadelphia   London   Toronto   Montreal   Sydney   Tokyo

W.B. SAUNDERS COMPANY
A Division of Harcourt Brace & Company

The Curtis Center
Independence Square West
Philadelphia, Pennsylvania 19106

Library of Congress Cataloging-in-Publication Data

Textbook of veterinary diagnostic radiology / [edited by] Donald E. Thrall.—
3rd ed.

p.   cm.

ISBN 0–7216–5092–9

1. Veterinary radiography.   I. Thrall, Donald E.

SF757.8.T48   1998   636.089′0757—dc21   97-6593

Textbook of Veterinary Diagnostic Radiology   ISBN 0–7216–5092–9

Printed in the United States of America.

Last digit is the print number: 9   8   7   6   5   4   3   2   1

Contributors

GRAEME ALLAN, B.V.Sc., M.V.Sc., FACVSc, Diplomate ACVR
Consultant Veterinary Radiologist, The University of
Sydney Veterinary Teaching Hospital, Sydney, New South
Wales, Australia
Radiographic Signs of Joint Disease

ROBERT J. BAHR, D.V.M., Diplomate ACVR
Associate Professor of Veterinary Radiology, Departments
of Medicine and Surgery, College of Veterinary Medicine,
Oklahoma State University; Instructor of Record,
Radiology Section, Boren Veterinary Medical Teaching
Hospital, Stillwater, Oklahoma
The Thoracic Wall; The Heart and Great Vessels

DON L. BARBER, D.V.M., M.S., Diplomate ACVR
Professor and Head, Department of Small Animal Clinical
Sciences, Virginia-Maryland Regional College of Veterinary
Medicine, Virginia Tech, Blacksburg, Virginia
The Peritoneal Space; The Stomach

CLIFFORD R. BERRY, D.V.M., Diplomate ACVR
Associate Professor, Department of Veterinary Medicine
and Surgery, College of Veterinary Medicine, University of
Missouri, Columbia, Missouri
*Anatomic and Physiologic Imaging of the Canine and Feline
Brain; Physeal Disorders of the Immature Horse*

DARRYL N. BIERY, D.V.M., Diplomate ACVR
Professor of Veterinary Radiology, School of Veterinary
Medicine, University of Pennsylvania, Philadelphia,
Pennsylvania
The Large Bowel

J. GREGG BORING, D.V.M., M.S., Diplomate ACVR
Professor of Radiology, Staff Radiologist; Director,
Biomedical Research Center, College of Veterinary
Medicine, Mississippi State University, Mississippi State,
Mississippi; Graduate Faculty Fellow, School of Dentistry,
Department of Periodontics, University of Alabama College
of Medicine, Birmingham, Alabama
The Carpus

CHARLES S. FARROW, D.V.M., B.S.(Zool.), Diplomate ACVR
Professor of Medical Imaging, Western College of
Veterinary Medicine, University of Saskatchewan,
Saskatoon, Saskatchewan, Canada
Larynx, Pharynx, and Proximal Airway; The Equine Lung

DANIEL A. FEENEY, D.V.M., M.S., Diplomate ACVR
Professor of Veterinary Imaging, College of Veterinary
Medicine, and Staff Radiologist, Lewis Hospital for
Companion Animals, University of Minnesota, St. Paul,
Minnesota
The Kidneys and Ureters; The Uterus, Ovaries, and Testes

PATRICK R. GAVIN, D.V.M., Ph.D., Diplomate ACVR
Professor, Veterinary Radiology, Radiobiology, Advanced
Radiation-Physics, Veterinary Clinical Sciences, College of
Veterinary Medicine, Washington State University,
Pullman, Washington
The Equine Vertebral Column

GARY R. JOHNSTON, D.V.M., M.S., Diplomate ACVR
Professor, Department of Veterinary Comparative
Anatomy, Pharmacology and Physiology, College of
Veterinary Medicine, Washington State University,
Pullman, Washington
The Kidneys and Ureters; The Uterus, Ovaries, and Testes

STEPHEN K. KNELLER, D.V.M., M.S., Diplomate ACVR
Associate Professor, College of Veterinary Medicine,
University of Illinois, Urbana, Illinois
*The Metacarpus and Metatarsus; The Larynx, Pharynx, and
Trachea*

LINDA J. KONDE, D.V.M., Diplomate ACVR
Veterinary Radiologist, Diagnostic Imaging, P.C., Aurora,
Colorado
*Aggressive Versus Nonaggressive Bone Lesions; Diseases of the
Immature Skeleton*

CHRISTOPHER R. LAMB, M.A., Vet.M.B., Diplomate ACVR
Lecturer in Radiology, Royal Veterinary College, London,
United Kingdom
The Canine Lung

JIMMY C. LATTIMER, D.V.M., M.S., Diplomate ACVR
Associate Professor, Veterinary Medicine and Surgery,
Section of Radiology, College of Veterinary Medicine,
Missouri University; Staff Radiologist, Veterinary Medical
Teaching Hospital, Columbia, Missouri
Equine Nasal Passages and Sinuses; The Prostate Gland

JOHN M. LOSONSKY, D.V.M., M.S., Diplomate ACVR
Associate Professor, Department of Veterinary Clinical
Medicine, College of Veterinary Medicine, University of
Illinois; Staff Radiologist, Veterinary Medical Teaching
Hospital, Urbana, Illinois
The Pulmonary Vasculature

MARY B. MAHAFFEY, D.V.M., M.S., Diplomate ACVR
Professor of Radiology, Department of Anatomy and
Radiology, College of Veterinary Medicine, University of
Georgia, Athens, Georgia
The Stifle and Tarsus; The Peritoneal Space; The Stomach

SANDRA V. McNEEL, D.V.M., Diplomate ACVR
Consulting Radiologist, Vet Care Animal Clinic, Dublin,
California
The Phalanges; The Small Bowel

WENDY MYER, D.V.M., M.S., Diplomate ACVR
Emeritus Associate Professor, College of Veterinary
Medicine, Ohio State University, Columbus, Ohio
*Cranial Vault and Associated Structures; Nasal Cavity and
Paranasal Sinuses*

MARC PAPAGEORGES, D.V.M., Ph.D., Diplomate ACVR
Veterinary Radiologist and President, Veterinary Diagnostic
Imaging, P.C., Gresham, Oregon
*Visual Perception and Radiographic Interpretation; The Equine
Vertebral Column*

RICHARD D. PARK, D.V.M., Ph.D., Diplomate ACVR
Professor, Department of Radiological Health Sciences,
Colorado State University; Section Chief, Radiology,
Veterinary Teaching Hospital, Ft. Collins, Colorado
The Diaphragm; The Urinary Bladder

ROBERT D. PECHMAN, Jr., D.V.M., Diplomate ACVR
Professor of Veterinary Radiology, Department of
Veterinary Clinical Sciences, School of Veterinary
Medicine, Louisiana State University, Baton Rouge,
Louisiana
The Liver and Spleen; The Urethra

ELIZABETH A. RIEDESEL, D.V.M., Diplomate ACVR
Associate Professor of Veterinary Clinical Sciences, College
of Veterinary Medicine, Iowa State University; Leader,
Radiology, Veterinary Teaching Hospital, Ames, Iowa
The Phalanges; The Small Bowel

GREGORY D. ROBERTS, D.V.M., M.S., Diplomate ACVR
Assistant Professor, Veterinary Radiology, College of
Veterinary Medicine, University of Florida, Gainesville,
Florida
The Equine Vertebral Column

CHARLES R. ROOT, D.V.M., M.S., Diplomate ACVR
Owner, Animal Medical Imaging, Redmond, Washington
*The Thoracic Wall; The Heart and Great Vessels; Abdominal
Masses*

RON D. SANDE, D.V.M., M.S., Ph.D., Diplomate ACVR
Professor, Veterinary Clinical Radiology, College of
Veterinary Medicine, Washington State University,
Pullman, Washington

*The Metacarpophalangeal (Metatarsophalangeal) Articulation;
The Pleural Space*

JAMES E. SMALLWOOD, D.V.M., M.S.
Professor of Anatomy, College of Veterinary Medicine,
North Carolina State University, Raleigh, North Carolina
Radiographic Anatomy of the Dog and Horse

KATHY A. SPAULDING, D.V.M., Diplomate ACVR
Associate Professor, Radiology, College of Veterinary
Medicine, North Carolina State University, Raleigh, North
Carolina
Radiographic Anatomy of the Dog and Horse

RUSS STICKLE, D.V.M., Diplomate ACVR
Associate Professor, College of Veterinary Medicine,
Michigan State University, East Lansing, Michigan
The Equine Skull

DONALD E. THRALL, D.V.M., Ph.D., Diplomate ACVR
Professor of Radiology, College of Veterinary Medicine,
North Carolina State University, Raleigh, North Carolina
*Radiation Physics, Radiation Protection, and Darkroom Theory;
Introduction to Radiographic Interpretation; Bone Tumors Versus
Bone Infections; The Mediastinum; The Pleural Space*

ROBERT L. TOAL, D.V.M., M.S., Diplomate ACVR
Associate Professor, Department of Large Animal Clinical
Sciences, College of Veterinary Medicine, University of
Tennessee, Knoxville, Tennessee
Fracture Healing and Complications; The Navicular Bone

MICHAEL A. WALKER, D.V.M., Diplomate ACVR
Professor of Radiology, College of Veterinary Medicine,
Texas A&M University, College Station, Texas
The Vertebrae

BARBARA JEAN WATROUS, D.V.M., Diplomate ACVR
Professor, College of Veterinary Medicine, Oregon State
University, Corvallis, Oregon
The Esophagus

WILLIAM R. WIDMER, D.V.M., M.S., Diplomate ACVR
Associate Professor of Diagnostic Imaging, School of
Veterinary Medicine, Purdue University, West Lafayette,
Indiana
*Radiation Physics, Radiation Protection, and Darkroom Theory;
Intervertebral Disc Disease and Myelography*

Preface

As the turn of the century approaches, diagnostic radiology remains the primary modality used to image most patients in veterinary medicine. Specialized techniques such as diagnostic ultrasound, computed tomography, nuclear medicine, and magnetic resonance imaging are becoming more widely available and used, but diagnostic radiology continues to be the mainstay of veterinary imaging. Thus, a firm understanding of the principles of diagnostic radiology is essential for students of veterinary medicine. Accordingly, the main emphasis of this book as a textbook of veterinary diagnostic radiology has not changed, and additions have been made to augment this goal. The dog, cat, and horse remain the species receiving the greatest coverage in the book, as they represent the majority of animals seen in private veterinary practices throughout the world.

Diagnostic ultrasound continues to grow as an imaging modality in veterinary medicine. Its use is widespread, and it is becoming widely available to private practitioners. Clearly, there is a need for veterinary students to have some basic information regarding the use of diagnostic ultrasound in veterinary medicine. However, it is difficult to include in-depth textbook-quality coverage of both radiology and ultrasound under one cover without the work's becoming massive, and other excellent sources of veterinary diagnostic ultrasonography are available. For reasons stated above, this book continues to emphasize diagnostic radiology, although newer specialized modalities have been introduced in a new chapter covering canine brain imaging. Material on brain imaging was added because brain imaging is becoming more common in academic veterinary institutions as well as in private practice, and because such information may not be conveniently available in one source. In the new chapter on brain imaging, the basic physical principles of computed tomography, magnetic resonance imaging, and nuclear imaging are discussed, with particular reference to canine brain disorders. This well-illustrated chapter provides a basis for understanding imaging abnormalities of a highly complex system in which diseases are being recognized with increased frequency as these sophisticated modalities become more widely available.

Another enhancement to the Third Edition is a new chapter on radiation safety and the physics of diagnostic radiology. Inclusion of safety issues was considered important because of the hazards associated with the use of ionizing radiation. Also, an understanding of the physical principles of radiology not only aids in the understanding of disease processes but also reinforces the value of using ionizing radiation in a safe manner. The physics of radiology is taught in most introductory veterinary radiology courses, and the new information contained in the Third Edition supplements instruction of this important topic.

Another new chapter deals with visual perception. Students are often mystified by how easily experienced film-readers extract information from an image. Much of this "ease of interpretation" is the result of experience, but proper perception of what the eye beholds is also necesssary. In this exciting new chapter, the subject of perception is explained, and some of the mystery associated with image interpretation is removed.

Recognition of normal anatomy remains perhaps the most important skill to be mastered prior to becoming an accomplished interpreter of images. A section on normal radiographic anatomy was a new addition to the Second Edition of this book, and this section has been revised and expanded in the Third Edition. Illustrations have been updated, and there is broader coverage of equine radiographic anatomy.

Self-assessment is becoming a widely used tool in higher education. In the Third Edition of this work, self-assessment questions have been added to each chapter. Some of these questions involve interpretation of images. The answers to the questions are found in the back of the book, to allow students of radiology to evaluate their progress or knowledge of imaging in a particular area.

As noted in the First and Second Editions, it would be a gargantuan task for any one person to produce a comprehensive, accurate, high-quality veterinary radiology textbook. It is truly an asset to have contributions made to this book by so many distinguished individuals. Without their cooperation, expertise, and hard work, this book would not have been possible.

DONALD E. THRALL

Contents

PRINCIPLES OF INTERPRETATION

Chapter 1

Radiation Physics, Radiation Protection, and Darkroom Theory

Donald E. Thrall • William R. Widmer

X-rays were discovered on November 8, 1895, by Wilhelm Conrad Roentgen, a German physicist.[1] These new "rays" were quickly put to use for medical purposes, and many sophisticated medical applications were soon devised. For example, angiography was first described in 1896, only 1 year after the discovery of x-rays. The discovery of x-rays revolutionized the diagnosis and treatment of disease in humans and animals. In 1901, Roentgen was awarded the first Nobel Prize for Physics in recognition of his discovery.

More than 100 years after their discovery, x-rays remain in widespread use for many aspects of medical imaging. Although valuable for medical purposes, the interaction of x-rays with tissue produces ionization, which, in turn, may produce significant biologic damage. Because x-rays are so widely applied and potentially harmful, it is important that their basic principles be understood.

BASIC PROPERTIES OF X-RAYS

X-rays and gamma rays are types of electromagnetic radiation. The major difference between x-rays and gamma rays is where they originate; x-rays are produced by electron energy transitions outside the nucleus, whereas gamma rays are emitted from unstable atomic nuclei. Other familiar types of electromagnetic radiation are radio waves, radar, microwaves, and visible light (Table 1–1).

Electromagnetic radiation is a combination of electric and magnetic fields that travel together. It is convenient to represent electromagnetic radiation as a "sine wave" model (Fig. 1–1). Sine waves are characterized by two related parameters, frequency and wavelength (see Fig. 1–1). The velocity of electromagnetic radiation, which is the speed of light, is the product of the frequency and wavelength.

Velocity (m/sec) = frequency (cycles per sec) × wavelength (m)

All types of electromagnetic radiation travel at the speed of light; thus, frequency is inversely proportional to wavelength. The energy of electromagnetic radiation is related to wavelength by the formula:

$$\text{Energy} = \text{Planck's constant} \times \frac{\text{speed of light}}{\text{wavelength}}$$

Energy, therefore, is also inversely proportional to wavelength.

The basic unit of photon (x-ray) energy is the electron volt (eV). An eV is the energy an electron achieves if it is accelerated by a potential voltage difference of 1 volt. Photons with energies greater than 15eV, a low quantity of energy, can cause ionizations within living cells. Because x-rays used for diagnosis have energies more than 1000 times this amount, the need to deal with x-rays safely and treat them with respect is clear.

Some of the physical properties of x-rays and gamma rays cannot be adequately explained by theories of wave propagation. The photon, or quantum concept, was developed to explain the apparent particulate behavior of x-rays and gamma rays and how they interact with their targets to create an image or to cause radiation damage. A photon is a discrete bundle of energy.

Properties of x-rays and gamma rays are given in Table 1–2. The ionizing property of x-rays and gamma rays renders them biologically hazardous. Ionization occurs when a photon strikes a molecule and ejects an electron creating an ion pair. Following ionization, the physical and functional characteristics of the molecule are changed (Fig. 1–2). Because DNA is involved in all metabolic and clonogenic cell processes, an ionization in DNA may result in *biologic amplification*. In other words, a lesion induced in one cell's DNA can affect many cells for future generations to come. An ionization in DNA can lead to (1) an increase in rate of mutations; (2) an increased rate of abortions or fetal abnormalities if irradiated in utero; (3) an increase in susceptibility to disease and shortened life span; (4) an increased risk of cancer,

Direction of Travel →

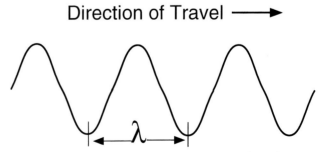

FIGURE 1–1. Sine wave model of electromagnetic radiation. The distance between crest separation, λ, is the wave length. Another characteristic of waves is their frequency, f, or the number of waves per unit time. The velocity (c) of a wave is related to wavelength and frequency by the formula, c = f × λ. Electromagnetic radiation travels at a constant speed, the speed of light.

Table 1–1
WAVELENGTH OF COMMON TYPES OF ELECTROMAGNETIC RADIATION

Type of Electromagnetic Radiation	Wavelength (cm)
Radio waves	30,000
Microwaves	10
Visible light	0.0001
X-rays	0.00000001

Table 1–2
PROPERTIES OF X-RAYS AND GAMMA RAYS

Have no charge
Have no mass
Travel at the speed of light
Are invisible
Cannot be felt
Travel in a straight line
Cannot be deflected by magnetic fields
Penetrate all matter to some degree
Cause certain substances to fluoresce
Can expose photographic emulsions
Can ionize atoms

particularly thyroid cancer, leukemia, and skin cancer; and (5) an increased risk of cataracts.[2] Such ionization interactions are exploited in radiation therapy with the intention of causing cell death. Because of the biologic damage that can be incurred by exposure to x-rays, it is necessary to have an understanding of principles of radiation protection.

RADIATION PROTECTION*

The object of diagnostic radiology is to obtain maximum diagnostic information with minimum exposure of the patient, radiology personnel, and general public. This section indicates the protection required in various circumstances and describes one or more methods by which the required protection may be achieved. The recommendations do not preclude alternative methods of achieving the radiation protection objectives. Because blind adherence to rules cannot substitute for the exercise of sound judgment, these recommendations may be modified in unusual circumstances on the professional advice of experts with recognized competence in radiation protection.

Radiation Units

For many years, the units roentgen, rad, and rem were used to quantify radiation exposure, radiation absorption, and equivalent dose. In 1977, the *International System of Units* (SI Units) was developed in keeping with the trend to universal adoption of the metric system.[3] The units roentgen, rad, and rem are not coherent with the SI system. The corresponding SI units for the roentgen and rad are coulomb per kilogram and joule per kilogram.

Because ionizing radiation has no mass and no charge, it can be detected only indirectly (i.e., it cannot be felt or weighed or detected by its perturbation of an electric field) (see Table 1–2). The amount of radiation exposure is commonly measured by detecting the number of ionizations (i.e., electrical charges) produced by the x-rays in air.

Exposure Quantity

Quantification of the amount of radiation striking a subject is often needed. This quantification is based on measurement of the number of ion pairs produced in air by the oncoming radiation and is expressed in the SI system as coulombs of charge per kilogram of air (C/kg). The old name used to describe exposure quantity was the roentgen. One roentgen is equal to production of 2.58×10^{-4} C/kg in air. No special name has been given to exposure quantity in the SI system, and exposure is quantified only in terms of C/kg.

Absorbed Dose

The efficiency by which various materials absorb x-rays varies considerably. Therefore, the radiation dose to objects with different absorption efficiencies is not constant when these objects are exposed to the same amount of radiation (Fig. 1–3). The SI unit for absorbed dose is the gray (Gy). The Gy is defined as the amount of radiation such that the absorbed energy is 1 joule/kg of tissue. Before SI units were accepted, the unit of absorbed dose was the rad, being equal to 100 ergs/g. By using appropriate conversion factors, it can be shown that 1 Gy = 100 rad. In soft tissue, exposure to 12.58 $\times$ 10^{-4} C/kg (1 roentgen) amounts to an absorbed dose of approximately 0.9 cGy (0.9 rad). Because bone is a more efficient absorber of x-rays than soft tissue, exposure of 12.58 $\times$ 10^{-4} C/kg (1 roentgen) results in a bone-absorbed dose of greater than 0.9 cGy. This differential between exposure and absorption in soft tissue versus bone may be as great as four to five times, depending on the energy of the radiation. The differential between exposure dose and absorbed dose is inversely proportional to photon energy.

Dose Equivalent

In living tissue, absorption of the same dose in Gy from different types of radiation does not necessarily produce the

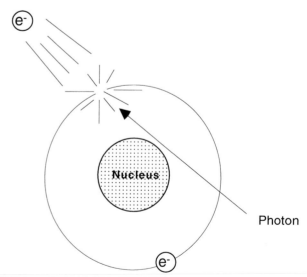

FIGURE 1–2. The principle of ionization. A quantity of electromagnetic radiation, often called a photon, interacts with a K-shell electron of an atom. The stippled circle represents the atomic nucleus. The electron is ejected; therefore, the atom is ionized. Ionization results in formation of an ion pair: the negatively charged electron and the positively charged atom. Subsequent to the ionization, the photon, depending on its energy, may be completely absorbed, or it may interact with other atoms to produce more ionizations. The ejected electron can interact with biologic molecules, such as DNA, and produce damage to macromolecules, resulting in cell death.

---

*Local, state, and national regulations supersede any recommendations given in this chapter.

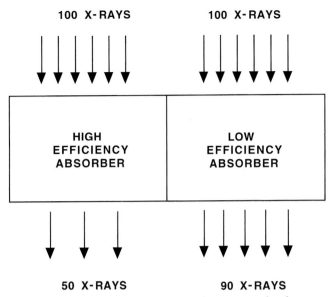

FIGURE 1–3. In this figure, two materials are exposed to 100 x-rays. Thus, the exposure dose, or dose in roentgens, is the same in each instance. However, the efficiency of x-ray absorption is not the same for each absorber. The absorber on the left absorbs 50 percent of x-rays hitting it, while the absorber on the right absorbs only 10 percent. Therefore, the absorbed dose will be higher in the absorber on the left, even though the exposure dose is the same. Bone is an efficient absorber of x-rays compared with soft tissues, such as fat and muscle.

same biologic effect. For example, the damage resulting from particulate radiations, such as alpha particles and neutrons, is higher on a Gy-for-Gy basis than the damage produced by the same dose of x-rays. This phenomenon is related to differences in *ionization density* for different types of radiation. For example, a high-mass, heavily charged particle, such as an alpha particle (a helium nucleus; two nuclear protons, two nuclear neutrons, no orbital electrons), creates many ionizations close to one another in tissue in comparison to a low-mass, lightly charged particle, such as an electron. Electrons set in motion by x-rays interacting with tissue (ionizations) are the major source of tissue damage resulting from x-ray exposure; this is described in greater detail later. Therefore, deposition of one Gy from alpha particle absorption does more biologic damage than deposition of one Gy from x-ray absorption. Damage from different types of radiation may be compared by use of a weighting factor, a numerical factor describing the relative effectiveness of a type of radiation to photons. The weighting factor for photons is 1.0 and is greater than 1.0 for charged or particulate types of radiation, such as neutrons or alpha particles. In the SI system of units, the unit of dose equivalency is the Sievert (Sv); the Sv is derived from the product of the absorbed dose in Gy and the weighting factor. Before SI units were accepted, the unit of dose equivalency was the rem. The rem was derived from the product of the absorbed dose in rads and the weighting factor. Because 1 Gy = 100 rads, 1 Sv = 100 rem. As a rule of thumb, an absorbed dose of 1 Gy from photons results approximately in an equivalent dose of 1 Sv.

Radiation Safety

The United States Nuclear Regulatory Commission (NRC) is the official source for establishing guidelines for radiation protection. The NRC has indicated that the annual occupational radiation dose to individual adults be limited to a maximum of 0.05 Sv (5 rem) per year.[4] The NRC has not established an upper limit for *cumulative* exposure. Previously

the NRC recommended that one's cumulative exposure be less than [5 rem/yr × (n − 18)], where *n* is the age of the individual; this recommendation has been overruled in favor of the ALARA principle (see below). Although the NRC is the official body regarding exposure limits for ionizing radiation, other groups also make recommendations regarding such. One other group is the National Council on Radiation Protection (NCRP), a governmental scientific group that meets regularly to review recent radiation research and update radiation safety recommendations. According to the NCRP, the objectives of radiation protection are:

1. To prevent clinically significant radiation-induced effects by adhering to dose limits that are below the apparent or practical threshold.

2. To limit the risk of cancer and heritable effects to a reasonable level in relation to societal needs, values, and benefits gained.[5]

These objectives can be met by adhering to the principle of ALARA—limiting exposure of radiation workers to a level As Low As Reasonably Achievable—and by applying established dose levels for controlling occupational and general public exposures.[6]

Maximum permissible dose is the maximum amount of absorbed radiation that can be delivered to an individual as a whole-body dose or as a dose to a specific organ and still be considered safe. The term *safe* in this context means there is no evidence that individuals receiving the maximum dose mentioned will suffer harmful immediate or long-term effects to the body as a whole or to any individual structure or organ of the body. Although the effect of very low doses of radiation is not known with certainty, it is safest to assume that any amount of radiation will have some effect on the subject. Thus, one should keep in mind that whenever an individual is exposed to ionizing radiation, some biologic damage may occur, and following the ALARA principle is of paramount importance. Analogy might be made to an individual smoking a cigarette only once a month. There is no evidence with this frequency of smoking that physical damage could result; however, with increasing frequency of smoking, the probability steadily escalates by virtue of its cumulative effect. Unfortunately, there is no established threshold for either cigarette smoking or radiation under which damage will not occur or over which damage will definitely result.

In December 1989, the National Academy of Sciences Committee on the Biological Effects of Ionizing Radiation (BEIR) produced its latest report, which concluded that radiation risks had until then been underestimated, specifically that the likelihood of cancer induction after exposure to low radiation doses is three to four times higher than previously thought.[7] Much of their data was derived from studies of survivors of the World War II atomic bomb explosions in Japan. Because few large human exposures to radiation have been documented, events such as Hiroshima/Nagasaki and Chernobyl have provided valuable information on tolerance to low-level radiation exposure. Also, the Department of Energy has released information of human radiation exposure experiments that were conducted during the cold war period of the 1950s and 1960s.

Even though ALARA is the official method of choice for limiting one's exposure to radiation dose, recommendations for upper limits of exposure have also been established by the NCRP to guide those involved in radiation work. The NCRP recommends the following:[8]

1. An individual worker's lifetime effective dose should not exceed age in years × 10 mSv (age in years × 1 rem),

and no occupational exposure should be permitted until age 18. Therefore, an individual's lifetime effective dose equivalent in rems should not exceed the value of his or her age in years.

2. The effective dose in any one year should not exceed 50 mSv (5 rem).

3. For the general public, radiation exposure (excluding from medical use) should not exceed 1 mSv (0.1 rem).

4. Once pregnancy is declared, the monthly limit to the embryo or fetus should not exceed 0.5 mSv (0.05 rem). Specific controls for occupationally exposed women are no longer recommended until a pregnancy is declared.

The difference in opinion between the NRC and NCRP regarding limits for cumulative exposure can be confusing. It is important to recognize that the NRC is the agency officially responsible for identifying Federal exposure standards. The NRC has elected to eliminate any recommendations regarding cumulative exposure limits, probably because of the uncertainty of such a prediction. The NCRP has elected to establish an estimate for acceptable cumulative exposure, which is much more conservative than that previously recommended by the NRC. Regardless, it is in the best interest of the radiation worker to adhere to the principle of ALARA regarding occupational exposure and to use the most conservative of any conflicting recommendations as a guideline.

In addition to occupational exposure, the population is continually exposed to very low levels of radiation, both natural and man-made. A breakdown of relative exposure of the United States public to radiation by various sources was published by the NCRP in 1987 (Fig. 1–4).[9] Briefly, the average United States citizen receives 3.6 mSv (360 mrem) annually; of this figure, more than 80 percent is due to inhalation of radon gas. The relative levels of different sources of exposure may vary based on geographic location. For example, because of greater altitude, exposure to cosmic radiation is higher in Colorado than in North Carolina, and in eastern Pennsylvania, household radon exposure is much greater than in most other areas in the United States. Table 1–3 shows typical radiation doses received from some familiar activities.

Biologic Principles

X-rays produce electron pairs (ionizations) in tissue. Because most tissue is 70 percent water, ionization of water molecules causes the formation of chemically active free radicals. These free radicals account for most of the damage to tissue. A smaller percentage of x-rays interact directly with DNA, resulting in several potential alterations, such as base nucleo-

Table 1–3
RADIATION DOSES RECEIVED FROM SOME FAMILIAR ACTIVITIES*

Event	Radiation Dose Received (mSv)
Flight from Los Angeles to Paris	.05
Thoracic radiograph	.22
Apollo X astronauts moon flight	4.8
Whole-mouth dental x-ray	9.1
Dose on Three Mile Island during accident	11.0
Mammography	15.0
Barium enema	80.0
Heart catheterization	450.0
Radiation therapy	70,000.0

*Doses are whole body in some instances and regional in others.

tide damage, DNA strand breakage, and DNA cross-linkage. These effects may be minimal and quickly repaired enzymatically or can result in lethal damage to the cell. DNA is uniquely sensitive because it is a large target relative to other intracellular structures and possesses little redundancy within any one cell. The principle of biologic amplification as described previously is another reason why DNA damage can have serious consequences.

Depending on the tissue involved, a given dose of x-rays can have effects varying in magnitude from imperceptible to lethality. The type of tissue irradiated has an impact on the effects of radiation. For example, a tissue that does not divide, such as muscle, may receive a high dose while exhibiting few side effects. Conversely, actively dividing tissues, such as intestinal epithelium and bone marrow, are quite responsive to radiation.

Two other tissues, gonadal and fetal, are of crucial importance with respect to radiation safety. Irradiation of these tissues at sensitive stages can result in biologic amplification of any damage caused. The younger the fetus/embryo, the greater the potential for damage, which may be manifested as embryonic death, congenital malformation, or growth defect.

Practical Considerations

To maximize their ability to protect themselves, radiation workers in veterinary practices must be aware of the risks of radiation. They should be skilled in proper patient positioning for radiography, machine operation, and darkroom techniques so that repeat radiographic studies are minimized. Workers should be instructed on proper use and care of radiation protection devices. Reduction of radiation exposure to an individual from external radiation sources may be achieved by any one or any combination of the following measures:

1. Distance—increasing the distance of the individual from the radiation source.

2. Time—reducing the duration of exposure.

3. Shielding—using protective barriers between the individual and radiation source.

With reference to x-ray equipment used by veterinarians, shielding and distance are the factors most readily controlled. Shielding may comprise permanent protective barriers and structural shielding, such as walls containing lead, concrete, or other materials in thickness sufficient to provide the required degree of attenuation. Shielding may also be a protective barrier incorporated into equipment, such as an alumi-

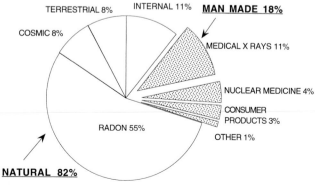

FIGURE 1–4. United States sources of exposure dose from ionizing radiation.

num filter to remove scattered radiation or a collimator to limit the size of the primary x-ray beam. Shielding may also consist of mobile or temporary devices used as the occasion demands, such as movable screens or lead-impregnated aprons or gloves.

Protective aprons and gloves are usually 0.5-mm Pb equivalent, and they must be worn when positioning patients for radiography. Although these devices are heavy and seemingly provide considerable protection, they are designed solely for protecting against scattered radiation and must never be placed in the primary beam. In addition, mishandling of this equipment results in it cracking and therefore affording less protection. Protective equipment should be treated with respect; it is used to protect the health of the radiation worker.

Pregnant and potentially pregnant women and individuals under 18 years of age should not hold animal patients during radiologic examination or treatment. A radiation protection supervisor (who may also be the user) should be designated for every installation to assume the responsibilities outlined next and to advise on the establishment of safe working conditions in compliance with all pertinent federal, state, and local regulations. The radiation protection supervisor should be familiar with the basic principles of radiation protection to carry out these responsibilities properly, although he or she may wish to consult with appropriate qualified experts for advice.

Suggested responsibilities of the radiation protection supervisor are the following:

1. To establish and supervise written operating procedures and to review them periodically to ensure their conformity with local regulations.

2. To instruct personnel in proper radiation protection practices.

3. To conduct or have conducted radiation surveys where indicated and to keep records of such surveys and tests, including summaries of corrective measures recommended or instituted.

4. To observe routinely and test periodically interlock switches and warning signals to ensure that they are working properly.

5. To ensure that warning signs and signals are properly located.

6. To determine the cause of each known or suspected case of excessive abnormal exposure and to take steps to prevent its recurrence.

Personnel Monitoring

Personnel monitoring is used to (1) check the adequacy of the radiation safety program, (2) to disclose improper radiation protection practices, and (3) to detect potentially serious radiation exposure situations. A film badge is commonly used as a personnel monitoring device. A film badge consists of a plastic holder that contains a paper-wrapped piece of photographic film. When struck by ionizing radiation, the film becomes exposed. Either monthly or quarterly the film is processed, and the degree of film blackening is equated to the amount of radiation reaching the film.

Personnel monitoring should be performed in controlled areas for each occupationally exposed individual for whom there is a reasonable possibility of receiving a dose exceeding one-fourth the applicable maximum permissible dose. A qualified expert should be consulted on establishment and evaluation of the personnel monitoring system. Devices worn for the monitoring of occupational exposure should not be worn by the individual when he or she is exposed as a patient for medical of dental examinations. Monitoring devices should be worn on the chest or abdomen except for special conditions. When a protective apron is worn, the monitoring device should be worn on the outside of the apron for monitoring the radiation environment but may be worn inside the apron when an estimate of the body exposure is desired.

Basic Radiation Safety Rules for Diagnostic Radiology

1. Remove personnel from the room who are not involved in the procedure.

2. Never permit anyone under the age of 18 or pregnant women in the room during the examination.

3. Rotate personnel who assist with radiographic examinations to minimize exposure to any one person.

4. Use sandbags, sponges, tapes, or other restraining devices for positioning the patient rather than manual restraint.

5. Use anesthesia or tranquilization for patient restraint when possible.

6. Never permit any part of the body to be in the primary beam, whether protected by gloves or aprons or not.

7. Never hold an x-ray tube, x-ray machine, or cassette in the hand.

8. Always wear protective aprons when assisting in positioning an animal.

9. Always wear protective gloves if hands are placed near the primary beam.

10. Consider use of protective goggles if work level is heavy. These glasses provide 0.25-mm Pb equivalent protection and offer protection to the lens of the eye.

11. Consider use of thyroid shields. These are mini-aprons that are worn around the neck and serve to protect the thyroid gland.

12. Use the collimator of the x-ray machine so there is an unexposed border on each film, proving that the primary beam does not exceed the size of the cassette.

13. Use the fastest film-screen combinations that are compatible with obtaining diagnostic radiographs.

14. All personnel should wear film badges outside the lead apron.

15. Plan the procedure carefully, and double-check machine settings.

PRODUCTION OF X-RAYS

Whenever high-speed electrons strike metal, x-rays are produced. X-ray tubes provide for acceleration of electrons and their subsequent interaction with a metal target. The initial step in producing x-rays is passage of an electric current through the filament (cathode) of the x-ray tube, much the same as an electric current is used to heat the filament of a light bulb. The heat allows electrons to "boil" off from the surface of the filament and to form an electron cloud around the filament (Fig. 1–5). The number of electrons in the cloud is controlled by the amount of electric current passing through the filament. This is determined by the mA (milliamperage) control on the panel of the x-ray machine. Increasing milliamperage is analogous to increasing the wattage of a light bulb. A 100-watt bulb has a hotter filament and emits more light rays per unit time than a 60-watt bulb. There is more current flowing through the filament of a 100-watt bulb than through a 60-watt bulb.

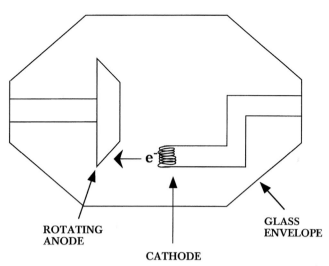

FIGURE 1–5. A schematic drawing of a rotating-anode x-ray tube. The anode rotates at high speed, dissipating heat over a large surface area.

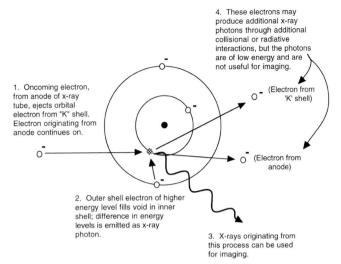

FIGURE 1–6. The collision model of x-ray production. An electron produced in an x-ray tube is accelerated to high speed through a potential difference and strikes an atom in the target of the x-ray tube. In some collisions, the oncoming electron will eject an orbital electron from the target atom and continue on at a different angle. Atoms with vacancies in electron shells are unstable, and the vacancy is quickly filled by a more peripheral electron, or a free electron. When this occurs, energy deposited by the original oncoming electron, which resulted in ejection of the target electron, is released in the form of electromagnetic radiation, called an x-ray. In general, electrons in shells near the nucleus are tightly bound and have less kinetic energy than those in peripheral shells. Electrons in the most peripheral shells are essentially "free" and have more energy owing to their weak attraction to the positively charged nucleus. Therefore, as an electron is ejected from the K shell, replacement electrons must give up energy before they can occupy the K shell.

The anode (target) is where x-rays are produced (see Fig. 1–5). X-rays are produced whenever high-speed electrons strike metal. Because electrons that have been produced at the filament remain stationary, there is a need to get them to strike the metallic target. This is done by applying a voltage differential between the anode and cathode. Electrons are negatively (−) charged. Therefore, if the target is positive (+) with respect to the filament of the cathode, the electrons are attracted to the target (opposite charges attract) and strike it. The energy of x-rays produced is a function of the energy of the electrons striking the anode. This energy is adjusted with the kilovoltage peak (kVp) control on the x-ray panel. Increasing kVp increases the voltage difference between the anode and cathode; thus, electrons are accelerated to higher velocities and have more energy when striking the anode. This provides for production of high-energy x-rays.

When electrons strike the metallic target, x-rays are produced by either collisional or radiative interactions.[10] Collisional interactions involve a collision between a high-speed electron and an atom in the target of the tube. The oncoming electron ejects an orbital electron from the atom with subsequent release of energy as an x-ray (Fig. 1–6). X-rays produced by this mechanism have specific energies, relating to the energy required to eject the target electron from its shell (the binding energy), and are therefore called characteristic x-rays. X-rays created by collisional interactions constitute only a small fraction of the total x-rays created in a diagnostic x-ray tube.

In a radiative interaction (Fig. 1–7), the oncoming high-speed electron passes close to the nucleus of the target atom (attracted by the opposite charge), but an electron is not ejected from the atom. As the electron slows as it bends around the nucleus, it releases energy in the form of electromagnetic radiation, called *braking radiation*, or bremsstrahlung. The energy released in the form of bremsstrahlung has a broad spectrum, depending on the amount of energy lost from electrons as they are deflected in various amounts by the nucleus. Most electrons have many interactions with atoms of the target as their kinetic energy is lost.

A range (spectrum) of energies of x-rays is produced for any given combination of mAs and kVp settings. This results from (1) most electrons undergoing multiple radiative interactions with each interaction resulting in production of an x-ray of different energy and (2) the wide range of energies of the electrons striking the anode (Fig. 1–8). The maximum x-

ray photon energy achievable is one with an energy equal to the kVp. For this to occur, an electron must be accelerated at maximal velocity (see next paragraph) and lose all of its energy in one interaction. As can be seen in Figure 1–8, the number of x-ray photons in the spectrum with an energy equal to the kVp is small.

At this time, it is important that the difference between the terms *kVp* and *keV** be understood. The kVp (kilovoltage peak) refers to the maximum voltage applied to the x-ray tube across the anode-cathode gap. In the United States,

---

*An electron vole (eV) is the amount of energy an electron gains as it is accelerated by a potential difference of 1 volt. 1 keV = 1000 eV.

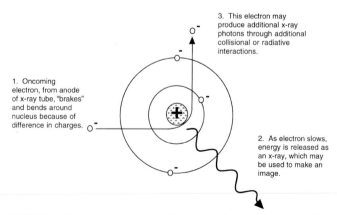

FIGURE 1–7. The radiative, or braking, model of x-ray production. An electron produced in an x-ray tube is accelerated to high speed through a large potential difference. Because of the difference in charge between the electron (negative) and the nucleus (positive), the electron is deflected as it nears the nucleus. As the deflected electron decelerates, it releases electromagnetic radiation in the form of an x-ray. Because deflected electrons may pass within various distances of the nucleus, braking radiation has a spectrum of energies.

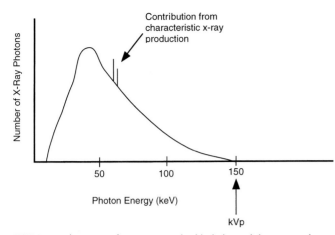

FIGURE 1–8. The spectrum of x-ray energy produced by braking and characteristic radiation. The maximal energy x-ray photon achievable is equal to the kVp. For this to occur, an electron must be accelerated at maximal velocity and release all of its energy in one interaction. As can be seen, the number of x-rays in the spectrum with an energy equal to the kVp is very small.

electric current is alternating; thus, for any given kVp setting, the voltage potential difference across the anode-cathode gap fluctuates between positive 110 volts and negative 110 volts (Fig. 1–9). The keV (kiloelectron volt) is a unit of energy, and keV can be used to describe the energy of either electrons or photons. If the kVp is set at 100 (100,000 volts maximum differential between the anode and cathode), electrons traveling from anode to cathode have energies equal to or less than 100 keV (100,000 electron volts). Few electrons achieve an energy of 100 keV because of the fluctuating nature of the voltage across the anode-cathode gap (i.e., the voltage is only at its maximum value for an instant during each cycle). If a 100-keV electron loses all of its energy in one interaction, it produces an x-ray photon with an energy of 100 keV. As noted previously, this is uncommon, and only a few x-ray photons in the beam have an energy equal to the kVp, and it is unusual for an electron to lose all of its energy in one interaction (see Fig. 1–8).

A basic discussion of problems relating to the use of alternating current for production of x-rays is necessary. If alternating current (see Fig. 1–9) were used for x-ray production, there would be times in the current fluctuation cycle when the cathode would be positive in relation to the anode. Any free electrons at the surface of the anode, present because of the high temperature of the anode, would be attracted to the cathode and damage it. To avoid this, alternating current is changed into direct current, and this process is called rectification. An in-depth discussion of rectification is beyond the scope of this book, but it is important to understand that rectification results in direct current application across the cathode-anode gap, and electrons therefore travel only from the cathode to the anode.

Much of the energy (>90 percent) of the electrons striking the anode is converted to heat. Therefore, x-ray tube targets are typically made of high melting–point substances, such as tungsten. Additionally, as an ancillary heat-dissipation mechanism, the anode may be designed to rotate to increase the effective surface area that is struck by the oncoming high-speed electrons. This rotation prevents the target from melting or becoming "pitted," as would happen if electrons struck the same small target region at all times. Targets in x-ray tubes are also typically made of a high atomic number material, such as tungsten, because the efficiency of x-ray production from electron interactions is directly related to atomic number.

The focal spot is the part of the target struck by electrons and thus the site of x-ray production. The smaller the focal spot, the better the detail on the radiograph. A practical example of this phenomenon is the sharpness of a shadow cast by a large versus small light source. A shadow cast by a small light source, assuming the distance from the light to the object is constant, is always sharper than a shadow cast by a large light source (see later section on image detail). Therefore, it is desirable to have the smallest focal spot possible. Angling the anode is one way to make the focal spot of the x-ray tube appear smaller than it really is, while maintaining a larger area on the anode being struck by electrons to facilitate heat distribution (Fig. 1–10).

Some x-ray tubes have two focal spots (filaments), which are operator selectable. The small filament is used to produce a small focal spot when greater image detail is necessary. One disadvantage of using the small filament is that one must also use low mA values or the filament will burn out.

It has already been stated that the mA controls the number of x-rays produced. Increasing mA increases the number of x-rays. The total number of x-rays produced can also be controlled by changing the length of time the x-ray tube is energized. A timer on the x-ray machine panel controls the length of time current is applied to the cathode and voltage is applied across the anode-cathode gap. X-rays are produced

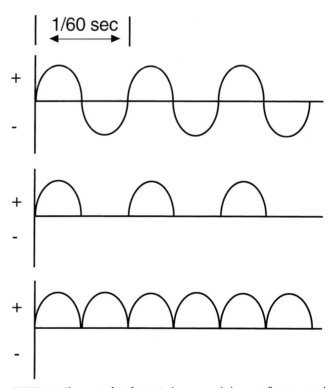

FIGURE 1–9. The concept of rectification. In the upper panel, the current fluctuation typical of alternating current is seen. There is one complete cycle every 60 seconds. If this current were used for voltage application in the x-ray tube, the cathode (filament) would be positive in relation to the anode (target) approximately half of the time. During this time, free electrons at the anode, created by heat build-up, would be attracted to the cathode and damage it. The middle panel illustrates the current pattern obtained when current is not allowed to flow during the negative phase of the cycle. In this instance, there is no tendency for electrons to flow from the anode to the cathode. One disadvantage of this type of current modification is a loss of potentially useful current during the negative phase of the cycle. Methods have been developed to reverse the direction of current flow in half of the cycle, and the resultant waveform is shown in the bottom panel. This is termed full-wave rectification and results in one useful pulse of current every 1/120 second. Many other modern methods provide direct and nearly nonfluctuating constant-potential current to the x-ray tube, but these are beyond the scope of this book.

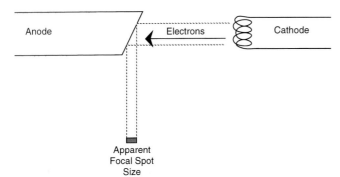

FIGURE 1–10. Angling the anode effectively decreases the size of the focal spot and ensures that a larger area on the anode will be struck by electrons to facilitate heat distribution.

only when there is a source of electrons and a voltage differential is present across the anode-cathode gap.

The concept of *mAs* (milliampere-seconds) is important in diagnostic radiology. It is a concept whereby the amount of radiation produced by the x-ray tube can be quantified. mAs is simply the product of mA (the setting on the control panel) and time, in seconds. The concept of mAs is analogous to allowing a 60-watt bulb to burn twice as long as a 120-watt bulb; in both instances, the total number of light rays emitted is the same, although the intensity at any one time is twice as great for the 120-watt bulb. A variety of combinations of mA and time can be used to produce the same number of x-rays (Table 1–4).

INTERACTION OF RADIATION WITH MATTER

To understand how radiographs are produced using x-rays, it is necessary to understand the ways in which radiation interacts with matter. There are five possibilities regarding interaction of a photon with matter: (1) coherent scattering, (2) photoelectric effect, (3) Compton scattering, (4) pair production, and (5) photodisintegration. Pair production and photodisintegration have no relevance to diagnostic radiology and are not discussed. A basic description of the coherent, photoelectric, and Compton processes is given, and sources for more detailed reading are available.[10]

Coherent Scattering

With coherent scattering, a photon interacts with an object and changes its direction, but there is no absorption of the photon by the subject and no change in photon energy. The percentage of x-rays striking a patient that undergo coherent scattering is small, approximately 5 percent. This type of interaction is not useful in terms of producing the radiograph and is in fact disadvantageous because these scattered photons may reach the x-ray film and degrade the image quality

Table 1–4

CONSTANT mAs CAN BE PRODUCED BY A VARIETY OF mA AND TIME COMBINATIONS

mA	Time (sec)	mAs
50	0.1	5
100	0.05	5
500	0.01	5
1000	0.005	5

(see later section), or they may strike the radiographer, increasing his or her exposure.

Photoelectric Effect

This type of interaction is important in diagnostic radiology. The x-ray striking the patient is totally absorbed in this absorption process (Fig. 1–11); thus, there is no scattered radiation to contend with. The x-ray photon ejects an electron, called a photoelectron, from an inner shell of a tissue atom. The photoelectron may produce multiple ionization events in the tissue and is eventually absorbed in the patient. When the vacancy created by ejection of the photoelectron is filled by a peripheral shell electron, or a free electron, a characteristic x-ray is given off (see Fig. 1–6). This is the same type of characteristic x-ray given off in the target of an x-ray tube when the oncoming electron from the cathode creates a vacancy in a target atom. The energy of characteristic radiation is related to the atomic number of the atom from which it arises. Thus, with a large atomic number atom such as tungsten (the target of the x-ray tube), the characteristic x-ray is actually a part, albeit small, of the useful x-ray beam. In the body, the energy of characteristic x-rays is so low that they are absorbed locally and therefore contribute to the absorbed dose in the patient being radiographed but not to production of the radiographic image. The probability of a photoelectric interaction is directly proportional to the cube of the atomic number and inversely proportional to the cube of the photon energy. The relationship between the photoelectric process and the atomic number of the absorber is important. This *magnifies* differences in absorption ability of various tissue types, such as bone versus soft tissue and soft tissue versus fat. If it were not for the atomic number dependence of the photoelectric effect, there would be insufficient differential absorption of x-ray photons between tissues for the resultant image to have any contrast (i.e., all

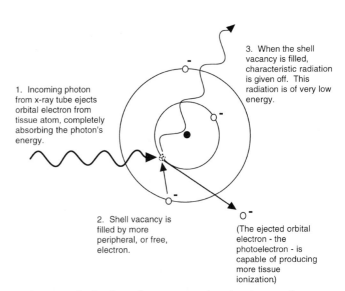

FIGURE 1–11. The photoelectric effect. An incoming photon from the x-ray tube ejects an electron, usually from an inner shell, of a tissue atom. The incoming photon is completely absorbed. Electrons in shells near the nucleus are tightly bound and have less kinetic energy than those in peripheral shells. Electrons in the most peripheral shells are essentially "free," owing to their weak attraction to the positively charged nucleus. Therefore, as a photoelectron is ejected from the K shell, replacement electrons must give up energy before they can occupy the shell. This energy is released in the form of a photon, called characteristic radiation, because shell energy levels are specific to the type of atom. In tissue, the characteristic radiation is of extremely low energy and is absorbed.

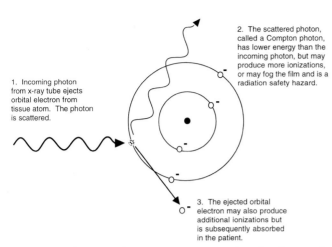

1. Incoming photon from x-ray tube ejects orbital electron from tissue atom. The photon is scattered.

2. The scattered photon, called a Compton photon, has lower energy than the incoming photon, but may produce more ionizations, or may fog the film and is a radiation safety hazard.

3. The ejected orbital electron may also produce additional ionizations but is subsequently absorbed in the patient.

FIGURE 1–12. The Compton absorption process. An incoming photon from the x-ray tube ejects an electron, usually from an outer shell, of a tissue atom. The incoming photon is scattered, not absorbed as in the photoelectric process. The ejected electron and scattered photon may continue and produce additional ionizations.

tissues would appear of similar opacity on the radiograph), and the radiograph would be useless. The differential absorption characteristics of the photoelectric process allow meaningful images to be produced. Another advantage of the photoelectric effect is the lack of unwanted exposure of the x-ray film because of scattered photons (film fog; see later section). Patient dose associated with the photoelectric effect is high, however, because all the energy of the oncoming photon is absorbed in the patient. Obviously the photoelectric interaction is good for the x-ray film but bad for the patient. The decrease in probability of photoelectric absorption as the energy of the photon beam increases results in a loss of contrast between tissues of various types when very high-energy (kVp) beams are used for radiography.

Compton Scattering

Almost all scattered radiation that is encountered in diagnostic radiology results from Compton scattering. In the Compton reaction, an oncoming x-ray photon interacts with a peripheral-shell electron of the patient. The electron is ejected, and the photon is scattered at a different angle; the scattered photon has lower energy than the original photon (Fig. 1–12). The scattered electron is termed either a *Compton electron* or a *recoil electron*. The probability of a Compton reaction depends on the total number of electrons in the absorber (patient), which, in turn, depends on its physical density (g/cm³) and number of electrons per gram. The probability of a Compton interaction increases as photon energy increases. Because most elements contain about the same number of electrons per unit mass, the probability of a Compton reaction is independent of atomic number. Such independence is disadvantageous. This pertains to the third-order (proportional to Z^3) dependence of photoelectric absorption on atomic number, which results in great differences in absorption (good tissue contrast) between tissues *versus* the first-order dependence (proportional to Z^3) of Compton absorption on physical density differences or electron density differences between tissues, which results in poor contrast. Thus, if the energy of the x-ray beam is such that Compton absorption predominates, there is little contrast in the image. This is why it is important to use x-ray beams with an energy in which the photoelectric absorption reaction predominates.

The photon scattering that occurs with Compton interactions is also disadvantageous because the scattered photons are radiation safety considerations, and they degrade the image by fogging it.

BASIC CONCEPT OF MAKING A RADIOGRAPH

In making radiographs, the patient is placed between the x-ray tube and an x-ray film (Fig. 1–13). In Figure 1–13, x-rays are emitted from the x-ray tube. As noted earlier, the spectrum of energy of x-rays produced by a diagnostic x-ray tube is broad. X-ray photons of low energy serve no useful purpose because they are absorbed in the patient and make no useful contribution to creation of the image. Therefore, filters are routinely placed in the x-ray tube housing to remove these low-energy x-rays. Some x-rays passing through the filter are absorbed by the beam-shaping collimator or tube housing and do not hit the patient. The collimator serves to limit the primary beam and prevent nonuseful radiation from leaving the tube housing. This nonuseful radiation serves only to (1) increase patient dose, (2) degrade image quality because of fogging (see later section on grids), and (3) increase dose to technical personnel. In Figure 1–13, three x-rays are seen leaving the collimator. The one on the left completely penetrates the patient and will be recorded on the x-ray film. It is necessary to have some x-rays penetrate the patient or no information would be recorded on the film. The middle x-ray hits a structure in the patient and is completely absorbed. This is also beneficial and emphasizes an important point: Radiographs are possible only because of differential absorption of x-rays by the patient. If absorption were uniform, it would be impossible to distinguish various structures in the patient. The x-ray on the right hits the patient and is scattered in another direction. In this instance, the x-ray will hit a technologist standing on that side of the patient. If the technologist is not wearing a protective apron and gloves, he or she will receive unnecessary radiation. If the angle of scatter had been different, the scattered x-ray might have hit the x-ray film. This would be disadvantageous

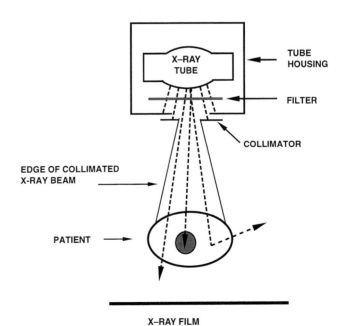

FIGURE 1–13. The schematic relationship between x-ray tube, patient, and cassette. The fate of three x-ray photons striking the patient is also shown.

because the x-ray no longer represents a structure in the patient. This x-ray would *fog* the film.

A radiograph is a visible image of the internal makeup of an object, usually a patient. The radiograph is used to assess internal structures. There must be some method of recording an image of an object if it is to be critically assessed. Fortunately, one of the important characteristics of x-rays is their ability to expose photographic emulsions. Therefore, x-rays passing through an object or patient can expose photographic emulsion in such a manner as to present a picture, or image, of the interior of the body. There are some important aspects of this process that must be understood now, although the radiographic image itself is dealt with in greater detail in Chapter 2.

Film Blackness/Opacity

X-ray film is basically photographic film, containing a light-sensitive emulsion. Crystals containing silver halide are present in the emulsion. Emulsion crystals exposed to x-rays or light are precipitated on the film during development as neutral silver deposits, which appear black to the eye, whereas unexposed crystals are removed during fixation, leaving clear areas on the film. Thus, the amount of precipitated silver in any particular part of the film determines how black, gray, or clear that part of the film appears to the eyes, and this is directly related to the number of x-rays which reach that part of the film from the patient. Precipitated silver creates film blackness. The degree of film blackness is affected by the number of x-rays striking the film, which, in turn, is affected by the x-ray machine output (mAs). The more x-rays emitted, the more that reach the film (Fig. 1–14).

Film blackness can also be affected by the energy of the x-ray beam (kVp). The higher the kVp, the higher the energy of x-rays in the beam, the larger the percentage of x-rays in the beam that penetrate the patient, and the greater the film blackness (Fig. 1–15).

The distance from the x-ray tube to the film also affects film blackness. This distance is referred to as the *focal spot-film distance* (FFD). As the FFD increases, film blackness decreases because the intensity of x-rays in the x-ray beam (x-rays/unit area) decrease (Fig. 1–16).

The amount of change in intensity of the x-ray beam as a function of distance is described by the inverse square law equation:

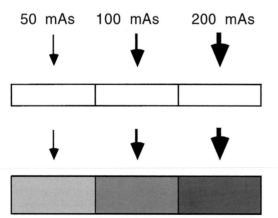

FIGURE 1–14. As mAs is increased, proportionally more x-rays will pass through the patient or object. Thus, as mAs is increased, film blackness (radiolucency) will also increase, and opacity will decrease.

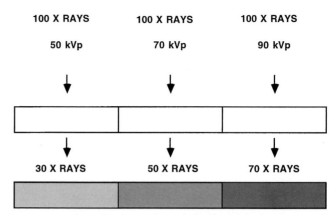

FIGURE 1–15. The number of x-rays that reach the film, and therefore opacity, can be controlled by changing the kVp setting on the control panel. Increasing kVp, while keeping mAs constant, will result in x-rays having more energy. As energy increases, the likelihood of penetration without interaction increases. This will result in more x-rays hitting the film and film blackness increasing.

$$\frac{I_1}{I_2} = \frac{(d_2)^2}{(d_1)^2}$$

where I is the intensity in terms of number of x-rays/unit area and d is distance, I_1 is the intensity at distance$_1$, and I_2 is the intensity at distance$_2$. Therefore, as FFD increases, intensity and film blackness decrease, and this decrease is a function of the square of the distance, not simply the distance (Fig. 1–17).

As an example, assume that at an FFD of 50 inches the intensity of the x-ray beam at the level of the film is 100 x-rays/cm². What will the intensity be if the FFD is decreased to 25 inches? Intuitively the intensity must be greater at a shorter distance, but the inverse square law equation can be used to obtain the exact solution. $I_1 = 100$ x-rays/cm², $d_1 = 50$ inches, $I_2 = ?$, $d_2 = 25$ inches. Substituting, the equation becomes:

$$\frac{100}{I_2} = \frac{(25)^2}{(50)^2};$$

$$\frac{100}{I_2} = \frac{625}{2500};$$

$$\frac{100}{I_2} = 0.25;$$

$$I_2 = 400 \ x\text{-}rays/cm^2$$

Therefore, by decreasing the distance from the x-ray source to the film by a factor of 2, the intensity increases not by a factor of 2, but by a factor of 4 (i.e., the square of the distance change).

The inverse square relationship has other practical implications. Suppose that an exposure of 100 mAs is needed for a radiograph of the abdomen using a 40-inch FFD. When using another x-ray machine, the maximum FFD that can be obtained is 30 inches. What mAs must be used to maintain the same radiographic opacity as that obtained at a 40-inch FFD? Common sense tells you that because the distance is shorter, a lower mAs must be used. The exact mAs value can be calculated from the inverse square principle. The inverse square law equation cannot be used for this calculation because it relates intensity change as a function of distance. In this example, we wish to maintain the same photon intensity at the film, which is now 10 inches closer to the x-ray tube. The question is: How much do we have to decrease the mAs to maintain the same intensity? In this situation, there is a

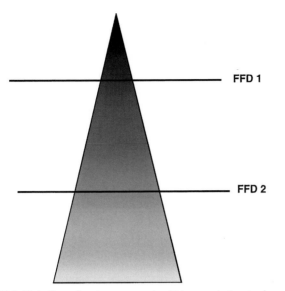

FIGURE 1–16. As distance from the x-ray source (anode) increases, the intensity of x-rays in the beam (x-rays/unit area) decreases because of beam divergence. It is clear in this example that as the FFD increases, the film blackness of the resultant radiograph also decreases. To obtain film blackness at FFD 2 similar to that at FFD 1 in this example, the number of x-rays produced at the anode (mAs) would have to be increased.

direct relationship between the mAs *needed* to maintain the same intensity and distance, so the equation is as follows:

$$\frac{mAs_1}{mAs_2} = \frac{(d_1)^2}{(d_2)^2}$$

and from the equation, $mAs_1 = 100$, $mAs_2 = ?$, distance$_1$ = 40 inches, distance$_2$ = 30 inches, and the proper relationship is:

$$\frac{100}{mAs_2} = \frac{(40)^2}{(30)^2};$$

$$\frac{100}{mAs_2} = \frac{1600}{900};$$

$$\frac{100}{mAs_2} = 1.77;$$

$$mAs_2 = \frac{100}{1.77};$$

$$mAs_2 = 56.25 \; mAs$$

Thus, the new mAs value at a 30-inch FFD is 56.25 and is lower than the original value of 100 mAs, which was needed at a 40-inch FFD. In this example, it is important to realize the intensity (x-rays per unit area) at the film is the same under either circumstance (i.e., 100 mAs at 40 inches or 56.25 mAs at 30 inches).

Therefore, FFDs are chosen as a compromise between long values to preserve radiographic detail (see later discussion) and short values that require lower mAs values. Use of a long FFD to preserve detail cannot be recommended because the large mAs values needed to maintain x-ray intensity at the film are potentially harmful to the x-ray tube, and to obtain high mAs values, longer exposure times are needed, which may result in patient motion, a cause of image unsharpness. FFD values are typically in the range of 40 to 60 inches.

FACTORS AFFECTING IMAGE DETAIL

Motion

Motion is the biggest enemy of detail in veterinary radiology. Animals cannot be made to be completely motionless, unless sedated or anesthetized, and any motion induces image unsharpness. Because of the problem of motion, it is necessary to use as fast an exposure time as possible. In some x-ray machines, the timer is capable of producing exposures in the millisecond range. To obtain mAs values satisfactory to obtain the necessary film blackness at these short exposure times, large mA values are needed. mA values up to 1500 can be obtained in some x-ray machines. In private practice, however, choice of mA values is more limited, and most machines have maximum mA values of 300. This means exposure times must be longer to obtain suitable mAs values and motion becomes more of a problem. Motion can be combated by (1) not using a long FFD (requires more mAs and, therefore, longer exposure times), (2) not using detail film, (3) by using high speed-screens (rare-earth), and (4) by using a grid with a medium grid ratio (e.g., 8:1). All of these factors are subsequently discussed.

Film Speed

X-ray film is available in a variety of types, which vary in the size of the silver halide crystals in the emulsion or the thickness of the silver halide layer. X-rays are more likely to interact with (hit) a large silver halide crystal or the increased number of silver halide crystals in a thicker crystal layer. Thus, degree of film blackness from a constant exposure is greater for films with larger silver halide crystals or thicker crystal layers. The variability in silver halide crystal size or thickness of the crystal layer is referred to as *film speed*. Fast films, or high-speed films, have larger silver halide crystals or thicker layers of silver halide crystals. Slow films have smaller crystals or thinner layers of crystals. The detail of the radiographic image is related to the speed of the film. Detail is inversely related to speed. Detail is greater with slow films (small crystals) because the area exposed by each x-ray is smaller (i.e., there is less amplification of information conferred by each x-ray) (Fig. 1–18).

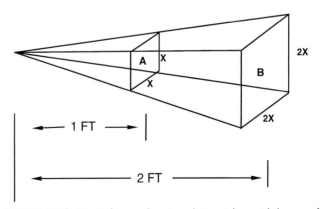

FIGURE 1–17. The intensity of an x-ray beam (x-rays/unit area) changes with the square of the distance. At a distance of 1 foot, the diverging x-ray beam covers an area represented by the square "A" with each side of dimension x, or an area of $(x) \cdot (x) = x^2$. At 2 feet, the diverging beam covers a square "B" in which each side is now twice as long as it was at 1 foot. The area covered by the beam at 2 feet is therefore $(2x) \cdot (2x) = 4x^2$, which is four times the area at 1 foot. Because the intensity of the beam originating at the anode is constant, the intensity falling on the small square must spread out over an area four times as large by the time the beam reaches the large square.

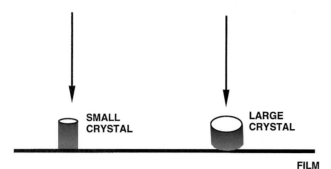

FIGURE 1–18. An x-ray carrying information from the patient is about to interact with an x-ray film crystal. On the left (small crystal, slow or detail film) the information from the patient will be deposited over a smaller area than on the right (large crystal, fast film). Therefore, detail will be better on the left, but more radiation will be necessary to make the radiograph, because the probability of an x-ray leaving the patient and hitting the crystal will be less with small crystals than with large crystals.

Focal Spot Size

Some x-ray tubes have a large and a small focal spot, which are operator selectable. Use of a small focal spot results in improved detail (Fig. 1–19). The disadvantage of using the small focal spot is that lower mAs values must be used to prevent the filament from burning out. With the small focal spot, edges of anatomic structures are projected much sharper than with the large focal spot. This edge unsharpness is termed *penumbra*. In practice, small focal spots are not used frequently because of the mAs limitations associated with them.

Focal Spot-Film Distance

Detail is also related to the FFD. Earlier the effect of FFD on film blackness was presented. It was also stated that FFD affected detail (Fig. 1–20). To summarize what is known about FFD values: (1) The advantage of keeping FFD long is optimization of detail. (2) The advantage of keeping FFD short is decreased radiographic technique (mAs) requirements. (3) One usually compromises, and 40- to 60-inch values are typical.

Object-Film Distance

The distance of the patient from the film also affects detail. This parameter is called object-film distance (OFD) (Fig. 1–21). Changes in OFD affect detail more than changes in FFD, although it should be obvious that both have some effect on

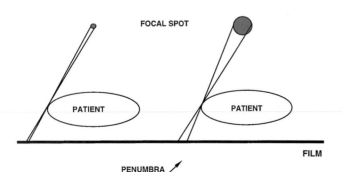

FIGURE 1–19. The effect of focal spot size on detail. With large focal spots, the edge unsharpness, or the penumbra, is larger. This contributes to image unsharpness.

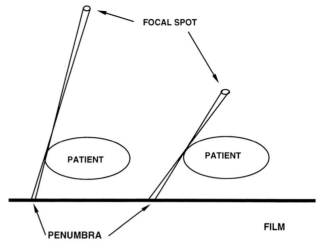

FIGURE 1–20. The effect of FFD on detail. At short FFDs, x-rays from either side of the focal spot will create a larger area of edge unsharpness (penumbra) on the film than at long FFDs. At short FFDs, information from the patient is spread out over a larger area of the film (magnification), resulting in loss of detail. This is synonymous with photographic enlargement. As a photograph is enlarged, detail decreases because the information is spread out over a larger area. The edge unsharpness associated with focal spot size and position is called *penumbra*.

detail. Therefore, when radiographing patients, it is important to keep the patient as close to the x-ray film as possible.

Intensifying Screens

In reality, the sensitivity of the emulsion to x-rays is much less than its sensitivity to visible light. Therefore, it is more efficient to turn the x-ray energy into visible light, with the visible light then exposing the x-ray film. This is possible because of the property of x-rays to cause certain compounds to fluoresce (see Table 1–2). Intensifying screens are used to convert x-rays into visible light. Intensifying screens are composed of layers of phosphorescent crystals, which emit light when struck by an x-ray (Fig. 1–22). The phosphorescent crystals of intensifying screens should not be confused with the silver halide crystals in the film emulsion.

For radiography, x-ray film is sandwiched between two

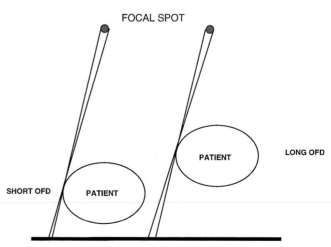

FIGURE 1–21. In this example, FFD is the same in both instances. The OFD is different, being short on the left and long on the right. As OFD increases, magnification and edge unsharpness increase, resulting in a decrease in radiographic detail. Note how much larger the image of the object is on the right in comparison to the left.

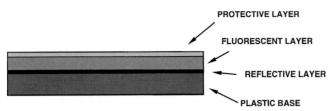

PROTECTIVE LAYER
FLUORESCENT LAYER
REFLECTIVE LAYER
PLASTIC BASE

FIGURE 1–22. The anatomy of an intensifying screen. Intensifying screens are covered with a protective layer. Beneath this is the phosphorescent layer, which fluoresces (converts x-rays into visible light) when struck by x-rays. There is a reflective layer deep to the fluorescent layer, which reflects light back in the direction of the x-ray film. The film contacts the protective layer. The plastic base provides support for the intensifying screen.

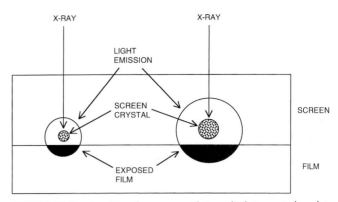

X-RAY   X-RAY
LIGHT EMISSION
SCREEN CRYSTAL
EXPOSED FILM
SCREEN
FILM

FIGURE 1–24. The effect of intensifying screen crystal size on detail. A screen is shown that contains crystals of two sizes. This is for illustration purposes only, as screens are never constructed with more than one size of phosphorescent crystal. The crystal on the left is smaller, and that part of the screen will be slower (will require more radiation to produce light because the chance of an x-ray hitting a small crystal is less) than the right side, where the crystals are bigger. An x-ray is shown hitting each crystal. A halo of light is emitted from each crystal. The halo is bigger on the right, resulting in a larger area of x-ray film being exposed. Therefore, detail on the right will be less because the information being recorded from the patient is spread over a larger area of the film. Screens for optimizing detail, so-called *detail screens*, have smaller crystals than do regular-speed screens, but require more radiation to produce an acceptable radiograph.

intensifying screens in a device called a cassette (Fig. 1–23). The cassette front is made from a low atomic number, low physical density material so as not to absorb a significant portion of the incident x-ray beam. The cassette is constructed in such a manner as to compress the film between the screens to ensure good film-screen contact. If there were not good contact between the film and screens, light from the screen would diffuse over a larger distance, and detail would be degraded. See the next section for details about light production by intensifying screens.

Regarding the intensifying screen, both the thickness of the phosphor layer and the size of the crystals in the phosphor layer can be varied (Fig. 1–24). As with x-ray film, there is an increased chance of interaction between an x-ray and the intensifying screen when the phosphor crystals are large or the phosphor layer is thick, but the radiographic detail is decreased considerably with large crystals or thicker phosphor layers because light produced in the screen diffuses over a wider area. In some intensifying screens, particularly those with a thick phosphor layer, a light-absorbing dye is added to the phosphor layer to reduce the amount of diffused light reaching the x-ray film; this leads to increased radiographic detail. These light-reducing dyes also result in more radiation being needed to produce a satisfactory radiographic image.

Intensifying screens are used because they can convert a few absorbed x-rays into many light rays, thereby decreasing the amount of radiation needed to make a radiograph. This results in less radiation exposure to the patient and to technical personnel and allows for use of relatively low-output x-ray machines to make radiographs of large body parts, such as the equine stifle or equine thorax.

Intensifying screens originally used calcium tungstate (CaWO$_4$) as the phosphor, but in the last few years new phosphors have been developed. These new phosphors are called *rare-earth* phosphors, not because the components are uncommon but because some of the components come from the rare-earth series of chemical elements, which includes elements of atomic numbers 57 through 71. The x-ray-to-light conversion of these rare-earth intensifying screens is

significantly greater than that of calcium tungstate. For example, one x-ray absorbed in calcium tungstate produces about 1000 light rays, and the same x-ray absorbed in a rare-earth phosphor produces about 4000 light rays. Thus, by using rare-earth intensifying screens, it is possible to produce radiographs at mAs settings lower than ever before.

In some instances, in which outstanding detail is desired, radiographs are produced without the use of intensifying screens. This so-called nonscreen technique requires much higher mAs values than screen techniques. Radiographic detail is superior in nonscreen techniques, however, because the distance light diffuses from a crystal in an intensifying screen is larger than the size of the silver-halide crystals in the film, which, in nonscreen techniques, are exposed directly by x-rays. Therefore, information from the patient is spread out over a larger area of film when screens are used than when nonscreen techniques are used.

Grids

Scattered radiation is a highly significant factor contributing to decreased detail. Scatter results from redirection of a portion of the primary x-ray beam either from coherent or Compton scattering. The effect of scattered radiation is to produce a generalized photographic fog on the film, which reduces contrast (see later section on factors affecting contrast) (Fig. 1–25). The amount of scattered radiation produced is directly related to the physical density of the patient, the total volume of tissue irradiated, and the energy of the x-ray beam (kVp). Scattered radiation is undesirable and can be removed from the x-ray beam by use of a grid. A grid is a flat rectangular plate with a series of lead and aluminum foil strips that improves diagnostic quality of radiographs by absorbing the majority of the scattered radiation (see Fig. 1–25). Some x-rays passing through the patient are aligned with the radiolucent aluminum strips and reach the x-ray film. Some x-rays hitting the patient are scattered, and the grid prevents these from reaching the film (see Fig. 1–25). These scattered x-rays represent useless information and would contribute only to fogging of the film if the grid were not present. Some primary x-rays not scattered by the patient

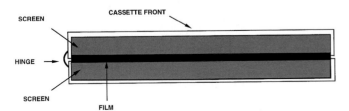

CASSETTE FRONT
SCREEN
HINGE
SCREEN
FILM

FIGURE 1–23. The anatomy of a cassette. X-ray film is placed in a cassette, sandwiched between two intensifying screens. This increases the efficiency of the entire system over that achieved if only one screen were used. Use of two screens decreases detail compared with only one screen, however.

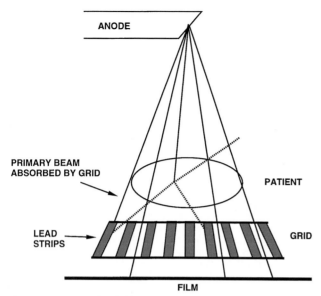

FIGURE 1–25. How a grid works. The grid is placed between the patient and the film, and its purpose is to absorb scattered radiation. The lead strips in the grid are shown as stippled regions. Between the lead strips are strips made from some low-atomic-number, low-physical-density material, such as aluminum or fiber. This allows a portion of the primary x-ray beam to reach the film, which is necessary for patient information to be recorded. The scattered photons, shown as dashed lines, that hit the grid are likely to be absorbed by the grid because their angle is such that they do not pass between the lead strips.

also hit the grid. Therefore, the number of x-rays generated must be increased when grids are used to compensate for this absorption of a portion of the primary x-ray beam. In general, two to three times as many x-rays must be generated when grids are used in comparison to when they are not. This means mAs values two to three times as large are needed when grids are used.

The amount of scatter by the patient is a function of the thickness of the patient. The larger the patient, the more scatter there is. Because small patients do not scatter many x-rays, grids are used only for patients with thicknesses greater than approximately 10 cm.

The size of each lead strip in Figure 1–25 has been exaggerated for diagrammatic purposes. Typically, there are on the order of 80 to 160 lead lines per linear inch of grid; thus, the lead strips are thin. In radiographs exposed with a grid, it may be possible to see the grid lines if the radiograph is examined closely. Notice that in Figure 1–25 the more peripheral lead strips are angled progressively steeper in such a way that planes drawn through each lead strip intersect at a point. The distance from the surface of the grid to the point of intersection of these planes is called the focal distance of the grid (see Fig. 1–29). The purpose of this focusing is to maximize the number of the diverging primary x-rays passing through the grid. If the lead strips were parallel, a large portion of the periphery of the diverging x-ray beam would be *cut off* by the grid.

The grid ratio is another parameter useful in describing a grid. Grid ratio is the relationship of the height of the lead strips to the distance between them (i.e., if lead strips are five times as high as the space between them, the grid ratio is 5:1) (Fig. 1–26). The larger the grid ratio, the more effective the grid is in absorbing scatter, but the more difficult it is for primary x-rays to pass through it. This phenomenon should be apparent by comparing the 8:1 and 12:1 grid in Figure 1–26. Thus, the higher the grid ratio, the more mAs needed to produce a diagnostic radiograph.

Whenever a grid is used in the making of a radiograph,

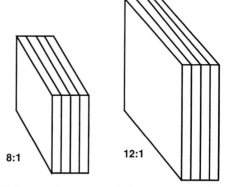

FIGURE 1–26. Illustration of grid ratio. The lead strips are represented as the thin black lines. The grid ratio is the ratio of the height of the lead strips to the distance between them.

each lead strip casts a linear opaque shadow. If the grid is stationary during the exposure, the shadows are easily detected on radiographs, particularly if there are few lead lines per inch of grid. If, however, the grid can be made to move during the exposure, the shadows cast by the lead strips are blurred and cannot be identified. One disadvantage of a moving grid is that it may make noise or vibrate during a radiographic exposure, causing the patient to move unexpectedly. When the primary x-ray beam is not properly aligned with the grid, particularly a focused grid, artifacts result (Figs. 1–27 to 1–30).

DISTORTION

Distortion is due to unequal magnification of the part being radiographed. This results from one part of the object being closer to the x-ray tube than the rest of the object (Fig. 1–31). Interpretation of radiographs can be compromised if the patient is not kept in proper relationship with the primary x-ray beam.

FACTORS AFFECTING CONTRAST

Contrast of a radiograph (radiographic contrast) refers to the difference in film blackness between areas in the radiograph.

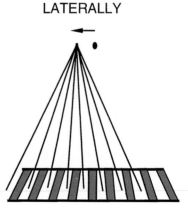

FOCAL SPOT DISPLACED LATERALLY

FIGURE 1–27. Lateral decentering. When the central ray is centered over the grid, the shadow of the lead strips will be very narrow. When the central ray is laterally decentered, the divergence of the beam no longer matches the divergence of the lead strips in the grid, and the lead strips will absorb more of the primary beam, reducing film blackness. Grid lines may also be visualized, depending on the grid ratio and number of grid lines per inch. Lateral decentering is the most common type of grid-induced artifact.

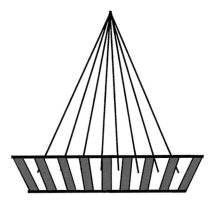

FIGURE 1–28. Upside-down grid. If a focused grid is used upside down, nearly complete absorption of the primary x-ray beam will occur, except in the exact center of the grid.

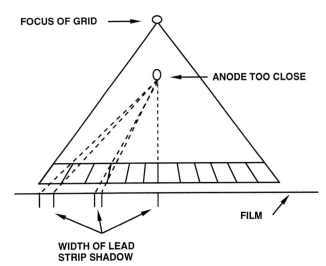

FIGURE 1–30. Because of the fixed relationship of the lead strips in a focused grid, the grid will function properly only over a small range of FFDs. The grid focus, the point from which the diverging x-rays match exactly the divergence pattern of the lead strips in the grid, is shown in this figure. The anode should be located near the grid focal point for proper use of the grid. If the focal spot is too close, the divergence of the x-ray beam will no longer match the divergence of the lead strips and cut-off will occur. Note even though the focal spot is too close, the shadows of the lead strips remain acceptable in the center of the grid. As one progresses toward the periphery of the grid, however, the shadows of the lead strips become progressively larger, and cut-off becomes severe.

Differing shades of grayness, or contrast, allow us to see the information contained in the image of the patient. If there were no contrast, all parts of the patient would be of the same opacity and no individual structures would be visible. Radiographic contrast depends on three factors: (1) subject contrast, (2) film contrast, and (3) fog and scatter.

Subject Contrast

Subject contrast is the difference in x-ray intensity transmitted through one part of the subject in comparison to another part. Subject contrast is affected by (1) thickness differences, (2) physical density differences, (3) atomic number differences, and (4) x-ray beam energy (kVp). Thickness, physical density, and atomic number effects on radiographic opacity and intensity have already been discussed. The effect of radiation energy, or quality, adjusted by the kVp control has not been discussed, but this is an extremely important factor that affects contrast.

The ability of an x-ray to penetrate tissue depends on its energy (see Fig. 1–15). X-rays generated at higher kVp values have higher energy. Selecting the proper kVp is one of the most important factors to consider in choosing the exposure technique. If the kVp is too low, almost all x-rays are attenuated in the patient and never reach the film (radiograph underexposed). If the kVp is too high, too many x-rays penetrate the patient and reach the film (radiograph overexposed). The kilovoltage selected also has a great effect on subject contrast, with contrast being inversely related to kVp

(i.e., a properly exposed radiograph made with low kVp and high mAs results in high contrast, whereas a properly exposed radiograph made with high kVp and low mAs results in low contrast). To understand how kVp affects contrast, it is extremely important to realize that there are numerous combinations of mAs and kVp that result in an acceptable radiograph. The major factor in producing an acceptable radiograph is there being just the right intensity of x-rays (x-rays/unit area) at the film. This can be achieved by many combinations of mAs and kVp; if high mAs values are used

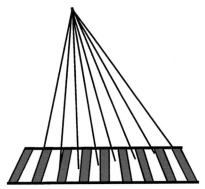

FIGURE 1–29. The primary x-ray beam is not perpendicular to the grid. This could occur if one uses a grid not affixed to the x-ray table, or if the x-ray tube housing is tilted. Absence of perpendicularity results in considerable cut-off of the primary beam and visualization of grid lines.

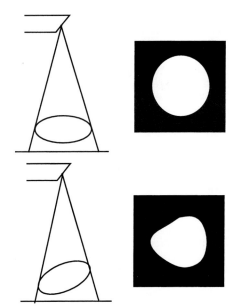

FIGURE 1–31. In the top part of this figure, a circular object is radiographed, and all parts of the circle are the same distance from the anode. The resulting radiograph represents the true shape of the object. In the lower part of this figure, some of the circle is closer to the anode than the rest of the circle. The resulting radiographic image of the object does not represent the true shape of the circle; it has been distorted and is now teardrop shaped.

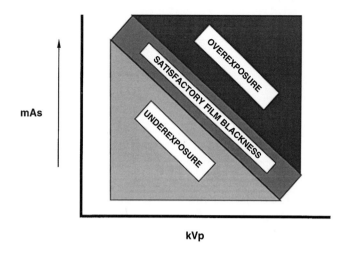

FIGURE 1–32. There is a range of mAs/kVp combinations that will produce a satisfactory radiograph. When low numbers of x-rays are generated, their energy must be high (high kVp) so that sufficient numbers reach the film. When many x-rays are generated (high mAs), their energy must not be too great, or too many will reach the film.

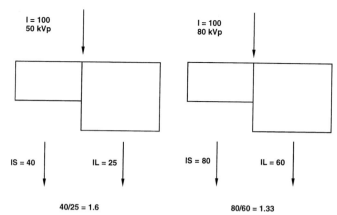

FIGURE 1–33. Assume that an x-ray beam with an intensity of 100 x-rays/unit area strikes an object made up of two distinct regions with different thicknesses. IS and IL are the intensities of the beam after being transmitted through small (thin, IS) and large (thick, IL) regions of the object, respectively. Contrast is defined as the ratio of the intensity of the x-ray beam after passing through the thin:thick regions of the object, i.e., IS/IL. On the left, most of the low-energy x-rays are attenuated by the thick part, but quite a few can penetrate the thin part. Therefore, subject contrast for 50 kVp is 40/25 = 1.6. This equation states that the thin part transmits 60 percent more x-rays than the thick part at 50 kVp. If the kVp is increased to 80, more x-rays will get through both the thick and the thin parts. Both IS and IL will increase, but IL will increase proportionally more than IS because the higher energy of the x-rays allows them to penetrate the thick part with greater ease. The ratio IS/IL becomes smaller, and subject contrast decreases, i.e., 80/60 = 1.33, or only 33 percent difference exists in the transmitted radiation intensity. Structures of high atomic number (bone) are also more easily penetrated by higher energy x-rays. Therefore, the thick part in the figure could also be something of high atomic number, and the same principle would apply.

(lots of x-rays generated), low kVp values must also be used to prevent too many of the x-rays from penetrating the patient and reaching the film. If low mAs values are used, higher kVp values must be used so that more of the x-rays penetrate the patient and reach the film (Fig. 1–32).

Even though there are many combinations of mAs and kVp that result in a satisfactory radiograph, the contrast of the image depends on whether the kVp is high or low relative to the mAs. As noted earlier, contrast refers to the magnitude of the gradation of film blackness in the radiograph. In a high-contrast radiograph, there are mostly black and white opacities and few shades of gray. High-contrast radiographs are also referred to as having a *short scale* of contrast because everything is either black or white. Low-contrast radiographs have few blacks and whites but many shades of gray; low-contrast radiographs are referred to as having a *long scale* of contrast because there is a long scale of shades of gray between the lighter and darker portions of the image.

In general terms, the reason low kVp produces greater subject contrast than high kVp can be explained by a simple example (Fig. 1–33). You should realize that the radiograph on the right in Figure 1–33 will have increased film blackness and will be overexposed if the radiograph on the left was satisfactory. This results from the intensity of x-rays (x-rays per unit area) being too high beneath the object on the right. This high intensity can be corrected by using a lower mAs with the higher kVp setting (Fig. 1–34).

Film Contrast

Radiographic contrast is also a function of the type of x-ray film in use. X-ray film exaggerates subtle changes in subject contrast. This is an inherent property of the film and cannot be varied. For general use, one should not purchase extremely high-contrast or low-contrast film; a midregion contrast film is satisfactory.

Fog and Scatter

The effect of fog is to reduce radiographic contrast. Fog produced by scattered radiation can be prevented by use of a

grid. Therefore, radiographs made with a grid have higher contrast than those that are made without a grid. Film can also become fogged by exposure to pressure, exposure to high temperature, or accidental exposure to light, such as a defective darkroom safelight or a defective light seal around the darkroom door. X-ray film also becomes fogged spontane-

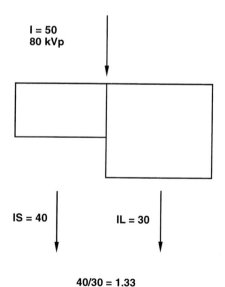

FIGURE 1–34. In Figure 1–33, the quality of the radiograph was acceptable when 50 kVp was used. When the kVp was increased to 80, contrast decreased, but the entire radiograph was overexposed. Thus, to obtain a satisfactory exposure, an intensity of 40 x-rays/unit area beneath the thin part of the object is needed, but we wish to continue to use 80 kVp because we desire lower contrast in this instance. To reduce the intensity under the thin part from 80 to 40, the original intensity (mAs) can be reduced by half. The intensity under the thin and thick parts of the object is thereby reduced to 40 and 30, respectively, and the contrast remains at 1.33, i.e., 40/30.

Table 1–5
RELATIONSHIP BETWEEN DEVELOPER TEMPERATURE AND TIME THAT RESULTS IN AN ADEQUATELY DEVELOPED RADIOGRAPH*

Developer Temperature (°F)	Time (min)
60	8.5
65	6.0
68	5.0
70	4.5
75	3.5

*Assumes that 5 minutes at 68°F is optimal.

ously over time; therefore, x-ray film is dated by the manufacturer.

FILM PROCESSING

The most common errors made in radiography of animals are related to the processing of exposed radiographic film. The area used as a darkroom should be clean, dry, lightproof, and uncluttered. It is difficult to encourage a technician to perform a radiographic examination carefully if the quality of the study is lowered by damaging the film in the darkroom. Despite the increased use of automatic processors, many radiographs in veterinary radiography are still processed manually in tanks.

Developing

The primary function of the developer is to reduce exposed silver halide crystals to metallic silver. This is done by supplying electrons to the positively charged silver ions that exist in exposed silver-halide crystals. A 5-minute developing time is recommended for film processing because it permits a

reduction of required radiation exposure factors (mAs). The process of film developing is a chemical process and is therefore dependent on both time and temperature. Because of this, a constant developer temperature is important in obtaining consistent film blackness. Generally, this is 68°F, but other times and temperatures can be used (Table 1–5).

Fixing

The purpose of the fixer is to convert undeveloped silver halide crystals on the film into a soluble compound and dissolve them. Fixer clears undeveloped, unexposed silver crystals from the film. This leaves the silver as a permanent image on the film. Areas where no or minimal silver halide exposure occurred are clear (radiolucent). Fixing time is approximately twice the development time. The film can stay in the fixer longer, but underfixing results in a cloudy or milky appearing radiograph.

Final Wash

The film should be washed after fixing to remove excess chemicals and any residual silver halide still on the film. Failure to wash adequately results in retained fixer chemicals reacting with silver in the film, forming silver sulfide, which causes the film to turn brown. When processing films by hand, films should wash for 30 to 40 minutes. Excessive washing results in the emulsion becoming soft and the entire image "slipping" off the film.

TECHNICAL ERRORS

Technical errors are commonplace in radiography. These errors at minimum are irritating when reviewing a radiograph

Table 1–6
APPEARANCE, CAUSE, AND CORRECTION FOR COMMON TECHNICAL ERRORS

Appearance	Cause	Correction
Too dark	Incorrect machine setting	Lower kVp, mA, or time
	FFD too short	Increase FFD
	Wrong screen/film	Check screen/film
	Overdeveloped	Check developer temperature/time
Too light	Incorrect machine setting	Raise kVp, mA, or time
	FFD too long	Decrease distance
	Wrong screen/film	Check screen/film
	Underdeveloped	Check developer temperature/time
Gray/loss of contrast	Film stored improperly	Check storage conditions
	Film exposed to light	Check storage conditions
	Old film	Discard film
	Incorrect machine setting	Decrease kVp, increase mAs
	Film processed improperly	Check age, temperature of chemicals
Crescent-shaped black marks	Film bent during handling	Handle film more gently
Sharp linear black marks	Film scratched before processing	Handle film more gently
Edge of film black	Film fogged	Check for light leak in cassette or film bin
Black water spots or fingerprints	Developer on film before development	Do not contaminate darkroom work surface or hands
White fingerprints	Fixer on hands before development	Do not contaminate darkroom work surface or hands
White "hair" marks	Hair in cassette	Clean cassette
Sharp white specks	Dirt in cassette	Clean cassette
Sharp white lines/marks	Emulsion scratched off	Handle film with care when wet
Blurred image	Patient motion	Use chemical restraint
	Tube motion	Secure tube
	Cassette motion	Secure cassette
Yellow-brown film	Insufficient washing	Wash completely
Tree-like black marks	Static electricity	Move film slowly

and at worst result in the radiograph being totally useless. A complete discussion of technical errors is beyond the scope of this book. In Table 1–6, the appearance, cause, and methods to correct some of the more common technical errors are presented.

References

1. Roentgen WC: December 28, 1895: On a new kind of rays. Vet Radiol & Ultrasound 36:371, 1995.
2. Widmer WR, Shaw SM, and Thrall DE: Effects of low-level exposure to ionizing radiation: Current concepts and concerns for veterinary workers. Vet Radiol & Ultrasound 37:227, 1996.
3. NCRP Report No. 82—SI units in radiation protection and measurements. Bethesda, MD, National Council on Radiation Protection and Measurements, 1985.
4. Title 10, Chapter 1, Code of Federal Regulations—Energy. Part 20, Standards for Protection Against Radiation. In: United States Nuclear Regulatory Commission Rules and Regulations. Washington, DC, 1995, pp 20–27.
5. Hall EJ: Radiation protection. In Hall EJ (Ed): Radiobiology for the Radiologist, 4th Ed. Philadelphia, JB Lippincott, 1994, pp 453–467.
6. NCRP Report No. 107—Implementation of the principle of As Low As Reasonably Achievable (ALARA) for medical and dental personnel. Bethesda, MD, National Council on Radiation Protection and Measurements, 1990.
7. Health Effects of Exposure to Low-levels of Ionizing Radiation. BEIR V. Washington, DC, National Academic Press, 1990
8. NCRP Report No. 91—Recommendations on limits for exposure to ionizing radiation. Bethesda, MD, National Council on Radiation Protection and Measurements, 1987.
9. NCRP Report No. 93—Ionizing radiation exposure of the population of the United States. Bethesda, MD, National Council on Radiation Protection and Measurements, 1987.
10. Curry III TS, Dowdey JE, and Murry Jr RC: The production of x rays. In Curry III TS, Dowdey JE, Murry Jr RC (Eds): Christensen's Physics of Diagnostic Radiology, 4th Ed. Philadelphia, Lea & Febiger, 1990, pp 10–35.

STUDY QUESTIONS

1. Which one of the following statements regarding x-rays and gamma-rays is correct?
   A. X-rays and gamma-rays originate in the atomic shells.
   B. X-rays and gamma-rays originate in the atomic nucleus.
   C. X-rays originate in the atomic shells, and gamma rays originate in the nucleus.
   D. X-rays originate in the atomic nucleus, and gamma rays originate in the atomic shells.

2. Which one of the following statements regarding the properties of x-rays is incorrect? X-rays are:
   A. also termed photons.
   B. a type of electromagnetic radiation.
   C. positively charged.
   D. devoid of mass.

3. Which one of the following statements regarding protective lead aprons and gloves is incorrect? Lead aprons and gloves:
   A. typically have 0.5 mm Pb equivalent.
   B. are designed to allow the shielded body part to be placed in the primary x-ray beam.
   C. have a finite useful life.
   D. are capable of protecting effectively against Compton scattered photons produced during diagnostic radiography.

4. Which one of the following statements regarding x-ray production is *true*? X-rays are produced in a diagnostic x-ray tube:
   A. primarily by radiative interactions.
   B. primarily by electrons interacting with the cathode.
   C. at just a few energies depending on kVp and mAs.
   D. only when the tube voltage approximates kVp.

5. Which one of the following statements regarding the anode of an x-ray tube is correct?
   A. The anode rotates to increase the efficiency of x-ray production.
   B. The anode is angled to improve image quality.
   C. The anode is made of low atomic number material to improve image quality.
   D. The anode is the primary source of electron production in the x-ray tube.

6. Fill in each blank with either photoelectric or Compton, depending on which type of interaction best fulfills the criterion.

Criterion	*Absorption Process*
Independent of atomic number	_____
Results in most exposure to radiographers	_____
The desirable process for diagnostic radiology	_____
Provides for differential absorption of x-rays by tissue	_____

7. To increase detail, the x-ray tube is moved from an FFD of 40 inches to an FFD of 60 inches. At 40 inches, a technique of 10 mAs and 70 kVp was suitable. What

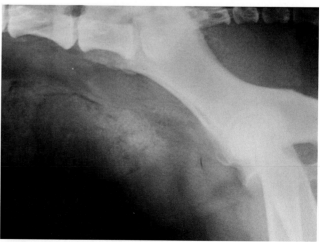

FIGURE 1–35

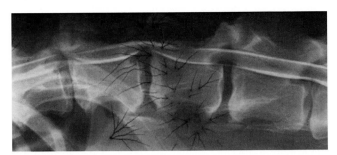

FIGURE 1–36

technique would be necessary at the new distance of 60 inches?

8. You have three intensifying screen techniques from which to choose: high-speed calcium tungstate screens, detail calcium tungstate screens, and no screens. Which screen would produce the following, assuming you use the same type of x-ray film and the same exposure factors?

Best inherent detail   _____

Poorest inherent detail   _____

Most film blackness   _____

Least film blackness   _____

9. If a radiograph is too light, which possibility out of each set could cause this?
   A. It was overexposed/ underexposed.
   B. A grid was/was not used.
   C. The grid was/was not aligned.
   D. The developer temperature was too low/too high.
   E. The developer was new/exhausted.

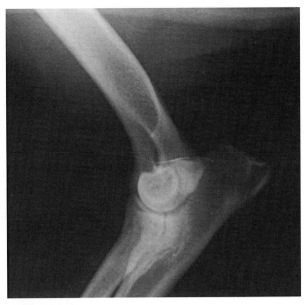

FIGURE 1–38

F. The film was in the developer too long/not long enough.
G. The film was fresh/old.
H. The screens had high/ low resolution.
I. The film was first placed in the developer/fixer.

10. (Fig. 1–35). What caused the black crescent mark just cranial to the pubic symphysis?

11. (Fig. 1–36). What caused the black arborizing artifacts superimposed over the lumbar spine?

12. (Fig. 1–37). What poor radiography practice is illustrated in this image?

13. (Fig. 1–38). What caused the linear white artifact superimposed over the distal humerus?

14. (Fig. 1–39). What caused the linear artifacts seen in this image?

(Answers appear on page 631.)

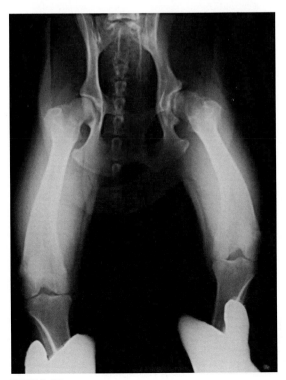

FIGURE 1–37

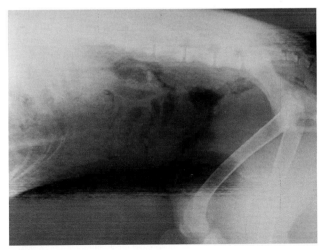

FIGURE 1–39

Chapter 2

Introduction to Radiographic Interpretation

Donald E. Thrall

X-RAYS AND RADIOGRAPHS

The science of radiology is based on the property of x-rays being able to penetrate matter. When a patient is struck by an x-ray beam, some x-rays are absorbed, and others pass through unchanged. A radiograph is an image of the number and distribution of x-rays passing through the patient. Jargon terms such as *x-ray, film, plate,* and *picture* are used in reference to a radiograph. This practice is incorrect and should be avoided.

The degree of blackness of a radiograph is directly related to the number of x-rays that reach the film or intensifying screen. Areas of the film emulsion struck by a large number of x-rays or a large amount of light from the intensifying screen are black after film processing. These film areas lie beneath parts of the patient that absorb few x-rays. Conversely, areas struck by no light or radiation are translucent or appear white (opaque). These film areas lie beneath parts of the patient that absorb many x-rays. Between these two extremes is a range of gray film tones, the blackness of which is directly related to the number of x-rays that reach the film or the intensifying screen (Figs. 2–1 and 2–2).

The degree of blackening of the x-ray film is measured in terms of optical density. Optical density and film blackness are directly related (Fig. 2–3). The term *density* is sometimes used to describe the degree to which a patient or object absorbs incident x-rays. For example, in Figure 2–2, some would refer to the ring, watch, and bones as denser than the adjacent soft tissue. Use of density in this context is confusing because the *optical* density of the film in these areas is low, whereas the *object* density is high. Further confusion arises when the added variable of physical density (g/cm³) of the patient or object is considered. As the physical density of the patient or object increases, the optical film density decreases, whereas the object or radiographic density increases. This confusing terminology can be avoided by *not* using the term *density* to describe radiographic changes. The degree of blackness or whiteness of the patient or object being radiographed should be referred to in terms of radiolucency or radiopacity. For example, in Figure 2–2, soft tissues of the hand are more radiolucent than the bones; both are more radiolucent than the watch and the ring. It may also be said that the watch and the ring are more radiopaque than the remainder of the hand. Describing radiographic appearance in terms of radiolucency (lucency) and radiopacity (opacity) avoids the confusion associated with the use of the word *density* for such purposes.

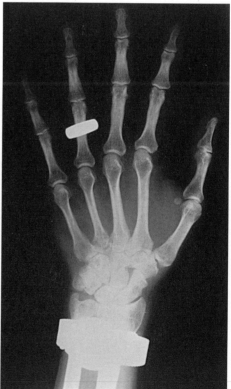

FIGURE 2–2. Radiograph of a human hand. Black regions represent film areas where no x-rays were absorbed from the x-ray beam before reaching the film. Homogeneously white areas, such as the watch and ring, are film areas where essentially *all* x-rays were absorbed from the x-ray beam before the beam reached the film. Between these two extremes are many shades of gray resulting from various degrees of x-ray absorption from the primary beam by the hand. It should be obvious that the bones absorbed more x-rays than fleshy parts of the hand.

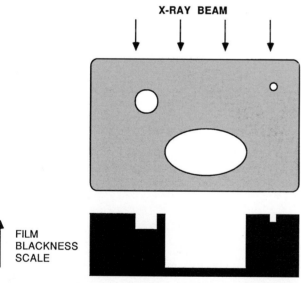

FIGURE 2–1. Diagram illustrating the principle of the effect of tissue composition on absorption of x-rays. A beam of x-rays strikes a large object containing three regions of higher physical density illustrated by the two circles and the ellipse. Beneath the object is a scale of film blackness. Where the x-ray beam does not hit one of the smaller objects, film blackness will be the greatest. Beneath the smaller objects, film blackness will be less because of absorption of x-rays by these objects. The degree to which film blackness will be less is, in this example, only a function of the thickness of the smaller objects, since they are all homogeneous and of the same physical density. The small circle on the right affects film blackness only minimally, while beneath the ellipse film blackness is decreased considerably. This decreased film blackness results because of absorption of more x-rays in the thicker ellipse, thereby reducing the number of x-rays that reach the film.

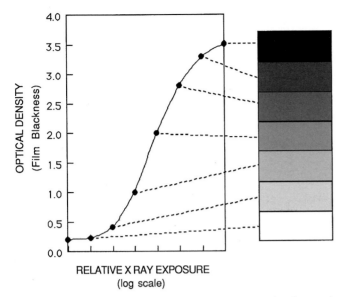

FIGURE 2–3. Relationship between relative radiation exposure (x-axis) and resulting optical film density (y-axis). As radiation exposure increases, so does optical film density (film blackness). (Adapted from the Fundamentals of Radiography, 12th ed. Rochester, NY, Eastman Kodak, 1980; reprinted courtesy of Eastman Kodak Company.)

IMAGE FORMATION AND DIFFERENTIAL ABSORPTION

It is possible to use x-rays to produce an image of a patient or an object on film because some x-rays are absorbed by the patient or object, and some pass through unchanged, producing film blackening (see Fig. 2–1). Of particular importance in patient radiography is the fact that x-rays are not absorbed homogeneously by the body; some tissues absorb x-rays more efficiently than others. This phenomenon is called *differential absorption*. If absorption of x-rays by the patient were uniform (no differential absorption), the resulting radiographic image would be gray or white. If no absorption occurred, the resulting radiograph would be homogeneously black. The effect of differential absorption is illustrated in Figure 2–2, in which the areas between the fingers and adjacent to the hand are black because no x-rays from the incident beam were absorbed before reaching the intensifying screen. Soft tissues of the hand are visible because they have absorbed some x-rays from the primary beam. Bones of the hand are more radiopaque than soft tissues; the bones have absorbed more x-rays, and thus that part of the intensifying screen under the bones was struck by fewer x-rays than the part under the fleshy parts of the hand. The watch and ring appear totally radiopaque because essentially no x-rays were able to pass through them. The degree of differential absorption of x-rays by a patient or an object depends on the energy of the x-rays and the composition of the patient or object. This was discussed in detail in Chapter 1.

IMPORTANCE OF TISSUE COMPOSITION

Although the effect of x-ray energy on differential absorption is important, it is the dependence of x-ray absorption on tissue or object composition that allows radiographic images of patients to be produced. X-ray absorption by a substance is affected by the effective atomic number of its elements and the physical density of the substance. Consider the physical density and effective atomic number of the substances listed in Table 2–1. If one recognizes the direct relationship between the absorption of x-rays, physical density, and effective atomic number, the substances in Table 2–1 may be ranked in order of increasing radiopacity. Air is the most radiolucent substance. The radiolucency of air and other gases results from their low physical density. Even though the effective atomic number of air is higher than that of fat, air is more radiolucent because of its lower physical density (i.e., there are many fewer molecules per unit area to absorb x-rays). If air could be compressed until its physical density equaled that of fat, it would be more radiopaque because of its greater atomic number.

The next more radiopaque substance in Table 2–1 is fat. Although the effective atomic number of fat is less than that of air, its physical density is greater, making fat more radiopaque than air. Next, consider the physical density and effective atomic number of water and muscle. It may be theorized that muscle would be more radiopaque than water because of its higher physical density and effective atomic number. The sensitivity of the radiographic imaging system, however, is not great enough to allow detection of differences in the radiopacity of substances with such small differences in physical density and effective atomic number. Thus, the radiopacity of most fluids (blood, urine, transudates, exudates, bile, and cerebrospinal fluid) and nonmineralized, nonadipose tissues (cartilage, muscle, fascia, tendons, ligaments, and parenchymal organs) is the same. The radiopacity of these fluids and tissues is referred to as soft-tissue radiopacity. The next most radiopaque substance in Table 2–1 is bone; its physical density and effective atomic number are higher than those of air, fat, water, and muscle. The most radiopaque substance is lead. Lead and other metals have high physical density and effective atomic number, making them extremely radiopaque. Thus, there are five perceivable degrees of inherent tissue radiopacity: air, fat, soft tissue, bone, and metal (Figs. 2–4 and 2–5).

In the discussion of relative inherent radiopacities, thickness was not mentioned. Thickness of the object and resulting radiopacity are interrelated; as thickness increases, radiopacity increases (Fig. 2–6). Thus, the different radiopacities discussed previously (air, fat, soft tissue, bone, and metal) are relative inherent radiopacities, assuming that the substance thickness is approximately the same. For example, although fat is inherently more radiolucent than bone, if a large piece of fat is placed on a cassette next to a small piece of bone, the fat would appear more radiopaque (i.e., its total radiopacity would be greater) (Fig. 2–7). Total radiopacity depends on thickness *and* inherent radiopacity.

RADIOGRAPHIC GEOMETRY AND THINKING IN THREE DIMENSIONS

It is extremely important to remember that a radiograph is a two-dimensional image of a three-dimensional object. Thus,

Table 2–1
PHYSICAL DENSITY AND EFFECTIVE ATOMIC NUMBER OF VARIOUS SUBSTANCES

Substance	Physical Density (g/cm³)	Effective Atomic Number
Air	0.001	7.8
Fat	0.92	6.5
Water	1.00	7.5
Muscle	1.04	7.6
Bone	1.65	12.3
Lead	8.70	82.0

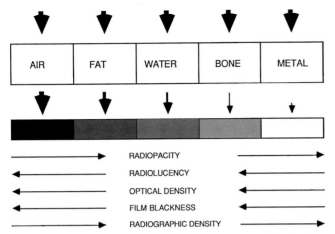

FIGURE 2–4. Identical thicknesses of five substances are struck by an equal number of x-rays. Not all substances absorb x-rays with the same efficiency. In this example, as the physical density and effective atomic number increase (from left to right), the number of x-rays passing through the substance decreases. This dependency of absorption on physical density and atomic number is what allows x-rays to be useful for producing radiographs. As the number of x-rays passing through the object changes, the blackness of the radiograph also changes. Note the changes in radiopacity that occur with each object above. Use of the term radiographic density is not recommended but is included in this figure for comparison.

the radiographic image of the object depends on its orientation with respect to the primary x-ray beam. There are four consequences of radiographs being two-dimensional images of three-dimensional objects: (1) magnification and distortion, (2) the image of a familiar object appearing unfamiliar, (3) a loss of depth perception, and (4) the presence of summation shadows.

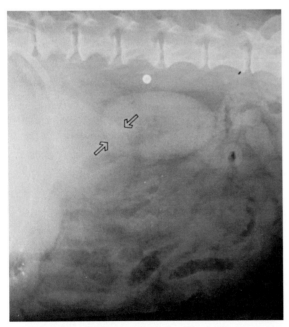

FIGURE 2–5. Lateral view of abdomen in which the five different radiopacities are represented. *Air:* gas in the bowel. *Fat:* adipose tissue in the retroperitoneal space. Fat is more radiopaque than gas, but less radiopaque than the kidneys. *Soft tissue:* the kidneys. Note the summation shadow created by the overlapping of the caudal pole of the right kidney and the cranial pole of the left kidney *(arrows). Bone:* the vertebrae. *Metal:* the shotgun pellet. The exact location of the pellet cannot be determined from this lateral view alone. It could be in the skin, intraperitoneal space, or retroperitoneal space, or lying on top of the x-ray table, under the dog. Two views, at 90 degrees to each other, are necessary for identifying the precise location of any object. The ventrodorsal abdominal radiograph of this dog is shown in Figure 2–19. By evaluating Figures 2–5 and 2–19, the location of the pellet may be determined.

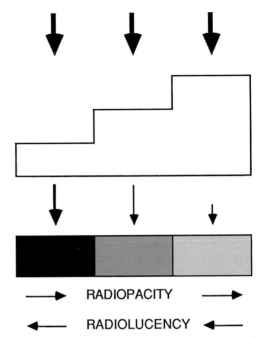

FIGURE 2–6. The effect of thickness on radiographic opacity. Increasing the thickness of the object in the path of the x-ray beam will reduce the number of x-rays that reach the film and, therefore, film blackness.

Magnification refers to the enlargement of the image relative to the actual object size. Magnification depends on the object-film distance and focal spot–film distance. In clinical practice, object-film distance affects magnification more than focal spot–film distance because focal spot distance is held constant. When object-film distance increases, magnification increases. In the magnified image, each bit of visual information is spread over a larger area of the film, which makes the

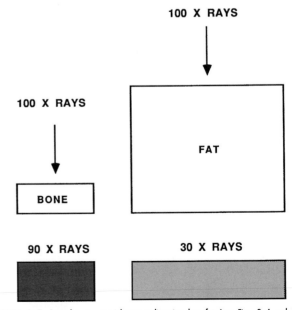

FIGURE 2–7. Bone has greater inherent radiopacity than fat (see Figs. 2–4 and 2–5). However, inherent radiopacities are relative to thickness, and thickness can cause substances with higher inherent radiopacity to appear less opaque. In this example, 100 x-rays hit a thin piece of bone and a thick piece of fat. More x-rays are absorbed in the fat because of its greater thickness, and in the resulting radiograph the fat will actually appear more opaque than bone even though its inherent radiopacity is less.

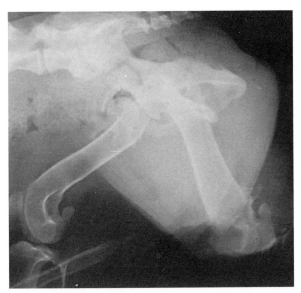

FIGURE 2–8. Lateral view of the pelvis of a dog in right lateral recumbency. The right pelvic limb was pulled cranially, the left pelvic limb caudally. Notice the increased diameter of the left femur in comparison with the right because of magnification—the left femur is farther from the cassette. Margins of the magnified left femur are also less sharp than those of the right.

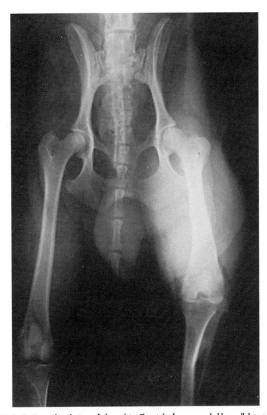

FIGURE 2–9. Ventrodorsal view of the pelvis. The right femur was held parallel to table top; the left femur was positioned with the stifle slightly flexed. This results in the left femur being angled in relation to the primary x-ray beam. Thus, the left femur appears shorter than the right and is asymmetrically magnified because of distortion; that is, it was not struck perpendicularly by the x-ray beam. The left thigh also appears more radiopaque than the right because the thickness of tissue traversed by the x-ray beam was greater on the left owing to the leg angulation.

image less sharp. It must be appreciated that some parts of the patient are always farther from the film than other parts (Fig. 2–8). Thus, whenever possible, the area of primary interest should be placed closest to the cassette to avoid having it magnified.

Distortion is present when the image misrepresents the true shape or position of the object. Distortion results from unequal magnification of different parts of the same object; it can be minimized by keeping the object and the film planes parallel. Some distortion occurs in every radiograph because there are always parts of the patient that are not parallel to the film plane. Severe distortion, however, may limit the diagnostic quality of the radiograph (Fig. 2–9).

An *unfamiliar image* of a familiar object sometimes results in the object not being identifiable (Fig. 2–10). Therefore, patient positioning for radiography is important and must be standardized. Clinicians become familiar with the radiographic appearance of patients as a result of positioning them in standard fashions.

Depth perception is lost in radiographs. To evaluate depth radiographically, it is necessary to make two radiographs of the object, with one view at a 90-degree angle to the other. Depth can then be mentally reconstructed (see Fig. 2–5). In addition, some lesions are apparent in only one radiographic projection (Fig. 2–11). Thus, for each patient, a minimum of two views at 90 degrees from each other, termed *orthogonal projections*, should be obtained. Views made at other than 90 degrees may also be necessary.

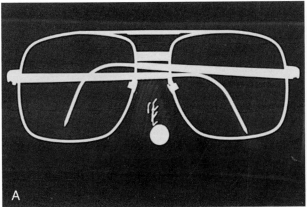

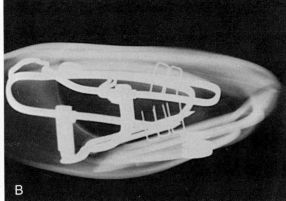

FIGURE 2–10. How recognizable an object, or a body part, is from its radiograph depends on its relationship to the primary x-ray beam. The object in *A* is easily recognizable. The object in *B* is difficult to recognize as the same pair of eyeglasses, unless one knew the identity of the object before radiography and that the glasses and their case were radiographed on end (parallel to the primary beam).

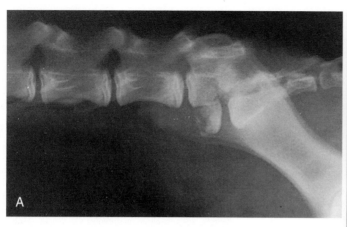

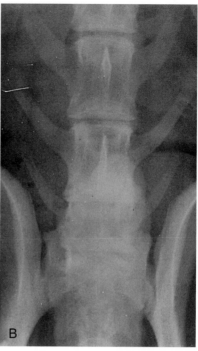

FIGURE 2–11. Lateral *(A)* and ventrodorsal *(B)* radiographs of a canine lumbar spine. *A,* There is a displaced fracture of L7. *B,* The fracture itself cannot be seen; however, L7 appears decreased in length. Some lesions are more apparent on one radiographic projection than on others. Thus, at least two projections of a body part should be made routinely.

Summation Effect

The summation effect results when parts of a patient or object in different planes are superimposed (see Fig. 2–5). The result is a summation image representing the degree of x-ray absorption by all superimposed objects. For example, consider the structure of a block of Swiss cheese. There are holes visible on the exterior of the block. These result from the cheese being sliced through gas cavities that formed as the cheese was made. Inside the block of cheese are more cavities, some of which overlap when viewed from the perspective of the x-ray tube. When a block of Swiss cheese is exposed to x-rays, fewer x-rays are absorbed by the cheese in areas where cavities overlap. The more cavities that over-

lap, the greater the number of x-rays that penetrate the cheese and reach the film (Figs. 2–12 and 2–13). In the instance of Swiss cheese, the resulting summation shadows are radiolucent because they represent summation of radiolucent images. Summation shadows can also be radiopaque (see Fig. 2–4). One must remember that radiographs are summation shadowgrams. When a suspicious radiopacity or radiolucency is identified, the possibility must be considered that it represents a summation shadow produced by the overlapping of structures.

Silhouette Effect

The silhouette principle is based on the fact that when two structures of the same radiopacity are in contact, their margin cannot be distinguished. Conversely, if two structures of the same radiopacity are not in contact and are separated by a

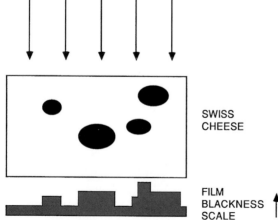

FIGURE 2–12. Illustration of the summation shadow effect. A block of Swiss cheese is struck by an x-ray beam. Gas cavities in the cheese may not be superimposed from the vantage point of the x-ray tube. The two on the left are not, and the resultant increase in film blackness beneath the bubbles is due to the individual absorption characteristics of each bubble. The two bubbles on the right, however, are partially overlapped from the perspective of the x-ray beam. In this region of overlap, there is an increase in film blackness as a result of decreased x-ray absorption in the region of bubble overlap.

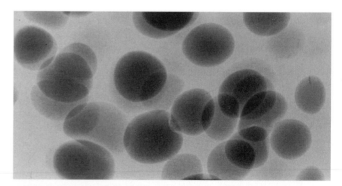

FIGURE 2–13. Radiograph of a block of Swiss cheese. Gas-filled cavities in the cheese are apparent. Areas in which gas cavities overlap are more radiolucent than areas in which no overlapping has occurred. Increased radiolucency is due to decreased x-ray absorption in areas where cavities overlap. There are areas where none, two, three, and four cavities have overlapped. Can you identify them? These summation shadows are negative, because they result in increased radiolucency. See Figure 2–5 for an example of a positive summation shadow.

X-RAY BEAM

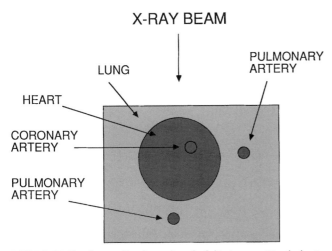

FIGURE 2–14. The silhouette effect. In a radiograph of this tissue containing the heart, a lung, a coronary artery, and two pulmonary arteries, the coronary artery will not be visible, but the two pulmonary arteries will be clearly seen. See text for more details.

substance of a differing radiopacity, their borders can be distinguished radiographically.

For example, consider Figure 2–14. This drawing represents a thoracic cavity containing the heart, a lung, a coronary artery, and pulmonary arteries. When radiographed, the coronary artery is not visible because it is of the same opacity as the heart, and there is no intervening tissue of another opacity. The pulmonary arteries are visible, however, because even though they are of the same radiographic opacity as the heart, they do not touch the heart, and there is an intervening tissue (lung) of another opacity (gas). The pulmonary artery positioned below the heart is superimposed on the cardiac silhouette in the radiograph but still is distinguishable as a distinct structure.

Because of the silhouette sign, diseases often mask normal radiographic structures. For example, in patients with pleural effusion radiographed in sternal recumbency, the pooling of fluid around the heart makes the heart margins invisible (see Fig. 29–10). Another example is the diminished bowel serosal margin seen in patients with peritoneal fluid.

IMPORTANCE OF A CONTRASTING SUBSTANCE

Just as the lack of a contrasting material prevents distinguishing between two structures of the same opacity, the presence of a contrasting material allows some structures to become exquisitely visible in radiographs. This is particularly true when the contrasting material is air, and the object in question is on the surface of the body. For example, in many patients, nipples and the prepuce are clearly visible in ventrodorsal radiographs of the body. These structures are not particularly large but seem to cast a disproportionately opaque shadow. The explanation for this phenomenon is that these structures both are surrounded by air and their margins are situated parallel to the central x-ray beam providing optimal geometry for their visualization (Fig. 2–15).

PERCEPTION

When interpreting radiographs, clinicians rely on their eyes to detect abnormalities. Unfortunately, the eyes and brain do not always perceive appearances accurately. For example, examine Figure 2–16. The two vertical lines appear to the

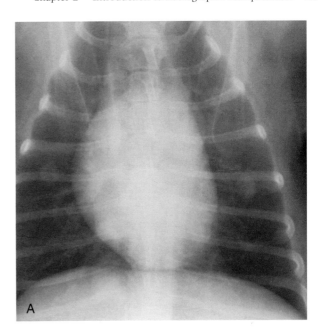

A

X-RAY BEAM DIRECTION

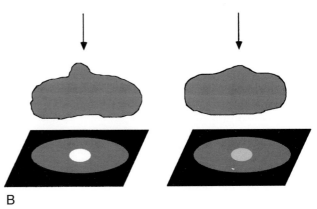

B

FIGURE 2–15. A, Ventrodorsal thoracic radiograph of a dog in which two soft tissue opacities are apparent lateral to the heart. These are nipples but could be confused with lung masses. Why should nipples be so opaque? B, Diagram illustrating why small superficial masses cast such apparent radiographic shadows. On the left, the mass has perpendicular sides and is surrounded on all sides by air. This creates a situation where the x-ray beam strikes the mass-air interface in a parallel fashion, making for optimization of contrast. On the right, a comparably sized mass has sloping sides that are not in a parallel relationship to the primary beam, and this mass, if seen at all, will not appear nearly as opaque because its sides will not be projected as distinctly.

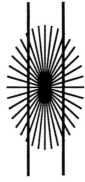

FIGURE 2–16. Perception artifact. The two vertical lines appear curved. Place a ruler next to them, and you will see they are straight. This optical illusion is created by the radiating lines on which the curved lines are superimposed. Perception can be a source of error in assessing radiographic abnormalities.

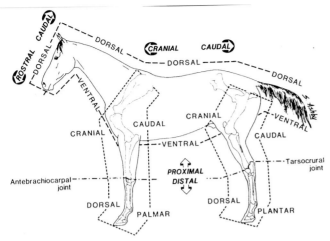

FIGURE 2–17. Proper anatomic directional terms as they apply to various parts of the body. (Courtesy of Dr. J. E. Smallwood.)

eyes to be curved, but when a straight edge is placed next to them, it is obvious that they are straight. The curving nature of these lines is an optical illusion created by the radiating lines on which they are superimposed. Therefore, what appears as concrete visual evidence is not always such. Perception is an important part of radiographic interpretation. What appears as an obvious finding to beginning radiologists may be an incorrect assessment because of perception. Only by viewing many radiographs, with the continual feedback of experienced interpreters, can perceptual inaccuracies be minimized. A more complete discussion of perception is given in Chapter 3.

RADIOGRAPHIC NOMENCLATURE

Radiographic projections are named according to the direction in which the central ray of the primary x-ray beam penetrates the body part of interest, from *point-of-entrance* to *point-of-exit*. Directional terms listed in the *Nomina Anatomica Veterinaria* should be used to describe radiographic views. An abdominal radiograph made with the dog in dorsal recumbency and the use of an overhead, vertically directed x-ray beam is called a ventrodorsal view; with the dog in ventral recumbency, it is called a dorsoventral view. The same method is used for other body parts, with the appropriate directional term applied (Fig. 2–17).

Oblique projections should be named by using the same method as standard views (i.e., by designating anatomically the points of entrance and exit) (Fig. 2–18). Angles of obliquity can also be designated by inserting the number of degrees of obliquity between the directional terms involved. If the dorsolateral-palmaromedial oblique (DL-PaMO) pro-

jection in Figure 2–18 were made by positioning the x-ray tube 60 degrees laterally with respect to dorsal, the designation would be D60L-PaMO. This term implies that, beginning dorsally, one proceeds 60 degrees to the lateral side to locate the point of entrance of the x-ray beam.

RADIOGRAPH VIEWING

To assist in developing a mental picture of normal radiographic anatomy, radiographs should always be placed on the illuminator in a standard manner. Random positioning of radiographs on the illuminator increases the difficulty in establishing a consistent mental picture of normal radiographic anatomy. Lateral views of any part should be viewed with the cranial (rostral) aspect of the animal to the viewer's left. Ventrodorsal or dorsoventral radiographs of the head, neck, or trunk should be placed with the cranial (rostral) part of the animal pointing up and with the left side of the animal to the viewer's right. Caudocranial (plantarodorsal, palmarodorsal) or craniocaudal (dorsopalmar, dorsoplantar) radiographs of the extremities should be placed on the illuminator with the proximal end of the extremity at the top. There is no convention regarding whether the medial or lateral side of the extremity is placed to the viewer's right or left.

When interpreting radiographs, an isolated, quiet environment should be sought; distractions cause one's diagnostic accuracy to decrease. Adequate illumination, such as a good-quality, evenly illuminated viewbox, is essential for accurate radiographic interpretation. At least two illuminators are desirable so that at least two views can be evaluated simultaneously. At all costs, the clinician should avoid interpreting radiographs by holding them toward an overhead light or a window. A valuable aid in interpreting radiographs, particularly of large animals, is a spotlight, sometimes referred to as a hot light. A spotlight is an intense light source that allows observation of overexposed areas on a radiograph, such as soft tissues adjacent to bone. Minimal new bone growth, which may be easily overlooked under normal illumination, can become apparent when the radiograph is viewed with a spotlight.

Radiographs should be viewed from distances of 6 inches and 6 feet. Often an abnormality is missed if the viewer is too close to the illuminator.

PRINCIPLES OF INTERPRETATION

Radiographic interpretation is neither mysterious nor difficult if certain basic procedures are followed. Interpreting a radiograph is a matter of compiling all the evidence, analyzing it, and arriving at reasonable conclusions. There are a number of important steps to this process.

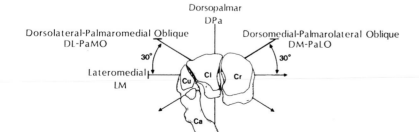

FIGURE 2–18. Description of radiographic projections by direction of the primary x-ray beam, from point-of-entrance to point-of-exit (proximal view of equine proximal carpal bones). (Courtesy of Dr. J. E. Smallwood.)

Step 1: Signalment and Case History

As in any phase of clinical diagnosis, the breed, gender, and age as well as complete knowledge of the medical history of the animal should be known for accurate radiographic assessment. Occasionally the history may be misleading, and historical information must never be taken for granted. Radiographs should never be interpreted, however, without access to history and signalment.

Step 2: Physical Examination

A radiographic examination should be performed only after a clinical opinion of the patient's health has been formed. Generally the purpose of a radiographic examination is to confirm a clinical diagnosis or impression, not to make the diagnosis. A detailed and complete physical examination is necessary to establish a reason for radiographic evaluation and to determine the part or parts of the animal to be examined radiographically.

Step 3: Correct Radiographic Procedure

No matter how astute the clinician becomes at radiographic interpretation, if a radiographic examination is technically inadequate because of an insufficient number of views, improper exposure factors, inadequate equipment such as cassettes and screens, or poor darkroom technique, important information may be overlooked, and the correct diagnosis may be missed. A poor-quality radiograph is at best inconclusive and at worst misleading.

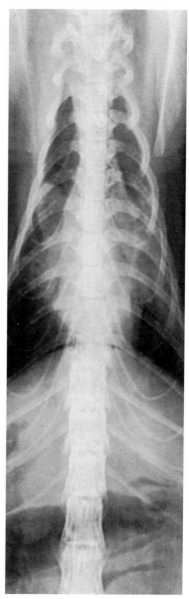

FIGURE 2–20. Roentgen sign example: number. There are 14 ribs on each side, rather than the normal 13.

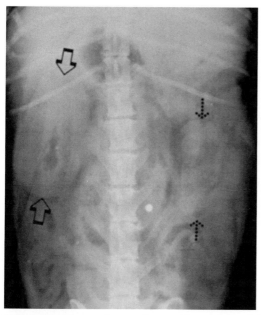

FIGURE 2–19. Roentgen sign example: size and position. The size of the right kidney is increased *(open arrows)*—compare it with the normal left kidney *(dotted arrows)*. The position of the caudal pole of the right kidney is abnormal; it is displaced laterally. This is the ventrodorsal view of the abdomen of the dog in Figure 2–5. Note the location of the shotgun pellet. By mentally reconstructing the third dimension after viewing both radiographs, one can deduce that the shotgun pellet is lodged in the retroperitoneal space medial to the caudal pole of the left kidney.

Step 4: Evaluating the Radiograph

Evaluating a radiograph consists of determining whether an abnormality exists, defining the anatomic location of the lesion, classifying the lesion according to its roentgen signs, and compiling a differential diagnosis.

In the process of trying to determine whether or not an abnormality exists, the entire radiograph must be evaluated. The *organ approach* or the *area approach* may be used. In the organ approach, the evaluator makes a conscious effort to evaluate every organ on the radiograph. In the area approach, the evaluator evaluates the radiograph by starting the analysis centrally and working toward the periphery or vice versa. Whether to use the organ or area approach is an individual decision. Nevertheless, whichever approach is adopted, the entire radiograph should be interpreted in a systematic manner.

Determining whether or not an abnormality exists is often the most difficult part of radiographic interpretation. One

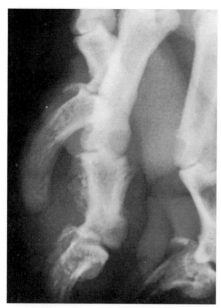

FIGURE 2–21. Roentgen sign example: margination. There is periosteal proliferation on the middle phalanx of the fourth digit.

reason for this difficulty is that the range of normal anatomic variation is broad. It is virtually impossible to remember, or even see in a lifetime, all of the anatomic variations present in domestic animals. This does not mean, however, that anatomic variation is always misinterpreted as abnormal. Published radiographic anatomy references are available for

comparison. In addition, if the suspected abnormality involves an extremity, the contralateral limb can be used for comparison. Also, individuals are encouraged to collect normal radiographs in a reference file, which can be consulted when needed. The importance of normal radiographic anatomy is so great that a complete section devoted to such is present in this book (see Chapter 47).

The value of experience in deciding if a radiographic abnormality is present cannot be underestimated. Clinicians just beginning to evaluate radiographs should not be discouraged by the relative ease with which more experienced clinicians discover radiographic abnormalities. The more radiographs one systematically analyzes, the easier is the detection of lesions. Positive reinforcement cannot be underemphasized. Questionable radiographic alterations should be reviewed with experienced radiograph interpreters as frequently as possible. During one's education, this is easy. In private practice, this is more difficult, but there are a large number of experienced radiologists in private practice, and radiographic consultation services are offered by most veterinary medicine programs.

Once a lesion has been identified, the next step is to determine its anatomic location. In certain instances, such as an abnormality involving a long bone, determination of lesion location is easier than when a more complex anatomic area is involved. Difficulty in identifying the location of an abnormality is compounded by the fact that the radiograph is a two-dimensional image of a three-dimensional object. Thus, a minimum of two radiographic projections at 90 degrees to each other is needed. Without two such views, the third dimension of depth cannot be mentally reconstructed, and it is impossible to locate accurately the lesion in question (see Fig. 2–5). Other projections may also be required. It is also necessary to have a thorough knowledge of gross anatomy. A skeletal model, particularly of complex areas such as the carpus and tarsus, is helpful.

After a lesion has been identified and located, the next step is to describe the lesion according to its roentgen signs. Roentgen signs have been defined as changes in *size, shape, number, location, margination,* and *radiopacity.* By describing the lesion according to its roentgen signs, the error-prone

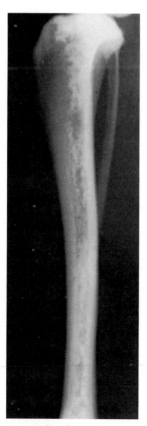

FIGURE 2–22. Roentgen sign example: radiopacity. There are multifocal areas of increased radiopacity in the medullary cavity of the tibia.

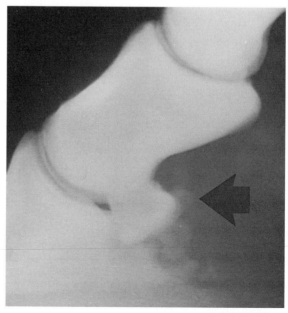

FIGURE 2–23. Roentgen sign example: shape. There is an enthesophyte on the proximal aspect of the navicular bone *(arrow).*

Table 2–2
GAMUTS FOR TWO COMMONLY OBSERVED ROENTGEN SIGNS

Increased Bronchial Wall Thickness	Increased Pulmonary Radiopacity—Alveolar, Patchy Distribution
Allergy	Pneumonia
Chronic inflammation	Hemorrhage
	Edema
	Allergy
	Thromboembolism
	Primary tumor
	Secondary tumor
	Toxicosis

method of immediately jumping to a diagnosis because the lesion looks like something the clinician may have seen or heard about before, the so-called *Aunt Minny* approach, can be avoided. The Aunt Minny approach to radiographic diagnosis can be impressive to beginning radiologists. Aunt Minny is a *charlatan,* however, and proponents of this method soon learn there is more than one possible cause for most radiographically detectable lesions. Thus, the roentgen sign approach is more reliable. By first describing a lesion according to its roentgen signs rather than immediately attempting to designate the cause for the detected abnormality, diagnostic accuracy increases considerably. Examples of roentgen signs are given in Figures 2–19 to 2–23.

Once roentgen signs have been defined, the next step is to consider what diseases can result in the production of these roentgen signs; this is called the *gamut* approach. A gamut is a list of diseases that may result in the production of a certain roentgen sign. Some gamuts are more extensive than others (Table 2–2). For radiographs in which more than one roentgen sign is present, gamuts for all roentgen signs should be considered collectively with the signalment, history, clinical signs, physical findings, and laboratory data so as to formulate a list of differential clinical diagnoses.

PITFALLS IN INTERPRETATION

There are a few circumstances in which the accuracy of radiographic interpretation decreases considerably. These are (1) the presence of *an obvious lesion* that distracts the evaluator, preventing the systematic evaluation of the remainder of the radiograph; (2) discovery of *a lesion that answers the clinical question* that prompted the radiographic examination, thereby distracting the evaluator from further analysis of the radiograph; (3) *tunnel vision,* which is a preconception of what will be found on the radiograph so that when the preconception is confirmed, the viewing of the radiograph ends.

Radiographic interpretation is both art and science. It is a skill that can be learned by most individuals. The more organized and analytic the approach to evaluating a radiograph, and the more feedback one obtains, the more astute the individual becomes in radiographic interpretation.

STUDY QUESTIONS

1. Describe a situation in which the relative radiopacity of two objects is not directly related to their effective atomic number and physical density.

2. What are the five basic radiopacities?

3. What are the six basic roentgen signs?

4. Obscuring of the radiographic detail of small intestinal serosal margin detail by the accumulation of peritoneal effusion is an example of which one of the following?

   A. summation effect
   B. silhouette sign
   C. Codman's triangle
   D. a perception artifact
   E. distortion

5. This lateral cervical radiograph (Fig. 2–24) was made of a dog who had been coughing for 3 days. Explain why the circular radiopacity is not a tracheal foreign body or tracheal wall mass.

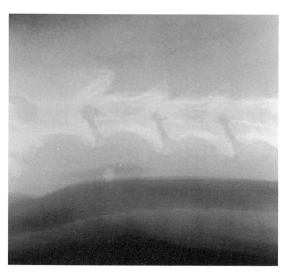

FIGURE 2–24

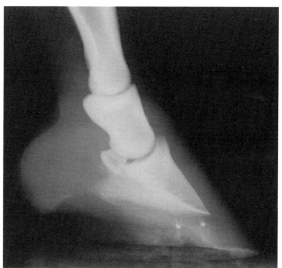

FIGURE 2–25

6. Is this lateral radiograph of the equine digit (Fig. 2–25) oriented correctly?

7. An x-ray tube is positioned directly in front of the left forelimb of a horse, at the level of the metacarpophalangeal joint. The cassette is positioned directly behind the metacarpophalangeal joint. The correct term for the view created by this configuration of tube and cassette is a(n):
   A. anteroposterior view
   B. craniocaudal view
   C. dorsoplantar view
   D. dorsopalmar view

8. Which one of the following structures would not be visible in a lateral thoracic radiograph of a normal dog?
   A. the left coronary artery
   B. the left cranial lobe pulmonary artery
   C. the caudal vena cava
   D. the descending aorta

9. In thoracic radiographs of a patient with respiratory distress, the cardiac silhouette is enlarged in size, round in shape, and homogeneous in opacity. Which one of the following conditions is least likely?
   A. intrapericardial lipoma
   B. pericardial effusion
   C. dilated cardiomyopathy
   D. hepatic peritoneopericardial hernia

10. It is essentially impossible to tell the difference between a craniocaudal and a caudocranial radiograph of a canine elbow joint. (True or False)

(Answers appear on pages 631 and 632.)

Chapter 3

Visual Perception and Radiographic Interpretation

Marc Papageorges

Vision is the most powerful sense, and we consider what we see to be an exact representation of the physical world. Numerous studies suggest, however, that often this confidence in what is seen is not justified.[1, 2] When one interprets medical images, it may be a good idea to think about how perception may be affecting the visual system.

VISUAL INACCURACIES

Slow dark adaptation and peripheral glare are widely recognized visual handicaps in radiographic interpretation. Their detrimental effects can be minimized with the use of optimal viewing conditions.[3–5] Poor performance in estimation of length, angle, and size (Figs. 3–1 to 3–4) is more difficult to acknowledge[1, 6] but, once conceded, is easily overcome with the use of measuring devices, such as a ruler. Other distortions of visual information, such as the Mach phenomenon (Fig. 3–5) and the contrast background effect (Fig. 3–6),

cannot be eliminated, but awareness of their existence reduces interpretation errors.[7, 8]

PERCEPTUAL DISTORTIONS

The most common and flagrant visual inaccuracies are difficult to detect and eliminate because they seem to involve perceptual mechanisms developed by the brain to make sense

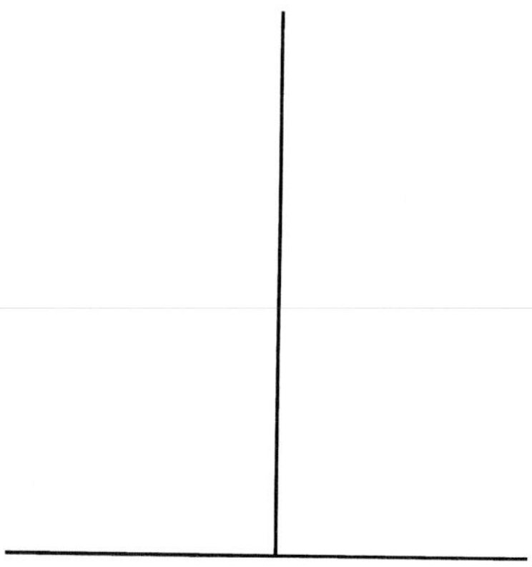

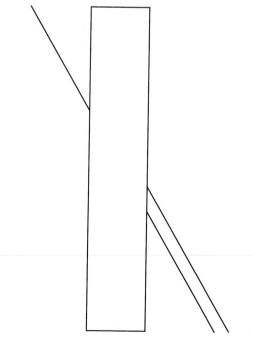

FIGURE 3–2. It is very difficult to align partially covered lines. Again, using a ruler or a straight paper edge may surprise you.

FIGURE 3–1. Which line is longer? Actual measurements may surprise you.

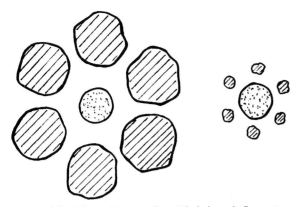

FIGURE 3–3. Which nodule *(stippled center)* is bigger? The background influences size perception.

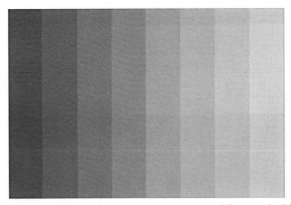

FIGURE 3–5. Mach lines (Mach phenomenon) are persistent optical illusions produced by a lateral inhibition neural network within the retina. They appear as false white or black lines at sharp boundaries. This illusion enhances boundary detection but can mimic lesions (fractures) or anatomic structures (bowel wall, bladder wall).

of sensory signals.[1, 2, 9] Many believe that the alarmingly high error rate reported in radiographic interpretation[10–12] is rooted in perceptual mechanisms. This hypothesis is supported by the fact that improving the quality of radiographs, even with digital manipulation of the image, does not seem to reduce the error rate.

Acknowledgment of the limitations of the visual system and familiarity with perceptual errors may be the only way of reducing the inconsistency of interpretation in radiology. To better understand perceptual mechanisms and their implication in radiology, the phenomena of subjective contours, multiplicity of perceptions, and visual search are examined.

SUBJECTIVE CONTOURS

Radiographs are two-dimensional images depicting exclusively the contour of objects. They are images of shadows. In contrast with the familiar shadows that surround us, however, radiographs are a summation of multiple types of shadows. This added complexity gives the false impression that the images are more than a collection of shadows, which leads to numerous perceptual errors. One should never forget that radiographs are merely images of shadows and that shadows depict only the contour of objects (Fig. 3–7).

Contours are perceived when there is an abrupt change in luminance or color of adjacent areas.[1] Under certain circumstances, the perception of contours can also occur where there is no edge (no change in brightness). Such subjective contours are the result of mental completion of partial lines to form familiar (expected) shapes.[13–15] Here is one example: When viewing three dots, most perceive a triangle. If there

are four dots, a square or a rectangle is perceived (Fig. 3–8). The objective visual information, however, is limited to three or four dots physically independent from one another; the dots could as well be part of a circle or a complex figure (Fig. 3–9). Yet, we perceive a triangle and a square. These figures give us a first clue about the difference between vision (what the eye sees) and perception (what the brain sees) and how previous knowledge—of triangles and squares—influences perception.

THEORY OF PERCEPTS

It is widely accepted that visual signals do not produce integral images in the brain: Transmission and reconstruction of

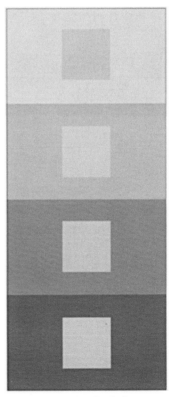

FIGURE 3–6. The eye is a poor judge of absolute brightness, as convincingly illustrated by the contrast background effect. All the small central squares are of identical brightness. The contrast background effect is a combination of the Mach phenomenon and subjective contours.

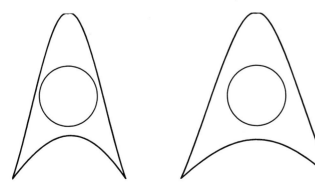

FIGURE 3–4. Apparent cardiomegaly on radiographs obtained during expiration is a very common perceptual error.

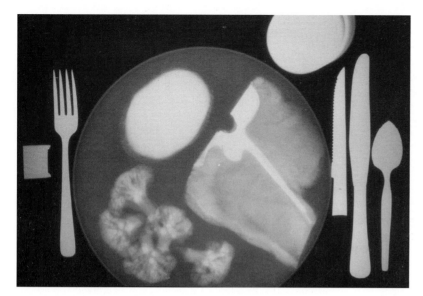

FIGURE 3–7. Examination of familiar objects reminds us that radiographs are images of shadows that show only contours.

integral visual information require too much computing power. Visual signals appear to be compared to mental images stored in memory. A meaningful image is perceived only when visual signals, after multiple comparisons, induce the emergence of a compatible mental image in the brain (Fig. 3–10). The mental images, called percepts, are continuously modified by experience.[1, 9, 14] Therefore, what we see is a mental image (percept) brought to consciousness and touched up by visual signals (shape, size, color, distance, motion). This theory explains the vivid images seen during dreams and hallucinations: They are percepts emerging spontaneously without control from visual signals. One could say that the purpose of the senses during waking hours is to induce a dream (series of percepts) and to make it as compatible as possible with physical reality.

Figure 3–11 is an example of a waking dream adrift. The objective visual information is limited to three black patches, each with a triangular defect. When viewing this figure, however, most of us perceive a large white triangle partially covering three black patches. Where is the white triangle coming from? The triangle has no physical reality other than in the brain. When the visual signals are compared to memorized mental images (percepts), our perception mechanisms conclude, based on our previous experience in the three-dimensional world, that the most likely explanation for the visual signals is the following percept: a white triangle partially covering three black patches. The image emerges in consciousness.[1, 14] The problem is that the dream is based as much (or more) on previous experience as it is on physical reality. For some of us, the illusion (mental image) is so strong that the triangle may appear lighter than the background, creating definite borders between the patches, even though the retinal stimulation is the same in both regions.

Would you perceive a triangle if you had never seen one and assimilated the concept before? Based on the experience of people who were blind at birth but gained sight later, the answer is no.[1] Would you perceive a megaesophagus on radiographs if you had never seen one with your mind's eye before?

When the brain has already been sensitized and expects a percept, limited information—or even unrelated information—can induce the mental image (Fig. 3–12). This phenomenon explains many radiographic errors.

If the amount of visual signals supporting the mental image increases, the compatibility with the percept builds, and the perception becomes stronger and more stable (Fig. 3–13). The opposite phenomenon occurs as well (i.e., when the brain does not expect or desire a certain discovery, sufficient information may not induce the perception). Everyone should be able to find a few examples of this phenomenon from personal experience.

On radiographs, subjective contours often appear as abdominal masses or false kidneys created by neighboring bowel loops or as cavitary lesions in the lungs produced by adjacent areas of increased opacity (Figs. 3–14 and 3–15). Superimposition of pulmonary blood vessels and ribs regularly mimics pulmonary nodules, particularly when blurred by motion or pulmonary opacifications.[13] Although persistent, a subjective contour is not an irreversible illusion; close examination of the radiograph often reveals that the contour is produced by unrelated opacities. The desire—or lack of desire—to find a lesion should never prevent clinicians from performing a close examination of the contour every time an abnormality is seen.

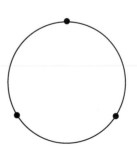

FIGURE 3–8. Seven black dots are perceived as a triangle and a square.

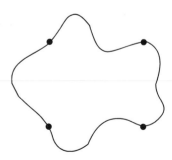

FIGURE 3–9. The same dots could as well be parts of a circle and a complex figure.

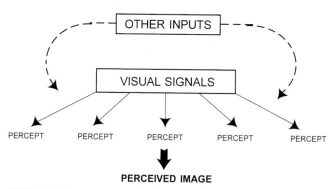

FIGURE 3–10. An image is perceived only when visual signals induce the emergence of a percept in our brain (mind).

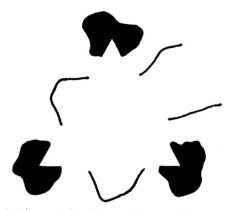

FIGURE 3–13. If more visual signals support the percept, the mental image becomes more stable.

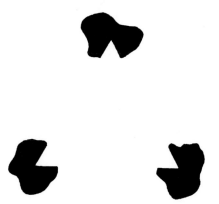

FIGURE 3–11. The visual information is limited to three black patches with small triangular defects. Where is the large white triangle coming from?

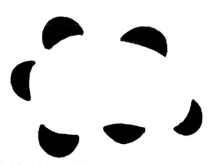

FIGURE 3–14. False kidneys or abdominal masses can be "created" by unrelated loops of bowel.

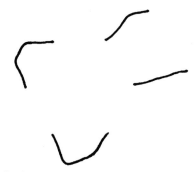

FIGURE 3–12. When the brain (mind) has been sensitized or expects the percept, limited—or unrelated—information can induce the mental image.

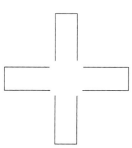

FIGURE 3–15. The perception of nodules or cavitary lesions can be induced by unrelated opacities. Note also how the nodule can appear as a square if you so desire.

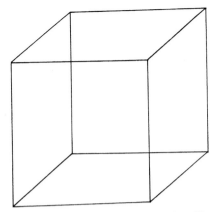

FIGURE 3–16. This image can trigger the perception of two different cubes.

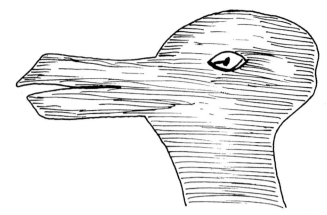

FIGURE 3–18. Different percepts triggered by the same image. If rabbits and seagulls are familiar to the observer, the perceptions alternate. Note that both are never "seen" at the same time.

MULTISTABILITY OF PERCEPTION

Multistability of perception is another phenomenon that illustrates the fundamental difference between vision and perception. Figures 3–16 and 3–17 provide classic examples. Such figures are called ambiguous, or reversible, because they represent images that may be perceived different ways.[1, 2, 16] If you look at Figure 3–16, you will most likely perceive a translucent cube seen from above. If you stare at it long enough, however, a similar but different cube appears, seen from below. Once both perceptions have been triggered, they alternate as if two different images were rapidly interchanged. Most of us perceive the cube from above first because based on our experience, we are more likely to find a cube resting on a surface than one floating weightlessly in midair. Note that only one perception is seen at any moment; the apparition of one forces the other out. Can you see the second image in Figure 3–17? It may help to turn the page upside down. Figure 3–18 is another example of different mental images triggered by the same visual signals. If one had never seen a seagull, the only image perceived would be that of a rabbit, and vice versa. If both animals are familiar to the observer, the perceptions alternate. Again, note that both animals are never seen at the same time; the emergence of percepts appears to be an all-or-nothing phenomenon. Brain mapping experiments suggest that perceptions arise from large-scale quantum changes in the collective activity of millions of neurons.[17] Figure 3–19 illustrates perceptual

errors caused by the gradual progression from one state to another (for example, from normal to pathologic in medicine). Because percepts appear to be an all-or-nothing phenomenon, we have a strong tendency to see things either one way or another (good or bad, masculine or feminine [see Fig. 3–19], normal or abnormal) even if we know that the criteria used to support the conclusion spread into a continuous range. In the midsection of the spectrum—a frequent occurrence in radiology—it is easy to understand how preconceptions have a definite effect on the percept triggered by the visual signals.

What is learned from those disconcerting figures is that two observers looking at the same radiograph or the same observer looking at one radiograph at two different times may have different perceptions. The plurality of perception has been suggested as the major explanation for the interobserver and intraobserver error rate of 20 to 30 percent in radiology.[10, 12, 18] If this hypothesis is true, multiple readings may be the only way of reducing inconsistency of interpretation.[10]

KNOWLEDGE, EMOTIONS, AND PERCEPTION

Knowledge and emotions change continuously, and both influence perception. We see more easily what is set or expected to be seen, and we are less likely to see what has no apparent connection with—or contradicts—the idea we have

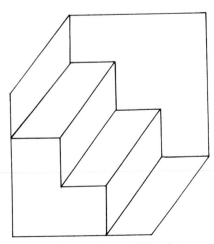

FIGURE 3–17. It is so unusual to see stairways upside down that you may feel upside down yourself when the second percept emerges into consciousness.

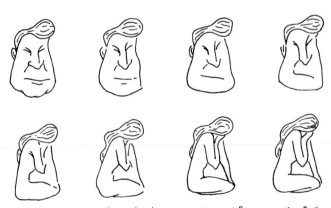

FIGURE 3–19. Progressive figures show how preconceptions can influence perception. Particularly in conditions of uncertainty, or if the phenomenon observed is part of a spectrum of possibilities.

in mind when we examine ambiguous medical images. This influence is unavoidable because perception is not the exact copying of an incoming stimulus: It is a fusion of sensory signals with past experience and expectations that identifies simultaneously the stimulus and its significance.[17] The plurality of perception is particularly apparent when radiologists have to make a diagnosis under conditions of uncertainty,[12] and this is not an uncommon situation. Interpretation of radiographs for evidence of progression, regression, or stability of disease is also grossly inconsistent.[10] The consequences are serious because many clinical decisions are based on the progression of lesions seen on serial radiographs. In such circumstances, the observer's attitude has a definite effect on radiographic interpretation. A pessimistic attitude, created, for example, by having missed pulmonary metastases in a previous patient, would make a clinician more likely to call an ill-defined shadow a nodule. Such an attitude would increase the number of true lesions detected but at the same time would increase the number of false-positive diagnoses.[12] A more optimistic attitude would decrease the number of true-positive lesions but would decrease the number of false-negative diagnoses. The ideal attitude should be determined by the number of false-positive diagnoses one is willing to accept.[12] The decision should also be based on the clinical significance of a positive finding as well as on the reliability and invasiveness of other tests likely to be used to confirm or rule out the radiographic diagnosis. Even with the best intentions, however, it is apparently impossible for human beings to maintain a constant attitude over a long period of time.

VISUAL PERCEPTION AND RADIOLOGY TEACHING

The theory of percepts should be considered in the design of radiology teaching.[19] To trained radiologists, the ability to integrate radiographic information is easy, automatic, and often taken for granted. The distress of students as they struggle to learn to *see* is a reminder of the complexity of image perception. For students, the radiology world is a hodgepodge from which they occasionally glean a useful bit of information. Perception occurs only after comparison between visual signals and memorized percepts. Because neophytes are faced with foreign visual signals, radiographs remain a confusing jumble of unconnected shades of gray until the brain has fully integrated into a unified explanation the separate visual cues of opacity, size, shape, location, and distortions associated with shadows. Such integration should be slowly developed with radiographic images of familiar objects because images cannot be interpreted without previous exposure and assimilation of the objects or concepts represented.[1, 19] Only then should tissues and pathologic processes be introduced, always keeping in mind that previous assimilation of the anatomic and pathologic concepts represented is necessary for perceptions to occur. One needs to know what to expect before *seeing* occurs. It takes years to become expert at interpreting the three-dimensional visual world. It also takes years to become expert at discovering the meaning of two-dimensional images of shadows showing the distribution and concentration of electrons in patients.

VISUAL SEARCH

All clinicians know that radiographs should be searched thoroughly, but how complete is a "complete" search? Studies have shown that large areas of radiographs are unexplored, even when interpreted by experienced radiologists.[20–22] For the most part, this is not the result of carelessness; it is the

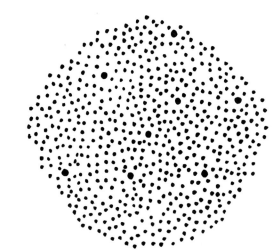

FIGURE 3–20. Lesions that stand out from the background are easily detected by the peripheral vision. How many larger dots do you find?

consequence of complex visual mechanisms, many of which are not under conscious control.[20] The area of acute vision is a lot smaller than most recognize. The fovea, the small area at the center of the retina densely packed with visual receptors, is the only structure of the eye capable of detailed vision. During interpretation of an image, eye movements temporarily fix the fovea on different parts of the image while the indistinct information gathered by the peripheral vision is used to trigger subjective contours and other percepts as well as to guide the eye movements via oculomotor reflexes.[20] A radiographic abnormality is easier to detect if it stands out from the background (high contrast) because it is more likely to be detected by the peripheral vision and attract visual attention (Figs. 3–20 and 3–21). The eyes move almost constantly from fixation to fixation in a succession of jumps. Each fixation lasts about one third of a second. Because vision is blurred during eye movements, we effectively see only when the eye is still, which can be as little as 30 percent of the time.[20, 23] We are unaware of this saccadic input of information because the process is efficiently smoothed in the visual perception centers. This smoothing of the visual input along with the filling of the peripheral field by mental images is dangerous in radiology because one has the impression of seeing in detail a large area at one glance, when the

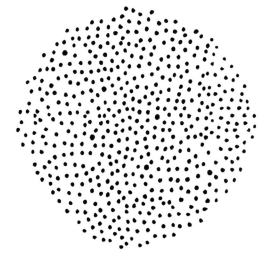

FIGURE 3–21. Lesions that do not stand out enough from the background to be detected by the peripheral vision are more difficult to find. Can you find six slightly larger dots?

actual area of acute vision is only about the size of a dime at a distance of 60 cm.[1, 20]

The apparently simple act of reading text displays the effectiveness and complexity of the filling mechanisms. An experienced reader makes three or four jumps per line (this is probably what you are doing at this moment). Even if you actually see in detail only 6 to 12 characters per line, you have the impression of having seen them all clearly. Fix your eyes on any word of this page for a few seconds. Most of the page will turn into a blur, and you will see clearly only two or three letters. This small surface of the page is the only one that is actually seen in detail at any given time. You might be able to identify one or two short words on either side of the fixation, but note how this identification is based more on extrapolation from word length and grammatical construction than on seeing the actual letters. When you resume reading, you have the impression of seeing every letter of every word again. The smoothing procedure is done by the brain, which fills in the missing information using our knowledge of the English language (as the triangle in Fig. 3–7 is filled in using our knowledge of triangles). The faster we read, the longer the jumps, and the more information is filled in by the mind. This is why we have such difficulty finding typos, particularly in a familiar text. Reading a text written in a foreign language makes one appreciate the effect of previous knowledge on perception: *De toute évidence, lire cette courte phrase en français vous prendra beaucoup plus de temps que si elle avait été écrite en anglais.*

The same phenomenon occurs with radiographs: The more familiar we are with the images, the more comfortable we become and the faster we can discover their meaning, but at the same time, the more information is filled in by the brain. Another interesting aspect of the eye jumps is that their dynamics is not under conscious control; we cannot change the length or direction of a jump once it is initiated. Therefore, we cannot be certain about what we actually see and what is filled in.[20, 23] The best we can do to control a search pattern is to concentrate on a certain area; the details of the search are always left to an unconscious part of the visual system.[20]

Try to find how many times the letter "F" is used in Figure 3–22 without reading any further. Most of us find four or five. The answer is seven. If you can't find them all after multiple attempts, try reading backwards (which suppresses the "fill-in" mechanisms). Do you still believe you have full control over your eye jumps?

Knowing that we see in detail only a surface the size of a dime, that it is impossible to control accurately where the "dime" will rest on the image, that we see only one third of the time we are actually looking, and that it is impossible to know how much we actually see and how much information the brain fills in makes it easier to understand how psychological factors, such as interest, motivation, training, and emotions, can modify the way we search, perceive, and interpret radiographs. It is also easier to understand how lesions can be missed. A systematic approach is important when interpreting radiographs to counterbalance the shortcomings of the visual system.

CONCLUSION

This chapter may give the impression that radiology is less reliable than other fields of medicine, but a similar error rate has been found regarding the ability to detect and describe lesions such as heart murmurs.[10] It appears that several aspects of medicine may be subject to a significant error rate rooted in the difference between sensory detection and perception.[10] Familiarity with perceptual mechanisms and with the limitations of the senses may be the only way of reducing perceptual errors. Rational knowledge, however, does not correct all perceptual errors, and they will remain a major challenge in radiology as well as in other fields of medicine. If you remain unconvinced, gather 25 radiographs for which you have generated reports and write new reports without looking at the previous ones. You will see things you did not see before and won't see others that you saw then. The inconsistencies are due to changes in subjective contours, multistability of perception, and visual search prompted by differences in patient information, pressure from the owner or other clinicians, other stresses influencing concentration, or simply the desire to prove that inconsistency of interpretation happens only to others.

FINISHED FILES ARE THE RESULT OF YEARS OF SCIENTIFIC STUDY COMBINED WITH THE EXPERIENCE OF MANY YEARS OF EXPERT OBSERVATION.

FIGURE 3–22. Counting how many times the letter "F" is used in one sentence proves more difficult than anticipated. Finding all pertinent lesions on one radiograph is likely to be a more arduous task.

References

1. Wandell BA: Foundations of Vision. Sunderland, MA, Sinauer Associates, Inc, 1995.
2. Hebb DO, and Favreau O: The mechanism of perception. Radiol Clin North Am 8:393, 1969.
3. Ravindra H, Normann RA, and Baxter B: The effect of extraneous light on lesion detectability: A demonstration. Invest Radiol 18:105, 1983.
4. Alter AJ, George MD, Kargas A, et al: The influence of ambient and viewbox light upon visual detection of low-contrast targets in a radiograph. Invest Radiol 17:402, 1982.
5. Baxter B, Ravindra H, and Normann RA: Changes in lesion detectability caused by light adaptation in retinal photoreceptors. Invest Radiol 17:394, 1982.
6. Jaffe CC: Medical Imaging, Vision, and Visual Psychophysics. Rochester, NY, Eastman Kodak Co, 1984.
7. Papageorges M, and Sande RD: The Mach phenomenon. Vet Radiol 31:274, 1990.
8. Papageorges M: How the Mach phenomenon and shape affect the radiographic appearance of skeletal structures. Vet Radiol 32:191, 1991.
9. Zeki S: The visual image. In Piel J (Ed.): Mind and Brain. New York, Scientific American, 1992, pp 69–76.
10. Yerushalmy J: The statistical assessment of the variability in observer perception and description of roentgenographic pulmonary shadows. Radiol Clin North Am 8:101, 1969.
11. Markus JB, Somers S, Slobodan EF, et al: Interobserver variation in the interpretation of abdominal radiographs. Radiology 17:69, 1989.
12. Lusted LB: Perception of the roentgen image: Application of signal detectability theory. Radiol Clin North Am 8:435, 1969.
13. Daffner RH, Gehweiler JA, and Rodan BA: Subjective contours and illusory roentgenographic images. Appl Radiol July/August: 95, 1984.
14. Kanizsa G: Subjective contours. Sci Am 234:48, 1976.
15. Ratliff F: Contour and contrast. Sci Am 226:90, 1972.
16. Attneave F: Multistability in perception. Sci Am 234:48, 1976.
17. Freeman WJ: The physiology of perception. Sci Am 264:78, 1991.
18. Fletcher CM, and Oldham PD: The use of standard films in the radiological diagnosis of coal workers' pneumonoconiosis. Br J Ind Med 8:138, 1954.
19. Squire LF: Perception related to learning radiology in medical school. Radiol Clin North Am 8:485, 1969.
20. Llewellyn-Thomas E: Search behavior. Radiol Clin North Am 8:403, 1969.
21. Llewellyn-Thomas E, and Lansdowne EL: Visual search patterns of radiologists in training. Radiology 81:288, 1963.
22. Tuddenham WJ, and Calvert WF: Visual search patterns in roentgen diagnosis. Radiology 76:694, 1961.
23. Kundel HL, and LaFollette PS: Visual search patterns and experience with radiological images. Radiology 103:523, 1972.

STUDY QUESTIONS

1. Radiographs are images of _____.

2. Radiographs show only the _____ of objects.

3. Visual signals are compared to _____ stored in memory.

4. On radiographs, subjective contours can appear as false _____, _____, _____ and _____.

5. The _____ of _____ has been suggested as the major explanation for the high error rate in radiology.

6. Images cannot be interpreted (or seen) without previous _____.

7. The area of acute vision is the size of a _____ at a distance of 60 cm.

8. Our eyes see only _____ percent of the time we are actually looking.

9. It is impossible to know how much we actually see and how much our brain _____.

10. Several fields of medicine may be subject to a significant error rate rooted in the difference between _____ and _____.

(Answers appear on page 632.)

Chapter 4

Aggressive Versus Nonaggressive Bone Lesions

Linda J. Konde

This chapter presents an overview of the radiographic appearance of normal bone, a general guideline for evaluating aggressive versus nonaggressive bone lesions, and a basic radiologic approach to use in the diagnosis of skeletal disorders.

RADIOGRAPHIC APPEARANCE OF NORMAL BONE

The four general anatomic regions present in long bones are the following:

1. The epiphysis, located at each end of the bone. In the young animal, ossification often proceeds at an uneven rate, and the articular surface of the epiphysis may have an irregular margin.

2. The physis, adjacent to the epiphysis. It is radiolucent in young animals owing to the presence of cartilage. In mature animals, the remnant of the physis is sometimes seen as a linear opacity.

3. The metaphysis, the region adjacent to the diaphyseal side of the physis. The boundary between the metaphysis and the diaphysis is not defined by an anatomic structure or radiographic landmark.

4. The diaphysis, the central shaft of the bone.

Cortical bone is structurally different from spongiosa. Cortical bone growth is intramembranous and extremely compact. Cortical bone surrounds the diaphysis and metaphysis and appears opaque on a radiograph. Arterial supply to a long bone enters via a nutrient foramen located in the diaphysis. When viewed lengthwise, these foramina are radiolucent channels penetrating obliquely through the cortex, and when viewed transversely, they are circular, centrally located radiolucencies. It is important to recognize a normal nutrient foramen so as not to mistake it for a fracture or a lytic lesion.

Trabecular bone is prominent in metaphyseal and epiphyseal regions. Discrete trabeculation is less apparent in the medullary canal because it contains elements that are less opaque than bone. In older animals, the major component of bone marrow is fat. Therefore, the radiographic appearance of the diaphysis is relatively homogeneous.

The diameter of bone is usually widest at the physis and metaphysis. In the young animal, the metaphyseal cortical margin is irregular owing to bone resorption and remodeling, which is necessary to achieve the more narrow diaphyseal diameter. The diaphysis should be of uniform diameter. When growth ceases, physeal cartilage is replaced by bone, uniting metaphysis and epiphysis. Often an opaque line is seen at the site of the physis; this is called the *physeal scar.*

The periosteum is a layer of fibroelastic connective tissue adherent to the external bone surface. The periosteum has two important functions: (1) Its rich supply of finely divided blood vessels penetrates the cortex, supplying nourishment to bone, and, (2) when stimulated, it is capable of producing reactive new bone. In the normal state, periosteum is not visible on a radiograph. Periosteal bone formation becomes visible only after trauma or in reaction to a disease process; therefore, periosteal new bone seen on a radiograph indicates an abnormal skeletal condition. Periosteal new bone is radiographically visible 7 to 10 days after injury.[1, 2]

GUIDELINES FOR EVALUATING AGGRESSIVE VERSUS NONAGGRESSIVE BONE LESIONS

In may be possible to reach a definitive diagnosis for a bone lesion based solely on signalment, history, and radiographic signs. Disorders such as fractures, canine panosteitis, and hypertrophic osteodystrophy are a few specific examples. Many bone disorders, however, have a similar radiographic appearance. Therefore, a logical approach in the evaluation of bony lesions is of paramount importance in formulating a differential diagnosis.

By determining if a lesion appears aggressive or nonaggressive, appropriate categories of disease may be considered that otherwise may be overlooked. The list of differential diagnoses, in combination with historical and clinical findings, may then be ranked in order of probability. In assessing aggressiveness, skeletal lesions should be evaluated by determining the following.

Location of a Lesion or Lesions

The lesion may be generalized (involving all bones in a similar manner), focal (involving a single bone in a defined area), or multifocal (involving multiple areas in the same bone or several different bones). Some examples of how lesion location may assist in diagnosis include the following:

1. Generalized bone involvement may indicate metabolic or nutritional disorders.
2. Primary bone tumors are usually solitary lesions most often located in metaphyses of long bones.[3-5]
3. Secondary metastatic neoplasias and fungal bone infection may be seen in multiple locations of different bones.[5]
4. Hematogenous bacterial osteomyelitis, a rare condition most often seen in younger animals, usually affects epiphyseal and metaphyseal regions.[6]
5. Secondary bacterial osteomyelitis usually results from penetrating wounds, soft-tissue infection, and surgical manipulation and is located at the site of the insult.[6]

Rate of Change in Appearance of Lesion

Rate of change in appearance of a lesion is determined by performing serial or follow-up radiographic examinations. Less aggressive lesions typically change little or not at all on follow-up examinations, whereas aggressive lesions appear dramatically different from one examination to the next. The appearance of lesions on follow-up examinations may also be used to document the effectiveness of treatment regimens.

Pattern of Bone Destruction

Bone lysis appears radiographically as a decrease in bone opacity. Approximately 30 to 50 percent of bone per unit area must be destroyed before lysis is radiographically visible.[1, 4, 7] Because of its compact structure, lysis of cortical bone is easier to detect than lysis of cancellous bone. Three patterns of bone destruction or lysis are recognized:[4, 7-9]

1. Geographic—benign or relatively nonaggressive.
2. Moth-eaten—moderately aggressive.
3. Permeative—highly aggressive.

Geographic bone destruction is characterized by a single, large, well-defined area of lysis or a few, large, confluent lytic areas in the bone (Fig. 4–1). The adjacent bone is uninvolved, and the border between normal and abnormal bone is relatively sharply defined. Often, there is a sclerotic bone reaction about the margin of the lesion, suggesting an attempt to wall it off. This type of pattern is usually confined to the medullary cavity; however, the cortex may become thinned and

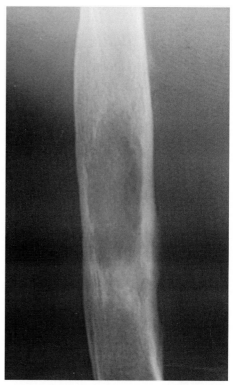

FIGURE 4–1. Geographic bone lysis (bone abscess). There is a single, circumscribed area of bone lysis in the midfemur with a relatively well-defined margin between normal and abnormal bone. Endosteal cortical bone lysis is present on the cranial and caudal aspects of the lesion. The margin of periosteal new bone is smooth and slightly lamellated (most apparent in the distocranial femur). These changes suggest a more benign bone lesion. The lucency extending across the cortex in the distocaudal aspect of this region is caused by a defect in the bone created surgically for drainage.

outwardly expanded. This pattern generally indicates a benign or less aggressive lesion, such as a bone cyst, enchondroma, or bone abscess.

Moth-eaten bone destruction is characterized by multiple areas of lysis of moderate and nonuniform size (Fig. 4–2). The lytic areas tend to coalesce. The lesion may be poorly circumscribed with an ill-defined margin or may have well-defined margins. Cortical destruction is usually present, and pathologic fractures may occur. Many aggressive primary and metastatic neoplasms, as well as acute bacterial osteomyelitis, have this pattern of bone lysis. The typical punched-out, lytic, multifocal bone lesions seen with multiple myeloma are another example of moth-eaten bone destruction.

Permeative bone destruction is characterized by multiple, uniformly pinpoint areas of bone lysis primarily involving cortical bone, although medullary bone is also affected (Fig. 4–3). The margin between normal and abnormal bone is poorly defined, with the lytic areas becoming smaller and more widely spaced near the edge of the lesion. This pattern correlates with a highly aggressive bone lesion, either neoplastic or infectious.

Cortical Involvement

An aggressive bone lesion causes partial or complete lysis of the cortex as it extends into surrounding soft tissues (Fig. 4–4A). Benign or less aggressive lesions may not involve cortical bone.[2, 4] If they do, the slow-growing lesion causes endosteal, cortical thinning and may expand the cortex out-

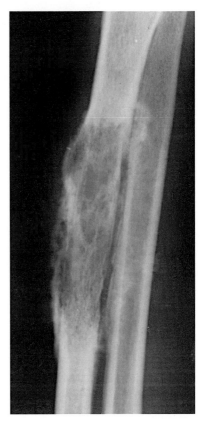

FIGURE 4–2. Moth-eaten bone lysis (osteosarcoma). Numerous lytic areas of variable size are present in the mid-diaphysis of the radius. The transition zone between normal and abnormal bone is irregular. It is poorly defined proximally and better defined distally. There is considerable cortical bone lysis. An interrupted, somewhat spiculated periosteal new bone formation is seen. These changes suggest a moderately aggressive bone lesion.

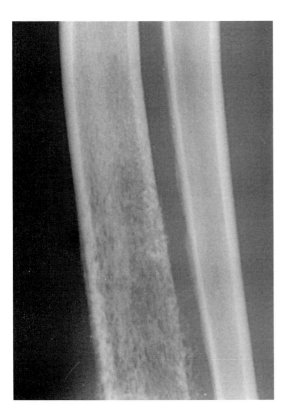

FIGURE 4–3. Permeative bone lysis (osteosarcoma). Multiple small areas of bone lysis are present in the cortex and medulla of the distal radial diaphysis. The transition zone between normal and abnormal bone is long and poorly defined. A minimal, interrupted periosteal new bone formation is seen at the distocaudal area of the lesion. These changes suggest a highly aggressive bone lesion.

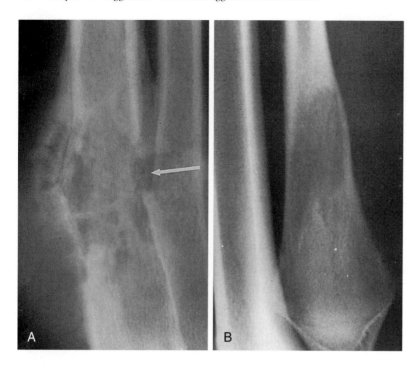

FIGURE 4–4. *A,* Cortical bone lysis (osteosarcoma). There is complete lysis of the caudal cortex *(arrow),* with endosteal cortical lysis distally. The cranial cortex contains numerous lytic areas and is pathologically fractured. Moth-eaten bone lysis is present, and edge margins between normal and abnormal bone are irregular and ill-defined. *B,* Endosteal bone erosion (enchondroma). There is smooth thinning of the endosteal cortical surface by a circumscribed region of geographic bone lysis in the distal ulna. The caudal ulnar cortex has a slight convexity from the slowly expanding bone lesion.

ward (see Fig. 4–4*B*). When the cortex is destroyed, there is a strong possibility of pathologic fracture.

Characteristic of Edge Margin Between Normal and Abnormal Bone

A *regular margin* has a smooth outline with no irregularity or scalloping. There is a distinct margin between normal and abnormal bone, and sclerosis may surround the lesion (Fig. 4–5). This is seen with benign or less aggressive lesions.

A *ragged margin* has an irregular or poorly defined edge (see Figs. 4–2 and 4–4*A*). The transition zone between normal and abnormal bone may be distinct or ill defined. This is seen with moderately aggressive lesions.

A *moth-eaten margin* has no clear distinction between normal and abnormal bone. There is a moth-eaten pattern of bone destruction in the transition zone, which may be small

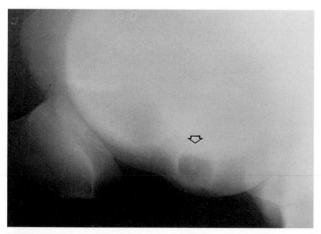

FIGURE 4–5. Regular edge margin (osseous cyst-like lesion) *(arrow).* There is a well-circumscribed lucency in the medial condyle of this equine stifle. The edge margin is sharply defined, and there is sclerosis surrounding the bone lesion.

or extensive (Fig. 4–6). This is seen with highly aggressive lesions.

Periosteal and Tumor New Bone Formation

Bone formation may originate from normal bone or from tumors. Both reactive new bone and tumor new bone may be formed within the medullary cavity, outside the bone, or both.[2, 9]

Internal Bone Formation

Intramedullary reactive new bone is usually organized and homogeneous in appearance (Fig. 4–7*A*). It results from thickening and increased opacity of normal trabeculae. This type of reaction is seen in disorders such as endosteal callus formation, canine panosteitis, bone infarction, and pyruvate kinase deficiency.

Tumor new bone usually creates focal bone opacities within the lesion that results in a nonhomogeneous appearance (see Fig. 4–7*B*). When this type of bone formation is identified, the list of differential diagnoses may be narrowed to osteogenic and chondrogenic neoplasia.

External Bone Formation

Periosteal reactive new bone may appear in many different ways, depending on the aggressive nature of the lesion. Periosteal new bone formation may be separated into two basic categories, *continuous* and *interrupted.*[1, 4, 5, 7, 9]

Continuous periosteal new bone formation is uniform in opacity and thickness. The degree of opacity is not significant, only that there is a uniform opacity. The free edge of the reactive new bone may be regular and solid or rough and undulating (Fig. 4–8). This pattern is considered an indicator of a benign process. Examples of this type of new bone are seen in callus formation, traumatic periosteitis, canine panosteitis, and hypertrophic osteopathy.

Interrupted periosteal new bone formation is extremely variable in radiographic appearance (Fig. 4–9). The proliferative re-

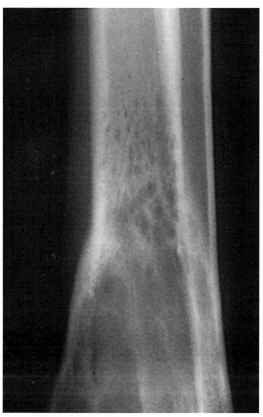

FIGURE 4–6. Moth-eaten edge margin (osteosarcoma). Multiple areas of bone lysis are present in the edge margin between normal and abnormal bone. This large, poorly defined transition zone is approximately 3 cm in length.

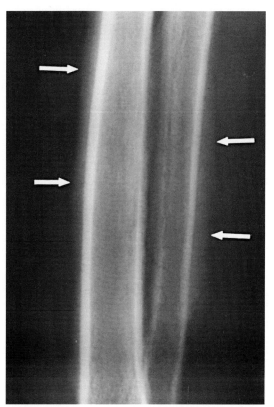

FIGURE 4–8. Continuous periosteal new bone formation (hypertrophic osteopathy). Periosteal new bone formation is present on the radial and ulnar diaphyses *(arrows)*. The free margin is slightly irregular, but the opacity of the periosteal new bone is homogeneous.

FIGURE 4–7. *A,* Intramedullary reactive new bone (panosteitis). There is a homogeneous increased opacity in the mid-diaphysis of the radius *(arrowheads).* Margins of the opacity are well defined. Mild periosteal new bone formation is seen between the radius and the ulna, which is probably related to strain of the interosseous ligament. *B,* Intramedullary tumor new bone (osteosarcoma). *Arrowheads* indicate multiple, ill-defined regions of increased opacity in the distal femur, suggestive of tumor new bone formation.

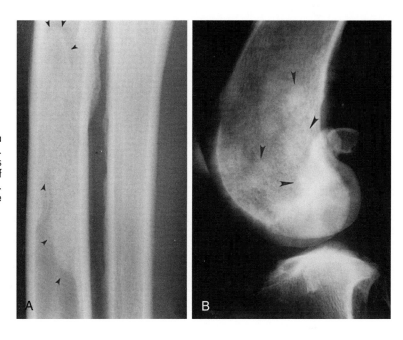

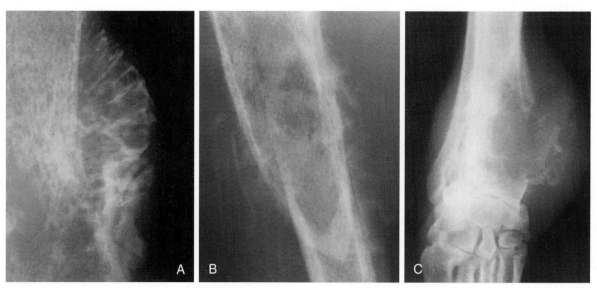

FIGURE 4–9. *A,* Interrupted periosteal new bone formation (osteosarcoma). The periosteal reaction is nonhomogeneous, with areas of lucency intermixed between spicules of new bone extending perpendicular to the cortex. Permeative and coalescing moth-eaten bone lysis is also seen. *B,* Interrupted periosteal new bone formation (osteosarcoma). Faint spicules of new bone are visible, especially arising from the caudal cortex. The new bone formation found proximally and cranially has a palisading, spiculated appearance, and craniodistally there is linear new bone formation seen in the soft tissues that is parallel to the cortex. Moth-eaten bone lysis with a pathologic fracture is present. *C,* Interrupted periosteal new bone formation (osteosarcoma). Complete cortical disruption is present on the distomedial radius. Extending into the soft tissues adjacent to this region is an amorphous, nonhomogeneous periosteal new bone formation.

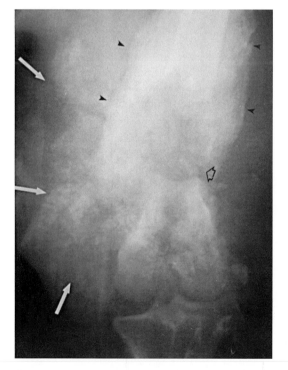

FIGURE 4–10. Tumor new bone formation (osteosarcoma). Extensive, amorphous mineral opacities are seen in the soft tissues surrounding the distal femur *(white arrows).* Interrupted periosteal new bone is seen adjacent to the cortex *(arrowheads).* There is a pathologic fracture in the distal femoral diaphysis in a region of complete bone lysis *(open arrow).*

sponse is disorganized and irregular. Often, wide separations exist between areas of new bone formation. Opacity of the new bone formation is nonhomogeneous, with areas or layers of decreased and increased opacity external to the cortex, and may not entirely surround the bone lesion. Spicules of reactive new bone may be seen extending perpendicular to the cortex into the surrounding soft tissues. This pattern is associated with an active, aggressive lesion, such as infectious and neoplastic processes. This type of reactive new bone may rapidly change in appearance on serial radiographs. Descriptive terms for this category of periosteal reactions, in order of increasing aggressiveness, include *lamellated* or *onionskin*, *spiculated*, and *amorphous*.

Peripheral tumor new bone varies in appearance but most commonly has an interrupted, spiculated, or amorphous reaction (Fig. 4–10). It is difficult to differentiate from periosteal new bone formation, but tumor new bone formation usually invades adjacent soft tissues far more extensively than does periosteal new bone formation.

BASIC RADIOLOGIC APPROACH IN THE DIAGNOSIS OF SKELETAL LESIONS

In clinical practice, the radiographic diagnosis of bone lesions may be readily apparent from the onset. Memorizing the appearance of each orthopedic disease (sometimes called the *Aunt Minnie* approach) should not be used, however, because that method is limited to the number of disease processes that can be remembered and because many diseases appear similar at first glance. Accurate radiographic interpretation depends on using a systematic approach to evaluate radiographs. A systematic approach to radiographic evaluation of bone lesions must be based on thorough knowledge of skeletal pathophysiology and radiographic patterns, coupled with a routine, careful film-reading technique. Systematic evaluation is based on the following accomplishments:

1. Demonstrating the bone lesion and its soft-tissue involvement on radiographs of high technical quality.
2. Describing in detail the radiographic changes, using the general guidelines given earlier for evaluating skeletal lesions.
3. Based on the radiographic changes, indicating the nature of the lesion (aggressive or nonaggressive). Many lesions have a combination of more and less aggressive changes. The lesion should be categorized by its most aggressive element.
4. If possible, establishing a specific diagnosis or determining the differential diagnoses in the order of probability.
5. When indicated, obtaining comparison studies, follow-up studies, or additional radiographic views.

Ideally, when formulating a diagnosis or differential diagnoses, all possible conditions involving bone and soft tissues should be considered. A survey of all rule-outs in skeletal disease is simplified if broad categories are used to narrow the possible differential diagnoses. If the following categories of skeletal disease are reviewed for every skeletal lesion, disease processes can be considered that may otherwise be overlooked:

1. Degenerative disease.
2. Anomalous developmental or congenital disorders.
3. Metabolic, endocrine, or nutritional disorders.
4. Neoplasia and tumor-like conditions.
5. Infectious or inflammatory diseases.
6. Traumatic incidents.

Once a category, or categories, is decided on, differential diagnoses may be determined. To help rank differentials in order of probability, the following additional factors should always be considered:

1. Signalment, including age, species, breed, and gender.
2. Historical findings, including duration of signs, pain pattern, and occupational or environmental conditions.
3. Physical and clinical findings.
4. Bone biopsy.

Integration of these factors with a basic approach to the radiographic evaluation of skeletal lesions allows an appropriate characterization of disorders affecting the skeletal system.

References

1. Kealy JK: Diagnostic Radiology of the Dog and Cat. Philadelphia, WB Saunders, 1987.
2. Park RD: Radiographic diagnosis of long bone neoplasms in the dog. Comp Contin Ed Vet Pract 3:922, 1981.
3. Ling GV, Morgan JP, and Pool RR: Primary bone tumors in the dog: A combined clinical, radiographic, and histologic approach to early diagnosis. J Am Vet Med Assoc *165*:55, 1974.
4. Hanlon GF: A radiologic approach to bone neoplasms. Vet Clin North Am [Small Anim Pract] *12*:329, 1982.
5. Morgan JP: Systematic radiographic interpretation of skeletal diseases in small animals. Vet Clin North Am [Small Anim Pract] *4*:611, 1974.
6. Morgan JP: Radiology in Veterinary Orthopedics. Philadelphia, Lea & Febiger, 1972.
7. Greenfield GB: Radiology of Bone Diseases. Philadelphia, JB Lippincott, 1985.
8. Lodwick GS, Wilson AJ, Farrell C, et al: Determining growth rates of focal lesions of bone from radiographs. Radiology *134*:577, 1980.
9. Edeiken J: Roentgen Diagnosis of Diseases of Bone. Baltimore, Williams & Wilkins, 1981.

STUDY QUESTIONS

1. Name two possible differential diagnoses for focal lytic and proliferative bone lesions seen at multiple skeletal sites.

2. You are presented with a 10-year-old dog who has a lameness of 3 weeks' duration in the right hind limb. There is a fracture of the distal fibula with poorly defined margins and minor, smooth periosteal bone reaction. It is uncertain if this is an old traumatic injury or a pathologic fracture. What course of action do you follow?

3. Name the three patterns of bone destruction.

4. Name three possible differential diagnoses for a well-circumscribed area of bone lysis.

5. A short transition zone between normal and abnormal bone indicates a benign bone lesion. (True or False)

6. Interrupted periosteal new bone formation indicates an active, aggressive lesion and can have a smooth or irregular margin. (True or False)

7. The location of a skeletal lesion is often helpful in determining a diagnosis. (True or False)

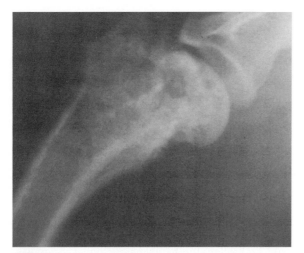

FIGURE 4–11

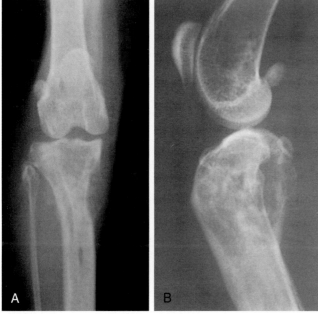

FIGURE 4–12

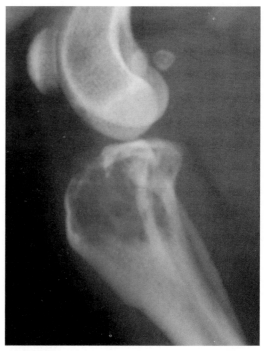

FIGURE 4–13

8. This radiograph (Fig. 4–11) of the shoulder is from a 5-year-old Terrier mix with a history of limping, shoulder pain, and tissue swelling about the shoulder for several months. Describe the type of bone destruction and periosteal bone reaction.

9. Radiographs of the tibia (Fig. 4–12) are from a 16-year-old domestic short hair cat who is limping on the right hind limb. Pain and swelling are palpated in the proximal tibia. How would you characterize this lesion?

10. This radiograph (Fig. 4–13) is from an older dog who has lameness in the right hind limb. How would you characterize this lesion?

(Answers appear on page 632.)

AXIAL SKELETON—COMPANION ANIMALS

Chapter 5

Cranial Vault and Associated Structures

Wendy Myer

RADIOGRAPHIC EVALUATION

Normal Anatomy

The skull houses the brain and the sense organs for hearing, equilibrium, sight, smell, and taste. Radiography is commonly used to evaluate abnormalities of these organs. In the dog, this evaluation is difficult because of differences in skull shape and size. Less pronounced breed differences are seen in the cat.[1]

Three head shapes have been described in the dog: dolichocephalic, mesaticephalic, and brachycephalic.[2] This classification is based on the relative proportions of the facial bones and the cranial vault. In addition to these differences, considerable change also occurs during miniaturization of the dog. As the dog's body size decreases, the occipital protuberance and frontal sinuses decrease in prominence, and there is progressive doming and cortical thinning of the calvaria. The more a breed digresses from the ancestral German shepherd type, the more pronounced are the changes in the shape and relative size of the calvaria.

When proper positioning is achieved, the bilateral symmetry of the skull allows comparison between a unilateral abnormality and the corresponding normal contralateral side. Even minor obliquity during positioning causes considerable anatomic distortion and superimposition. Routine positions include the lateral and dorsoventral, or ventrodorsal, views. In addition, depending on the area to be evaluated, oblique, rostrocaudal, and open-mouth views are often used.[3] Detailed descriptions of these special views may be found elsewhere.[4]

Alterations in Size, Shape, and Margination

Congenital alterations in calvarial shape and margination are most commonly associated with hydrocephalus and malformations of the occipital portion of the skull. Internal hydrocephalus is excess fluid in the cerebral ventricles. It is most often found in small breeds, such as the Yorkshire terrier and Chihuahua. Only rarely has hydrocephalus been documented in the cat.[5, 6]

Radiographic signs suggestive of hydrocephalus are doming of the calvaria with cortical thinning, decreased prominence of the normal calvarial convolutional markings, persistent fontanelles, and a brain that appears homogeneous (Fig. 5–1).[7] The degree of resultant calvarial distortion depends on the rate at which fluid accumulates, the severity of ventricu-

lar enlargement, and the stage of ossification of the cranial sutures at the onset of disease.[8] The most severe radiographic changes occur in congenital hydrocephalus, with less severe alterations in animals that acquire hydrocephalus after calvarial ossification.

In the past, pneumoventriculography was necessary to assess ventricular size and shape accurately.[9] Ultrasonography, magnetic resonance imaging (MRI), and computed tomography (CT) now provide less invasive methods for evaluating the brain. The normal ultrasonographic appearances of the neonatal and adult canine ventricular system have been described.[10, 11] The mean height of the normal lateral ventricle in these studies was 0.15 cm. Lateral ventricles were considered to be enlarged if their height exceeded 0.35 cm.[12] Another author has used the percentage of brain occupied by the dorsoventral dimension of the lateral ventricle as a method of assessing ventriculomegaly. The following categories were established: normal (0 to 14 percent), moderate (15 to 25 percent) or severe (greater than 25 percent) ventriculomegaly.[13]

Occipital dysplasia, an abnormal dorsal extension of the foramen magnum, was first described in 1965 and usually occurs in toy and miniature breeds, such as Poodles, Yorkshire terriers, and Chihuahuas.[14] The size of the foramen magnum is best evaluated in a rostrodorsal-caudoventral skull radiograph. The anesthetized animal is placed on its back with its neck flexed so the nose moves toward the

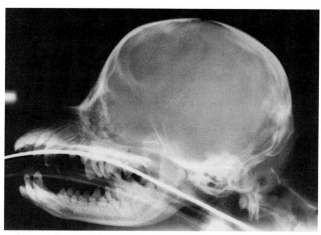

FIGURE 5–1. Lateral radiograph of a 1-year-old male Chihuahua with severe hydrocephalus. Note the loss of normal convolutional skull markings and resulting homogeneous appearance of the calvaria.

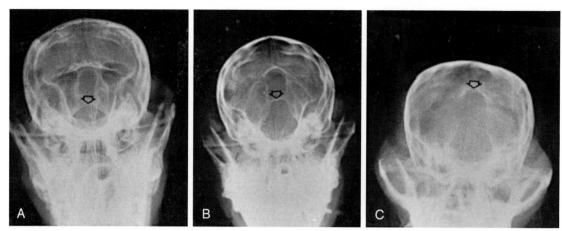

FIGURE 5–2. Rostrodorsal-caudoventral oblique views of the skull in three small-breed dogs. Note the appearance of the foramen magnum. *Arrows* indicate the dorsal extent of the foramen magnum. *A,* A normal foramen. *B,* Moderate occipital dysplasia. *C,* Severe occipital dysplasia.

sternum. The central x-ray beam passes between the eyes and exits through the foramen magnum. The angle of the beam from the vertical axis varies from 25 to 40 degrees, depending on the shape of the calvaria.[15] Figure 5–2 illustrates the normal and abnormal appearances of the foramen magnum. Two studies suggest that occipital dysplasia is relatively common in smaller dogs. A 100 percent incidence was found in 15 asymptomatic small-breed dogs.[16] In another study, a 50 percent incidence was found in 45 normal Beagles.[17] Most of these animals had only a minor dorsal extension of the foramen magnum, and it is unlikely that the occipital dysplasia was clinically significant. Occipital dysplasia is often accompanied by other abnormalities, such as hydrocephalus and atlantoaxial malformation, which may cause neurologic dysfunction.

Several congenital calvarial malformations have been described in the cat.[18–20] Mucopolysaccharidosis, which has been described in Siamese and domestic shorthair cats, is caused by inborn errors in glycosaminoglycan metabolism. Although the metabolic error in these two breeds is not identical, the clinical appearance of the cats is similar. Characteristically the cats have a broad, short maxilla with aplastic or hypoplastic frontal and sphenoid sinuses and abnormal nasal conchal development. Concurrent dysplasias of other areas of the skeleton are often present. In people and in the Siamese cat, this condition appears to be inherited as an autosomal recessive trait. The mode of inheritance in the domestic shorthair cat has not been determined.

Trauma is the most common cause of acquired alterations in skull shape and margination in the dog and cat. Automobile accidents, wounds inflicted by other animals, and injuries of unknown causes accounted for approximately 75 percent of traumatic lesions in one report.[21]

Maxillary and mandibular fractures are more common than fractures of the calvaria (Fig. 5–3).[22] Oblique and open-mouth views are especially helpful when maxillary and mandibular fractures are being evaluated. Fractures of the facial bones are often accompanied by soft-tissue swelling and are generally displaced enough to be readily evident on routine radiographs. If the nasal passages or frontal sinuses are involved, subcutaneous air accumulation is a frequent finding; this appears as a radiolucent area in the soft tissues surrounding the fracture or fractures.

A common mandibular injury in the cat is symphyseal separation.[23] In urban areas, where multiple-story housing is common, cats may sustain severe injuries after falls from

heights. Because cats usually land on all four feet, these falls result in a uniform pattern of fractures. The force of the landing results in the maxilla striking the ground, with resultant fracture of the mandibular symphysis and splitting of the hard palate. Femoral fractures and carpal dislocations with or without forelimb fractures also often occur.[24] This pattern of injuries is called the *high-rise syndrome.*

The exposed portion of the calvaria is more prone to injury than is the more protected base of the skull. Fractures of the calvaria are not as common in dogs as in people, suggesting

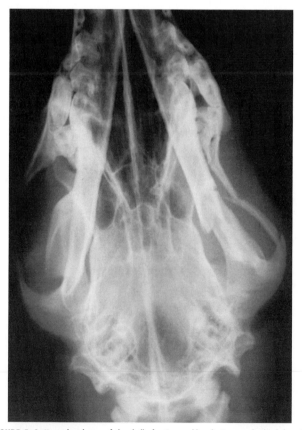

FIGURE 5–3. Ventrodorsal view of the skull of a 2-year-old male German shepherd dog with comminuted fractures of the left zygomatic arch and mandible. Note the severe depression of the zygomatic arch fragments.

that there is some protection owing to the thicker calvaria and heavy overlying musculature. Smaller dogs have a greater risk of injury because of their domed, relatively thin calvaria (Fig. 5–4).[25]

Alterations in Radiographic Opacity

Focal losses in bone opacity may occur secondary to traumatic, inflammatory, infectious, or neoplastic processes. Generalized loss of radiographic opacity may be caused by primary or secondary hyperparathyroidism as well as other metabolic causes of deficient osteoid synthesis or mineralization.[26]

One of the first radiographic signs of hyperparathyroidism is the loss of the lamina dura, the bone that forms the dental alveolus. The disappearance of the lamina dura causes teeth to appear to float in the demineralized maxilla and mandible (Fig. 5–5). Concomitant fibrous osteodystrophy may result in thickening of the maxilla and filling of the nasal cavity with soft tissue (Fig. 5–6). Teeth may become displaced, and in the young animal, eruption of the permanent teeth may be impaired, especially in subhuman primates.[27]

The degree of cortical thinning and decreased bone opacity depends on the severity of the mineral imbalance and the duration of the disease. Age also affects the relative severity of skull changes compared with those in long bones. Skull demineralization tends to predominate in secondary renal hyperparathyroidism, whereas cortical thinning of the long bones is most severe in the secondary nutritional form of the disease. This difference may be because the nutritional disease occurs more often in young animals in whom there is rapid skeletal turnover. The nutritional form of the disease occurs infrequently because of the widespread use of balanced commercial rations.

Increases in bone opacity may result from a number of factors. One acquired cause of increased bone opacity in the dog is craniomandibular osteopathy. The cause of this proliferative bone disease is unknown; however, in the West Highland White terrier, it appears to be inherited as an autosomal recessive trait. It occurs most often in West Highland White, Scottish, and Cairn terriers, but isolated instances in other breeds have been reported.[28] The disease affects young,

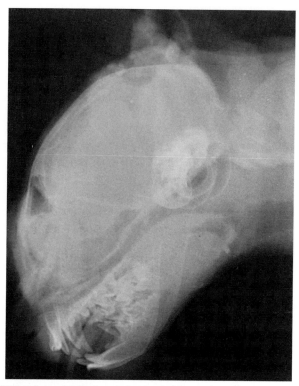

FIGURE 5–5. Lateral skull radiograph of a 12-week-old kitten with severe secondary nutritional hyperparathyroidism. Note the overall loss of bone opacity, the loss of the lamina dura, and the severe cortical thinning of all the bones of the skull.

growing animals between 4 and 11 months of age. Affected animals may have fever, anorexia, atrophy of the temporal and masseter muscles, and mandibular pain, especially during mastication.[29]

Craniomandibular osteopathy usually involves the occipital, parietal, and temporal portions of the calvaria, especially the tympanic bullae and the mandibular rami. One or more of these bones may be affected, and the involvement is often symmetric. Bony proliferation near the temporomandibular joints may result in bridging and ankylosis of these joints, thus interfering with the ability of the dog to open its mouth (Fig. 5–7). Proliferative changes on the long bones, which

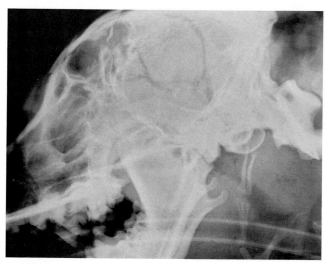

FIGURE 5–4. Lateral skull radiograph of a 3-year-old male cocker spaniel. Multiple fractures of the maxilla, frontal sinuses, and calvaria are present. There is severe swelling of the soft palate and occlusion of the nasopharynx. An endotracheal tube is in place.

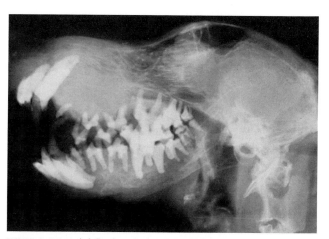

FIGURE 5–6. Lateral skull radiograph of a 12-year-old female Scottish terrier with primary hyperparathyroidism and severe fibrous dysplasia (proliferation of fibrous tissue in nasal cavity) with thickening of the maxilla and displacement of the teeth. Note the absence of the lamina dura around the teeth.

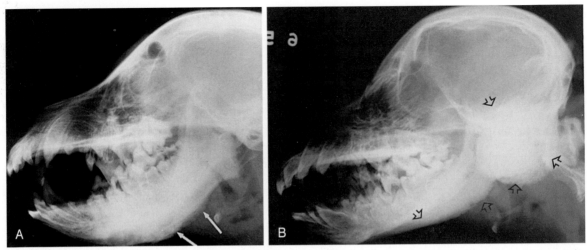

FIGURE 5–7. Lateral skull radiographs of two West Highland white terriers with craniomandibular osteopathy. *A,* The proliferation is primarily on the mandibular ramus *(arrows). B,* The proliferation involves the tympanic bullae and temporomandibular joints in addition to the mandibular ramus *(arrowheads).*

resemble those seen in hypertrophic osteodystrophy, have also been reported. Bony proliferation ceases when the animal reaches skeletal maturity.

In the past, radiographic diagnosis of brain disease was limited to conditions that resulted in parenchymal mineralization or alterations in size, shape, opacity, or margination of the calvaria. Most brain tumors do not produce bone changes in the calvaria, although meningiomas may calcify and, therefore, be visible on survey radiographs.[30] Focal hyperostosis of the calvaria has also been reported in the cat secondary to meningiomas. Detection of most brain tumors is dependent on CT and MRI (see Chapter 7).[31] The normal CT and MRI anatomic features of the dog have been described.[32–36]

Bone destruction involving the calvaria usually results from primary bone neoplasia or from neoplasia of surrounding soft tissue. Malignant neoplasms of bone occur more frequently in the dog than in the cat.[37] The most common neoplasm of bone in both species is osteosarcoma.[38] Between 10 and 15 percent of all osteosarcomas are found in the skull. In one report concerning the distribution of osteosarcomas in the dog skull, it was found that 37 percent of neoplasms arose from the cranial vault, 36 percent from the facial bones, and 27 percent from the mandible.[39]

Radiographically, osteosarcomas arising from the cranial vault do not resemble those arising from the appendicular skeleton or from other areas of the skull. Cranial vault osteosarcomas tend to be osteoblastic, have well-defined borders, and contain granular areas of calcification. Facial and mandibular osteosarcomas more closely resemble osteosarcomas of the extremities, being characterized by osteolysis, cortical destruction, and new bone formation in surrounding soft tissues (Fig. 5–8).

When compared with osteosarcomas, other primary bone neoplasms of the skull are rare. Osteomas are composed of dense, homogeneous bone; they have a smooth, well-defined margin and a slow growth rate (Fig. 5–9). Osteomas may arise from the mandible, the cranial vault, or the sinuses; do not cause bone destruction at their attachment site; and often are amenable to surgical removal. Those lesions that arise from the cranial vault may predispose to neurologic signs because of compression. Osteochondromas resemble osteomas radiographically but characteristically occur in immature dogs and usually involve multiple areas of the skeleton, especially the spine and ribs.

Another relatively uncommon neoplasm is multilobular

osteochondrosarcoma. Synonyms include *multilobular osteoma, chondroma rodens, juvenile aponeurotic fibroma,* and *calcifying aponeurotic fibroma.* Lesions in the dog most often involve the temporo-occipital area of the skull, although involvement of the orbit has been reported.[40] The neoplasm occurs most often in medium-breed to large-breed dogs, at an average age of 7 years (range of 15 months to 12 years); no gender predilection has been reported. Multilobular osteochondrosarcomas appear as multilobular soft-tissue masses that contain stippled areas of mineralization with lysis of underlying bone (Fig. 5–10). Histologically the neoplasm consists of a lobulated mass with islands of partially calcified or ossified cartilage, or both, surrounded by dense fibrous tissue. The neoplasm is locally invasive and may cause neurologic signs owing to brain compression. Metastasis is more common than originally thought.[41] Surgical excision, with or without radiation therapy, appears to be the treatment of choice.[41, 42]

Malignant soft-tissue neoplasms of the skull often invade adjacent bone with varying amounts of destruction and proliferation.[43] Bone destruction is more common than bone

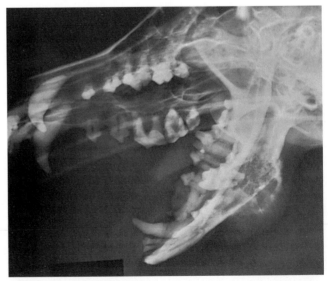

FIGURE 5–8. Open-mouth oblique skull radiograph of a 12-year-old Afghan with a mandibular osteosarcoma. Note the severe cortical destruction and irregular new bone proliferation indicating a highly aggressive lesion.

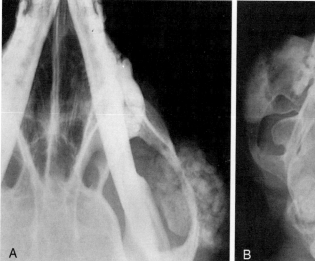
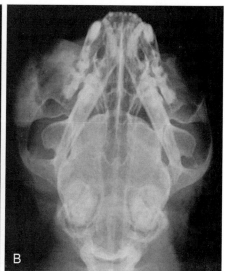

FIGURE 5–9. *A,* Ventrodorsal radiograph of a 9-year-old female mixed-breed dog with an osteoma of the left zygomatic arch. *B,* Ventrodorsal radiograph of an aged cat with an osteoma of the rostral portion of the right zygomatic arch. Note the well-ossified, smoothly margined, nondestructive appearance of these neoplasms, which suggests their benign etiology.

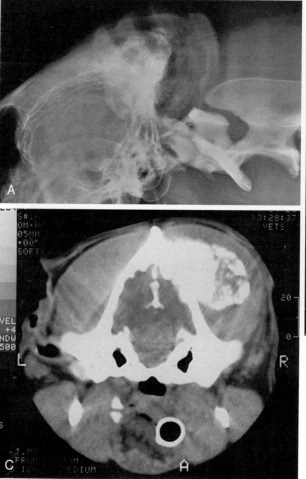

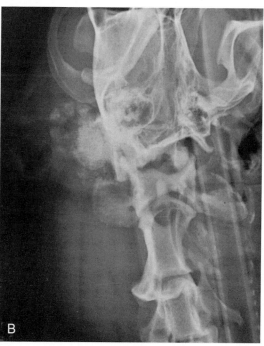

FIGURE 5–10. Lateral *(A)* and right ventral–left dorsal *(B)* radiographs and computed tomography (CT) image *(C)* of the skull of a 9-year-old Boxer with a multilobular osteochondrosarcoma of the right occipital region of the skull. Note the improved estimation of tumor size and cortical involvement apparent in the CT image. Minimal brain compression was evident in this animal.

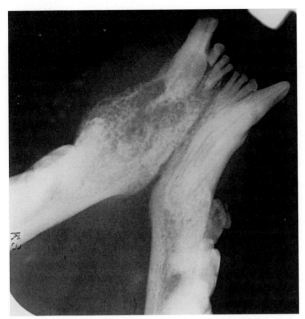

FIGURE 5–11. Occlusal ventrodorsal view of the mandible of a 15-year-old male domestic shorthair cat with squamous cell carcinoma of the rostral mandible. There is a moth-eaten bone lysis with enlargement of the rostral mandibular body and destruction of the root of the right canine and lateral incisor.

produce a sclerotic bone reaction. *Cryptococcus neoformans* is a saprophytic fungus that usually involves the respiratory or central nervous systems, although ulcerated skin lesions on the head with lysis of the underlying bone may also result.[45]

ABNORMALITIES OF THE MIDDLE AND INNER EAR

Conditions of the middle ear that may be evaluated radiographically include craniomandibular osteopathy, otitis media, inflammatory polyps, and neoplasia. Although sclerosis of the petrous temporal bone may be seen, otitis interna does not produce readily apparent radiographic signs in most animals, and diagnosis of otitis interna must be based on clinical signs.[45]

As mentioned earlier, craniomandibular osteopathy may result in severe bone proliferation involving the tympanic bullae. Differential diagnosis is based on the age and breed of the animal as well as on the absence of clinical signs of otitis. In addition, involvement with craniomandibular osteopathy is often bilateral with concurrent mandibular periostitis.

Radiography may be useful in the evaluation of otitis media. Oblique and open-mouth projections of the skull usually require the use of general anesthesia, but these views are necessary for adequate radiographic evaluation of the tympanic bullae. Although the anatomy of the petrous temporal bone is complex, most animals have unilateral involvement, allowing comparison of the affected and unaffected sides.

Otitis media is generally a sequel to chronic otitis externa, and thus narrowing of the external ear canal may be seen on the ventrodorsal radiograph. Radiographic signs of otitis media include thickening and sclerosis of the wall of one or both tympanic bullae and filling of these normally well-aerated structures with soft-tissue material (Fig. 5–14). In advanced disease, bony proliferation may involve the remaining petrous temporal bone, the temporomandibular joint, or both. In a discussion of surgical versus radiographic diagnosis of otitis media, all patients with positive radiographic signs were confirmed at surgery; however, 25 percent of the surgically confirmed patients had false-negative radiographic findings.[46]

production (Figs. 5–11 through 5–13). Neoplasms of the nasal cavity region are especially common and are discussed in Chapter 6. Metastatic neoplasms of the skull and mandible occur rarely.

Alterations in bone opacity may also occur with osteomyelitis. Bacterial and fungal infections of the skull in the dog and cat usually involve the teeth, sinuses, or tympanic bullae. Radiographic signs related to these areas are described elsewhere. Bacterial osteomyelitis may occur secondary to fractures or their surgical repair. Osteomyelitis generally causes a combination of bone destruction and proliferation. The presence and degree of proliferation depend on the virulence of the infectious organism; thus, low-grade infections tend to

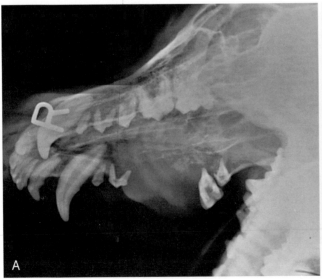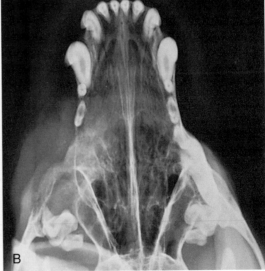

FIGURE 5–12. Left ventral–right dorsal *(A)* and open-mouth ventrodorsal *(B)* views of the maxilla of a 3-year-old male German shepherd dog with a rapidly enlarging right maxillary melanoma of 2 months' duration. The right maxillary third and fourth premolars are absent, with cortical destruction of the maxilla and a suggestion of tumor extension into the nasal cavity.

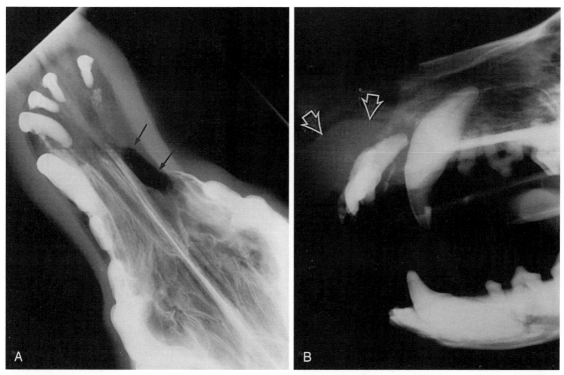

FiGURE 5–13. Open-mouth ventrodorsal *(A)* and lateral *(B)* views of the maxilla of a 10-year-old female mixed-breed dog made 5 months after partial maxillectomy and radiation therapy for a squamous cell carcinoma of the left maxilla. The tumor has recurred at the rostral margin with extensive lysis of the incisive bone and rostral maxilla. An oronasal fistula *(black arrows)* is seen in *A* at the previous surgery site. A soft-tissue mass *(open arrows)* that was interfering with normal respiration is seen extending into the nasal passages on the lateral view *(B)*.

Nasopharyngeal polyps are an uncommon condition in cats. A nasopharyngeal polyp, however, should be considered in young cats presenting with signs of nasal discharge, sneezing, or stridor. In one series of 31 cats with nasopharyngeal polyps, 30 had a soft-tissue pharyngeal mass radiographically, whereas 26 had thickening of one or both tympanic bullae suggestive of otitis media (Fig. 5–15). Twenty-seven of these cats had single polyps, whereas four had bilateral polyps.[47] The cause of the polyps is unknown, although histologically they appear to be inflammatory. It is also unknown whether otitis media is a precursor to or a sequel of the polyp.[48]

Malignant soft-tissue neoplasms of the ear canal, most notably squamous cell carcinoma and mucinous gland adenocarcinoma, may result in extensive bone destruction, proliferation, or both and may involve the bulla or base of the calvaria with occasional extension to the temporomandibular joint. This occurrence is more common in cats than in dogs (Fig. 5–16).

EVALUATION OF THE TEETH

A tooth is composed of the root, which is embedded in the cancellous bone of the skull, and the crown, that part within the oral cavity. The bone between adjacent teeth is called the *alveolar crest*. The dentin, enamel, and lamina dura are radiopaque, whereas the pulp cavity and periodontal membrane are of soft-tissue opacity. Special radiographic positions and film types recommended for optimal evaluation of teeth have been described elsewhere.[49, 50]

Changes in the appearance of the teeth may occur owing to age, trauma, infection, or neoplasia. Congenital adontia (complete absence of the teeth) is rare, whereas oligodontia (partial absence of the teeth) is common, especially in

brachycephalic dogs. Supernumerary teeth also occur. Rarely are congenital alterations in the number of teeth clinically significant.[51]

The appearance of the teeth changes considerably during normal development and maturation.[52, 53] The apical foramina of the teeth in the young animal are open (Fig. 5–17). The permanent teeth develop beneath or to one side of their deciduous precursors. All the permanent teeth usually erupt by 7 months of age. Shortly after this eruption, the apical foramina close, and the size of the pulp cavity gradually decreases. Regression of the alveolar crest, decreased prominence of the lamina dura, and coarsening of the bony trabeculation surrounding the teeth are normal changes that occur with age.[54]

Periodontal disease is a common form of dental disease in dogs and cats. Radiographic signs include resorption of the alveolar crest, rounding of the amelocemental junction, widening of the periodontal space with loss of the lamina dura, and lysis of the bone surrounding the teeth. Loss of bone opacity around the teeth also occurs with primary or secondary hyperparathyroidism. Bone lysis in hyperparathyroidism is more generalized and is not restricted to the periodontal area.

Periapical infections are common in older animals and may be secondary to periodontal disease. Other causes include fracture of the tooth or of the adjacent bone, neoplasia, and hematogenous infections. Periapical abscesses may arise in more than one tooth concurrently and may be found incidentally in asymptomatic aging dogs and cats that are examined radiographically for other reasons. In the dog, infection of the fourth upper premolar (carnassial tooth) often results in an externally draining fistulous tract just below the eye. Open-mouth oblique views of the teeth are necessary for complete evaluation of this condition. Radiographic signs of

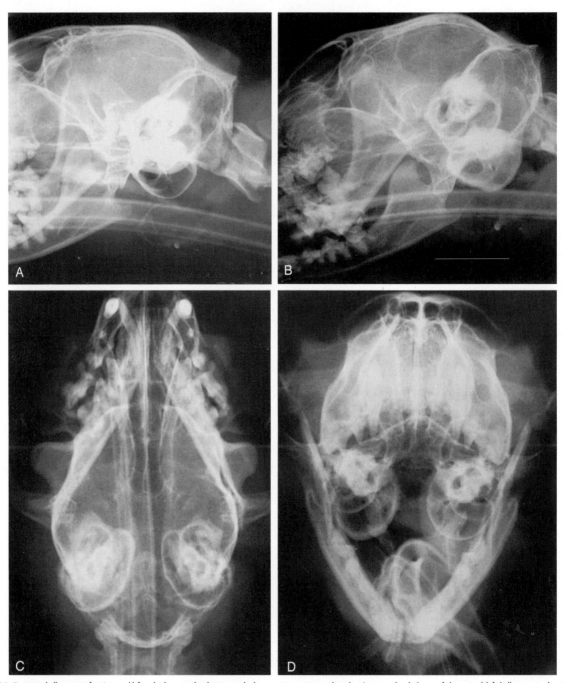

FIGURE 5–14. Tympanic bulla series of a 6-year-old female domestic shorthair cat with chronic otitis externa and media. Compare the thickness of the normal left bulla seen in the right dorsal–left ventral view *(A)* with the thickened right bulla seen in the left dorsal–right ventral *(B)*, ventrodorsal *(C)*, and open-mouth rostrocaudal *(D)* views.

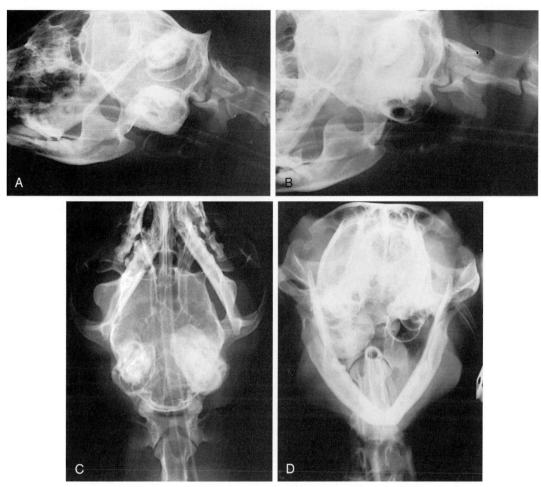

FIGURE 5–15. Left dorsal–right ventral *(A)*, right dorsal–left ventral *(B)*, dorsoventral *(C)*, and open-mouth rostrocaudal *(D)* views of a 2-year-old male domestic shorthair cat with chronic otitis media and a nasopharyngeal polyp. The right tympanic bulla appears fluid-filled and severely thickened. The left tympanic bulla is normal.

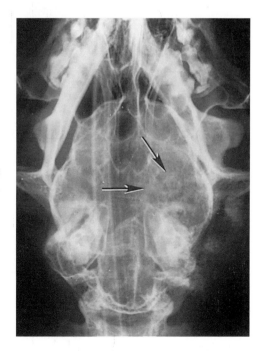

FIGURE 5–16. Ventrodorsal skull radiograph of a 12-year-old domestic shorthair cat with squamous cell carcinoma of the left ear canal. There is lysis of the base of the skull *(arrows)* as well as of the lateral aspect of the left tympanic bulla.

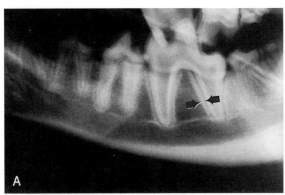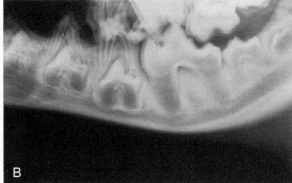

FIGURE 5–17. *A,* Close-up lateral view of the mandible of a mature dog. Notice the well-defined lamina dura *(arrows)* marking the dental alveolus. *B,* Close-up lateral view of the mandible of a 4-month-old dog. Notice the open apical foramina of the teeth and the location of the permanent premolars ventral to their deciduous precursors.

periapical disease include widening of the periodontal space surrounding the apex, bone lysis or sclerosis adjacent to the apex, resorption of the tooth root, and osteomyelitis of the adjacent bone (Fig. 5–18). Complications, such as delayed gingival healing and nasal discharge after dental extractions, may occur as a result of retained roots or the presence of sequestered fragments of alveolar bone.[55] Structural injury to the teeth, especially fractures with pulpal exposure, may lead to bacterial pulpitis, pulp necrosis, and endodontic resorption, Radiographically, this appears as mild to severe enlargement of the pulp cavity and most commonly affects the canine teeth. Periapical abscessation and external fistulation may also occur concurrently (Fig. 5–19).

Focal destruction of bone adjacent to teeth may also occur with neoplasia arising from the dental elements themselves or from the adjacent bone or soft tissues. Malignant neoplasms tend to be more lytic, whereas benign processes tend to have a more sclerotic, well-demarcated border, reflecting their slower growth rate.

Periodontal epulides are the most common type of benign oral neoplasm in the dog. Epulides arise from the periodontal membrane. Three types of epulides have been described: fibromatous, ossifying, and acanthomatous. Only the acanthomatous epulis has the potential to infiltrate locally into the bone.[56] Aggressive surgical excision or radiation therapy is the treatment of choice for these tumors.

Odontogenic neoplasms in dogs are rare.[57] These neoplasms arise from the dental laminar epithelium and usually contain enamel inclusions, dental pulp stroma, or organized dental structures, which distinguish them from the epulides. One classification scheme outlines the odontogenic neoplasms as ameloblastomas, keratinizing ameloblastomas, ameloblastic fibro-odontomas, compound odontomas, and complex odontomas.[58]

Ameloblastomas occur most commonly in the dog. These lesions often cause osteolysis around involved tooth roots but may also be accompanied by an osteoblastic reaction.

Odontomas typically occur in immature animals who often present with a nonpainful facial swelling and expansion of the affected portion of maxilla or mandible. Odontomas appear as multiloculated radiolucent masses that contain multiple teeth or tooth-like structures (Fig. 5–20). Surgical curettage or radiation therapy has been used for treatment.[59]

A rare odontogenic neoplasm that was described in young cats (younger than 14 months of age) is the fibroameloblastoma. This neoplasm contains ameloblastic epithelial tissue and dental pulp–like stroma and causes bone lysis and proliferation of the maxilla. Wide surgical excision is the most successful form of treatment because these neoplasms are not radioresponsive.[60]

DISORDERS OF THE TEMPOROMANDIBULAR JOINT

The temporomandibular joint is a condylar joint that allows considerable lateral sliding movement. The transversely elongated mandibular condyle does not correspond exactly with the shape of the articular surface of the temporal bone. In addition, the synchondrosis at the mandibular symphysis allows independent motion between the mandibular rami, which, in turn, permits congenital or traumatic luxations of the temporomandibular joint to occur without fracture.[61]

Disorders of the temporomandibular joint in the dog and cat include congenital dysplasias, traumatic luxations, fractures, and osteoarthritis. Involvement of this joint in craniomandibular osteopathy has been discussed. Radiographic examination is often the only method of reaching a definitive diagnosis of temporomandibular region abnormalities. In addition to the standard ventrodorsal and lateral views, oblique views with the animal under anesthesia or sedation are gen-

FIGURE 5–18. Close-up lateral view of a periapical abscess around the rostral root of the first mandibular molar. Note the severe lysis of the alveolus with loss of the normal lamina dura and the erosion of the dental enamel.

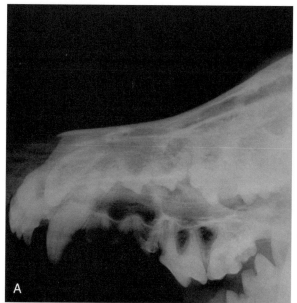

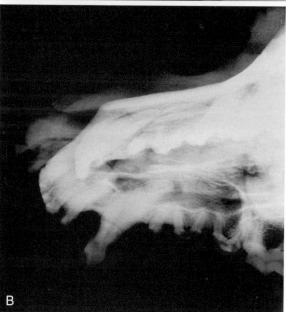

FIGURE 5–19. *A,* Open-mouth oblique view of the right maxilla of a 3-year-old male Scottish terrier presented with a draining fistula over the left maxillary canine tooth. The right upper canine tooth (projected ventrally) has a normal-diameter pulp cavity. The diseased left upper canine tooth (superimposed over the maxilla) has a severely enlarged pulp cavity, indicating pulpitis and pulp necrosis. A small amount of radiopaque contrast medium was injected into the external fistula and is seen around the periapical area of the tooth, verifying a periapical abscess. *B,* Open-mouth oblique view of the right maxilla of a 6-year-old male Akita presented for evaluation of a fractured tooth. Note the abnormal shape of the tip of the right maxillary canine tooth due to the fracture and the enlargement of the pulp cavity, indicating pulpitis and endodontic resorption. Compare the appearance of the pulp cavity of this tooth to the normal diameter seen in the right maxillary canine in Figure 5–19*A.*

erally required for adequate evaluation of these joints. These views are described elsewhere.[62]

Open-mouth jaw locking is a prominent clinical sign of congenital dysplasia of the temporomandibular joint. Jaw locking is precipitated by yawning or excessive opening of the mouth. The condition is uncommon but is most often reported in the Basset hound.[63] In this breed, the condition appears to be the result of abnormal angulation of the condyloid processes with resulting subluxation. Stretching of the

lateral ligament of the affected joint and excessive lateral movement of the condyloid process allow the coronoid process to become entrapped lateral to the zygomatic arch. Jaw locking usually occurs on the contralateral side from the joint with the most severe dysplastic changes (Fig. 5–21). This condition has been treated successfully by removal of the proximal portion of the coronoid process of the mandible of the ventral portion of the zygomatic arch.[64] A similar problem with jaw locking may result from callus formation after fracture of the zygomatic arch.[65]

Traumatic injuries that affect the temporomandibular region are especially common in the cat, perhaps as a result of the relative frequency of mandibular symphyseal injury as well as the lack of structural support for the mandibular fossa. Traumatic dislocations generally result in rostrodorsal displacement of the mandibular condyle (Fig. 5–22). Dislocations may be unilateral or bilateral and may occur alone or in combination with a variety of fractures, including fractures of the condylar portion of the joint, the base of the condylar portion, the mandibular fossa or retroarticular process, and the zygomatic process.[66] Oblique and ventrodorsal views are especially helpful in the characterization of these lesions. Malocclusion is a prominent feature of temporomandibular joint injuries. Radiography is helpful in eliminating a diagnosis of rostral mandibular fractures as the cause of the malocclusion.

Other less common conditions that result in abnormal temporomandibular joint function include osteoarthritis, myositis, retrobulbar abscesses, tetanus, and neoplasia. Causes of osteoarthritis include extension of otitis media, craniomandibular osteopathy, congenital malformation with secondary joint laxity, and trauma. Benign or malignant neoplasms of either bone or soft tissue that occur adjacent to the temporomandibular joints may interfere with normal joint motion and may produce localized bone destruction or proliferation. Radiographic evaluation in patients with myositis, retrobulbar abscess formation, and tetanus is normal.

Radiographic evaluation of the eye is of limited value except in instances of disruption of the bony orbit. Ultrasonography and CT have added to the diagnosis of ocular and retrobulbar disease.[67, 68] The normal anatomic features of the orbit using these modalities have been described.[69, 70]

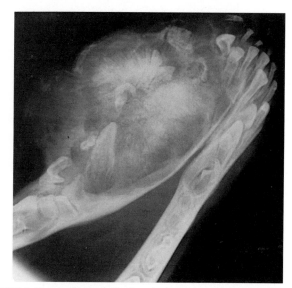

FIGURE 5–20. Ventrodorsal occlusal radiograph of a 3-month-old male collie with complex odontoma. This irregularly margined, mineralizing mass has caused destruction of the rostral portion of the mandible and displacement of the teeth. The soft-tissue component of the tumor extended across the midline.

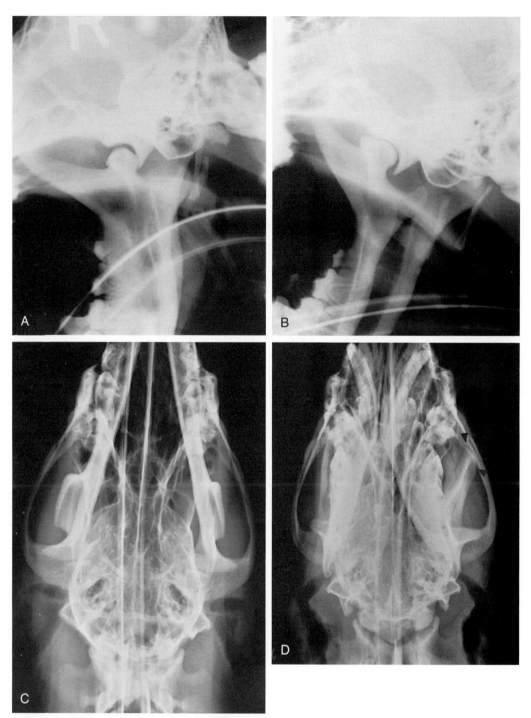

FIGURE 5–21. Open-mouth left dorsal–right ventral *(A)*, open-mouth right dorsal–left ventral *(B)*, closed-mouth ventrodorsal *(C)*, and open-mouth ventrodorsal *(D)* views of the temporomandibular joints of a 2-year-old female Gordon setter with a history of chronic, intermittent jaw locking. There is subluxation of the right temporomandibular joint *(A)* compared with the more normal appearance of the left joint *(B)*. These views were taken after the jaw was locked; subluxation was not evident on the routine lateral oblique views. Note the difference in the relationship of the coronoid process of the mandible and the zygomatic arch on the closed-mouth *ventrodorsal* view *(C)* compared with the open-mouth ventrodorsal view *(D)* after the jaw has been locked in the open position. When the jaw is locked, the coronoid process shifts laterally and is in contact with the zygomatic arch *(arrowheads)*.

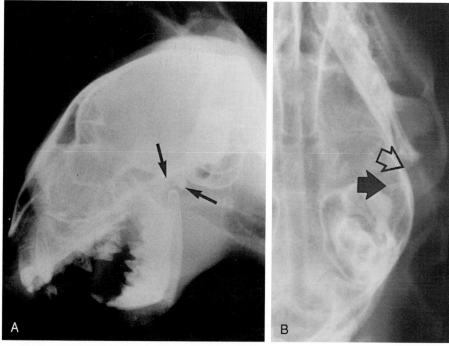

FIGURE 5–22. *A,* Lateral skull radiograph of a 4-year-old domestic shorthair cat with bilateral temporomandibular luxations, mandibular symphyseal fracture, and some fractured teeth. The mandible is displaced in a rostroventral direction with severe malocclusion. *Arrows,* The temporal portion of one of the joints. *B,* Dorsoventral radiograph of a 6-month-old domestic shorthair cat with left temporomandibular luxation. The condylar process (articular surface) of the mandible *(open arrow)* is distracted rostrally from the mandibular fossa (articular surface) of the temporal bone *(solid arrow).*

References

1. Hare WCD: Radiographic anatomy of the feline skull. J Am Vet Med Assoc *134*:349, 1959.
2. Miller EA, Christensen GC, and Evans HE: Anatomy of the Dog. Philadelphia, WB Saunders, 1964, p 8.
3. Ticer JW: Radiographic Technique in Veterinary Practice. Philadelphia, WB Saunders, 1984, pp 231–259.
4. Morgan JP, and Silverman S: Techniques of Veterinary Radiography. Davis, CA, Veterinary Radiology Associates, 1982, pp 169–174.
5. Krum S, Johnson K, and Wilson J: Hydrocephalus associated with the noneffusive form of feline infectious peritonitis. J Am Vet Med Assoc *167*:745, 1975.
6. Burt JK, Bhargava AK, and Prynn RB: Unilateral hydrocephalus with cranial distortion in a cat. Vet Med Clin North Am [Small Anim Pract] *65*:745, 1970.
7. Becker SA, and Selby LA: Canine hydrocephalus. Comp Contin Ed Pract Vet *2*:647, 1980.
8. Ettinger SJ: Textbook of Veterinary Internal Medicine. Philadelphia, WB Saunders, 1983, pp 487–490.
9. Hoerlein BF: Canine Neurology. Philadelphia, WB Saunders, 1978, pp 560–569.
10. Hudson JA, Cartee RE, Simpson ST, et al: Ultrasonographic anatomy of the canine brain. Vet Radiol *30*:13, 1989.
11. Hudson JA, Simpson ST, Cox NR, et al: Ultrasonographic examination of the normal canine neonatal brain. Vet Radiol *32*:50, 1991.
12. Hudson JA, Simpson ST, Buxton DF, et al: Ultrasonographic diagnosis of canine hydrocephalus. Vet Radiol *31*:50, 1990.
13. Spaulding KA, and Sharp NJH: Ultrasonographic imaging of the lateral cerebral ventricles in the dog. Vet Radiol *31*:59, 1990.
14. Bardens JW: Congenital malformation of the foramen magnum in dogs. SW Vet *18*:295, 1965.
15. Ticer JW: Radiographic Technique in Veterinary Practice. Philadelphia, WB Saunders, 1984, p 256.
16. Wright JA: A study of the radiographic anatomy of the foramen magnum in dogs. J Small Anim Pract *20*:501, 1979.
17. Watson AG: The phylogeny and development of the occipitoatlas-axis complex in the dog. MS Thesis, Cornell University, Ithaca, NY, 1981.
18. Haskins ME, Jezyk PF, Desnick RJ, et al: Mucopolysaccharidosis in a domestic short-haired cat—a disease distinct from that seen in the Siamese cat. J Am Vet Med Assoc *175*:384, 1979.
19. Konde LJ, Thrall MA, Gasper P, et al: Radiographically visualized skeletal changes associated with mucopolysaccharidosis VI in cats. Vet Radiol *28*:223, 1987.
20. Cornell Feline Health Center: Veterinary News. Ithaca, NY, Cornell University, Winter, 1983.
21. Kolata RJ: Trauma in dogs and cats: An overview. Vet Clin North Am [Small Anim Pract] *10*:515, 1980.
22. Phillips IR: A survey of bone fractures in the dog and cat. J Small Anim Pract *20*:661, 1979.
23. Gibbs C: Traumatic lesions of the mandible. J Small Anim Pract *18*:51, 1977.
24. Roush JC: Orthopedic problems of the cat—a review. Feline Pract *10*:10, 1980.
25. Gibbs C: Traumatic lesions of the skull. J Small Anim Pract *17*:551, 1976.
26. Ettinger SJ: Textbook of Veterinary Internal Medicine. Philadelphia, WB Saunders, 1983, pp 1565–1572.
27. Morgan JP: Radiology in Veterinary Orthopedics. Philadelphia, Lea & Febiger, 1972, pp 332–335.
28. Watson ADJ, Adams WM, and Thomas CB: Craniomandibular osteopathy in dogs. Comp Contin Ed Vet Pract *17*:911, 1995.
29. Riser WH, Parkes LJ, and Shiver JF: Canine cranio-mandibular osteopathy. J Am Vet Radiol Soc *8*:23, 1967.
30. Lawson C, Burk RL, and Prate RG: Cerebral meningioma in the cat: Diagnosis and surgical treatment of 10 cases. J Am Anim Hosp Assoc *20*:33, 1984.
31. Turrel JM, Fike JR, LeCouter RA, et al: Computed tomography characteristics of primary brain tumors in 50 dogs. J Am Vet Med Assoc *188*:851, 1986.
32. Fike JR, Druy RM, Zook BC, et al: Canine anatomy as assessed by computerized tomography. Am J Vet Res *41*:1823, 1980.
33. George TF, and Smallwood JE: Anatomic atlas for computed tomography in the mesaticephalic dog: Head and neck. Vet Radiol Ultrasound *33*:217, 1992.
34. Feeney DA, Fletcher TF, and Hardy RM: Atlas of Correlative Imaging Anatomy of the Normal Dog, Ultrasound and Computed Tomography. Philadelphia, WB Saunders, 1991.
35. Kraft SL, Gavin PR, Wending LR, et al: Canine brain anatomy on magnetic resonance images. Vet Radiol *30*:147, 1989.
36. Thomsom CE, Kornegay JN, Burn RA, et al: Magnetic resonance imaging—general overview of principles and examples of veterinary neurodiagnosis. Vet Radiol Ultrasound *34*:2, 1993.
37. Liu SK, Dorfman HD, and Patnaik AK: Primary and secondary bone tumors in the cat. J Small Anim Pract *15*:141, 1974.
38. Turrel JM, and Pool RR: Primary bone neoplasms in the cat. Vet Radiol *23*:152, 1982.
39. Hardy WD, Brodey RS, and Riser WH: Osteosarcoma of the canine skull. J Am Vet Radiol Soc *8*:5, 1967.
40. Pletcher JM, Koch SA, and Stedhem MA: Orbital chondroma rodens in a dog. J Am Vet Med Assoc *175*:187, 1979.

41. Straw RC, LeCouter RA, Powers BE, and Withrow SJ: Multilobular osteo-chondrosarcoma of the canine skull: 16 cases (1978–1988). J Am Vet Med Assoc 195:1764, 1989.
42. Selcer BA, and McCracken MD: Chondroma rodens in dogs. J Vet Orthop 2:7, 1981.
43. Richardson RC, Jones MA, and Elliott GS: Oral neoplasms in the dog: A diagnostic and therapeutic dilemma. Comp Contin Ed Pract Vet 5:441, 1983.
44. Rutman MA, Rickardo DA, and Chandler FW: Feline cryptococcosis. Feline Pract 53:36, 1975.
45. Gibbs C: The head: III. Ear disease. J Small Anim Pract 19:539, 1978.
46. Remedios AM, Fowler JD, and Pharr JW: A comparison of radiographic versus surgical diagnosis of otitis media. J Am Anim Hosp Assoc 27:183, 1991.
47. Kapatkin AS, Matthiesen DT, Noone KE, et al: Results of surgery and long-term follow-up in 31 cats with nasopharyngeal polyps. J Am Anim Hosp Assoc 26:387, 1990.
48. Parker NR, and Binnington AG: Nasopharyngeal polyps in cats: Three case reports and a review of the literature. J Am Anim Hosp Assoc 21:473, 1985.
49. Zontine WJ: Canine dental radiology: Radiographic technic, development, and antomy of the teeth. Vet Radiol 16:75, 1975.
50. Roman FS, Llorens MP, Pena MT, et al: Dental radiography in the dog with a conventional x-ray device. Vet Radiol 31:235, 1990.
51. Kealy JK: Diagnostic Radiology of the Dog and Cat. Philadelphia, WB Saunders, 1979, pp 400–404.
52. Hooft J, Mattheeuws D, and Van Bree P: Radiology of deciduous teeth resorption and definitive teeth eruption in the dog. J Small Anim Pract 20:175, 1979.
53. Morgan JP, and Miyabayashi T: Dental radiography: Ageing changes in permanent teeth of Beagle dogs. J Small Anim Pract 32:11, 1991.
54. Zontine WJ: Dental radiographic technique and interpretation. Vet Clin North Am [Small Anim Pract] 4:741, 1974.
55. Gibbs C: The head: Dental disease. J Small Anim Pract 19:701, 1978.
56. Dubielzig RR, Goldschmidt MH, and Brodey RS: The nomenclature of periodontal epulides in dogs. Vet Pathol 16:209, 1979.
57. Gorlin RJ, Barren CN, Chandhry AP, et al: The oral and pharyngeal pathology of domestic animals: A study of 487 cases. Am J Vet Res 79:1032, 1959.
58. Dubielzig RR: Proliferative dental and gingival diseases of dogs and cats. J Am Anim Hosp Assoc 18:577, 1982.
59. Valentine BA, Lynch MJ, and May JC: Compound odontoma in a dog. J Am Vet Med Assoc 186:177, 1985.
60. Dubielzig RR, Adams WM, and Brodey RS: Inductive fibroameloblastoma, an unusual dental tumor of young cats. J Am Vet Med Assoc 174:720, 1979.
61. Lane JG: Disorders of the canine temporomandibular joint. Vet Annu 21:175, 1982.
62. Ticer JW: Radiographic Technique in Veterinary Practice. Philadelphia, WB Saunders, 1984, p 232.
63. Robins G, and Grandage J: Temporomandibular joint dysplasia and open-mouth jaw locking in the dog. J Am Vet Med Assoc 171:1072, 1977.
64. Thomas RE: Temporo-mandibular joint dysplasia and open-mouth jaw locking in a Bassett hound: A case report. J Small Anim Pract 20:697, 1979.
65. Bennett D, and Campbell JR: Mechanical interference with lower jaw movement as a complication of skull fractures. J Small Anim Pract 17:747, 1976.
66. Ticer JW, and Spencer CP: Injury of the feline temporomandibular joint: Radiographic signs. J Am Vet Radiol Soc 19:146, 1978.
67. Morgan RV: Ultrasonography of retrobulbar diseases of the dog and cat. J Am Anim Hosp Assoc 25:393, 1989.
68. Dziezyc J, Hager DA, and Millichamp NJ: Two-dimensional real-time ocular ultrasonography in the diagnosis of ocular lesions in dogs. J Am Anim Hosp Assoc 23:501, 1987.
69. Hager DA, Dziezyc J, and Millchamp NJ: Two-dimensional real-time ocular ultrasonography in the dog: Technique and normal anatomy. Vet Radiol 28:60, 1987.
70. Fike JR: Anatomy of the canine orbital region: Multiplanar imaging by CT. Vet Radiol 25:32, 1984.

STUDY QUESTIONS

1. What are the radiographic signs of congenital hydro-cephalus? What breeds of dogs are most commonly affected?

2. What injuries are most commonly seen in cats following a fall from a great height, the so-called high-rise syndrome?

3. What are the radiographic signs seen in the skull of an animal with hyperparathyroidism, regardless of cause?

4. What radiographic features help to differentiate benign from malignant neoplasms of the skull?

5. What are the clinical and radiographic features that would suggest the presence of a nasopharyngeal polyp in a cat?

6. What are the radiographic features of otitis media? What special views are useful in the radiographic assessment of this condition?

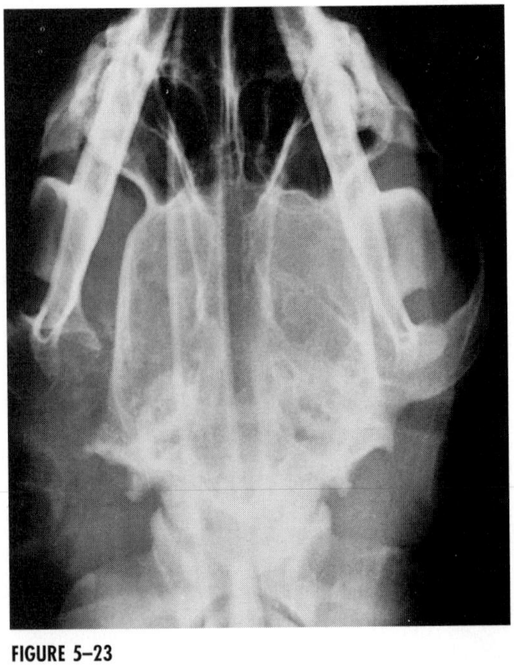

FIGURE 5–23

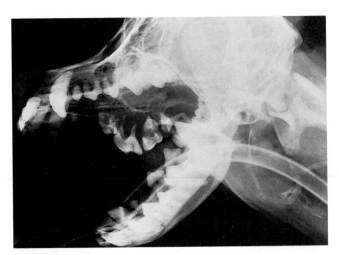

FIGURE 5–24

7. What are the radiographic signs associated with a periapical tooth root abscess?

8. What are the three types of epulides described in the dog? Which of these is considered the most aggressive and why?

9. You are presented with a 12-year-old Cocker spaniel with a history of chronic otitis externa involving the right ear. On physical examination, the tissues of the right ear canal are thickened and you are not able to evaluate the deeper structures of the ear with an otoscope. The animal seems painful around the right ear and has some difficulty and pain on opening its mouth. You decide to radiograph the dog and obtain the ventrodorsal view shown here (Fig. 5–23). What are the radio-

graphic findings? What is the assessment of these findings, and what would you recommend next to the owner?

10. You are presented with a 9-year-old terrier with a soft swelling just ventral to the right eye. The dog is reluctant to allow you to examine its mouth, and you suggest general anesthesia and skull radiographs. On oral examination, you notice that the tissue around the right fourth maxillary premolar appears thickened and irregular in contour and that the tooth is displaced ventrally and appears loose. What are the radiographic findings (Fig. 5–24)? What is the assessment of these findings, and what would you recommend next to the owner?

(Answers appear on page 633.)

Chapter 6

Nasal Cavity and Paranasal Sinuses

Wendy Myer

RADIOGRAPHIC EVALUATION

Conventional radiography is a noninvasive and relatively effective method for evaluating the extent and location of diseases within the nasal passages. General anesthesia is necessary for achieving good positioning. Comparison between the normal and the affected sides of the skull facilitates an evaluation of the complex nasal passages and the recognition of minor alterations in contour and opacity. The routine examination should begin with lateral and open-mouth ventrodorsal or dorsoventral occlusal views of the nasal cavity. These views are preferred to the routine dorsoventral or ventrodorsal view because they allow an obstructed view of the nasal conchae. A rostrocaudal view of the frontal sinuses is also advisable.

Although radiographic signs tend to be nonspecific, some assessment of the aggressiveness of a disease process may be made. A tentative differential diagnosis may be reached based on the location of the radiographic lesion, that is, unilateral versus bilateral and rostral versus caudal, and on the radiographic pattern of bony destruction or proliferation. Because radiographic changes are nonspecific, however, definitive diagnoses should be based on nasal flushes and cytologic studies, biopsies, or cultures.

Alterations in Shape and Contour

There are wide variations in the shape, size, and contour of the normal nasal passages and sinuses as a result of breed and species differences. For example, changes in the conchal size and shape occur as the facial portion of the skull is shortened, that is, in brachycephalic dog breeds and in the cat.[1] Clinically significant congenital abnormalities involving the nasal passages are rare. Malformation of the conchae and nasal septum may occur with congenital defects in the hard palate.

Trauma is the most common cause of acquired facial deformity in the dog and cat. Fractures of the facial portion of the skull often involve multiple bones and are more common than fractures of the calvaria. The fractures usually appear as straight or curved radiolucent lines. Occasionally, however, they appear radiopaque owing to overlapping bone fragments. Overlying soft-tissue swelling and subcutaneous emphysema are common. Resulting nasal hemorrhage may appear as patchy or widespread areas of increased radiopacity in the nasal fossae.

Facial deformity also may result from neoplastic processes of the nasal cavity. Benign processes, such as dentigerous cysts and odontomas, tend to cause cortical expansion, whereas malignant tumors, which are generally poorly confined and highly aggressive, cause cortical lysis and irregular periosteal new bone formation.

Alterations in Radiographic Opacity

The normal radiographic appearance of the nasal passages is due to the delicate bony scrolls of the nasal conchae and the air surrounding them. On the open-mouth view, the nasal conchae appear as fine, semiparallel radiopaque lines that extend caudally from the canine teeth to the level of the third premolars. Although the rostral portion of the nasal septum is radiolucent, its location on the open-mouth radiograph is marked by the sagittal groove of the vomer bone. The ethmoidal conchae form a fine linear bone pattern fanning out from the cribriform plate to their junction with the nasal conchae.[2] The conchal pattern may also be seen on the lateral radiograph, but it is not as prominent.

Virtually all chronic diseases that affect the nasal passages and sinuses result in alterations in their radiographic opacity.[3] Radiographic findings generally conform to one of the following patterns:

1. Normal radiographic appearance of both nasal passages.
2. Areas of increased soft-tissue opacity superimposed over the normal conchal pattern.
3. Areas of increased soft-tissue opacity superimposed over areas of conchal destruction.
4. Areas of decreased opacity owing to conchal destruction *without* accompanying soft-tissue opacity.
5. A mixed pattern with areas of conchal destruction and superimposed soft-tissue opacity interspersed with areas of conchal destruction alone.

Although some radiographic changes are more common in certain diseases, the aforementioned radiographic patterns are more a reflection of the aggressiveness and duration of the disease process than an indication of a specific cause. In some animals, however, establishing the location of an abnormality within the nasal cavity may be helpful in formulating a differential diagnosis. For instance, most nasal neoplasms originate from the region of the ethmoid conchae and cribriform plate.[4] In contrast, destructive rhinitis and hyperplastic rhinitis involve the middle and rostral segments of the nasal passages with equal or greater frequency than they involve the middle and caudal segments. Obliteration of the air passages in one or both nostrils is a common finding in animals with nasal discharge from any cause. In a study of intranasal neoplasia and chronic rhinitis in 29 cats, unilateral aggressive lesions were more suggestive of neoplasia, whereas bilaterally symmetric lesions were more suggestive of chronic rhinitis.[5]

Animals with acute rhinitis often have nasal passages that are normal radiographically. Possible causes for rhinitis include foreign bodies, viruses, bacteria, and allergies. Nasal foreign bodies are uncommon in the dog and cat but should be considered in patients with acute onset of violent sneezing, head shaking, and nose rubbing. Unless the foreign body is radiopaque, however, radiographic examination may be unrewarding (Fig. 6–1). Plant awns and other vegetable materials often lodge in the rostral portion of the nasal passages. In chronic rhinitis secondary to a foreign body, a focal area of increased soft-tissue opacity may be seen owing to the presence of mucopurulent exudate or to a local inflammatory response. In some animals, foreign body rhinitis is due to congenital or traumatic defects in the palate coupled with the introduction of food into the nasal passages.

Chronic rhinitis is often characterized by areas of increased soft-tissue opacity superimposed over the normal conchal pattern. This opacity tends to involve the rostral portion and midportion of the nasal passages and is often bilateral.[5] This increased opacity may be due to the presence of nasal exudate or to swelling and proliferation of the nasal mucosa (Fig. 6–2). In the cat, chronic rhinitis and concurrent frontal sinusitis are common sequelae to viral upper respiratory infections. Post-traumatic hemorrhage may produce similar opacities.

Nasal conchal destruction is an indication of a more aggressive disease process and occurs primarily with destructive rhinitis or neoplasia. Destructive rhinitis is generally due to fungal infections and most commonly affects mesocephalic or dolichocephalic dogs younger than 4 years of age.[6] *Aspergillus* species (especially *Aspergillus fumigatus*) are the most common causative agents.[7–9] Infections caused by *Penicillium* species and other fungal agents are noted less often.[10, 11] Most patients with destructive rhinitis have focal radiolucent areas of conchal destruction. These lesions vary in size from small punctate holes to large, poorly marginated areas of lysis (Fig. 6–3). A mixed pattern of destruction and soft-tissue proliferation may be seen, but it is less common. Erosion or deviation of the nasal septum is unusual except in advanced disease. Partial to complete increase in frontal sinus opacity with mottled thickening of the frontal bone is also seen.[12] *Cryptococcus neoformans* also may infect the nasal passages, especially in the cat, but this organism usually causes hyperplastic rather than destructive rhinitis.[13]

Increased soft-tissue opacity superimposed over areas of conchal destruction and a mixture of radiopaque areas interspersed with well-defined areas of radiolucency are patterns typically seen with neoplasia, although they may also occur in destructive rhinitis (Fig. 6–4). In many animals, these areas of increased opacity are due to accumulated nasal secretions. Opacification of the ipsilateral frontal sinus is generally due to impaired sinus drainage, although neoplastic extension into the sinus also occurs.[14]

Neoplasms of the nasal cavity and paranasal sinuses are rare, representing approximately 1 percent of all neoplasms in the dog and cat.[15, 16] Studies concerning the biologic behavior of these lesions and their response to various treatment modalities are ongoing.[17, 18] It has been reported that 80 percent of nasal neoplasms in dogs are malignant; in cats, 91 percent are malignant.[19, 20] Of these malignant neoplasms, 60 to 75 percent are carcinomas, with adenocarcinomas predominating over other cell types.[21] Older animals are most frequently affected, with a mean age at diagnosis of 8 to 10 years. A marked gender predisposition appears in the cat; males are nearly twice as likely to be affected as females.[22, 23]

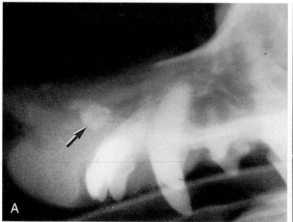
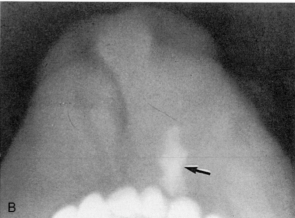

FIGURE 6–1. Lateral *(A)* and close-up ventrodorsal open-mouth *(B)* radiographs of a 9-year-old female poodle with a history of unilateral nasal discharge and sneezing for 3 weeks. A radiopaque foreign body *(arrows)* can be seen in the left nostril; note the loss of normal aeration of that nostril.

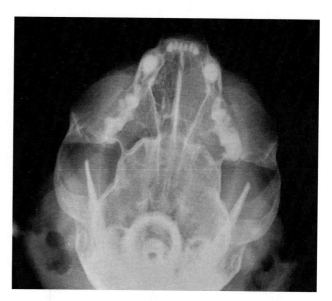

FIGURE 6–2. Open-mouth ventrodorsal radiograph of a 13-year-old castrated male domestic shorthair cat with a 4-week history of primarily left-sided nasal discharge and anorexia. There is a diffuse increase in opacity of the left nasal passage with decreased definition of the nasal conchi. Severe subacute pyogranulomatous rhinitis due to *Pasteurella multocida* was diagnosed following nasal curettage and culture.

No gender predilection has been identified for adenocarcinomas in the dog, although tumors of nonepithelial origin, such as chondrosarcomas, appear to have a male predilection.

The radiographic appearance of nasal neoplasms varies depending on the type of neoplasm, its duration, and any previous surgical or medical treatment. The more aggressive the neoplasm, the more destructive and less confined it appears. Early nasal neoplasms may appear similar radiographically to rhinitis and therefore are difficult to diagnose. A unilateral increase in nasal opacity with attenuation or obliteration of the normal conchal pattern is a consistent finding in early nasal tumors of epithelial origin. This homogeneous appearance is due to cellular debris and fluid silhouetting with the conchae. Opacification of the ipsilateral frontal sinus is often present and may be due to the presence of a tumor or obstruction with accumulation of mucus. As the neoplasm grows, the radiographic appearance becomes more heterogeneous owing to progressive conchal destruction (Fig. 6–5).

Disruption of the nasal septum is often seen with malignant neoplasms. As mentioned previously, the integrity of the nasal septum is difficult to assess radiographically. Large areas of the nasal septum may be destroyed, and this destruction may not be evident radiographically.[24] Recognition of septal penetration is most likely to occur in those animals with destruction of the vomer or deviation of the nasal septum (Fig. 6–6).

Peripheral signs of soft-tissue swelling, facial bone destruction, and periosteal new bone formation are usually associ-

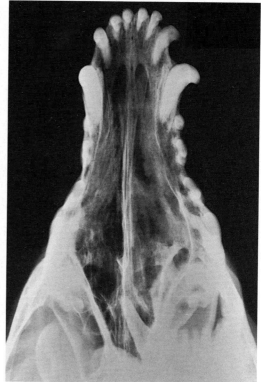

FIGURE 6–3. Open-mouth ventrodorsal radiograph of a 6-year-old male Doberman pinscher presented for chronic weight loss and a bilateral mucopurulent nasal discharge. There is severe bilateral destruction of the normal nasal conchal pattern in the midportion of the nasal cavity. Destructive rhinitis secondary to *Aspergillus fumigatus* was diagnosed by culture.

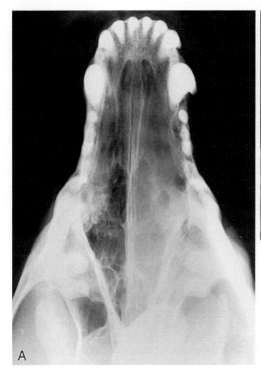

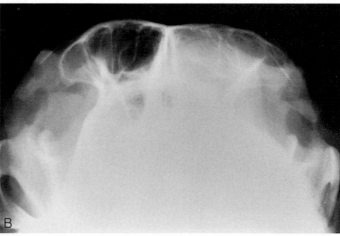

FIGURE 6–4. Open-mouth ventrodorsal maxillary *(A)* and rostrocaudal skull *(B)* radiographs of a 10-year-old mixed-breed dog with chronic unilateral epistaxis. There is a diffuse increase in soft-tissue opacity of the left nasal passage with decreased conchal definition *(A)* and opacity of the left frontal sinus on the rostrocaudal view *(B)*. Osteosarcoma was diagnosed; however, this appearance is also typical of other epithelial and mesenchymal nasal cavity tumors.

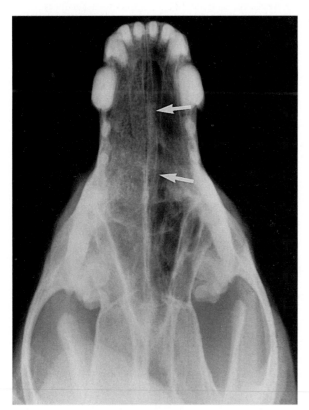

FIGURE 6–5. Open-mouth ventrodorsal view of a 6-year-old male German shepherd dog with a 4-month history of unilateral epistaxis. There is diffuse opacification of the right nasal passage with many punctate areas of calcification in the middle and rostral portions. There is thinning and deviation of the vomer *(arrows)*. The diagnosis of chondrosarcoma was made histologically.

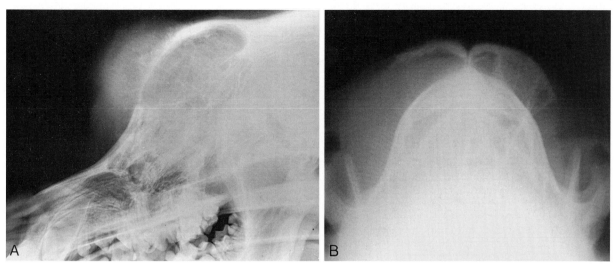

FIGURE 6–6. Lateral *(A)* and rostrocaudal *(B)* views of the frontal sinuses of a 7-month-old male Great Dane with a rapidly enlarging mass over the right frontal sinus of 4 weeks' duration. There is extensive destruction of the dorsal and lateral cortices of the right frontal sinus with diffuse soft-tissue opacification extending outside of the sinus and irregular periosteal new bone formation. Histologic diagnosis was a highly anaplastic mucoepidermoid carcinoma.

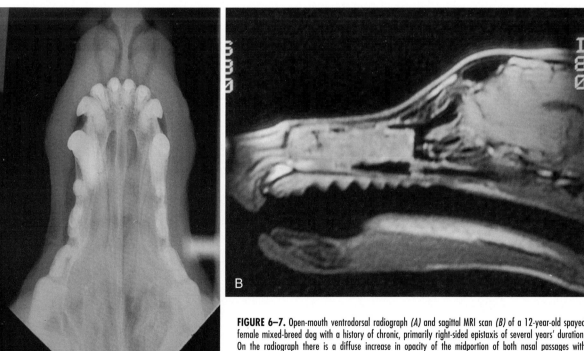

FIGURE 6–7. Open-mouth ventrodorsal radiograph *(A)* and sagittal MRI scan *(B)* of a 12-year-old spayed female mixed-breed dog with a history of chronic, primarily right-sided epistaxis of several years' duration. On the radiograph there is a diffuse increase in opacity of the midportion of both nasal passages with conchal destruction that appears more severe on the right side. On the MRI scan, made just to the right of the midline plane, a solid mass is seen filling most of the rostral and midportions of the nasal passage. A chondrosarcoma was identified on biopsy of the mass.

ated with highly aggressive neoplasms.[25] These areas of bone destruction may be evident on palpation or may cause obvious facial swelling. Superimposition of disrupted overlying bone often contributes to the mixed opacity seen on the open-mouth view (Fig. 6–7). Oblique projections may help demonstrate defects in the maxillae, the palate, and the nasal and frontal bones.

Despite the use of multiple views and improved film-screen combinations, accurate radiographic assessment of the extent of nasal cavity involvement in patients with nasal tumors remains extremely difficult. One group of investigators has developed an objective radiographic scoring system that quantifies the severity of radiographic changes and uses this score to assess patient prognosis in terms of disease-free interval and survival time regardless of the histologic tumor type.[26] The increasing interest in using radiation therapy for treatment of nasal tumors in companion animals has necessitated the use of more sophisticated imaging modalities. Computed tomograpy (CT) and magnetic resonance imaging (MRI) have become more widely used and allow improved assessment of the intracranial and extracranial extension of nasal cavity neoplasia. The normal CT anatomy of the canine nasal passages has been presented elsewhere.[27]

Both CT and MRI provide tomographic images of the skull that allow improved anatomic information concerning many regions difficult to assess with conventional radiography. Even in those patients with radiographic evidence of nasal malignancies, CT and MRI are more accurate in identifying unilateral versus bilateral disease and providing precise anatomic information concerning the extent of malignant nasal cavity disease than is possible with the use of conventional radiography.[28, 29] Extension to adjacent structures, such as the cribriform plate, cranium, and hard palate, are also more easily assessed.[30-33] Routine use of CT and CT-based radiation therapy planning should improve the homogeneity of the delivered radiation dose and in that way, it is hoped, improve patient response and survival. Their use has greatly improved diagnosis and staging of nasal tumors as well as improving the ability to assess response to different treatment modalities.

References

1. Hare WCD: Radiographic anatomy of the feline skull. J Am Vet Med Assoc 134:349, 1959.
2. Sande RD, and Alexander JE: Turbinate bone neoplasms in dogs. Mod Vet Pract 51:23, 1970.
3. Harvey CE, Biery DN, Morello J, et al: Chronic nasal disease in the dog: Its radiographic appearance. Vet Radiol 20:91, 1979.
4. Bright RM, and Bojrab MJ: Intranasal neoplasia in the dog and cat. J Am Anim Hosp Assoc 12:806, 1976.
5. O'Brien RT, Evans SM, Wortman JA, et al: Radiographic findings in cats with intranasal neoplasia or chronic rhinitis: 29 cases (1982–1988). J Am Vet Med Assoc 208:385, 1996.
6. Bedford PG: The differential diagnosis of nasal discharge in the dog. Vet Annu 18:232, 1978.
7. Lane JG, and Warnock DW: The diagnosis of Aspergillus fumigatus infection of the nasal chambers of the dog with particular reference to the value of the double diffusion test. J Small Anim Pract 18:169, 1977.
8. Bright RM: Nasal aspergillosis in the dog. Comp Contin Ed Pract Vet 1:664, 1979.
9. Hargis AM, Liggitt HD, Lincoln JD, et al: Noninvasive nasal aspergillosis (fungal ball) in a six-year-old Standard poodle. J Am Anim Hosp Assoc 22:504, 1986.
10. Harvey CE, O'Brien JA, Felsburg PJ, et al: Nasal penicilliosis in six dogs. J Am Vet Med Assoc 178:1084, 1981.
11. Sharp JH, Harvey CE, and Sullivan M: Canine nasal aspergillosis and penicilliosis. Comp Contin Ed Pract Vet 13:41, 1991.
12. Sullivan M, Lee R, Jakovljevic S, et al: The radiological features of aspergillosis in the nasal cavity and frontal sinuses of the dog. J Small Anim Pract 27:167, 1986.
13. Wilkinson GT: Feline cryptococcosis: A review and seven case reports. J Small Anim Pract 20:749, 1979.
14. Gibbs C, Lane JG, and Denny HR: Radiological features of intranasal lesions in the dog: A review of 100 cases. J Small Anim Pract 20:515, 1979.
15. Norris AM: Intranasal neoplasms in the dog. J Am Anim Hosp Assoc 15:231, 1979.
16. Evans SM, and Hendrick M: Radiotherapy of feline nasal tumors. Vet Radiol 30:128, 1989.
17. Patnaik AK: Canine sinonasal neoplasms: Clinicopathological study of 285 cases. J Am Anim Hosp Assoc 25:103, 1989.
18. Patnaik AK: Canine sinonasal neoplasms: Soft-tissue tumors. J Am Anim Hosp Assoc 25:491, 1989.
19. Reznik G, and Stinson SF: Nasal Tumors in Animals and Man. Boca Raton, FL, CRC Press, 1983.
20. Madewell BR, Priester WA, Gillette EL, et al: Neoplasms of the nasal passages and paranasal sinuses in domesticated animals as reported by 13 veterinary colleges. Am J Vet Res 37:851, 1976.
21. Brodey RS: Canine and feline neoplasia. Adv Vet Sci Comp Med 14:309, 1970.
22. Legendre AM, Krahwinkel DJ, and Spaulding KA: Feline nasal and paranasal neoplasms. J Am Anim Hosp Assoc 17:1038, 1981.
23. Cox NR, Brawner WR, Powers RD, et al: Tumors of the nose and paranasal sinuses in cats: 32 cases with comparison to a national database (1977–1987). J Am Anim Hosp Assoc 27:339, 1991.
24. Harvey C: The nasal septum of the dog: Is it visible radiographically? Vet Radiol 20:88, 1979.
25. Legendre AM, Spaulding KA, and Krahwinkel DJ: Canine nasal and paranasal sinus neoplasms. J Am Anim Hosp Assoc 19:115, 1983.
26. Morris JS, Dunn KJ, Dobson JM, et al: Radiological assessment of severity of canine nasal tumors and relationship with survival. J Small Anim Pract 37:1, 1996.
27. Burk RL: Computed tomographic anatomy of the canine nasal passages. Vet Radiol Ultrasound 33:170, 1992.
28. Thrall DE, Robertson ID, McLeod DA, et al: A comparison of radiographic and computed tomographic findings in 31 dogs with malignant nasal cavity tumors. Vet Radiol 31:92, 1989.
29. Burk RL: Computed tomographic imaging of nasal disease in 100 dogs. Vet Radiol Ultrasound 33:177, 1992.
30. Koblik PD, and Berry CR: Dorsal plane computed tomographic imaging of the ethmoid region to evaluate chronic nasal disease in the dog. Vet Radiol 31:92, 1990.
31. Berry CR, and Koblik PD: Evaluation of survey radiography, linear tomography, and computed tomography for detecting experimental lesions of the cribriform plate in dogs. Vet Radiol 31:146, 1990.
32. Moore MP, Gavin PR, Kraft SL, et al: MR, CT, and clinical features from four dogs with nasal tumors involving the rostral cerebrum. Vet Radiol 32:19, 1991.
33. Voges AK, and Ackerman N: MR evaluation of intra and extracranial extension of nasal adenocarcinoma in a dog and cat. Vet Radiol Ultrasound 36:196, 1995.

STUDY QUESTIONS

1. What radiographic views are most helpful in assessing diseases of the nasal cavity and paranasal sinuses?

2. What are common radiographic signs seen following fractures of the facial portion of the skull?

3. What is the normal radiographic appearance of the nasal passages, and what anatomic structures account for this appearance?

4. What are four common causes of acute rhinitis? What are their radiographic features?

5. What are the most common radiographic features of chronic bacterial rhinitis?

6. What is the most common causative agent of destructive rhinitis in the dog? What radiographic features help to differentiate this infection from chronic bacterial rhinitis?

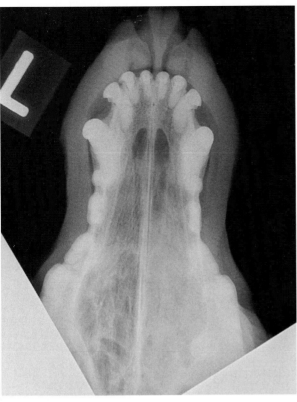

FIGURE 6–8

7. What is the predominant type of malignant tumor seen in the nasal cavity of the dog?

8. What factors affect the radiographic appearance of malignant nasal tumors?

9. You are presented with a 9-year-old male mixed-breed dog with a 1-month history of a right-sided, blood-tinged nasal discharge. You decide to radiograph the dog and obtain a dorsoventral occlusal radiograph (Fig. 6–8). What are the radiographic findings? What is your assessment of these findings, and what would you recommend next to the owner?

10. You are presented with a 12-year-old male Doberman pinscher who has a history of a chronic nasal discharge and right-sided epistaxis. Over the last few weeks, the owner has noticed a swelling over the top of the nose and extending down the right side of the dog's face. You decide to take radiographs and obtain the lateral and open-mouth ventrodorsal radiograph shown here (Fig. 6–9). The aforementioned soft-tissue swelling is indicated on the figure by the long white arrows. What is indicated by the short white arrow? What are the radiographic findings? What is your assessment of these findings, and what would you recommend next to the owner?

(Answers appear on pages 633 and 634.)

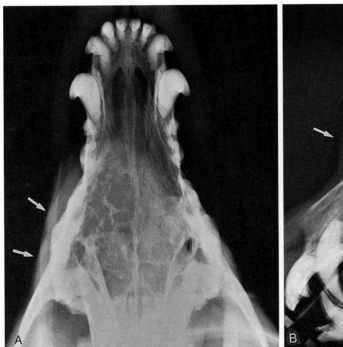
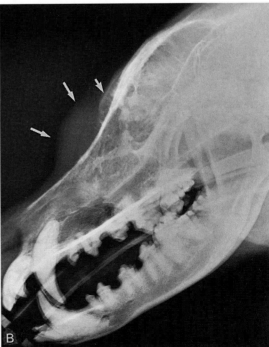

FIGURE 6–9

Chapter 7

Anatomic and Physiologic Imaging of the Canine and Feline Brain

Clifford R. Berry

Transcranial ultrasonography, computed tomography (CT), and magnetic resonance imaging (MRI) can be used for anatomic imaging of the canine and feline brain, whereas magnetic resonance spectroscopy and nuclear medicine techniques can be used for obtaining functional information. Advances in the use of cross-sectional imaging have allowed techniques that are routinely applied in humans to be available in veterinary medicine. This chapter introduces the use of these modalities for imaging the canine and feline brain. The physical basics of image acquisition and principles of interpretation are reviewed for CT, MRI, and computed nuclear medicine techniques. Common abnormalities are emphasized rather than specifics about a particular disorder because overlap exists among the various disease processes.

PRINCIPLES OF IMAGE FORMATION

The physical principles of image formation for cross-sectional imaging techniques share the common use of a computer system that takes raw data and reconstructs it into various imaging planes (i.e., transverse, dorsal, sagittal, and oblique).[1–5] For nuclear medicine (single-photon emission CT [SPECT]), MRI, and CT, a volume of information is obtained, thereby allowing reconstruction into any of the desired imaging planes. The physics of each of these techniques are well described and only the basics are covered here.[1, 3–5]

Computed Tomography

CT has dramatically changed the way the anatomy of a particular subject is viewed. Before CT, survey radiographs were used to evaluate a three-dimensional subject as a two-dimensional image. By obtaining orthogonal radiographs, one could try to triangulate where a particular structure was within the subject (i.e., nodule in a particular lung lobe). CT allows one to obtain a cross-sectional image of a subject so that the inside of the subject can be visualized. The basic principles of CT are similar to those of radiography, in that x-rays are used to create an attenuation map of the patient.[1] The technique of CT is dependent on the rotation of an x-ray tube around the patient and acquiring a series of x-ray projections with the use of rotating (third generation) or stationary (fourth generation) x-ray detectors.[1] As in conventional radiography, the x-rays either pass through the patient or are attenuated. This attenuation depends on the density (physical and electron) of the material in the patient, the thickness of the patient, and the effective atomic number of a particular substance in the patient. This transverse raw data set is then reconstructed with the use of a computer algorithm, and an image is produced (Fig. 7–1).

A CT image is a matrix of squares, each square having a unique degree of blackness depending on the attenuation of photons from a given location in the patient. Each individual square is called a picture element or *pixel*. Standard CT scan-

ners acquire data from a certain thickness with each transverse slice. Because there is a slice thickness, each pixel has a certain depth or volume associated with it, and this volume-element is termed a *voxel*. All of the attenuation information that is collected within a given voxel is averaged and the average gray scale value is then displayed. This averaging can lead to erroneous interpretation because of *volume averaging* owing to the volume or thickness of a given slice of information. If a voxel contains a very opaque and a very lucent structure, the overall end-result is an intermediate shade of gray. Thus, volume averaging can artificially raise or lower a structure's attenuation value and thereby the appearance on the image.[1, 2] When the computer reconstructs the images, the image voxel values are normalized to the linear attenuation coefficient of water. These values are expressed in *Hounsfield units* (HU).* Water has an HU of zero, whereas cortical bone has an HU of $+3000$ and air has an HU of -1000. The HU of different organs and structures within the body are characteristic for that organ or structure (Table 7–1).

One can manipulate the values of the gray scale that are assigned to the CT image. The window width describes the range of CT values assigned to the gray scale within the image. A wide window width is 1000, whereas a narrow window width is 250. A wide window width is used when there are extreme spectrums of physical density (and thereby of HU) that are being imaged (i.e., the lung). A narrow window width is used when there is a smaller spectrum of

---

*CT value (Hounsfield Unit) $= [(\mu material - \mu water)/(\mu water)] \times 1000$, where $\mu = $ linear attenuation coefficient

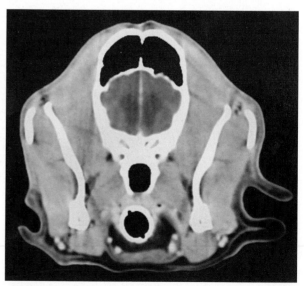

FIGURE 7–1. Transverse computed tomography image (window width = 260; window level = 60) from an 8-year-old male Golden retriever. The reconstructed data are presented as a transverse image, the plane of data acquisition. In this dog, the slice thickness was 5 mm. The lateral ventricles are dilated secondary to a glioma.

Table 7–1

REPRESENTATIVE CT VALUES (IN HOUNSFIELD UNITS) OF DIFFERENT PARTS WITHIN THE BODY

Body Part	CT Value
White matter	30 (35*)
Gray matter	35 (42*)
Cerebrospinal fluid	6–10
Hemorrhage, acute (whole blood)	52
Blood clot	50–80
Plasma	25
Water	0

*CT values of white and gray matter increase after contrast enhancement. Gray matter receives four times the blood flow as white matter, so gray matter is more attenuated just after delivery of the contrast medium to the brain. Edema decreases the attenuation coefficient of the affected area proportional to the amount of water within the edematous structure.

physical densities (HU) that are close to one another (i.e., differentiating gray and white matter within the brain). The window level is a midpoint for the range of window width values. For example, if a window level of 50 is used and window width of 200, the range of HU values that would be displayed would include −50 to 150 HU.

Magnetic Resonance Imaging

In MRI, the mechanism for acquisition of data is completely different from any other imaging modality.[3, 4] The fundamentals of MRI depend on several inherent nuclear phenomena. The nucleus is made of protons and neutrons, which exist in pairs. Both protons and neutrons have a property called a *spin* or *angular momentum*. The proton behaves like a magnet and because of its positive electric charge and spin establishes a small magnetic field about itself. This property is called a *magnetic dipole*. If there is an odd number of protons, the unpaired proton exerts a magnetic dipole with a discrete strength and direction (a vector quantity). The hydrogen atom is found in high concentrations in the body and thereby is the nucleus most commonly imaged with the use of MRI. Other potential nuclei with odd proton numbers that could be used in MRI include ^{13}C, ^{23}Na, and ^{19}F.

With the patient in an MRI scanner, a high field strength magnet is turned on, and the proton magnetic dipoles align themselves with the long axis of the magnetic field (usually along the axis of the patient's body and defined as the z-axis). A *net magnetic moment* is then established (Fig. 7–2). Another property of the individual protons is that they can absorb radiofrequency waves. This absorbed energy causes the individual proton's vector direction to move out of alignment with the external magnetic field (Fig. 7–3). The excited proton then starts to rotate around its original spin state and return to its original position over time, through a process called *precession*. This rotation of the magnetization vector or magnetic moment induces an electric signal in receiver coils present in the x-y plane. This electric signal oscillates as the magnetization vector points toward and away from the receiver coil. The amplitude of the electric signal decreases over time as the individual protons lose phase coherence with each other and return to the lower energy state. The speed with which each proton (individual magnetic moments) loses coherence depends on the relaxation properties described later in this chapter. The electric signal that is induced in the receiver coil is called the *free induction decay (FID)*. Each term in FID is meaningful for understanding the process of obtaining the MRI signal. *Free* refers to the fact that the net magnetization vector (protons) is no longer under the influence of the radiofrequency pulse. *Induction*

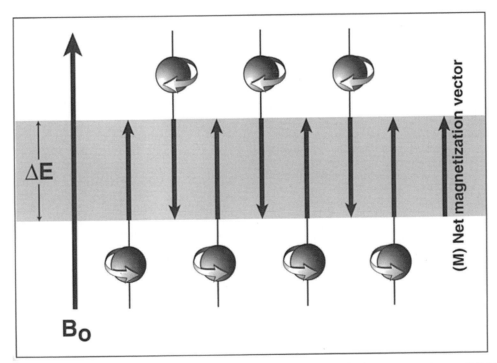

FIGURE 7–2. Schematic representation of individual protons that exhibit a given spin and energy state. Once they are placed within a strong external magnetic field (B$_0$), the individual magnetic moments will align themselves along the axis or direction of B$_0$ (z-axis). A majority of the protons will align themselves in the parallel or lower energy state, whereas some of the protons will align themselves in the antiparallel or higher energy state. The net magnetization vector is determined by the summation of all of the individual protons within the area of interest. Conceptually, it is easier to think in terms of large net magnetic moment when one explains the effects of radiofrequency pulses on the net magnetic moment (M) versus the individual protons, although the imaging magnet takes into account discrete numbers of individual protons within the field of view.

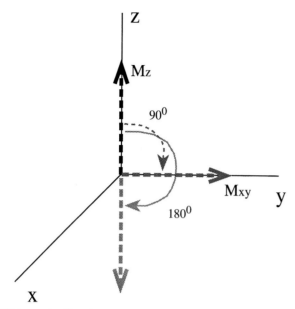

FIGURE 7–3. The effects of a 90-degree or a 180-degree radio frequency pulse on the net magnetization vector (Mz). In this example, the radio frequency pulses serve to excite the net magnetization vector out of the parallel state (aligned with the z-axis) into an excited state along the x-y plane (90 degrees) or opposite to the z-direction (180 degrees). The "excited" Mz will then lose energy as it returns to the parallel, resting z-axis.

means that the oscillating magnetic field that is being created by the precession of the net magnetization vector within a closed coil system induces an electric current that represents the MRI signal. *Decay* means that the signal decreases over time.[3]

The intensity of a given signal that is released from the excited protons is complex and is dependent on four essential components: the concentration of the protons (^{1}H) or proton density, the intermolecular interactions for a given proton that is defined by two different relaxation times (defined as *T1* and *T2 relaxation times*, which are discussed later), and the bulk flow of the protons.

MRI is different from CT in that the types of physical and chemical bonds and amounts of chemical elements that are present, their individual thermal motions, and the chemical interactions strongly affect the relaxation characteristics of excited protons and thereby the signal that is given off. In fact, because of these environmental interactions, along with the inherent resolution of MRI equipment, excellent soft-tissue contrast can be achieved between structures that have only minor differences in physical density with decreased contrast resolution on CT, as seen in the brain.

These magnetic dipoles that are exerted by the protons are randomly arranged in tissues. Once an external magnetic field is turned on, the dipoles align themselves into specific energy states within the body. As described, their orientations include either parallel (lower energy) or an antiparallel (higher energy) state. Because the lower energy state is preferred, when the protons are placed in a static magnetic field (B_0), a *net magnetic moment* is created and is aligned parallel with the external magnetic field (typically denoted as the z-direction in MRI nomenclature). In reality, the torque of the external magnetic field causes the net magnetic moment to rotate around the axis of B_0 at a characteristic frequency called the *angular frequency*. This angular frequency is directly proportional to the magnetic field strength, B_0, by the equation:

$$w_0 \text{ (angular frequency)} = g \text{ (gyromagnetic ratio)} \times B_0 \text{ (external field strength in Tesla)}$$

Because angular frequency is measured in radians per second and there are 2π radians in a complete rotation, the equation can be rewritten in terms of the precessional frequency expressed in cycles per second or Hertz as follows: f_0 (*precessional frequency*) $= g/2\pi \times B_0$ (external field strength in Tesla), where the frequency of precession (f_0) is also called the *resonance frequency* or the *Larmor frequency*. For protons, $g/2\pi$ is equal to 42.58 MHz/Tesla. This means that in a static magnetic field of 1.5 Tesla, the protons precess with a frequency of 63.87 MHz (1.5 × 42.58).

The *net magnetic moment (Mz)* is aligned with the external magnetic field. If electromagnetic radiation is applied as a short radiofrequency pulse, the magnetic moment can be reoriented to a new direction out of the z or longitudinal plane and into the x-y or transverse plane. For the protons within the subject to absorb the radiofrequency photons (and thereby move from a parallel to the higher energy and less stable antiparallel state), the radiofrequency pulse must be equal to the precession frequency of the protons in the subject. Once the proton has been reoriented in a different plane owing to the absorption of the radiofrequency pulse, it will try to reach the lower energy state again. This process of relaxation depends on several factors, including magnetic field strength, spin interactions, magnetic field inhomogeneities, presence of paramagnetic materials, and the environmental lattice within which the proton is found.

One can think of the simplest MRI experiment as the patient being placed inside the magnet and the magnet being turned on; a series of radiofrequency waves (pulses) are then used to excite the given nuclei; then the excitation pulse is turned off and the receiver coils are turned on to listen for the free induction decay signal generated by the excited protons as they lose phase coherence and return to their lower energy state. These latter two steps are repeated a number of times, and the volume of raw data information is available for reconstruction into a given imaging plane. This represents an oversimplification of the process, and further explanation is warranted for defining the MRI characteristics of different tissues.

T1 Relaxation (Spin-Lattice or Longitudinal Relaxation)

T1 relaxation is the time (milliseconds or seconds) required for the protons to recover 63 percent of the original magnetization in the z direction after the application of a radiofrequency pulse that rotates the original net magnetic moment by 90 degrees. Because this involves the release of energy from the protons moving from the excited (antiparallel) state to the lower energy (parallel) orientation, the longitudinal (z-direction) magnetization is gradually recovered, so T1 relaxation is also referred to as *longitudinal relaxation*. Additionally, the T1 relaxation is dependent on the energy exchange between the excited protons and the surrounding molecular lattice, so another name for T1 relaxation is *spin-lattice relaxation*.

T1 relaxation is dependent on several factors, including molecular motion, the molecule being bound to other substances or found in a free state, and the size of the molecule. The interactions among these three factors are complex. In general, T1 relaxation is enhanced (shortened) by molecular motions with moderate speeds or medium-sized molecules that are partially bound. T1 relaxation is lengthened by very slow or very fast moving molecules and larger, bound and smaller, unbound molecules. For example, water is a small, fast-moving molecule that is not bound (free) and has a T1 relaxation of 3000 msec, whereas protein-bound water has a shorter T1 relaxation.

When reviewing an MRI image, structures are referred to

Table 7–2

REPRESENTATIVE MRI T1 AND T2 RELAXATION VALUES OF DIFFERENT PARTS WITHIN THE BODY*

Structure	T1 Value (msec)	T2 Value (msec)
White matter	589	76
Gray matter	1215	106
Cerebrospinal fluid	2000	1200
Water	3000	>2000

*As measured by a GE Signa, 1.5 Tesla MR Imager.
Data from Smith Hans J, and Ranallo FN: A Non-Mathematical Approach to Basic MRI. Madison, WI, Medical Physics Publishing Corporation, 1989.

by the intensity of signal that is produced, with white being considered hyperintense and black being considered hypointense. On T1-weighted images, a structure with a prolonged T1 relaxation (e.g., cerebrospinal fluid) appears hypointense (black), whereas a structure with a short T1 relaxation (e.g., fat) appears hyperintense (white).

Differences in intensity on a T1-weighted image that influence soft-tissue contrast include proton density and the differences in the T1 between two different tissues. Factors that influence T1 relaxation include the strength of the magnetic field and the use of paramagnetic contrast media. Low-field strength magnets (0.5 Tesla) increase the soft-tissue contrast differences based on T1 relaxation. Intravenous paramagnetic substances, such as gadolinium-DTPA (Magnevist®), decrease T1 relaxation times. The normal range of T1 relaxation times in the body is between 100 and 2500 msec. Some representative T1 relaxation times are shown in Table 7–2.

T2 Relaxation (Spin-Spin or Transverse Relaxation)

T2 relaxation can be defined as the time required to reduce the net transverse magnetization to 37 percent of its original value. Therefore, a short T2 means a rapid loss of transverse

magnetization (after the net magnetic moment has been excited or flipped from the z orientation into the x-y or transverse plane). As protons release the excess energy and change to the more stable form, the energy released can interact in several ways. The first is that the energy is absorbed by the lattice or environment and directly impacts the thermal molecular motions of the tissue. This process is responsible for T1 relaxation. Second, the energy released could be absorbed by another proton that is then shifted from the low energy to the higher energy state. T2 relaxation is based on direct proton-proton interactions in which the released energy is absorbed by another proton. This energy exchange results in changes in spin orientation of the proton and is thereby called *spin-spin relaxation*. The T2* is the actual relaxation time that is initially measured (Fig. 7–4) because of imperfections in the magnetic field that result in altered T2 relaxation characteristics.

T2 relaxation occurs after the net magnetization vector has been rotated into the transverse plane. Now the large magnetization vector in the x-y plane loses coherence because of the local interference of the proton's own minute magnetic field and inherent inhomogeneities in the large applied magnetic field, B_0. The protons exchange their energy with neighboring protons by interactions with their spin states. Protons that are found in fluid state have decreased spin interactions with their neighbors and thereby longer T2 relaxation times (milliseconds). The range of T2 relaxation times in the body is between 20 and 1500 msec (see Table 7–2).

In contrast to T1 relaxation, structures with longer T2 relaxation characteristics produce a higher signal intensity (appear white on T2-weighted images). Additionally, increasing the field strength has little effect on T2, and the T2 values are less than the T1 values for a given body tissue. Additionally, paramagnetic substances decrease the T2 relaxation time and thereby produce decreased signal (appear darker on T2-weighted images) in areas where the paramagnetic substance localizes. The appearance of different structures on T1-weighted and T2-weighted images is summarized in Table 7–3.

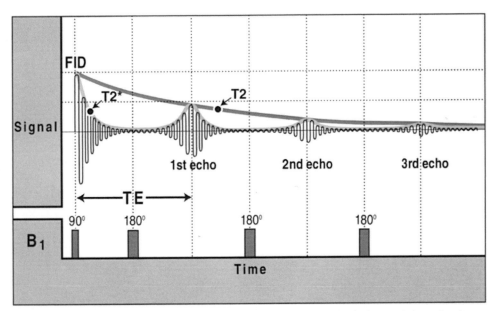

FIGURE 7–4. Schematic representation of free induction decay (FID) and echo signals that would be induced in the receiver coils after a standard spin-echo pulse sequence that uses an initial 90-degree pulse and repetitive 180-degree pulses to produce multiple echoes. The exponential decay of the FID from each echo represents the T2*, while the exponential decay line that intersects the peak of the FID from each echo represents the true T2 relaxation time. The reason for the more rapid decay as seen in the T2* decay curves is due to magnetic field inhomogeneities. The TE represents the echo time or time from the initial 90-degree pulse to the first peak echo signal that will be used for image formation.

Table 7–3

REPRESENTATIVE DIFFERENTIAL DIAGNOSTIC CONSIDERATIONS FOR INTENSITY PATTERNS SEEN ON T1-WEIGHTED AND T2-WEIGHTED IMAGES

T1 Image	T2 Image	Differential Diagnosis
Hypointense (dark)	Hyperintense (bright)	Cerebrospinal fluid, fluid collections, edema
Hyperintense	Hypointense	Fat, some protein solutions, calcium deposits, or transient blood flow
Hyperintense	Hyperintense	Paramagnetic solutions/contrast medium, extracellular methemoglobin, proteins, mucopolysaccharide solutions
Hypointense	Hypointense	Dense calcium deposits, bone, air, rapid flow, hemosiderin, metallic artifacts

Physical Basis of Spin-Echo Imaging

There are different pulse sequences that can be applied to MRI of the patient that directly affect the type of image that is obtained. A basic pulse sequence can be defined as the application of an excitation pulse followed by a time for listening for the FID signal given off by the tissues. In some sequences, rephasing pulses can be applied that allow for maximization of the initial excitation pulse by being able to read smaller signals, called echoes. Some of these pulse sequences emphasize just T1 relaxation (called *saturation-recovery* and *inversion-recovery*). Some pulse sequences can be used to emphasize fluid in vessels or de-emphasize fat in the tissues. The most common pulse sequence used today for routine MRI is the *spin-echo sequence*. Using spin-echo techniques, one can obtain three different image types (T1-weighted images, proton density images, and T2-weighted images) of a tissue by altering the pulse sequence within the spin-echo imaging protocol.

As previously stated, the timing of an MRI sequence is critical as to which relaxation characteristics are emphasized. One can think of these sequences as a series of repetitive experiments that are done to increase the signal-to-noise ratio. As one increases the number of pulse sequences performed (experiments), the signal-to-noise ratio increases. The number of excitations (NEX) is the number of pulse sequences that are done with the same x, y, and z gradients. A pulse sequence is made up of (1) an initial 90-degree radiofrequency pulse (along with an application of a z gradient for slice localization), (2) application of a y-gradient, (3) a rephasing 180-degree radiofrequency pulse, and (4) an echo time for recording of the FID signal (along with application of an x or readout gradient) (Fig. 7–5).

As mentioned, these pulse sequences are centered around an initial excitation radiofrequency pulse of the area or slice that is being imaged. The initial FID signal is ignored in this process, and a second radiofrequency pulse is applied that rephases the protons so that a signal is created that is called the echo. The time between the application of the initial 90-degree pulse and the peak of the echo signal is called the *echo time (TE)*. This time is actually the time when the signal induced in the receiver coils is recorded and used for producing the MRI image. Additional 180-degree pulses can be applied that result in smaller echoes from the original FID. To differentiate T2* from true T2 relaxation, an exponential curve can be fit to the peaks of the FID echoes that gives the true time constant that is equal to T2. An initial 90-degree pulse is used to create an initial FID signal that is not used. A series of 180-degree radiofrequency pulses are applied that result in multiple echoes that can be used for the creation of the MRI image. The time between successive applications of 90-degree pulses is called the *repetition time (TR)*. The *delay time (TD)* represents the delay between the recording of the final echo and the initiation of the next 90-degree radiofrequency pulse.

By varying the TR and TE, one can selectively use specific relaxation features that enhance T1-weighted, T2-weighted,

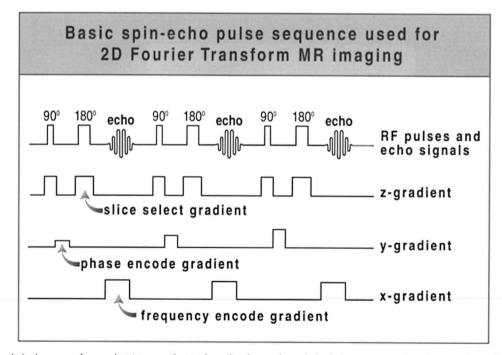

FIGURE 7–5. The standard pulse sequence for spin-echo MR imaging. The RF pulses and readout signals are displayed along the top line. The different encoding gradients are applied in three different directions for object or area localization within the patient. Each of these different gradients takes advantage of an established gradient in the x, y and z directions so that signals from the volume of data can be oriented correctly in three-dimensional space in the final data set for image reconstruction.

or proton density images. A short TR (400 msec) and short TE (20 msec) emphasize T1 relaxation of the tissues and proton density. A long TR de-emphasizes the T1 relaxation and emphasizes T2 relaxation. A long TR (2000 msec) and short TE (20 msec) emphasize just the proton density, whereas a long TR (2000 msec) and long TE (100 msec) emphasize T2 relaxation and proton density.

Image localization is accomplished by creating a strength gradient of the static B_0 magnetic field along the x, y and z directions of the magnetic field. This is done by specially designed gradient coils within the bore of the magnet. These gradients are applied during different times of the spin-echo pulse sequence so that the echo signal given off can be accurately localized to a given voxel with the volume of tissue or a given slice of tissue being imaged. The z-gradient (also called slice-select gradient) is applied at the time of the 90-degree and 180-degree radiofrequency pulses. The y-gradient (phase-encode gradient) is applied after the initial 90-degree pulse and before the 180-degree pulse is applied. The x-gradient (frequency-encode gradient) is applied at the time of the echo, so it is also called the readout gradient. As protons precess at different frequencies owing to differences in the local magnetic field strength (B_0), different signal frequencies result based on the Lamor equation. The frequency of these signals can be localized to the known location of where the protons are located that are precessing with that given frequency. The signal strength gives rise to the intensity of the gray-scale value that is assigned to that given voxel.

Two-dimensional and three-dimensional imaging are available in most MRI scanners. In two-dimensional imaging, specific transverse slices are excited (usually two to three slices at a time), and, somewhat similar to a CT scanner, data are acquired slice by slice. In three-dimensional imaging, a volume of information is obtained, which can then be reformatted into any of the anatomic or oblique planes desired. In the latter case, the entire volume or area to be imaged is excited and undergoes the MRI experiment.

Image contrast depends on the spin-echo pulse sequence selected and the relaxation properties of the tissue in question. In general, the effects of T1 and T2 changes are opposite. Increasing the T1 (presence of peritumoral edema) makes the image darker (hypointense or decreased signal), whereas increasing the T2 (peritumoral edema) makes the image brighter. Paramagnetic contrast media decrease both T1 and T2, which increases signal intensity on the T1 images while decreasing the signal intensity on T2 images.

Nuclear Medicine

Nuclear medicine is based on the radiotracer principle, in which a radioactive pharmaceutical is injected into a patient and that *radiopharmaceutical* traces or mimics a certain physiologic process without disrupting the process itself.[5] Once the radiopharmaceutical localizes to the given organ or area of interest, the patient is placed on or next to a scintillation detector made of a large *sodium iodide (Tl-activated) crystal*. The radionuclide emits gamma rays as part of the nuclear radioactive decay process. The gamma rays then interact with the crystal and are converted to light flashes, which, in turn, are converted to electric signals by photomultiplier tubes. These electric signals are then recorded into computer memory for display or image manipulation. Planar scintigraphy can be thought of as the x-ray equivalent of survey radiographs. It is a two-dimensional presentation of a three-dimensional structure.

SPECT is the CT equivalent in nuclear medicine except that a volume of information is acquired with each acquisition and each acquisition lasts 15 to 30 minutes rather than the acquisition of individual 1.5-second slices as in CT.[5] The volume of raw data information is then reconstructed into certain imaging planes for visual display. The radiopharmaceuticals that are used in SPECT must localize to an organ system, and because of the low photon flux (small numbers of gamma rays that are actually imaged), temporal resolution is poor. Therefore, dynamic studies are difficult to perform with the use of SPECT.

The most common radionuclide used in nuclear medicine is technetium 99m (^{99m}Tc), which can be tagged to a number of pharmaceuticals that localize to specific organs or areas in the body. In general, nuclear medicine provides primarily physiologic information and only a sketch of the anatomy (Fig. 7–6). The common radiopharmaceuticals used for brain scintigraphy are ^{99m}Tc-glucoheptonate and ^{99m}Tc-DTPA. Both of these are routinely used for renal imaging and localize to brain lesions because of disruption of the normal blood-brain barrier. Other agents that have been used for physiologic imaging include specific receptor imaging (^{123}I-L-dopa, ^{123}I-iodoamphetamine) and radiopharmaceuticals used for cerebral perfusion imaging (^{99m}Tc-hexamethylpropyleneamine oxime).

Another branch of nuclear medicine that provides the basis for metabolic imaging is called *positron emission tomography (PET)*.[5] In PET imaging, positrons are emitted by the radioactive nucleus as it decays. These positrons (within millimeters of being released) come to rest near an electron and undergo an *annihilation reaction*, in which the positron and electron are converted from matter into energy in the form of two 511 keV photons emitted at 180 degrees to each other. These *annihilation photons* are imaged with the use of a complete ring of bismuth germanate detectors around the patient and a specialized circuitry for *coincidence detection*. Common positron emitters include ^{18}F, ^{11}C, ^{15}O, and ^{13}N. The disadvantages of these radionuclides are that they require an on-site cyclotron for their production and they have short physical half-lives. The most common radiopharmaceutical used in PET is *^{18}F-fluorodeoxyglucose (^{18}F-FDG)*, which is used as a glucose analogue and localizes to areas that are metabolically active (Fig. 7–7).

PRINCIPLES OF INTERPRETATION

Computed Tomography

Deviations from normal require an understanding of how expected normal variants might appear and knowing the normal anatomy in the region of interest.[6-11] CT images of the brain are usually displayed with a window width of 200 to 250 and a window level of 45 to 60. If bone erosion is suspected or identified, additional images with wide window width (2000) and high window level (650 to 800) should be reviewed to assess the degree of bone involvement. A precontrast study is done, then an iodinated contrast medium is injected (Conray 400 or Renograffin 76, 0.5 mL/kg intravenously) and a second image set acquired. Slice thickness usually varies from 2 mm for cats and small dogs up to 10 mm for large dogs.

The roentgen sign approach can be applied to interpreting CT images (i.e., recognition of alterations in size, shape, opacity, location, and contours or margins). Additionally, the symmetry of the intracranial structures should be evaluated. The degree of contrast enhancement within structures in question and the attenuation characteristics of areas that surround intracranial lesions can provide clues as to the possible makeup of a given mass or lesion. Complete evaluation of

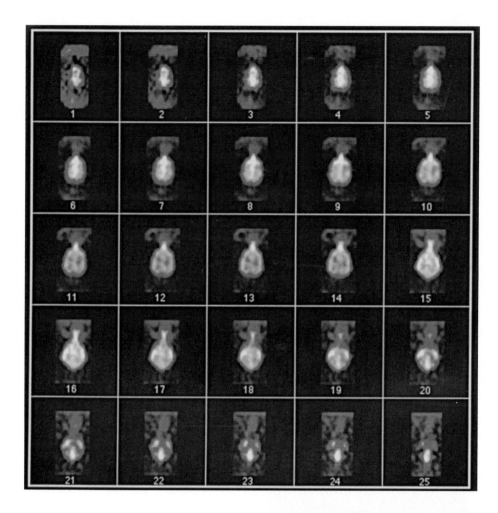

FIGURE 7–6. Dorsal plane reconstructed SPECT images from a normal dog obtained 60 minutes after intravenous administration of ^{99m}Tc-hexamethylpropyleneamine oxime (HMPAO), a cerebral blood flow agent. There is increased distribution of ^{99m}Tc-HMPAO in the gray matter of the cerebral cortex, reflecting normal increased blood flow to these areas.

FIGURE 7–7. Coronal reconstructed images from a human who was imaged with a PET scanner 30 minutes after intravenous administration of ^{18}F-FDG. There is increased metabolism normally noted in the cerebral cortex and the basal ganglia. Additionally, a small hypermetabolic area is noted in the left posterior aspect of the temporal lobe inferiorly *(arrow)*, in an area of a known neoplasm. (Courtesy of Dr. R. Edward Coleman, Duke University Medical Center.)

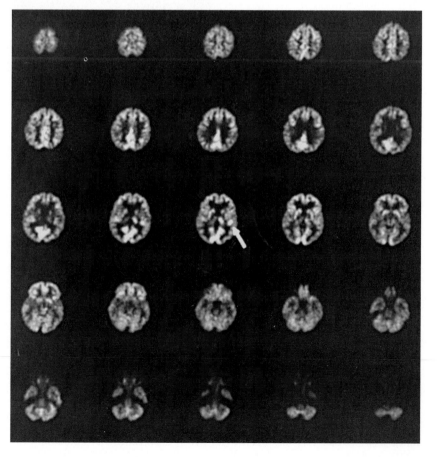

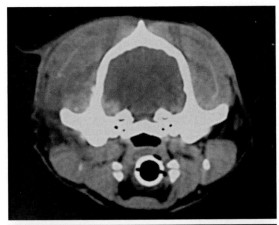

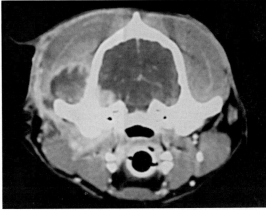

FIGURE 7–8. Transverse CT image from a 13-year-old, neutered male mixed-breed dog. There is a partially mineralized mass on the non–contrast-enhanced image *(top)* that is seen in the left ventral temporal lobe area. On the contrast-enhanced images *(bottom)*, the mass is seen to contrast-enhance. Additionally, there are mixed opacities with partial contrast enhancement lateral to the temporal bone in the region of the brain lesion. Biopsy of this mass documented an aggressive, undifferentiated sarcoma with invasion of the muscle, temporal bone, and temporal lobe of the brain.

areas outside the skull should also be done (Fig. 7–8). Other areas that need evaluating include presence of ventricular enlargement; ventricular asymmetry; degree and pattern of contrast enhancement; and presence of shifting of the central, dorsal falx cerebri (Fig. 7–9).

The characteristics of enhancement of a mass lesion following contrast medium administration may provide some indication as to the disease process that is involving the brain. Extensive work has validated that certain ring enhancement patterns are not pathognomonic for brain tumors. Certain tumor types, such as pituitary gland tumors and meningiomas, tend to have specific locations of occurrence and homogeneous patterns of contrast enhancement.

Magnetic Resonance Imaging

When evaluating MRI images, the same principles of interpretation hold true as described for CT images.[4] The main problem in reviewing MRI images is the number of images that one has to evaluate. When the standard spin-echo sequence is used, there are at least three different image sets (T1-weighted, T2-weighted, and proton density images), and if a contrast study is used, a fourth data set is also acquired (T1-weighted with contrast). For reformatting, all studies are displayed in the transverse plane. One of the image sets typically is reconstructed into the sagittal and dorsal planes.

In general, T1-weighted images are used for anatomic detail. Peritumoral edema may not be readily detected, but as for CT, the presence of ventricular asymmetry, enlargement, and collapse can all be used to determine a mass effect within the brain. Additionally the lack of visualization of normal structures on any of the image planes can give one a clue as to where a lesion might be. On T2-weighted images, because water is hyperintense (white), areas with edema or increased permeability are readily identified. Use of contrast medium (Magnevist) and repeated T1-weighted images allow identification of areas of neovascularization and increased permeability, but the images may still be dramatically different from the T2-weighted images because contrast medium may not mix completely in areas of increased tumor water (Fig. 7–10).

Nuclear Medicine

Radiopharmaceutical localization in planar scintigraphy is based on extravasation into an area with capillary breakdown or neovascularization such as with an intracranial neoplasm. Routinely, ^{99m}Tc-DTPA and ^{99m}Tc-glucoheptonate are used as screening agents for intracranial lesions. Lateral, dorsal, and caudal views of the skull are then obtained. Each image is evaluated for additional radioactivity (hot spot) within the boundary of the skull. A lesion should be triangulated as being intracranial on all three images for a diagnosis of a lesion to be made. On a normal brain scintigraphic study, no additional radioactivity is present within the calvaria.[12–15]

SPECT imaging has allowed for different agents, such as ^{201}thallium, to be used for evaluating intracranial lesions.[16, 17] SPECT allows for better target-to-background contrast, and the sensitivity of the procedure should increase, although studies in animal patients have not been published. Human studies have shown areas of increased ^{201}thallium uptake in metabolically active tumors because ^{201}thallium is a potassium analogue and taken up by normal cells that have an active sodium-potassium pump at the cell membrane surface. ^{201}Thallium has been used for differentiating tumor recurrence from radiation-induced necrosis in humans.[17]

PET allows one to measure quantitatively metabolic activity within the brain.[18] A variety of functional neurologic and psychiatric disorders have been evaluated with the use of ^{18}F-FDG in humans. Metabolic imaging has been used to differentiate metabolically active residual tumors from scar tissue or radiation necrosis.[18] All three of these lesions may have similar appearances on CT and MRI images.

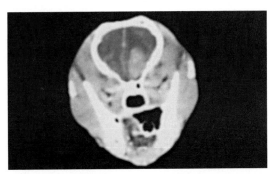

FIGURE 7–9. Transverse, contrast-enhanced image from the rostral brain region of an 11-year-old, female Golden retriever. A primary nasal tumor (adenocarcinoma) is seen as a contrast-enhancing mass that extends into the olfactory lobe region of the brain. There is a marked mass effect with a falx cerebri shift.

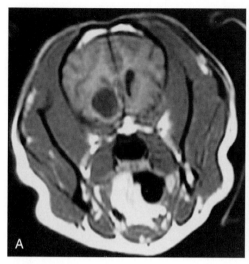
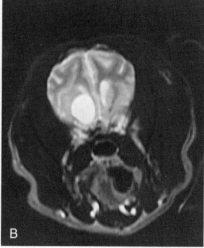

FIGURE 7–10. Transverse T1-weighted *(A)* and T2-weighted *(B)* pre–contrast-enhanced spin-echo MR images from an 8-year-old, male miniature Dachshund with a large right forebrain contrast-enhancing lesion. There is an area of hyperintensity noted throughout the tumor on the T2-weighted image. Histologically, this lesion was a glioma.

DIAGNOSTIC NEUROIMAGING

As with many other areas of radiology, overlap exists between the diagnostic features of particular intracranial disorders, and ultimately biopsy is required for a specific diagnosis to be reached. The areas of overlap between the various disorders and the unique or common features of a given disorder are emphasized in the following review of various central nervous system disorders. Keep in mind that the initial intent of an imaging study is the identification of an abnormality that might explain the particular clinical signs a patient is exhibiting. Then a differential or primary diagnosis can be arrived at when taking all of the information regarding the patient and imaging abnormalities into consideration. A major difference in the imaging of a patient using CT and MRI includes the possible neurologic localization before the study. If a caudal fossa lesion (cerebellum or brain stem) is suspected, MRI may be the better choice for imaging. CT suffers from beam hardening artifacts in these regions of the brain, where the brain stem region appears hypoattenuated owing to artificial hardening of the x-ray beam as it passes through the thicker areas of the skull (e.g., petrous temporal bone) (Fig. 7–11).

Congenital Abnormalities

Congenital anomalies such as feline cerebellar hypoplasia, arachnoid cysts, hydrocephalus, hydranencephaly, and vascular anomalies have been diagnosed in small animals with the use of MRI and CT.[4, 19, 20] Use of sagittal MRI images clearly delineates feline cerebellar hypoplasia.[4] Contrast enhancement has not been shown to be helpful in evaluating these congenital anomalies. Arteriovenous malformations have been evaluated in humans with the use of magnetic resonance angiography. The imaging findings of an intracranial arachnoid cyst in a cat have been described.[20] The cyst was hypointense on T1 images and hyperintense on T2 images as would be expected with a fluid-filled structure.[20]

Inflammatory Disorders

In a retrospective study that used CT to evaluate dogs and cats with primary inflammatory disorders, it was found that certain CT findings were suggestive of inflammation, but CT could not be used by itself to establish clearly a diagnosis

of inflammatory brain disease.[21] CT abnormalities included ventricular abnormalities (asymmetry, compression, or dilation), deviation of the dorsal falx cerebri, perivascular edema, and a variety of contrast-enhancing patterns that were usually inhomogeneous and occasionally had ring patterns of enhancement. In a CT-neuropathologic study, the appearance of ring enhancement of the contrast medium was found not to correlate with a specific pathology but was seen in many inflammatory and neoplastic disorders.[22] Abnormalities could, however, be identified on CT examinations, but other causes of these CT abnormalities cannot be ruled out. In the acute stages of encephalitis, contrast enhancement of the ventricular system may be seen.[1, 4, 21]

In a large retrospective nuclear medicine study, a pattern of generalized, intracranial uptake of the radiopharmaceutical was found not to be a sensitive or specific indicator for generalized inflammatory diseases of the brain.[13] In an earlier study, planar scintigraphic techniques were only 17 percent sensitive for detecting inflammatory lesions.[15]

In humans, MRI has been shown to be sensitive for identifying focal central nervous system infections.[23] Inflammation

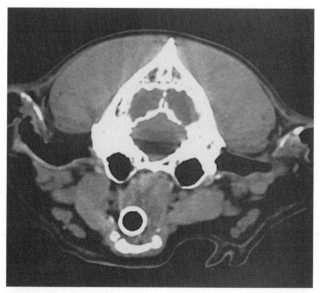

FIGURE 7–11. An area of hypoattenuation is present between the petrous temporal bones in this 8-year-old, female Newfoundland. This artificially lowered area of opacity is due to beam hardening.

within the brain results in prolongation of the T1 and T2 values so that on T1 images, the lesion appears hypointense, while on T2 images the lesion appears hyperintense.[23]

Neoplasia

The most common CT and MRI abnormality is usually an intracranial, solitary mass lesion.[24–27] Depending on the location of the lesion, presence or absence of mineralization, pattern of mass effect seen, and pattern of contrast medium enhancement, a reasonable differential diagnosis can be formulated. The CT and MRI patterns of specific abnormalities in animals have been described.[24–27] Meningiomas typically are peripheral mass lesions that have a marked uniform to slightly nonuniform uptake pattern of contrast medium.[27] On MRI images, meningiomas have increased signal intensity on T2 images and decreased signal intensity on T1 images.[27] Peripheral edema and patterns of mass effect may be present. Additionally, cystic lesions within or adjacent to the tumors may be present as well. In cats, variable degrees of mineralization have been reported.

Pituitary tumors are ventrally located, contrast-enhancing masses that are seen originating in the region of the pituitary gland at the sella turcica (Fig. 7–12).[25] Decreased to isointense characteristics are seen on T1 images, and the lesions appear hyperintense on T2 images. Mild edema or ventricular changes (or both) may be seen.

Gliomas originate from within the neural tissue itself (i.e., astrocytoma or oligodendroglioma).[25] These tumors are located deep within the brain parenchyma and have heterogeneous CT and MRI appearances.[23–25] There is a significant mass effect, peritumoral edema, and variable patterns of contrast enhancement, including homogeneous uptake of contrast or ring patterns of enhancement (Figs. 7–13 and 7–14).

Choroid plexus tumors are located in or around the ventricular system.[25] The tumors are hypointense on T1 images and hyperintense on T2 images with a marked homogeneous pattern of contrast enhancement. Obstructive hydrocephalus is commonly associated with choroid plexus tumors (Fig. 7–15).

Metastatic neoplasia to the brain is much less common in dogs and cats than are primary tumors of the nervous system. Metastatic carcinomas, lymphomas, and sarcomas have been reported in the dog.[28] The identification of multiple, contrast-enhancing circular lesions within the brain should be considered consistent with metastatic neoplasia, although granulomatous or parasitic inflammatory conditions cannot be ruled out (Fig. 7–16).

Vascular Abnormalities

Vascular abnormalities are uncommon causes of brain disease in the small animal. Possible causes for vascular disease include acute trauma (subdural hematoma), coagulopathies with intracranial bleeding, vasculitis, immune-mediated vasculitis, arteriovenous malformations, and cerebrovascular accidents (infarcts).[29, 30]

Acute trauma can lead to hemorrhage from associated depression skull fractures or deceleration injuries (Fig. 7–17). Bleeding can be intraparenchymal, subdural, subarachnoid, or epidural in location.[29, 30] Typical CT findings in acute subdural hemorrhages include displacement of the cerebral cortex away from the cranium by hypoattenuating or hyperattenuating material.[29, 30] If hemorrhage is severe, tentorial herniation of the occipital lobe or cerebellar herniation through the foramen magnum may occur. As a hematoma organizes, the CT opacity of the lesion becomes iso-opaque or hyperopaque relative to the cerebral cortex. Subdural or epidural intracranial collections can also result from coagulopathies with a fluid level pattern being seen between the exudate and cerebrospinal fluid or plasma (Fig. 7–18).

Cerebrovascular accidents, strokes, or infarcts are relatively uncommon in dogs and cats.[29, 31–34] Predisposing disorders in humans include systemic idiopathic hypertension and atherosclerosis.[31–34] These two disorders rarely occur in dogs and cats. The CT and MRI characteristics of cerebrovascular accidents have been well described in humans.[31] Acutely, T1 and T2 relaxation times increase within the infarcted region because of increased water content.[29, 31] MRI can accurately detect cerebrovascular accidents within 3 hours of the initial event. Chronically, cavitation of the lesion occurs with surrounding parenchymal atrophy.[29, 31] MRI images can be followed according to the iron and hemoglobin degradation products that are seen within the area of hemorrhage (Table 7–4). Dogs with cerebrovascular disease usually have an underlying cause, such as hypothyroidism, of the atherosclerosis and hypercholesterolemia (Fig. 7–19).[31–34] On CT images, the presence of hyperopaque peripheral lesions on noncontrast images usually indicates hemorrhage, mineralization, or a lesion with increased cellularity or fibrosis. The HU ranges of 55 to 90 HU within regions of acute hemorrhage in the brain are due to the attenuation of the globin within the hemoglobin. Over time the lesion decreases in density and ultimately becomes hypo-opaque with fluid cavitation.

SUMMARY

Alternative imaging modalities allow for noninvasive evaluation of intracranial disorders in dogs and cats. Contrast me-

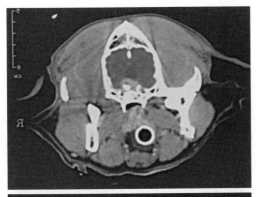
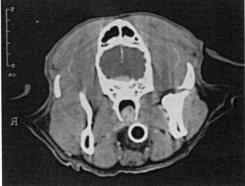

FIGURE 7–12. Transverse, contiguous, 10-mm, contrast-enhanced CT images from an 8-year-old, female Newfoundland with a pituitary adenoma. Note the ventral location and marked, homogeneous contrast enhancement.

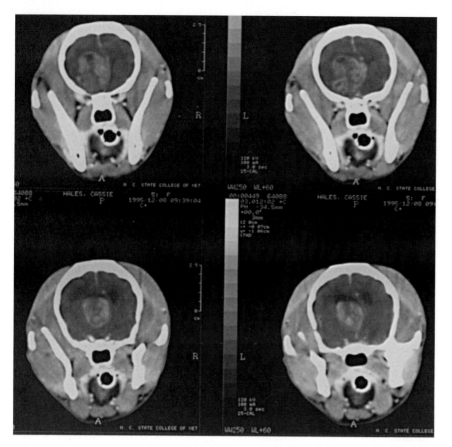

FIGURE 7–13. Four transverse, contrast-enhanced CT images from a 6-year-old, female Miniature Schnauzer that has a ventral left-sided mass with nonhomogeneous contrast enhancement. There is peritumoral edema characterized by a band of decreased attenuation around the mass lesion. Additionally, a shift in the dorsal falx cerebri, obstructive hydrocephalus, and ventricular asymmetry are present. The histologic diagnosis was a glioma.

FIGURE 7–14. T1-weighted precontrast *(A)* and postcontrast *(B)* transverse images from a 10-year-old, neutered male mixed-breed dog with a contrast-enhancing mass lesion noted. Histologic diagnosis was an oligodendroglioma.

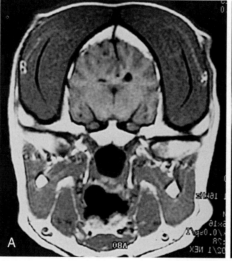
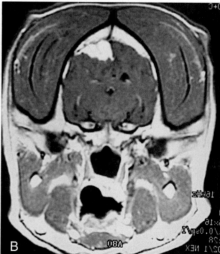

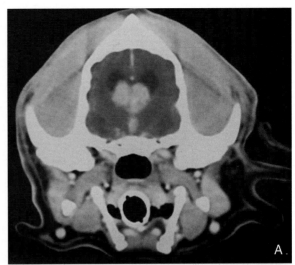

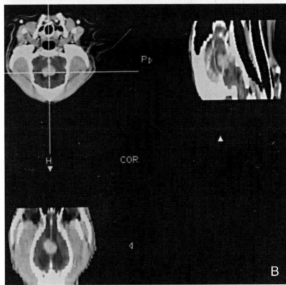

FIGURE 7–15. A transverse CT image *(A)* from an 8-year-old male Golden retriever with a contrast-enhancing mass located along the floor of the lateral ventricles. There is extension of the mass ventrally into the third ventricle. Reconstructed dorsal and sagittal plane images *(B)* from the same dog. Obstructive hydrocephalus is present. The histologic diagnosis was choroid plexus tumor.

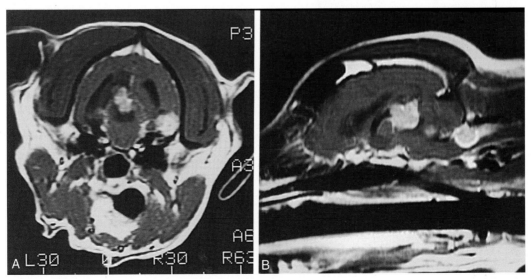

FIGURE 7–16. Transverse *(A)* and sagittal *(B)* T1-weighted, contrast-enhanced images from a 10-year-old, mixed-breed dog with three contrast-enhancing circular lesions located within the brain parenchyma. These findings are consistent with metastatic neoplasia. At necropsy, metastatic carcinoma was identified.

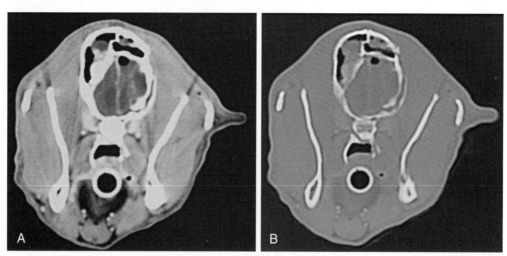

FIGURE 7–17. Transverse CT images from a 2-year-old, male Golden retriever that had been hit by a car 5 days earlier. The CT images are from the same location with brain *(A)* and bone *(B)* windowing. There are multiple compression fractures with soft-tissue opacity noted within the caudal aspect of the frontal sinuses and frontal bone. Gas is also seen within the calvaria. Compression calvarial fractures were also present ventrally in the region of the sphenoid and sphenofrontal suture.

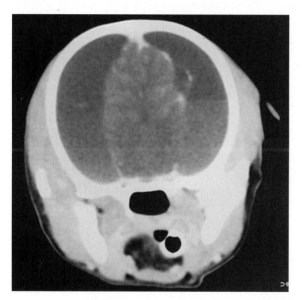

FIGURE 7–18. Transverse, contrast-enhanced, midbrain CT image from a 5-year-old, mixed-breed dog with an idiopathic hemorrhagic diathesis that could not be characterized. On the CT image there is separation of the cerebral cortices from the calvaria bilaterally, with a hypoattenuating/hyperattenuating fluid level interface. Aspiration of the fluid was consistent with chronic hemorrhage.

Table 7–4
STAGES OF THE MRI APPEARANCE OF HEMORRHAGE OVER TIME*

Stage	Time After Injury	Degradation Products	T1	T2
Hyperacute	0–6 hr	Oxyhemoglobin	Equal or decreased	Increased
Acute	7–72 hr	Deoxyhemoglobin	Equal or decreased	Decreased
Early subacute	4–7 d	Intracellular methemoglobin	Increased	Decreased
Late subacute	1–4 wk	Extracellular methemoglobin	Increased	Increased
Chronic	Months	Hemosiderin	Equal or decreased	Decreased

*The T1-weighted and T2-weighted values are signal-intensity relative to normal gray matter.

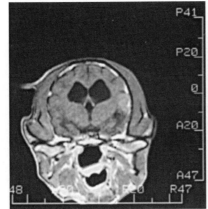
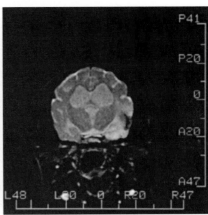

FIGURE 7–19. T1-weighted, contrast-enhanced and T2-weighted transverse MR images from a 15-year-old Dachshund that had presented for disorientation 4 weeks prior to the MR examination. The dog was noted to have hypercholesterolemia and hypothyroidism on biochemical work-up. The MR images document a peripheral change in the cerebral cortex consistent with parenchymal atrophy and cavitation that can be seen after a cerebrovascular accident.

dium is required to increase the sensitivity and specificity of these imaging modalities; however, changes are nonspecific, and a wide range of overlap exists among the various groups of diseases. Surgical biopsy is often required to make a definitive diagnosis. Use of these imaging modalities can be helpful not only for detecting disease but also for determining the response of a particular disease to treatment. When identifying intracranial lesions, CT and MRI changes consistent with a mass effect are often used. For differentiating types of intracranial neoplasms, location appears to be the single best determinant for predicting tumor type.

References

1. Miraldi F, and Mieson EJ: Imaging principles in computed tomography. *In* Haaga JR, and Alfidi RJ (Eds): Computed Tomography of the Whole Body, 2nd Ed. St. Louis, CV Mosby, 1988.
2. Barthez PY, Koblik PD, Hornof WJ, et al: Apparent wall thickening in fluid filled versus air filled tympanic bulla in computed tomography. Vet Radiol Ultrasound 37:95, 1996.
3. Smith Hans-J, and Ranallo FN: A Non-Mathematical Approach to Basic MRI. Madison, WI, Medical Physics Publishing Corporation, 1989.
4. Thomson CE, Kornegay JN, Burn RA, et al: Magnetic resonance imaging: A general overview of principles and examples in veterinary neurodiagnosis. Vet Radiol Ultrasound 34:1, 1993.
5. Sorenson JA, and Phelps ME: Physics in Nuclear Medicine, 2nd Ed. Orlando, Grune & Stratton, 1987.
6. Fike JR, LeCouteur RA, and Cann CE: Anatomy of the canine brain using high resolution computed tomography. Vet Radiol 22:6, 1981.
7. George TF, and Smallwood JE: Anatomic atlas for computed tomography in the mesaticephalic dog: Head and neck. Vet Radiol Ultrasound 33:4, 1992.
8. Voorhout G: Cisternography combined with linear tomography for visualization of the pituitary gland in healthy dogs: A comparison with computed tomography. Vet Radiol 31:2, 1990.
9. De Haan CE, Kraft SL, Gavin PR, et al: Normal variation in size of the lateral ventricles of the labrador retriever dog as assessed by magnetic resonance imaging. Vet Radiol Ultrasound 35:2, 1994.
10. Hudson LC, Cauzinille L, Kornegay JN, et al: Magnetic resonance imaging of the normal feline brain. Vet Radiol Ultrasound 36:4, 1995.
11. Morgan RV, Daniel GB, and Donnell RL: Magnetic resonance imaging of the normal eye and orbit of the dog and cat. Vet Radiol Ultrasound 35:2, 1994.
12. Dijkshoorn NA, and Rijnberk A: Detection of brain tumors in dogs by scintigraphy. J Am Vet Radiol Soc 18:5, 1977.
13. Dykes NL, Warnick LD, Summers BA, et al: Retrospective analysis of brain scintigraphy in 116 dogs and cats. Vet Radiol Ultrasound 35:1, 1994.
14. Daniel GB, Twardock AR, Tucker RL, et al: Brain scintigraphy. Prog Vet Neurol 3:25, 1994.
15. Kallfelz FA, deLahunta A, and Allhands RV: Scintigraphic diagnosis of brain lesions in the dog and cat. J Am Vet Med Assoc 172:589, 1978.
16. Van Heertum RL, Miller SH, and Mosesson RE: SPECT brain imaging in neurologic disease. Radiol Clin North Am 31:881, 1993.
17. Scott AM, and Larson SM: Tumor imaging and therapy. Radiol Clin North Am 31:859, 1993.
18. Hoffman JM, Hanson MW, and Coleman RE: Clinical positron emission tomography imaging. Radiol Clin North Am 31:935, 1993.
19. Karkkainen M: Low- and high-field strength magnetic resonance imaging to evaluate the brain in one normal dog and two dogs with central nervous system disease. Vet Radiol Ultrasound 36:6, 1995.
20. Milner RJ, Engela J, and Kirberger RM: Arachnoid cyst in cerebellar pontine area of a cat—diagnosis by magnetic resonance imaging. Vet Radiol Ultrasound 37:1, 1996.
21. Plummer SB, Wheeler SJ, Thrall DE, et al: Computed tomography of primary inflammatory brain disorders in dogs and cats. Vet Radiol Ultrasound 33:5, 1992.
22. Wolf M, Pedroia V, Higgins RJ, et al: Intracranial ring enhancing lesions in dogs: A correlative CT scanning and neuropathologic study. Vet Radiol Ultrasound 36:1, 1995.
23. Stark DD, and Bradley WG (Eds): Magnetic Resonance Imaging. St. Louis, CV Mosby, 1988.
24. LeCouteur RA, Fike JR, Cann CE, et al: Computed tomography of brain tumors in the caudal fossa of the dog. Vet Radiol 22:6, 1981.
25. Thomas WB, Wheeler SJ, Kramer R, et al: Magnetic resonance imaging features of primary brain tumors in dogs. Vet Radiol Ultrasound 37:1, 1996.
26. Fike JR, Cann CE, Turowski K, et al: Differentiation of neoplastic from non-neoplastic lesions in the dog brain using quantitative CT. Vet Radiol 27:4, 1986.
27. Hathcock JT: Low field magnetic resonance imaging characteristics of cranial vault meningiomas in 13 dogs. Vet Radiol Ultrasound 37:4, 1996.
28. Jubb KVF, and Huxtable CR: The nervous system. *In* Jubb KVF, Kennedy PC, and Palmer N (Eds): Pathology of Domestic Animals, 4th Ed, Vol I. San Diego, Academic Press, 1993.
29. Tidwell AS, Mahony OM, Moore RP, et al: Computed tomography of an acute hemorrhagic cerebral infarct in a dog. Vet Radiol Ultrasound 35:4, 1994.
30. Hopkins AL, and Wheeler SJ: Subdural hematoma in a dog. Vet Surg 20:413, 1991.
31. Virapongse C, Mancuso A, and Quisling R: Human brain infarcts: Gd-DTPA-enhanced MRI imaging. Radiology 161:785, 1986.
32. Liu S, Tilley LP, Tappe JP, et al: Clinical and pathologic findings in dogs with atherosclerosis: 21 cases (1970–1983). J Am Vet Med Assoc 189:227, 1986.
33. Patterson JS, Rusley MS, and Zachary JF: Neurologic manifestations of cerebrovascular atherosclerosis associated with primary hypothyroidism in a dog. J Am Vet Med Assoc 186:5, 1985.
34. Joseph RJ, Greelee PG, Carillo JM, et al: Canine cerebrovascular disease: Clinical and pathological findings in 17 cases. J Am Anim Hosp Assoc 24:569, 1988.

STUDY QUESTIONS

1. This image (Fig. 7–20) is a transverse plane CT image from a 9-year-old intact female mixed-breed dog that presented for acute onset of seizures. The most significant CT abnormality that suggests a mass effect in the brain of this dog is:
   A. Falx cerebri shift.
   B. Ventricular asymmetry.
   C. Contrast enhancement.
   D. Lack of visualization of the third ventricle.

2. All of the following imaging modalities are considered currently acceptable imaging modalities for anatomic imaging of the brain *except*:
   A. MRI.
   B. CT.
   C. Transcranial ultrasonography.
   D. Planar scintigraphy.

3. MRI is dependent on which of the following principles:
   A. Inherent unequal nuclear spin state of the hydrogen proton.
   B. Creation of a net magnetic moment when the subject is placed in a large field strength external magnet.
   C. Ability of the individual spins (protons) to absorb radiofrequencies at their respective Lamor frequency.
   D. All of the above.

4. In CT images, volume averaging is a result of:
   A. Metallic artifacts created by high atomic number materials.
   B. Third-generation CT scanner artifacts created by faulty detectors.
   C. Inherent attenuation differences of the objects located within the volumetric slice being imaged.
   D. Artificially lowered CT values assigned within a structure with high attenuation characteristics.

5. Postcontrast MRI image that is T1 weighted from a 10-year-old mixed-breed dog (Fig. 7–21). The most likely neoplasm would be a(n):
   A. Oligodendroglioma.
   B. Choroid plexus tumor.
   C. Pituitary tumor.
   D. Meningioma.

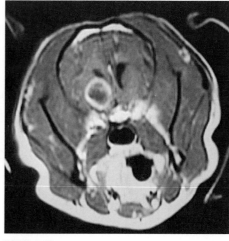

FIGURE 7–21

6. The radiofrequency pulse of an MRI sequence is used to:
   A. Depolarize the protons.
   B. Oxidize methemoglobin.
   C. Excite the net magnetization moments.
   D. Induce the actual MRI signal within the receiver coils.

7. On T1-weighted and T2-weighted images, bone appears _____ relative to normal brain (gray matter).
   A. hypointense
   B. isointense
   C. hyperintense
   D. none of the above

8. A peripherally located solitary lesion over the left frontal lobe that appears partially mineralized on noncontrast images and undergoes marked, homogeneous contrast enhancement in a 9-year-old cat most likely represents a(n):
   A. Oligodendroglioma.
   B. Choroid plexus tumor.

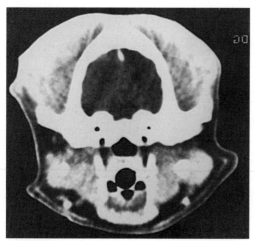

FIGURE 7–20

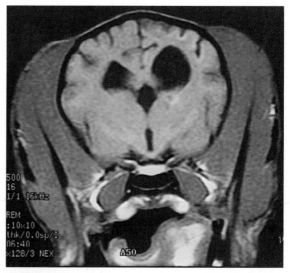

FIGURE 7–22

C. Pituitary tumor.

D. Meningioma.

9. The most common radiopharmaceutical used for imaging intracranial lesions in planar nuclear medicine is:

A. ^{123}I-iodoamphetamine.

B. ^{99m}Tc-glucoheptate.

C. ^{99m}Tc-methylene diphosphonate.

D. ^{18}F-fluorodeoxyglucose.

10. This transverse MR image (Fig. 7–22) is from a 6-year-old neutered female Boston terrier that presented for evaluation of seizures. The most marked MRI change that suggests a mass effect elsewhere in the brain is:

A. Dorsal falx cerebri shift.

B. Sella turcica displacement.

C. Ventral deviation of the corpus callosum.

D. Ventricular dilation and asymmetry.

(Answers appear on page 634.)

Chapter 8

The Vertebrae

Michael A. Walker

ANATOMIC PRINCIPLES

The following are important basic anatomic principles regarding the canine or feline spine:

1. There are 7 cervical, 13 thoracic, 7 lumbar, and 3 sacral vertebrae.

2. The dorsal spinous process of C2 should be adjacent to or overlap the arch of C1.

3. On a lateral view, the cervical articular processes are positioned obliquely across and superimposed on the intervertebral foramina and vertebral canal.

4. C6 has a large lamina ventral to its transverse process. This is an important distinguishing radiographic landmark.

5. Rib heads are cranial to their corresponding vertebrae.

6. T11 is the anticlinal vertebra.

7. The T10–T11 intervertebral disc space is normally more narrow than other disc spaces.

8. In general, adjacent intervertebral disc spaces should be of approximately equal width.

9. Adjacent vertebrae should be approximately equal in size, shape, and radiopacity.

10. The intervertebral foramina serve as windows to the vertebral canal.

11. The ventral cortex of the L3 and L4 vertebral bodies may appear poorly defined owing to origins of the diaphragmatic crura. This is particularly true in large dogs.

12. The lumbosacral angle is variable among individuals and varies with flexion or extension of the lumbosacral joint.

13. The vertebral canal should be smoothly aligned.

14. Bony hemal arches may be present ventral to caudal vertebrae.

Proper radiographic positioning may require the use of sedation or general anesthesia. In instances of suspected spinal fracture, however, loss of the patient's pain perception because of general anesthesia may allow for hazardous manipulation of the unstable spine. Good judgment is necessary in every instance. An improperly positioned, exposed, or processed radiograph of the spine is often nondiagnostic and should be repeated (Fig. 8–1).

BASIC ROENTGEN SIGNS RELATING TO THE SPINE

The roentgen signs that apply to the spine are (1) number, (2) alignment, (3) size, (4) shape, and (5) radiopacity. Each roentgen sign is discussed, followed by examples and listings of abnormalities that may result in that roentgen sign being expressed.

Number

Number abnormalities (Table 8–1) imply an excess or a deficiency of parts. In many instances, number changes are clinically insignificant. Excessive vertebrae are usually manifest as an extra lumbar vertebra. A false impression of excessive lumbar vertebrae may occur if there is agenesis or incomplete formation of the 13th ribs or if there is lack of fusion of the

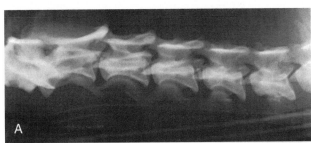

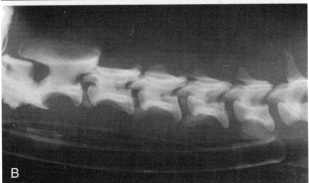

FIGURE 8–1. *A,* Malpositioned lateral view of the cervical spine illustrating the difficulty of accurate interpretation introduced by poor positioning. *B,* Correctly positioned lateral view of same cervical spine. The vertebrae, their articular processes, and the intervertebral disc spaces are clearly seen.

Table 8–1
ABNORMALITIES IN THE NUMBER OF VERTEBRAE

> **Increased**
>   Anomalous excess
>   Pseudoincrease due to transitional vertebrae
> **Decreased**
>   Anomalous lack of normal number
>   Pseudodecrease due to transitional vertebrae
>   Manx cat
>   Tail docking or trauma

first sacral vertebra with the sacrum. Lack of fusion of the first sacral vertebra to the remainder of the sacrum is referred to as *lumbarization* of the sacrum.

Occasionally, there is a decreased number of vertebrae in either the thoracic or the lumbar spine. It is helpful to count the ribs and determine the location of the anticlinal vertebra when deciding which part of the spine is anatomically deficient. L7 may be partially or completely fused with the first sacral vertebra or with the wing of one or both ilia. This condition is referred to as *sacralization*. Lumbosacral transitional vertebrae are most often encountered in German shepherds, Brittany spaniels, Rhodesian Ridgebacks, Doberman pinschers, Great Danes, Labrador retrievers, and St. Bernards.[1] It has been thought that the condition is inherited and familial in German shepherds.[1, 2]

A decreased number of caudal vertebrae may be the result of tail docking or trauma. Because of congenital defects, Manx cats may possess decreased numbers of caudal and occasionally sacral vertebrae. Spina bifida and spinal cord abnormalities, such as meningocele, myelomeningocele, syringomyelia, and spinal dysraphism, may accompany sacrococcygeal abnormalities in Manx cats.[3]

Alignment

Although the bony spine does not lie in one single dorsal plane, the vertebral canal should always be smoothly aligned from one vertebra to the next. Numerous causes of abnormal spinal alignment are listed in Table 8–2. Abnormal curvatures of the spine are *scoliosis,* a lateral bowing; *kyphosis,* a dorsal arching; and *lordosis,* a ventral deviation. Such abnormal contour of the spine may be congenital, idiopathic, or related to another spinal abnormality. Congenital alterations in spinal contour may result from some form of wedge-shaped hemivertebra, including unilateral hemivertebra, causing scoliosis; ventral hemivertebra, causing lordosis; and dorsal hemivertebra, causing kyphosis. The abnormal contour may also be

Table 8–2
ABNORMAL SPINAL ALIGNMENT

> Scoliosis—lateral deviation
> Kyphosis—dorsal deviation
> Lordosis—ventral deviation
> Subluxation/luxation
> Atlantoaxial subluxation (odontoid agenesis, fracture,
>   fusion failure; ligament rupture)
> Fracture
> Anomaly (hemivertebra)
> Transitional vertebrae (sacralization, lumbarization)
> Muscle spasm—back or abdominal pain
> Malunion fracture
> Cervical spondylopathy
> Lumbosacral instability

postural as a manifestation of a pain response or as a result of other deforming spinal abnormalities.[4, 5]

Fractures may involve any part of the spine. The most common sites of fracture are the vertebral body, the transverse process, and the spinous process. Fractures of the vertebral bodies may be accompanied by abnormal spinal alignment, especially when the fracture involves the lumbar spine and less so with involvement of the thoracic or cervical spine.[6] Fractures may be accompanied by subtle narrowing of the adjacent intervertebral disc space. Orthogonal views to determine the degree of fracture displacement should be made. Horizontal-beam radiography may be needed to prevent unsafe manipulation of the spine.

Subluxation and luxation, with or without fracture of the spine, may be evident on one radiographic view but less apparent on the orthogonal view. Subluxation may be accompanied by narrowing of the adjacent intervertebral disc space.

Atlantoaxial (C1–C2) subluxation (Fig. 8–2) may be caused by agenesis, fracture, or fusion failure of the odontoid process or by rupture of the stabilizing ligaments between C1 and C2. Normally the spinous process of C2 lies adjacent to or overlaps the caudal aspect of the arch of C1, and the odontoid process lies on the ventral midline of the vertebral canal of C1. Subluxation of C2 appears radiographically as caudodorsal displacement of C2. The position and appearance of the odontoid process varies with the aforementioned pathologic conditions. An oblique lateral radiograph may be necessary to offset the wings of the atlas to the degree that the odontoid process may be seen. A lateral view obtained during flexion can be used to visualize the subluxation, but care should be taken so as not to overflex the neck because if the odontoid process is present, it could compress the spinal cord.[7]

Cervical vertebral malformation-malarticulation, also-called *canine wobbler syndrome* and *caudal cervical spondylopathy,* may result in abnormal alignment of affected cervical vertebrae to a degree that spinal cord compression results (Fig. 8–3). C4–C5, C5–C6, and C6–C7 are the most frequently involved sites, and multiple lesions are often present. Young Great Danes and adult Doberman pinschers are the breeds most often affected. Dorsal subluxation of the cranial end of a cervical vertebra may be dynamic or adynamic. Dynamic changes are related to cervical flexion-extension. Adynamic changes occur owing to stabilization in malalignment by sec-

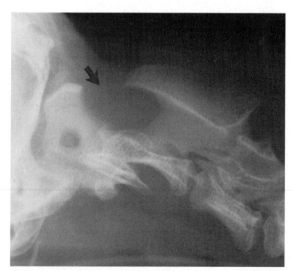

FIGURE 8–2. Atlantoaxial subluxation. Distance between laminae of C1 and C2 is increased *(arrow).* The odontoid process is hypoplastic.

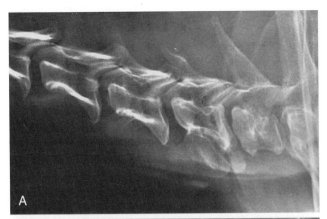

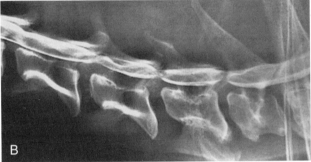

FIGURE 8–3. *A*, Cervical instability with narrowing of the C6–C7 intervertebral disc space, remodeling of the cranioventral margin of C7 vertebral body, and spondylosis at C6–C7. *B*, Myelogram of dog in A. There is extensive extradural compression of the spinal cord at C4–C5, C5–C6, and C6–C7. Note the large normal ventral lamina on C6, characteristic of this vertebra.

Table 8–3
VARIATIONS IN VERTEBRAL SIZE

Increased	Decreased
Block vertebrae	Fractures (traumatic or pathologic)
	Anomaly (hemivertebra)
	Dwarfism

lumbosacral joint. Dynamic malalignment is often seen best on flexed views in which the sacrum subluxates ventral to L7. Static malalignment may be evident on survey as well as on flexed or extended lateral views. Concurrent lumbosacral spondylosis has been associated with increased dynamic malalignment, rather than with stabilization of the lumbosacrum. Spondylosis alone may not be indicative of degenerative lumbosacral stenosis. Collapse of the lumbosacral disc space and dorsal herniation of disc may occur. There may be narrowing of the central vertebral canal or neural foramina by hypertrophied or degenerate bone, protruding degenerate disc, or fibrous tissue (Fig. 8–4). Infrequently, there may be stenosis of the sacral vertebral canal. A lumbosacral transitional vertebra may be present and has been considered a causative factor for degenerative lumbosacral stenosis in some dogs.[2, 11–15] The optimum imaging method for assessment of the lumbosacral space has yet to be defined, but epidurography and discography, computed tomography, and magnetic resonance imaging appear to hold the most promise.

Size

Vertebrae may be larger or smaller than normal (Table 8–3). One possibility for a vertebra appearing longer than normal is block vertebra (Fig. 8–5). In congenital block vertebra, two or possibly more vertebral bodies, arches, or spines may be fused (Fig. 8–6). The fusion, which may be partial or complete, results from improper segmentation of embryonal somites.[4, 5] Regions of fused vertebrae often appear osteopenic because of disuse atrophy involving the fused segments.

Vertebrae may appear smaller than normal owing to traumatic or pathologic fractures, anomaly, or dwarfism. Because of the compacting nature of compression fractures, the vertebrae are often increased in opacity in addition to being short. Hemivertebrae are anomalously short and misshapen, as previously described. Primordial dwarfism, manifest by proportionate skull, spine, and limb size decrease, has resulted in

ondary changes, such as spondylosis deformans. Standard lateral views and lateral views during flexion may be helpful when assessing dynamic instability. Other roentgen findings may include misshapen articular processes, flattening of the cranioventral aspect of an affected vertebral body, stenosis of the cranial end of the vertebral canal of the affected vertebrae, myelographically determined hyperplasia of the ligamentum flavum, and secondary intervertebral disc calcification and herniation.[8–10]

In the dog, degenerative lumbosacral stenosis and its associated cauda equina syndrome may result from lumbosacral malalignment. Because the malalignment can be dynamic or static, lateral radiographs should be made in a nonstressed position and with hyperextension and hyperflexion of the

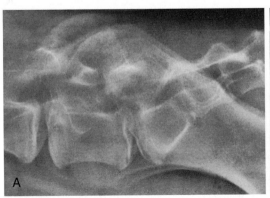

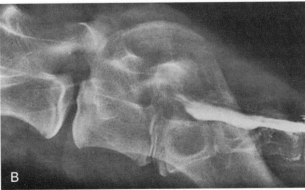

FIGURE 8–4. *A*, Lateral view of the lumbosacral spine of a dog with cauda equina syndrome in which slight ventral malpositioning of the sacrum is apparent. The first sacral segment appears to be incompletely fused to the remainder of the sacrum, suggestive of a partial transitional vertebra. *B*, Epidurogram of dog in A. There is complete obstruction to flow of contrast medium, with dorsal displacement of the contrast medium column. This is consistent with herniation of the L7–S1 disc.

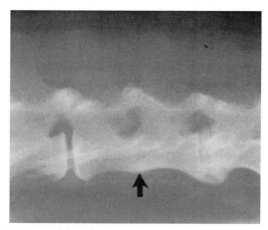

FIGURE 8–5. Block vertebrae *(arrow)* from two fused lumbar vertebral bodies.

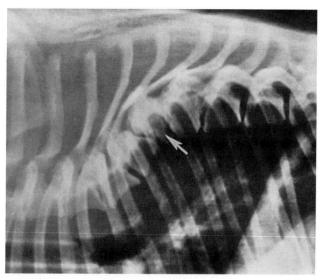

FIGURE 8–7. Hemivertebra in the midthoracic spine *(arrow)* resulting in malalignment.

distinct miniature breeds. Chondrodystrophic dwarfs have a disproportionate form, with short, thick limbs, short cranial base, and short vertebrae.

Shape

There are numerous types and causes of abnormally shaped vertebrae (Table 8–4). Block vertebrae are congenitally fused in part or in whole and when anatomically junctional, as in lumbarization or sacralization, are called *transitional vertebrae.* An anomalously shaped transverse process may result from fusion of a rib with a transverse process at the thoracolumbar junction. A wedge-shaped hemivertebra (Fig. 8–7) may result embryonically from improper vascularization and therefore incomplete ossification of the dorsal or ventral portion of the vertebral body; hence, the term *dorsal* or *ventral hemivertebra* is used. Hemimetameric displacement results in unilateral, left, and right hemivertebrae. The persistence of sagittal cleavage of the embryonic notochord results in the vertebral end plates having a funnel shape grossly and a butterfly appearance radiographically in the ventrodorsal view. The shapes of the bodies of the butterfly vertebrae and hemivertebrae may be compensated for by adjacent vertebral bodies, but spinal malalignment may also result. Hemivertebrae and

butterfly vertebrae occur most often in bulldogs, Pugs, and Boston terriers.[4, 5]

Other shape anomalies and developmental defects include a dorsally angled odontoid process, dwarfism, and spina bifida. Abnormal dorsal angulation of the odontoid process may result in signs that are similar to those of atlantoaxial subluxation. Chondrodystrophic dwarfism may result in short vertebral bodies that appear to have accordion-like bony protrusions from the ventral surface. Spina bifida is a midline cleavage in the vertebral arch or dorsal spinous process. The arch may be incompletely fused or absent, and the dorsal spinous process may appear in duplicate (Fig. 8–8). Associated spinal cord changes may include meningocele and myelomeningocele. Spina bifida is reported most often in brachycephalic dogs and Manx cats.[4, 5, 16] Fractures and malunion fractures of vertebrae may result in innumerable distorted shapes.

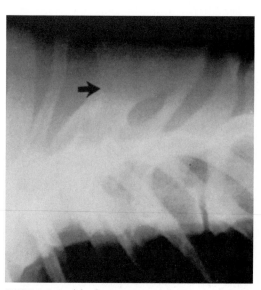

FIGURE 8–6. Fused dorsal spinous processes *(arrow)*.

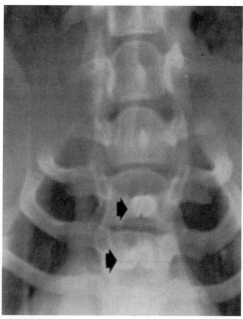

FIGURE 8–8. Ventrodorsal view of the cervicothoracic spine in which spina bifida with duplication of the T1 and T2 spinous processes can be seen *(arrows)*.

Table 8-4
ABNORMALITIES IN THE SHAPE OF VERTEBRAE

General Shape Alteration	Articular Process Changes
Block vertebrae	Bony proliferation
Transitional vertebrae	Degenerative joint disease
Fused processes	Bone destruction
Hemivertebrae	Neoplasia—primary bone, cord, meningeal,
Hemimetameric displacement	metastases, marrow
Dwarfism	Osteomyelitis
Spina bifida	Hemilaminectomy/dorsal laminectomy
Fracture	**Expansile-Appearing Bone Lesions**
Malunion fracture	Multiple cartilaginous exostoses
Osteomyelitis/discospondylitis	Chondroma/chondrosarcoma
Spondylosis	**Intervertebral Foramen**
Neoplasia, primary and secondary	Enlarged
Cervical spondylopathy	Meningeal or nerve sheath neoplasia—
Lumbosacral stenosis (acquired, congenital)	meningioma, neurilemoma
Previous surgery	Small
Healed previous disease	Intervertebral disc herniation
Mucopolysaccharidosis	**Vertebral Canal**
Spondylosis	Widened
Spondylosis deformans	Spinal cord tumor—astrocytoma, ependymoma
Lumbosacral instability/degenerative lumbosacral stenosis	Narrowed
Cervical spondylopathy	Cervical spondylopathy
Spirocerca lupi infection	Lumbosacral stenosis
Hypervitaminosis A	Healing reaction
Periosteal Reaction	Subluxated vertebra
Neoplasia, primary and secondary	Space-occupying mass in the canal—herniated
Osteomyelitis—bacterial, actinomycotic, coccidioidomycotic	disc, neoplasm
Spirocerca lupi infection	
Healing reaction	

Vertebral osteomyelitis, discospondylitis, vertebral physitis, and spondylosis deformans alter the shape of affected vertebrae. *Vertebral osteomyelitis* is a general term for sepsis manifest as irregular, poorly marginated bone lysis and production on any or all parts of one or more affected vertebrae. An irregularly shaped periosteal reaction is often present (Fig. 8–9). Bacterial and mycotic vertebral osteomyelitis may occur. Hematogenous infections are often the cause, but secondary contiguous infection from migrating foreign bodies or other soft-tissue infection is possible.

Discospondylitis is sepsis of the intervertebral disc space and adjacent ends of the adjoining vertebral bodies (Fig. 8–10). The hallmark sign of discospondylitis is lysis of the vertebral body end plates. Areas of bone production (sclerosis) in the vertebral bodies adjacent to the end plate lysis are common. Spondylosis may develop from the adjacent ends of the affected vertebrae. Discospondylitis most often affects the thoracic and lumbar vertebrae of young to middle-aged, large-breed male dogs. Multiple-site lesions occur, but single-site lesions are reported more often.[17–20] *Staphylococcus aureus* and *Brucella* species are common isolates.

Vertebral physitis has been proposed as a disease entity distinct from discospondylitis. Roentgen signs of vertebral physitis include bone lysis, initially of the caudal physeal region of the affected vertebral body, with sparing of the vertebral end plates. Eventual collapse of the caudoventral portion of the vertebral body may occur.[21]

Spondylosis deformans is a noninflammatory vertebral body remodeling that may vary in extent from formation of small spurs to complete bridging of adjacent vertebrae (Fig. 8–11). Spondylosis may occur secondary to several spinal abnormalities, including ventral disc protrusion, but often it is idiopathic and clinically insignificant. The new bone formation may be limited to the vertebral body epiphyses or may extend over the entire length of affected and adjacent verte-

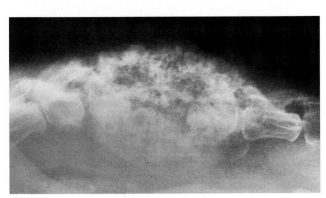

FIGURE 8–9. Osteomyelitis of the caudal spine. There is destruction of two vertebrae and active new bone formation at multiple sites.

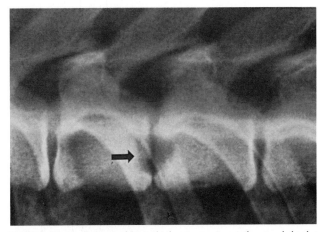

FIGURE 8–10. *Brucella* discospondylitis in the thoracic spine *(arrow)*. There is end plate lysis, the hallmark sign of discospondylitis, affecting two vertebrae.

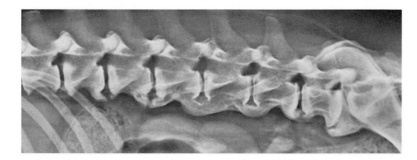

FIGURE 8–11. Spondylosis of the lumbar and lumbosacral spine. Some of the ventral new bone has fused in this patient.

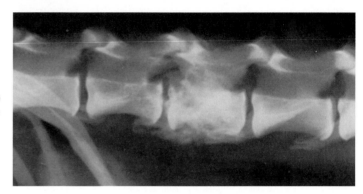

FIGURE 8–12. Metastatic neoplasia (squamous cell carcinoma) involving L2 and L3. There is destruction of the craniodorsal aspect of the body of L3 and irregular new bone formation.

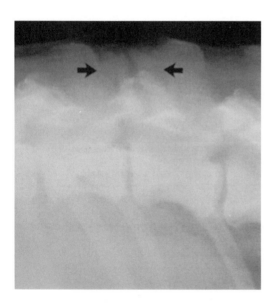

FIGURE 8–13. Degenerative joint disease of articular processes at T13–L1 *(arrows).* The joint space is irregular, and there are osteophytes on the articular processes.

FIGURE 8–14. Lateral view of the lumbar spine of an African lion with nutritional hyperparathyroidism. The overall opacity of the skeleton is decreased, and vertebrae are misshapen.

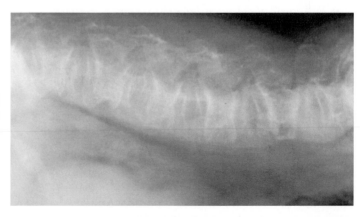

Table 8–5
ALTERATIONS IN RADIOPACITY

Increased
    Radiographic technique—underexposure, short scale of contrast
      (relative)
    Compression fracture
    Healing fracture/reaction
    Osteoblastic metastasis
    Osteomyelitis
    Discospondylitis
Decreased
    Radiographic technique—long scale of contrast (relative)
    Excessive scatter radiation; obesity
    Disuse atrophy
    Hyperparathyroidism—primary, secondary
    Paraneoplastic syndrome
    Neoplasia—primary, secondary, myeloma
    Osteomyelitis
    Discospondylitis
    Cushing's syndrome
    Diabetes mellitus
    Hypothyroidism/hyperthyroidism

brae. Radiographically the new bone formation is best seen ventral to the affected vertebrae, but it may occur along the lateral and dorsolateral margins of vertebral bodies. The dorsolateral new bone may extend to the intervertebral foramina, but it does not usually encroach on the spinal cord.

Spondylosis is most often reported in the thoracic, lumbar, and lumbosacral spine of middle-aged to old male dogs.[22, 23] Spondylosis in the caudal cervical spine of Doberman pinschers and in the lumbosacral spine of all dogs may be associated with, but is not diagnostic of, cervical or lumbosacral instability. Idiopathic spondylosis deformans should not be confused with the ventral vertebral body bony proliferation that may occur in dogs with *Spirocerca lupi* infection or in cats with hypervitaminosis A. In *S. lupi* infection, bony proliferation may occur across the ventral surfaces of T8 to T11, and an esophageal mass is often present. In hypervitaminosis A, ankylosing bony proliferation may occur on the arches and lateral aspects of the bodies of the cervical vertebrae. In addition, bony proliferation may occur on thoracic and lumbar vertebrae, on some of the long bones, and around limb joints.[24] Mucopolysaccharidosis, a lack of degradation of acid mucopolysaccharides before their excretion from the body, may cause multiple bony changes, including partial fusion of cervical vertebrae, irregularly shortened and misshapen vertebrae, partial fusion of lumbar vertebrae, widened intervertebral spaces, and a seemingly widened spine, owing to bony proliferation.[25, 26]

Most primary vertebral neoplasms are osteosarcomas, although other sarcomas occur; most secondary vertebral neoplasms are carcinomas, although sarcomas occur. Most primary vertebral neoplasms reside within one vertebra; secondary vertebral neoplasms may reside in one or more vertebrae. Large breeds of dogs are more likely to have vertebral neoplasms than smaller breeds. Primary or secondary vertebral neoplasia may alter the shape of vertebrae by destroying bone, producing bone, or both (Fig. 8–12). The bone destruction often affects the cortical bone of the vertebra, and there may be collapse of the adjacent disc space. A paraspinal, soft-tissue mass may be present. In contrast with discospondylitis, spinal neoplasia does not routinely result in end plate lysis occurring simultaneously cranial and caudal to an intervertebral disc. Radiographically the differentiation of neoplasia from osteomyelitis may be difficult if the tumor is producing bone.[27–29]

Alterations in the shape of the articular processes result most often from degenerative joint disease. Bony proliferation on the articular processes gives them an irregularly shaped appearance typical of degenerative joint disease (Fig. 8–13).

The intervertebral foramen may become enlarged when occupied by a growing neoplasm, such as a meningioma and a neurofibroma. Although these neoplasms may occur at any location, they most often involve the cervical spine.[30] A decrease in the size of the intervertebral foramen may be the result of vertebral shifting secondary to intervertebral disc herniation.

The vertebral canal may appear widened as a result of soft-tissue expansion from a spinal cord neoplasm, such as an astrocytoma and an ependymoma.[30] Localized narrowing of the vertebral canal may result from cervical spondylopathy, lumbosacral stenosis, subluxation, or a space-occupying mass, such as a mineralized herniated disc and neoplasm in the vertebral canal.

Radiopacity

Causes of alterations in radiopacity of the spine are listed in Table 8–5. Increased radiopacity may be artifactual as a result of underexposure or relative as a result of an excessively short scale of contrast (mAs too high, kVp too low). Because compression fractures compact a given mass of bone into a smaller volume, the radiopacity of the affected vertebra is increased. Bony callus in a healing fracture and the reactive bone in osteomyelitis, discospondylitis, vertebral physitis, or neoplasia may also increase radiopacity.

Decreased radiopacity of the spine may be relative as a result of an excessively long scale of contrast. Scatter radiation and obesity diminish radiographic contrast and give the appearance of decreased bone radiopacity. Primary or secondary hyperparathyroidism may result in a poorly mineralized and weakened spine (Fig. 8–14).[31] Focal, well-defined regions of decreased bone opacity in the spine may result from lymphoreticular neoplasms, such as myeloma and lymphoma; these are usually multiple. Solitary radiolucent lesions may be due to primary or metastatic solid tumors.

References

1. Larsen JS: Lumbosacral transitional vertebrae in the dog. J Am Vet Radiol Soc 18:3, 1977.
2. Morgan JP, Bahr A, Franti CE, et al: Lumbosacral transitional vertebrae as a predisposing cause of cauda equina syndrome in German shepherd dogs: 161 cases (1987–1990). J Am Vet Med Assoc 202:1877, 1993.
3. James CM, Lassman LP, and Tomlinson BE: Congenital anomalies of the lower spine and spinal cord in Manx cats. J Pathol 97:269, 1969.
4. Bailey CS: An embryological approach to the clinical significance of congenital vertebral and spinal cord abnormalities. J Am Anim Hosp Assoc 11:426, 1975.
5. Colter SB: Congenital anomalies of the spine. In Bojrab MJ (Ed): Pathophysiology in Small Animal Surgery. Philadelphia, Lea & Febiger, 1981, p 729.
6. Feeney DA, and Oliver JE: Blunt spinal trauma in the dog and cat: Insight into radiographic lesions. J Am Anim Hosp Assoc 16:805, 1980.
7. Oliver JE, and Lewis RE: Lesions of the atlas and axis in dogs. J Am Anim Hosp Assoc 9:304, 1973.
8. Chambers JN, and Betts CW: Caudal cervical spondylopathy in the dog: A review of 20 clinical cases and the literature. J Am Anim Hosp Assoc 13:571, 1977.
9. Raffe MR, and Knecht CD: Cervical vertebral malformation—a review of 36 cases. J Am Anim Hosp Assoc 16:881, 1980.
10. Trotter EJ, de Lahunta A, Geary JC, et al: Caudal cervical vertebral malformation-malarticulation in Great Danes and Doberman pinschers. J Am Vet Med Assoc 168:10, 1976.
11. Denny HR, Gibbs C, and Holt PE: The diagnosis and treatment of cauda equina lesions in the dog. J Small Anim Pract 23:425, 1982.

12. Oliver JE, Selcer RR, and Simpson S: Cauda equina compression from lumbosacral malarticulation and malformation in the dog. J Am Vet Med Assoc 173:2 1978.
13. Tarvin G, and Prata RG: Lumbosacral stenosis in dogs. J Am Vet Med Assoc 177:2, 1980.
14. Mattoon JS, and Koblik PD: Quantitative survey radiographic evaluation of the lumbosacral spine of normal dogs and dog with degenerative lumbosacral stenosis. Vet Radiol Ultrasound 34:194, 1993.
15. Adams WH, Daniel GB, Pardo AD, et al: Magnetic resonance imaging of the caudal lumbar and lumbosacral spine in 13 dogs (1990–1993). Vet Radiol Ultrasound 36:3, 1995.
16. Wilson JW, Kurtz HJ, Leipold HW, et al: Spina bifida in the dog. Vet Pathol 16:165, 1979.
17. Hurov L, Troy G, and Turnwald G: Discospondylitis in the dog: 27 cases. J Am Vet Med Assoc 173:3, 1978.
18. Johnston DE, and Summers BA: Osteomyelitis of the lumbar vertebrae in dogs caused by grass-seed foreign bodies. Aust Vet J 47:289, 1971.
19. Kornegay JN, and Barber DL: Discospondylitis in dogs. J Am Vet Med Assoc 177:4, 1980.
20. Walker TL, and Gage ED: Vertebral osteomyelitis, discospondylitis, and cauda equina syndrome. In Bojrab MJ (Ed): Pathophysiology in Small Animal Surgery. Philadelphia, Lea & Febiger, 1981, p 474.
21. Jimenez MM, and O'Callaghan MW: Vertebral physitis: A radiographic diagnosis to be separated from discospondylitis. Vet Radiol Ultrasound 36:188, 1995.
22. Wright JA: A study of vertebral osteophyte formation in the canine spine: I. Spinal survey. J Small Anim Pract 23:697, 1982.
23. Wright JA: A study of vertebral osteophyte formation in the canine spine: II. Radiographic survey. J Small Anim Pract 23:747, 1982.
24. Morgan JP: Radiology in Veterinary Orthopedics. Philadelphia, Lea & Febiger, 1972.
25. Cowell KR, Jezyk PF, Haskins ME, et al: Mucopolysaccharidosis in a cat. J Am Vet Med Assoc 169:3, 1976.
26. Haskins ME, Jezyk PF, Desnick RJ, et al: Mucopolysaccharidosis in a domestic short-haired cat—a disease distinct from that seen in the Siamese cat. J Am Vet Med Assoc 175:4, 1979.
27. Luttgen PJ, Braund KG, Brawner WR Jr, et al: A retrospective study of twenty-nine spinal tumors in the dog and cat. J Small Anim Pract 21:213, 1980.
28. Morgan JP, Ackerman N, Bailey CS, et al: Vertebral tumors in the dog: A clinical, radiologic, and pathologic study of 61 primary and secondary lesions. Vet Radiol 21:5, 1980.
29. Wright JA, Bell DA, and Jones DG: The clinical and radiological features associated with spinal tumors in thirty dogs. J Small Anim Pract 20:461, 1979.
30. Gilmore DR: Intraspinal tumors in the dog. Comp Contin Ed Vet Pract 5:1, 1983.
31. Smith HA, and Jones TC: Veterinary Pathology, 3rd Ed. Philadelphia, Lea & Febiger, 1966.

STUDY QUESTIONS

1. Normally, there are seven lumbar vertebrae in the dog. How might one explain what appears to be eight lumbar vertebrae on a radiograph?

2. Scoliosis is a lateral bowing of the spine, kyphosis is a dorsal bowing of the spine, and lordosis is a ventral bowing of the spine. (True or False)

3. List four potential causes for atlantoaxial subluxation.

4. Vertebral malformation-malarticulation may result in abnormal alignment, either dynamic or adynamic, of which vertebrae in young Great Dane and adult Doberman pinscher dogs?

5. List the most common roentgen signs of degenerative lumbosacral stenosis and its associated cauda equina syndrome.

6. Distinguish between the terms *discospondylitis* and *spondylosis deformans*.

7. List one roentgen sign to differentiate vertebral neoplasia from discospondylitis.

8. List two potential differences between primary and secondary malignant neoplasia of the spine.

9. What is/are the preferential radiographic diagnosis/diagnoses based on this lateral radiograph of a canine spine (Fig. 8–15)?

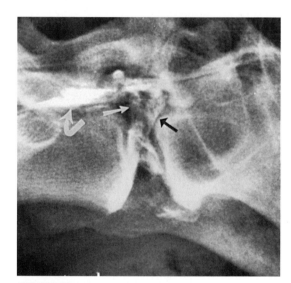

FIGURE 8–16

10. What is the preferential radiographic diagnosis/diagnoses based on this lateral view of a canine lumbosacral junction, subsequent to an epidurogram (contrast medium indicated by curved white arrow) and a discogram (black and white straight arrows) (Fig. 8–16)?

(Answers appear on page 634.)

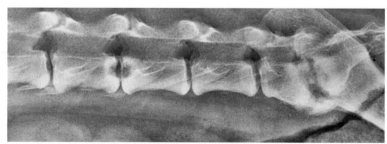

FIGURE 8–15

Chapter 9

Intervertebral Disc Disease and Myelography

William R. Widmer

OVERVIEW

Intervertebral disc disease is a degenerative condition of unknown cause that results in protrusion of the disc or disc material into the vertebral canal, compressing the spinal cord or spinal nerve roots.[1-3] Although other diseases affect the intervertebral disc, this chapter considers only disc protrusion.

Intervertebral disc disease affects all breeds of dogs; the chondrodystrophic breeds are overrepresented with the highest prevalence in the Dachshund (45 to 65 percent of dogs with intervertebral disc disease).[1-4] Beagles, Cocker spaniels, toy Poodles, and Pekingese are also considered to have a high prevalence. Doberman pinschers afflicted with cervical vertebral instability-malformation,[5] German shepherds,[6] and mixed-breed dogs also develop intervertebral disc disease.

Neural signs of intervertebral disc disease generally manifest after 3 years of age; however, in chondrodystrophic breeds, disc degeneration begins before 1 year of age. No sex predilection has been identified.[1] Common sites of disc protrusion are T12–T13 and T13–L1 in the thoracolumbar region and C2–C3 and C3–C4 in the cervical region.[1, 3] Although clinical signs of intervertebral disc disease are uncommon in cats, cervical disc degeneration frequently occurs in cats over 6 years old.[1, 2]

Suspected intervertebral disc disease is one of the most important indications for radiographic evaluation of the vertebral column of small animals. Accurate radiographic examination can establish the presence and severity of disc disease, allowing clinicians to determine prognosis and proceed with treatment. Because many radiographic signs of disc disease are subtle and other spinal conditions may be the cause of clinical signs, accurate radiographic interpretation requires a thorough knowledge of anatomy, physiology, and neurology.

ANATOMIC AND PHYSIOLOGIC CONSIDERATIONS

The intervertebral disc is composed of a tough outer annulus fibrosus, which contains the gelatinous, inner nucleus pulposus (Fig. 9–1).[7, 8] The annulus has several concentric fibrocartilaginous layers, which are firmly attached to adjacent vertebral end plates and centra.[1, 8] The nucleus pulposus is eccentrically located; thus, the annulus is thin dorsally and thick ventrally. This fact partially explains the tendency for dorsal herniation of diseased discs. A mixture of proteoglycans, collagen fibers, mesenchymal cells, and water makes up the normal jelly-like nucleus. Only the outermost layers of the annulus have a neurovascular supply.[1] The disc forms a cartilaginous joint between each vertebral segment (excluding C1–C2 and the sacrum), functioning as a hydraulic shock absorber. Shock absorption is dependent on a hydrated, deformable nucleus and an intact, elastic annulus.[7]

The longitudinal ligaments of the vertebral column provide dorsal and ventral support for the intervertebral discs.[8] The dorsal longitudinal ligament joins the dorsum of the vertebral centra and lies on the floor of the vertebral canal (see Fig. 9–1). In the cervical region, the dorsal ligament is wide and thick; consequently, lateral extrusion of disc material and radiculopathy (root signature) are more common than dorsal extrusion and severe cord compression.[9] In comparison, the dorsal longitudinal ligament is thin in the thoracolumbar region, predisposing to dorsal protrusion and cord compression. The ventral longitudinal ligament spans the ventral surface of the vertebral column, offering ventral support. The intercapital ligaments are short, transverse fibrous bands that lie ventral to the dorsal longitudinal ligament, joining the rib heads between T2 and T11. These ligaments buttress the dorsal part of the annulus and help resist dorsal disc protrusion cranial to T11.[8, 10, 11]

The vertebral canal of the dog is crowded, and the epidural space is small. Thus, the canine spinal cord is subject to compression by epidural masses (e.g., disc protrusion). The Dachshund, compared to the German shepherd, has a high spinal cord:canal ratio (i.e., a small epidural space).[12] Possibly, this explains the severe neurologic signs seen in the Dachshund following disc protrusion. Owing to a larger epidural space, small protrusions causing minimal cord compressions are less significant in large dog breeds. The ratio of spinal cord to vertebral canal is lowest in the cervical area; therefore, neurologic signs tend to be less severe with cervical versus thoracolumbar disc protrusion.[3, 9, 11]

The spinal cord and spinal nerve roots lie within the bony vertebral canal, which consists of the individual vertebral foramina (see Fig. 9–1). Paired intervertebral foramina serve as windows allowing exit of the spinal nerves and blood vessels. The meninges surround the spinal cord and consist of the inner pia-arachnoid membrane and the tough, outer dura (Fig. 9–2). The cervical and lumbar intumescences are normal enlargements of the cord and should not be confused with cord swelling. The spinal cord begins at the foramen magnum and, depending on the breed of dog, terminates at the conus medullaris, near the level of L6. In small dog breeds, the cord ends caudal to L6 and in large breeds cranial to L6, an important factor to consider when performing lumbar subarachnoid puncture. In the cat, the spinal cord extends slightly beyond L6.[13]

The spinal cord segments and vertebra have the same numerical designation (with the exception of cord segment C8), but the location of each cord segment is rarely found within the corresponding vertebra.[10] The reason is twofold. First, the spinal cord is shorter than the vertebral column because of differential fetal growth rates. Second, many of the cord segments are shorter than the vertebral segments. Therefore, cord segments are usually located cranial to their respective vertebra, and the spinal nerves must course obliquely within the vertebral canal a short distance before exiting via the intervertebral foramina. The collection of spinal nerve roots in the lumbosacral region is known as the caudal equina. These nerves, similar to the spinal cord, are subject to compressive injury by disc protrusion.

The subarachnoid space lies between the arachnoid membrane and the pia mater, surrounding the spinal cord and spinal nerve roots. Cerebrospinal fluid fills the subarachnoid space, displacing the lacy, arachnoid membrane peripherally against the dura. The spinal subarachnoid space begins at the foramen magnum, where it communicates with the rostral subarachnoid space and ends caudally at the filum terminale,

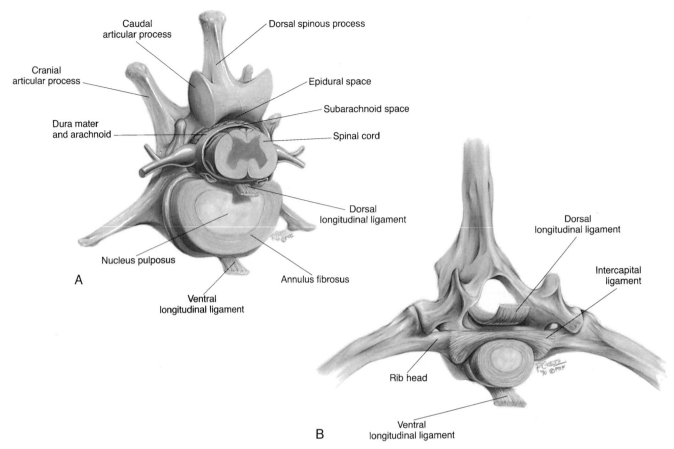

FIGURE 9–1. *A*, Anatomic components of a typical lumbar vertebra and intervertebral disc. *B*, Anatomic components of a typical thoracic vertebra and intervertebral disc. (Courtesy Dr. J.P. Toombs, copyright Purdue University, 1996.)

near the lumbosacral junction.[8] The central canal of the spinal cord is filled with cerebrospinal fluid and communicates rostrally with the ventricular system. In most dogs, the central canal terminates blindly at the cons medullaris; however, in a small percentage of dogs, the canal is continuous with the lumbar subarachnoid space.

PATHOPHYSIOLOGIC CONSIDERATIONS

The terminology used to describe intervertebral disc lesions is confusing and inconsistent.[1] *Protrusion* is a nonspecific term that defines any discal mass that is impinging on the spinal cord or spinal nerve roots. *Herniation (bulging disc)* implies that the nucleus pulposus is causing a bulge by stretching an intact annulus. An *extruded, prolapsed,* or *blown-out* disc is one in which the nucleus has broken through the annulus, into the epidural space. Unfortunately, these terms have been used interchangeably throughout the literature. A simpler classification might describe disc material to be either contained or noncontained (extruded) with respect to the annulus. The distinction between herniation and extrusion is not always evident with conventional radiography; therefore, the term *disc protrusion* is preferred.

Two forms of disc degeneration have been described and result in different types of protrusion.[1, 7] *Chondroid* degeneration occurs in chondrodystrophic breeds and is typified by dehydration and mineralization of the nucleus pulposus. The annulus fibrosus also degenerates and loses its capacity to contain the diseased nucleus. Consequently the weakened disc cannot withstand dynamic forces that are applied by the vertebral column, and protrusion ensues. Type I protrusion

follows chondroid degeneration and is a result of extrusion of dehydrated nuclear material into the vertebral canal. *Fibroid* degeneration is frequently recognized in old, nonchondrodystrophic breeds and is characterized by fibrous metaplasia of the nucleus pulposus. The annulus fibrosus may stretch, partially rupture, or hypertrophy and protrude into the vertebral canal, compressing the cord. Type I lesions tend to be acute, forceful extrusions that cause compressive myelopathy and severe neurologic signs.[9] Type II lesions are associated with a chronic, progressive course and mild neurologic signs, even though significant cord compression may be present.[9] This is because the spinal cord can better sustain the slow deformation of a type II lesion than the explosive concussion and compression of a type I lesion.[7]

Spinal cord compression by protruded discs causes a closed type of injury that alters cord function and structure.[7, 9, 11, 14–16] Two main factors contribute to the pathologic changes of closed cord injury: (1) mechanical disruption caused by compression and concussion and (2) chemical and vascular changes within the cord. Severity depends on the dynamic force, duration and amount of compression, and degree of concussion associated with the initial injury. Spinal cord compression restricts the local arteriovenous supply, and severe arterial compromise may cause infarction. Ischemia of the spinal cord induces the release of potent vasoactive amines, including norepinephrine, serotonin, and dopamine, which leads to hematomyelia and myelomalacia.[14]

SURVEY RADIOGRAPHY

Good technique for radiography of the vertebral column includes the use of detail film-screen combinations, strict

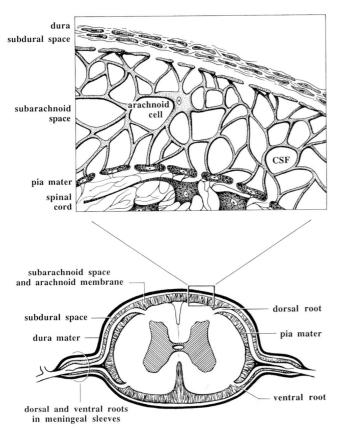

FIGURE 9–2. Anatomic relationship (transverse plane) of spinal cord, meningeal layers, and subarachnoid space. *Inset* shows microscopic structure of a segment of the meninges and cord. (Adapted from Hoerlein BF: Canine Neurology: Diagnosis and Treatment. 3rd Ed. Philadelphia, WB Saunders, 1978; with permission.)

collimation, and multipoint centering (only disc spaces in the central region of the primary beam can be assessed for size because of the divergent nature of the x-ray beam). The animal should be anesthetized to prevent movement, and

close attention should be paid to positioning. Dependent regions of the vertebral column should be supported with radiolucent pads to keep it parallel to the cassette.

Radiographic signs consistent with intervertebral disc protrusion include (1) narrowing of the disc space; (2) narrowing of the dorsal intervertebral articular process joint space; (3) small intervertebral foramen; (4) increased opacity in the intervertebral foramen; and (5) extruded, mineralized disc material within the vertebral canal (Figs. 9–3 and 9–4). Shifting of the vertebra as the disc space narrows also results in narrowing of the articular process joint, decreasing the size of the intervertebral foramen; hence, three survey radiographic signs are typically present with most protrusions. Increased foramen opacity is a result of extruded disc material and inflammation of epidural fat. Careful patient positioning for the lateral radiograph is necessary to align the right and left intervertebral foramina; otherwise the foramen may falsely appear small or opaque.

Disc space narrowing must be assessed in view of the animal's age and presence of secondary bony changes.[17] Narrowing may be due to acute (type I) disc protrusion in young to middle-aged dogs when there are no secondary bony changes. In old dogs, narrowing may represent chronic (type II) disc disease, and only a bulging annulus fibrosus is present. End plate sclerosis and ventrolateral enthesophyte formation (e.g., spondylosis deformans) often accompany chronic protrusion and reflect poor shock absorption by the diseased disc. Many dogs with radiographic evidence of spondylosis deformans have chronic disc changes but remain asymptomatic.[17]

Discal mineralization is indicative of intervertebral disc degeneration but not always disc protrusion.[17] Dystrophic mineralization of a degenerating disc usually begins in the center of the nucleus pulposus and extends peripherally. The annulus may undergo mineralization separately. Contained, mineralized disc material is not a sign of disc prolapse (see Fig. 9–4A). Not all mineralized discs prolapse, and not all prolapsed disc material is mineralized. Noncontained (extruded), mineralized disc material can be seen on survey radiographs (see Fig. 9–4B and C) and is a sign of disc prolapse. With acute prolapse, mineralized disc material is dis-

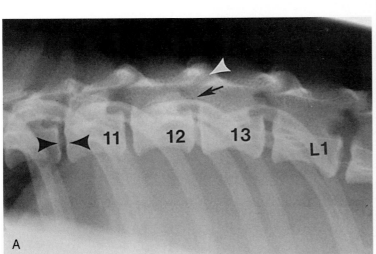
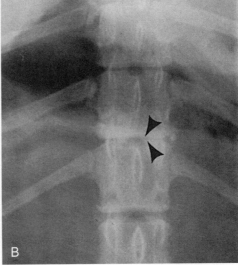

FIGURE 9–3. Survey radiographic signs of intervertebral disc disease. *A*, At T12–T13, the intervertebral disc space and dorsal intervertebral articular process joint are narrow *(white arrowhead)*, and the intervertebral foramen is small and cloudy *(arrow)*. The anteclinal disc space at T10–T11 is normally narrow compared with adjacent spaces *(black arrowheads)*. *B*, Ventrodorsal radiograph of dog in *A*. There is a narrow disc space at T12–T13 *(arrowheads)*. Because of overlap of the vertebral end plates, the ventrodorsal projection is less accurate than the lateral projection for evaluating disc spaces.

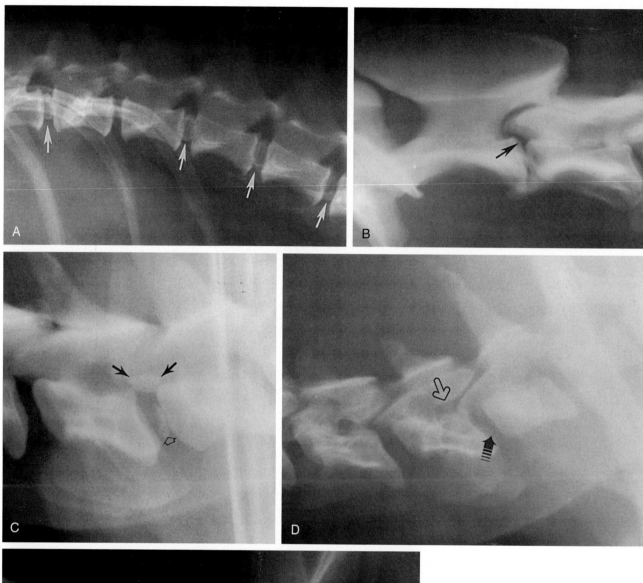

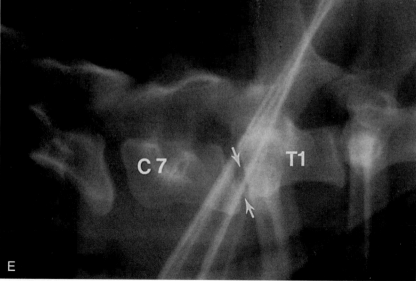

FIGURE 9–4. Patterns of intervertebral disc mineralization. *A,* Contained, mineralized disc material at multiple sites *(arrows)* in a dog without neurologic signs. *B* and *C,* Mineralized, extruded discs in a dog with cervical pain. The intervertebral foramen at C2–C3 *(B)* is small, and diffusely mineralized disc material is causing slight opacity within the canal *(arrow).* These findings are typical of an acute prolapse. The button-like mineralized disc material at C6–C7 *(C)* is consistent with chronic prolapse *(closed arrows).* Note narrow disc space at C6–C7 and mineralized material remaining within the disc *(open arrow). D,* Mineralized, empty annulus fibrosus *(striated arrow)* following extrusion of the nucleus pulposus *(open arrow). E,* False mineralization at C7–T1 is caused by overlap of the first rib pair *(arrows).* The intervertebral disc space at C7–T1 is normally narrower than adjacent spaces.

persed by local inflammation. Therefore, the opacity of disc material in the vertebral canal is nearer that of soft tissue than mineral. After extrusion of nuclear material, an empty, hollow shell of the annulus may remain (see Fig. 9–4D). As the inflammation subsides, the extruded mass of disc material contracts and becomes more opaque. In addition, chronically extruded disc material may undergo mineralization or ossification. This information can be used to help distinguish acute from chronic disc protrusion.

Normal variants should be kept in mind when interpreting survey radiographs of animals with suspected intervertebral disc disease. In the cervical region, the disc spaces become progressively wider from C2–C3 to C6–C7. Superimposition of the rib heads may cause the disc space at C6–C7 to appear mineralized (see Fig. 9–4E). The anteclinal disc space at T10–T11 is narrow, and the spaces at C7–T1 and L4–L6 are often narrower than the adjacent spaces. Assessment of disc space width is best accomplished with accurate lateral radiographic projections. The curvature of the vertebral column always causes some degree of overlap of the vertebral end plates on the ventrodorsal projection, making disc spaces appear falsely narrowed (see Fig. 9–3B). This is most apparent at the periphery of a radiograph where beam parallax is maximal.

Lateral and intraforaminal protrusions of the cervical discs may escape detection by use of standard, 90-degree orthogonal projections. Because of the relatively large extradural space in the cervical region, protrusions may not cause an extradural myelographic lesion. Oblique radiographic projections (ventral 45-degree left-dorsal right or ventral 45-degree right-dorsal left) allow assessment of the left and right foramina, enabling identification of an opaque foramen. This procedure aids the surgeon because the animal may otherwise fall into the nonsurgical treatment category.[18]

Following hemilaminectomy, the disc space often remains narrow. The hemilaminectomy site can be identified by unilateral absence of the articular processes (Fig. 9–5A). The thoracolumbar region should always be scrutinized for this finding because historical information regarding previous surgical decompression may be lacking. If complete laminectomy has been performed, the absence of the lamina and spinous processes is easily recognized (see Fig. 9–5B). Fenestrations generally result in disc space narrowing and occasionally discospondylitis.[17]

MYELOGRAPHY

Myelography, radiography following injection of contrast medium into the spinal subarachnoid space, is useful for evaluating the spinal cord and cauda equina. Indications for myelography include (1) confirming a spinal lesion seen or suspected on survey radiographs, (2) defining the extent of a survey lesion, (3) finding a lesion not observed on survey radiographs, and (4) distinguishing between surgical and nonsurgical lesions. Myelography increases anesthesia time and may cause intensification of pre-existing neurologic signs.[19] When the clinical presentation is consistent with a diagnosis of intervertebral disc protrusion and unequivocal survey radiographic signs are present, the surgeon may elect to perform decompression without myelographic evaluation. In studies of dogs with surgically confirmed disc disease, however, survey radiographs were only 68 to 72 percent accurate in identifying the site of disc protrusion, whereas the accuracy of myelography was 86 to 97 percent.[4, 20] Myelography also provides evidence for whether a hemilaminectomy should be performed on the left or the right side of the affected disc space.

Technique

Myelographic technique is well described[18–27]; therefore, only a brief description of the procedure is presented here. Myelography is always performed under aseptic conditions with the animal subjected to general anesthesia. An accurate survey radiographic study serves as a baseline and must precede myelography. Iohexol (Omnipaque, 240 mgI/mL) and iopamidol (Isovue, 200 mgI/mL) are safe and efficacious and are the nonionic contrast media of choice for small animal myelography. The full-spine dose is 0.45 mL/kg, and the regional dose is 0.30 mL/kg. A 22-gauge spinal needle and stylet should always be used for myelography because it has a short bevel, which increases the likelihood of positioning the needle in the narrow subarachnoid space. Keeping the stylet in place while making a puncture reduces the damage that might occur if the spinal cord is accidentally pierced.

Cervical myelography is performed by injecting contrast medium into the cerebellomedullary cistern through the at-

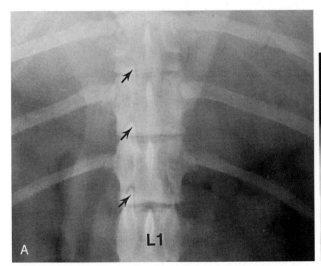

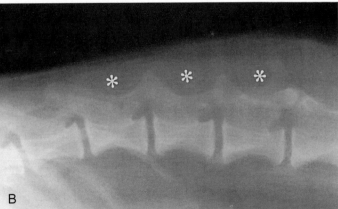

FIGURE 9–5. Radiographic appearance after surgical decompression. A, Unilateral absence of articular processes following left hemilaminectomy; compare to intact processes on the right (arrows). B, Laminectomy site is easily recognized because the lamina and the spinous process have been removed (asterisks).

lanto-occipital space (Fig. 9–6). Puncture can be accomplished with the animal in either sternal or lateral recumbency. The head is flexed ventrally, and the needle is carefully inserted on the midline near the center of a triangle formed by the external occipital protuberance and the wings of the atlas.[21] A distinct *pop* immediately followed by loss of resistance is often felt as the needle traverses the dorsal atlanto-occipital membrane and dura. This classic sensation is less obvious or absent in small dogs and should not be relied on as evidence of cisternal entry. During puncture, the myelographer should frequently stop, withdraw the stylet, and check for evidence of cerebrospinal fluid to determine needle location. With the animal in sternal recumbency, needle placement is less risky because the occipital plate is used to find the proper depth before entering the cerebellomedullary cistern (see Fig. 9–6A).

Lumbar myelography is performed by puncture of the subarachnoid space, preferably at L5–L6, but L4–L5 can be used if necessary (Fig. 9–7A and B). The animal is placed in lateral recumbency, and either of two methods can be used to puncture the subarachnoid space.[18] With the paramedian approach, the needle is inserted slightly caudolateral to the spinous process of L5 or L6 and directed cranioventrally at a 45-degree angle, through the interarcuate space. The median approach requires insertion of the needle just cranial to the spinous process of L5 or L6, at a 90-degree angle to the vertebral column. Because the lumbar subarachnoid space ends blindly in most dogs, contrast medium can be forced past an area of intramedullary swelling, revealing both sides of a compressive lesion. With cervical injection, contrast medium tends to flow rostrally into the ventricular system when cord swelling is present; thus, only the cranial margin of a compressive lesion is often identified. Cervical myelography is rarely of value when severe thoracolumbar cord swelling is present. In some instances, a lumbar study is the best way to evaluate a caudal cervical cord lesion.

The pros and cons of dorsal versus ventral lumbar subarachnoid injection are open to debate. Because it is difficult to locate the dorsal subarachnoid space, most myelographers choose to position the needle bevel in the ventral subarachnoid space instead (see Fig. 9–7A and B). There is also less risk of intramedullary injection of contrast medium with ventral puncture. Positioning the needle bevel in the dorsal subarachnoid space is technically more difficult but causes

less mechanical damage to the spinal cord (see Fig. 9–7C). Transmedullary passage of the needle is necessary for ventral subarachnoid puncture and invariably damages the cord. (This can be minimized by keeping the stylet in place and avoiding horizontal movement of the needle during puncture.) It has been shown, however, that the dorsal aspect of the cord is compressed 2 to 3 mm ventrally as the needle tip is resisted by the tough dura (Fig. 9–8).[28] Therefore, the cord can be injured by compression as well as mechanical disruption by the needle. Obviously, with dorsal needle placement, there is only compression of the cord. With either ventral or dorsal puncture, correct needle placement should be confirmed by fluoroscopy or radiography after a test injection of contrast medium; otherwise, intramedullary injection may occur. Dorsal subarachnoid entry is technically superior because only one puncture of the subarachnoid space is made, decreasing the likelihood of extradural leakage of contrast medium. Regardless of the approach used, multiple needle punctures should be avoided because the risk of epidural leakage is increased with each attempt.[21]

Interpretive Principles

Knowing the relationship of the spinal cord to the meninges, epidural space, and vertebral canal is essential for accurate myelographic interpretation (see Fig. 9–2). The normal myelogram is typified by sharply marginated, thin columns of contrast medium within the subarachnoid space (Fig. 9–9A and B).[21–23] Small-breed dogs and cats (see Fig. 9–9C and D) tend to have relatively large cords and, as a result, thin contrast medium columns.[22] The ventral epidural (extradural) space is normally wide in the caudal cervical region, giving the false impression of cord displacement. The dorsal subarachnoid space is widest at the C1–C2 level and tends to be wider than the corresponding ventral subarachnoid space in the thoracolumbar region. Normal epidural soft tissues cause a filling defect in the ventral contrast medium column at C1–C2 and should not be confused with an extradural lesion. Smaller filling defects often seen dorsal to the remaining cervical discs are caused by hypertrophy of the ligamentum flavum or the annulus fibrosus. Clinically significant subarachnoid filling defects should be accompanied by thinning of the opposite contrast medium column or evidence of

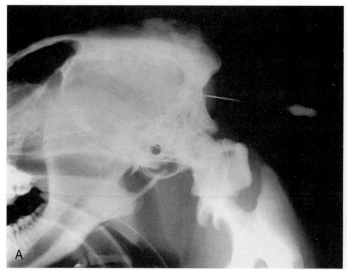
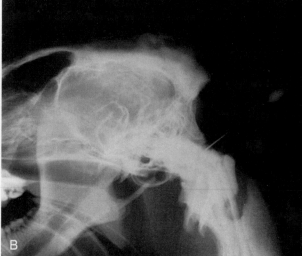

FIGURE 9–6. Technique of cervical myelography. A, Lateral radiograph; the spinal needle is in contact with the occipital bone, establishing proper depth for cerebellomedullary puncture. B, After the occipital bone is located, the needle can be "walked" caudally and inserted into the cerebellomedullary space. Contrast medium has been injected into the subarachnoid space.

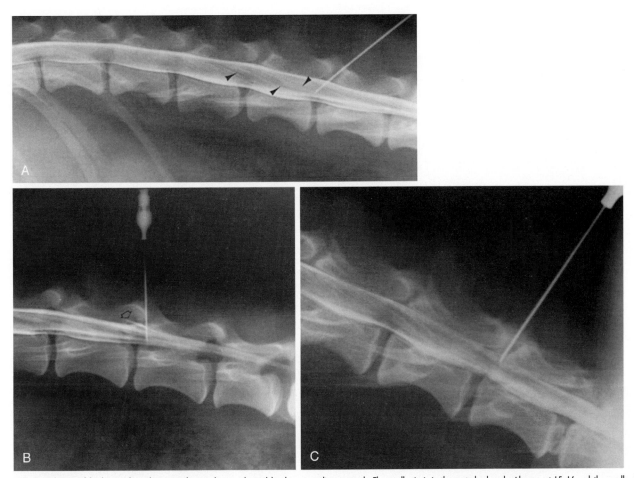

FIGURE 9–7. Technique of lumbar myelography. *A,* Lumbar myelogram obtained by the paramedian approach. The needle tip is in the ventral subarachnoid space at L5–L6 and the needle shaft is approximately 45 degrees to the spinal cord and parallel to the plane of the dorsal intervertebral articular process joints. Filling defects *(arrowheads)* are caused by the spinal nerve roots of the lumbar cord segments. Note the sharply marginated contrast medium columns indicative of subarachnoid injection. *B,* Lumbar myelogram obtained by the median approach at L5–L6. The needle tip is in the ventral subarachnoid space, and the needle shaft is perpendicular to the spinal cord. Slight epidural leakage has occurred around the needle tract *(arrow).* The dural sac is opacified, ending at L7–S1. *C,* Lumbar myelogram with the needle tip in the dorsal subarachnoid space at L5–L6; note disc mineralization at L6–L7.

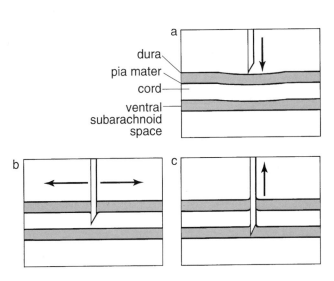

FIGURE 9–8. Lumbar puncture causes mechanical damage to the cord. *A,* Compression of the cord by resistance of the tough dura. *B,* The compression is released as the needle tip passes through the dura, entering the cord. Horizontal movement should be minimized to avoid cord damage. *C,* The needle is retracted slightly (1 to 2 mm) after it has reached the ventral aspect of the vertebral canal, reducing the chance of epidural injection. (From Widmer WR, and Blevins WE: Veterinary myelography: A review of contrast media, adverse effects and technique. J Am Anim Hosp Assoc *19:*755, 1991; with permission.)

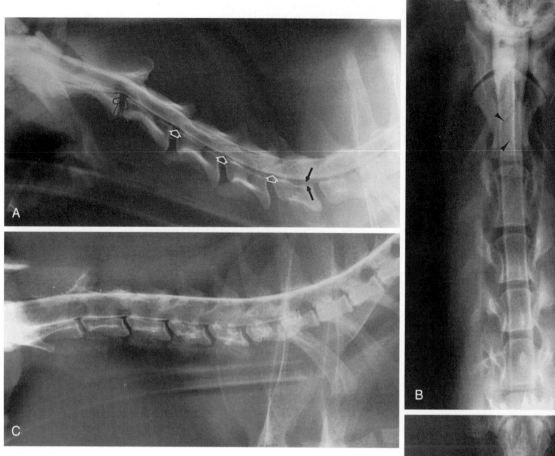

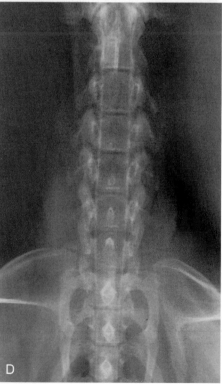

FIGURE 9–9. Normal cervical myelogram. *A,* In the dog, on the lateral radiograph, the contrast medium columns are wide cranially and thin caudally. Soft tissues (dorsal longitudinal ligament or annulus) normally cause thinning of the ventral subarachnoid space at C2–C3 *(open black arrow)* and should not be confused with disc prolapse. Smaller indentations *(open white arrows)* are also seen in normal dogs. The epidural space is widest dorsal to C6–C7 *(closed black arrows).* *B,* In the dog, on the ventrodorsal radiograph, a serpentine subarachnoid filling defect is caused by the basilar artery *(arrowheads).* Contrast medium columns are also wider cranially. Note poor subarachnoid filling in the caudal cervical region as a result of the effect of dependency. *C* and *D,* In the cat, the cord is relatively wide and occupies a large percentage of the vertebral canal. As a result, the contrast medium columns are thin and conform closely to the margins of the vertebral canal, giving a false impression of cord swelling.

cord compression. The thoracic cord lacks an intumescence and is smaller than the cervical and lumbosacral segments. Although the canine spinal cord terminates at L5–L6, the contrast medium–filled dural sac may extend beyond the lumbosacral junction (see Fig. 9–7B).[38]

The abnormal myelogram is characterized by changes in the size and location of the subarachnoid contrast medium columns and the width and opacity of the spinal cord. Myelographic lesions can be grouped into the following patterns:

VENTRODORSAL

LATERAL

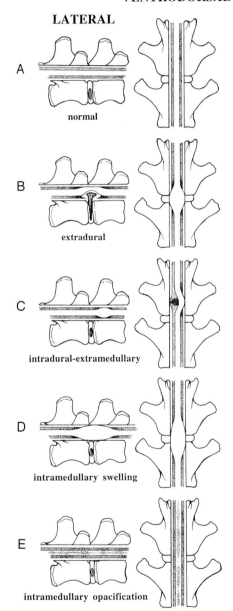

A
normal

B
extradural

C
intradural-extramedullary

D
intramedullary swelling

E
intramedullary opacification

FIGURE 9–10. Classification of myelographic lesions. *A,* Normal. *B,* Extradural. The contrast medium columns are displaced and thin or absent (subarachnoid filling defect) on one radiographic projection, whereas cord swelling may be evident on the orthogonal projection. *C,* Intradural-extramedullary. A mass lesion within the subarachnoid space causes a filling defect on the orthogonal projection; cord swelling may be present, depending on the size of the mass. *D,* Intramedullary swelling. The spinal cord is swollen, causing thinning and obliteration of the contrast medium columns on both myelographic projections. *E,* Intramedullary opacification. Opacification of the cord parenchyma is caused by uptake of contrast medium and is consistent with myelomalacia. Opacification of the central canal differs and should not be confused with myelomalacia (see Fig. 9–12).

Table 9–1

DIAGNOSTIC POSSIBILITIES ASSOCIATED WITH MYELOGRAPHIC PATTERNS

Pattern	Diagnosis
Extradural	Intervertebral disc protrusion Ligamentous hypertrophy Hematoma/hemorrhage Neoplasia (vertebral or epidural soft tissue) Vertebral fracture/dislocation
Intradural extramedullary	Neoplasia (neurofibroma, neurofibrosarcoma, and meningioma) Granuloma
Intramedullary swelling	Spinal cord edema Neoplasia (neural, metastatic discrete cell, e.g., granulomatous meningoencephalitis) Ischemic myelopathy
Intramedullary opacification	Myelomalacia Hematomyelia
Normal	Degenerative myelopathy* Ischemic myelopathy Myelitis Meningitis

*It is the author's opinion that spinal cord size may be decreased in dogs with degenerative myelopathy; however, this has not yet been proven by scientific investigation.

extradural, intradural-extramedullary, intramedullary swelling, and intramedullary opacification (Fig. 9–10; Table 9–1).[21, 31, 32]

Several technical factors affect myelographic quality and interpretation (Fig. 9–11).[26] Air bubbles cause circular or oval filling defects that are potentially confusing; however, their location is usually variable on subsequent radiographs.[21] Subdural leakage may occur if the needle bridges the subdural and the subarachnoid spaces causing irregular margination and poor filling of the contrast medium columns. Epidural leakage of contrast medium should be avoided because it adds unwanted opacity, obscuring the subarachnoid contrast columns.[27] Gravity affects distribution of contrast medium, reducing subarachnoid opacification in nondependent regions. On the ventrodorsal projection, dependency causes contrast medium to pool cranially, reducing the opacity of the caudal cervical subarachnoid space. The opposite situation occurs with the dorsoventral projection; therefore, both projections should be routinely obtained. On the lateral projection, contrast medium pools cranial and caudal to the thoracic region. The effect of pooling can be overcome by padding dependent body regions or elevating the rear and forequarters of the animal, filling the thoracic subarachnoid space. Pooling becomes more of a problem with hyperosmolal–high iodine content contrast media.[26]

Injection into the normal central canal of the spinal cord (*canalogram*) occurs when the needle shaft is within the central canal or if the canal communicates with the subarachnoid space at the level of the conus medullaris (Fig. 9–12A).[29] In the former instance, contrast medium is presumed to leak back along the needle, especially during rapid injection.[29] Canalograms are most likely to occur when puncture is made at L4–L5, where the cord:vertebral canal ratio is large. The presence of a normal canalogram should not be confused with cord opacification caused by myelomalacia (see Fig. 9–12B). Large central canals are associated with hydromyelia. The central canal may also become opacified when the cord parenchyma is disrupted by severe trauma or neoplasia.

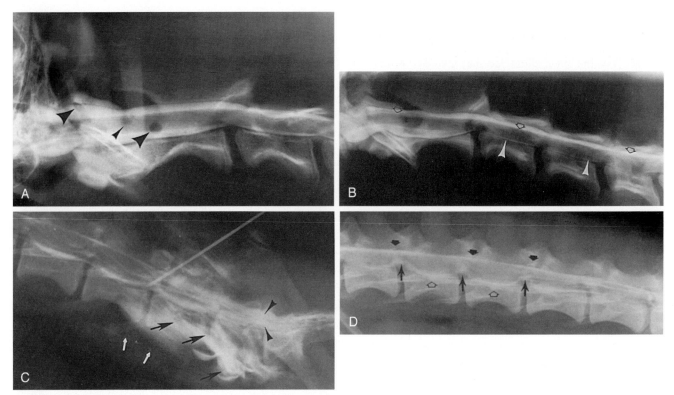

FIGURE 9–11. Myelograms with artifacts caused by technical errors. *A,* Air bubbles *(arrowheads)* create circular or oval filling defects; their location varies from radiograph to radiograph, in comparison to a filling defect caused by a lesion. Air bubbles can be eliminated by attaching a contrast medium–filled extension set to the needle. *B,* Injection of contrast medium into the subdural space may occur if the needle bevel bridges the subdural and subarachnoid spaces. Note wavy and irregularly marginated dorsal contrast column *(open arrows)* and incomplete filling of the ventral subarachnoid space *(arrowheads). C,* Severe epidural leakage caused by improper needle placement. Contrast medium has spilled into the epidural space of the intervertebral canal *(arrowheads)* and that which surrounds the sacral nerve roots *(black arrows).* White arrows depict opacified ventral external veretebral venous plexus. *D,* Moderate epidural leakage following lumbar myelography at L5–L6. Epidural contrast medium columns can be recognized ventrally by the appearance of opacified vertebral venous sinuses *(large closed arrows)* and dorsally by opacification dorsal to the subarachnoid contrast medium column *(small closed arrows).* Opacified depressions in the centra contain the basivertebral veins *(open black arrows).*

Intervertebral Disc Protrusion

Either extradural or intramedullary patterns may result from disc protrusion (Table 9–2).[21, 22, 33–35] Disc protrusion typically causes an extradural lesion characterized by thinning and dorsal deviation of the ventral subarachnoid contrast medium column (lateral radiograph) and compensatory widening of the cord (ventrodorsal radiograph) (Fig. 9–13*A* and *B*).[26] On the lateral radiograph, the cord is compressed and deviated away from the site of disc protrusion. The contrast medium column adjacent to the protrusion tends to be dome shaped, and the opposite contrast medium column is narrowed by the displaced spinal cord. When disc protrusion is slightly lateral to the ventral midline, a forked contrast medium column may be seen on the lateral projection (see Fig. 9–13*C*). This finding should not be confused with an intradural-extramedullary lesion (see Fig. 9–10).[4, 26] Both extruded disc material and a bulging annulus can deviate the subarachnoid contrast medium column and the cord.

Frequently in type I protrusion, an intramedullary pattern owing to severe cord swelling predominates and masks classic extradural signs of extrusion. Cord swelling is caused by edema of one to three vertebral segments cranial or caudal to the site of protrusion secondary to acute injury but is

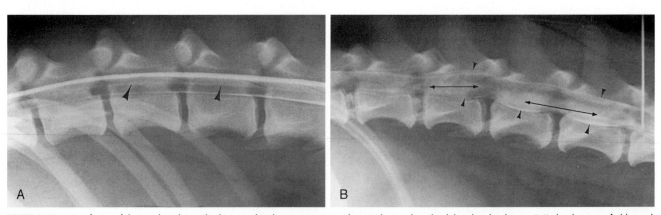

FIGURE 9–12. *A,* Opacification of the central canal *(arrowheads)* occurs when there is communication between the central canal and the subarachnoid space. *B,* Myelomalacia is typified by uptake of contrast medium by the cord parenchyma *(double-headed arrows).* Intramedullary swelling is also present, and the subarachnoid contrast medium columns are thin *(arrowheads).*

Table 9–2
MYELOGRAPHIC SIGNS OF INTERVERTEBRAL DISC DISEASE

Extradural Pattern
    Deviation and thinning of subarachnoid contrast column at
       intervertebral disc space (ventral, dorsal, or lateral)
    Forked subarachnoid contrast column
    Spinal cord displacement
    Spinal cord compression (compensatory displacement
       flattens cord due to extradural mass, mimics cord swelling)
    Hourglass subarachnoid filling defect

Intramedullary Pattern
    Uniform spinal cord swelling due to edema, subarachnoid
       contrast columns displaced, thin or absent
    Opacification of spinal cord parenchyma

not a feature of chronic disc protrusion. The subarachnoid displacement of intramedullary swelling differs from that of extradural compression. With intramedullary swelling, the contrast medium column is thin and displaced abaxially (Fig. 9–14A and B). In some instances, severe swelling may completely obliterate the subarachnoid space (see Fig. 9–14C). Evidence of intramedullary swelling is found on lateral and ventrodorsal radiographic projections. Compensatory extradural compression of the cord causes focal intramedullary swelling (shorter length than intramedullary swelling) on a single radiographic projection (usually the ventrodorsal), and extradural signs of disc protrusion are seen on the orthogonal projection. In some instances, acutely extruded disc material may disperse around the cord and cause a subarachnoid filling defect that mimics cord swelling.[36]

If intramedullary swelling is present and there are no obvious extradural signs, careful scrutiny of the myelogram may identify the site of disc protrusion. Slight axial deviation of the contrast medium column at the site of cord swelling suggests the site of an extradural discal mass (see Fig. 9–14B). This important clue is often found on only one radiographic projection but can help determine the site for surgical exploration and decompression. Hemorrhage from rupture of the ventral vertebral veins is a complication of acute disc disease and may cause an extradural lesion. Whenever there is doubt about the location of disc protrusion on the myelogram, the survey radiographs should be re-evaluated to be certain nothing has been overlooked.

Technical considerations play an important role in the myelographic diagnosis of intervertebral disc disease. Because subarachnoid distention is maximal during the injection of

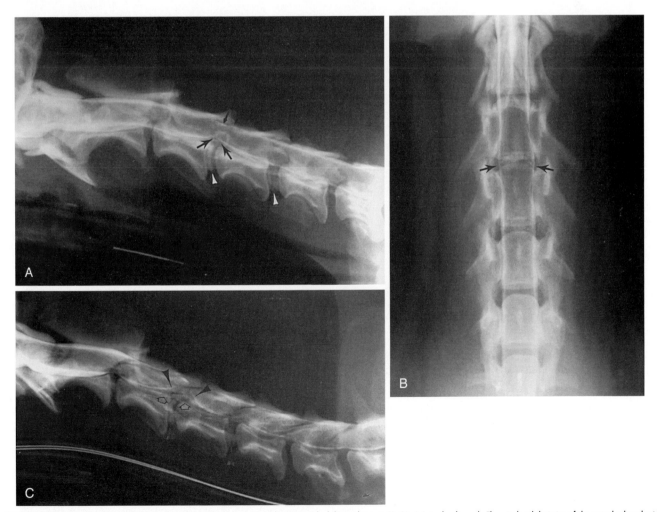

FIGURE 9–13. Cervical myelogram. There are typical extradural lesions caused by intervertebral disc prolapse at C3–C4. *A,* Lateral radiograph. There is dorsal deviation of the ventral subarachnoid contrast medium column *(large arrows).* The dorsal contrast medium column is thin because of displacement of the spinal cord *(small arrow).* Note mineralized disc material *(white arrowheads). B,* On the ventrodorsal radiograph, cord swelling is typified by thinning and abaxial deviation of the contrast columns at C3–C4 *(arrows). C,* Forked appearance of the ventral contrast medium column is caused by the x-ray beam striking two tangents of the ventral subarachnoid space. The extruded disc material is located just lateral to the midline, causing the ventral contrast medium column to appear as a double line on the lateral radiograph *(open arrows).* The double line is not seen in *A* because of a slight difference in patient positioning.

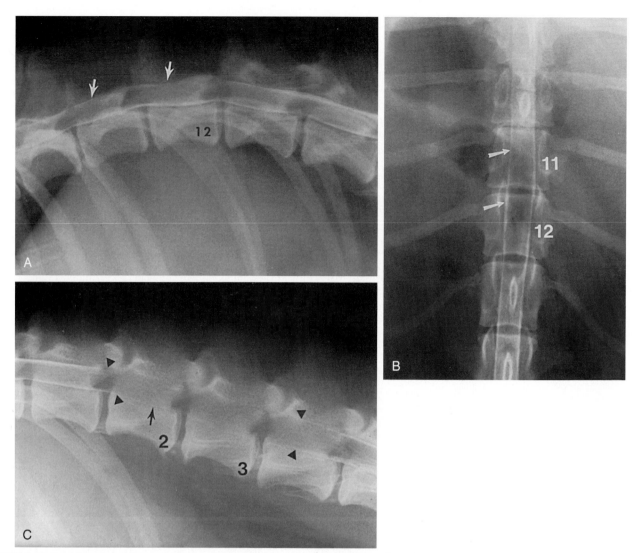

FIGURE 9–14. Type I disc prolapse with intramedullary pattern. *A,* Lateral myelogram. There is intramedullary swelling and thin contrast medium columns *(arrows)* at T11–T12. *B,* Ventrodorsal myelogram of same dog as in *A.* The cord is wide at T11–T12; note axial shift of the right contrast medium column *(arrows),* which indicates lateralization of the prolapse. In this instance, the surgeon may elect to perform a right hemilaminectomy. Intervertebral disc prolapse at T11–T12 was confirmed at surgery. *C,* With severe intramedullary swelling, the contrast medium columns may be obliterated *(arrowheads),* masking the extradural component of the lesion. Faint opacification of the ventral contrast column can be seen at L2 *(arrow).* Intervertebral disc prolapse at L2–L3 was confirmed at surgery.

contrast medium, the simultaneous use of videofluoroscopy may allow detection of an extradural lesion when none is found on conventional radiographs. If videofluoroscopy is not available, radiographs made immediately after rapid injection of contrast medium may enhance the extradural component of disc protrusion and the extent of cord swelling.[4, 33] The use of oblique radiographic projections should be considered on every myelographic study because they frequently provide useful information. If disc material is located significantly lateral to the ventral midline, the lateral and ventrodorsal radiographs show only cord swelling, whereas in oblique radiographic projections (ventral left-dorsal right and ventral right-dorsal left), an extradural pattern is seen (Fig. 9–15).

The gradual onset of type II disc protrusion tends to minimize cord swelling, resulting in an extradural myelographic pattern (Fig. 9–16). Chronic changes, including hypertrophy of the annulus fibrosus, ligamentum flavum, and joint capsule of the dorsal intervertebral articular process joint, cause circumferential compression of the spinal cord (*hourglass appearance*). Type II protrusion is part of the cervical vertebral malformation-instability (wobbler) and lumbosacral stenosis-instability (caudal equina) syndromes of large-dog breeds.[5, 6]

In dogs with cervical vertebral malformation-instability syndrome, dynamic compression of the cord may be detected with radiographic projections made with the head and neck in flexion or extension. Many radiologists, however, choose to rely solely on information obtained from radiographs made with the neck in neutral position. Stress radiography may be of value if surgical decompression (*ventral slot*) is being considered to correct cord compression caused by cervical disc protrusion. By placing steady traction on the forelimbs and hindlimbs, extradural signs of disc protrusion noted on the pretraction lateral myelogram should be reduced. If the post-traction myelogram does not show improvement of extradural compression, ventral slot decompression may be ineffective.

Diagnosis of lumbosacral disc protrusion presents a special problem to the radiologist. Although disc space narrowing, end plate sclerosis, and spondylosis deformans are associated with L7–S1 disc protrusion, these changes can also occur in asymptomatic dogs.[6] In addition, some dogs with L7–S1 protrusion have no radiographic changes.[21] Lateral radiographic projections of the lumbosacrum in flexion and extension help demonstrate the dynamics of lumbosacral instability, but results are often misleading.[6] A method using quantitative

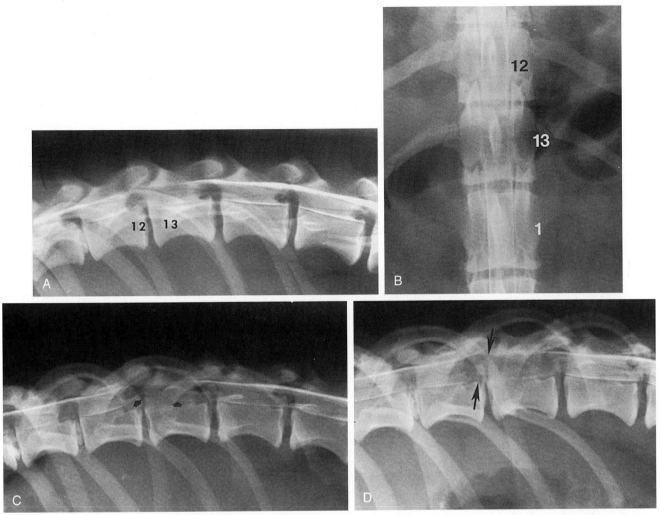

FIGURE 9–15. Ventrolateral disc protrusion. *A* and *B,* Lateral and ventrodorsal myelograms. There are mild signs of cord swelling, but the site of disc protrusion is not evident. *C,* In a ventral 65-degree right-dorsal left oblique projection, there is an extradural lesion typified by subarachnoid thinning and deviation owing to disc prolapse *(arrows).* *D,* In a ventral 65-degree left-dorsal right oblique projection (orthogonal to *C*), there is marked cord swelling *(arrows).* The extradural and intramedullary lesions are best recognized on the oblique projections because the x-ray beam is striking each lesion tangentially.

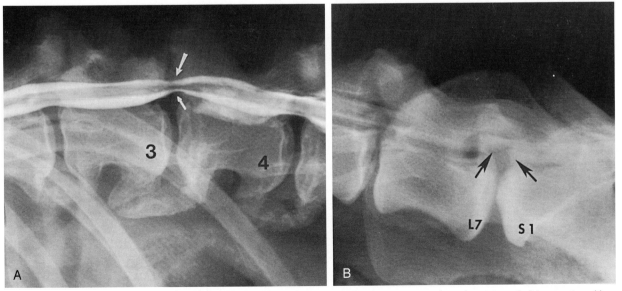

FIGURE 9–16. Type II disc protrusion. *A,* Extradural lesion caused by disc protrusion at L3–L4 *(arrows).* The hourglass appearance, a chronic change, is a result of disc protrusion and hypertrophy of the ventral longitudinal ligament, annulus fibrosus, and ligamentum flavum. Chronic degenerative changes of the vertebra are also present (spondylosis and spondylarthritis). *B,* Disc protrusion at L7–S1. Note narrowed intervertebral disc space and filling defect in the dural sac *(arrows).*

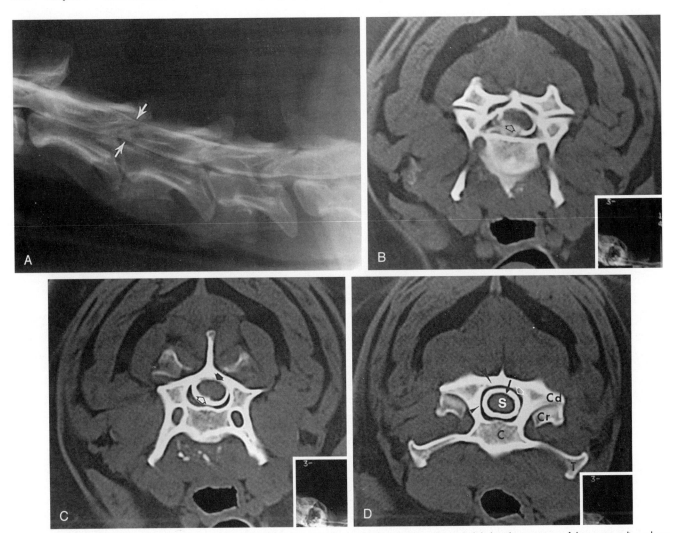

FIGURE 9–17. Myelography and computed tomography (CT) of a cervical disc prolapse. *A,* In the lateral cervical myelogram, there is a slight hourglass appearance of the contrast medium columns at C3–C4 *(arrows). B,* In a transverse CT image, there is ventrolateral cord compression at C3–C4 *(open arrow)* due to extruded disc material. Dorsolaterally the subarachnoid space is thin. Only a small margin of the intervertebral disc can be seen because the image plane is oblique with respect to the disc space. *C,* A contiguous 3-mm slice caudal to *B;* there is cord compression *(open arrow)* and thinning of the dorsolateral aspect of the contrast medium column *(closed arrow). D,* A slice made at the caudal aspect of C4 is within normal limits. S, spinal cord; Cd, caudal articular process; Cr, cranial articular process; C, centrum of vertebra; *open arrow,* epidural space; *black arrow,* subarachnoid space with contrast medium; *small black arrowhead,* vertebral pedicle; *large black arrowhead,* vertebral lamina.

radiographic evaluation of the lumbosacrum was 86 percent accurate in identifying dogs with stenosis at L7–S1.[37]

Radiographic contrast procedures routinely used to evaluate the lumbosacral region include flexion extension–myelography[38] and epidurography.[39] Myelography may reveal evidence of disc protrusion, provided that the dural sac extends beyond the lumbosacral joint and the myelogram is technically correct. Epidurography is performed by placing a spinal needle into the vertebral canal between S3 and Cd3 and injecting contrast medium into the epidural space.[39] Dorsal displacement of the ventral epidural space and complete obstruction to cranial flow of contrast medium are the most consistent epidurographic findings of lumbosacral stenosis (compression).[39] The normal contour of the epidural space, compared to the subarachnoid space, is undulating and subject to misinterpretation. Myelography should always precede epidurography because the latter obscures the subarachnoid space.

Computed Tomography

Computed tomography (CT) and CT myelography are useful when conventional myelography does not clearly demon-

strate a suspected extradural lesion caused by disc protrusion (Fig. 9–17).[40, 41] Because the contrast resolution of CT is superior to that of conventional radiography, extradural compressive lesions caused by lesions other than disc protrusion (e.g., ligamentous hypertrophy, hematoma, tumor) can be identified. Cord swelling and intervertebral foraminal changes are accurately diagnosed with CT myelography, especially when there is minimal subarachnoid distention. In Doberman pinschers with caudal cervical vertebral malformation-instability, CT findings provide prognostic information about paraspinal soft-tissue structures and the cord parenchyma that cannot be obtained with conventional radiography.[42] High-resolution CT provides excellent spatial resolution and image contrast and is used to diagnose lesions of the caudal equina of human beings. A technique using this modality has been proposed for evaluation of the canine lumbosacral region.[43]

References

1. Hoerlein BF: Canine Neurology: Diagnosis and Treatment, 3rd Ed. Philadelphia, WB Saunders, 1978.

2. DeLahunta A: Veterinary Neuroanatomy and Clinical Neurology, 2nd Ed. Philadelphia, WB Saunders, 1983.
3. Trotter EJ: Canine intervertebral disc disease. *In* Kirk RW (Ed): Current Veterinary Therapy VI. Philadelphia, WB Saunders, 1977, pp 841–848.
4. Kirberger RM, Roos CJ, and Lubbe AM: The radiological diagnosis of thoracolumbar disc disease in the Dachshund. Vet Radiol *33*:255, 1992.
5. Seim HB, and Withrow SJ: Pathophysiology and diagnosis of caudal cervical spondylo-myelopathy with emphasis on the Doberman pinscher. J Am Anim Hosp Assoc *18*:241, 1982.
6. Wheeler SJ: Lumbosacral disease. Vet Clin North Am [Sm Anim Pract] *22*:859, 1992.
7. Thatcher CT: Neuroanatomic and pathophysiologic aspects of intervertebral disc disease in the dog. Prob Vet Med Intervertebral Disc Dis *1*:337, 1989.
8. Evans HE, and Christensen JC: Miller's Anatomy of the Dog, 2nd Ed. Philadelphia, WB Saunders, 1979.
9. Toombs JP: Cervical intervertebral disc disease in dogs. Compend Contin Ed Pract Vet *14*:1477, 1992.
10. Shores A: Intervertebral disc syndrome in the dog: Part I. Pathophysiology and management. Compend Contin Ed Pract Vet *7*:639, 1981.
11. Simson S: Intervertebral disc disease. Vet Clin North Am [Sm Anim Pract] *22*:889, 1992.
12. Morgan JP, Atilola M, and Bailey CS: Vertebral canal and spinal cord mensuration: A comparative study and its effect on lumbosacral myelography in the Dachshund and German shepherd dog. J Am Vet Med Assoc *191*:951, 1987.
13. Pardo AD, and Morgan JP: Myelography in the cat: A comparison of cisternal versus lumbar puncture, using metrizamide. Vet Radiol *29*:89, 1988.
14. Shores A: Spinal trauma: Pathophysiology and management of traumatic spinal injuries. Vet Clin North Am [Sm Anim Pract] *22*:859, 1992.
15. Prata R: Neurosurgical treatment of thoracolumbar discs: The rationale and value of laminectomy and concomitant disc removal. J Am Anim Hosp Assoc *17*:17, 1981.
16. Griffiths IR: The extensive myelopathy of intervertebral disc protrusion in dogs ('the ascending syndrome'). J Sm Anim Pract *13*:425, 1972.
17. Morgan JP, and Miyabayashi T: Degenerative changes in the vertebral column of the dog: A review of radiographic findings. Vet Radiol *29*:72, 1988.
18. Felts JF, and Prata RG: Cervical disc disease in the dog: Intraforaminal and lateral extrusions. J Am Anim Hosp Assoc *19*:755, 1983.
19. Widmer WR, and Blevins WE: Veterinary myelography: A review of contrast media, adverse effects and technique. J Am Anim Hosp Assoc *27*:163, 1991.
20. Olby NJ, Dyce J, and Houlton JEF: Correlation of plain radiographic and lumbar myelographic findings in thoracolumbar disc disease. J Sm Anim Pract *35*:345, 1994.
21. Roberts RE, and Selcer BA: Myelography and epidurography. Vet Clin North Am [Sm Anim Pract] *23*:307, 1993.
22. Burk RL: Problems in the radiographic interpretation of intervertebral disc disease in the dog. Prob Vet Med *1*:381, 1989.
23. Sande R: Radiography, myelography, computed tomography and magnetic resonance imaging of the spine. Vet Clin North Am [Sm Anim Pract] *22*:811, 1992.
24. Wood AKW: Iohexol and iopamidol: New non-ionic contrast media for myelography in dogs. Comp Contin Ed Pract Vet *10*:32, 1988.
25. Widmer WR, Blevins WE, Cantwell HD, et al: Iohexol and iopamidol myelography in the dog: A clinical trial comparing adverse effects and myelographic quality. Vet Radiol *33*:327, 1992.
26. Lamb CR: Common difficulties with myelographic diagnosis of acute intervertebral disc disease in the dog. J Sm Anim Pract *35*:549, 1994.
27. Weber WJ, and Berry CR: Radiology corner: Determining the location of contrast medium on the canine lumbar myelogram. Vet Radiol *35*:430, 1994.
28. Tilmant L, Ackerman N, and Spencer CP: Mechanical aspects of subarachnoid space puncture in the dog. Vet Radiol *25*:227, 1984.
29. Kirberger RM, and Wrigley R: Myelography in the dog: A review of patients with contrast medium in the central canal. Vet Radiol *34*:253, 1993.
30. Wright JA, and Jones DGC: Metrizamide myelography in sixty-eight dogs. J Sm Anim Pract *22*:415, 1981.
31. Adams WM: Myelography. Vet Clin North Amer *12*:295, 1971.
32. Suter PF, Morgan JP, Holliday TA, et al: Myelography of the dog: Diagnosis of tumors of the spinal cord and vertebrae. Vet Radiol *12*:29, 1971.
33. Funquist B: Thoraco-lumbar myelography with water-soluble contrast medium in dogs: I. Technique of myelography; side effects and complications. J Sm Anim Pract *3*:53, 1962.
34. Funquist B: Thoraco-lumbar myelography with water-soluble contrast medium in dogs: II. Appearance of the myelogram in disc protrusion and its relation to functional disturbances and pathoanatomic changes in the epidural space. J Sm Anim Pract *3*:67, 1962.
35. Ticer J, and Brown SJ: Water-soluble myelography in canine intervertebral disc protrusion. Vet Radiol *15*:3, 1974.
36. Morgan JP, Suter PF, and Holliday TA: Myelography with water-soluble contrast medium: Radiographic interpretation of disc herniation in dogs. Acta Radiol *319*(suppl):217, 1972.
37. Mattoon JS, and Koblik PD: Quantitative survey radiographic evaluation of the lumbosacral spine of normal dogs and dogs with degenerative lumbosacral stenosis. Vet Radiol *34*:194, 1993.
38. Lang J: Flexion-extension myelography canine caudal equina. Vet Radiol *29*:242, 1988.
39. Selcer BA, Chambers JN, Schwensen K, et al: Epidurography as a diagnostic aid in canine lumbosacral compressive disease: 47 cases (1981–1986). Vet Comp Orthop Trauma *29*:97, 1988.
40. Stickle RL, and Hathcock JT: Interpretation of computed tomographic images. Vet Clin North Am [Sm Anim Pract] *23*:417, 1993.
41. Feeney DA, Fletcher TF, and Hardy RM: Atlas of Correlative Imaging Anatomy of the Normal Dog. Philadelphia, WB Saunders, 1991.
42. Sharp NJ, Cofone M, Robertson ID, et al: Computed tomography in the evaluation of caudal cervical spondylomyelopathy of the Doberman pinscher. Vet Radiol *36*:100, 1995.
43. Jones JC, Wilson ME, and Bartels JE: A review of high resolution computed tomography and a proposed technique for regional examination of the lumbosacral spine. Vet Radiol *35*:339, 1994.

STUDY QUESTIONS

Perform the indicated operation. For multiple choice questions, choose the best answer.

1. In nonchondrodystrophic breeds, intervertebral disc disease is typified by:
   A. chondroid degeneration.
   B. fibroid degeneration.
   C. severe neurologic signs.
   D. disc prolapse at T12–T13 and T13–L1.
   E. all of the above.
   F. none of the above.

2. Which of the following is correct with respect to the canine spinal cord?
   A. The conus medullaris ends caudal to L6 in large-dog breeds.
   B. In the lumbar region, the cord segments lie caudal to the corresponding vertebral segment.
   C. The pia is the thinnest meningeal layer and covers the spinal cord.
   D. The ratio of spinal cord to vertebral canal is highest in the cervical region.
   E. none of the above.
   F. all of the above.

3. Regarding pathophysiology of intervertebral disc herniation, which of the following is correct?
   A. The cord can better withstand slow deformation than explosive concussion.
   B. Type I lesions tend to cause more acute injury than type II lesions.
   C. Type II lesions are a result of fibroid degeneration.
   D. Pathologic changes are caused by mechanical disruption of the cord and by chemical and vascular alterations.
   E. all of the above.
   F. none of the above

4. Name three technical considerations that engender good-quality radiographs of the vertebral column.

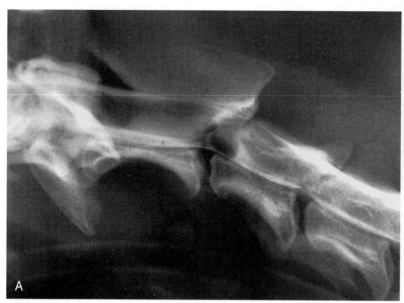
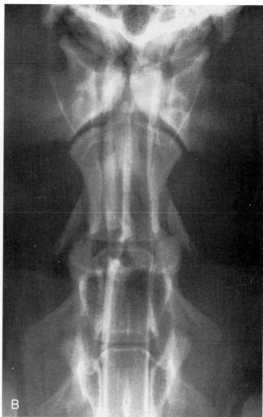

FIGURE 9–18

5. What are four survey radiographic signs of intervertebral disc disease?

6. Which is true regarding disc mineralization?
   A. Disc mineralization begins peripherally and extends centrally.
   B. Disc mineralization is a dystrophic change.
   C. Disc mineralization and disc prolapse are synonymous.
   D. Only the annulus fibrosis undergoes mineralization.
   E. all of the above.
   F. none of the above.

7. Which is true regarding myelographic technique?
   A. Iodinated ionic contrast media such as meglumine diatrizoate are safe and efficacious for myelography.
   B. Cervical myelography is best accomplished by puncture of the ventral subarachnoid space.
   C. Lumbar myelography can be most easily accom-
   plished by puncture of the dorsal subarachnoid space at L4–L5 or L5–L6.
   D. The normal myelogram is characterized by uniform, thin contrast columns and uniform cord width except at the cervical and lumbar regions.
   E. all of the above.
   F. none of the above.

8. The myelogram shown (Fig. 9–18) was obtained from a 7-year-old, female, mixed-breed dog with neck pain. What type of myelographic pattern is present?

9. What is the cause of the opacification just dorsal to the dorsal subarachnoid space at L5–L6 of Figure 9–7C?

10. Type I disc lesions often cause intramedullary swelling as well as an extramedullary pattern. Which type of myelographic pattern is most typical of type II disc herniation?

(Answers appear on page 634.)

AXIAL SKELETON—EQUIDAE

Chapter 10

The Equine Skull

Russ Stickle

This chapter reviews the major radiographic lesions of the equine skull, excluding the nasal cavity and sinuses (see Chapter 11 for those conditions). A review of the complex anatomy of the skull, which often creates problems in diagnosis, is recommended.[1–3]

Many areas of the head lend themselves to radiographic examination with the use of relatively low-capacity equipment.[4–6] The rostral portions of the mandible, the calvaria, and the facial bones do not have much soft-tissue covering, and the facial bones are relatively thin. The normal presence of air in structures such as the nasal cavity, sinuses, pharynx, and guttural pouches enhances their radiographic examination.

TRAUMA

Mandibular fractures are usually obvious, especially when they are complete or bilateral. Certain injuries, such as mandibular symphysis separation in foals and trauma to the incisor teeth, are more easily diagnosed by physical examination than radiographically. Fractures that involve the caudal mandible as well as unilateral and fissure fractures of the mandible are difficult to visualize radiographically. Oblique, ventrodorsal, and intraoral views are more useful than lateral views in these horses (Figs. 10–1 and 10–2). It is important to

evaluate for fracture complications, such as tooth alveolar involvement, tooth root fracture, and sequestra formation, because these can lead to problems during healing.

Fractures of the maxilla or calvaria may be characterized by displacement, soft-tissue swelling, or evidence of hemorrhage into the sinuses. Nondisplaced fractures are often difficult to visualize radiographically, and normal sutures in young horses should not be mistaken for fracture lines (Fig. 10–3). Oblique views are particularly useful in the evaluation of trauma of the maxilla, orbit, and zygomatic arches.[7] When available, computed tomographic imaging may provide valuable information in horses with head trauma (Fig. 10–4).

Basilar skull fractures are most common in horses that fall over backward.[8, 9] These fractures occur, in part, from tension on the muscle insertions at the base of the skull. Radiographically, displacement between the basisphenoid and the basioccipital bones may be seen on the lateral view (Fig. 10–5). This displacement is an important diagnostic criterion because the normal suture line between these bones may be visible radiographically until the horse is 3 years of age.[10] Avulsion of a portion of the longus capitis muscle from its attachment site on the basisphenoid bone has also been reported; extensive guttural pouch hemorrhage may also accompany this condition.[11, 12]

Fractures of the petrous temporal bone have also been seen in association with, and possibly secondary to, osseous

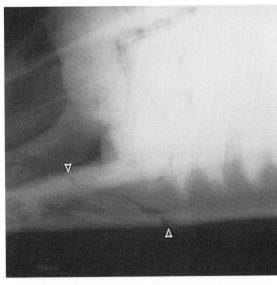

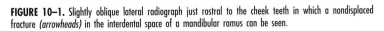

FIGURE 10–1. Slightly oblique lateral radiograph just rostral to the cheek teeth in which a nondisplaced fracture *(arrowheads)* in the interdental space of a mandibular ramus can be seen.

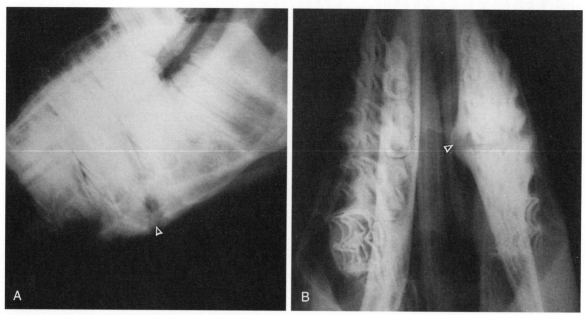

FIGURE 10–2. *A,* Lateral radiograph of the tooth region in which bone remodeling with a central area of radiolucency can be seen *(arrowhead).* Superimposition of both mandibular rami obscures detail. *B,* Ventrodorsal view allows better visualization of this chronic fracture *(arrowhead)* and confirms that only one mandibular ramus is involved.

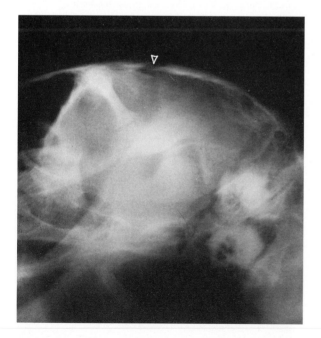

FIGURE 10–3. Lateral skull radiograph of a young foal with possible head trauma. The wide lucent line *(arrowhead)* is a normal suture, not a fracture.

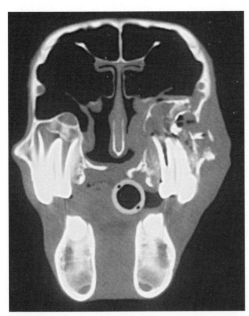

FIGURE 10–4. Transverse computed tomographic image of the caudal tooth region. There is a comminuted fracture of one maxilla (viewer's right). The extent of the fracture could not be ascertained from multiple radiographic views.

fusion of the cartilaginous joint between the stylohyoid and the temporal bones. Fractures of the stylohyoid bone may accompany these lesions. Facial and vestibular neuropathy may occur secondary to these injuries. Radiographic signs include periosteal reactivity, which is sometimes accompanied by bone lysis, involving the proximal portion of the stylohyoid bone and the tympanic bulla (Fig. 10–6).[13, 14] Septic otitis media or interna is suspected to be the inciting cause of the hyoid-temporal fusion,[13, 14] although guttural pouch mycosis may also cause fusion of this joint.[8] Stylohyoid fractures have also been reported as primary injuries. Stylohyoid fractures usually involve the distal portion of the bone and are associated with falling or excessive traction on the tongue during examination of the mouth.[8] Temporomandibular joint

luxations occasionally occur in horses, with or without accompanying mandibular fractures.[15, 16]

BONE INFECTIONS

Osteomyelitis of the bones of the head often accompanies penetrating wounds, open fractures, tooth root abscesses, and lesions of adjacent soft tissue (e.g., lymph node abscess formation and guttural pouch infection). Radiographically, osteomyelitis is aggressive and usually characterized by bone lysis accompanied by varying degrees of sclerosis and periosteal new bone production. Chronic fistulas associated with the mandible suggest sequestra and tooth root involvement. Fistulography may be useful in the evaluation of these infections (Fig. 10–7).

NEOPLASIA

Primary bone tumors in the horse are relatively rare. Osteomas are usually osteoblastic and well marginated and often involve the rostral portion of the mandible (Fig. 10–8). Tumors of dental germ origin appear most often in the mandible. These lesions may have irregular areas of osseous opacity within the mass and appear polycystic (see Fig. 10–11).[8, 17, 18] Ameloblastic odontomas have been reported in the maxilla of young horses; these tumors may contain radiopaque, tooth-like structures.[19]

CONGENITAL LESIONS

Malformations of the occipital bone and the first two cervical vertebrae (occipitoatlantoaxial malformations) are common in the Arabian breed (Fig. 10–9). Several variations are reported, but there is usually hypoplasia of the atlas with fusion to the occiput (occipitalization of the atlas) accompanied by hypoplasia of the axis, which may resemble an atlas. These defects are associated with a variety of clinical signs owing to compressive myelopathy.[20, 21]

Dentigerous cysts (temporal teratomas) usually develop at

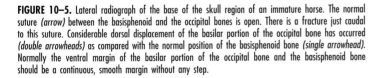

FIGURE 10–5. Lateral radiograph of the base of the skull region of an immature horse. The normal suture *(arrow)* between the basisphenoid and the occipital bones is open. There is a fracture just caudal to this suture. Considerable dorsal displacement of the basilar portion of the occipital bone has occurred *(double arrowheads)* as compared with the normal position of the basisphenoid bone *(single arrowhead).* Normally the ventral margin of the basilar portion of the occipital bone and the basisphenoid bone should be a continuous, smooth margin without any step.

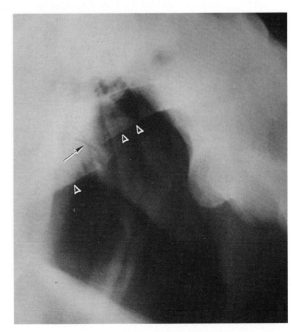

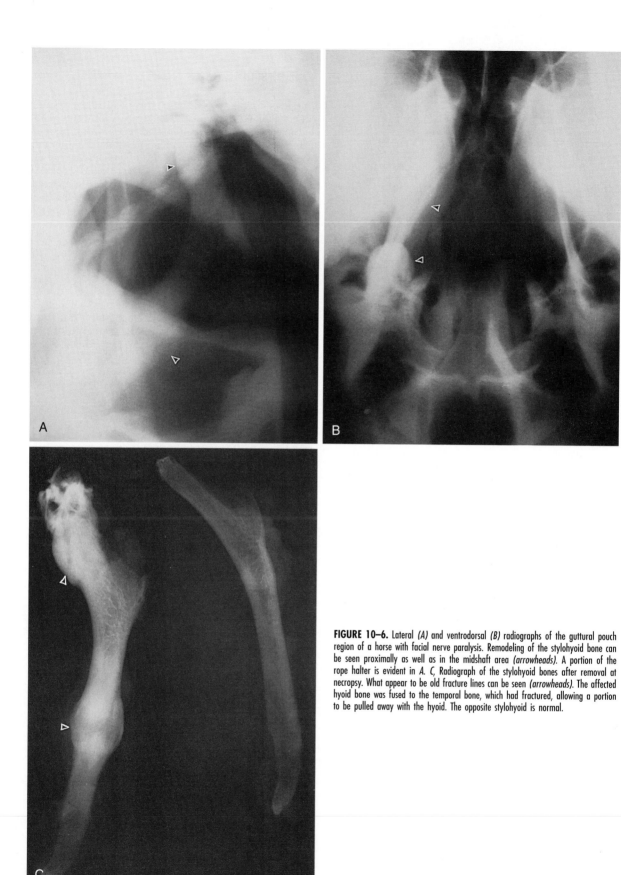

FIGURE 10–6. Lateral *(A)* and ventrodorsal *(B)* radiographs of the guttural pouch region of a horse with facial nerve paralysis. Remodeling of the stylohyoid bone can be seen proximally as well as in the midshaft area *(arrowheads)*. A portion of the rope halter is evident in *A. C,* Radiograph of the stylohyoid bones after removal at necropsy. What appear to be old fracture lines can be seen *(arrowheads)*. The affected hyoid bone was fused to the temporal bone, which had fractured, allowing a portion to be pulled away with the hyoid. The opposite stylohyoid is normal.

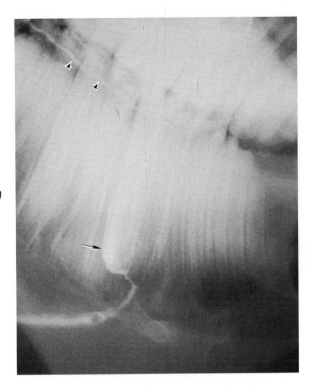

FIGURE 10–7. Positive-contrast fistulogram. Contrast medium can be seen around the tooth root *(arrow)* and in the mouth *(arrowheads)*. Diagnosis was alveolar periostitis with a secondary draining tract.

the base of the ear from misplaced dental germinal cells. A fistula forms near the ear. Radiography may reveal a tooth-like radiopaque structure within the soft-tissue mass (Fig. 10–10).[22]

Polycystic lesions are occasionally seen in the mandible or maxilla in young horses and are believed to be congenital, non-neoplastic cysts. They may attain considerable size and grossly distort the affected bone. Differentiation of these lesions from dental germ neoplasms is not possible radiographically (Fig. 10–11).[22]

Retained deciduous premolars (caps) often cause undulating swellings along the ventral ramus of the mandible. Retained deciduous premolars are easily seen radiographically (Fig. 10–12).

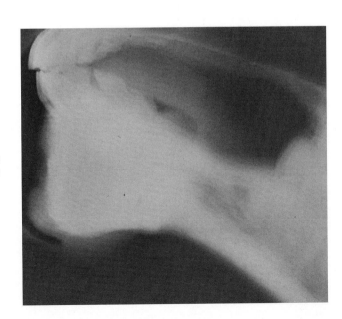

FIGURE 10–8. Lateral view of the rostral mandible in which a smooth-margined mandibular mass canbe seen. Diagnosis was osteoma. Long-standing inflammatory disease can also produce this radiographic appearance.

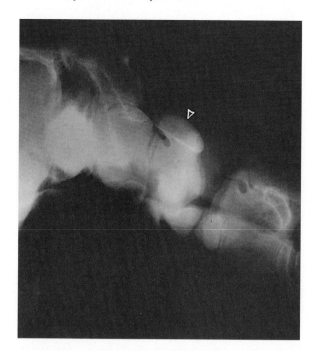

FIGURE 10–9. Lateral radiograph of the atlanto-occipital region of an Arabian foal. The normal occipital condyles are not present, and there is fusion of the atlas to the occipital bone *(arrowhead).*

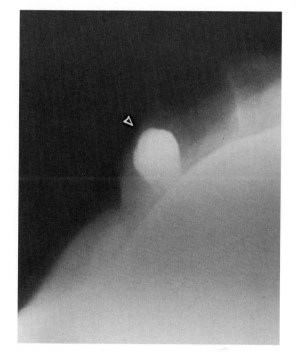

FIGURE 10–10. Oblique radiograph of the temporal region of a young horse. The radiopaque object *(arrowhead)* just rostral to the base of the ear is a dentigerous cyst, which contains a vestigial tooth.

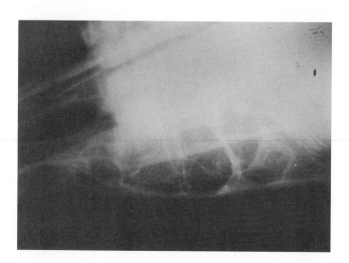

FIGURE 10–11. Oblique lateral view of the mandible of a young horse. A large polycystic lesion is present in the mandible. The major diagnoses to rule out in a lesion of this appearance in a young horse include congenital polycystic bone lesions or a dentigerous neoplasm. A biopsy is necessary for definitive diagnosis.

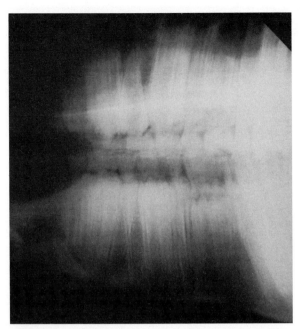

FIGURE 10–12. Lateral radiograph of the midportion of the maxilla and mandible in a 3-year-old horse. The typical irregular outlines of retained deciduous premolars (caps) can be seen on all premolar teeth.

References

1. Getty R (Ed): Sisson and Grossman's The Anatomy of the Domestic Animals, 5th Ed. Philadelphia, WB Saunders, 1975.
2. Schebitz H, and Wilkens H: Atlas of Radiographic Anatomy of the Horse, 3rd Ed. Philadelphia, WB Saunders, 1978.
3. Butler JA, Colles CM, Dyson SJ, et al: Clinical Radiology of the Horse. Oxford, Blackwell Scientific Publications, 1993.
4. Gibbs C: The equine skull: Its radiological investigation. J Am Vet Radiol Soc 15:70, 1974.
5. Lane JG, Gibbs C, Meynink SE, et al: Radiographic examination of the facial, nasal and paranasal sinus regions of the horse: I. Indications and procedures in 235 cases. Equine Vet J 19:466, 1987.
6. Gibbs C, and Lane JG: Radiographic examination of the facial, nasal, and paranasal sinus regions of the horse: II. Radiological findings. Equine Vet J 19:474, 1987.
7. Caron JP, Barber SM, Bailey JV, et al: Periorbital skull fractures in five horses. J Am Vet Med Assoc 188:280, 1986.
8. Cook WR: Skeletal radiology of the equine head. J Am Vet Radiol Soc 11:35, 1970.
9. Stick JA, Wilson T, and Kunze D: Basilar skull fractures in three horses. J Am Vet Med Assoc 176:228, 1980.
10. Ackerman N, Coffman JR, and Corley EA: The spheno-occipital suture in the horse: Its normal radiographic appearance. J Am Vet Radiol Soc 15:79, 1974.
11. Darien BJ, Watrous BJ, Huber MJ, et al: What is your diagnosis? J Am Vet Med Assoc 198:1799, 1991.
12. Sweeney CR, Freeman DE, Sweeney RW, et al: Hemorrhage into the guttural pouch (auditory tube diverticulum) associated with rupture of the longus capitis muscle in three horses. J Am Vet Med Assoc 202:1129, 1993.
13. Power HT, Watrous BJ, and de Lahunta A: Facial and vestibulocochlear nerve disease in six horses. J Am Vet Med Assoc 183:1076, 1983.
14. Blythe LL, Watrous BJ, Schmitz JA, et al: Vestibular syndrome associated with temporohyoid joint fusion and temporal bone fracture in three horses. J Am Vet Med Assoc 185:775, 1984.
15. Hurtig BM, Barber SM, and Farrow CS: Temporomandibular luxation in a horse. J Am Vet Med Assoc 185:78, 1984.
16. Shiroma JT: What is your diagnosis? J Am Vet Med Assoc 198:1663, 1991.
17. Hanselka DV, Roberts RE, and Thompson RB: Adamantinoma of the equine mandible. Vet Clin North Am [Small Anim Pract] 69:57, 1974.
18. Vaughan JT, and Bartels JE: Equine mandibular adamantinoma. J Am Vet Med Assoc 153:454, 1968.
19. Roberts MC, Groenendyk S, and Kelly WR: Ameloblastic odontoma in a foal. Equine Vet J 10:91, 1978.
20. Mayhew IG, Watson AG, and Heissan JA: Congenital occipitoatlantoaxial malformations in the horse. Equine Vet J 10:103, 1978.
21. Mayhew IG, and MacKay RJ: The nervous system. In Mansmann RA, McAllister ES, and Pratt PW (Eds): Equine Medicine and Surgery, 3rd Ed, Vol 2. Santa Barbara, CA, American Veterinary Publications, 1982, pp 1159–1252.
22. Baker GJ: Diseases of the teeth and paranasal sinuses. In Mansmann RA, McAllister ES, and Pratt PW (Eds): Equine Medicine and Surgery, 3rd Ed, Vol 1. Santa Barbara, CA, American Veterinary Publications, 1982, pp 437–458.
23. Jackman BR, and Baxter GM: Treatment of a mandibular bone cyst by use of a corticocancellous bone graft in a horse. J Am Vet Med Assoc 201:892, 1992.

STUDY QUESTIONS

1. This slightly oblique radiograph of the rostral mandible (Fig. 10–13) was made of an 8-year-old horse with soft tissue swelling ventral to the mandible. What abnormal radiographic signs are present, and what is the assessment?

2. This ventrodorsal skull radiograph (Fig. 10–14) was made of a 6-year-old horse with unilateral left chronic facial nerve paralysis. There was a possibility of previous head trauma. What abnormal radiographic signs are present, and what is the assessment?

3. This lateral skull radiograph (Fig. 10–15) was made of an 11-year-old horse with acute head trauma. The horse was cast in the stall, and the head was trapped against the wall. What abnormal radiographic signs are present, and what is the assessment? (The metallic opacity adjacent to the occipital condyle is an artifact and not clinically significant.)

4. Radiography of the equine skull is aided by
   A. lack of extensive soft tissue covering.
   B. relative thinness of certain bones.
   C. air in the nasal passages and sinuses.
   D. all of the above.
   E. none of the above.

5. In a horse that has fallen backwards, a transverse lucent line seen on a lateral radiograph between the basisphenoid and the basioccipital bones always indicates a fracture. (True or False)

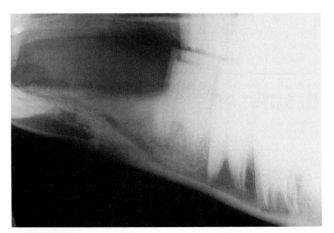

FIGURE 10–13

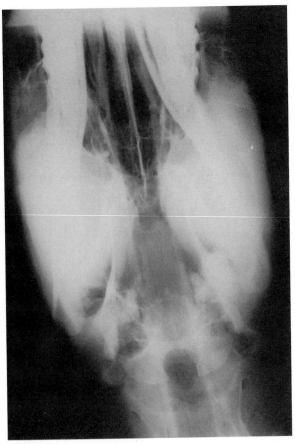

FIGURE 10-14

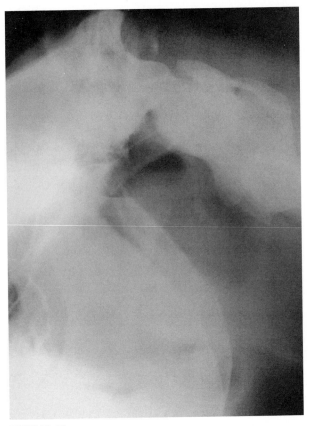

FIGURE 10-15

6. Lateral radiographs are usually the most useful views for evaluation of mandibular trauma or tooth root infection. (True or False)

7. Fusion of the stylohyoid-temporal joint:
   A. may result from infection of the middle ear or guttural pouch.
   B. usually is not characterized by radiographic abnormalities.
   C. may be diagnosed only with the use of computed tomography.
   D. is normal.
   E. none of the above.

8. Dentigerous cysts would most probably occur on the:
   A. mandible.
   B. maxilla.
   C. temporal bone.
   D. occipital bone.
   E. none of the above.

9. Primary bone tumors in horses occur most frequently on the limbs and almost never on the head. (True or False)

10. "Caps" in regard to equine teeth are _____.

(Answers appear on page 634 and 635.)

Chapter 11

Equine Nasal Passages and Sinuses*

Jimmy C. Lattimer

Radiographic examination is a useful technique for assessing disease of the paranasal sinuses and nasal cavity in the horse. In one report, radiography was useful in establishing a diagnosis in 90 percent of patients.[1] The decision to make radiographs should be based on the need to answer specific questions indicated by the clinical and physical findings, such as nasal discharge, nasal airway obstruction, facial swelling, epistaxis (particularly unilateral), dental defects, draining tracts, epiphora, and facial deformity.[2]

The task of radiographing the head of a conscious horse may be formidable. Many horses are frightened by the proce-

*See Chapter 33 for discussion of the guttural pouches.

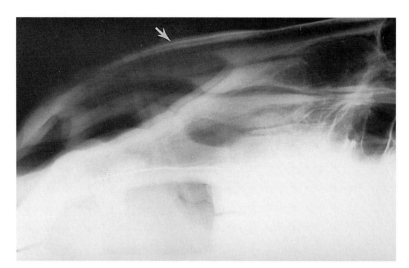

FIGURE 11–1. Lateral view, rostral portion of the nasal passage. Note that the only bone support for the nares is ventral. *Arrow* shows the long narrow rostral projection of the nasal bone.

dure. There is also the problem that most horses, while standing, are in motion from respiration and postural shifting. Thus, anesthesia has been recommended for radiographic projections other than the lateral projection.[2] The need to induce general anesthesia to obtain satisfactory radiographs makes the decision to radiograph the skull difficult, especially in a clinically ill animal. Generally, more margin for technical error exists if high kVp, low mAs techniques are used; they also result in reduced exposure times.

One of the greatest deterrents to radiography of the equine head is the complexity of the image. When radiographic anatomy is so complex, it is easy to overlook even relatively major lesions. It is therefore imperative that a systematic method of evaluating the radiograph be used. It is also necessary that some type of radiographic anatomy reference be consulted because comparison of the radiograph with a known normal image usually resolves any questions regarding whether or not a structure in question is abnormal. Remember, however, that there are slight individual variations in anatomic structure, and minor differences in positioning may radically alter these radiographic and anatomic relationships, making comparisons with reference material difficult.

Many possible radiographic projections of the skull may be made, but it is not necessary to perform them all in any given patient. The clinical signs of the patient dictate the radiographic projections to be made. This is especially true when facial trauma or distortion is present. Radiographs should be made in such a way that any visible alteration in the shape of the head is projected tangentially. Occasionally, especially in instances of dental disease, the disease is best evaluated by positioning the central ray of the x-ray beam perpendicular to the area of the lesion, that is, en face. As a rule, however, the tangential projection is usually more rewarding. When there are no externally visible defects, the standard lateral, ventrodorsal, and oblique views should be made initially. Once abnormalities are detected on these views, further projections may be tailored to evaluate the disease process more completely if necessary.

NORMAL ANATOMY

Nasal Cavity

The minimal radiographic examination of the equine nasal passages should include right and left lateral and ventrodorsal

views. Because of the thickness of the head, two lateral views are needed to help differentiate on which side unilateral lesions are located. The ventrodorsal view is used to make this determination on lesions near the midline, but this view cannot be used for lesions away from the midline because the mandible and teeth obscure much of these areas in the ventrodorsal projection.

On the lateral view, the most rostral part of the nasal passage in the horse is composed principally of soft tissue. The rostral one fourth of the nasal passage either is surrounded completely by soft tissue or is supported ventrally only by bone (Fig. 11–1). The rostral nasal passage is usually more easily examined by palpation and endoscopic examination.

The nasal passage caudal to the second maxillary premolar is surrounded by and contains bony structures. The maxillary, nasal, palatine, and vomer bones form the limits of the nasal passage; the dorsal, middle, ventral, and ethmoid turbinates are contained within the passage.[3] Contained within the alveolar recesses of the maxilla are the large maxillary premolars and molars. Usually, it is not possible to delineate the individual bones of the skull. Likewise, it is difficult to identify specific turbinates, other than the ethmoid, as individual structures. A number of external and internal landmarks, however, serve as reference points (Fig. 11–2).[4]

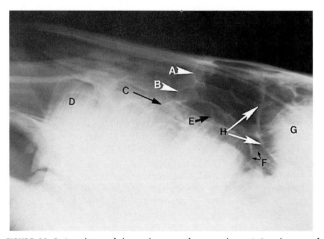

FIGURE 11–2. Lateral view of the nasal passage of a young horse. *A,* Rostral margin of dorsal conchal sinus. *B,* Rostral margin of ventral conchal sinus. *C,* Rostral margin of maxillary sinus. *D,* First maxillary cheek tooth. *E,* Intermaxillary septum. *F,* Intraorbital canal. *G,* Ethmoid turbinates. *H,* Rostral margin of the frontal sinus.

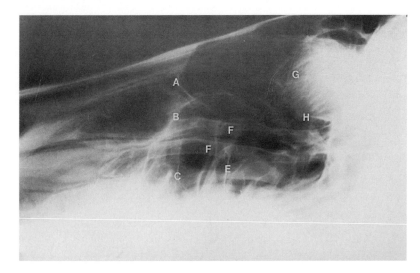

FIGURE 11–3. Slightly oblique, lateral view of the caudal nasal passage in a 12-year-old horse. *A,* Rostral margin of dorsal conchal sinus. *B,* Rostral margin of ventral conchal sinus. *C,* Rostral margin of maxillary sinus. *E,* Intermaxillary septum. *F,* Infraorbital canal. *G,* Ethmoid turbinates. *H,* Rostral margin of the frontal sinus.

The most obvious extranasal landmarks on the lateral view of the nasal passage are the large molars and premolars, although they are partially surrounded by the sinuses. These teeth provide a constant point of reference for lesion localization. It is always advisable to use a field of view of sufficient size so that either the second premolar or the third molar is identifiable. Another external structure that is usually evident over the caudal portion of the nasal passage is the zygomatic arch, which is also superimposed over the orbit. The zygomatic arch continues rostrally as a linear region of bone opacity, which represents the facial crest. Depending on the exact cassette orientation and exposure factors used, the facial crest may or may not be apparent. Identification of the facial crest and first maxillary molar is important in that their rostral limits define the rostral limits of the caudal and rostral maxillary sinuses. Because the two compartments of the maxillary sinus do not usually communicate except in mules and donkeys, it is important to determine which of the cavities is affected.[3, 5]

Internal nasal cavity landmarks include the rostral limits of the dorsal and ventral conchal sinuses, the rostral limits of the maxillary sinus, and the ethmoid turbinates (see Fig. 11–2). These landmarks basically define the limits of the paranasal sinuses, making it possible to determine if the disease process being observed involves the sinuses, the nasal cavity, or both.

The ethmoid turbinates are the most consistently placed of the internal landmarks. They mark the caudal limit of the nasal cavity and are, for radiographic purposes, interposed between the maxillary and the frontal sinuses on the lateral projection. The finely scrolled bones of the ethmoid turbinates are readily visible as numerous fine, linear opacities that rise from the cribriform plate (Fig. 11–3).

The rostral limit of the maxillary sinus is immediately dorsal to the root of the fourth premolar and may vary somewhat in position from horse to horse and with age; it may be completely obscured in young horses owing to tooth overlap. The dorsal and ventral conchal sinuses do not extend as far rostrally as the maxillary sinuses. The thin plates of bone that define their rostral margins are usually seen dorsal to the first maxillary molar. The dorsal sinus is located just below the nasal bone; the ventral sinus is just beneath the dorsal sinus and extends slightly more rostrally.[4, 6, 7] The middle conchal sinus in the horse is small, and landmarks attributable to it are not usually observed. The nasal turbinates are not recognized as well-defined structures and are represented only as multiple scalloped opacities in the dorsal caudal portion of the nasal passage.

In young horses, the long roots of premolars two through four and the molars overlap and obscure much of the ventral portion of the nasal passage and paranasal sinuses when seen on the lateral view (see Fig. 11–2). Continuous tooth wear as the animal ages results in shortening of these roots. By the time the horse is 15 to 20 years old, the roots of the teeth do not obscure as much of the nasal passage and sinuses (Fig. 11–4). Thus, abnormalities of the nasal passage may be more readily apparent in older animals.

On the ventrodorsal projection, much of the nasal passage and paranasal sinuses are obscured by the mandible and the teeth. Therefore, the usefulness of the ventrodorsal view is limited principally to evaluating midline structures. The nasal septum and common meatus are well visualized on the ventrodorsal view. In contrast to in the dog,[8] the nasal septum in the horse, along with its attached mucosa, contributes markedly to the midline opacity of the nasal cavity.[9] The septal structures are represented by a linear but slightly bulging radiopacity bordered on either side by the radiolucent common nasal meatus (Fig. 11–5). Slight obliquity of the projection affects both the projected width of the septum and the relative widths of the common nasal meati, making detection and description of disease difficult. Therefore, good positioning on the ventrodorsal view is mandatory.

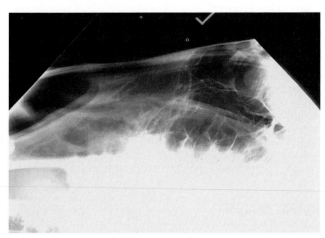

FIGURE 11–4. Lateral view of the nasal passages in a 21-year-old horse. The teeth have almost completely receded from the nasal passage allowing a clear view of the maxillary and ventral conchal sinuses. Only the fourth premolar has any significant overlap with the nasal passage.

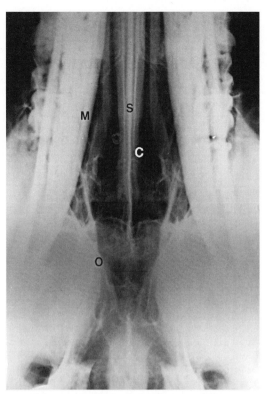

FIGURE 11–5. Ventrodorsal view of the nasal passage. M, medial border of mandible; S, nasal septum; O, medial wall of orbit; C, common nasal meatus.

Paranasal Sinuses

The paranasal sinuses of the horse are large and complex. Together with the nasal cavity, they account for most of the volume of the skull. There are six pairs of sinuses in the horse. The dorsal, middle, and ventral conchal sinuses are within the turbinates of the same name. Lateral to the nasal cavity is the maxillary sinus, which is divided into rostral and caudal compartments. Dorsal and caudal to the nasal cavity is the frontal sinus. Ventral and caudal to the nasal cavity and the ethmoid turbinates is the sphenopalatine sinus. All of the sinus cavities on one side of the skull communicate freely, with one exception. The rostral maxillary sinus generally does not communicate with the remaining paranasal sinuses except in some mules or donkeys.[3, 5] The frontal sinus communicates with the dorsal conchal and caudal maxillary sinuses; the caudal maxillary sinus communicates with the frontal, middle conchal, sphenopalatine, and ventral conchal sinuses.

More precise delineation of the dimensions and limits of the paranasal sinuses with the use of positive-contrast sinusography has been described as a more sensitive means of detecting small lesions of the paranasal sinuses.[6, 11] This technique is potentially useful in differentiating between normal anatomic structures and abnormalities within the sinuses, especially when the lesions are small. Description of large lesions should be possible without resort to sinusography.

The maxillary sinuses are relatively larger in the mule and the donkey than in the horse.[5] The septum between the two compartments of the maxillary sinus is usually visible as a thin, angled (vertically to slightly caudally) bone plate dorsal to the first molar (see Figs. 11–3 and 11–8B).[4] In mules and donkeys, the septum is more irregular and less laminar in appearance than is seen in horses. This septum may not be seen if there is obliquity to the radiograph because the thin

plate is easily overpenetrated unless it is oriented parallel to the x-ray beam. The septum is also visible on oblique projections of the maxillary sinus (see Fig. 11–18), that is, a ventral 15-degree lateral-dorsal medial view (Fig. 11–6). This view allows most of the lateral portion of the maxillary sinus to be seen in profile without the interference of the overlying teeth. Both sides of the skull must be examined radiographically to serve as an internal control. It is easy to interpret the opacity of the overlying masseter muscle incorrectly as fluid in the sinus if the angle of the projection is not optimal. The 15-degree oblique projection usually provides better evaluation of the maxillary sinus than does the lateral view or the more conventional 30- to 40-degree oblique view, which is designed to project the roots of the molars and premolars rather than the sinuses.

Identification of the septum between the compartments of the maxillary sinus allows the determination of which of the two compartments is affected by disease. Fluid is more readily retained within the rostral compartment because the nasomaxillary opening of the sinus is located at the highest point in the sinus.[3] The nasomaxillary opening of the sinus is common to both the rostral and the caudal maxillary sinuses, but it is divided by the septum. This aperture, which empties into the middle nasal meatus, is usually the sole site of drainage of the paranasal sinus system into the nasal cavity; it is not radiographically visible.

The rostral limit of the maxillary sinus is just dorsal to the fourth premolar and is often obscured on the lateral projection by the molars and premolars in younger animals. This cranial extremity is more readily seen on the ventral 15-degree lateral-dorsal medial view of the maxillary sinus (see Figs. 11–6 and 11–19).

The infraorbital canal passes longitudinally through the maxillary sinus, dividing it into lateral and medial portions. The caudal medial compartment communicates with the sphenopalatine and middle conchal sinuses. The infraorbital canal is located immediately dorsal to the roots of the teeth; in the young animal, it is virtually in contact with them as they project into the maxillary sinus. The canal is usually seen as a band of increased opacity that runs longitudinally just above the teeth on the lateral view (see Figs. 11–3 and 11–4) but is not readily seen on oblique and ventrodorsal

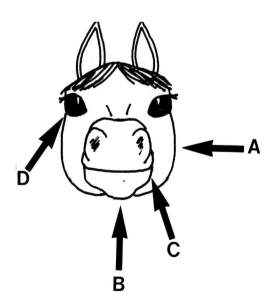

FIGURE 11–6. Projections for examination of the nasal passages and sinuses. A, Lateral view. B, Ventrodorsal view. C, Ventral 15-degree lateral-dorsomedial view of maxillary sinus. D, Ventral 30-degree lateral-dorsomedial view of orbit.

projections.[3, 7, 12] The normal root shortening occurring with aging results in better visibility of the maxillary sinus and leaves the infraorbital canal more obviously in the middle of the sinus on the lateral view (see Fig. 11–4).

The caudal limits of the maxillary sinus are difficult to recognize radiographically. Its communication with the sphenopalatine sinus, the overlying teeth and ethmoid turbinates, and the vertical mandibular ramus makes the caudal limits indistinct. Fortunately, identification of the caudal limit is not usually necessary. For the purposes of radiographic interpretation, the maxillary sinus ends at the level of the ethmoid turbinates caudally and at the level of the frontal sinus caudodorsally. It should be recognized that the third molar projects into the caudal part of the caudal maxillary sinus.

The frontal sinus is dorsocaudal to the nasal cavity; its radiographic limits are not as extensive as its anatomic limits because of the presence of overlying bone. It is relatively larger in the donkey than in the horse and mule.[5] Radiographically, there are two parts to the frontal sinus: the roughly triangular dorsocaudal portion and the portion rostral to the orbit (see Fig. 11–3). The triangular part is dorsal and caudal to the ethmoid turbinates on the lateral view and tends to be radiolucent in the normal horse. The marked radiolucency is due to the relatively great width of the sinus at this point. This part of the frontal sinus communicates with the maxillary sinus through the frontomaxillary opening.[3] The rostral portion of the sinus is rostrodorsal to the ethmoid turbinates and has a scalloped cranial margin that is dorsal to the second molar; this margin is readily seen on many radiographs.[3] The rostral portion of the frontal sinus communicates openly with and is continued forward by the dorsal conchal sinus. The dorsal conchal sinus usually terminates at the rostral margin of the first molar; it is superimposed over the dorsal one half of the nasal passage and is somewhat tubular. Other than the most caudal portion of the frontal sinus, the dorsal conchal sinus is the most medial of the paranasal sinuses. It virtually touches the midline, owing to the small size of the dorsal nasal meatus. Because it is located so close to the midline, it is superimposed over the nasal passage on the ventrodorsal projection. Filling of the dorsal conchal and frontal sinuses with fluid or tissue causes increased opacity in these areas, and incomplete filling may lead to the formation of a fluid level in standing lateral radiographs.

The sphenopalatine sinuses are relatively small in the horse and usually are not recognized as separate entities. This fact is due in part to their size as well as to the marked opacity of the vertical rami of the mandibles. If recognized, they are small radiolucent areas just ventral to the cranial vault and caudal to the ethmoid turbinates. Their caudal termination is usually at about the level of the temporomandibular joint.[7]

RADIOGRAPHIC ABNORMALITIES

Diseases of the Nasal Passage

Clinical signs of nasal disease consist of nasal discharge, noisy or restricted respiration, facial distortion, dental defects, sinus tracts, epiphora, and epistaxis, in any combination.[1, 2] The list of possible differential diagnoses indicated by these clinical signs is long and includes both local and systemic diseases. Diseases such as infectious rhinitis, purpura hemorrhagica, congestive heart failure, emphysema, and pneumonia may cause nasal discharge or epistaxis, but these conditions are unlikely to result in significant radiographic abnormalities, unless there is fluid collection in the sinuses.[12–15]

Fractures of the nasal bones are common. Any visible facial deformity is frequently less pronounced than the underlying bone injury. Profuse epistaxis is usually associated with the acute injury.[17] A chronic mucopurulent discharge may develop if the fracture is untreated and a piece of depressed bone triggers an infectious or foreign body reaction. Radiographically and clinically a fracture of the nasal region is usually recognized as a depressed area in the bone (Fig. 11–7). Occasionally a large piece of bone is depressed into the nasal passages or into a sinus (Figs. 11–8 and 11–9).[17] The true extent and severity of the fracture are usually difficult to delineate on radiographs, and the fracture is almost invariably found to be more extensive at surgery. When the nasal passage is examined radiographically, it is a good idea to obtain at least one projection that is tangent to the surface of suspected fracture. The nasal bones are quite thin, and if a fracture fragment is not struck edge-on by the x-ray beam, it may not be recognized. Tangential projections have the best chance of allowing displaced fragments to be detected. It may be difficult to recognize a fracture on one view, whereas it is obvious on another. Therefore, standard lateral and ventrodorsal projections should also be obtained.

Foreign bodies are another source of trauma to the nasal passage, but they are uncommon. Small foreign bodies are often not problematic, but large objects, such as sticks, wire, and bullets, may lodge within the nasal passage and cause a foreign body reaction (Fig. 11–10). Foreign bodies in the ventral and common meatus may be detected and removed by endoscopic procedures. In other instances, however, radiography may be needed to localize the problem, especially if the foreign body is in the dorsal or lateral portion of the nasal cavity. A foreign body reaction within the nasal passage usually appears as a poorly defined area of increased radiopacity. If the foreign body is radiopaque, it is generally visible in the middle of the area of increased opacity. Objects such as sticks are usually not recognizable radiographically. Because foreign bodies are usually unilateral, their location may be detected on the ventrodorsal view.

Uncomplicated rhinitis is unlikely to result in radiographic change. Only if rhinitis is associated with sinusitis or some other abnormality, such as a foreign body and a nasal deformity, is it likely to be radiographically obvious. The most one may expect to perceive is a slight increase in opacity of the nasal passage and perhaps a slight narrowing of the airways on the ventrodorsal view. These are subtle findings that are highly susceptible to aberrations in technique and positioning

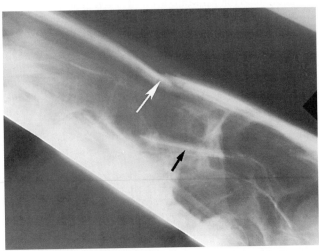

FIGURE 11–7. Depressed nasal bone fracture. Direct trauma resulted in slight depression of the nasal bone (white arrow). A larger fragment of the maxilla (black arrow) was displaced into the nasal cavity.

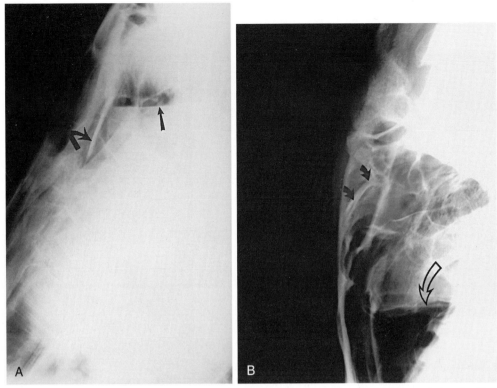

FIGURE 11–8. *A,* Depressed maxillary bone fracture with displacement of sharp cortical fragments into the maxillary sinus *(curved arrow)*. Note gas-fluid interface (fluid line) within the maxillary sinus *(straight arrow)*. *B,* Fluid in the caudal maxillary sinus. This animal suffered a fracture into the maxillary sinus *(black arrows)* and subsequently developed sinusitis. This radiograph clearly indicates the division between the rostral and caudal maxillary sinus along the air-fluid interface *(open arrow)*.

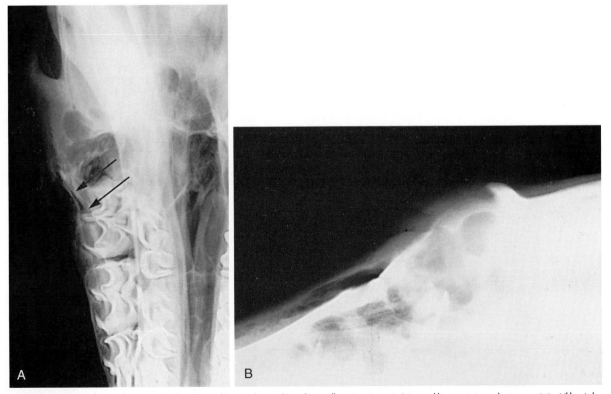

FIGURE 11–9. Blunt trauma to the maxillary sinus. *A,* A large piece of bone is depressed into the maxillary sinus *(arrows)*. *B,* In an oblique projection, subcutaneous air is visible; air has migrated from the sinus into the subcutaneous tissues. The likelihood of infection is high in such an instance.

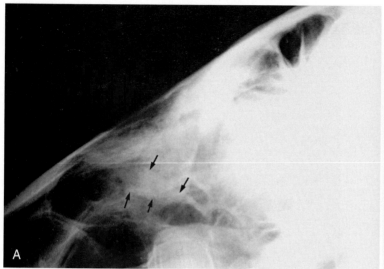

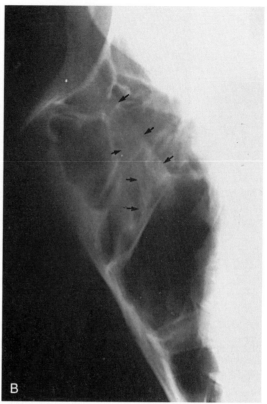

FIGURE 11–10. Foreign body (wood) in the maxillary sinus. *A,* Lateral view. *B,* Oblique view. After a collision with a fence, this horse had a skin wound over the face and profuse unilateral epistaxis. There is a well-marginated foreign opacity in the maxillary sinus *(arrows)*. Two fragments of lumber and bone fragments were removed from the sinus.

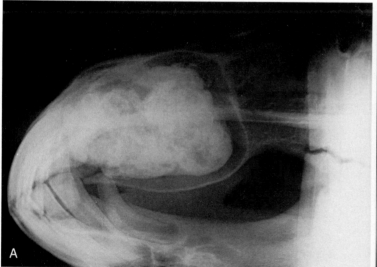

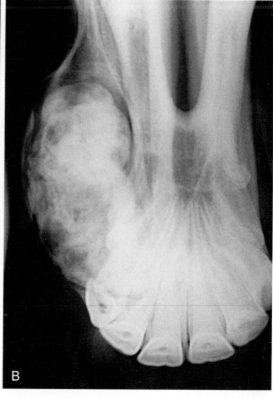

FIGURE 11–11. Osteoma. *A,* Lateral view. *B,* Ventrodorsal view. A large amorphous bone opaque mass is located in the left maxilla. The mass is contained within a larger radiolucent space, which is the result of expansion of the space between the inner and outer layers of the maxilla. This mass was causing substantial distortion of the maxilla.

and should be supported by other diagnostic procedures before a diagnosis of rhinitis is made.

Nasal tumors are uncommon in the horse but occasionally occur. The nasal passage may be the primary site of the tumor, or it may be secondarily invaded from one of the sinuses. Benign lesions are usually osteomas or adamantinomas and occur in young animals.[17, 19] These neoplasms may present as expansile radiolucent lesions (adamantinoma) or as well-defined bony expansile lesions (osteoma or odontoma) (Figs. 11–11 and 11–12). Benign tumors such as these may not produce clinical signs and therefore may be large before a diagnosis is made.

Malignant lesions, usually adenocarcinomas, occur in older animals and are invasive, grow rapidly, and are ill-defined.[1, 12, 14, 19] The clinical signs are usually unilateral mucopurulent nasal discharge, epistaxis, facial deformities, and upper airway obstruction. The severity and characteristics of the clinical signs depend on the stage and location of the disease when first evaluated. Radiographically, malignancies are of soft-tissue opacity and are ill defined (Fig. 11–13). There may be lysis of the turbinate and facial bones and in rare instances invasion of the cranial vault through the cribriform plate.[20] Distortion or destruction of the nasal septum may be obvious on the ventrodorsal view, and advanced tumors may have bilateral involvement or may project caudally into the nasopharynx.

Intranasal cysts usually occur in young animals and may be congenital.[1] These lesions are large, fluid-filled structures within the nasal passage or sinuses. They may cause facial deformity and nasal discharge, but because of their benign nature, intranasal cysts are usually large when detected. Radiographically, these cysts appear as large, well-defined areas of increased opacity in the nasal passage; they may be single or multiple, unilateral or bilateral (Fig. 11–14). As they grow, these lesions displace bone structures, especially turbinates. The nasal septum often appears displaced. There is nothing radiographically that distinguishes a cyst from a large, well-defined soft-tissue tumor or ethmoid hematoma, other than possibly the location of the lesion. A well-defined dental structure or aberration in dentition, however, may be evident, as with an intranasal dentigerous cyst (Fig. 11–15). Fluid accumulation in both the sinuses and the nasal cavity may result from occlusion of the drainage pathway by large cysts.

Non-neoplastic polyps are often seen in the nasal passage of young horses. These lesions are usually composed of granulation tissue and are probably associated with chronic inflammation.[15, 21] Polyps may be recognized radiographically as relatively well-defined areas of increased opacity in the nasal passage; they vary in size and number. Clinical signs may be delayed until the polyps are of sufficient size or number to interfere with respiration.

Deviation of the nasal septum is easily detected on the ventrodorsal projection. This deviation may result from an intrinsic disease, such as cyst formation, or from pressure by a mass within the nasal passage or may be present as a benign anatomic variation with no clinical significance (Fig. 11–16). The degree and site of deviation are usually obvious, but the underlying cause may be difficult to determine.

A special form of cystic disease occurs in the nasal septum. Varying amounts of the nasal septum in the young horse may undergo cystic degeneration because of trauma or infection.[22] The nasal septum widens substantially and interferes with respiration. Both radiographic and endoscopic examinations of the nasal passages are needed to evaluate the extent and severity of the problem adequately. Cystic disease of the septum is one condition for which the ventrodorsal projection is mandatory. The lateral radiograph is of minimal help in determining the severity of the thickening of the septum, although it may aid in establishing the caudal limit of the thickening. Accurate evaluation of the extent of the lesion is imperative because surgical resection of the affected septal portion is the only effective treatment. Postoperative radiographic evaluation must wait until after the removal of the packing used to control the profuse hemorrhage induced by surgery. When the postoperative radiograph is evaluated, consideration must be given to the fact that although the nasal septum is a major contributor to the midline opacity of the nasal passages, it is not the only midline opacity.[9] Persistence of some midline opacity, therefore, does not indicate inadequate resection.

Progressive ethmoid hematoma is a slowly enlarging hematoma containing granulomatous reactions that originates from the submucosa of an ethmoid endoturbinate.[21, 23, 24] It is not known why the mass continues to enlarge because it is not neoplastic. Extension into the maxillary, frontal, and sphenopalatine sinuses as well as into the nasal cavity is common, as are distortion and destruction of the ethmoid and nasal turbinates and the nasal septum. The clinical signs of inspiratory stridor, coughing, choking, excessive salivation,

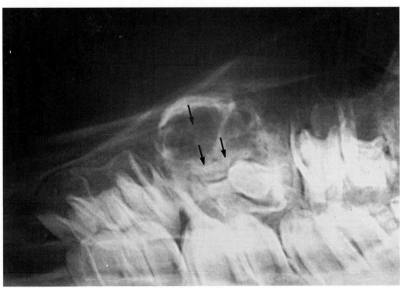

FIGURE 11–12. Oblique view of the maxilla. There is expansion of the alveolus of the fourth maxillary premolar. The premolar is decreased in size, and multiple tooth opacities *(arrows)* are noted within the expanded alveolus. Distortion of the maxilla is present. The diagnosis was maxillary odontoma.

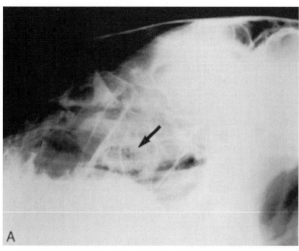

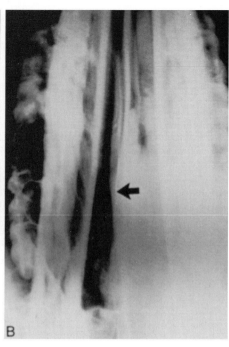

FIGURE 11–13. *A,* Lateral view. A large, poorly marginated soft-tissue opacity is present in the caudal left nasal cavity of this horse. Note the relative radiolucency *(arrow)* within the mass, representing myxomatous tissue heterogeneity. *B,* Ventrodorsal view. Slight displacement of the nasal septum to the right *(arrow)* is present. Diagnosis was nasal adenocarcinoma.

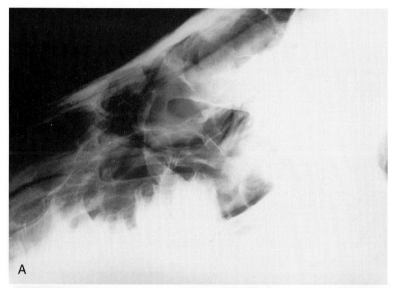

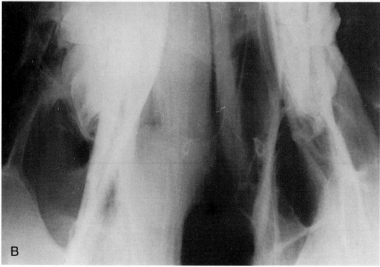

FIGURE 11–14. Large epithelial cyst in the right nasal passage. *A,* Lateral view. The mass is sharply marginated but appears to have less than fluid opacity because of its superimposition over the air-filled maxillary sinus and left nasal passage. Note the thickening of the frontal bone dorsal to the cyst as a reaction to pressure on the bone by the cyst. *B,* Ventrodorsal view. The cyst is completely occluding the right nasal passage and appears more radiopaque in *B* than in *A* owing to the relatively small amount of air superimposed over it.

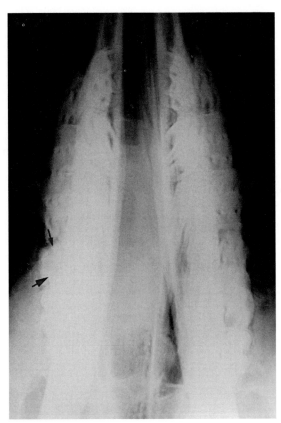

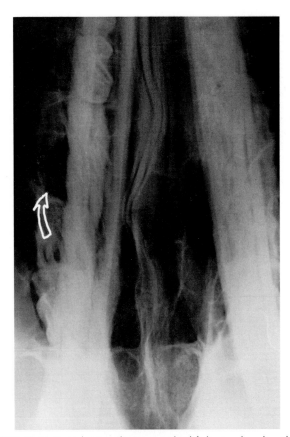

FIGURE 11–15. A large soft-tissue mass is displacing the nasal septum to the left and occluding the nasal passage on the right in a 3-year-old horse. Malformation of the right fourth maxillary premolar *(arrows)* is evident. A dentigerous cyst was found at surgery. This is an unusual manifestation of dentigerous cyst because most are not within the maxilla.

FIGURE 11–16. Deviated septum. This was an incidental finding in radiographs made for evaluation of the teeth. There was no nasal discharge or other clinical abnormality. The right first maxillary molar is missing *(arrow).*

purulent nasal discharge, halitosis, and head shaking are characteristic findings. Facial deformity may or may not be seen. There is often a history of chronic epistaxis. Endoscopically, there may be a large, smooth-walled, greenish mass in the caudal part of the nasal passage.[21, 23] A hematoma in the dorsal caudal portion of the nasal passage may not be visible endoscopically. Although the differential diagnosis for these clinical signs is extensive, a thorough physical examination combined with the result of endoscopic and radiographic examinations should make the diagnosis easy to establish.[24]

The radiographic examination of progressive ethmoid hematoma should consist of lateral, ventrodorsal, and oblique maxillary sinus projections. Single lesions are usually confined to one side of the nasal passage, but the lesion may deform the septum and the ethmoid turbinates. Multiple lesions are occasionally seen and may be on both sides of the septum. Ethmoid hematomas are usually seen as round, smooth-walled, soft-tissue masses arising from the region of the ethmoid turbinates (Fig. 11–17).[21, 23, 24] Calcification and air trapping within the lesion have not been described, and overt destruction of dense cortical bone is not a feature of this disorder. This may help distinguish it from malignant neoplasms, which also occur in the same areas. Because recurrence is common (40 to 50 percent), it is advisable to re-examine the animal at 6-month intervals for at least 2 years after the hematoma is removed.[24]

Diseases of the Paranasal Sinuses

Lesions in the paranasal sinuses tend to parallel those seen in the nasal cavity—fractures, cysts, tumors, and empyema. Ethmoid hematomas also invade the sinuses.[21, 23]

Fractures of the sinuses are similar to nasal bone fractures. Once again, the physical appearance of the head may not indicate the true extent of the lesion. When fracture fragments are depressed into a sinus, there is a great likelihood that infection will develop because of reduced drainage and air exchange. The radiographic approach to the diagnosis of paranasal sinus fractures is the same as for fractures of the nasal passage. Whenever it appears that a fracture line enters a sinus, special attention should be given to any increased opacity within the sinuses. Because of the interconnecting

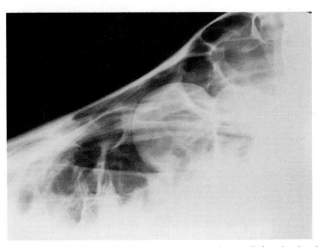

FIGURE 11–17. This large, round, well-margined mass protruding rostrally from the ethmoid region is an ethmoid hematoma.

nature of the sinuses and their limited drainage (see Fig. 11–2), infection or injury to a sinus may affect all of the sinuses on that side, and fluid lines and increased opacity within the sinuses may be seen quite removed from the actual site of injury.

As with the nasal cavity, benign sinus tumors are usually osteomas or adamantinomas that arise from or around the roots of the teeth within the maxillary sinus.[25] Malignant neoplasms are either primary (adenocarcinoma and fibrosarcoma) or secondary (extension or a squamous cell carcinoma from the orbit).[16, 21, 26] Malignant tumors are ill-defined, lobulated to diffuse, soft-tissue lesions. Lysis of cortical bone and deformity of the facial bones are common, as is periosteal new bone growth. Focal calcifications, radiolucencies, or both within the tumor mass may be seen (Fig. 11–18).[19] With primary tumors, much of the opacity within the sinuses may be the result of trapped secretions because the neoplasm obstructs the outflow from the nasomaxillary opening,[19] and encroachment on the nasal passage with displacement of the nasal septum may block the nasal passage. Thus, the area of increased opacity may be substantially larger than the true area of neoplastic involvement. The trapped secretions may also silhouette with the tumor and result in fluid lines on standing lateral projections mimicking the radiographic appearance of sinusitis.

Secondary invasion of the frontal sinus by squamous cell carcinoma of the orbit is an unusual but serious finding. There is usually obvious bone destruction of the orbit. Because of the possibility of orbital tumors extending through the bone into the frontal or maxillary sinus, it is advisable to make radiographic projections designed to project the orbital margins (see Figs. 11–6 and 11–18). Most orbital neoplasms do not invade the sinuses, but the markedly poorer prognosis in that event justifies the examination.

The most common disease of the sinuses necessitating radiographic evaluation is empyema,[27] and the most common cause of accumulation of exudate within a sinus is a periapical abscess of one of the premolar or molar teeth. The most commonly affected tooth is the first maxillary molar. Other causes include trauma, fungal granulomas, and neoplasms.[1, 21, 27] The clinical signs of sinusitis are poor condition, fetid nasal discharge, halitosis, and, occasionally, head shaking. There may be evidence of facial deformity if the infection is secondary to trauma. On physical examination, it may be possible to percuss a dull area in the region of fluid accumulation.

Endoscopic examination of the sinuses, other than to observe the nasomaxillary opening for drainage of exudate, is not possible.[27] Therefore, radiography is usually the primary means to evaluate sinus empyema. Sinus fluid is recognized

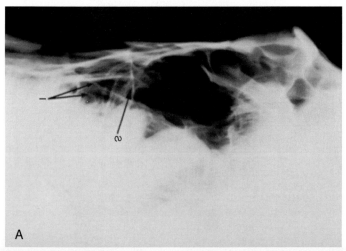

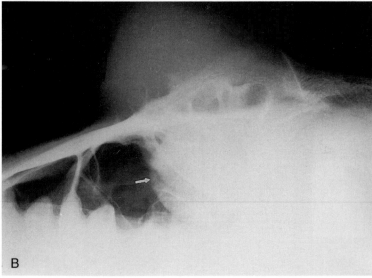

FIGURE 11–18. Ventral 15-degree lateral-dorsomedial projection of the maxillary sinus. *A,* Normal appearance. *B,* Invasion of sinus by a large squamous cell carcinoma arising from third eyelid. I, infraorbital canal; S, intermaxillary septum. *Arrow* shows margin of the invading neoplasm within the maxillary sinus.

by the presence of a homogeneous fluid opacity in the area of the suspected sinus; it is often possible to identify a fluid line within the sinus on horizontal-beam radiographs (Fig. 11–19).[15, 27] If the sinus is completely filled with fluid, no fluid line is present. It is then necessary to perform oblique projections of both sinuses to establish that one sinus is of greater radiopacity and therefore fluid filled. Left and right sinuses should be examined to avoid misdiagnosis of sinus empyema because of the mild increase in opacity caused by overlying muscles. In some instances, inspissated exudate within the ventral conchal sinus may result in a well-circumscribed, soft-tissue opacity overlying the nasal passages and teeth. Expansion of the sinus may result in encroachment on the nasal passages.[28] This radiographic appearance mimics that of paranasal sinus cysts and ethmoid hematomas, mandating histologic confirmation of the diagnosis. If sinusitis is the result of dental disease, there may also be sclerosis around the tooth root, if that is the source of the problem (see Fig. 11–19).[17] Correct identification of the tooth involved, however, is possible from radiographs in fewer than 50 percent of affected patients.[27] The periodontal membrane of the tooth is usually widened and decreased in definition. The alveolar bone over the root of the cheek teeth may be absent as a result of lysis, with no evidence of proliferation or sclerosis.[27] It is difficult to establish that a tooth is the source of the problem in these horses.

Cysts of congenital, dentigerous, or unknown origin occasionally occur in the paranasal sinuses.[2, 21, 28, 29] The maxillary sinus is the most commonly affected sinus, but cysts may occur in any sinus. Radiographically, opacification of the sinus is a consistent finding. Depending on the size of the cyst, discrete margins may or may not be seen. When the cysts are large, distortion of the facial bones and encroachment on the nasal passages may be seen. Free fluid accumulation, distortion of dentition, and mineralization and fragmentation of the frontal or maxillary bones are less common findings.[30] Definitive diagnosis from radiographs is not possible but is dependent on aspiration and analysis of fluid from the affected sinus.

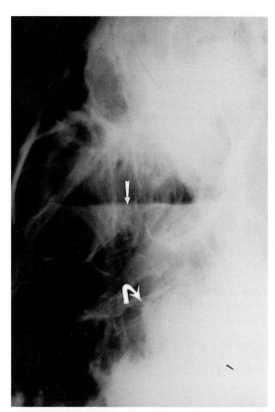

FIGURE 11–19. Fluid in the maxillary sinus secondary to a periapical abscess of the second maxillary molar. *Straight arrow* shows gas-fluid interface (fluid line). *Curved arrow* shows slight increase in opacity around the root of the second maxillary molar.

References

1. Boulton CH: Equine nasal cavity and paranasal sinus disease: A review of 85 cases. Equine Vet Sci 5:268, 1985.
2. Lane JG, Gibbs C, Meynink SE, et al: Radiographic examination of the facial, nasal and paranasal sinus regions of the horse: I. Indications and procedures in 235 cases. Equine Vet J 19:466, 1987.
3. Hillman DJ: Equine osteology. In Getty R (Ed): Sisson and Grossman's The Anatomy of the Domestic Animals. Philadelphia, WB Saunders, 1975, pp 344–348.
4. Schebitz H, and Wilkens H: Horse: head. In: Atlas of Radiographic Anatomy of Dog and Horse. Berlin, Paul Parey, 1968, pp 123–146.
5. El-Guindy MH, and Selim SM: Anatomical and radiological studies on the frontal and maxillary sinuses of the farm animals: I. Family Equidae. Assuit Vet Med J 15:185, 1985.
6. Behrens J, Schumacher J, Morris E, et al: Equine paranasal sinusography. Vet Radiol 32:98 1991.
7. Nickel R, Schummer A, Seiferle E, et al: Respiratory system. In: The Viscera of the Domestic Mammals. Berlin, Paul Parey, 1973, pp 211–225.
8. Harvey DE: The nasal septum of the dog: Is it visible radiographically? Vet Radiol 20:88, 1978.
9. Stilson AE Jr, Herring DS, and Robertson JT: Contribution of the nasal septum to the radiographic anatomy of the equine nasal cavity. J Am Vet Med Assoc 186:590, 1985.
10. Heffron CJ, Baker GJ, and Lee R: Fluoroscopic investigation of pharyngeal function in the horse. Equine Vet J 11:148, 1979.
11. Behrens J, Schumacher J, and Morris E: Contrast paranasal sinusography for evaluation of disease of the paranasal sinuses of five horses. Vet Radiol 32:105 1991.
12. Bayly WM, and Robertson JT: Epistaxis caused by foreign body penetration of the guttural pouch. J Am Vet Med Assoc 180:1232, 1982.
13. Ferraro GL: Epistaxis in race horses. Mod Vet Pract 63:395, 1982.
14. Larson VL, and Sorenson DK: The respiratory system. In Catcot EJ, and Smithcors JF (Eds): Equine Medicine and Surgery, 2nd Ed. Wheaton, IL, American Veterinary Publications, 1972, pp 363–375.
15. Coumbe KM, Jones RD, and Kenward JH: Bilateral sinus empyema in a six-year-old mare. Equine Vet J 19:559, 1987.
16. Cook WR: Skeletal radiology of the equine head. J Am Vet Radiol Soc 11:35, 1970.
17. Wyn-Jones G: Interpreting radiographs: VI. Radiology of the equine head (Part 2). Equine Vet J 17:417, 1985.
18. Kold SE, Ostblom LC, and Philipsen HP: Headshaking caused by a maxillary osteoma in a horse. Equine Vet J 14:167, 1982.
19. Hilbert BJ, Huxtable CR, and Brighton AJ: Erosion of the internal carotid artery and cranial nerve damage caused by guttural pouch mycosis in a horse. Aust Vet J 57:346, 1981.
20. Zaruby JF, Levesey MA, and Percy DH: Ethmoid adenocarcinoma perforating the cribriform plate in the horse. Cornell Vet 83:283, 1993.
21. Boles C: Abnormalities of the upper respiratory tract. Vet Clin North Am [Large Anim Pract] 1:89, 1979.
22. Tulleners EP, and Raker CW: Nasal septum resection in the horse. Vet Surg 12:41, 1983.
23. Cook WR, and Littlewort MCG: Progressive haematoma of the ethmoid region in the horse. Equine Vet J 6:101, 1974.
24. Specht TE, Colahan PT, Nixon AJ, et al: Ethmoidal hematoma in nine horses. J Am Vet Med Assoc 197:613, 1990.
25. Schmotzer WB, Hultgren BD, Watrous BJ, et al: Nasomaxillary fibrosarcomas in three young horses. J Am Vet Med Assoc 191:437, 1987.
26. Gibbs C, and Lane JG: Radiographic examination of the facial, nasal and paranasal sinus regions of the horse: II. Radiological findings. Equine Vet J 19:474, 1987.
27. Schumacher J, Honnas C, and Smith B: Paranasal sinusitis complicated by inspissated exudate in the ventral conchal sinus. Vet Surg 5:373, 1987.
28. Cook WR: The auditory tube diverticulum (guttural pouch) in the horse: Its radiographic examination. J Am Vet Med Assoc 14:51, 1973.
29. Beard WL, Robertson JT, and Leeth B: Bilateral congenital cysts in the frontal sinuses of a horse. J Am Vet Med Assoc 196:435, 1990.
30. Lane JG, Longstaffe JA, and Gibbs C: Equine paranasal sinus cysts: A report of 15 cases. Equine Vet J 19:537, 1987.

STUDY QUESTIONS

1. At what level is the septum separating the rostral and caudal compartments of the maxillary sinus?

2. What structure surrounds the roots of maxillary premolars three and four and the molars?

3. Why is it important to make multiple views (especially oblique views) in horses suspected of having trauma to the nasal passages?

4. What are the two major radiographic lesions evident on this lateral radiograph of the nasal passages (Fig. 11–20) in a horse presented with a nasal discharge?

5. What radiographic projection of the nasal cavities would best visualize lesions of the nasal septum?

6. What structure overlies the maxillary sinus on the straight ventral dorsal view of the nasal passages and can give the false impression of sinusitis?

7. Considering a large soft-tissue lesion in the nasal passages or sinuses, what radiographic finding would be virtually confirmatory of a neoplastic process?

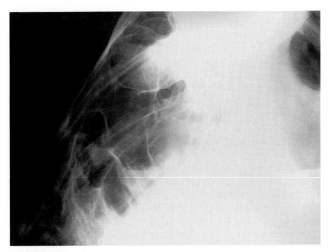

FIGURE 11–20

8. In Figure 11–17, what is the linear opacity extending rostrally from the ventral margin of the hematoma?

(Answers appear on page 635.)

Chapter 12

The Equine Vertebral Column

Patrick R. Gavin • Gregory D. Roberts • Marc Papageorges

Radiography is useful for the diagnosis of spinal diseases in horses, but only if one appreciates the indications, limitations, and importance of proper positioning, which often requires general anesthesia. High-quality radiographs of the equine cervical spine may be made with the use of portable x-ray machines and fast intensifying screens, and many referral centers have equipment capable of imaging the entire vertebral column. Lateral views of the cervical and thoracic spine may be obtained with the patient standing in a normal position, but if a long exposure time is required because of thick body parts, motion blurring often decreases the amount of information obtained from the examination. Personnel and patient safety, radiographic quality, and the likelihood of finding a lesion should always be weighed carefully before an examination of a standing or an anesthetized horse is performed.

RADIOGRAPHIC ANATOMY

The vertebral formula of the horse is 7 cervical, 18 thoracic, 6 lumbar, 5 sacral, and about 15 to 20 caudal vertebrae.[1] As in other species, it is not unusual for the first or last vertebra of a segment to take characteristics from the next or preceding one. This feature is seen more commonly at the thoraco-

lumbar and lumbosacral junctions (e.g., sacralization of L6) and should be considered as a normal variant.

Four cervical vertebrae (C1, C2, C6, and C7) have characteristic shapes and are used as landmarks to identify individual vertebrae when no other reference point (skull or first rib) is included on a radiograph. C3, C4, and C5 are nearly identical in appearance and cannot be recognized individually from their shape.

The atlas (C1) has no radiographically visible dorsal spinous process but does have two large articular fossae enclosing most of the occipital condyles and two large lateral processes (wings), each one with two foramina. The atlas originates from four ossification centers, but only three remain separate at birth. The suture between the separate ossification centers of the dorsal arch should not be mistaken for a fracture on the ventrodorsal view in a young horse (younger than 6 months).

The axis (C2) has a large dorsal spinous process that extends to the caudal articular processes, and a cranial extension of its body (the dens or odontoid process) articulates with the ventrocaudal portion of the atlas. The axis originates from six or seven ossification centers: one or two for the dens, in addition to the usual five for a vertebra. The suture between the two separate ossification centers of the dens is visible on the lateral view in young horses and should not be misinterpreted as a fracture. Small osseous projections are present at the cranial aspect of the dorsal spinous process in immature horses. They fuse with the dorsal arch by 2 years of age, forming the lateral vertebral foramina. A tortuous vascular channel is sometimes seen within the dorsal spinous process and should not be mistaken for a fracture. The authors have also occasionally seen discrete areas of increased opacity within the medullary cavity of the dorsal spinous process that they believe are analogous to "bone islands" considered as normal variants in people.[2]

The sixth cervical vertebra has large lateral processes with three projections, the caudal one having a separate ossification center at birth. This caudal projection is seen ventrally to the caudal aspect of the vertebral body, which is the distinctive feature of C6 (Fig. 12–1). The authors have seen similar lateral processes on C7 instead of C6 in about 1 percent of horses, and it is good practice to use a second landmark, such as the first rib, to confirm their exact location if surgery is contemplated.

The seventh cervical vertebra has a more prominent dorsal spinous process than the other cervical vertebrae, but the process is smaller than that on the first thoracic vertebra. Its caudal endplate is situated just cranial to the first rib.

The hypoplastic dorsal spinous processes of the other caudal cervical vertebrae are thin and irregular and may mimic periosteal new bone formation on lateral views. The articular surfaces of the articular processes are usually not seen distinctly because they are not oriented tangentially to the x-ray beam.

The cranial endplates of C3 to C7 fuse at about 2 years of age. The caudal endplates fuse at their dorsal aspect initially, but the ventral portion may still be open at 5 years of age.[1]

During flexion of the neck, apparent subluxation of adjacent vertebral bodies is commonly seen, even in neurologically normal horses. Although this radiographic sign may be associated with a spinal cord compressive lesion, it is unreliable and leads to a high incidence of false-positive diagnoses.[3]

Investigators have reported measurements of the vertebral canal in neutral and flexed position at various sites.[4] Radiographic measurements have to be corrected for magnification, parallax, and anatomic or individual variations. Measurement of the minimum sagittal diameter, minimum flexion diameter, and flexion angle were attempted at Washington State University, but subjective evaluation proved to be as reliable.

Thoracic vertebrae are surrounded by thick soft tissues, and their visualization is considerably impaired either by lack of penetration of the x-ray beam or by excessive amounts of scattered radiation. The bodies of the midthoracic vertebrae, particularly the ventral portion, may be seen more clearly because they are bordered by the dorsal aspect of the lungs. Closure of the thoracic vertebrae endplates occurs between 3 and 4 years of age. The dorsal spinous processes of T2 to T10 are long (the longest is T4, T5, or T6) and may be seen on lateral projections. The anticlinal vertebra is usually T16.

It is difficult to obtain good radiographs of the entire length of the dorsal spinous processes without a wedge filter because the thickness of overlying soft tissues varies tremendously. Separate ossification centers appear at the dorsal aspect of the dorsal spinous processes of the cranial thoracic vertebrae at about 1 year of age and usually never fuse; their normal irregular appearance may be mistaken for an inflammatory process.

Although portions of the cranial lumbar vertebrae may be seen on a lateral view, a ventrodorsal view under general anesthesia is necessary to visualize the caudal lumbar, sacral, and caudal vertebrae because, again, the muscle mass superimposed over the spine on the lateral view prevents adequate penetration of the beam and produces excessive amounts of scattered radiation.

POSITIVE-CONTRAST MYELOGRAPHY

Although its use is virtually limited to the cervical spine in adult horses, positive-contrast myelography is the only method of obtaining an antemortem diagnosis of cervical vertebral instability—malformation syndrome, the most common cause of ataxia in horses.[5]

Myelography is a relatively safe procedure and may result in identification of compressive spinal cord lesions more accurately than survey radiography.[3, 6–11] The dynamic aspects of the vertebral column and its relationship to the spinal cord are important to recognize, and myelography should always include multiple positional views.[3, 6] Equivocal myelographic findings should always be correlated with clinical and laboratory findings before a final diagnosis is made.

Cervical myelography is performed by injecting a nonionic, iso-osmolar, water-soluble, iodinated contrast medium in the subarachnoid space at the occipitoatlantal junction with the patient under general anesthesia. Iopamidol has a lower rate of complications than metrizamide.[3, 12] The morbidity and mortality rates associated with myelography were 15 percent for metrizamide and 1 percent for iopamidol at the authors' institution.[3] Morbidity and mortality rates for iopamidol myelography in a large number of horses have not yet been reported.

On neutral lateral projections, the dorsal contrast medium column is slightly wider than the ventral column, which normally narrows to a thin line at the dorsal aspect of the intervertebral disc space on flexion of the neck (Fig. 12–2). During hyperextension of the neck, the contrast medium columns should appear similar to those in the neutral position.

Myelograms should be examined for narrowing of the contrast medium columns within the subarachnoid space, as for other species. Most compressive lesions of the cervical spinal cord in horses, however, are dynamic[3]; the dorsal contrast medium column may be normal in the neutral position but narrowed during flexion of the neck with cranial

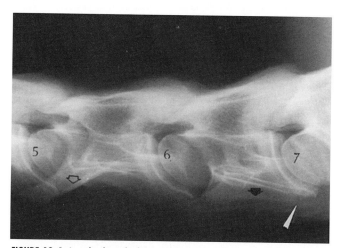

FIGURE 12–1. Lateral radiograph of the caudal cervical vertebral column. Transverse process of C5 with only one cranial projection *(open arrowhead)*. Ventral portion of the lateral process of C6 between the cranial and the caudal projections *(solid black arrowhead)*. Separate ossification center of the caudal projection of the lateral process *(solid white arrowhead)*. The numbers 5, 6, and 7 mark the cranial end plate of C5, C6, and C7.

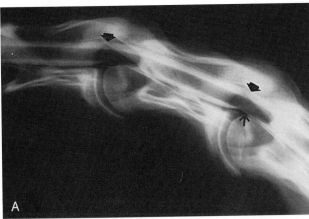 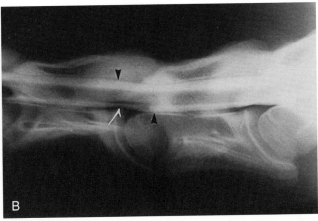

FIGURE 12–2. *A,* Lateral myelogram of the midcervical area in flexed position. *Large arrows* show dorsal contrast medium column. *Small arrow* shows normal thinning of the ventral contrast medium column during flexion. There is no evidence of spinal cord compression because the dorsal column is wide at the same location (the vertebrae are C3 through C5). *B,* Lateral myelogram of the caudal cervical area in extended position. The ventral column dorsal to the intervertebral disc space at C5–C6 *(arrow)* is thinner than the ventral and dorsal columns at other sites *(arrowheads),* but the dorsal column is wide at the same location.

cervical lesions or during extension with caudal cervical lesions.

The major problem in equine myelography arises from the fact that the degree of subarachnoid space narrowing that indicates a spinal cord lesion is undetermined. The authors have used a diametrically opposed narrowing of the dorsal and ventral contrast medium column of at least 50 percent compared with the same location in other positions,[3] and others suggest that narrowing of the dorsal contrast medium column to less than 2 mm confirms the diagnosis.[13] These criteria, however, have never been validated in a controlled study.

Because the width of the subarachnoid space may vary among individuals[3] and because narrowing of the contrast medium columns depends on the degree of flexion or extension of the neck, measurements as well as subjective evaluation of the width of the contrast medium columns should be interpreted with caution. One should avoid excessive flexion and extension until a severe compressive lesion is ruled out to avoid further damage to the spinal cord. However, attempts should be made to get maximum flexion or extension of a particular segment of the spine if an equivocal lesion is found. Unfortunately the degree of flexion and extension necessary to confirm a dynamic cord compression as well as the variations in the width of the subarachnoid space in normal horses is unknown.

CONGENITAL ANOMALIES

Most congenital anomalies of the vertebral column have little or no clinical significance. Prominent dorsal spinous processes of the cervical vertebrae, cervical ribs, fusion of the dorsal spinous processes of the thoracolumbar spine, block (fused) vertebrae, and hemivertebrae may be clinically silent and often remain undetected. Block vertebrae and fused vertebrae may occasionally be associated with scoliosis, lordosis, or kyphosis.[14]

Occipitoatlantoaxial malformation is an apparently inherited syndrome, more common in Arabian horses, characterized by varying degrees of hypoplasia and fusion of the occiput, atlas, and axis.[17] Clinical signs of cranial cervical compressive myelopathy may be recognized shortly after birth or later as acute or progressive ataxia. This condition is also discussed in Chapter 10.

INFECTIOUS LESIONS

The most common infectious lesion of the spine in horses is osteomyelitis of the dorsal spinous processes of the cranial thoracic vertebrae as an extension of infectious supraspinous bursitis (fistulous withers). Often the infection is limited to the supraspinous bursa and surrounding soft tissues, and it is difficult to determine whether osteomyelitis is present because the separate ossification centers of the dorsal spinous processes in the affected area are normally irregular and mottled, which mimics bone inflammation. In addition, there is often periosteal bone proliferation at the insertion of tendons and ligaments on the spinous processes. Therefore, one should search carefully for lysis of the body of the spinous process or aggressive periosteal reaction to confirm a diagnosis of osteomyelitis in that area. If available, bone scintigraphy is more sensitive and specific than radiography for the detection of osteomyelitis (Fig. 12–3). *Brucella* species, as a possible zoonosis, should be ruled out with appropriate tests.

The diarthrodial joints of the spine may become secondarily involved during septicemia in foals, and vertebral osteomyelitis (spondylitis) may result from direct extension or hematogenous spread of bacterial or fungal infections. If such conditions are suggested by the clinical findings, one should look carefully for osteolysis, bone proliferation, and swelling of the surrounding soft tissues. Bone lysis rarely becomes visible on radiographs before 10 days from the onset of an infectious process and periosteal new bone formation even later, 4 or 5 more days. Discospondylitis has also been reported, but its incidence is unknown.[16]

TRAUMATIC LESIONS

Fractures may occur anywhere along the vertebral column but are more common in the cervical area, particularly in foals with cartilaginous physes.[14] In other segments of the spine, fractures are a diagnostic challenge if the displacement of bone fragments is minimal, which is common because of the strong paraspinal musculature. The complex shape of the vertebrae and the excessive thickness of a horse's back additionally reduce the sensitivity of radiography for the detection of fractures. Fractures of the dorsal spinous processes of the withers after a backward fall have been described and are usually not associated with neurologic deficits (Fig.

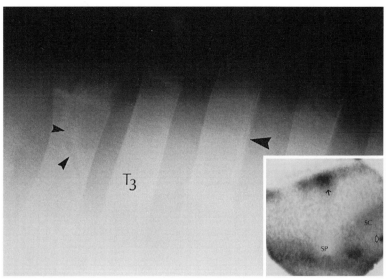

FIGURE 12-3. Lateral radiograph of the thoracic spinous processes of a horse with fistulous withers. There is a curvilinear area of decreased opacity superimposed over the spinous process of T2 *(small arrowheads).* This area may be a bone lesion as well as a fistulous tract in the soft tissues. The caudal aspect of the spinous process of T4 is irregular *(large arrowhead)* at the attachment of epaxial musculature tendons. *Inset,* Left lateral technetium 99m methylene diphosphonate (Tc 99m-MDP) bone scintigram of the same area. The area of increased uptake of the radiopharmaceutical product *(solid arrow)* indicates involvement of a spinous process (determined as T2 with the use of a radioactive marker *[open arrow]* during the study). The spinous process of T1 also appears to be involved to a lesser degree. SP, cranial thoracic spine; SC, scapula.

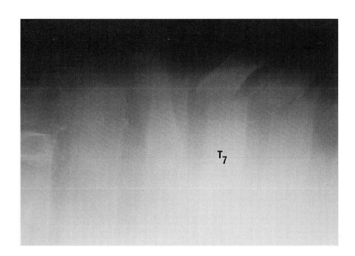

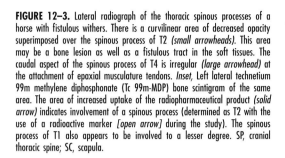

FIGURE 12-4. Lateral radiograph of the dorsal midthoracic area of a horse following a fall on the withers. The dorsal extremities of the spinous processes of T4 through T8 are fractured.

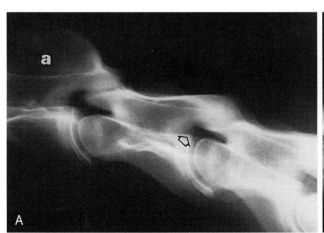

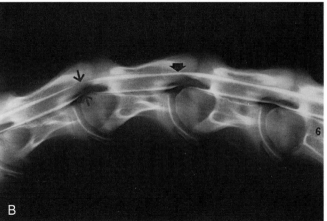

FIGURE 12-5. *A,* Lateral radiograph of the cranial cervical area of an ataxic Arabian filly. The axis is easily recognized by its large dorsal spinous process (a). There is mild remodeling of the caudal aspect of the floor of the vertebral canal of C3, apparently reducing its dorsoventral diameter *(open arrow). B,* Lateral myelogram of the midcervical area of the same horse during flexion of the neck. Both dorsal and ventral contrast medium columns are narrowed at the level of the cranial end plate of C4 *(small arrows),* indicating dynamic spinal cord compression (there was no narrowing of the columns on other views). At C4–C5 *(large arrow),* there is no alteration of the dorsal contrast medium column; thus, the apparent ventral compression is likely insignificant.

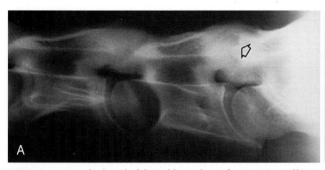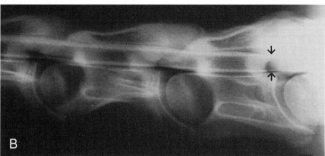

FIGURE 12–6. A, Lateral radiograph of the caudal cervical area of an ataxic 2-year-old Hanover stallion. There is periarticular bone proliferation at the articular processes at C6–C7 (open arrow). B, Lateral myelogram of the same area during extension of the neck. Both ventral and dorsal contrast medium columns are narrowed at C6–C7 (small arrows). The width of the columns was within normal limits on other views, which is typical of a caudal cervical lesion.

12–4).[14] If the history and clinical signs suggest a spinal fracture at a location that could be difficult to confirm radiographically, bone scintigraphy may be used to support the diagnosis and guide further radiographic examination.

ACQUIRED LESIONS AND LESIONS OF UNKNOWN ETIOLOGY

Sacroiliac subluxation is reported as a cause of back pain in horses.[14, 17] The sacroiliac joint cannot be seen clearly on radiographs because of its obliquity relative to the x-ray beam on conventional projections. The sensitivity and specificity of radiography for the detection of this condition are low.

Thoracolumbar spondylosis has been observed in old horses, with or without clinical signs of back pain.[14, 18, 19] As in dogs and people, the clinical significance of this finding is difficult to determine.

Overlapping of the dorsal spinous processes of the thoracolumbar segment has been suggested as a cause of back pain, particularly in jumpers.[14, 18] Radiographic signs include narrowing of the interspinous space with remodeling of adjacent dorsal spinous processes and pseudoarthrosis. Fusion of adjacent dorsal spinous processes is rare.[18] Although these radiographic signs are easily identified, their clinical significance is more difficult to determine because they are also seen in clinically normal horses.[18, 19] Soft-tissue injury is undoubtedly the most common cause of back pain in the horse,[19] and there may be a tendency to place too much significance on radiographically visible osseous changes. As in most instances, the clinical significance of any radiographic finding should be determined clinically.

ATAXIA

The differential diagnosis of ataxia in horses is extensive and includes compressive and noncompressive myelopathies.[4, 5] The cervical vertebral malformation-instability syndrome (wobbler disease) is the most common cause of equine ataxia,[5] and antemortem confirmation of the diagnosis is based on radiographic examination.[3, 6–11, 14]

Cranial cervical and caudal cervical radiographs in neutral and flexed positions should be included in both survey and myelographic examinations. Myelographic examination should also include a caudal cervical view in extended position because dorsal compressive lesions are seen at C6–C7 and C7–T1.

Survey radiographs are examined for the following changes: (1) remodeling of the caudal aspect of the floor of the vertebral canal; (2) proliferative response at the articular processes; and (3) apparent narrowing of the vertebral canal in neutral, flexed, or extended positions (Figs. 12–5 and 12–6).[3] Significant bone remodeling of the vertebrae may

occur without myelographic evidence of spinal cord compression, and soft-tissue lesions, including synovial cysts and hypertrophy of the dorsal longitudinal ligament, may cause spinal cord compression without abnormality visible on survey radiographs.[3] Therefore, myelography is always necessary to confirm a diagnosis of spinal cord compression.[3, 14]

In a study including 309 ataxic horses, 58 percent had myelographic evidence of a compressive spinal cord lesion.[3] In decreasing order of frequency, the most common sites of compression were C3–C4, C6–C7, C5–C6, and C4–C5, in 32 percent, 17 percent, 14 percent, and 11 percent of all horses, respectively. Two compressive lesions were seen in 17 percent of these 309 ataxic horses, and 1 percent had evidence of spinal cord compression at three sites.

The mechanisms leading to the myelopathy in cervical vertebral malformation-instability syndrome are not fully understood. In many patients, repetitive trauma to the spinal cord appears to be caused by positional narrowing of the vertebral canal, which supports the authors' belief that evaluation of dynamic changes is extremely important in myelography. Stretching of the spinal cord against remodeled bone may also be incriminated in the pathogenesis of the myelopathy, and absence of myelographic signs of cord compression may not preclude a diagnosis of cervical vertebral malformation-instability syndrome.[13]

Although intervertebral disc herniation has been reported in horses, the authors have not recognized one after performing more than 600 myelograms at Washington State University. In the authors' experience, lateral compressive lesions are exceedingly rare. They should cause widening of the spinal cord as well as narrowing of the contrast medium columns on the lateral view; they are more difficult to confirm with ventrodorsal views, in which numerous superimpositions and increased scattered radiation reduce radiographic detail.[20]

A large proportion of ataxic horses (42 percent in one of the authors' studies[3]) do not show radiographic signs of cervical vertebral malformation-instability syndrome; therefore, the numerous other causes of cervical spinal cord diseases should always be considered in the differential diagnosis.

References

1. Getty R: Equine osteology. In Getty R (Ed): Sisson and Grossman's The Anatomy of Domestic Animals, 5th Ed. Philadelphia, WB Saunders, 1975.
2. Keats TE: Atlas of Normal Roentgen Variants That May Simulate Disease, 4th Ed. Chicago, Year Book Medical Publishers, 1988.
3. Papageorges M, Gavin PR, Sande RD, et al: Radiographic and myelographic examination of the cervical vertebral column in 306 ataxic horses. Vet Radiol 28:53, 1987.
4. Mayhew IG, Whitlock RH, and deLahunta A: Spinal cord disease in the horse. Cornell Vet 6(suppl):13, 1978.

5. Reed SM, Bayly WM, Traub JL, et al: Ataxia and paresis in horses: I. Differential diagnosis. Comp Contin Ed Vet Pract 3:88, 1981.
6. Rantanen NW, Gavin PR, Barbee DD, et al: Ataxia and paresis in horses: II. Radiographic and myelographic examination of the cervical vertebral column. Comp Contin Ed Vet Pract 3:161, 1981.
7. Nyland TG, Blythe LL, Pool RR, et al: Metrizamide myelography in the horse: Clinical, radiographic, and pathologic changes. Am J Vet Res 41:204, 1980.
8. Beech J: Metrizamide myelography in the horse. J Am Vet Radiol Soc 20:22, 1979.
9. Nixon AJ, Stashak TS, and Ingram JT: Diagnosis of vertebral malformation in the horse. Proceedings of the Annual Convention of the American Association of Equine Practitioners, Vol 28, 1983, pp 253–266.
10. Conrad RL: Metrizamide myelography of the equine cervical spine. Vet Radiol 25:73, 1984.
11. Foley JP, Gatlin SJ, and Selcer BA: Standing myelography in six adult horses. Vet Radiol 27:54, 1986.
12. May SA, Wyn-Jones G, and Church S: Iopamidol myelography in the horse. Equine Vet J 18:199, 1986.
13. Moore BR, Holbrook TC, Stefanacci JD, et al: Contrast-enhanced computed tomography and myelography in six horses with cervical stenotic myelopathy. Equine Vet J 24:197, 1992.
14. Nixon AJ: The wobbler syndrome. In Stashak TS (Ed): Adams' Lameness in Horses, 4th Ed. Philadelphia, Lea & Febiger, 1987, pp 772–785.
15. Mayhew LG, Watson AG, and Heissan JA: Congenital occipitoatlantoaxial malformations in the horse. Equine Vet J 10:103, 1978.
16. Adams SB, Stickel R, and Blevins W: Diskospondylitis in five horses. J Am Vet Med Assoc 186:270, 1985.
17. Jeffcott LB: Pelvic lameness in the horse. Equine Pract 21:1, 1982.
18. Jeffcott LB: Disorders of the thoracolumbar spine of the horse—a survey of 443 cases. Equine Vet J 12:197, 1980.
19. Jeffcott LB: Diagnosis of back problems in the horse. Comp Contin Ed Pract Vet 4:S134, 1981.
20. Foss RR, Genetzky RM, Riedesel EA, et al: Cervical intervertebral disc protrusion in two horses. Can Vet J 24:188, 1983.

STUDY QUESTIONS

1. The axis (C2) has:
   A. five to six centers of ossification.
   B. one to two centers of ossification for the dens.
   C. small osseous projections from the dorsal spine that form a foramen by 2 years of age.
   D. a tortuous vascular channel in the spinous process that may be mistaken for a fracture.
   E. all of the above.

2. The sixth cervical vertebra (and rarely) the seventh vertebra have large lateral processes and the (cranial, caudal) projection has a separate center of ossification that may be mistaken for a fracture in young horses.

3. The cranial end plates of C3–C7 fuse at _____ years of age, and the ventral portion of the caudal end plates fuses last at _____ years of age.

4. Of metrizamide or iopamidol, which is the best nonionic iso-osmolar, water-soluble iodinated contrast agent for equine myelography?

5. Flexed and extended position views are used in equine cervical myelography because most compressive lesions in the horse are dynamic. (True or False)

6. Occipitoatlantoaxial malformation is an apparently inherited syndrome in:
   A. Arabians.
   B. Quarter horses.
   C. Thoroughbreds.
   D. Walking horses.
   E. Draft horses.

7. The bacteria _____ must be considered in horses with fistulous withers because of the zoonotic potential.
   A. *Staphylococcus* species
   B. *Pseudomonas* species
   C. *Escherichia coli*
   D. *Brucella* species
   E. *Streptococcus* species

8. In a study of 309 ataxic horses, 58 percent had compressive lesions on myelography. The most common sites in order of frequency were:
   A. C3–C4, C6–C7, C5–C6, and C4–C5.
   B. C4–C5, C6–C7, C5–C6, and C3–C4.
   C. C3–C4, C4–C5, C5–C6, and C6–C7.

9. A 2-year-old Thoroughbred horse with signs of ataxia was examined. Survey films of the cervical spine were normal. A contrast myelogram was performed. What is

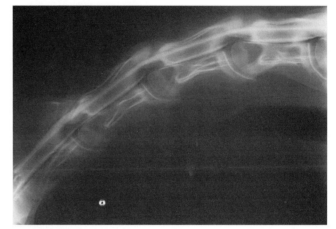

FIGURE 12 –7

your assessment of the myelogram (Fig. 12–7), in which C2 through C5 are depicted?

10. A 3-year-old Thoroughbred with ataxia was examined with survey and contrast myelography. What is your assessment of the portion of the contrast myelogram shown (Fig. 12–8)? Which vertebra is designated by the arrow?

(Answers appear on page 635.)

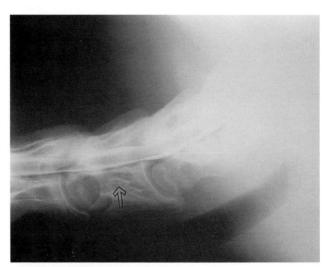

FIGURE 12–8

APPENDICULAR SKELETON—COMPANION ANIMALS

Chapter 13

Diseases of the Immature Skeleton

Linda J. Konde

JOINT DISORDERS

Osteochondrosis and Osteochondritis Dissecans

Osteochondrosis is a major cause of lameness in young, rapidly growing, large-breed dogs. Clinical signs usually develop between 6 and 9 months of age. Osteochondrosis is caused by a disturbance of normal enchondral ossification that results in an abnormal thickening of articular cartilage.[1–3] Vascularization around the affected area may lead to resumption of normal ossification superficial to the lesion and spontaneous resolution of the disease process. If revascularization does not occur, progressive chondromalacia leads to development of cartilage fissures and the formation of cartilage flaps and free cartilage fragments in the joint.[4] When cartilage flaps or fragments are present, the disorder is referred to as *osteochondritis dissecans*.[1]

Osteochondrosis occurs in specific locations. It is most commonly seen in the caudal aspect of the humeral head (Fig. 13–1).[1, 2] Other locations include the distomedial aspect of the humeral condyle (Fig. 13–2), the lateral and medial femoral condyles (Fig. 13–3), the femoral trochlea, and the medial and lateral trochlear ridges of the talus (Fig. 13–4).[3–6] The condition often occurs bilaterally, but affected animals may have clinical signs in only one limb.

Roentgen Signs of Osteochondrosis

1. Irregularity and flattening of subchondral bone are present.
2. Bony sclerosis may surround the lesion.
3. Mineralized cartilage flap or free mineralized cartilage fragment may be visible.
4. Degenerative joint disease usually develops.

The size of shoulder osteochondrosis lesions typically correlates with the severity of pain and lameness. Large subchondral defects are also more likely to be associated with the presence of cartilage flaps. Quantification of the relative size of osteochondral defects may be helpful as a guide for determining the necessity of surgical treatment and prognosis. The length of the defect can be measured and expressed as a percentage of the length of the humeral head from the intertubercular groove to the caudal humeral head. Mean size of osteochondral lesions associated with clinical signs is 27.4 ± 7.3 percent versus dogs without clinical signs where the mean size was 21.3 ± 7.1 percent. Mean size of osteochondral lesions with a cartilage flap was 27.38 ± 7.0 percent;

the mean size of lesions in dogs with intact cartilage was 20.3 ± 8.3 percent.[7]

Vacuum phenomenon is the accumulation of gas in a joint caused by negative intra-articular pressure induced by joint traction. The intra-articular gas primarily consists of nitrogen, and it provides negative contrast to outline the articular cartilage (see Fig. 13–1). Vacuum phenomenon has been associated with osteochondrosis lesions in the shoulder, and a majority of these dogs have a cartilage flap.[8] The vacuum phenomenon has also been described in normal dogs and in dogs with radiographic evidence of degenerative joint disease without osteochondrosis.[9] Therefore, the presence of intra-articular gas seems to be a nonspecific finding, but if it is seen, the shoulder should be scrutinized for possible osteochondrosis lesions.

A cartilage flap is not visible on radiographs unless it is mineralized. If a nonmineralized cartilage flap is present, an arthrogram has a high probability of outlining the flap if contrast medium dissects between the flap and the humeral head. Arthrography may also allow identification of nonmineralized cartilage fragments (joint mice) in the caudal humeral joint capsule and the bicipital tendon sheath.[10] Newer nonionic and low osmolar contrast media provide significantly better arthrographic quality than the hyperosmolar, ionic contrast media that have been used routinely for arthrograms.[11] Arthroscopy of the shoulder joint is more sensitive than arthrography in detecting cartilage flaps, fissures, and caudal humeral head joint mice.[12] Joint mice in the bicipital tendon sheath cannot be visualized arthroscopically.

Fragmentation of the medial malleolus of the tibia has been described as another possible site of osteochondrosis in the tarsus.[13] This theory is speculative at this time because histopathology has not been performed to determine if osteochondrosis is present. Medial malleolar fragmentation is seen concurrently with medial trochlear ridge osteochondrosis of the talus and as a solitary lesion. Solitary medial malleolar fragmentation may lead to degenerative joint disease, but lameness is not a common finding.

Osteochondrosis-Like Lesion of the Sacrum

A lesion resembling osteochondrosis has been seen involving the craniodorsal margin of the first sacral vertebra.[14] This lesion is primarily seen in the German shepherd and is more common in males. The presence of this lesion can lead to degenerative disc disease and result in signs of cauda equina compression. Dogs with sacral osteochondrosis may develop cauda equina signs at a younger age than dogs with cauda

131

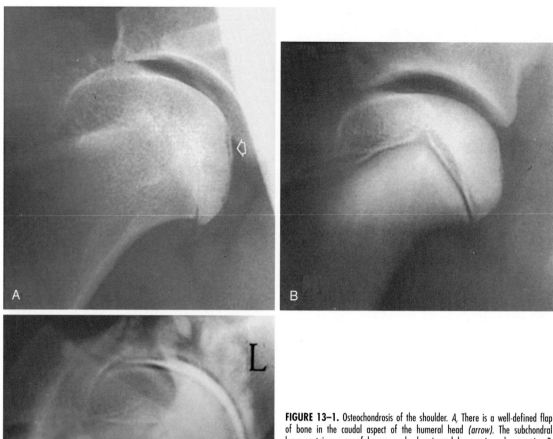

FIGURE 13–1. Osteochondrosis of the shoulder. *A,* There is a well-defined flap of bone in the caudal aspect of the humeral head *(arrow).* The subchondral bone contains areas of lucency and sclerosis and has an irregular margin. *B,* There is a slightly flattened caudal humeral head, but no obvious flap is seen. *C,* In an arthrogram on the same shoulder as in *B,* there is contrast medium outlining a linear, dissecting lesion in the caudal humeral head *(arrows).* In *A* and *B,* the vacuum phenomenon has resulted in visualization of the articular cartilage.

equina compression and no sacral osteochondrosis. The lesion has been seen in clinically normal dogs.

Roentgen Signs of Sacral Osteochondrosis

1. Flattened or deformed dorsocranial margin of the first sacral vertebra (S1) is present.

2. A small bone spur off the dorsal margin of S1 may be seen extending into the vertebral canal (Fig. 13–5). Some dogs may show a radiolucent line at the base of the bone spur.

3. Sclerosis of the sacral end plate and vertebral body is present, especially around the deformed area of S1.

4. One or more bone fragments may be seen adjacent to the flattened craniodorsal end plate. These are usually paramedian on the ventrodorsal view.

5. Possible sequelae include L7–S1 degenerative disc disease, narrowed disc space, spondylosis, and vacuum phenomenon on extension of the lumbosacral joint.

Elbow Dysplasia

Elbow dysplasia is an inclusive term referring to developmental disorders causing pain and lameness of the elbow joint that usually progress to degenerative joint disease. Disorders that are implicated include ununited anconeal process, fragmented medial coronoid process, and osteochondrosis of the distomedial aspect of the humeral condyle. Osteochondrosis has been implicated as an underlying cause of all three of these disorders.[3, 4, 15–17] More recently, it has been theorized that maldevelopment of the ulnar trochlear notch, and resulting joint incongruity, is the major cause of these disorders.[4, 18, 19] Joint incongruity between the proximal ulna and the humerus places abnormal stress on the anconeus, medial coronoid process, and humeral trochlea.

Ununited anconeal process affects large-breed dogs that have a separate center of ossification of the anconeus. It occurs most often in the German shepherd. The anconeus should be fused to the ulna by 4 to 5 months of age. In ununited anconeal process, the anconeal center of ossification fails to fuse to the ulna. The disorder is often bilateral, so it is

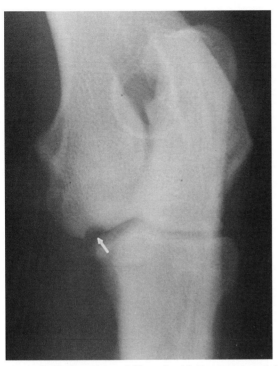

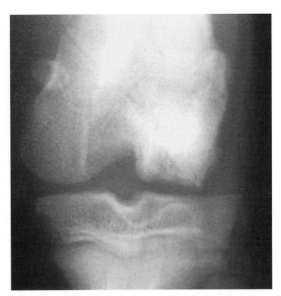

FIGURE 13–3. Osteochondrosis of the lateral femoral condyle. The subchondral bone in the lateral femoral condyle is flattened. Irregular lucent areas in the condyle are surrounded by marked sclerosis.

FIGURE 13–2. Osteochondrosis of the medial humeral condyle. There is a circumscribed lucent concavity seen in the subchondral bone of the medial humeral condyle *(arrow)*.

recommended that radiographs of both elbows be obtained if this condition is suspected or confirmed in one ulna. A flexed lateral radiograph as well as routine lateral and craniocaudal views should be made. The flexed lateral view displaces the

medial epicondylar physis away from the anconeus, thereby eliminating the possibility of confusing an overlying epicondylar physis with an ununited anconeal process.

Roentgen Signs of Ununited Anconeal Process

1. There is a radiolucent line between the anconeal process and the ulna after 5 to 6 months of age (Fig. 13–6).

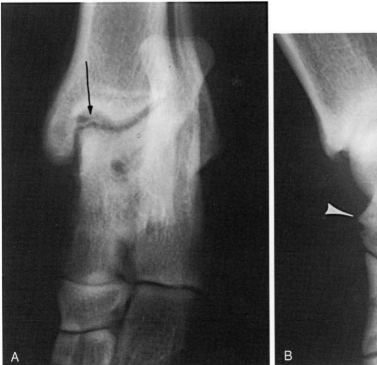

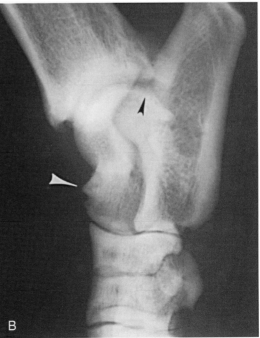

FIGURE 13–4. Osteochondritis of the talus. *A,* On the dorsoplantar view, a small bone flap is seen proximal to the medial trochlear ridge of the talus *(arrow)*. Adjacent to the flap, the bone is irregular in contour, with bone lucency surrounded by sclerosis. *B,* Flattening of the trochlear ridge and concurrent widening of the tarsocrural joint *(black arrow)* are seen on the lateral view. Osteophyte formation is seen on the cranial and caudal margins of the distal tibia and on the dorsal surface of the talus *(white arrow)*.

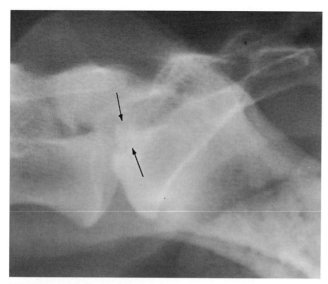

FIGURE 13–5. Osteochondrosis-like lesion of the sacrum. A large bone fragment is seen off the dorsocranial margin of the first sacral vertebra *(arrows)*. Sclerosis is seen on the sacral cranial end plate and adjacent to the bone fragment.

2. The radiolucent line may be sharply defined or may appear irregular and widened.

3. Degenerative joint disease develops and may obscure the ununited anconeus.

Fragmented medial coronoid process is the most common disorder involving the elbow joint.[4] It primarily affects medium-breed and large-breed dogs and is often bilateral. Clinical signs may be apparent as early as 4 to 6 months of age. Radiographic visualization of the coronoid fragment is often not possible owing to its superimposition on the radius or its superimposition on osteophytes and proliferative new bone. In addition, some coronoid fragments consist mostly of cartilage and are not radiopaque. Therefore, it is important to be able to recognize secondary bone changes associated with fragmented medial coronoid process. Lateral and craniocaudal radiographs of both elbow joints should be made. In addition, a flexed lateral radiograph helps identify degenerative changes that commonly form on the proximal anconeus. A cranial 25-degree lateral-caudomedial oblique view best highlights the medial coronoid region and fragmented coronoid.[20] Computed tomography is also used to diagnose fragmented medial coronoid process and has a higher diagnostic accuracy than survey radiography.[21]

Roentgen Signs of Fragmented Coronoid Process

1. Coronoid fragmentation may be visible (Fig. 13–7).
2. Proliferative bone may develop on the proximal anconeus.
3. Sclerosis of subchondral bone is present along the trochlear notch of the ulna and adjacent to the proximal radioulnar articulation near the lateral coronoid process.
4. Medial coronoid process appears abnormal on the lateral view; it may be enlarged, blunted, or absent. On the craniocaudal view, the medial coronoid process may appear blunted or have a large osteophyte.[22]
5. Widened humeroulnar and humeroradial joint spaces may be present.
6. Lack of congruity or a step between the lateral coronoid process and the radial head may occur and is best seen on the lateral view.
7. Degenerative joint disease develops.

Aseptic Necrosis of the Femoral Head (Legg-Calvé-Perthes Disease)

Aseptic necrosis of the femoral head occurs in adolescent, toy, and small-breed dogs. An undetermined cause of compromised blood supply to the femoral capital epiphysis results in necrosis of subchondral bone while overlying articular cartilage continues to grow. Initially the necrotic bone may not have an abnormal radiographic appearance. Revascularization occurs in an attempt to repair the defect, and removal of necrotic bone causes decreased opacity in the affected femoral head. Incomplete removal of necrotic bone and an invasion of granulation tissue interfere with healing.[4, 23, 24] Secondary pathologic fractures are also common.

Roentgen Signs

1. Linear radiolucencies deep to subchondral bone in the femoral head are an early change (Fig. 13–8).
2. Areas of decreased opacity are usually seen in the femoral epiphysis and metaphysis.
3. Flattening and irregularity of the femoral head and neck occur.
4. The coxofemoral joint is widened; subluxation of the femoral head may occur.
5. Fragmentation of the femoral head may develop.
6. Muscle atrophy and degenerative joint disease usually develop.

Incomplete Ossification of the Humeral Condyle in Spaniels

A higher than normal incidence of humeral condylar fractures associated with normal activity has been found to occur in spaniels.[25] It is believed that some spaniels have a heritable condition that results in incomplete ossification of the distal humeral condyle, which predisposes to humeral condylar fracture. There are normally two separate centers of ossification in the humeral condyle that appear at 14 ± 8 days after birth and should fuse by 70 ± 14 days after birth. The radiolucent line seen in the humeral condyle, representing incom-

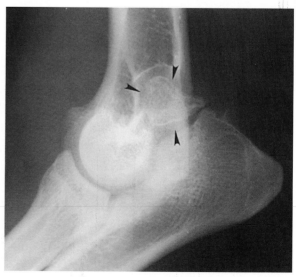

FIGURE 13–6. Ununited anconeal process. *Arrows* outline the anconeal process, which is separate from the proximal ulna. The bone margins at the site of separation are smooth and sclerotic, suggesting chronicity.

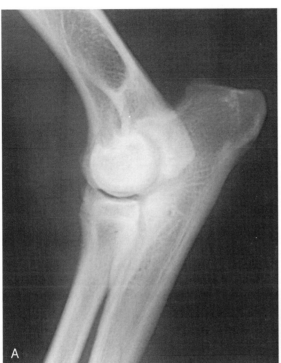

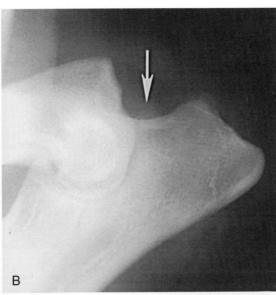

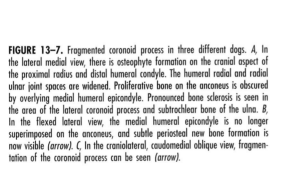

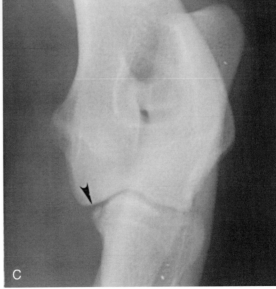

FIGURE 13–7. Fragmented coronoid process in three different dogs. *A,* In the lateral medial view, there is osteophyte formation on the cranial aspect of the proximal radius and distal humeral condyle. The humeral radial and radial ulnar joint spaces are widened. Proliferative bone on the anconeus is obscured by overlying medial humeral epicondyle. Pronounced bone sclerosis is seen in the area of the lateral coronoid process and subtrochlear bone of the ulna. *B,* In the flexed lateral view, the medial humeral epicondyle is no longer superimposed on the anconeus, and subtle periosteal new bone formation is now visible *(arrow).* *C,* In the craniolateral, caudomedial oblique view, fragmentation of the coronoid process can be seen *(arrow).*

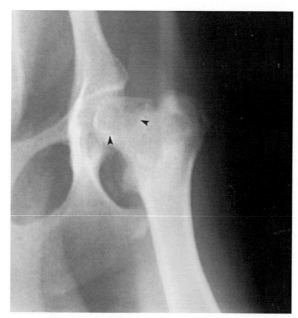

FIGURE 13–8. Aseptic necrosis of the left femoral head. The femoral head contains two large radiolucent areas with surrounding sclerosis *(arrows)*. There is flattening of the weight-bearing surface of the femoral head, and the joint space is widened. Osteophyte formation is present on the femoral neck.

plete ossification, is seen only on a craniocaudal view with the radiographic beam oriented from 15 degrees craniomedial to caudolateral, with no greater than 5 degrees rotation. There may be a higher incidence of incomplete ossification in male spaniels. If a spaniel presents with a humeral condylar fracture, especially if it occurs with normal activity, a craniocaudal radiograph of the opposite elbow should be obtained to check for incomplete ossification of the humeral condyle.

Roentgen Signs

1. Radiolucent line in the intercondylar area may have partial or complete extension to the physeal scar or trochlear notch (Fig. 13–9).
2. There may be a smooth periosteal proliferation along the lateral and caudal aspect of the humeral condyle.
3. Fragmented coronoid process may be seen in association with incomplete ossification or fractured humeral condyles.
4. Degenerative elbow joint disease may develop.

DISEASES OF UNDETERMINED ETIOLOGY

Panosteitis

Panosteitis is a self-limiting disease that affects the long bones of primarily young large-breed dogs and is common in the German shepherd. Dogs between the ages of 5 and 12 months are most often affected; however, affected dogs from 2 months to 7 years of age have been reported.[4] Histologically the bone marrow undergoes excessive osteoblastic activity that results in the increased opacity seen on radiographs.[4, 26, 27] Panosteitis lesions may be solitary, affect multiple sites in a single bone, or be multifocal in multiple bones. Bone involvement is often sequential and may be protracted over several months.

Roentgen Signs

1. Early in the disease, there is blurring and accentuation of trabecular bone.
2. Circumscribed, nodular opacities (similar in opacity to cortical bone) form in the diaphysis of long bones, often located near nutrient foramina (Fig. 13–10).
3. Medullary opacities become diffuse and homogeneous; a smooth, continuous periosteal new bone may develop.
4. Late in the disease, opacities resolve, leaving coarse, thickened trabecular bone that eventually assumes a normal appearance. Cortical thickening may be apparent as periosteal new bone remodels.

Hypertrophic Osteodystrophy

Hypertrophic osteodystrophy affects large-breed and giant-breed dogs between the ages of 2 and 7 months. The cause is unknown, but oversupplementation of minerals and vitamins, hypovitaminosis C, and suppurative inflammation (without isolation of infectious agents) have been implicated.[4, 28, 29] Metaphyseal regions of long bones, particularly the distal radius, ulna, and tibia, are common locations for the disease. The mandible, metacarpal bones, and costochondral ribs may also be involved.[4, 29] Radiographic changes are usually bilaterally symmetric in the forelimbs and hindlimbs.

Roentgen Signs

1. Metaphyseal lucent zone is present adjacent to the physis, known as the *double-physis* sign (Fig. 13–11).

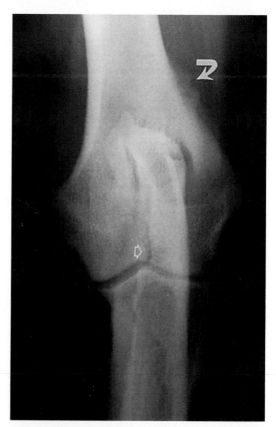

FIGURE 13–9. Incomplete ossification of the humeral condyle. A vertical radiolucent line is seen in the intercondylar area of the distal humerus *(open arrow)*. Periosteal new bone formation is present on the distal lateral humerus *(curved arrow)*, probably secondary to motion from a fracture extending laterally from the supracondylar foramen.

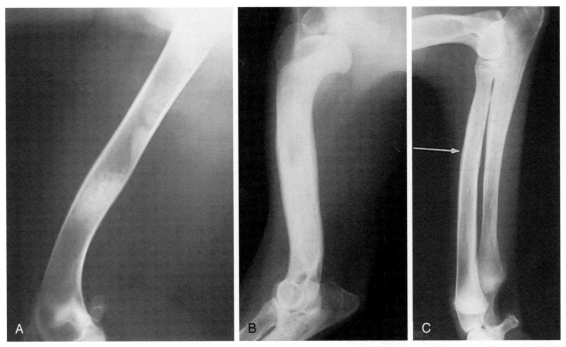

FIGURE 13–10. Stages of panosteitis. *A,* Early stage in a lateral femur. There is circumscribed increased opacity in the middle and proximal diaphysis. *B,* Middle stage in a lateral humerus. There is diffuse increased opacity of the entire diaphysis and continuous periosteal new bone formation surrounding the diaphysis. *C,* Later stage in a lateral radius-ulna. There is less intense but still apparent increased opacity primarily in the proximal radius and ulna. There is a suggestion of mild, continuous periosteal new bone on the cranial radius *(arrow).*

2. Bone sclerosis develops adjacent to the lucent zone.

3. A cuff of periosteal new bone develops around the metaphysis that is usually separate from the cortex.

4. Proliferative bone response may involve the diaphysis in severely affected patients.

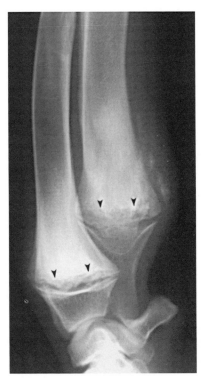

FIGURE 13–11. Hypertrophic osteodystrophy. Irregular radiolucent zones are seen in the radial and ulnar metaphyses, proximal to the physis *(arrows).* Proximal to the lucent zones are regions of increased opacity. Caudal to the distal ulnar metaphysis, there is a cuff of periosteal new bone formation.

5. Diffuse soft-tissue swelling is present about the metaphyseal regions.

Retained Cartilage Cores

Retained cartilage cores are seen primarily in the distal ulnar metaphysis of large-breed dogs, although they may also be seen in the lateral femoral condyle.[4, 30] Retained cartilage may cause angular limb deformity, although the exact cause is unknown.

Roentgen Signs

1. There is a cone-shaped radiolucent area in the distal ulnar metaphysis or lateral femoral condyle (Fig. 13–12).

2. A small zone of sclerosis may surround the radiolucent area.

3. Angular limb deformities may result.

METABOLIC DISEASE

Nutritional Secondary Hyperparathyroidism

Nutritional secondary hyperparathyroidism is a metabolic disorder caused by feeding a diet that either is low in calcium or has low to normal calcium levels and increased levels of phosphorus. This improper diet causes an increase in circulating parathyroid hormone levels that results in calcium resorption from bone and generalized osteoporosis (Fig. 13–13). The skeletal changes are diffuse and generalized.[31, 32]

Roentgen Signs

1. Generalized, decreased bone opacity with thin cortices is seen; bones may be almost the same opacity as soft tissues.

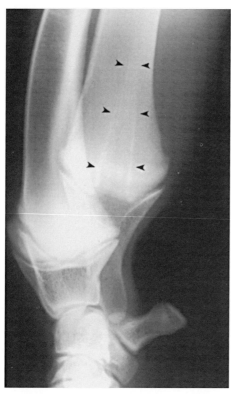

FIGURE 13–12. Retained cartilage core in the distal ulna. A triangular radiolucent shape is seen in the distal ulnar metaphysis *(arrows)*. A thin rim of bone sclerosis is present next to the radiolucency. Slight cranial bowing of the radius and a thick caudal radial cortex suggest the possibility of mild angular limb deformity owing to delayed ulnar growth.

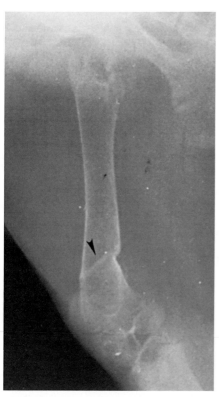

FIGURE 13–13. Nutritional secondary hyperparathyroidism. Overall bone opacity of the femur is decreased, and cortices are thin. An opaque line in the distal femur *(arrow)* with angulation at this site indicates a pathologic folding fracture.

2. There is loss of visualization of lamina dura (see Chapter 3).

3. Pathologic folding fractures and malunion of fractures occur.

Mucopolysaccharidosis

This genetically transmitted disorder is related to lysosomal enzyme deficiencies involved in the degradation of glycosaminoglycans. Ten forms are recognized in humans, and three forms are seen in dogs and cats.[4, 33] The disorder affects the musculoskeletal, ocular, neurologic, and circulatory systems.

Animals present with facial dysmorphia, including broad maxilla, widespread eyes, flat nose, and short ears. In most instances, affected animals are smaller than normal and experience pain in multiple joints. Radiographic changes of mucopolysaccharidosis affect the axial and appendicular skeletons (Fig. 13–14).[34]

Roentgen Signs

1. The maxilla is short and flattened; the frontal sinus may be absent.

2. Hip subluxation or luxation with eventual development of degenerative joint disease occurs.

3. There is generalized epiphyseal dysplasia with delayed ossification of epiphyses and progressive degenerative joint disease.

4. Ventral, bridging spondylosis is seen in older animals.

INHERITED DISORDERS

Chondrodysplasia in Alaskan Malamutes

Chondrodysplasia is transmitted by an autosomal recessive gene that causes affected dogs to be smaller than their normal littermates. Cranial and lateral deviation of the forelimbs and

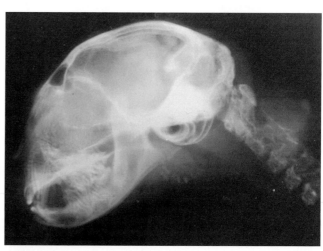

FIGURE 13–14. Mucopolysaccharidosis. Lateral skull of a Siamese kitten. There is marked foreshortening of the maxilla with decreased turbinate detail. The cervical vertebrae are shorter than normal, and marked irregularity of epiphyses is seen.

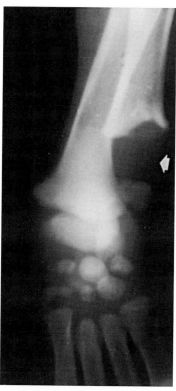

FIGURE 13–15. Chondrodysplasia in an Alaskan Malamute. The distal ulnar metaphysis is flattened, and the physis is much wider than normal *(arrow)*. The carpal bones are smaller in size than those in normal littermates.

enlarged carpi are common clinical signs.[35] All growth plates are affected, but the most obvious changes are seen in the distal ulnar physis and the metaphysis (Fig. 13–15). Radiographic changes have been described in the forelimbs and may be detected in dogs as early as 7 to 10 days of age.[36]

Roentgen Signs

1. There is a flattened distal ulnar metaphysis.
2. There is an irregular, flared distal radial metaphysis with narrow zone of increased opacity.
3. Decreased size of carpal bones and other forelimb epiphyses is seen.
4. There is a decreased length of the radius and ulna when compared with normal littermates.
5. Cranial and lateral deviation of the forelimbs develops.

Pseudoachondroplasia

Pseudoachondroplasia has been reported in young miniature Poodles, and a similar form of epiphyseal dysplasia has been seen in Beagle puppies.[37, 38] Puppies are presented with stunted growth and difficulty in walking. Histologically the hyaline cartilage is abnormal, and delayed enchondral ossification results in small bony foci present in the epiphyses. As the animal matures, the bones become well mineralized but remain shorter than normal, and angular limb deformities may be present.

Roentgen Signs

1. Opaque foci are seen in long-bone epiphyses (stippling); they may not be seen in all epiphyses (Fig. 13–16).
2. The long bones are shorter and wider than normal; the cortices are thinned.
3. Cuboidal bones are delayed in ossification.

Multiple Cartilaginous Exostoses

Multiple cartilaginous exostoses is a benign proliferative disease of bone and cartilage. A hereditary transmission of the disease is suspected in dogs.[39] Any bone that develops by enchondral ossification may be affected, and simultaneous

FIGURE 13–16. Epiphyseal dysplasia in a 2-month-old Beagle. The distal humeral epiphysis consists of rounded, sclerotic centers of bone formation. The proximal radial and olecranon physes have a normal appearance.

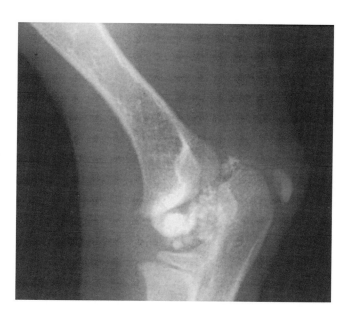

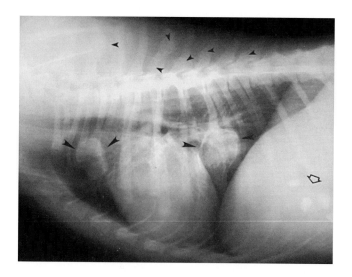

FIGURE 13–17. Multiple cartilaginous exostosis. Two large expansile lesions are present involving the third and seventh ribs *(large arrowheads)*. The opacity is mixed bone and soft tissue. Multiple nodular bone masses are seen deforming the shape of the dorsal spinous processes of the thoracic vertebrae *(small arrowheads)*. An incidental finding is the presence of rocks in the stomach *(open arrow)*.

involvement in multiple bones is common. Chondrocytes are pushed into the metaphyses and do not differentiate into osteoblasts. Instead, these cartilage islands continue to proliferate as cartilaginous masses that eventually ossify. Growth usually ceases once the animal has reached maturity, resulting in nonpainful bony protuberances present throughout the skeleton (Fig. 13–17). The bone lesions are of no clinical significance unless they arise in an area that might compromise function, such as the spinal canal and the trachea. A similar disorder is seen in mature cats, and a viral cause has been proposed.[40] Most exostoses remain inert once the dog has matured, but malignant transformation has been reported.[41, 42] Two atypical examples of multiple cartilaginous exostoses have been reported.[43] One was a 2-year-old Great Dane that developed multiple cartilaginous exostoses after reaching skeletal maturity. The exostoses continued to grow,

with some bridging of physeal regions and irregular margins. The other was a 4-month-old Border collie that had tumors with a stippled appearance that were not contiguous with adjacent bone. Histologic appearance in both dogs was consistent with multiple cartilaginous exostoses.

Roentgen Signs

1. Rib masses are an amorphous mixture of radiolucency and bone opacity with irregular contours.

2. Long-bone and vertebral masses tend to be more organized in appearance with radiolucent cartilage and trabecular bone.

3. Cortical bone in the area of the lesion may be present or absent; the bone may be deformed, or the exostosis may project externally.

4. The size and shape of exostoses are variable.

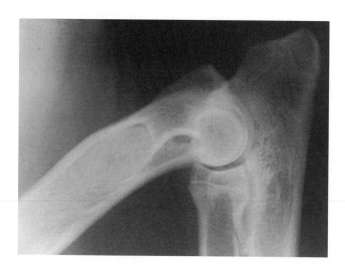

FIGURE 13–18

References

1. Poulos PW: Canine osteochondrosis. Vet Clin North Am [Small Anim Pract] *12*:313, 1982.
2. Smitach LW, and Stowater TL: Osteochondritis dissecans of the shoulder joint: A review of 35 cases. J Am Anim Hosp Assoc *11*:658, 1975.
3. Olsson S-E: The early diagnosis of fragmented coronoid process and osteochondritis dissecans of the canine elbow joint. J Am Anim Hosp Assoc *19*:616, 1983.
4. Pedersen NC, Wind A, Morgan JP, et al: Joint diseases of dogs and cats. *In* Ettinger DJ (Ed): Textbook of Veterinary Internal Medicine, Vol 2. Philadelphia, WB Saunders, 1989.
5. Alexander JW, Richardson DC, and Selcer BA: Osteochondritis dissecans of the elbow, stifle and hock—a review. J Am Anim Hosp Assoc *17*:51, 1981.
6. Denny HR, and Gibbs C: Osteochondritis dissecans of the canine stifle joint. J Small Anim Pract *21*:317, 1980.
7. van Bree H: Evaluation of subchondral lesion size in osteochondrosis of the scapulohumeral joint in dogs. J Am Vet Med Assoc *204*:1472, 1994.
8. van Bree H: Vacuum phenomenon associated with osteochondrosis of the scapulohumeral joint in dogs: 100 cases (1985–1991). J Am Vet Med Assoc *201*:1916, 1992.
9. Weber WJ, Berry CR, and Kramer RW: Vacuum phenomenon in twelve dogs. Vet Radiol Ultrasound *36*:493, 1995.
10. van Bree H: Comparison of the diagnostic accuracy of positive-contrast arthrography and arthrotomy in evaluation of osteochondrosis lesions in the scapulohumeral joint in dogs. J Am Vet Med Assoc *203*:84, 1993.
11. van Bree H, van Ryssen B: Positive contrast shoulder arthrography with iopromide and diatrizoate in dogs with osteochondrosis. Vet Radiol Ultrasound *36*:203, 1995.
12. van Bree H, van Ryssen B, and Desmidt M: Osteochondrosis lesions of the canine shoulder: Correlation of positive contrast arthrography and arthroscopy. Vet Radiol Ultrasound *33*:342, 1992.
13. Newell SM, Mahaffey MB, and Aron DN: Fragmentation of the medial malleolus of dogs with and without tarsal osteochondrosis. Vet Radiol Ultrasound *35*:5, 1994.
14. Lang J, Hani H, and Schawalder P: A sacral lesion resembling osteochondrosis in the German Shepherd dog. Vet Radiol Ultrasound *33*:69, 1992.
15. Boudrieau RJ, Hohn RB, and Bardet JF: Osteochondritis dissecans of the elbow in the dog. J Am Anim Hosp Assoc *19*:627, 1983.
16. Goring RL, and Bloomberg MS: Selected developmental abnormalities of the canine elbow: Radiographic evaluation and surgical management. Comp Contin Ed Vet Pract *5*:178, 1983.
17. Mason TA, Lavelle SC, Skipper SC, et al: Osteochondrosis of the elbow joint in young dogs. J Small Anim Pract *21*:641, 1980.
18. Wind AP: Elbow incongruity and developmental elbow diseases in the dog: I. J Am Anim Hosp Assoc *22*:711, 1986.
19. Wind AP: Elbow incongruity and developmental elbow diseases in the dog: II. J Am Anim Hosp Assoc *22*:725, 1986.
20. Berzon JL, and Quick CB: Fragmented coronoid process: Anatomical, clinical, and radiographic considerations with case analyses. J Am Anim Hosp Assoc *16*:241, 1980.
21. Carpenter LG, Schwarz PD, Lowry JE, et al: Comparison of radiologic imaging techniques for diagnosis of fragmented medial coronoid process. J Am Vet Med Assoc *203*:78, 1993.
22. Berry CR: Evaluation of the canine elbow for fragmented medial coronoid process. Vet Radiol Ultrasound *33*:273, 1992.
23. Lee R: Legg-Perthes disease in the dog: The histological and associated radiological changes. J Am Vet Radiol Assoc *15*:24, 1974.
24. Lee R: A study of the radiographic and histological changes occurring in Legg-Calvé-Perthes disease (LCP) in the dog. J Small Anim Pract *11*:621, 1970.
25. Marcellin-Little DH, DeYoung DJ, Ferris KK, et al: Incomplete ossification of the humeral condyle in Spaniels. Vet Surg *23*:475, 1994.
26. Stead AC, Stead MCP, and Galloway FH: Panosteitis in the dog. J Small Anim Pract *24*:623, 1983.
27. Bohning RH, Suter PF, Hohn RB, et al: Clinical and radiologic survey of canine panosteitis. J Am Vet Med Assoc *156*:870, 1970.
28. Woodward JC: Canine hypertrophic osteodystrophy: A study of the spontaneous disease in littermates. Vet Pathol *19*:337, 1982.
29. Alexander JW: Hypertrophic osteodystrophy. Can Pract *5*:48, 1978.
30. Riser WH, Lincoln JP, Rhodes WH, et al: Genu valgum: A stifle deformity of giant dogs. J Vet Radiol Soc *10*:28, 1969.
31. Riser WH: Radiographic differential diagnosis of skeletal diseases of young dogs. J Vet Radiol Soc *5*:5, 1964.
32. Bojrab MJ: Nutritional secondary hyperparathyroidism. *In* Bojrab MJ (Ed): Pathophysiology in Small Animal Surgery. Philadelphia, Lea & Febiger, 1981, pp 677–680.
33. Haskins ME, Jezyk PF, Desnick RJ, et al: Alpha-L-iduronidase deficiency in a cat: A model of mucopolysaccharidosis: I. Pediatr Res *13*:1294, 1979.
34. Konde LJ, Thrall MA, Gasper P, et al: Radiographic changes associated with mucopolysaccharidosis in the cat. Vet Radiol *28*:223, 1987.
35. Fletch SM, Smart ME, Pennock PW, et al: Clinical and pathologic features of chondrodysplasia (dwarfism) in the Alaskan Malamute. J Am Vet Med Assoc *162*:357, 1973.
36. Sande RD, Alexander JE, and Padgett GA: Dwarfism in the Alaskan Malamute: Its radiographic pathogenesis. J Vet Radiol Soc *15*:10, 1974.
37. Riser WH, Haskins ME, Jezyk PF, et al: Pseudoachondroplastic dysplasia in Miniature Poodles: Clinical, radiologic, and pathologic features. J Am Vet Med Assoc *176*:335, 1980.
38. Rasmussen PG: Multiple epiphyseal dysplasia in a litter of Beagle puppies. J Small Anim Pract *12*:91, 1971.
39. Gambardella PC, Osborne CA, and Stevens JB: Multiple cartilaginous exostoses in the dog. J Am Vet Med Assoc *166*:761, 1975.
40. Pool RR, and Harris JM: Feline osteochondromatosis. Feline Pract *5*:24, 1975.
41. Doige CE, Pharr JW, and Withrow SJ: Chondrosarcoma arising in multiple cartilaginous exostoses in a dog. J Am Anim Hosp Assoc *14*:605, 1978.
42. Owen LN: Multiple cartilaginous exostoses with development of a metastasizing osteosarcoma in a Shetland Sheepdog. J Small Anim Pract *12*:507, 1971.
43. Jacobson LS, and Kirberger RM: Canine multiple cartilaginous exostoses: Unusual manifestations and a review of the literature. J Am Anim Hosp Assoc *32*:45, 1996.

STUDY QUESTIONS

1. Vacuum phenomenon in the shoulder joint has been associated with osteochondrosis. (True or False)

2. The size of an osteochondrosis lesion in the shoulder joint correlates positively with the presence of a cartilage flap and clinical signs. (True or False)

3. The anconeal process is considered ununited if separation of the anconeus from the ulna is present after what age?

4. Radiographic diagnosis of fragmented coronoid process depends on visualizing a bone fragment off the medial coronoid process of the ulna. (True or False)

5. A 4-month-old Great Dane is presented with soft-tissue swelling about the carpi and tarsi. The puppy has a high fever and painful forelimbs. Radiographs show lucent zones in the metaphyses adjacent to the physes with sclerosis adjacent to the lucencies. Periosteal new bone formation is present around the metaphyses. What is the most likely diagnosis?

6. Panosteitis is typically located in
   A. Diaphysis.
   B. Metaphysis.
   C. Epiphysis.

7. What is an important potential sequela of multiple cartilaginous exostoses?

8. This elbow (Fig. 13–18) is from an 8-month-old German shepherd with lameness and pain isolated to the elbow region. Describe the radiographic changes.

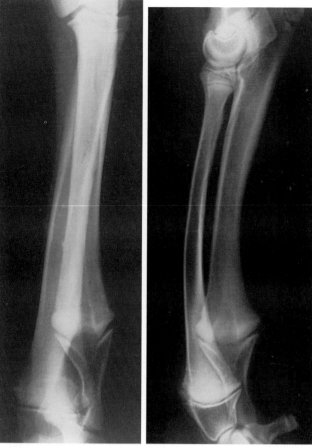

FIGURE 13–19

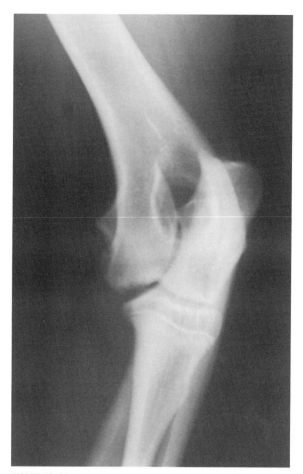

FIGURE 13–20

9. These are forelimb radiographs of a 5-month-old Irish wolfhound who presented with an angular limb deformity (Fig. 13–19). Describe the radiographic findings.

10. This elbow is from a 6-month-old Labrador retriever

with lameness and pain in the elbow joint (Fig. 13–20). What is the radiographic diagnosis?

(Answers appear on pages 635 and 636.)

Chapter 14

Fracture Healing and Complications

Robert L. Toal

INITIAL RADIOGRAPHS

If a limb fracture is suspected, at least two radiographs should be made at a 90-degree angle to each other. The joints above and below the affected bone should be included in the field of view; this allows for the assessment of joint involvement and degree of fragment rotation. The use of sedation or anesthesia is helpful so the animal may be positioned properly. A horizontal-beam craniocaudal radiograph may be obtained when the patient's condition, limb swelling, or decreased range of motion prevents viewing the limb in

extension with a vertically directed x-ray beam.[1] Stressed, oblique, and opposite-limb comparison radiographs are helpful in some patients.

FRACTURE RECOGNITION

Radiographically a fracture is a disruption in bone continuity. One or more radiolucent fracture lines may be seen, or there may be a sclerotic line or zone where overlapping fragment ends summate. Alterations in bone size, shape, position, and function are usually present to some degree.

Occasionally a fracture may be present, but bone distraction is minimal, making radiographic detection difficult. Reasons for fracture nonvisualization include poor-quality radiographs, a fracture line not tangential to the x-ray beam, early cortical stress fractures, minimal displacement, and obscured visualization by overlying structures (Fig. 14–1). Repeat radiographs obtained with the use of proper technique or oblique projections may help. In some instances, a more apparent fracture line or early callus formation is apparent in radiographs made 1 or 2 weeks later. In instances such as early cortical stress fractures, nuclear scintigraphy is indicated because of its inherent sensitivity in detecting bone lesions.

Occasionally, normal or variant anatomic structures may simulate fracture. This situation occurs with normal or ectopic nutrient foramina,[2] normal and accessory ossification centers, inconstant and multipartite sesamoid bones, open physes, and syndesmoses.

FRACTURE EVALUATION

Radiographic evaluation plays a role in helping to determine the method of fracture fixation. A radiographic assessment begins with the fracture type, the bone involved, and the location within the bone.[3] The direction of fissure fractures, the presence of joint involvement, and the presence of intra-articular fragments is carefully assessed. Intra-articular fragments may be associated with luxations, subluxations, or any joint trauma. Next, the positional changes of the major distal fragment relative to the proximal fragment should be characterized. The direction of displacement and angulation of the fracture fragments should be evaluated. Alterations in bone length are described as overriding (bone shortening) or distraction (bone lengthening). Rotational deformities should be noted, although unstable distal fragments that are fully movable vary markedly in rotational direction. Lastly, the amount of soft-tissue change should be characterized in terms of size (swelling or atrophy) and opacity (e.g., emphysema and opaque foreign objects).

FRACTURE TYPE

Fracture type may influence the (1) therapeutic plan, (2) rate of fracture healing, (3) appearance of fracture callus, and (4) possibility of postoperative complications. Most fractures may be classified according to one or more of the types.

Open Versus Closed

Open fractures have a skin defect in the region of the fracture. The defect may result in wound contamination and possible infection. Radiographically the bone may or may not protrude from the skin. Occasionally, foreign debris, metallic opacities, or tissue emphysema is identified. Often, no radiographic clues are seen, making clinical assessment important. A closed fracture does not have a skin defect in the region of the fracture. The categorization of a fracture as open or closed is a basic first step in fracture classification. The method of fracture repair, patient management, and prognosis is directly influenced by this information.[4]

Number and Extent of Fracture Lines

Simple *complete* fractures have one fracture line that extends through the bone. The direction may be characterized as transverse, spiral, or oblique. *Comminuted* fractures have multiple fracture lines that communicate to a single plane or point (Fig. 14–2). *Multiple fractures* have more than one fracture line within a bone, and the fracture lines do not communicate.

In an *incomplete* fracture, only a portion of the bone or a single bone cortex has a fracture line. Incomplete fractures are often seen as fissure fractures, which may originate with the main fracture site and radiate into the major fragments or even a joint (see Fig. 14–2). Other examples of incomplete fractures include greenstick fractures in immature animals, folding fractures in demineralized bone, and stress fractures. *Stress* (fatigue) fractures are microfractures in the bone cortex from cyclic loading, resulting in local strain of bone tissues.[5] Initially, no radiographic signs are found, although increased

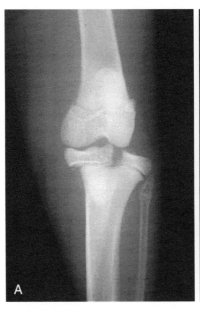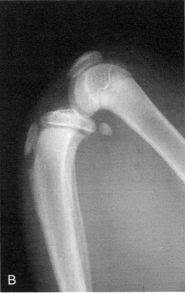

FIGURE 14–1. *A and B*, Fractured proximal tibial epiphysis. In the lateral view, there is no abnormality, but in the craniocaudal view, there clearly is a fracture. If only a lateral radiograph had been made, this fracture would have not been detected. This emphasizes the importance of making a minimum of two radiographic projections at right angles to each other.

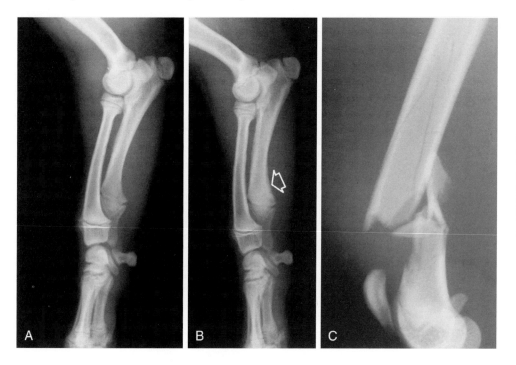

FIGURE 14–2. *A,* An incomplete fracture of the ulna was suspected in this young dog but was not seen in the radiograph. *B,* The fracture (arrow) was confirmed with a follow-up radiograph. *C,* There is an obvious comminuted femoral fracture in this cat, with several fissure fractures radiating into the proximal fragment. The full extent of fissure fractures is sometimes difficult to detect radiographically.

radiotracer uptake may be seen scintigraphically. When present, roentgen signs include focal increases in bone opacity, faint periosteal reaction, and oblique to dish-shaped fracture lines that involve a single cortex. Impacted fractures result from compression forces that shorten bone length by crushing bone tissue. Impacted fractures occur most commonly in vertebral bodies or open physes.

Avulsion Versus Chip Fractures

Avulsion and chip fractures result in fragments of variable size with a defect or fracture bed in the parent bone. Avulsion fractures are associated with excessive traction by a muscle, ligament, or tendon; they are usually periarticular or intra-articular or involve traction epiphyses. Chip fractures are small fragments that usually result from direct bone trauma or hyperextension. Periarticular chip fractures should be distinguished from accessory ossification centers and soft-tissue dystrophic mineralization. Differentiation is not always possible radiographically; findings should thus be correlated with the clinical signs.

Fracture-Luxation

Some luxations occur only in association with a nearby fracture. These are sometimes referred to as *fracture-luxations.* This term is often reserved for sacroiliac luxations because sacroiliac displacement is almost always accompanied by fracture of the pubis and ischium or separation along the pelvic symphysis. Obviously, fractures with secondary luxations-subluxations involving other joints also occur, particularly if the fracture involves a collateral ligament attachment site or another joint component. These include fractures of the ulnar styloid, malleolar fractures of the distal tibia, shearing injuries that destroy collateral ligament support, and proximal ulnar fractures with cranial dislocation of the radial head. In the last instance, if the radial annular ligament ruptures and separation of the radius from the ulna also occurs, it is termed *Monteggia's fracture.*

Salter Fractures

The various combinations of metaphyseal-physeal-epiphyseal fractures in growing bone are called *Salter fractures.* Six classes have been described (Fig. 14–3).[6–8] Prognosis for Salter fractures is related to Salter type, the degree of initial displacement, and the exactness of reduction. Serious complications of Salter fractures include clinically evident growth disturbances and joint abnormalities. Type II injuries are the most common type of Salter fracture (Fig. 14–4). Salter type V injuries most often result in growth deformities, especially when the distal ulnar physis is involved.

Some physeal fractures are minimally displaced, making initial detection difficult (see Fig. 14–1). Radiographs of the opposite normal limb are helpful for comparison purposes

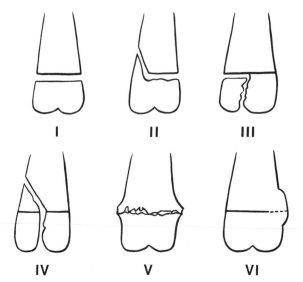

FIGURE 14–3. Six types of Salter fractures: I, physeal; II, physeal-metaphyseal; III, physeal-epiphyseal; IV, physeal-epiphyseal-metaphyseal; V, impacted physis; VI, eccentric physeal impaction resulting in transphyseal bridging.

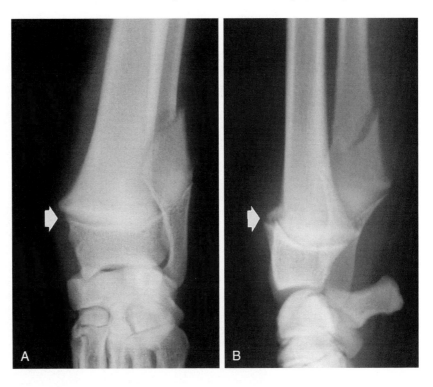

FIGURE 14–4. Craniocaudal *(A)* and lateral *(B)* views of a distal ulnar metaphyseal fracture and a distal radial Salter II physeal fracture. Minimal displacement of the epiphysis makes detecting the physeal fracture *(arrows)* difficult.

when subtle fractures are suspect. Fractures of the growing physis usually involve the zone of hypertrophied chondrocytes. Regional trauma may be sufficient to compromise the epiphyseal vasculature or to disrupt the germinal layer directly. Growth deformities may then result, especially if the distal radius and ulna are involved. Angulation deformity of the lower extremity with or without rotation may occur. Variable degrees of elbow subluxation may also be present. Insufficient longitudinal growth of the *ulna* can result in carpal valgus, radial bowing, and humeroulnar subluxation (Fig. 14–5). Insufficient longitudinal *radial* growth can result in distal subluxation of the radius and proximal subluxation of the ulna from the humerus (see Fig. 14–5). Physeal growth disturbances may occur after soft-tissue trauma alone, without the presence of a fracture.[20] The clinician should be aware of this fact. Follow-up radiographs of the entire antebrachium and elbow obtained after 2 to 4 weeks should be considered if growth deformity is suspected.

Pathologic Fractures

A pathologic fracture is a spontaneous fracture that occurs without history of overt trauma in bone weakened by a pre-existing lesion. Pathologic fractures are most often seen in bones weakened by tumor. An aggressive bone lesion in conjunction with a fracture is indicative (Fig. 14–6). Metabolic bone disease, especially hyperparathyroidism, as a cause of pathologic fracture is suspect when a fracture occurs in bone that radiographically is less opaque and has thin cortices and scant trabeculae (Fig. 14–7).

FRACTURE HEALING

Three distinct histologic patterns of bone healing have been identified: (1) direct healing of bone by osseous tissue, called *primary bone healing*, and (2) secondary bone healing, histologically seen as two patterns—union of fragments by fibrous

connective tissue, which is later converted to bone (intramembranous ossification), and callus formation that matures through a sequence of granulation tissue, cartilage, mineralized cartilage, and, finally, replacement by bone (endochondral ossification).[9]

Primary Bone Healing

Direct healing of a fracture by the initial formation of bone has been termed *primary bone healing*.[10, 11] Primary bone healing may occur under conditions of rigid fixation, which is usually achieved only by anatomic reduction and compression fixation. In areas of stable bone contact, direct extension of haversian osteons unites the fragments. In minute fracture gaps that are rigidly stabilized, lamellar bone forms after granulation tissue or woven bone deposition. The process in each instance is bony union through direct bone formation; callus formation is not involved in the process. Although this repair is exclusively of bone tissue, initially, it is mechanically inferior to normal cortical bone. Normal strength is attained through extensive remodeling, which may take months to complete.

Primary bone healing is characterized radiographically by a lack of periosteal callus, a gradual loss in opacity of the fragment ends, and a progressive disappearance of the fracture line. The re-establishment of cortex and medullary cavity continuity occurs quickly (Fig. 14–8).

Secondary Bone Healing

The process of secondary bone healing involves fibrous connective tissue or fibrocartilaginous callus that is replaced by bone. This is the most frequently encountered form of bone healing clinically. The cells participating in the healing process are pluripotential mesenchymal elements, which differentiate into osteoblasts, fibroblasts, or chondroblasts, depending on the specific microenvironment at the time. Bone

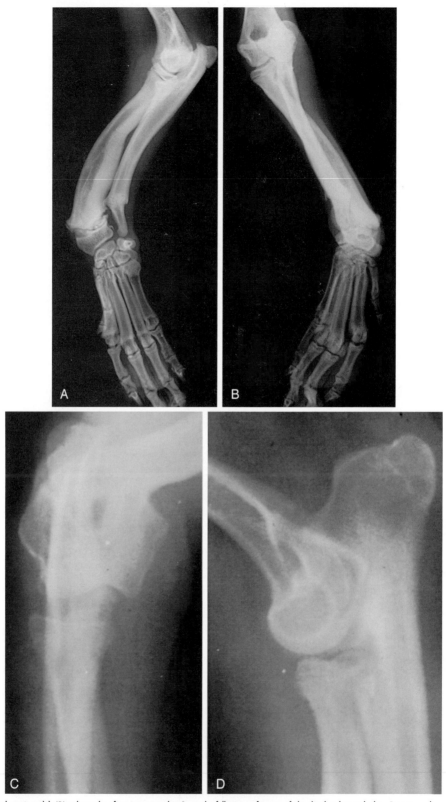

FIGURE 14–5. Lateral *(A)* and craniocaudal *(B)* radiographs of an immature dog 2 months following a fracture of the distal radius and ulna. Premature closure of the distal ulnar physis has resulted in a valgus and rotational deformity of the forelimb. There is proximal subluxation of the humeroulnar joint with remodeling of the anconeal process and semilunar notch of the ulna. Lateral *(C)* and craniocaudal *(D)* radiographs of the elbow of a young dog with insufficient longitudinal radial growth. There is distal subluxation of the radius and proximal subluxation of the ulna from the humerus.

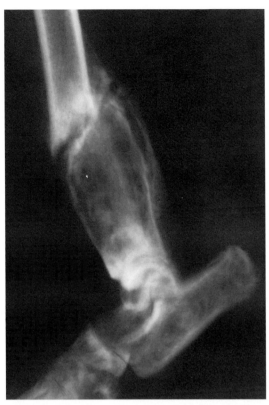

FIGURE 14–6. Lateral radiograph in which an expansile lesion of the distal tibia with cortical thinning and generalized osteolysis can be seen. There is a pathologic fracture at the junction of the expansile lesion and the tibial shaft. A cuff of periosteal bone is present subjacent to the fracture. Histologic diagnosis was fibrosarcoma.

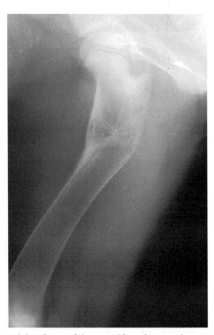

FIGURE 14–7. Pathologic fracture of the proximal femur from secondary nutritional hyperparathyroidism. Mineral resorption with subsequent bone weakening resulted in the fracture. The cortices are thin, the trabeculae are scant, and the bone is less opaque than normal.

Clinical Union

Clinical union refers to the point in fracture healing when the fixation or stabilization device can be removed and the animal returned to some degree of normal activity. A combina-

cannot form in an unfavorable environment (motion). Therefore, under conditions of instability, the mesenchymal cells of the periosteum respond by the production of a fibrous-to-fibrocartilaginous callus. With time, this callus bridges the fragments and increases stability. The stable environment permits vascularization of the callus, resulting in callus ossification and thus bony union. Callus size is determined by a host of factors: fracture type, degree of stability, width of the fracture gap, and vascularity of the regional soft tissues.

The following radiographic description of uncomplicated secondary bone healing is of a simple long-bone diaphyseal fracture that has been stabilized with an intramedullary pin (Table 14–1).[12] By the first week, fragment ends begin to lose their sharp margins, and the fracture gap increases slightly in width. These changes result from a combination of interfragmentary motion, resorption of necrotic bone ends, and vascular ingrowth. Within the next 2 weeks, variable amounts of periosteal, endosteal, and intercortical callus appear. Initial periosteal callus is faintly mineralized and has irregular margins; it is located subjacent to the cortex on each fragment a slight distance from the fracture gap. By 4 weeks, the callus is smoother and more opaque and is visualized as a cuff of bone beginning to bridge the fracture gap; the fracture line should be smaller in size. After 4 weeks, the fracture line is slowly obliterated, and the bony callus bridges the fracture area. At this point, the callus should be as opaque as normal bone. After 12 weeks, the external callus remodels until the continuity of the cortex and medullary cavity is re-established. This final process may take several months to years. Healing in individual patients varies from this description, depending on several factors (Fig. 14–9).

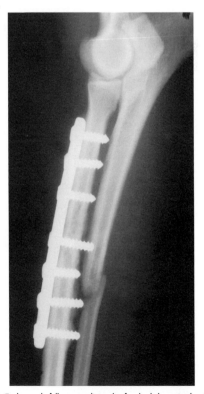

FIGURE 14–8. Twelve-week follow-up radiograph of a healed proximal radial fracture. The fracture line is no longer evident, and there is continuity of the cortex and medullary cavity. Anatomic reduction and stable fixation resulted in bone healing without the formation of a periosteal callus. The ulnar fracture is not healed.

Table 14-1
RADIOGRAPHIC SIGNS OF SECONDARY BONE HEALING

5–10 days after reduction
  Fracture fragments loose sharp margins
  Demineralization of fracture fragment ends results in slight
    fracture line widening
10–20 days after reduction
  Formation of endosteal and periosteal callus
  Decreasing size of fracture gap
  Variable loss in opacity of free fracture fragments
30 days after reduction
  Fracture lines gradually disappear
  External callus increases in opacity and remodels
3 months after reduction
  Continued remodeling of external callus
  Trabecular pattern may develop within the callus
  Cortical shadow becomes visible through the callus
  Medullary cavity continuity re-established gradually
  Cortical remodeling along the lines of stress

tion of radiographic, clinical, and historical evidence is used to arrive at this assessment. Knowledge of the factors that modify fracture healing is important in this regard.

Factors That Modify Fracture Healing

In the evaluation of fracture healing, many factors that influence healing or contribute to complications must be considered. Understanding their role partially explains the radiographic appearance in follow-up evaluations.

Vascular Integrity

The normal blood supply of a long bone is derived from several sources (Fig. 14–10). Although the degree of vascular compromise to a fractured bone is not detectable radiographically, vascular disruption can be estimated based on the type and location of the fracture and the degree of separation and overriding of the fragments (Fig. 14–11).

Normal vascular ingrowth at the fracture site occurs within the first 10 days after injury. Radiographically, this ingrowth is seen as slight demineralization of fragment ends that results in slight widening of the fracture gap and fuzzy fragment margins. Isolated bone fragments that are revascularizing respond similarly. Regional vascular status also influences callus characteristics because of the effects of relative tissue hypoxia on stem cell differentiation.[13] A rich vascular network results in pluripotential daughter cells that become osteoblasts. Decreased vascularity below a critical point results in chondroblasts or fibroblasts. The produced bone or fibrocartilage differs in radiographic opacity. Because of compromised circulation, the initial callus formation at the fracture site is fibrocartilaginous (soft-tissue opacity). Initial mineralized callus forms at a slight distance from the fracture gap where the circulation is less compromised. With increasing stability and subsequent vascular ingrowth, the entire callus mineralizes.

The temporal sequence of revascularization after a fracture and the associated roentgen findings vary for each fracture. This variation is the result of differences in the extent of the initial circulatory compromise, postreduction fragment stability, and available soft tissue in the region, which is a principal source of neovascularization for healing bone (extraosseous blood supply of healing bone).[14]

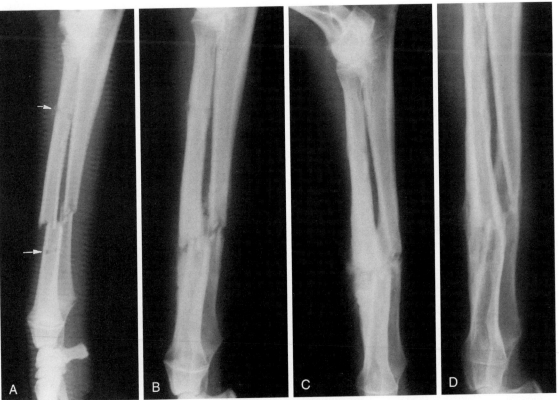

FIGURE 14–9. Sequential lateral radiographs of a midshaft antebrachial fracture, which healed by secondary bone healing. *A,* In the initial postreduction radiograph, there is approximately 50 percent purchase of the fracture fragments. A cast has been placed on the limb. Pins were used with a reduction apparatus, causing the pin tracts in the radius *(arrows). B,* Poorly mineralized immature callus (2-week follow-up). *C,* Mature callus begins to bridge the fracture (4-week follow-up). *D,* Healed fracture (10-week follow-up).

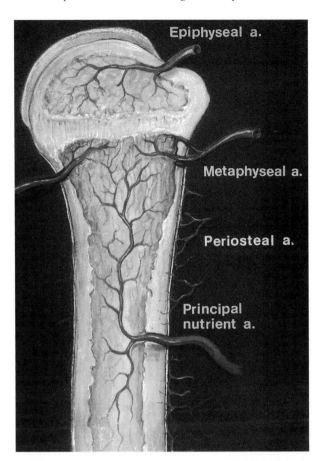

FIGURE 14–10. The blood supply to long bones is derived from several sources. This diagram depicts a long bone with an open physis. Following physeal closure, vascular tufts of the epiphyseal and metaphyseal arteries unite.

Fracture Location

The anatomic location of a fracture may influence the healing response. For example, metaphyseal fractures have an early onset of mineralized callus when compared with diaphyseal

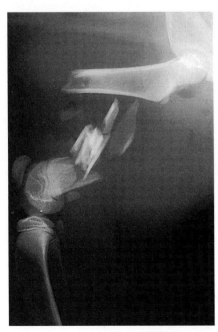

FIGURE 14–11. Severe comminution and fragment displacement in this femoral fracture probably resulted in damage to the nutrient artery and periosteal blood supply. What impact would this have on fracture healing and the appearance of future follow-up radiographs?

fractures; this is due to the rich blood supply in the metaphyseal region and to the abundant trabecular bone with its increased surface area. In general, metaphyseal fractures heal more rapidly than diaphyseal fractures. Antebrachial diaphyseal fractures in miniature breeds and tibial shaft fractures in mature dogs heal more slowly and have a greater incidence of complication than other diaphyseal fractures because there is decreased soft-tissue support and poor vascular supply in the region.[15, 16] Healing capital femoral physeal fractures and femoral neck fractures undergo rapid revascularization if they are adequately reduced and stabilized. In some instances, an exuberant fibrovascular response may occur, which causes local osteolysis of the femoral neck.[17] Radiographically, this response results in femoral neck narrowing, which may proceed to an "apple-core" appearance (Fig. 14–12). Narrowing of the femoral neck may occur in as many as 70 percent of the healing capital physeal repairs. In most dogs, this narrowing is not associated with complications.[18]

Degree of Motion

Stability and adequate blood supply are related factors that are essential for normal fracture healing. An unstable fracture results in damage to the microvasculature in the region. Radiographically, fracture fragments may retain their sharp margins longer than usual. Initial callus at the fracture site is usually poorly mineralized and nonbridging (Fig. 14–13). Periosteal stimulation due to fragment motion may result in callus formation at a point distant from the fracture site. The callus initially presents as ill-defined, poorly marginated periosteal new bone that extends over a large portion of the diaphysis. This latter finding, however, is not specific for fragment motion; it may occur secondary to periosteal strip-

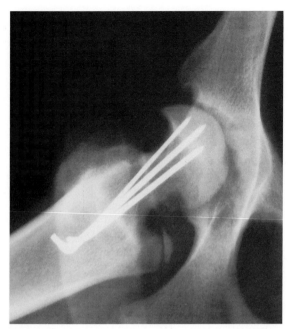

FIGURE 14–12. Follow-up radiograph of a capital femoral physeal fracture 1 month after repair. There is considerable bone resorption in the femoral neck. An exuberant fibrovascular healing response resulted in local osteolysis, producing an "apple-core" appearance of the femoral neck.

ping at the time of injury or surgery or to early osteomyelitis. Clinical signs may help in this distinction.

Persistent motion results in exuberant fibrocartilaginous callus formation, which is an attempt by the body to provide stability. If the callus later mineralizes, it usually does not bridge the fracture gap. Intramedullary pin migration may also be present (Fig. 14–14). If motion is severe, complications such as delayed union or nonunion may result.

Adequate stabilization and vascular integrity lead to the early formation of a well-mineralized callus. The callus is small to moderate in size, sharply marginated, and limited to the fracture site. Rigid fixation with an external fixator or plate results in minimal to no callus formation (see Fig. 14–8). Radiographic assessment of fracture healing in this instance may be difficult. In this situation, one may have to rely more heavily on clinical assessment.

Fracture Type and Degree of Postreduction Apposition

The type of fracture, the degree of initial displacement, and the accuracy of reduction influences fracture-healing characteristics. Spiral and long, oblique diaphyseal fractures heal with more callus than do transverse fractures. Comminuted fractures with multiple fragments may heal more slowly and with more variable callus than do simple fractures. Gunshot fractures with severe soft-tissue injury are often associated with delayed union (Fig. 14–15).[19] Open fractures have a greater tendency for osteomyelitis and complications than do closed fractures.

Severe displacement of fragments with marked overriding indicates severe disruption of the periosteum and regional vasculature. Periosteal stripping alone may stimulate the production of new bone. In these instances, the extent of the periosteal reaction often exceeds the anatomic limit of the fracture itself. Damaged regional vasculature regenerates with time as stability improves.

Poor postreduction apposition may adversely affect stability and thus callus characteristics and healing time. Large fracture gaps require more callus and time to bridge the frag-

ments. Good reduction and alignment minimize the callus requirement and promote anatomic restoration. Good alignment is also important for proper joint function and helps prevent fracture disease and osteoarthrosis. Cancellous bone grafts to augment fracture healing may result in visible islands of ill-defined soft tissue mineralization at the fracture site. As time progresses, these mineralized areas become more uniform in opacity and begin to incorporate fracture fragments.

Age

Juvenile bone heals more rapidly (2 to 4 weeks) and with more exuberant callus formation than mature bone. This is because the immature skeleton is rapidly growing and has a more extensive blood supply than the adult skeleton. Young animals also exhibit a periosteal reaction after injury that is especially evident at sites where heavy fascial attachments are stripped from bone, such as the adductor muscle attachment to the caudal femur. In this instance, a prominent spike of new bone formation coursing proximally in the caudal musculature may occur. This finding is seen to a variable degree in all dogs but seems to be more prominent in younger animals (Fig. 14–16).

POSTREDUCTION AND FOLLOW-UP RADIOGRAPHIC EVALUATION

Initial Postoperative Evaluation

The immediate postoperative radiographs should be evaluated for the quality of fracture reduction, fragment apposi-

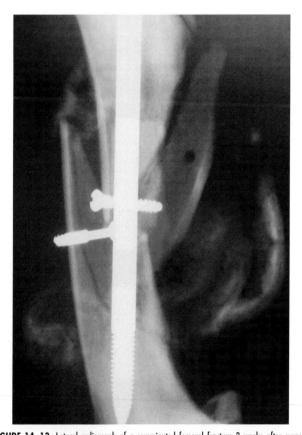

FIGURE 14–13. Lateral radiograph of a comminuted femoral fracture 3 weeks after surgery. The surgical devices have not maintained stability, and the main fracture fragments are telescoping. There is a mineralized periosteal reaction in the soft tissue typical of stripped periosteum. Radiographically the fracture fragments are sharply marginated, suggesting nonhealing because of poor regional microvasculature.

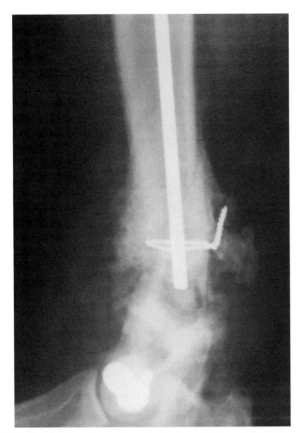

FIGURE 14-14 Follow-up lateral radiograph of a Y-type distal humeral fracture 2 months after repair. There is migration of a large intramedullary pin in a proximal direction. An exuberant nonbridging periosteal and endosteal callus is visualized. These changes suggest instability at the fracture site and infection.

tion, fragment alignment, and proper placement of fixation devices. The degree of fracture reduction refers to the amount of fragment ends that are in contact with one another. For simple fractures, 50 percent contact is the acceptable minimum for adequate healing, but more is desirable. Joint fractures require more accurate reduction for adequate function. Joint incongruities are identified as step deformities or fracture gaps that disrupt articular contour (Fig. 14–17).

Fragment alignment and rotation should also be assessed. Exact anatomic alignment is desirable but impossible to accomplish in all fractures for all fragments. Rotation of the distal fragment relative to the proximal fragment is an important finding that may have serious consequences if not identified and corrected. The accurate assessment of alignment and rotational deformities, however, requires the use of good radiographic positioning. Excess abduction or torsion of the distal limb by the holder during radiography may simulate rotational or angular malalignment of the distal fragment in the postoperative radiograph. In addition, changes in the angle of the x-ray beam relative to the fracture may project fragments differently. These artifacts may be avoided if the animal is carefully positioned.

Next the orthopedic fixation device is evaluated for placement and the ability to maintain reduction and to prevent motion throughout the healing phase. Weakness in fixation placement, if caught early, may be corrected, and disastrous complications may be avoided. Intramedullary pins should be seated deeply and should span the fracture gap adequately. The pins should be of sufficient size for the bone involved and should not penetrate the joint. The far and near pins of a two-pin external fixator apparatus should be properly angled toward the bone, just penetrating both cortices. Wires should be of adequate size, they should not be kinked or broken, and each arm should be twisted equally. The wire should be seated snugly against the cortex with a minimum of space between it and the bone. Bone plate size is important to evaluate. Excessively large plates may result in stress protection of the bone and bone atrophy-demineralization. Implants that are too small may result in instability at the fracture site, with delayed union or nonunion as a possible sequela. Bone plates should be anchored securely to the bone, with a minimum of six cortices engaged by the bone screws above and below the fractures. Bone screws should be solidly seated and fully engaged in each cortex. The orthopedic devices should not cause fragment distraction or be interposed between major fragments.

Follow-Up Evaluations

The limb should be remeasured during each radiographic evaluation, and appropriate kVp and mAs factors should be selected on the basis of an established technique chart. Limb atrophy changes the thickness measurement significantly during fracture healing. Follow-up studies in which the same exposure factors were used as for the initial fracture radiograph may vary markedly in tissue opacity.

Bandages, casts, and external fixation rods should be removed if possible before radiography. A clear, unobstructed view of the fracture area is then ensured. If cast removal is impractical, the following technical alterations are suggested.

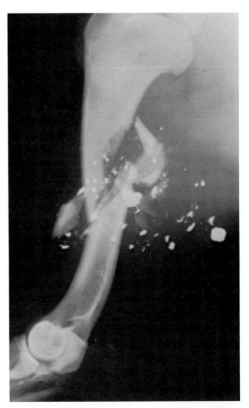

FIGURE 14-15. Lateral radiograph of a severely comminuted gunshot-induced fracture of the humerus. Multiple metallic fragments are identified within the soft tissues. Gunshot fractures are open fractures that usually have extensive regional soft-tissue trauma owing to the projectile. Both of these factors contribute to complications in the healing process. This fracture was stabilized by using an external fixator and eventually healed 1 year later.

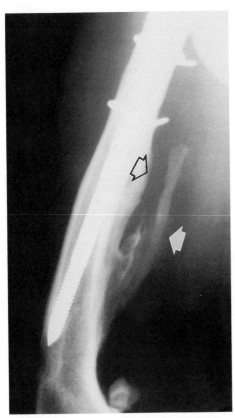

FIGURE 14–16. Lateral radiograph of a pinned femoral fracture. There is mineralization in the area of attachment of the adductor muscle *(solid arrow)*. Mature callus is present at the fracture site *(open arrow)*.

For plaster casts, the cast limb is measured, and the normal kVp is increased by 10 percent. For fiberglass casts and heavy bandages, the cast limb is measured, and the normal kVp for that measurement is used.

The protocol for repeat radiographs in fracture healing varies with the clinician and with the circumstances of each patient. Obviously, every follow-up office visit of a fracture patient need not include a radiographic examination. Good clinical judgment should be exercised in this regard. In general, a basic radiographic plan should be followed and modified when appropriate.[21] Radiographs should be made immediately after initial fracture reduction or after any major alterations (removal, adjustments, or additions) of stabilization devices. Routine follow-up radiographs are made every 3 or 4 weeks (or longer) to assess healing. If the clinical signs and history suggest complications, immediate re-examination is indicated. Revision of the routine follow-up schedule may be necessary if complications are seen that necessitate more frequent monitoring.

Follow-up radiographs should be evaluated for progression in the fracture healing process or the possible development of complications. This evaluation is facilitated by comparing current radiographs with previous studies, especially the immediate postoperative and the most recent follow-up examination.

Radiograph Evaluation Scheme

To ensure that vital information is not overlooked, the ABCDS mnemonic system may be used when evaluating postreduction films. The five letters in the mnemonic stand for *A*lignment, *B*one, *C*artilage (joints), *D*evice (orthopedic appliance or device), and *S*oft tissues. When this system is used, a complete radiographic evaluation is ensured.

Alignment

The major and minor fracture fragments should be evaluated for any changes in alignment, reduction, or rotation since the previous study. This evaluation is especially important for poorly reduced fractures or for those stabilized with intramedullary pins in which rotational forces are not adequately controlled.

Bone

The bone should be evaluated for the progression of fracture healing and callus formation. All fragments should be involved in the healing response and should be in the same location as in previous radiographs. Fragments that are

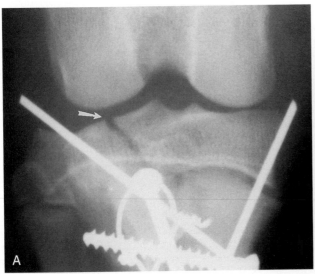

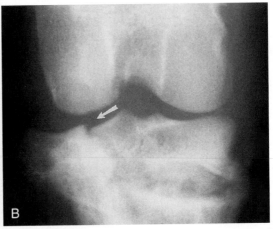

FIGURE 14–17. *A,* Immediate postreduction radiograph of a proximal tibial fracture. A small fracture gap of the tibial articular surface is present *(arrow)*. The joint surface is still congruent; therefore, this is acceptable reduction. *B,* Follow-up radiograph showing a *step deformity* of the proximal tibial articular surface *(arrow)*. The incongruity can lead to degenerative joint disease.

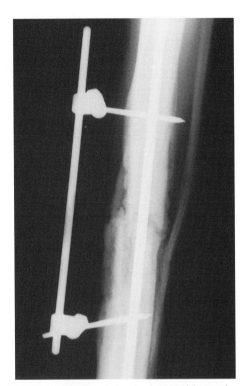

FIGURE 14–18. Craniocaudal radiograph 4 weeks after internal fixation of a midshaft tibial fracture. There is a smoothly marginated, continuous periosteal reaction surrounding the fragments distal to the fracture site. Periosteal stripping at the time of injury and slight rotational instability could account for the finding. The smooth margins suggest chronicity. When the fracture site was examined 2 weeks later, there was complete fragment union, and the orthopedic devices were removed.

poorly vascularized retain their sharp margins radiographically. With time, they may revascularize and become incorporated into the healing process, or they may become ischemic and develop into a sequestrum. Persistence of sharp margins and an increased opacity of the fragment on subsequent radiographs indicate sequestrum formation.

Fragments removed surgically create defects in the region of the fracture. Large defects seldom fill in completely and may serve as a point of stress concentration, rendering the implant vulnerable to bending or breaking. The bone may also be weaker at this site when the implant is removed.

The overall bone opacity and architecture should also be evaluated. Complications such as osteomyelitis and disuse atrophy, if gone unsuspected, may be well advanced by the next follow-up examination. The routine evaluation of bone opacity and architecture may help identify suspect areas and, thus, treatment planning.

Excessive periosteal reactions are often seen either at or distant from the fracture site. These reactions may result from a number of possibilities: normal callus for that fracture, rotational instability, infection, and periosteal avulsion or stripping at the time of injury or surgery (Fig. 14–18; see Fig. 14–16). On follow-up studies, many plated bones have a variably sized callus. This finding may suggest some instability, but other possibilities include interfragmentary callus formation owing to the size of the fracture gap, cancellous grafting with new bone production, and periosteal trauma during surgery.

Situations in which no to minimal callus formation is evident are occasionally encountered. Possibilities for such scant formation include too short an interval since fixation, primary bone healing (must have anatomic reduction and rigid fixation), rigid fixation resulting in minimal callus formation,

compromised vascularity with poorly mineralized callus, and atrophic nonunion. Clinical signs, history, and serial radiographs are helpful in distinguishing among these possibilities.

Cartilage

It is important to evaluate the joint spaces near the fracture. For articular fractures, the apposition of fragments should be carefully evaluated on standard and oblique views. Joints should be scrutinized for evidence of migration of the orthopedic device into the joint space. The development of joint effusion, an irregular periosteal reaction, and subchondral bone lysis may signal septic arthritis. Joint effusion in the presence of osteophytes is suggestive of degenerative joint disease. The range of motion of the joint is better evaluated clinically than radiographically.

Orthopedic Device

The placement and position of the orthopedic implants should be compared with those on previous radiographs. Always check for movements, bending, or breakage of pins, wires, plates, and screws. Minimal implant bending may be detected by placing a straight edge on the radiograph. A loose implant is painful and does not provide the structural support for which it was intended. A radiolucency is often noted in bone at the point where a metallic device is located (Fig. 14–19). The list of radiographic diagnoses to be ruled out for this finding includes motion of the implant or fracture fragments, osteomyelitis, and bone necrosis secondary to heat generated by high-speed drills. Bone loss around an implant may be sufficient to result in loosening but not in detectable radiopacity changes because 50 percent of bone matrix must be lost before a lytic area is detectable radiographically.

The time to remove a surgical implant (clinical union) varies with each patient and should depend on a blend of clinical and radiographic information but mostly good clinical judgment. Clinically the limb should be palpably firm and nonpainful, and some weight bearing should be present. Radiographically, pin implants are removed if the fracture line is not visible and normal callus bridges all or most of the fracture. Removal of plate implants follows similar principles, although callus is more variable, depending on the type and severity of the fracture and the rigidity of fixation. Suggested timetables for plate removal have been published.[22, 23] In one study, 3 to 5 months for young animals and 5 to 14 months

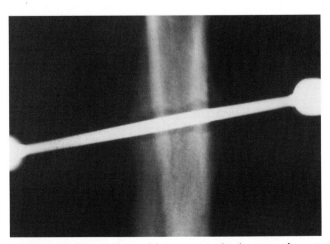

FIGURE 14–19. There is an obvious radiolucent tract surrounding this transverse fixator pin. This amount of bone loss is sufficient to result in implant loosening. Many of these pin tracts are infected, albeit subclinically.

for adults were the recommended intervals.[24] Removal of screws and pins penetrating the cortex leaves defects in the bone. Although these areas fill with bone, the new bone is less opaque, and thus the defect may remain radiographically apparent for months to years.[24] If an implant is removed prematurely or physical activity is too vigorous shortly after removal, refracture through the original fracture site may occur.

Soft Tissues

Postoperative emphysema and soft-tissue swelling are usually gone or are significantly decreased within 7 to 10 days. Subcutaneous and fascial emphysema is recognized as rounded or linear air opacities within the soft tissues. Soft-tissue swelling is characterized by the loss of fascial plane visualization and increased limb size. Air pockets with soft-tissue swelling that recurs after initial subsidence indicate infection. Chronically, soft-tissue atrophy results in loss of fascial plane visualization with a decrease in muscle mass. Calcification of soft tissues in animals with a fracture is occasionally seen, possibly resulting from an isolated bone fragment or cancellous grafts within the soft tissue, dystrophic mineralization, mineralization of hematoma, and myositis ossificans. Soft-tissue mineralization may also occur in conjunction with an aggressive bone lesion secondary to osteomyelitis or fracture-associated sarcoma.

FRACTURE COMPLICATIONS

Malunion is defined as bone healing in an abnormal position. In long bones, malunion may be characterized as end to end, side to side, end to side, and cross-union with adjacent bones. These configurations are associated with variable degrees of angular and rotational deformities (Fig. 14–20). If deformity is severe, functional impairment may ensue, or abnormal weight bearing may result in joint arthrosis. When malunion occurs within a joint, the incongruity quickly leads to degenerative changes.

Delayed union is present when a fracture has not healed in the time that would be expected for the bone involved and the type of fracture (Table 14–2). Radiographically, fracture lines remain evident with minimal callus bridging the fracture gap. In addition, there may be minimal change in the sharpness of fragment margins. Fragment motion due to instability is the most common cause of delayed union. If the underlying cause is adequately corrected, healing ensues. If the situation is not remedied, nonunion may result (Fig. 14–21).

Nonunion is the situation in which all evidence of fracture healing has ceased and the fragment ends have not united. Sequential radiographs are helpful in making this assessment. Radiographically, nonunion has been classified as hypertrophic and atrophic (Fig. 14–22). Clinically, it may be important to distinguish between the two.[25] Hypertrophic nonunion has a well-defined fracture gap; a small to large (elephant foot) nonbridging callus; sclerotic fracture ends with a closed marrow cavity; and fragment ends that are smooth, rounded, and well defined. Atrophic nonunion has minimal if any callus formation, a well-defined fracture gap, and sharply marginated to tapered fragment ends with a sclerotic marrow cavity. Demineralization of bone and soft-tissue atrophy may be present in each instance to varying degrees.

In some nonunion fractures, a pseudoarthrosis (false joint) may form. Bone ends are connected by a fibrous tissue structure resembling a joint capsule that contains mucinous synovium-like fluid. Radiographically, presumptive evidence of

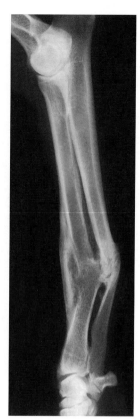

FIGURE 14–20. Lateral antebrachial radiograph in which a malunited fracture of the distal radius and ulna is apparent.

a joint may be seen as a soft-tissue mass at the fracture site with focal bone fragments appearing in a flexed position.

Osteomyelitis as a complication in bone healing is usually due to a combination of local contamination with bacteria, local avascular bone, and instability (Fig. 14–23). Potential causes include contamination from open fractures, long surgical procedures with wide exposure, excessive tissue damage from the trauma or during surgery, and foreign objects (sequestra, sutures and sponges, and occasionally the implant itself) (see Fig. 14–23). The diagnosis of osteomyelitis at a fracture site is usually suspected clinically before the radiographic changes are positive. Clinical signs of acute osteomyelitis are fever, local heat, swelling, and pain. Soft-tissue swelling with or without subcutaneous emphysema may be the only abnormality seen on initial radiographs. In repeat radiographs 7 to 10 days after the onset of clinical signs, a generalized, irregular periosteal reaction is a common finding. As the bone infection progresses, radiographic signs of

Table 14–2

APPROXIMATE TIME TO REACH CLINICAL UNION IN A NONCOMPLICATED DIAPHYSEAL FRACTURE

Age of Animal	External Skeletal and Intramedullary Pin Fixation	Fixation with Plates
Under 3 mo	2–3 wk	4 wk
3–6 mo	4–6 wk	2–3 mo
6–12 mo	5–8 wk	3–4 mo
Over 1 yr	7–12 wk	5–8 mo

From Brinker WO, Hohn RB, and Prieur WD (Eds): Manual of Internal Fixation in Small Animals. New York, Springer-Verlag, 1984; with permission.

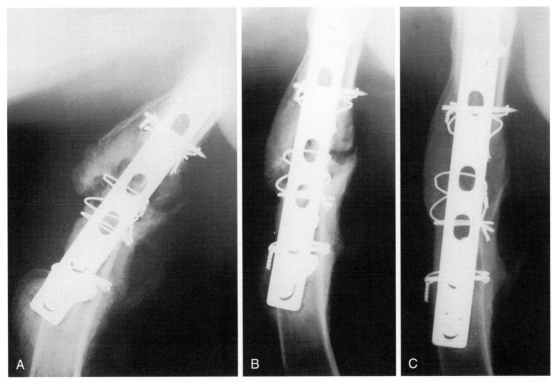

FIGURE 14–21. Sequential lateral radiographs of a delayed union, comminuted midshaft femoral fracture. *A,* Four-month follow-up radiograph shows malalignment of fragments, reactive nonbridging callus formation, and a visible fracture gap. *B,* Five months later, there is an organized callus. Clinically the limb was stable and not painful; the animal was bearing weight. *C,* Nine months later, bridging callus obliterates the fracture gap. The fracture has healed.

an aggressive bone lesion may develop (see Fig. 14–23) (see Chapters 4 and 15). A combination of corticomedullary osteosclerosis with areas of osteolysis surrounding metallic pin implants is highly suggestive of motion or pin tract osteomyelitis. Pin tract osteomyelitis is frequently associated with external fixator pins (see Fig. 14–19). Irregular periosteal reactions are often at the pin-cortex junction.

A *sequestrum* is a dead bone fragment. It may be paraosteal,

cortical, or intramedullary in location. Classically an infected sequestrum is recognized as a sharply marginated sclerotic fragment separated from the parent bone by a zone of radiolucency and an outer rim of sclerotic bone (involucrum) (Fig. 14–24). In some instances, the draining tract is evident (cloaca). Bone sequestra may be associated with infections or draining tracts. Failure of any isolated bone segment to be resorbed or revascularized may result in a sterile sequestra.

FIGURE 14–22. *A,* Hypertrophic nonunion. In this lateral view of a chronic distal humeral fracture, there is a well-defined fracture gap, nonbridging callus formation, and a sclerotic marrow cavity of the fragment ends. *B,* An atrophic nonunion is evident in a 3-month follow-up radiograph of a proximal tibial fracture. There is fragment distraction with a well-defined fracture gap, no visible callus formation, sharply marginated fragment ends, and a sclerotic marrow cavity.

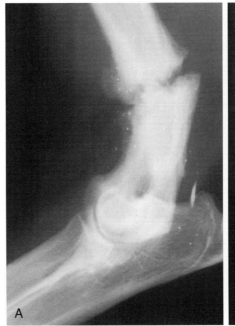
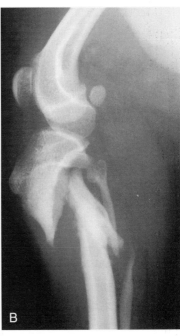

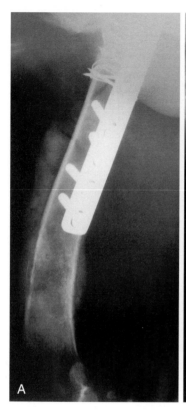

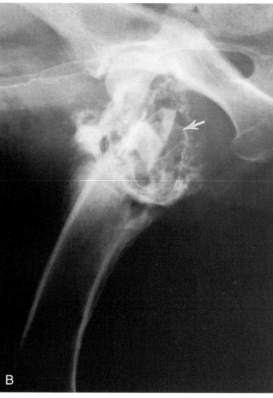

FIGURE 14–23. *A,* Lateral view 4 weeks after repair of a proximal femoral fracture. There is abundant periosteal reaction, cortical thinning, and permeative osteolysis of the distal femoral fragment. Minimal callus formation is associated with the fracture site. Radiographic diagnosis was osteomyelitis. *B,* Lateral view of a previous proximal femoral fracture in which a sponge was left postoperatively. There is bone discontinuity, cortical destruction, ill-defined periosteal reaction, and soft-tissue mineralization; these signs suggest osteomyelitis. A shell-like mineralization developed around the sponge *(arrow).*

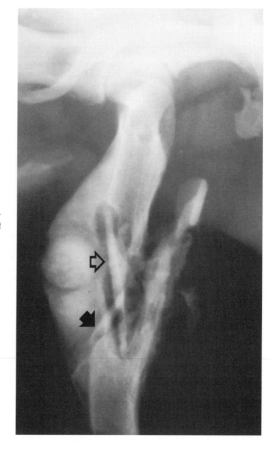

FIGURE 14–24. Chronic midshaft femoral fracture had an associated draining tract for several months. Two well-marginated radiopaque cortical fragments (sequestra) were identified *(solid and open arrows).* The largest fragment *(open arrow)* is surrounded by a zone of radiolucency and an outer rim of sclerotic bone (involucrum).

In these instances, reaction of surrounding bone tissue is less exuberant, and clinical signs of osteomyelitis are not present.

Nerve injury may be associated with the initial fracture (e.g., the radial nerve in spiral humeral fractures) or with fracture repair and healing (sciatic nerve in femoral fracture pinning). Fracture-related sciatic palsy may occur with medially displaced caudal iliac shaft fractures or sacroiliac fracture-luxation with cranial displacement of the ilium.[26] It may also occur secondary to surgically induced trauma, scar formation in the region of the nerve, and the proximal placement of the pin in the femur.[27] The more medial that the exit of the pin relative to the greater trochanter is and the longer the exposed proximal portion of the pin, the more likely is the occurrence of sciatic entrapment (Fig. 14–25). Thus, postoperative femoral radiographs should be evaluated for proximal pin location.

Bone atrophy-demineralization may result from chronic disuse of the limb or from stress protection by the orthopedic device. A generalized decrease in bone opacity with coarse trabeculation involving the entire limb signifies disuse atrophy-demineralization. The bone may become hypoplastic. Demineralization may occur within 2 or 3 weeks in young animals but takes longer in the adult. A focal decrease in bone opacity and cortical thickness subjacent to an orthopedic implant suggest demineralization due to stress protection by the implant. Stress protection is related to increased implant size and stiffness and not to implant type (plate or pin)

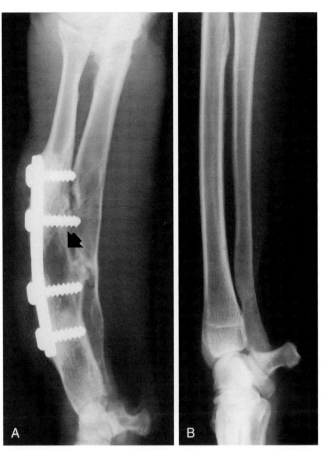

FIGURE 14–26. *A,* Lateral view of the antebrachium of a 2-year-old dog 1 year after corrective osteotomy for radius curvus. The dog was moderately lame and exhibited elbow pain. A large bone plate with four bone screws is affixed to the radius. There is medullary sclerosis surrounding the bone screws and a focal area of decreased bone opacity involving the radius beneath the bone plate and two innermost screws *(arrow).* These findings are compatible with demineralization secondary to stress protection. In addition, the entire distal limb exhibits a generalized decrease in bone opacity, cortical thinning, and coarse texture of the trabecular bone. *B,* The distal antebrachium of a normal dog. Compare the cortical thickness and trabecular bone with those in *A.*

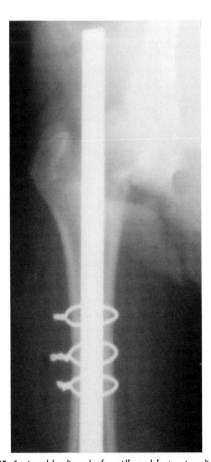

FIGURE 14–25. Craniocaudal radiograph of a midfemoral fracture immediately after repair with three full cerclage wires and a large intramedullary pin. There is a more medial exit of the proximal pin relative to the greater trochanter than desired. Additionally, there is a long, exposed proximal portion of the pin. Both of these factors contribute to a reactive tissue scar that could entrap the sciatic nerve. The therapeutic plan includes cutting the pin to decrease its length.

(Fig. 14–26). In this instance, sequential removal of implants or parts of implants results in increased bone stress and mineral deposition, which may be monitored radiographically.

Joint complications after fractures include degenerative joint disease, ankylosis, and soft-tissue muscular and capsular contracture. Physeal growth deformities may follow direct trauma to the physis or may result from radioulnar synostosis (see Fig. 14–5).

Fracture-associated sarcomas in the dog have been described.[28] The cause is unknown, but theories include coincidental spontaneous osteosarcomas, carcinogenesis owing to corrosion byproducts of metallic implants, and the cocarcinogenic effects of chronic inflammation in an environment in which stem cells are proliferating (fracture healing). Current evidence suggests that the last is the most likely cause. The overall incidence is low, and a variable postfracture latency period is usually present (mean, 5.8 years). The femoral diaphysis is the most frequently involved site of fracture-associated sarcoma (Fig. 14–27). The roentgen signs are those of an aggressive bone lesion with soft-tissue mineralization, which occurs in the location of a previous fracture that had experienced serious postoperative complications, such as infection, delayed union, implant loosening, and draining

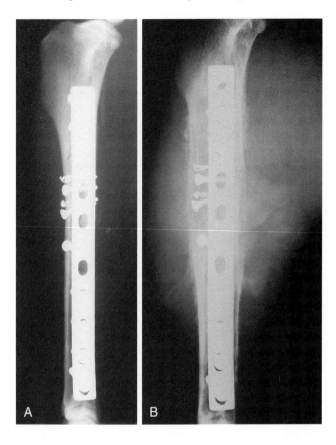

FIGURE 14–27. *A,* Lateral view of a midshaft tibial fracture repair using a bone plate. *B,* Same limb 5 years later. There is a midshaft aggressive bone lesion with extensive periosteal reaction and soft-tissue mineralization. Histologic diagnosis was undifferentiated sarcoma.

tracts.[29] A draining fistula may be present in some instances, and thus osteomyelitis may be present simultaneously. The lungs should always be examined radiographically for potential metastatic disease when limb neoplasia is suspected.

References

1. Walker M: Horizontal-beam radiography as a diagnostic aid for trauma of the abdomen and extremities. *In* Scientific Proceedings, Vol II, 42nd Annual Meeting of American Animal Hospital Association, Cincinnati, OH, 1975, pp 254–256.
2. Orsini PG, Rendano VT, and Sack WO: Ectopic nutrient foramina in the third metatarsal bone of the horse. Equine Vet J *13*:132, 1981.
3. Pitt M, and Speer D: Radiologic reporting of orthopedic trauma. Med Radiogr Photogr *15*:14, 1982.
4. Nunamaker D: Management of infected fractures—osteomyelitis. Vet Clin North Am [Small Anim Pract] *5*:259, 1975.
5. Carter D, and Spengler D: Biomechanics of fracture. *In* Sumner-Smith G (Ed): Bone in Clinical Orthopedics. Philadelphia, WB Saunders, 1982, pp 315–316.
6. Salter RB, and Harris WR: Injuries involving the epiphyseal plate. J Bone Joint Surg *45*:587, 1963.
7. Llewellyn HR: Growth plate injuries: Diagnosis, prognosis and treatment. J Am Anim Hosp Assoc *12*:77, 1976.
8. Marretta SM, and Schrader SC: Physeal injuries in the dog: A review of 135 cases. J Am Vet Med Assoc *182*:708, 1983.
9. Peacock E, and Van Winkle W: Wound Repair. Philadelphia, WB Saunders, 1976, pp 547–606.
10. Perren SM: Primary bone healing. *In* Bojrab MJ (Ed): Pathophysiology in Small Animal Surgery. Philadelphia, Lea & Febiger, 1981, pp 519–528.
11. Rahn B: Bone healing: Histologic and physiologic concepts. *In* Sumner-Smith G (Ed): Bone in Clinical Orthopedics. Philadelphia, WB Saunders, 1982, p 366.
12. Braden TD, and Brinker WO: Radiologic and gross anatomic evaluation of bone healing in the dog. J Am Vet Med Assoc *169*:1318, 1976.
13. Dingwall JS: Fractures. *In* Archibald J (Ed): Canine Surgery, 2nd Ed. Santa Barbara, CA, American Veterinary Publications, 1974, pp 949–956.
14. Rhinelander FW, and Wilson JW: Blood to developing, mature, and healing bone. *In* Sumner-Smith G (Ed): Bone in Clinical Orthopedics. Philadelphia, WB Saunders, 1982, pp 81–158.
15. Lappin MR, Aron DN, Herron HL, et al: Fracture of the radius and ulna in the dog. J Am Anim Hosp Assoc *19*:643, 1983.
16. Heppenstall RB: Fractures of the tibia and fibula. *In* Heppenstall RB (Ed): Fracture Treatment and Healing. Philadelphia, WB Saunders, 1980, pp 777–802.
17. Hulse DH, Abdelbaki YZ, and Wilson J: Revascularization of femoral capital physeal fractures following surgical fixation. J Vet Orthop *2*:50, 1981.
18. DeCamp CE, Probst CW, and Thomas MW: Internal fixation of femoral capital physeal injury in dogs: 40 cases (1979–1987). J Am Vet Med Assoc *194*:1750, 1989.
19. Swan KG, and Swan RC: Gunshot Wounds: Pathophysiology and Management. Littleton, MA, PSG Publishing, 1980, p 211.
20. O'Brien TR, Morgan J, and Suter P: Epiphyseal plate injury in the dog: A radiographic study of growth disturbance in the forelimb. J Small Anim Pract *12*:19, 1971.
21. Morgan JP: Radiographic diagnosis of fractures and fracture repair in the dog. Bi-weekly Small Anim Vet Med Update Series *19*:1, 1978.
22. DeAngelis M: Causes of delayed union and nonunion of fractures. Vet Clin North Am [Small Anim Pract] *5*:251, 1975.
23. Brinker W, Flo G, Braden T, et al: Removal of bone plates in small animals. J Am Anim Hosp Assoc *11*:577, 1975.
24. Rahn B: Bone healing: Histologic and physiologic concepts. *In* Sumner-Smith G (Ed): Clinical Orthopedics. Philadelphia, WB Saunders, 1982, p 377.
25. Brinker WO, Hohn RB, and Prieur WD: Manual of Internal Fixation in Small Animals. New York, Springer-Verlag, 1983, p 243.
26. Jacobson A, and Schrader S: Peripheral nerve injury associated with fracture or fracture-dislocation of the pelvis in dogs and cats: 34 cases (1978–1982). J Am Vet Med Assoc *190*:569, 1987.
27. Fanton JW, Blass CE, and Withrow SJ: Sciatic nerve injury as a complication of intramedullary pin fixation of femoral fractures. J Am Anim Hosp Assoc *19*:687, 1983.
28. Stevenson S, Hohn R, Pohler O, et al: Fracture-associated sarcoma in the dog. J Am Vet Med Assoc *180*:1189, 1982.
29. Vasseur P, and Stevenson S: Osteosarcoma at the site of a cortical bone allograft in a dog. Vet Surg *16*:70, 1987.

STUDY QUESTIONS

Select the single best response to each question.

1. Fractures of the growing physis usually involve what cellular layer?
   A. The reserve layer of chondrocytes.
   B. The zone of proliferating chondrocytes.
   C. The zone of hypertrophied chondrocytes.
   D. The zone of provisional calcification.
   E. The zone of osseous replacement.

2. Which of the following would result in fracture healing with a minimum of callus?
   A. Poor postreduction apposition.
   B. Persistent motion at the fracture site.
   C. Extensive periosteal stripping.
   D. Comminuted fracture with numerous fragments.
   E. Rigid fracture fixation.

3. Which of the following is true about an avascular bone fragment in a comminuted fracture?
   A. Undergoes permeative osteolysis.
   B. Is a sign of osteomyelitis.
   C. Retains sharp margins radiographically.
   D. Is a sign of nonunion.
   E. Indicates excessive motion of the fragment.

4. Blood supply to the diaphysis of normal bone comes from
   A. Epiphyseal vessels, periosteal vessels, and endosteal vessels.
   B. Telangiectatic vessels, recrudescent vessels, and lacunar vessels.

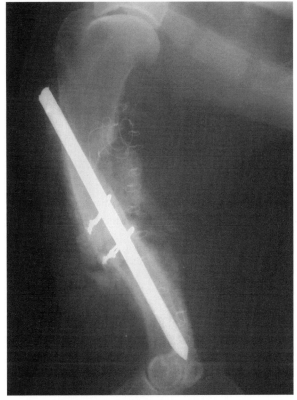

FIGURE 14–29

C. Periosteal vessels, metaphyseal vessels, and nutrient vessels.
D. Articular vessels, joint capsule vessels, and capillary loops.
E. None of the above.

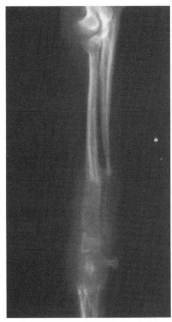

FIGURE 14–30

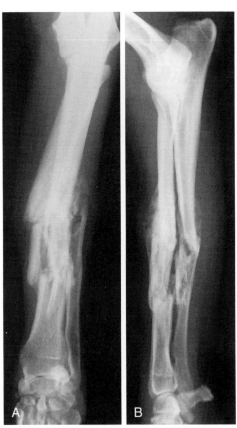

FIGURE 14–28

5. Excessive periosteal reaction seen at or distant from the fracture site may be due to:
   A. Rotational instability of the fragments.
   B. Periosteal stripping at the time of injury or surgery.
   C. Osteomyelitis/bone infection.
   D. All of the above.
   E. None of the above.

6. Which of the following is a radiographic warning sign that a fracture is not healing normally? (Assume that a visible fracture gap is present.)
   A. Demineralization of the fragment ends at the fracture site.
   B. Smooth periosteal reaction located a slight distance from the fracture gap.
   C. A linear radiolucency surrounding the shaft of an external fixator pin.
   D. Sclerotic fragment ends and a closed marrow cavity.
   E. Minimal callus noted in a fracture with rigid fixation.

7. Examine the 3-month follow-up radiographs (Fig. 14–28) of a comminuted radius/ulna fracture repaired with the use of external coaptation. Which statement best describes the healing status at this time?
   A. Nonunion; atrophic type.
   B. Osteomyelitis with possible sequestrum.
   C. Healing fracture but fragments malaligned.
   D. Fracture-induced sarcoma is highly likely.
   E. No evidence of healing—a bone plate should be applied.

8. Examine the 6-week follow-up lateral radiograph of an oblique humeral fracture that has been pinned (Fig. 14–29). Using this single view, which statement best describes the healing status at this time?
   A. Nonunion; hypertrophic type.
   B. Osteomyelitis is highly likely.
   C. The fracture has healed—remove the pin.
   D. Healing but incompletely healed fracture.
   E. None of the above.

9. Examine the 10-week follow-up lateral radiograph of a radius and ulnar transverse fracture repaired with the use of a metasplint (Fig. 14–30). Using this single view, which statement best describes the healing status at this time?
   A. Permeative osteomyelitis is present.
   B. Healed with poorly mineralized callus.
   C. Atrophic nonunion is present.
   D. Healed fracture with bone atrophy-demineralization.
   E. None of the above.

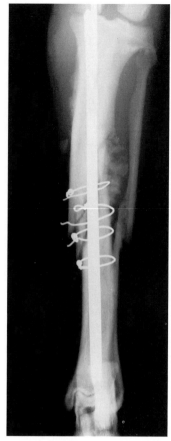

FIGURE 14–31

10. Examine this 4-week follow-up craniocaudal radiograph of a pinned tibial fracture (Fig. 14–31). Using this single view, which statement best summarizes the healing status at this time?
    A. Fragment distraction with probable low-grade osteomyelitis.
    B. Healing but incompletely healed fracture, loose wire.
    C. Delayed union is present.
    D. Malunion with probable cerclage wire–induced ischemia.
    E. None of the above.

(Answers appear on page 636.)

Chapter 15

Bone Tumors Versus Bone Infections

Donald E. Thrall

Neoplastic and infectious bone lesions typically have an aggressive radiographic appearance. The radiographic signs of aggressive bone lesions were discussed in Chapter 4. It is impossible to make a definitive distinction between neoplastic and infectious bone lesions by radiographic means alone. By consideration of the radiographic features of the bone lesion with the signalment, history, and physical and laboratory findings, however, one may often rule in or rule out neoplasia versus infection with a high degree of accuracy.

SOLITARY METAPHYSEAL AGGRESSIVE LESIONS

The most common cause of a solitary metaphyseal aggressive bone lesion is a primary bone tumor.[1] Any solitary aggressive metaphyseal bone lesion in dogs or cats should be considered to be a primary bone tumor until proved otherwise. Osteosarcomas are the most common primary bone tumor in dogs; they originate most commonly in the metaphysis of long tubular bones in large-breed and giant-breed dogs. Common osteosarcoma sites are the proximal humerus, distal radius, distal femur, and proximal and distal tibia. Osteosarcomas may appear primarily lytic (Fig. 15–1); primarily sclerotic (blastic or productive) (Fig. 15–2); or mixed, with lytic and productive features being present (Fig. 15–3). The degree of lysis versus sclerosis is not a feature that should be used to decide whether a lesion is aggressive or not (see Chapter 4).

Osteosarcomas in dogs may also be characterized by a range of periosteal reactions, varying from active (Fig. 15–4) to inactive (see Figs. 15–1 and 15–2). Although bone infections may result in an active periosteal reaction, extremely aggressive and amorphous types of periosteal reactions are more commonly associated with tumors.

Osteosarcoma is also the most common type of primary bone tumor in cats, but it is less common than in the dog. Typically the hindlimbs are affected more often than the forelimbs.[2–4] Feline osteosarcomas are also aggressive radiographically, but primary osteolytic lesions are the most common manifestation.[4] Pulmonary metastasis from feline osteosarcoma is less common than that from canine osteosarcoma.[4]

In both cats and dogs, most osteosarcomas begin in the metaphysis, but they may readily involve the epiphysis or diaphysis, or both. The belief that primary bone tumors do not cross joints or invade adjacent bones is false because both are possible as the tumor enlarges. Such invasion, however, occurs late in the disease process after the primary tumor has grown to a large size. Additionally, primary bone tumors may metastasize to parenchymal organs and other parts of the skeleton.

There are two specific situations in which the development of osteosarcoma is associated with another bone abnormality: (1) bone infarction and (2) fracture-associated osteosarcoma. Idiopathic polyostotic bone infarction is uncommon. Radio-

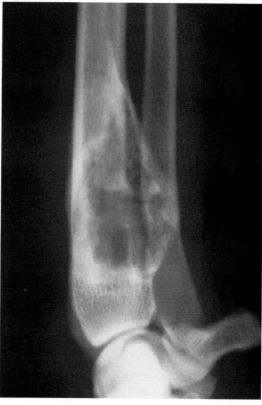

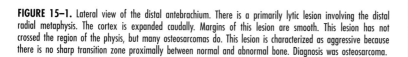

FIGURE 15–1. Lateral view of the distal antebrachium. There is a primarily lytic lesion involving the distal radial metaphysis. The cortex is expanded caudally. Margins of this lesion are smooth. This lesion has not crossed the region of the physis, but many osteosarcomas do. This lesion is characterized as aggressive because there is no sharp transition zone proximally between normal and abnormal bone. Diagnosis was osteosarcoma.

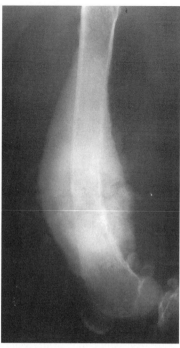

FIGURE 15–2. Lateral view of the femur. A predominantly sclerotic (blastic) lesion is present. The periosteal reaction is smooth, and there is little evidence of cortical destruction. The lesion is classified as aggressive, however, because of the lack of a sharp transition zone proximally between normal and abnormal bone. Diagnosis was osteosarcoma.

graphically, it is characterized by multifocal increases in opacity within the medullary cavity of tubular bones (Fig. 15–5). Dogs with bone infarction are prone to the development of bone sarcoma.[5] The specific cause-and-effect relationship between bone infarction and bone sarcoma is unknown. Dogs developing idiopathic polyostotic bone infarction and subsequent osteosarcoma are occasionally small breeds (shelties and terriers) in comparison with the large breeds usually affected by primary bone neoplasia. Bone infarction resulting from a known cause, such as previous physical insult to the bone, may also result in the development of subsequent osteosarcoma (Fig. 15–6).

The association of tumorigenesis and a fracture or internal fixation device occurs occasionally. Case history reports have been published in which the development of malignant tumors in association with previous skeletal trauma has been documented. This association is discussed in Chapter 14.

Primary bone tumors of the appendicular skeleton other than osteosarcoma are uncommon, but when they do occur, they are typically mesenchymal tumors and include fibrosarcoma, chondrosarcoma, and hemangiosarcoma. These neoplasms generally have a similar radiographic appearance to osteosarcoma and may be differentiated only on the basis of biopsy results. Identification of these alternate tumor types may alter the prognosis because metastatic incidence may be different than from osteosarcoma.

Other than neoplasia, the major diagnosis to be ruled out for a monostotic aggressive bone lesion is mycotic osteomyelitis. Occasionally a mycotic bone lesion is monostotic and metaphyseal-epiphyseal in location. Based strictly on radiographic criteria, such lesions may appear identical to a primary bone tumor (Fig. 15–7). There may be other radiographic evidence, such as pulmonary infiltrates or thoracic lymphadenopathy, or clinical signs of systemic debilitation that support the diagnosis of an infectious process, but a biopsy of the bone lesion is necessary for a definitive diagnosis. Solitary metaphyseal mycotic bone lesions are uncommon, but they do occur, and any monostotic metaphyseal aggressive lesion should be biopsied before a course of therapy is selected.

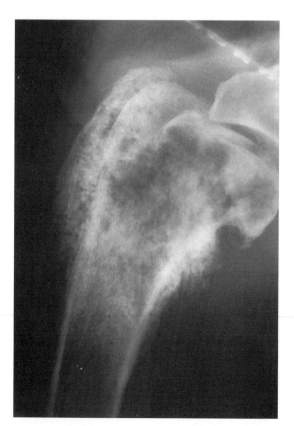

FIGURE 15–3. Lateral view of the proximal humerus. There is a mixed lytic and blastic lesion in the proximal metaphysis and epiphysis. There is cortex destruction cranially, an active periosteal reaction, and no evidence of a transition zone distally between normal and abnormal bone. Diagnosis was osteosarcoma.

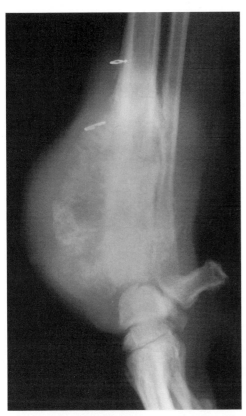

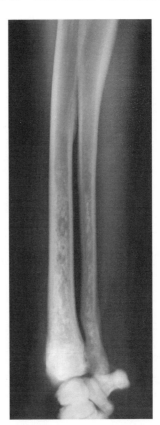

FIGURE 15–4. Lateral view of the distal antebrachium. There is a mixed lytic and blastic lesion in the distal radius. The cortex is destroyed cranially and caudally, there is an active periosteal reaction, and an indistinct transition zone is seen proximally between normal and abnormal bone. The metallic wires were inserted after a biopsy. Diagnosis was osteosarcoma.

FIGURE 15–5. Lateral view of the antebrachium. There are multifocal regions of opacity within the medullary cavity of the distal radius and ulna. The most likely cause for this appearance is bone infarction.

Bacterial osteomyelitis may also result in a monostotic aggressive lesion. Bacterial osteomyelitis is most often the result of direct contamination of the bone, such as by surgery and trauma, rather than being hematogenous. Thus, the location of bacterial osteomyelitis in the bone is more variable than the location of primary tumors, and there is usually a history of previous trauma or surgery. Additionally the signalment and radiographic distribution of the lesion are often sufficient for bacterial infection to be distinguished from neoplasia (Fig. 15–8).

MULTIPLE AGGRESSIVE BONE LESIONS

The major diagnoses to be ruled out for polyostotic aggressive bone lesions are metastatic neoplasia and mycotic osteomyelitis. Mycotic osteomyelitis is more common in dogs than in cats. In general, patients with mycotic osteomyelitis tend to be younger than patients with metastatic solid tumors. Mycotic osteomyelitis is generally of hematogenous origin, accounting for its polyostotic nature. Another consequence of mycotic osteomyelitis being of hematogenous origin is a metaphyseal distribution of the lesions because of the rich blood supply in this region of bone. Diaphyseal lesions, however, do occur.

Identification of mycotic osteomyelitis is most common in geographic regions where predisposing fungi are endemic, for example, the Southeast (blastomycosis) and the Southwest (coccidioidomycosis). Infected dogs, however, may relocate to nonendemic areas, where they may be examined by veterinarians who do not have a high index of suspicion for fungal infections. As noted earlier for solitary mycotic bone lesions,

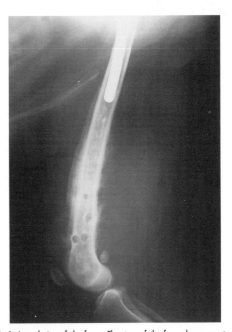

FIGURE 15–6. Lateral view of the femur. The stem of the femoral component of a total hip prosthesis is visible. The prosthesis had been present for 5 years. Focal opacities in the medullary cavity of the femur developed shortly after implant insertion and were interpreted as bone infarcts. The dog became acutely lame, and in this radiograph, a lamellar-appearing periosteal reaction is present cranially, but an irregular, active periosteal reaction is present caudally. There is also soft tissue swelling, which contains regions of mineralization, and no obvious distal transition between normal and abnormal bone. These radiographic signs are indicative of an aggressive process. Multiple biopsy specimens of the femur were obtained; circular biopsy sites are visible. The histologic diagnosis was osteosarcoma, and there is a possibility that the tumor resulted from the long-standing infarcts.

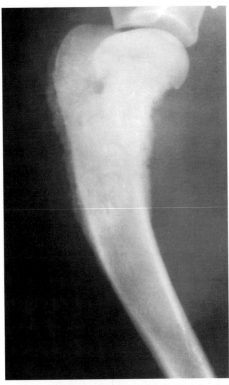

FIGURE 15–7. Lateral view of the proximal humerus. There is a predominantly proliferative lesion in the metaphysis and epiphysis. There is cortex destruction, active periosteal reaction, and an indistinct transition zone distally between normal and abnormal bone. Therefore, the lesion is aggressive. Other bone lesions were not detected. The appearance of the lesion is consistent with neoplasia. The focal lytic region was produced by a biopsy. *Actinomyces* was identified. The bone lesion resolved after appropriate chemotherapy.

there may be other clinical or radiographic evidence supporting an infectious cause of polyostotic aggressive bone lesions, but this is not always true. Mycotic osteomyelitis should be considered in any dog in which polyostotic aggressive bone lesions are identified (Fig. 15–9).

With animal cancer patients being treated more aggressively and living longer, it has become apparent that metastatic bone cancer is common. Any malignant tumor has the potential to metastasize to the skeleton, but, in general, bone metastases from epithelial tumors are more common than bone metastases from mesenchymal tumors.[6] In dogs, mammary, lung, liver, thyroid, and prostate cancers are primary tumors from which it is not uncommon for bone metastases to result.[7, 8] Metastatic tumor sites in the skeleton arise hematogenously. Therefore, they tend to have a polyostotic distribution (Fig. 15–10); ribs, vertebrae, femur, and humerus are commonly affected sites.[7, 8] In long bones, both diaphyseal and metaphyseal locations are common. Metastatic bone tumors are aggressive radiographic lesions, and, as with primary bone tumors, they may be sclerotic, mixed, or predominantly osteolytic. Patients with metastatic bone tumors are generally older and also usually have a history of primary tumor, making the index of suspicion higher for tumor than for mycotic infection.

Bacterial osteomyelitis may also cause polyostotic aggressive lesions. Hematogenous bacterial osteomyelitis is rare in dogs and cats. As for monostotic bacterial osteomyelitis, surgery and trauma are the most common causes. Therefore, bacterial osteomyelitis usually involves only one limb, but more than one bone may be involved. Polyostotic bacterial osteomyelitis affecting one limb may be confused with neo-

plasia. As stated previously, however, the signalment, history, and clinical findings are usually sufficient to separate infectious from neoplastic processes (Fig. 15–11).

AGGRESSIVE DIGITAL BONE LESIONS

The digit is another location where it may be difficult to differentiate radiographically between infectious and neoplastic causes for an aggressive lesion. Subungual tumors are relatively common in the dog, with the most common type being squamous cell carcinoma.[9] Most subungual squamous cell carcinomas involve large-breed dogs with black-hair coats.[9, 10] Melanomas are another common canine subungual tumor.[11] Inflammatory conditions of the digit (i.e., pododermatitis) also occur, and these may be difficult to differentiate radiographically from tumors. Radiographic changes in dogs with pododermatitis and digital tumors were compared.[12] It was found that tumors and pododermatitis were fairly evenly distributed between the manus and the pes. Also, the frequency of bone involvement was similar between subungual tumors and pododermatitis: 25 of 48 (52.1%) for pododermatitis and 33 of 52 (63.5%) for digital tumors. Regarding radiographic changes, it was concluded that pododermatitis could not be differentiated from malignant tumors because both conditions resulted in aggressive bone lesions. Lesions

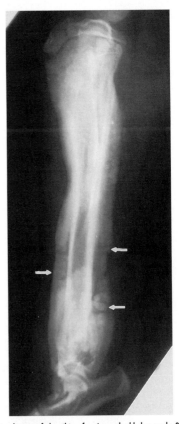

FIGURE 15–8. Lateral view of the tibia of a 6-month-old dog made 3 weeks after external fixation of an open distal tibial physeal fracture. The limb is swollen, warm, and painful. There is extensive periosteal reaction along the bone. In some areas, the periosteal reaction has a palisade appearance *(arrows)*, which is highly suggestive of bacterial osteomyelitis. The combination of the age of the patient, the history, the extension of the periosteal reaction along the entire shaft of the bone, and the palisade appearance of the periosteal reaction is most consistent with bacterial osteomyelitis. Tumor is not a likely diagnosis in this patient. Diagnosis was bacterial osteomyelitis.

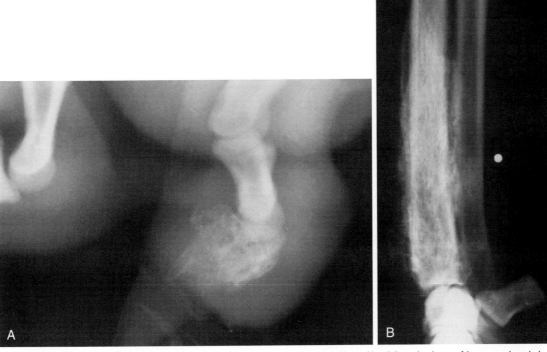

FIGURE 15–9. Lateral radiographs of a rear-limb distal phalanx *(A)* and the distal antebrachium *(B)* of a 5-year-old mixed-breed dog with a history of lameness and weight loss. The phalanx is characterized by multifocal regions of bone destruction, with some evidence of new bone formation. The cortex of the phalanx is destroyed. The distal radius is characterized by mottled regions of increased and decreased bone opacity. The cortex is destroyed cranially and caudally, and there is an active periosteal reaction. There is no sharp transition zone proximally between normal and abnormal bone. The phalanx and radial lesions are both aggressive. Taken alone, both are consistent with primary neoplasia. Taken collectively, a more likely diagnosis is mycotic osteomyelitis or metastatic solid tumor. This dog is relatively young, lives in a blastomycosis endemic area, and had no identifiable primary tumor. Blastomycosis titers were high, and *Blastomyces* was isolated from a bone biopsy. Diagnosis was blastomycosis.

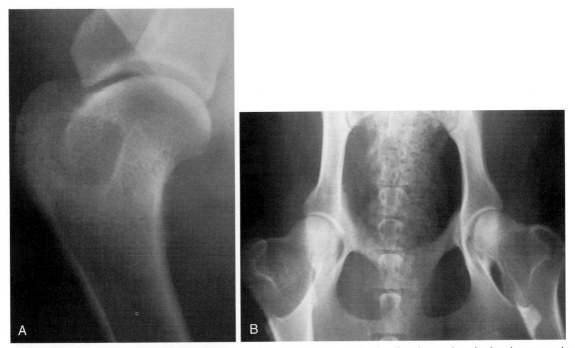

FIGURE 15–10. Lateral view of the proximal humerus *(A)* and ventrodorsal view of the pelvis *(B)* of a 10-year-old Border collie with previously irradiated nasal carcinoma and recent onset of lameness. In the humerus, there is a focal region of decreased bone opacity that has indistinct margins; thus, this lesion is considered aggressive. Additionally, there is active periosteal reaction on the caudal humeral metaphysis. In the pelvis, there is a region of mixed increased and decreased opacity in the right proximal femur, medial to the greater trochanter. The femoral lesion also has indistinct margins and is therefore aggressive. Polyostotic aggressive lesions in an older dog with a known malignant tumor are most likely caused by metastatic cancer. Although malignant nasal tumors rarely metastasize to bone, such occurred in this dog. Diagnosis was metastatic nasal carcinoma.

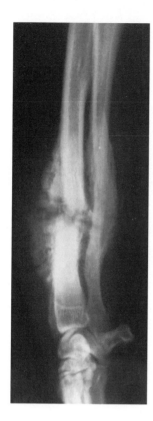

FIGURE 15–11. Lateral view of the antebrachium of a 2-year-old dog that had been bitten by another dog 2 months previously. The dog was lame, and there was swelling of the limb. The radius is characterized by increased opacity in the distal diaphysis and metaphysis, an active periosteal reaction, and a fracture. The periosteal reaction has a palisade appearance in some areas; as mentioned previously (see Fig. 15–7), this is strongly suggestive of osteomyelitis. The ulna is characterized by a relatively smooth periosteal reaction, increased bone opacity, and apparent bending around the radial lesion. There are no sharp transition zones proximally or distally in either the radius or the ulna. Both the radial and the ulnar lesions are aggressive. Although pathologic fractures occasionally develop through primary bone tumors, the history and signalment and the fact that both the radius and the ulna are extensively involved suggest infection as the most likely diagnosis. Diagnosis was radial fracture and bacterial osteomyelitis.

FIGURE 15–12. Lateral view of the distal phalanx of the fifth digit of a dog with a subungual melanoma. There is extensive lysis of the distal phalanx; the lesion is aggressive. This radiographic appearance is more consistent with neoplasia than with pododermatitis, but histopathologic assessment is needed for a definitive diagnosis. (From Voges AK, Neuwirth L, Thompson JP, et al: Radiographic changes associated with digital, metacarpal and metatarsal tumors, and pododermatitis in the dog. Vet Radiol Ultrasound *37*:327, 1996; with permission.)

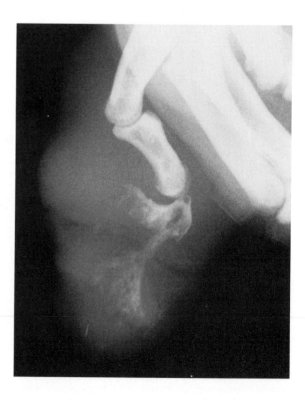

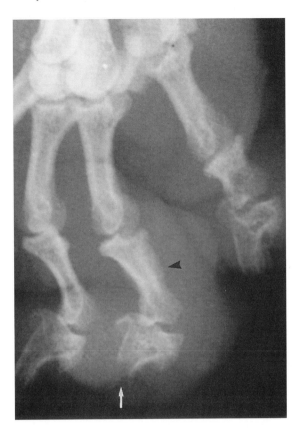

FIGURE 15–13. Pododermatitis involving the third digit. There is lysis of the most distal aspect of the distal phalanx *(white arrow)* and periosteal proliferation on the palmar aspect of the middle phalanx *(black arrowhead).* The entire digit is swollen. These radiographic changes could result from either a tumor or an inflammatory disease, and a biopsy is needed for a definitive diagnosis. (From Voges AK, Neuwirth L, Thompson JP, et al: Radiographic changes associated with digital, metacarpal and metatarsal tumors, and pododermatitis in the dog. Vet Radiol Ultrasound *37:*327, 1996; with permission.)

characterized primarily by osteolysis, however, were more likely to be due to a malignant neoplasm.[12] In another study of dogs with digit masses, digit osteolysis was seen in dogs with all types of digit masses but was more commonly associ-ated with squamous cell carcinoma (Figs. 15–12 and 15–13).[13] Digital tumors typically involve a single digit, but syndromes of multiple digit tumors have been described in dogs[14, 15,] and cats (Fig. 15–14).[16–19]

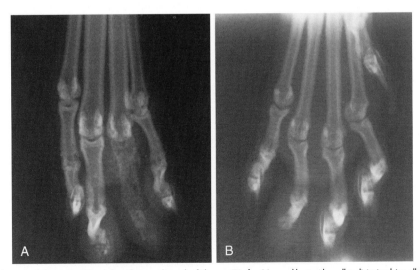

FIGURE 15–14. Dorsopalmar radiograph of the manus *(A)* and dorsoplantar radiograph of the pes *(B)* of a 14-year-old cat with swollen digits involving all feet. In the manus, there is swelling of the fourth digit with lysis of the distal phalanx of that digit. In the pes, there is lysis of the distal phalanx of the third digit and lysis of the proximal, middle, and distal phalanges of the fourth digit; some reactive bone is present on the proximal phalanx of the fourth digit. In radiographs of the thorax, multiple lung masses were present. Histologic diagnosis of the lung and digital lesions was squamous cell carcinoma. Presumably, the digital tumors represent metastatic sites.

References

1. Alexander JW, and Patton CS: Primary tumors of the skeletal system. Vet Clin North Am [Small Anim Pract] 13:181, 1983.
2. Bitetto WV, Patnaik AK, Schrader SC, et al: Osteosarcoma in cats: 22 cases (1974–1984). J Am Vet Med Assoc 190:91, 1982.
3. Quigley PF, and Leedale AH: Tumors involving bone in the domestic cat: A review of 58 cases. Vet Pathol 20:670, 1983.
4. Turrel JM, and Pool RR: Primary bone tumors in the cat: A retrospective study of 15 cats and a literature review. Vet Radiol 23:152, 1982.
5. Dubielzig RR, Biery DM, and Brodey RS: Bone sarcomas associated with multifocal medullary bone infarction in dogs. J Am Vet Med Assoc 179:64, 1981.
6. Russell GR, and Walker M: Metastatic and invasive tumors of bone on dogs and cats. Vet Clin North Am [Small Anim Pract] 13:163, 1983.
7. Geodegebuure SA: Secondary bone tumors in the dog. Vet Pathol 16:520, 1979.
8. Brodey RS, Reid CF, and Sauer RM: Metastatic bone neoplasms in the dog. J Am Vet Med Assoc 148:29, 1966.
9. Vail DM, and Withrow SJ: Tumors of the skin and subcutaneous tissues. In Withrow SJ, MacEwen EG (Eds): Small Animal Clinical Oncology, 2nd Ed. Philadelphia, WB Saunders, 1996, pp 167–191.
10. O'Brien MG, Berg J, and Engler SJ: Treatment by amputation of subungual squamous cell carcinomas in dogs: 21 cases (1987–1988). J Am Vet Med Assoc 201:759, 1992.
11. Aronsohn MG, and Carpenter JL: Distal extremity melanocytic nevi and malignant melanomas in dogs. J Am Anim Hosp Assoc 26:605, 1990.
12. Voges AK, Neuwirth L, Thompson JP, et al: Radiographic changes associated with digital, metacarpal and metatarsal tumors, and pododermatitis in the dog. Vet Radiol Ultrasound 37:327, 1996.
13. Marino DJ, Matthiesen DT, Stefanacci JD, et al: Evaluation of dogs with digit masses: 117 cases (1981–1991). J Am Vet Med Assoc 207:726, 1995.
14. O'Rourke M: Multiple digital squamous cell carcinomas in 2 dogs. Mod Vet Pract 66:644, 1985.
15. Paradis M, Scott DW, and Breton L: Squamous cell carcinoma of the nail bed in three related giant schnauzers. Vet Rec 125:322, 1989.
16. Brown PJ, Hoare CM, and Rochlitz I: Multiple squamous cell carcinoma of the digits in two cats. J Small Anim Pract 26:323, 1985.
17. Pollack M, Martin RA, and Diters RW: Metastatic squamous cell carcinoma in multiple digits of a cat: Case report. J Am Anim Hosp Assoc 20:1984, 1984.
18. May C, and Newsholme SJ: Metastasis of feline pulmonary carcinoma presenting as multiple digital swelling. J Small Anim Pract 30:302, 1989.
19. Scott-Moncrief JC, Elliott GS, Radovsky A, et al: Pulmonary squamous cell carcinoma with multiple digital metastases in a cat. J Small Anim Pract 30:696, 1989.

STUDY QUESTIONS

1. Which one of the following is the most common cause of a solitary metaphyseal aggressive bone lesion in a dog?
   A. Osteogenic sarcoma.
   B. Lymphosarcoma.
   C. Fibrosarcoma.
   D. Chondrosarcoma.
   E. Osteoma.

2. Which radiographic appearance best describes the most common appearance of primary bone tumors in the dog?
   A. Primarily lytic.
   B. Primarily sclerotic.
   C. Mixed lysis and sclerosis.
   D. No bone changes, only soft-tissue swelling.
   E. Multifocal medullary opacities.

3. Which radiographic appearance best describes the most common appearance of primary bone tumors in the cat?
   A. Primarily lytic.
   B. Primarily sclerotic.
   C. Mixed lysis and sclerosis.
   D. No bone changes, only soft-tissue swelling.
   E. Multifocal medullary opacities.

4. Primary bone tumors in the dog and cat primarily originate in the
   A. Diaphysis.
   B. Metaphysis.
   C. Epiphysis.
   D. Joint surface.
   E. Periosteum.

5. Which radiographic appearance best describes the most common appearance of bone infarcts in the dog?
   A. Primarily lytic.
   B. Primarily sclerotic.
   C. Mixed lysis and sclerosis.

   D. No bone changes, only soft-tissue swelling.
   E. Multifocal medullary opacities.

6. Other than primary bone tumor, the major diagnosis to be ruled out for a monostotic aggressive bone lesion is:
   A. Bone infarcts.
   B. Bacterial osteomyelitis.
   C. Osteoma.
   D. Metastatic neoplasia.
   E. Mycotic osteomyelitis.

7. Which of the following tumors would be least likely to metastasize to the skeleton?
   A. Mammary adenocarcinoma.
   B. Prostate adenocarcinoma.
   C. Thyroid adenocarcinoma.
   D. Acanthomatous epulis.
   E. Nasal adenocarcinoma.

8. Hematogenous bacterial osteomyelitis is (more, less) common than hematogenous mycotic osteomyelitis in dogs in the United States.

9. The most common type of digital tumor in dogs is the:
   A. Squamous cell carcinoma.
   B. Melanoma.
   C. Fibrosarcoma.
   D. Osteosarcoma.
   E. Hemangiosarcoma.

10. Which one of the following radiographic changes is most suggestive of primary subungual neoplasia?
    A. Periosteal proliferation.
    B. Multiple bone involvement.
    C. Soft-tissue swelling.
    D. Osteolysis.
    E. Soft-tissue calcification.

(Answers appear on page 636.)

Chapter 16

Radiographic Signs of Joint Disease

Graeme Allan

Signs of joint disease that may be distinguished radiographically are listed in Table 16–1 and illustrated in Figure 16–1. Many of these signs are seen in more than one type of joint disease; that is, they are not specific. Animals with joint diseases that are progressive may have different signs when examined during different phases of the disease.

The examining clinician must determine whether lameness is due to a monoarticular or a multiarticular problem. A hallmark of immune-mediated joint diseases is their polyarticular distribution. The same finding applies to hematogenously disseminated septic arthritis. Most other joint diseases involve one or only a few joints.

Are there systemic signs of illness? Cats with feline chronic progressive polyarthropathy or mycoplasma arthritis have systemic signs of illness, including transient fever, malaise, and stiffness as well as lameness. Animals with signs of bleeding disorders and concurrent joint pain should be examined for signs of hemarthrosis. Systemic lupus erythematosus (SLE) is a multiorgan disease, of which polyarthropathy may be a mild clinical sign. These points are mentioned only to underscore that sound knowledge of joint pathophysiology is as important in the diagnosis of joint diseases as is the ability to make and interpret radiographs of joints.

SIGNS OF JOINT DISEASE

Increased Synovial Mass

Any moderate increase in joint capsular or intracapsular soft-tissue mass may be detected on good-quality radiographs. The joint cartilage, synovial fluid, synovial membrane, and joint capsule cannot be differentiated on survey radiographs because they are of the same radiopacity and therefore silhouette with each other. In most joints, any increase in synovial mass appears as periarticular soft-tissue swelling, which is identified radiographically by the increased radiopacity of affected soft tissues.

When the stifle is involved, the infrapatellar fat pad sign may be used. The normal infrapatellar fat pad is readily identified on lateral stifle radiographs as a triangular radiolucent region immediately caudal to the patellar ligament. When stifle synovial mass increases, a combination of in-

flammatory response, edema, and compression causes the fat pad to become less visible.

If necessary, the joint cartilage and the synovium may be evaluated with the use of contrast arthrography. This technique has been used to aid in the identification of chondral flaps and tears in osteochondritis dissecans in dogs and in synovial hypertrophy in villonodular synovitis in horses.[1]

Altered Thickness of the Joint Space

The joint space is the region of soft-tissue opacity between the subchondral bone of opposing weight-bearing surfaces of a joint. This space consists of two layers of articular cartilage separated by a microfilm of synovial fluid. In early stages of joint disease, synovial effusion may cause widening of the joint space. As joint disease progresses, attrition of articular cartilage results in the joint space appearing thinner. Radiographs made while the patient is weight bearing on an affected joint are required if changes in the thickness of the joint space are to be properly assessed. Radiographs made of the recumbent animal are not adequate for this purpose. The one exception to this rule may be when muscle contracture is present, compressing the joint space. Contracture of the infraspinatus and quadriceps muscles has been reported to reduce the shoulder[2] and stifle[3] joint spaces.

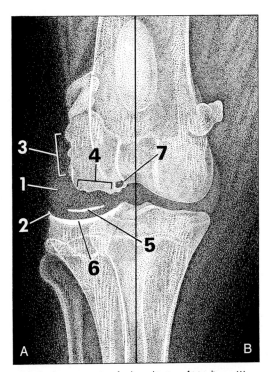

FIGURE 16–1. Graphic representation of radiographic signs of joint disease *(A)* compared with a normal joint *(B)*. Increased synovial mass (1), perichondral osteophyte (2), and enthesophyte formation (3) are commonly observed radiographic changes. Erosion of the subchondral bone surface (4) and joint mice (5) are signs seen less often, whereas increased subchondral bone opacity (6) and subchondral bone cyst formation (7) are signs of chronic joint disease.

Table 16–1
RADIOGRAPHIC SIGNS OF JOINT DISEASE

Increased synovial mass
Altered thickness of the joint space
Decreased subchondral bone opacity
Increased subchondral bone opacity
Subchondral bone cyst formation
Altered perichondral bone opacity
Perichondral bony proliferation
Mineralization of joint soft tissues
Intra-articular calcified bodies
Joint displacement
Joint malformation

Decreased Subchondral Bone Opacity

The subchondral bone is separated from the synovial fluid by an intact layer of joint cartilage. Any disease process that changes the character of the synovial fluid, causing the joint cartilage to erode, potentially threatens the integrity of the subchondral bone. In inflammatory joint diseases, inflammatory exudates may cause pronounced subchondral bone loss. Infectious arthritis may extend into subchondral bone. Subchondral bone loss initially appears as a ragged margin of subchondral bone, but it may extend to cause marked destruction of bone. When bone loss affects smaller carpal and tarsal bones, these small cuboidal bones may be dramatically reduced in mass.

Increased Subchondral Bone Opacity

In benign joint diseases, such as degenerative joint disease, the subchondral bone may be more opaque than normal. Increased subchondral bone opacity appears as a subchondral zone of opacity that is 1 to 2 mm wide.

Subchondral Bone Cyst Formation

Subchondral bone cysts, a feature of degenerative joint disease in humans, are occasionally encountered in young dogs with osteochondrosis[4] and in mature dogs with degenerative joint disease.[5]

Altered Perichondral Bone Opacity

At the chondrosynovial junction, articular cartilage merges with the synovial membrane. The highly vascular membrane is sensitive to inflammation. Synovial inflammation, or hypertrophy, may result in erosion of the bone adjacent to the synovium. Early inflammation causes the adjacent bone to appear ragged and spiculated. Long-standing or severe synovial inflammation or hypertrophy may cause pronounced bone erosion. Perichondral bone erosion is characteristic of some immune-mediated joint diseases and of villonodular synovitis.

Perichondral Bone Proliferation

In degenerative joint disease, fibrocartilage elements form at the chondrosynovial junction. Gradual ossification of this fibrocartilaginous periarticular collar produces osteophytes. Progressive enlargement of osteophytes may result in their incorporation in the adjacent joint capsule.[5]

Articular Soft-Tissue Mineralization

As a consequence of many chronic joint diseases, mineralization may occur within the joint capsule, within the synovial membrane, or free within the synovial fluid. Occasionally, large accumulations of articular or periarticular calcific material may be observed.[6] Large osteochondromas have been reported within the joints of dogs[7, 8] and cats,[9] and intrameniscal calcification and ossification have been observed in the stifle joints of cats.[10] Pseudogout, or calcium pyrophosphate deposition disease, has been reported in dogs causing mineralization of articular and periarticular soft tissues.[11, 12]

Table 16–2
SOME COMMON CAUSES OF INTRA-ARTICULAR CALCIFIED BODIES

Joint	Etiology
Shoulder	Osteochondritis dissecans of the head of the humerus
	Mineralization of the bicipital tendon
	Synovial osteochondroma
Elbow	Un-united anconeal process
	Fragmented coronoid process
	Osteochondritis dissecans of the humeral medial condyle
	Avulsion fractures of the humeral medial epicondyle
Hip	Avulsion epiphyseal fractures after femoral luxation
	Avascular necrosis of the femoral head
Stifle	Osteochondritis dissecans of the femoral condyles
	Avulsion fractures of the
	origin of the long digital extensor tendon
	origin or insertion of the cruciate ligaments
	origin of m. popliteus
	Meniscal calcification
	Synovial osteochondroma
Tarsus	Osteochondritis dissecans of the talus

* In all joints, soft-tissue periarticular mineralization may occur secondary to degenerative joint disease.

Intra-articular Calcified Bodies

Small, well-defined articular and periarticular calcific opacities are occasionally observed in dogs and cats. Such mineralized fragments are sometimes called *joint mice*. Not all such fragments are free within the joint, although they may appear so radiographically. As in humans, intra-articular calcified bodies usually fall into three fairly distinct categories: avulsed fragments of articular or periarticular bone, osteochondral components of a disintegrating joint surface, or small synovial osteochondromas (Table 16–2). They must be differentiated from sesamoid bones.[13] Sesamoid bones are commonly present adjacent to the elbow, stifle, tarsus, and metacarpophalangeal and metatarsophalangeal joints. Some causes of joint mice are listed in Table 16–3.

Table 16–3
SESAMOID AND OTHER SMALL BONES VISIBLE ON RADIOGRAPHS OF JOINTS OF THE CANINE APPENDICULAR SKELETON

Joint	Name and/or Location
Shoulder	Clavicle (medial end of tendinous intersection in m. brachiocephalicus)
Elbow	Tendon of origin of m. supinator[10]
Carpus	Tendon of m. abductor pollicis longus
Metacarpophalangeal	Paired palmar sesamoid bone
	Single dorsal sesamoid bone
Coxofemoral	None*
Femorotibial	Patella (tendon of insertion of m. quadriceps femoris)
	Sesamoid bone of m. gastrocnemius (fabellae)
	Medial head
	Lateral head
	Popliteal sesamoid (tendon of m. popliteus)
Tarsus	Lateral plantar tarsometatarsal sesamoid bone[11]
	Intra-articular tarsometatarsal sesamoid bone[11]
Metatarsophalangeal	Paired plantar sesamoid bone
	Single dorsal sesamoid bone

* Sesamoid bone located in the iliopubic cartilage may be seen cranial to the iliopubic eminence.[12]

Joint Displacement

When the normal spatial relationship between the adjacent osseous components of a joint is disturbed, some type of displacement has occurred. A good example is the cranial drawer sign in a stifle with a ruptured cranial cruciate ligament. Clinically detectable displacement is not always easy to demonstrate radiographically. Stress radiography may be employed to reproduce displacement so that it can be recorded radiographically. Joint displacement is usually a consequence of trauma to fibrous or ligamentous supporting structures.

Joint Malformation

Joint malformation represents the end product of osseous remodeling and is usually the result of malunion of bones of traumatized joints, chronic degenerative joint disease, or congenital joint disease.

CONTRAST RADIOGRAPHY OF JOINTS

Radiographs using added contrast material enhance visualization of important intra-articular structures, such as the articular cartilage and synovium. Contrast radiography has been most useful in evaluation of the canine shoulder joint for evidence of osteochondritis dissecans. Other applications include evaluation of capsular trauma, documentation of synovial hypertrophy, and identification of radiolucent joint mice. Interest in methods of evaluating dogs with bicipital tenosynovitis and fragmented coronoid processes has seen renewed enthusiasm for contrast arthrography.[18–20] When compared with sonography, arthrography was considered a more sensitive method of identifying abnormalities in the bicipital tendon and intertubercular groove of the humerus.[21]

Either positive-contrast or negative-contrast medium may be used (Fig. 16–2). A diluted mixture of an isotonic positive-contrast medium, such as iohexol (Omnipaque, Nycomed, New York, NY) is recommended for positive-contrast studies, the concentration being reduced to 100 mg/mL of iodine by the addition of sterile diluent. For average-sized dogs, an optimal volume of 2 to 4 mL is injected into the shoulder joint.[17] This dose can be varied for studies that evaluate the bicipital tendon, in which the objective is to fill the bicipital tendon sheath; 0.4 mL/kg body weight can be used for this application.[18] For elbow arthrography in dogs, the optimal volume was 2 mL in one report; in that study, low volumes were preferred to higher volumes[19] (Table 16–4). Strict adherence to sterile technique is mandatory. When iodine concentrations greater than 100 mg/mL are used, the radiopaque contrast medium may camouflage underlying articular structures, rendering them invisible.

Air or carbon dioxide may be used for negative-contrast arthrography. When gas is used, it should be injected into

Table 16-4
VOLUME OF CONTRAST MEDIUM USED FOR ARTHROGRAPHY*

Canine elbow	2 mL
Canine shoulder for osteochondritis dissecans	2–4 mL
Canine shoulder for bicipital tendinitis	0.4 mL/kg
Canine stifle	5–10 mL

* Using sterile organic iodine solutions, diluted to a final concentration of 100 mg I/mL.

the joint space through a Millipore filter to ensure that it contains no particulate matter or microorganisms.

DEGENERATIVE JOINT DISEASE

Degenerative joint disease is the most common joint abnormality seen in small animal practice. The disease occurs most frequently in the large, weight-bearing joints of medium-sized to large-sized dogs, but it may afflict any synovial joint. The best example of canine degenerative joint disease is that occurring secondary to canine hip dysplasia. The incidence of hip dysplasia varies from breed to breed. In many large breeds, the incidence exceeds 50 percent. The next most frequent locations are the canine shoulder and stifle joints. Signs of shoulder degenerative joint disease were identified in 33 percent of a group of dogs examined at necropsy,[22] whereas in another study, radiographic evidence of degenerative changes was identified in the shoulders of 78 dogs out of a colony of 149 Beagles.[5] It has been reported that in a necropsy survey of 150 dogs, 20 percent of the dogs had stifle degenerative joint disease.[23]

Degenerative joint disease may be primary (idiopathic) or secondary to a developmental or acquired disorder. Examples of developmental disorders include osteochondrosis, fragmented coronoid process, ununited anconeal process, hip dysplasia, patellar luxation, achondroplasia, and conformational disorders such as valgus and varus deformities of the carpus. Acquired disorders capable of causing degenerative joint disease include trauma, joint instability, epiphyseal aseptic necrosis, and acquired postural or conformational defects such as joint malalignment after fracture repair.[24]

The initial stages of degenerative joint disease are asymptomatic and escape radiographic detection. The first pathologic change is a mild nonsuppurative synovitis, accompanied by a significant increase in the volume of synovial mass. Focal articular degeneration follows. The joint space may appear widened during this stage.[25–27] In the coxofemoral joint, the increased synovial mass may appear radiographically as joint laxity or subluxation.[27] The presence of passive hip laxity is a powerful indicator of the risk of developing coxofemoral degenerative joint disease.[28] Workers studying passive coxofemoral joint laxity, as quantified by a unitless distraction index (DI), reported a strong correlation between the DI and subsequent development of degenerative joint disease. In four breeds studied (Borzoi, German shepherd, Rottweiler, and Labrador retriever), the likelihood of coxofemoral degenerative joint disease varied with the breed and with the DI. Interestingly the threshold DI, below which coxofemoral degenerative joint disease is unlikely to occur, is different for the different breeds. For the German shepherd, the threshold DI is 0.3; it appears to be higher for the Labrador retriever and Rottweiler.[28–31]

Radiographic changes vary according to the stage of the disease. As the joint cartilage becomes thinner, several pathologic changes take place. The most readily recognizable change is osteophyte formation, which follows neovascularization of the chondrosynovial junction with resultant fibrocartilage formation. This fibrocartilage collar gradually ossifies with the formation of characteristic perichondral new bone (Fig. 16–3). Enthesophytes develop on non–weight-bearing surfaces and are eventually incorporated into adjacent ligamentous or capsular attachments.[25, 32, 33]

Continued attrition of the articular cartilage may be detected on radiographs obtained during weight bearing as thinning of the radiolucent joint space. Pathologic alteration of the subchondral bone shelf, including eburnation, com-

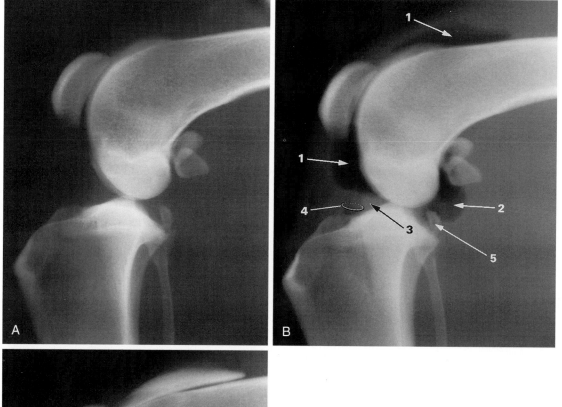

FIGURE 16–2. Contrast arthrography. *A,* Lateral noncontrast radiograph of a normal stifle. *B,* Negative-contrast arthrography of the stifle illustrated in *A.* Ten milliliters of air was injected into the cranial aspect of the joint space (1). Note the caudal joint sac (2), the menisci (3), and air in the bursa surrounding the tendon of the extensor digitorum longus (4). Air is also visible in the bursa of the popliteus adjacent to the popliteal sesamoid (5). *C,* A positive-contrast arthrogram of the contralateral stifle was achieved by injecting 10 mL of iohexol (60 mg/mL of iodine). Additional intra-articular features demonstrated by this technique include the cranial (6) and caudal (7) cruciate ligaments (linear filling defects) and the articular cartilage (8).

pression, and necrosis, may be detected radiographically as increased subchondral opacity of the weight-bearing surface.[34, 35] Subchondral cyst formation, a feature of degenerative joint disease of the human femoral head, has also been observed in joints of small animals.[5, 33]

Affected joints exhibit decreased range of movement, which results in increased loading of the diminished weight-bearing surface. The combination of increased load, diminished subchondral strength, and loss of shock-absorbing cartilage results in alteration in the shape of the subchondral bone table. This remodeling of the subchondral bone is complemented by the addition of peripheral new bone in the form of perichondral osteophytes. The altered shape of the osseous components of affected joints is readily identified

radiographically.[33] The gamut of the radiographic changes seen in degenerative joint disease is outlined in Table 16–5.

HIP DYSPLASIA

The term *hip dysplasia* means abnormally formed hip joints. Hip dysplasia occurs principally in large dogs but also affects small dogs and cats. The incidence in males and females is similar. Usually the condition is bilateral, but unilateral hip dysplasia has been reported in about 11 percent of dogs radiographed with the use of the extended ventrodorsal projection.

Hip dysplasia is an inherited disorder. Heritability estimates

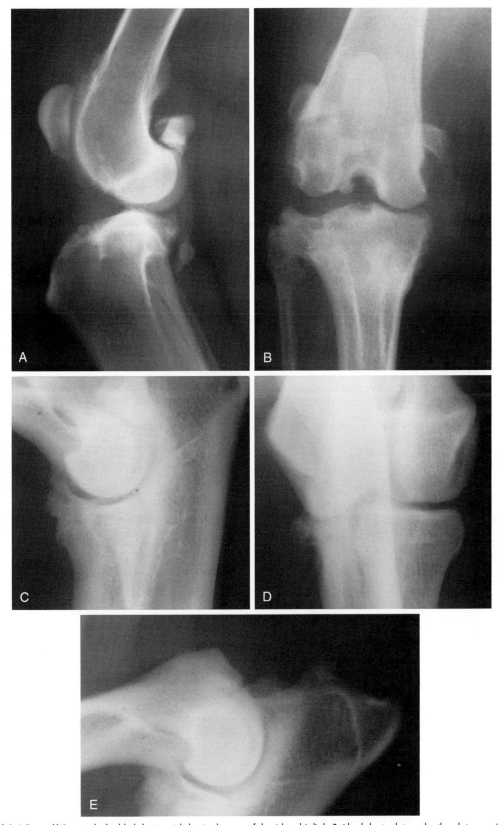

FIGURE 16–3. *A* and *B,* A 7-year-old German shepherd had chronic weight-bearing lameness of the right pelvic limb. Perichondral osteophytes and enthesophytes are visible on the distal femur and the proximal tibia. Synovial effusion and subchondral bone erosion (lateral tibial articular surface) are also evident. The presence of a prominent osteophyte at the origin of the cranial cruciate ligament suggests that these changes are secondary to chronic joint instability originally caused by cruciate ligament trauma. *C* to *E,* Degenerative joint disease in the elbow of a 2-year-old Rottweiler. Osteophytes on the dorsal surface head of the radius *(C)* and the medial portion of the coronoid process of the ulna *(D)* and enthesophyte formation on the anconeal process *(E)* are degenerative changes often seen secondary to fragmented medial coronoid process.

Table 16–5
RADIOGRAPHIC SIGNS OF DEGENERATIVE JOINT DISEASE

Synovial effusion
Initial widening then thinning of the radiolucent joint space
Perichondral osteophyte formation of non–weight-bearing surfaces
Enthesophyte formation
Increased subcondral bone opacity
Remodeling of subchondral bone
Mineralization of intra-articular and periarticular soft tissues
Subchondral cyst formation (rare)
Subluxation (of the coxofemoral joint)

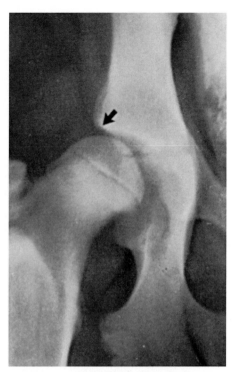

FIGURE 16–5. Moderate hip dysplasia. Subluxation of the femoral head is accompanied by remodeling of the acetabulum. The cranial effective acetabular margin is rounded *(arrow)*, and the acetabulum is shallow. Note the wedge-shaped joint space.

range from 0.2 to 0.6. With the use of more sensitive radiographic techniques, the estimated heritability in German shepherds has been raised from 0.46[36] to 0.61.[37] Environmental factors influence the phenotypic expression of hip dysplasia.[38] The role of nutrition has been studied extensively. Overnutrition is regarded as one of the principal nongenetic factors that influence the expression of canine hip dysplasia.[39] Hip dysplasia is a developmental, age-related disorder; it is not present at birth. A variable amount of time must elapse before radiographic changes are manifest. Once present, these radiographic changes usually progress as the affected animal ages.

The earliest recognizable change in the coxofemoral joints is joint laxity. This may be palpated (the Ortolani sign, Barden's lift method) or visualized radiographically (Figs. 16–4 and 16–5).[26, 46, 47] Subsequent radiographic changes are those of degenerative joint disease (Fig. 16–6). The order of subsequent changes is (1) perichondral osteophyte formation,[48, 51] (2) remodeling of the femoral head and neck, (3) remodeling of the acetabulum, and (4) sclerosis of subchondral bone of the femoral head and acetabulum. An early and sensitive sign of new bone formation has been described.[48] Solitary bony osteophytes present on the caudal aspect of the

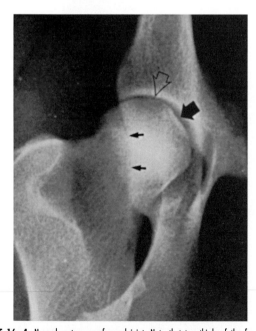

FIGURE 16–4. Normal mature coxofemoral joint. Note that two thirds of the femoral head lies medial to the shadow of the dorsal effective acetabular margin *(small arrows)*. The cranial margin of the femoral head is separated from the adjacent acetabulum by a fine radiolucent line, which represents the radiolucent joint cartilage and a microfilm of synovial fluid *(open arrow)*. The flattened portion of the femoral head is normal and represents the fovea capitis femoris *(solid arrow)*.

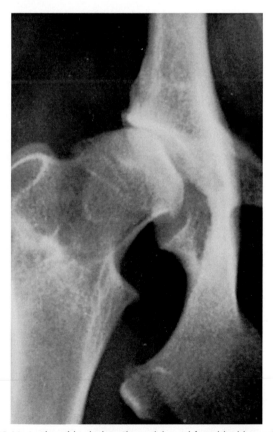

FIGURE 16–6. Advanced hip dysplasia. The acetabulum and femoral head have undergone advanced remodeling. Osteophytes are forming on the femoral neck and head as well as on the cranial effective acetabular margin. New bone formation has filled the acetabular fossa, and the subchondral bone of the acetabular articular surface is sclerotic. These are easily recognized signs of degenerative joint disease.

femoral neck may be visualized as an opaque line (Fig. 16–7) directed distally rather than around the femoral neck. Because it is sometimes evident in animals without signs of coxofemoral joint laxity on the extended view, it should be regarded as an early and significant sign of coxofemoral degenerative joint disease. As the degenerative phase advances, the femoral head loses its spheroidal shape and becomes flattened along its articular surface. The femoral neck becomes thickened, and the surface of the neck becomes irregular, owing to a growth of a collar of perichondral osteophytes. The acetabulum loses its cup-like shape and becomes shallow. Increased bone opacity of the subchondral articular surfaces represents bone sclerosis, a response to cartilage thinning. A variable degree of coxofemoral subluxation is always present, and coxa valga is common. Subchondral cyst formation is an infrequent manifestation of degenerative joint disease in small animals but may occasionally be observed.[49, 50]

The optimal method of radiographic evaluation to quantify hip joint changes is disputable. Screening programs used around the world have persisted with the extended ventrodorsal projection (Fig. 16–8), although it has been long recognized that it is an insensitive indicator of coxofemoral joint laxity. Work[39] has revealed that coxofemoral joint laxity can be identified with the use of a ventrodorsal projection with the femurs placed in a distracted neutral position (Fig. 16–9). These workers claim that laxity detected by their method is a reliable indicator of future degenerative changes in the coxofemoral joints. This information can be obtained at a much earlier age than with the standard extended ventrodorsal projection.

Most screening programs require the extended ventrodorsal radiograph of the coxofemoral joints be made and submitted for evaluation. The method of obtaining the projection required by the Orthopedic Foundation for Animals (OFA), which is similar to the projections used by other screening programs internationally, has been described in detail[40] (see Fig. 16–8). With the dog in dorsal recumbency, the hindlegs are extended with the femurs parallel and the stifles rotated inward so that the patellae are located over the middle of

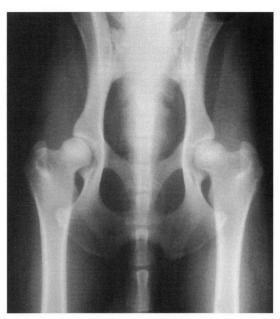

FIGURE 16–8. Extended ventrodorsal projection of the coxofemoral joints (Orthopedic Foundation for Animals [OFA] preferred view). Note bilateral symmetry of the pelvis and parallel femurs. The coxofemoral joints appear normal. (Courtesy of Dr. Ian Robertson.)

the cranial surface of the distal femur. The x-ray beam should be centered over the coxofemoral joints, and the radiograph should include the entire pelvis and the femurs. The pelvis must appear symmetric in the radiograph, without evidence of pelvic rotation. Although satisfactory radiographic quality may be achieved without the assistance of chemical restraint,[41] failure to anesthetize the subject may decrease radiographic sensitivity for signs of coxofemoral joint laxity.[42] Because the extended ventrodorsal projection is an insensitive method of detecting signs of coxofemoral subluxation,[43–45] care must be taken to ensure accurate subject positioning and radiographic quality.

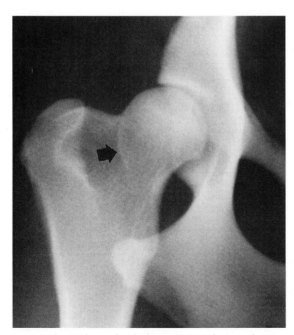

FIGURE 16–7. A sentinel sign of early degenerative joint disease is the Morgan line, representing osteophyte formation on the femoral neck adjacent to the trochanteric fossa *(arrow)*.

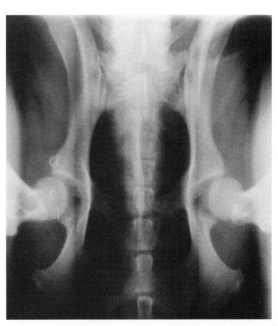

FIGURE 16–9. Neutral ventrodorsal distraction projection (PennHip view). Bilateral coxofemoral subluxation (laxity) is evident. This radiograph is of the same dog as in Figure 16–8. (Courtesy of Dr. Ian Robertson.)

The so-called PennHip method[28, 29, 45] also requires the dog to be placed in dorsal recumbency (see Fig. 16–9). The femurs are placed in a neutral position, to duplicate standing. This neutral position avoids spiral tensioning of the joint capsule, a significant disadvantage of the OFA projection. With the hindlimbs held with the femurs neutrally positioned, a radiograph is made while the coxofemoral joints are compressed, to obtain an image of the coxofemoral joints at their most congruent position. A distraction device is then placed between the femurs for the second radiograph. When the femurs are pressed against the bars of the distracter, any coxofemoral laxity that is naturally present is visualized radiographically. The two views of the hips are compared, and any coxofemoral laxity is quantified by a unitless measure, the DI. A third (OFA) projection is made, so that secondary signs of hip dysplasia, such as degenerative joint disease, can be identified.

The PennHip method has several inherent advantages over the traditional (OFA) method of evaluating the coxofemoral joints (Table 16–6). First, it quantifies joint laxity, which is generally accepted as the beginning, and probably the cause, of subsequent dysplastic changes. Second, the examination can be done on young dogs. The predictive value of the DI is constant after 6 months of age, providing invaluable information to breeders when selecting their stock. Third, the technique predicts a DI below which degenerative changes are unlikely to occur. Conversely, there appears to be a direct relationship between the DI and the subsequent development of degenerative joint disease when the DI is greater than 0.3 (for German shepherds) or 0.4 (for Labrador retrievers and Rottweilers).

TRAUMA THAT INVOLVES THE OSSEOUS COMPONENTS OF JOINTS

Any fracture that communicates with a joint space is an articular fracture (Fig. 16–10). Articular fractures must be accurately diagnosed to ensure appropriate surgical reduction and stabilization. Radiographic examinations should include two projections made at right angles to one another. To these should be added oblique views and projections during flexion and stress, when needed. These additional projections are of most value when chip or avulsion fractures are suspected or when the osseous structures of interest are superimposed on other osseous structures.[52, 53]

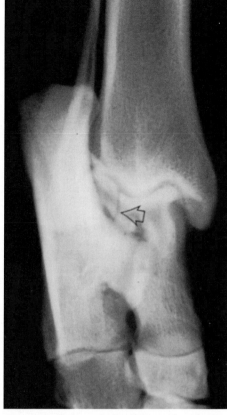

FIGURE 16–10. A 3-year-old German shorthaired pointer with acute onset of non–weight-bearing lameness of the left pelvic limb. There is a fracture through the lateral trochlear ridge of the talus (arrow). Diagnosis was articular fracture of the talus. (Courtesy of University of Sydney.)

Articular fractures occur frequently in immature animals because of the high incidence of physeal and epiphyseal trauma in these patients. Physeal fractures that are articular are usually classified as Salter type III or IV fractures.[54] Because the proximal femoral physis is intracapsular, all proximal femoral physeal fractures are articular fractures. In a retrospective study of femoral head and neck fractures, 77 percent of lesions were intracapsular, 59 percent of which were physeal.[55]

Table 16–6
COMPARISON OF OFA AND PennHip METHODS FOR HIP DYSPLASIA RADIOGRAPHY

Extended Ventrodorsal Projection	PennHip Distraction Projection
Advantages	
Currently the most popular screening program internationally	A valuable screening method for breeders before litters are placed in homes (as early as 16 wk)
Does not require special training or any accessory equipment	
Only one radiograph required	Most sensitive method of identifying joint laxity
Has amassed a large database of information about the coxofemoral phenotype	Generates a unitless index (distraction index) that can be used to predict whether or not degenerative joint disease will develop
Animals can be radiographed without personnel exposure	Has a greater heritability than the OFA method
An accurate method of predicting dysplastic changes in young animals, from 6 mo	
Disadvantages	
Inaccurate in young animals; accuracy increases with age; optimal time to radiograph is 24–36 mo	Requires special training for users to become certified
An insensitive method of identifying coxofemoral joint laxity	Requires special equipment
Technique of extending the femurs camouflages signs of joint laxity by spiral tensioning of the joint capsule	Multiple radiographic projections required
	Personnel exposure during radiographic exposure difficult to avoid

OFA, Orthopedic Foundation for Animals.

Premature physeal closure sometimes follows repair of Salter fractures and may be observed within 2 or 3 weeks of surgery.[55, 56] It should be regarded as an expected finding, regardless of the type of physeal trauma, and it should be included in the prognosis. Although many dogs in the aforementioned study had significant growth potential remaining at the time of injury, clinical signs related to premature physeal closure were rare.

The proportion of physeal trauma that is articular is lower for joints other than the coxofemoral joint. It has been reported that 9 of 57 distal femoral physeal fractures were classified as Salter type III or IV.[57] Distal humeral fractures are classified as condylar or intercondylar. Lateral condylar fractures predominate and are most frequently reported in immature dogs.[58] Fractures that involve the carpal and tarsal bones occur frequently, particularly in racing Greyhounds.

SPRAINS: CAPSULAR, LIGAMENTOUS, AND TENDINOUS INJURY TO JOINTS

Supporting soft-tissue structures of joints are of soft-tissue opacity and silhouette with each other and with adjacent soft tissues and therefore are not visualized clearly on a radiograph. Mild to moderate sprains, such as partial rupture of the cranial cruciate ligament,[59] may be difficult to diagnose because the only radiographic sign is minimal soft-tissue swelling. The radiographic features of severe sprains include: (1) periarticular soft-tissue swelling; (2) avulsion fractures at points of attachment of ligaments, tendons, and capsules to bone; (3) joint instability or subluxation; and (4) spatial derangement of the osseous components of a joint.[2] It is important to diagnose sprains promptly. In many instances, appropriate medical or surgical therapy ensures normal joint function in moderate to severe sprain injuries.[60, 61] Many patients with profound sprains, such as carpal hyperextension injuries, may be effectively treated, thus allowing the affected animal to ambulate satisfactorily instead of surviving with a disability.[62]

The clinical assessment (palpation and manipulation) of a sprained joint is usually the best diagnostic tool. Radiographic examination adds information that is useful for treatment planning while documenting the presence and magnitude of the sprain and identifying avulsed osseous fragments. A useful technique for radiographic assessment of a sprained joint is stress radiography (Figs. 16–11 and 16–12). In practice, this technique involves application of force to the joint in question to demonstrate displacement of its osseous components. The forces applied are the same stresses to which the joint would be subject in normal daily activity and are defined as compressive, rotational, traction, shear, and wedge forces (Fig. 16–13).[63]

An excellent example of a compressive stress is a radiograph of a joint during weight bearing. Ligamentous trauma, as in carpal hyperextension injuries, is readily demonstrated by this technique. The cranial drawer sign seen in cranial cruciate ligament trauma is a practical example of a shearing stress. It is stress that is used routinely in clinical examination of the stifle. The same manipulative procedure may be applied to the stifle during radiography. Traction stress involves pulling the osseous components of the joint away from one another. One useful application of traction stress involves capital physeal fractures of the femoral head. By applying traction to the femur in the extended ventrodorsal position, capital physeal fractures are easy to identify.

A technique employing traction stress has been described for identifying medial scapulohumeral joint instability in

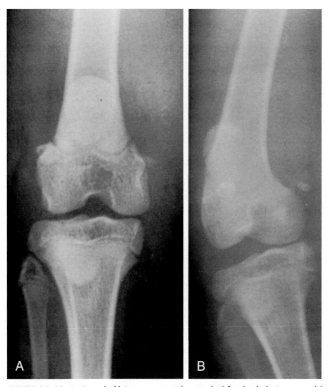

FIGURE 16–11. An 8-month-old Burmese cat was lame in the left pelvic limb. A craniocaudal radiograph (A) was normal. In a stressed craniocaudal radiograph (B), widening of the lateral aspect of the joint space was apparent. Diagnosis was ruptured lateral collateral ligament. (Courtesy of University of Sydney.)

small dogs. With the patient in lateral recumbency, nontraction and traction radiographs are made of the shoulder joint. A significant increase in the shoulder joint space has been identified as a sign of medial shoulder joint instability.[64] Traction and wedge stresses are useful for examining joints for small avulsion fractures and intra-articular joint mice. Unilateral trauma to collateral ligaments of the elbow and stifle are lesions that may be uncovered with the use of wedge stresses. Because stress radiography involves personnel holding the patient during x-ray exposure, utmost care must be taken to ensure that such persons wear appropriate protective clothing.

HEMARTHROSIS

Intra-articular hemorrhage may occur in dogs with coagulopathies or after joint trauma. Hemarthrosis was reported in a dog with suspected warfarin toxicosis.[65] Other coagulopathies in the dog that may cause hemarthrosis include hemophilia A and B; von Willebrand's disease; deficiencies in factors VII, X, and XI; and liver disease.[66] Isolated, infrequent episodes of intra-articular bleeding do not significantly alter the articular cartilage. Repeated hemorrhage may lead to severe damage to the cartilage as well as the subchondral bone.[67]

Affected animals suffer severe non–weight-bearing lameness of affected limbs, and affected joints are swollen and painful. Radiographic examination in acute hemarthrosis reveals joint soft-tissue swelling, which may be extensive.[65] With chronic intra-articular hemorrhage, the joint cartilage may be eroded and thin, causing the appearance of decreased articular joint space on weight-bearing radiographs. The subchondral bone appears irregular if it is involved in the destructive process. Remodeling of bones adjacent to affected

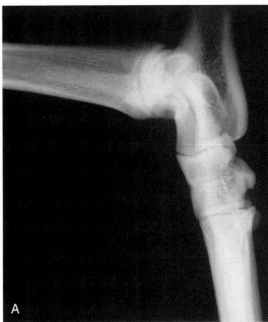

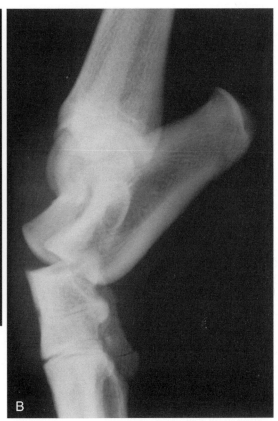

FIGURE 16–12. *A,* A neutral lateral radiograph of a racing Greyhound appears normal. *B,* Stress radiography was performed, and this allowed identification of instability of the proximal intertarsal joint.

stifles was reported in dogs after repeated intra-articular injections of whole blood.[67] In advanced hemarthrosis, signs similar to degenerative joint disease may be present.

INFECTIOUS ARTHRITIS

Infectious arthritis is a relatively infrequently diagnosed joint disease in small animals, the incidence being lower than that of immune-mediated joint disease. Infectious arthritis is difficult to diagnose radiographically. Initial radiographic changes are similar to those seen in any effusive, nonerosive joint disease. Irreversible joint damage has occurred by the time a definitive radiographic diagnosis can be made. Ideally

the patient should be diagnosed and successfully treated without definitive radiographic changes becoming apparent.[68]

Polyarticular infectious arthritis may occur secondary to bacteremia caused by an isolated focus of infection (endocarditis, discospondylitis, or omphalophlebitis) or in conjunction with some systemic diseases (mycoplasma arthritis, canine leishmaniasis, or feline caliciviral lameness).[69] Monoarticular infectious arthritis most likely results from an extension of focal osteomyelitis into an adjacent joint, direct joint trauma, or foreign body penetration (grass seed awns), or it may occur after joint surgery or intra-articular therapy.[34, 70] Polyarticular infectious arthritis must be differentiated from immunologic joint disease.

The earliest radiographic changes are synovial effusion and increased synovial mass, which represent an inflammatory

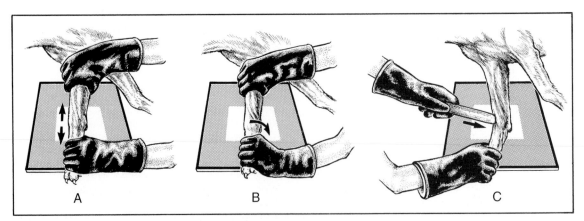

FIGURE 16–13. Stress radiography of joints employs the application of traction *(A)*, rotational *(B)*, and wedge *(C)* forces to demonstrate subluxation that may not be appreciated on standard radiographic projections. (Adapted from Farrow CS: Stress radiography: Applications in small animal practice. J Am Vet Med Assoc *181:*777, 1982; with permission.)

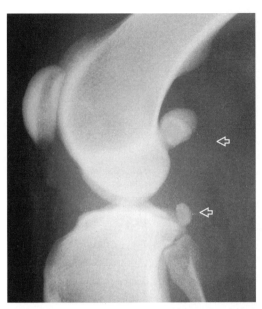

FIGURE 16–14. An 8-year-old male Australian cattle dog had neurologic signs related to the hindquarters as well as pain in the right stifle. In the lateral view of the right stifle, it is apparent that the infrapatellar fat pad is compressed by synovial effusion. Note the bulging caudal compartment of the stifle joint *(arrows).* Discospondylitis was identified in radiographs of the thoracic spine. Laboratory diagnosis was septic arthritis, based on isolation of *Staphylococcus aureus* from the synovial fluid.

response of the synovium (Fig. 16–14). Soft-tissue swelling is usually demarcated by the distended joint capsule. Joint capsular distention is best identified in carpal, tarsal, and stifle joints. A useful landmark in the stifle is the infrapatellar fat pad. When the fat pad silhouette becomes unclear or is lost, synovial effusion is present (see Fig. 16–14). In untreated infectious arthritis, joint cartilage destruction follows synovial effusion and is followed by subchondral and perichondral bone destruction (Figs. 16–15 and 16–16).

Specific radiographic features of infectious arthritis become prominent after the articular cartilage is destroyed and subchondral osteomyelitis is established. It has been reported that destruction of the femoral head was noted radiographically 4 weeks after the onset of clinical signs of coxofemoral infectious arthritis.[71] The width of the radiolucent joint space is progressively reduced as the articular cartilage is destroyed. Radiographs obtained during weight bearing are needed to demonstrate this change. Destruction of the subchondral

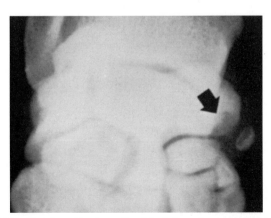

FIGURE 16–15. A 2-year-old male mixed-breed dog had acute lameness of the right carpus. Radiographically, subchondral osteolysis of the radial carpal bone *(arrow)* can be identified adjacent to the carpal sesamoid bone. Laboratory diagnosis was septic arthritis.

Table 16–7
PROGRESSION OF RADIOGRAPHIC SIGNS OF INFECTIOUS ARTHRITIS

Increased synovial mass, indicating synovial effusion, and widened radiolucent joint space
Diminished radiolucent joint space, indicating destruction of articular cartilage
Loss of the smooth surface of the subchondral bone plate, an early sign of infectious penetration of subchondral bone
Osteolytic destruction of subchondral and perichondral bone, which is usually highlighted by a peripheral border of osteosclerosis
In advanced infectious arthritis, weight-bearing surfaces may collapse, causing distortion of joint architecture

bone plate and subsequent subchondral osteomyelitis cause the margins of the joint space to appear uneven or ragged. Continued subchondral bone destruction produces large cystic subchondral radiolucent spaces. Bone sclerosis adjacent to the osteolytic bone is a sign of osseous inflammatory response to the infection (Table 16–7).

Increasingly, septic arthritis is being identified in joints that have well-established degenerative joint disease. Initial radiographs reveal changes consistent with degenerative joint disease, often leading to inappropriate therapy for this condition. Radiographs taken 2 to 4 weeks later reveal more aggressive signs of periosteal new bone formation and intra-articular bone destruction.[71] Septic arthritis should be suspected when acute lameness and joint pain are identified in individual animals whose degenerative joint disease has previously been well controlled.

RHEUMATOID ARTHRITIS

Rheumatoid arthritis is a severe, progressive, erosive polyarthritis that has been reported in dogs.[72] Diagnostic criteria for human rheumatoid arthritis have been established and have been modified for the dog.[73] Nine criteria must be evaluated; six of the nine criteria should be satisfied for a diagnosis of classic rheumatoid arthritis to be made in the dog (Table 16–8).

Radiographic changes usually occur in distal joints of the extremities. The more proximal large joints (stifle and elbow) are occasionally affected. Synovial effusion occurs initially. Radiographs made early in the course of the disease detect nonspecific soft-tissue swelling around affected joints. The joint capsule may be distended. The first radiographic signs of an osseous pathologic process may be detected several weeks after the onset of clinical signs. Initial changes are mild, but as expected in a progressive disease, the magnitude of radiographic abnormalities becomes more obvious as the disease advances.[34]

Table 16–8
DIAGNOSTIC GUIDELINES IN CANINE RHEUMATOID ARTHRITIS

Morning stiffness
Pain or tenderness in one or more joints
Soft-tissue swelling or effusion in one or more joints
Swelling of any other joints
Symmetric onset of joint symptoms and swelling
Radiographic signs consistent with rheumatoid arthritis
Positive rheumatoid factor test
Poor mucin precipitate of synovial fluid
Characteristic histologic changes in the synovium

From Barrett RE: Canine polyarthritis. *In* Kirk RW (Ed): Current Veterinary Therapy 7. Philadelphia, WB Saunders, 1980, p 800; with permission.

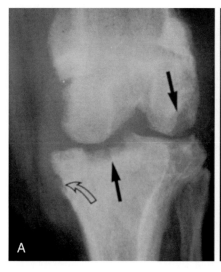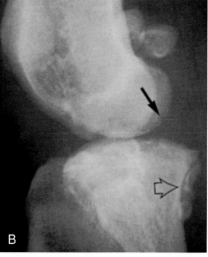

FIGURE 16–16. An 8-year-old male Australian cattle dog had stifle swelling and pain that persisted after repair of a ruptured cranial cruciate ligament. *A* and *B,* Subchondral bone erosion involves the medial condyle of the tibia and the femoral condyles *(solid arrow).* Periarticular new bone formation is also evident *(open arrow).* Note the concurrent medial patellar luxation. Laboratory diagnosis was septic arthritis, based on isolation of *Staphylococcus aureus* from the synovial fluid.

The progression of radiographic changes includes (1) perichondral decreased bone opacity, (2) subchondral bone destruction and cyst formation (Fig. 16–17*A*), (3) perichondral osteolysis and erosion (see Fig. 16–17*B*), (4) narrowing of the joint space, (5) progressive decreased opacity of epiphyses adjacent to affected joints, (6) destruction of subchondral and perichondral bone, (7) mushrooming of the ends of the metacarpi and metatarsi (which occurs in advanced cases and represents collapse of subchondral bone), and (8) varying degrees of joint subluxation and luxation in advanced cases. Other changes, more characteristic of degenerative joint disease (perichondral osteophytes, subchondral sclerosis, and calcified periarticular tissues) may also be present at this stage.[72]

SYSTEMIC LUPUS ERYTHEMATOSUS

SLE is a multisystemic disease of unknown origin. It affects dogs of all breeds as well as cats. The disorder has a variety of clinical manifestations, including polyarthritis, anemia, nephropathy, skin disease, pericarditis and myocarditis, and lymphadenopathy.[74] The diagnosis of SLE is complicated, being based on the concurrence of clinical manifestations and serologic evidence of the disease. The most valuable serologic screening test for SLE is the antinuclear antibody test (Table 16–9). Animals with nonerosive polyarthritis that return negative tests for serum antinuclear antibodies may still have a polyarthropathy of immune-based origin. An immune-based idiopathic polyarthritis and a polyarthritis-polymyositis syndrome in dogs have been described, neither of which fully satisfy criteria for SLE (see Table 16–9).[75, 76]

The relative frequency of the different clinical manifestations seen in SLE varies according to different authors. In one study, 121 patients were reviewed, and it was reported that joint disease was the most frequent clinical sign (69 percent), followed by hematologic (53 percent), renal (50 percent), cutaneous (33 percent), and intrathoracic (17 percent) manifestations.[74]

Arthritis that occurs in SLE is described as nonerosive and effusive. Polyarthritis (five or more joints affected) is usual, but monoarticular and pauciarticular arthritis have been reported. Clinically, affected animals are reluctant to move because they often have a shifting lameness. Affected joints may be swollen, painful, and warm. The joints most commonly affected are the carpus, tarsus, metatarsus, stifle, and elbow.

Radiographic signs are usually absent or are minimal. In chronic SLE, the joint space of affected joints may be narrowed, and the joint capsule is distended. A mild periosteal response has been reported at the junction of the joint capsule and the bone. Contrast arthrography has been used to demonstrate distention of the joint capsule. The synovial margin outlined by arthrography was reported as being irregular and indistinct.

FELINE NONINFECTIOUS POLYARTHRITIS

Feline noninfectious polyarthritis is a disease of male cats, aged 1 to 5 years.[77–79] Affected animals are categorized as erosive or nonerosive.[80] There are two types of erosive polyarthritis—the periosteal proliferative form and the erosive form—the latter more commonly referred to as *feline rheumatoid arthritis.* Nonerosive, effusive polyarthropathies that are thought to be immune mediated may be associated with a variety of conditions.

Periosteal Proliferative Form

Affected cats display clinical signs characterized by fever, malaise, and stiffness, which are followed by periarticular

Table 16–9

DIAGNOSTIC CRITERIA FOR CANINE SYSTEMIC LUPUS ERYTHEMATOSUS[75]

There should be involvement of more than one body system, the main features being
  Polyarthritis
  Immune-based thrombocytopenia
  Immune-based leukopenia
  Glomerulonephritis
  Polymyositis
  Skin disease
  Central nervous system
  Gastrointestinal disease
Serum antinuclear antibodies should be detectable at a significantly high titer
Immunopathologic features consistent with the clinical involvement should be demonstrated, e.g., if arthritis is present, immune complexes should be demonstrable in tissue biopsy samples.

Data from Bennett D: Immune-based non-erosive inflammatory joint disease of the dog: I. Canine SLE. J Small Anim Pract *28*:871, 1987.

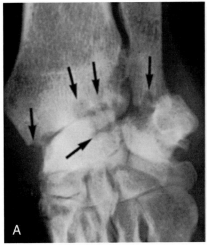
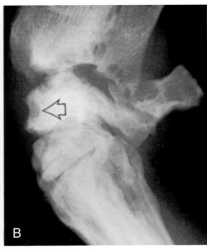

FIGURE 16–17. An 8-year-old male (neutered) Corgi cross-breed had non–weight-bearing lameness of the right forelimb, valgus deviation of the left manus, and left carpal joint swelling and crepitus. A, Dorsolateral-palmaromedial projection (right carpus). There is extensive subchondral erosion of the styloid process of the ulna and of the articular surfaces of the distal radius and radial carpal bone *(arrows)*. B, Lateral projection during flexion. In addition to the changes seen in A, note the lysis of the non–weight-bearing dorsal surface of the radial carpal bone *(arrow)*. Laboratory diagnosis was canine rheumatoid arthritis. (Courtesy of University of Sydney.)

soft-tissue swelling and regional lymphadenopathy. Radiographic changes may be identified in affected joints after a few weeks of clinical illness. The joints most commonly affected are the carpi and tarsi. The stifle, elbow, shoulder, and hip joints are affected to a lesser extent.

During the first month, periarticular soft-tissue swelling is the predominant sign. Swelling may be either intracapsular or extracapsular. One to 3 months after the onset of clinical signs, periosteal new bone production at points of joint capsular attachment may be identified. During this phase, the bone adjacent to affected joints may have decreased bone opacity and a coarse trabecular pattern. Perichondral new bone formation is pronounced 2 or 3 months after onset of the disease.

Extensive osteophytes may bridge smaller joint spaces. More severe radiographic manifestations include perichondral bone erosion and formation of subchondral cysts. Narrowing of affected joint spaces may occur late in the disease.[78] The radiographic signs of the periosteal proliferative form of feline chronic progressive polyarthritis include periarticular soft-tissue swelling, periosteal new bone formation, perichondral osteophyte production, perichondral and subchondral erosion, subchondral cysts, osteopenia of bone adjacent to affected joints, and narrowed joint spaces (Fig. 16–18).

Erosive Form

A second, more erosive form has been described; it resembles human rheumatoid arthritis[78] and is seen in older cats.[79] This form of the disease is characterized radiographically by severe subchondral bone erosion, perichondral bone erosion, and subchondral cyst formation. Perichondral osteophyte formation, bone destruction at points of ligamentous insertion to bone, and subluxation of small joints of the extremities also occur.

A diagnosis of feline rheumatoid arthritis requires a positive rheumatoid factor test, characteristic histologic changes seen on a synovial biopsy, or both. Both of these test results are negative in cats with feline proliferative polyarthritis.[80]

Feline Nonerosive Polyarthritis

Radiography is used to separate the erosive from the nonerosive forms of feline polyarthritis. The latter group is identified as having periarticular soft-tissue swelling, joint capsule dis-

tention, and synovial fluid accumulation. Five categories of nonerosive polyarthritis have been described in cats.[80] They are feline SLE and four types of idiopathic polyarthritis: (1) uncomplicated polyarthritis; (2) reactive polyarthritis, associated with a disease process elsewhere in the body; (3) enteropathic polyarthritis, associated with gastrointestinal disease; and (4) malignant-related idiopathic polyarthritis, associated with myeloproliferative disease.

HYPERTROPHIC OSTEOPATHY

Hypertrophic osteopathy is a generalized osteoproductive disorder of the periosteum that affects the long bones of the

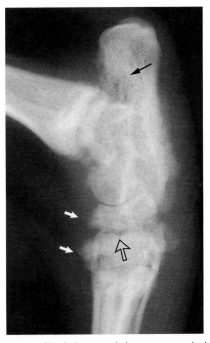

FIGURE 16–18. A 2-year-old male domestic cat had progressive generalized lameness, which was preceded by fever and lassitude. Regional lymph nodes were palpably enlarged. Radiographs made 1 month after onset of the clinical illness revealed periosteal new bone formation on many tarsal bones *(small arrows)*. Subchondral osteolysis is pronounced in the centrodistal articulation *(open arrow)*. Some tarsal bones have foci of osteolysis *(large arrow)*. Peritarsal soft-tissue swelling is evident. Laboratory diagnosis was feline chronic progressive polyarthritis. (Courtesy of University of Sydney.)

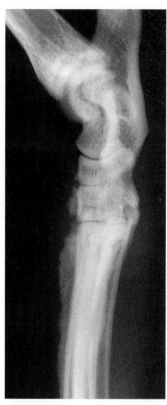

FIGURE 16–19. A 4-year-old female domestic cat had swollen paws and progressive lameness for 6 weeks. Radiographically, there was periosteal new bone formation on the dorsal aspect of the central and fourth tarsal bones as well as on the dorsal surface of the metatarsal bones. Histologic diagnosis was hypertrophic osteopathy secondary to bronchogenic carcinoma.

extremities (Fig. 16–19). Hypertrophic osteopathy is usually seen secondary to cardiopulmonary disease or neoplasia.[81] Most neoplasms are pulmonary (primary or secondary), but hypertrophic osteopathy is also reported in animals with primary intra-abdominal neoplasia without pulmonary involvement.[82–84] Non-neoplastic causes include inflammatory lung disease (e.g., blastomycosis), intrathoracic foreign bodies, *Dirofilaria immitis* infestation, and spirocercosis.

The pathogenesis of hypertrophic osteopathy is incompletely understood. The most consistent pathologic finding in affected animals is increased blood flow to the extremities. This increased flow results in an overgrowth of vascular connective tissue with subsequent fibrochondroid metaplasia and subperiosteal new bone formation. New bone formation typically commences on the digits and progressively extends toward the axial skeleton.

Periosteal new bone formation results in cortical thickening. The periosteal surface appears nodular or spiculated when visualized radiographically. When joints are involved, the bone surfaces that are not covered with cartilage are roughened, and large perichondral osteophytes form.

VILLONODULAR SYNOVITIS

Villonodular synovitis is an intracapsular joint disorder characterized by nodular synovial hyperplasia, which is thought to represent a response of the synovium to trauma. Experimentally, villonodular synovitis has been reproduced in dogs by repeated intra-articular injections of whole blood. Villonodular synovitis is an established, although uncommon, disor-

der of humans that has also been reported in horses and dogs.[1, 85, 86]

The radiographic signs of the disease may be nonspecific but include articular soft-tissue swelling and erosion of cortical bone at the chondrosynovial junction. These cortical erosions may appear cyst-like, with slightly sclerotic borders. In severe proximal femoral villonodular synovitis in humans, the femoral neck has been described as looking like an apple core. The articular cartilage and subchondral bone are not involved in the disease process.

Arthrography has been used to identify the intracapsular nodular masses of hypertrophied synovium in humans and horses.[1, 87] Arthrographic examination also allows visualization of the expanded synovial sac. The differential diagnosis for perichondral erosive lesions, characteristic of villonodular synovitis, should include synovial osteochondromatosis, rheumatoid arthritis, and amyloidosis.[88]

SYNOVIAL OSTEOCHONDROMAS

Synovial osteochondromas have long been recognized in the joints of humans. These lesions are described as islands of cartilage that are produced by the synovial membrane. Foci of cartilage become pedunculated and may become separated from their pedicles to form loose bodies within the joint.

The radiographic appearance of mineralized synovial osteochondromas varies. These lesions are usually well-defined, rounded, often multiple intra-articular nodules of a calcific opacity (Fig. 16–20). Not all chondromas become calcified, in which instance contrast arthrography may be necessary for their diagnosis.[5] Synovial osteochondromas may also arise from extra-articular foci of synovial tissue (Fig. 16–21).

Synovial osteochondromas have been reported in the dog[7, 89] and the cat.[9, 90] Their cause is unknown, but the theory of synovial metaplasia is generally accepted.[7] These lesions have

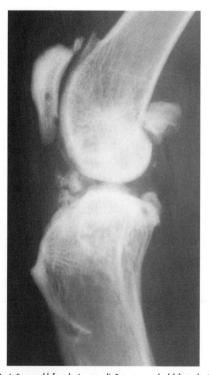

FIGURE 16–20. A 5-year-old female (neutered) Burmese cat had bilateral stifle enlargement. Mineralization of the infrapatellar fat pad and within the stifle joint compartment was evident radiographically. Histologic diagnosis was synovial osteochondroma.

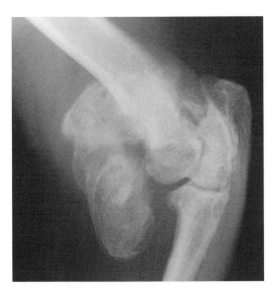

FIGURE 16–21. A 6-year-old male (neutered) Burmese cat had progressive lameness of the right forelimb for 6 weeks. Radiographically, there was a large, well-defined, ossified mass on the craniomedial aspect of the right elbow. Histologic diagnosis was extra-articular synovial osteochondroma.

been reported to cause severe lameness in some dogs. Surgical removal of synovial osteochondromas relieves clinical signs of joint pain and lameness.[89]

Intrameniscal calcification and ossification have been reported in the stifle joint of cats.[10] Radiographically, these lesions appear similar to the reported appearance of osteochondromas within the feline stifle joint.[9, 90]

SYNOVIAL SARCOMA

Synovial sarcomas arise from primitive mesenchymal precursor cells outside the synovial membrane of joints and bursa.[95] These tumors are uncommon in the dog and are rare in the cat.[91, 92] They occur most frequently in middle-aged, medium-sized to large-sized dogs. The most commonly affected joints are the stifle and the elbow. Synovial sarcomas grow slowly and are first noticeable as a homogeneous soft-tissue mass that involves or is near to a joint. Initially, radiographs reveal a mass of soft tissue. Portions of the tumor may be calcified, with mineral deposits appearing as hazy and punctate or as linear streaks (Fig. 16–22).

Canine synovial sarcomas are more likely to invade adjacent bone than their counterpart in humans.[93] Initial bone involvement appears as a spiculated periosteal response, followed by ragged erosion of the cortical bone adjacent to the tumor. Destruction of cancellous bone may be extensive and most commonly occurs on both sides of the joint[91, 93] (Fig 16–23). The tumor is locally invasive with an unpredictable capacity to metastasize,[94] although distant metastasis, particularly to the lungs, occurs in as many as one half of reported patients.[91, 95] Radiographic examination of the thorax is therefore mandatory in patients with suspected synovial sarcoma.

Before the appearance of cortical and cancellous bone destruction, synovial sarcomas must be differentiated from primary tumors of soft-tissue origin, fibrosarcomas or chondrosarcomas of the periosteum, parosteal sarcoma, periosteal hematoma, ossifying myositis, and metastatic disease. The location of an osteodestructive lesion on both sides of a joint, associated with an adjacent soft-tissue mass, is strong presumptive radiographic evidence of synovial sarcoma.[91] Pri-

FIGURE 16–22. A 14-year-old female (neutered) Golden retriever had progressive lameness of the right forelimb for 4 weeks. In addition, the elbow was swollen. *A* and *B,* Active periosteal proliferation is present on the distal humerus and the proximal ulna. Punctate areas of radiolucency are evident in the proximal ulna and olecranon. Histologic diagnosis was synovial sarcoma.

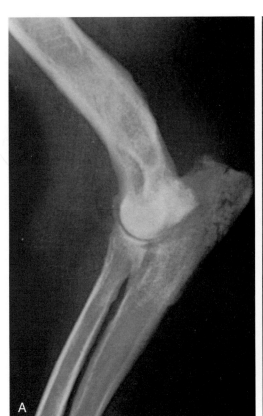
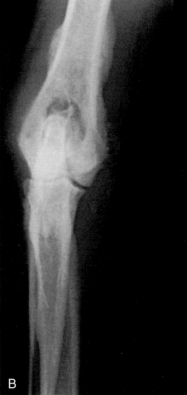

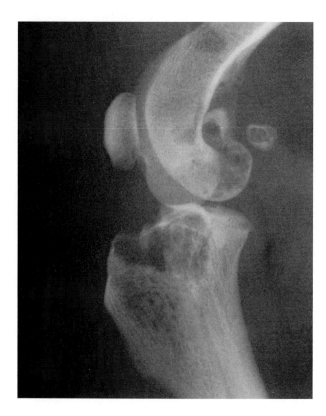

FIGURE 16–23. Multiple radiolucent lesions are evident on both sides of this dog's stifle. Histologic diagnosis was synovial sarcoma.

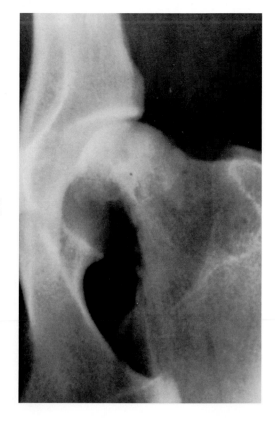

FIGURE 16–24. A 10-year-old female Doberman pinscher had acute-onset pain and non–weight-bearing lameness referable to the left hip. Osteolysis of the left femoral head and neck was evident radiographically. Histologic diagnosis was pancreatic adenocarcinoma metastasis to the left femoral head and neck.

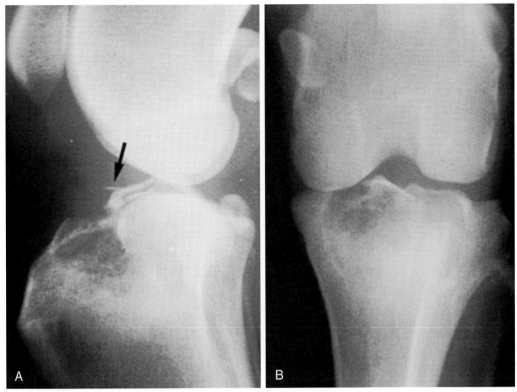

FIGURE 16–25. A 2-year-old female Great Dane had gradual enlargement of the proximal left tibia and subsequent acute onset of non–weight-bearing lameness of the left hindlimb. A and B, A focus of osteolysis within the medial condyle of the proximal tibia extends to involve the joint space. A small bone fragment is free within the joint space *(arrow)*. Histologic diagnosis was hemangiosarcoma. (Courtesy of University of Sydney.)

mary and metastatic bone tumors occasionally invade joints (Figs. 16–24 and 16–25).

References

1. Nickels FA, Grant BD, and Lincoln SD: Villonodular synovitis of the equine metacarpophalangeal joint. J Am Vet Med Assoc *168*:1043, 1976.
2. Vaughan LC: Muscle and tendon injuries in dogs. J Small Anim Pract *20*:711, 1979.
3. Bardet JF, and Hohn RB: Quadriceps contracture in dogs. J Am Vet Med Assoc *183*:680, 1983.
4. Basher AWP, Doige CE, and Presnell KR: Subchondral bone cysts in a dog with osteochondrosis. J Am Anim Hosp Assoc *24*:321, 1988.
5. Morgan JP, Pool RR, and Miyabayashi T: Primary degenerative joint disease of the shoulder in a colony of Beagles. J Am Vet Med Assoc *190*:531, 1987.
6. Ellison CW, and Norrdin RW: Multicentric periarticular calcinosis in a pup. J Am Vet Med Assoc *177*:542, 1980.
7. Schawalder von P: Die synoviale osteochondromatose (synoviale chondrometaplasie) beim hund. Schweiz Arch Tierheilk *122*:673, 1980.
8. Flo GL: Synovial chondrometaplasia in five dogs. J Am Vet Med Assoc *200*:943, 1992.
9. Kealy JK: Diagnostic Radiology of the Dog and Cat. Philadelphia, WB Saunders, 1979, p 371.
10. Whiting PG, and Pool RR: Intrameniscal calcification and ossification in the stifle joints of three domestic cats. J Am Anim Hosp Assoc *21*:579, 1985.
11. de Haan JJ, and Anderson CB: Calcium crystal associated arthropathy in a dog. J Am Vet Med Assoc *200*:943, 1992.
12. Short RP, and Jardine JE: Calcium phosphate deposition disease in a Fox Terrier. J Am Anim Hosp Assoc *29*:363, 1993
13. Mahoney PN, and Lamb CR: Articular, periarticular and juxtaarticular calcified bodies in the dog and cat: A radiologic review. Vet Radiol Ultrasound *34*:325, 1993.
14. Wood AKW, and McCarthy PH: Radiologic and anatomic observations of plantar sesamoid bones at the tarsometatarsal articulations of greyhounds. Am J Vet Res *45*:2158, 1984.
15. Wood AKW, McCarthy PH, and Howlett CR: Anatomic and radiographic appearance of a sesamoid bone in the tendon of origin of the supinator muscle of dogs. Am J Vet Res *46*:2043, 1985.
16. McCarthy PH, and Wood AKW: Anatomical and radiological studies of the iliopubic cartilage in adult Greyhounds. Anat Histol Embryol *15*:73, 1986.
17. Muhumnza L, Morgan JP, Miyabayashi T, et al: Positive-contrast arthrography: A study of the humeral joints in normal Beagle dogs. Vet Radiol *29*:157, 1988.
18. Barthez PY, and Morgan JP: Bicipital tenosynovitis in the dog—evaluation with positive contrast arthrography. Vet Radiol Ultrasound *34*:325, 1993.
19. Lowry JE, Carpenter LG, Park RD, et al: Radiographic anatomy and technique for arthrography of the cubital joint in clinically normal dogs. J Am Vet Med Assoc *203*:72, 1993.
20. Muir P, and Johnson KA. Supraspinous and biceps brachii tendinopathy in dogs. J Am Anim Pract *35*:239, 1994.
21. Rivers B, Wallace L, and Johnson GR: Biceps tenosynovitis in the dog: Radiographic and sonographic findings. Vet Comp Orthop Traumatol *5*:51, 1992.
22. Ljunggren G, and Olsson S-E: Osteoarthrosis of the shoulder and elbow joints in dogs: A pathologic and radiographic study of a necropsy material. J Am Vet Radiol Soc *16*:33, 1975.
23. Tirgari M, and Vaughan LL: Arthritis of the canine stifle joint. Vet Rec *96*:394, 1975.
24. Marshall JL: Peri-articular osteophytes—initiation and formation in the knees of the dog. Clin Orthop *62*:37, 1969.
25. Alexander JW: Pathogenesis and biochemical aspects of degenerative joint disease. Comp Contin Ed Vet Pract *2*:96l, 1980.
26. Lust G, and Summers BA: Early, asymptomatic stage of degenerative joint disease in canine hip joints. Am J Vet Res *42*:1849, 1981.
27. Olsewski JM, Lust G, Rendano VT, et al: Degenerative joint disease: Multiple joint involvement in young and mature dogs. Am J Vet Res *44*:1300, 1983.
28. Smith GK, Popovitch CA, Gregor TP, et al: Evaluation of risk factors for degenerative joint disease associated with hip dysplasia in dogs. J Am Vet Med Assoc *206*:642, 1995
29. Smith GK, Gregor TP, Rhodes WH, et al: Coxofemoral joint laxity from distraction radiography and its contemporaneous and prospective correlation with laxity, subjective score, and evidence of degenerative joint disease from conventional hip-extended radiography in dogs. Am J Vet Res *54*:1020, 1993.
30. Popovitch CA, Smith GK, Gregor TP, et al: Comparison of susceptibility for hip dysplasia between Rottweilers and German Shepherd Dogs. J Am Vet Med Assoc *206*:648, 1995.

31. Lust G, Williams AJ, Burton-Worster N, et al: Joint laxity and its association with hip dysplasia in Labrador Retrievers. Am J Vet Res 54:1990, 1993.

32. Marshall JL, and Olsson S-E: Instability of the knee: A long-term experimental study in dogs. J Bone Joint Surg (Am) 53:1561, 1971.

33. Sokoloff L: The pathology of osteoarthritis and the role of ageing. In Nuki J (Ed): The Aetiopathogenesis of Osteoarthritis. Tunbridge Wells, UK, Pitman Medical Publishing, 1980, pp 1–15.

34. Owens JM, and Ackerman N: Roentgenology of arthritis. Vet Clin North Am [Small Anim Pract] 8:460, 1978.

35. Pedersen NC, Pool RR, and Morgan JP: Joint diseases of dogs and cats. In Ettinger SJ (Ed): Textbook of Veterinary Internal Medicine. Philadelphia, WB Saunders, 1983, pp 2187–2235.

36. Hedhammar A, Olsson S-E, Andersson S-A, et al: Canine hip dysplasia: Study of heritability in 401 litters of German shepherd dogs. J Am Vet Med Assoc 174:1012, 1979.

37. Leighton EA, Smith GK, McNeil M, et al: Heritability of the distraction index in German Shepherd dogs and Labrador Retrievers (abstr). In Proceedings, American Kennel Club Conference on Molecular Genetics and Genetic Health, 1994.

38. Lust G, Rendano VT, and Summers BA: Canine hip dysplasia: Concepts and diagnosis. J Am Vet Med Assoc 187:638, 1985.

39. Hedhammar A, Wu F-M, Krook L, et al: Overnutrition and skeletal disease. Cornell Vet 64:9, 1974.

40. Rendano VT, and Ryan G: Canine hip dysplasia evaluation. Vet Radiol 26:170, 1985.

41. Farrow CS, and Back RT: Radiographic evaluation of non-anesthetized and non-sedated dogs for hip dysplasia. J Am Vet Med Assoc 194:524, 1989.

42. Aronson E, Kraus KH, and Smith J: The effect of anesthesia on the radiographic appearance of the coxofemoral joints. Vet Radiol 32:2, 1991.

43. Madsen JS, and Svalastoga E: Effect of anesthetics and stress on the radiographic evaluation of the coxofemoral joint. J Small Anim Pract 32:64, 1991.

44. Belkoff SM, Padgett G, and Soutas-Little RW: Development of a devise to measure canine coxofemoral joint laxity. Vet Comp Orthop Traumatol 1:31, 1989.

45. Smith GK, Biery JN, and Gregor TP: New concepts of coxofemoral joint stability and the development of a clinical stress radiographic method for quantitating hip joint laxity in the dog. J Am Vet Med Assoc 196:59, 1990.

46. Lust G, Beilman WT, Dueland DJ, et al: Intra-articular volume and hip joint instability in dogs with hip dysplasia. J Bone Joint Surg (Am) 62:576, 1980.

47. Lust G, Beilman WT, and Rendano VT: A relationship between degree of laxity and synovial fluid volume in coxofemoral joints of dogs predisposed for hip dysplasia. Am J Vet Res 41:55, 1980.

48. Morgan JP: Canine hip dysplasia: Significance of early bony spurring. Vet Radiol 28:2, 1987.

49. Riser WH: The dysplastic hip joint: Its radiographic and histologic development. J Am Vet Radiol Soc 14:35, 1973.

50. Shively MJ, and Van Sickle DC: Developing coxal joint of the dog: Gross morphometric and pathologic observations. Am J Vet Res 42:185, 1982.

51. Brooymans-Schallenburg JHC: Diagnosis of hip dysplasia and selection against this trait. Vet Q 5:8, 1983.

52. Rendano VT, Quick CB, Allan GS, et al: Radiographic evaluation of femoral head and neck fractures: The value of the flexed ventrodorsal and oblique projections in diagnosis. J Am Anim Hosp Assoc 16:485, 1980.

53. Robins GM: Some aspects of the radiographic examination of the canine elbow joint. J Small Anim Pract 21:417, 1980.

54. Salter RB, and Harris WR: Injuries involving the epiphyseal plate. J Bone Joint Surg 45:587, 1963.

55. Daly WR: Femoral head and neck fractures in the dog and cat: A review of 115 cases. Vet Surg 7:29 1978.

56. Marretta SM, and Schrader SC: Physeal injuries in the dog: A review of 135 cases. J Am Vet Med Assoc 182:708, 1983.

57. Grauer CF, Banks WJ, Ellison CW, et al: Incidence and mechanisms of distal femoral physeal fractures in the dog and cat. J Am Anim Hosp Assoc 17:579, 1981.

58. Denny HR: Condylar fractures of the humerus in the dog: A review of 133 cases. J Small Anim Pract 24:185, 1983.

59. Scavelli TD, Schrader SC, Matthiesen DT, et al: Partial rupture of the cranial cruciate ligament of the stifle in dogs: 25 cases. J Am Vet Med Assoc 196:1135, 1990.

60. Culvenor JA, and Howlett CR: Avulsion of the medial epicondyle of the humerus in the dog. J Small Anim Pract 23:83, 1982.

61. Pond MJ: Avulsion of the extensor digitorum longus muscle in the dog: A report of four cases. J Small Anim Pract 14:785, 1973.

62. Gambardella PC, and Griffiths RC: Treatment of hyperextension injuries of the canine carpus. Comp Contin Ed Vet Pract 4:127, 1982.

63. Farrow CS: Stress radiography: Applications in small animal practice. J Am Vet Med Assoc 181:777, 1982.

64. Puglisi TA, Tangner CH, Green RW, et al: Stress radiography of the canine humeral joint. J Am Anim Hosp Assoc 24:235, 1988.

65. Bellah JR, and Weigel JP: Hemarthrosis secondary to suspected warfarin toxicosis in a dog. J Am Vet Med Assoc 182:1126, 1983.

66. Dodds WJ: Hemostasis and coagulation. In Kaneko JJ (Ed): Clinical Biochemistry of Domestic Animals, 3rd Ed. New York, Academic Press, 1980, pp 671–718.

67. Hoaglund FT: Experimental haemarthrosis: The response of canine knees to injection of autogenous blood. J Bone Joint Surg 49:285, 1967.

68. Bennett D, and Taylor DJ: Bacterial infective arthritis in the dog. J Small Anim Pract 29:207, 1988.

69. Moise NS, Crissmam JW, Fairbrother JF, et al: Mycoplasma gateae arthritis and tenosynovitis in cats: Case report and experimental reproduction of the disease. Am J Vet Res 44:10, 1983.

70. Roberts RE: Osteomyelitis associated with disseminated blastomycosis in nine dogs. Vet Radiol 20:124, 1979.

71. Schrader SC: Septic arthritis and osteomyelitis of the hip of six mature dogs. J Am Vet Med Assoc 181:894, 1982.

72. Bennett D: Immune-based erosive inflammatory joint disease of the dog: Canine rheumatoid arthritis: I. Clinical, radiological and laboratory investigations. J Small Anim Pract 28:779, 1987.

73. Barrett RE: Canine polyarthritis. In Kirk RW (Ed): Current Veterinary Therapy, Vol 7. Philadelphia, WB Saunders, 1980, pp 800–802.

74. Grindem CB, and Johnston KH: Systemic lupus erythematosus: Literature review and report of 42 new canine cases. J Am Anim Hosp Assoc 19:489, 1983.

75. Bennett D: Immune-based non-erosive inflammatory joint disease of the dog: I. Canine SLE. J Small Anim Pract 28:871, 1987.

76. Bennett D: Immune-based non-erosive inflammatory joint disease of the dog: II. Polyarthritis/polymyositis syndrome. J Small Anim Pract 28:891, 1987.

77. Moise NS, and Crissman JW: Chronic progressive polyarthritis in a cat. J Am Anim Hosp Assoc 18:965, 1982.

78. Pedersen NC, Pool RR, and O'Brien T: Feline chronic progressive polyarthritis. Am J Vet Res 41:522, 1980.

79. Carro T: Polyarthritis in cats. Comp Contin Ed Vet Pract 16:57, 1994.

80. Bennett D, and Nash AS: Feline immune-based polyarthritis: A study of thirty-one cases. J Small Anim Pract 29:501, 1988.

81. Brodey RS: Hypertrophic osteoarthropathy. In Andrews EJ, Ward BC, and Autman NH (Eds): Spontaneous Animal Models of Human Disease. New York, Academic Press, 1979, p 153.

82. Caywood DD, Osborne CA, Stevens JB, et al: Hypertrophic osteoarthropathy associated with an atypical neuroblastoma in a dog. J Am Anim Hosp Assoc 16:855, 1980.

83. Nate LA, Herron AJ, and Burk RL: Hypertrophic osteopathy in a cat associated with renal papillary adenoma. J Am Anim Hosp Assoc 17:659, 1981.

84. Rendano VT, and Slauson DO: Hypertrophic osteopathy in a dog with prostatic adenocarcinoma and without thoracic metastasis. J Am Anim Hosp Assoc 18:905, 1982.

85. Kusba JK, Lipowitz AJ, Wize M, et al: Suspected villonodular synovitis in a dog. J Am Vet Med Assoc 182:390, 1983.

86. Somer T, Sittnikow K, Henriksson K, et al: Pigmented villonodular synovitis and plasmacytoid lymphoma in a dog. J Am Vet Med Assoc 197:877, 1990.

87. Doeken WP: Pigmented villonodular synovitis: A review with illustrated case reports. Semin Arthr Rheum 9:1, 1979.

88. Goldberg RP, Weissman BN, Naimark A, et al: Femoral neck erosions: Sign of hip joint synovial disease. AJR 141:107, 1983.

89. Flo GL, Stickle RL, and Dunstan RW: Synovial chondrometaplasia in five dogs. J Am Vet Med Assoc 191:1417, 1987.

90. Hubler M, Johnson KA, Burling RT, et al: Lesions resembling osteochondromatosis in two cats. J Small Anim Pract 27:181, 1986.

91. Madewell BR, and Pool RR: Neoplasms of joints and related structures. Vet Clin North Am [Small Anim Pract] 8:511, 1978.

92. Silva-Krott IU: Synovial sarcoma in a cat. J Am Vet Med Assoc 203:1430, 1993.

93. Lipowitz AJ, Fetter AW, and Walker MA: Synovial sarcoma in the dog. J Am Vet Med Assoc 174:76, 1978.

94. McGlennon NJ, Houlton JEF, and Gorman NT: Synovial sarcoma in the dog—a review. J Small Anim Pract 29:139, 1988.

95. Vail DM, Powers BE, Getzy DM, et al: Evaluation of prognostic factors for dogs with synovial sarcoma: 36 cases (1986–1991). J Am Vet Med Assoc 205:1300, 1994.

STUDY QUESTIONS

1. List three types of stress that can be applied to a joint during stress radiography.

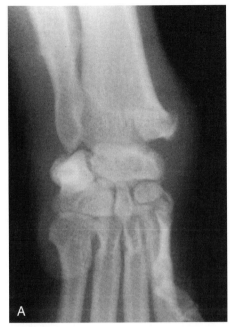

FIGURE 16–26. *A*

2. What is the earliest radiographic sign of canine hip dysplasia?

3. What concentration of contrast medium is recommended for canine arthrography?

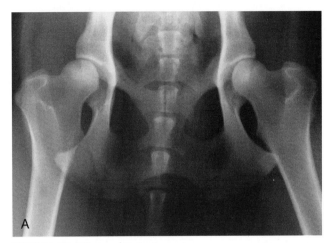

FIGURE 16–27. *A* (Courtesy of Dr. Ray Ferguson.)

4. List six radiographic signs of joint disease.

5. List two causes of an erosive arthropathy.

6. Name the primary joint neoplasm.

7. List the origin of intra-articular calcified bodies that may be seen in the stifle.

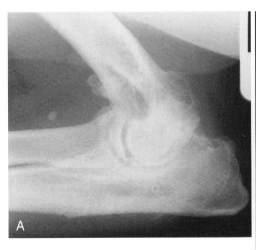

FIGURE 16–28. *A* and *B*

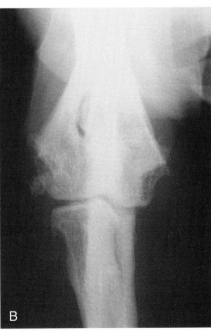

8. An 18-month-old Beagle sustained carpal trauma. Look at Figure 16–26A—a dorsopalmar carpal radiograph. Describe the pathology evident on this radiograph. What could be done to evaluate the joint further (other than make the lateromedial, and possibly oblique, views)?

9. An extended ventrodorsal radiograph was made of the pelvis of an 18-month-old Labrador retriever to assess for hip dysplasia. Look at Figure 16–27A. Does this image reveal any signs of hip dysplasia? What are they? What else could be done to further evaluate the coxofemoral joints?

10. The elbow of an 8-year-old Boxer was radiographed because of lameness. Look at Figure 16–28A and B. What are the likely causes of the changes seen in this elbow?

(Answers appear on page 636.)

APPENDICULAR SKELETON—EQUIDAE

Chapter 17

Physeal Disorders of the Immature Horse

Clifford R. Berry

In the equine neonate, radiographic anatomy is complicated by incomplete mineralization of cartilaginous structures and the number of growth plates or physes. Early detection of bone changes may require serial radiographs for complete evaluation. In fact, by the time bony changes are identified, the prognosis for the given disease process is usually poorer, owing to the potential for abnormal joint or bone development in the future.

Another peculiarity to the horse, as compared with small animals (dog and cat), is that transphyseal blood vessels exist, so direct extension of disease can occur across the physis from the metaphysis to the epiphysis. This chapter reviews physeal abnormalities of the equine neonate and weanling.

DISEASE PROCESSES

Infectious Physitis and Arthritis

It is not uncommon for foals to develop a lameness during the first 2 to 7 days after birth. Typically the lameness is associated with hematogenous spread of bacteria from an infected umbilicus (omphalophlebitis), pneumonia, or enteritis. Bacterial emboli lodge in the capillary loops and small vessels of the metaphysis, physis, epiphysis, and joint capsule, so infections are typically polyostotic and involve multiple joints. Other risk factors for the development of these hematogenous infections include poor farm management, failure of passive transfer, and presence of an unclean environment at the time of foaling. The initial sites of septic emboli are in the metaphyseal capillary loops at the physis and in the developing subchondral bone of the articular surfaces of long and cuboidal bones. The factors that have been suggested to contribute to the bacterial colonization in these regions include (1) high capillary density in these areas, (2) neovascularization at the sites undergoing endochondral ossification, and (3) rapid changes in blood flow from the arterial to sluggish flow within sinusoids.

Radiographic changes associated with septic physitis, metaphysitis, epiphysitis, and arthritis are highly variable and depend on how long the infection has been localized to the bone and joint. The earliest radiographic feature may be only soft-tissue swelling. Classically, bone destruction initially precedes and is more advanced than bone production or medullary sclerosis (Figs. 17–1 to 17–3). Multiple joints are invariably involved, and radiographic changes can progress rapidly over several days. In the author's experience, the

tarsus, stifle, carpus, metacarpophalangeal, and metatarsophalangeal joints are the most commonly affected. A classification system has been proposed as to different types of infectious arthritis based on location and age of the horse and is summarized in Table 17–1.

Physeal Dysplasia

The radiographic features of physitis, *aseptic* physitis, or physeal dysplasia are similar to the lucencies one might expect in a foal that develops an infectious physitis. Several features regarding physeal dysplasia may help distinguish these two from each other; however, one may not be able to do so radiographically. Physeal dysplasia is usually seen in weanling

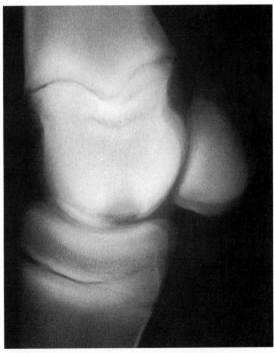

FIGURE 17–1. Lateromedial view of the right metacarpophalangeal joint from a foal with an infected umbilicus and multiple swollen joints. There is soft-tissue swelling and a destructive lesion identified in the distal end of third metacarpus. A small sequestrum is also present. *Escherichia coli* was cultured from the joint.

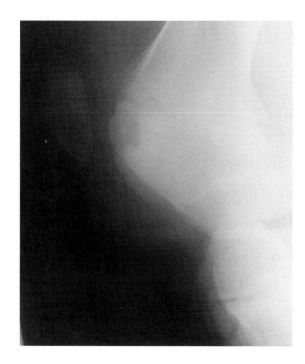

FIGURE 17–2. Lateromedial radiograph of the distal right femur from a foal with an infectious arthritis and pneumonia. There is osteolysis within the trochlear groove between the medial and lateral femoral trochlea. *Klebsiella pneumoniae* was cultured from the joint.

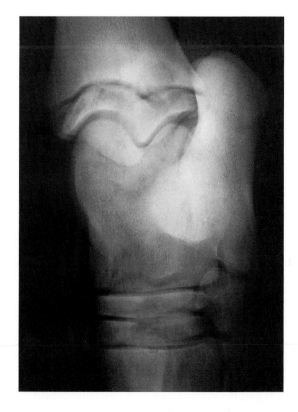

FIGURE 17–3. Dorsolateral—45 degree—plantaromedial oblique radiograph of the left tarsus from a 3-week-old Thoroughbred foal. There are multiple areas of bone lysis without surrounding reaction. These changes involve the central and third tarsal bones, the calcaneus, talus, metaphysis, and epiphysis of the distal tibia. *Escherichia coli* was cultured from the joint.

Table 17–1
SKELETAL DISTRIBUTION ASSOCIATED WITH THE PATTERN OF INFECTIOUS POLYARTHRITIS-POLYOSTOTIC OSTEOMYELITIS COMPLEX OF FOALS

Type	Location	Age	Bacterial Agents
S type	Multiple large joints*	1–3 days	*E. coli, Klebsiella,* beta-hemolytic *streptococci*
E type	Arthritis epiphyseal†	Older foals	*E. coli, Salmonella,* beta-hemolytic *streptococci*
P type	1 or 2 joints, metaphyseal sequestration‡	Older foals	Beta-hemolytic *streptococci, Salmonella* type B and *Rhodococcus equi*
T type	Carpal/tarsal bones	1–3 days	*E. coli, Klebsiella,* beta-hemolytic *streptococci*

*Stifle, hock, shoulder, and hip joints.
†Epiphyses from the medial and lateral femoral condyle, lateral facet of the distal radius, distal tibia, and patella.
‡Physes of the distal radius, distal tibia, and third metacarpi and third metatarsi.

or yearling horses during the 3- to 6-month age category. Radiographically, there is an indistinct area noted to the distal physis of the radius, tibia, or third metacarpus and third metatarsal (Fig. 17–4). These bones are the only bones involved. All or only one bone may be affected. Metaphyseal or epiphyseal periosteal new bone formation occurs that is smooth and chronic in appearance. This periosteal reaction is a late development, with the physeal lucencies, widening, and irregularity being the earliest radiographic change. Soft-tissue swelling may or may not be present.

These horses are typically rapidly growing and on high-protein feed additives. Although the exact pathogenesis of this disease is not known, several theories have suggested an underlying hereditary (osteochondrosis) or developmental (nutritional, metabolic) abnormality. Decreasing the amount of calcium and phosphorus supplements and high crude protein diets may help. The physeal abnormality can lead to unequal physeal growth, possible premature closure of one side of the physis, and angular limb deformities. Over time, the radiographic changes regress, particularly as the physis comes close to closing.

Traumatic Physeal Injuries

Often a foal is stepped on by other horses in the paddock or stall, and radiographs are used to evaluate the extent of bone injury. Salter-Harris fractures can occur in horses, and type I and type II physeal injuries are common (Fig. 17–5). Initial radiographic evaluation may not indicate an abnormality, particularly if the fracture is nondisplaced. Over time, however, the physis becomes irregular and takes the appearance of an infected physis as it heals. As with other physeal injuries, the possibility of premature closure of the physis is great as the physeal fracture heals.

SUMMARY

Radiographic evaluation of the equine neonate is complicated by incomplete cartilage mineralization (large cartilage models still present) and increased numbers of separate centers of ossification. A knowledge of the normal closure times of the long bones of the equine front and rear leg is required for making accurate interpretations regarding physeal appearances. Bone lysis is one of the earliest changes (aside from soft-tissue swelling) that can be identified radiographically when a bone is infected. Polyostotic infectious arthritis and osteomyelitis of the neonate is usually spread from a hematogenous infection, the most common site being the umbilicus. Physeal dysplasia (aseptic physitis) is usually seen in older horses before skeletal maturity. The most common

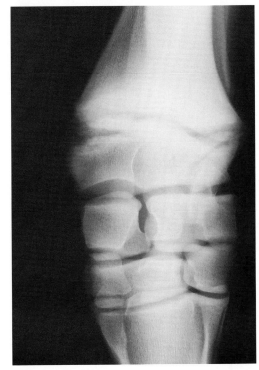

FIGURE 17–4. Dorsopalmar radiograph of the left carpus from a 4-month-old Quarter horse. There is widening and irregular lucency associated with the medial aspect of the distal radial physis. These changes were bilateral and are consistent with physitis or physeal dysplasia.

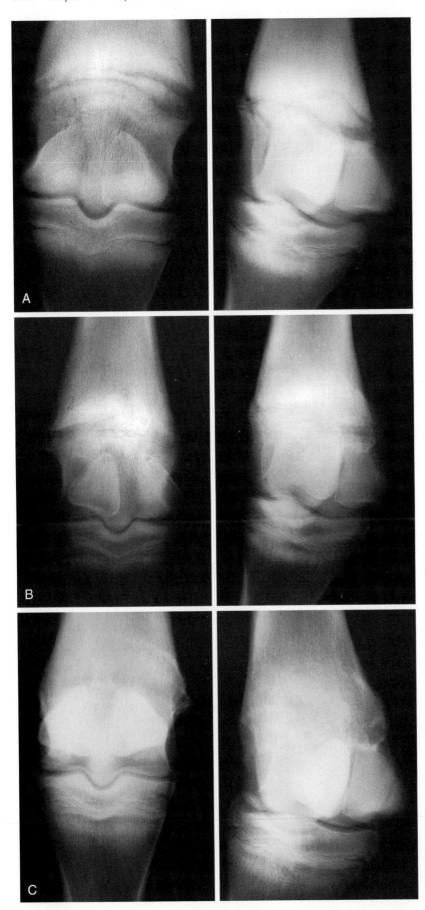

FIGURE 17–5. Dorsopalmar and dorsomedial–45 degree—palmarolateral oblique radiographs of the left third metacarpus of a 4-month-old Thoroughbred made at the time of injury (A), 3 weeks (B), and 6 weeks (C) after a type I Salter-Harris fracture. There is marked physeal irregularity with metaphyseal and epiphyseal flaring and periosteal reaction that resulted in premature closure of the physis 6 weeks after the injury.

bones involved include the distal tibial, radial, and metacarpal and metatarsal physes. Radiographs can be useful for evaluating these changes over time and monitoring the response of a particular horse to therapy.

References

1. Bertone AL, and McIlwraith CW: A review of current concepts in the therapy of infectious arthritis in the horse. *In* Proceedings of the American Association of Equine Practitioners, 1986, pp 323–339.

2. Frith EC: Current concepts of infectious polyarthritis in foals. Equine Vet J *15*:5, 1983.
3. Firth EC: Hematogenous osteomyelitis in the foal. *In* Proceedings American Association of Equine Practitioners, 1987, pp 795–803.
4. Morgan JP, Van de Watering CC, and Kersjes AW: Salmonella bone infection in colts and calves: Its radiographic diagnosis. J Am Vet Radiol Soc 1974; 15:66–76.
5. Kobluk CN, Ames TR, and Goer RJ. The Horse: Diseases and Clinical Management. Philadelphia, WB Saunders, 1995.
6. Butler JA, Colles CM, Dyson SJ, et al: Clinical Radiology of the Horse. London, Blackwell Scientific Publications, 1993.

Study Questions

1. Common sources of infection resulting in septic arthritis and physitis in the neonatal foal include:
   A. Umbilical vein.
   B. Lungs.
   C. Intestinal tract.
   D. All of the above.

2. All of the following physeal areas are commonly involved in physeal dysplasia *except*:
   A. Distal radius.
   B. Distal femur.
   C. Distal tibia.
   D. Distal third metacarpus.

3. In the E type of septic arthritis and osteomyelitis, the most common bone manifestion is involvement of the:
   A. Metaphysis.
   B. Physis.
   C. Epiphysis.
   D. Apophysis.

4. Irregularity and lucency within the physis of a foal could represent:
   A. Infectious physitis.
   B. Osteochondritis dessicans.
   C. Epiphyseal dysplasia.
   D. Premature closure of the physis.

5. This lateromedial radiograph (Fig. 17–6) of the tarsus is from a 7-month-old yearling that has been lame in the right hindlimb for several weeks. Your radiographic diagnosis is:
   A. Osteochondrosis of the lateral trochlear ridge of the talus.
   B. Osteochondrosis of the intermediate ridge of the distal tibia.

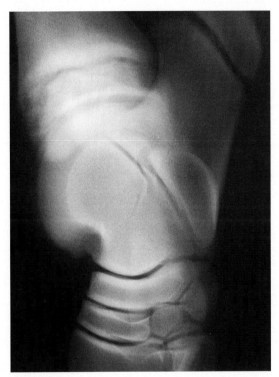

FIGURE 17–6

   C. Physeal dysplasia of the distal tibia.
   D. Tarsal dysmaturity of the third and central tarsal bones.

(Answers appear on page 637.)

Chapter 18

The Stifle and Tarsus

Mary B. Mahaffey

THE STIFLE

Radiographic Technique

For routine evaluation, caudocranial and lateromedial projections of the stifle should be made. Occasionally, craniolateral-caudomedial or caudolateral-craniomedial oblique views are useful to project other surfaces of the joint. Because of the thickness of the stifle area, the use of a grid increases radiographic detail considerably. Disadvantages of grid use are the need for alignment of the primary x-ray beam so that it strikes the grid perpendicularly and the necessity for larger exposure factors.

Radiographic Abnormalities

Osteochondrosis and Osseous Cyst–Like Lesions

Osteochondrosis is a relatively common disorder in young horses. It is a cartilage maturation failure in which the proliferating cartilage model is not completely replaced by bone. The persistent cartilage appears radiographically as a radiolucent bone defect, which is usually adjacent to an articular surface.

In the equine stifle, osteochondrosis may affect the lateral trochlear ridge of the femur (Fig. 18–1), in which instance the periphery of the lateral trochlear ridge has an irregular appearance owing to multiple areas of cartilage that have not matured into bone.[1] Occasionally, free or partially detached osteochondral fragments are observed adjacent to the periph-ery of the trochlea. Osteochondrosis is often bilateral; therefore, a radiograph of the opposite stifle should be made if osteochondrosis is identified.

Bone cysts have been described as occurring in many locations in horses.[2] One location is the medial femoral condyle. In some reports, it has been suggested that these cystic lesions are a manifestation of osteochondrosis; this conclusion is unproved. In addition, there is still debate as to whether these lesions are true cysts. Therefore, it seems prudent to refer to them as *osseous cyst–like lesions*. In the stifle, these lesions are found primarily in the medial condyle and may be observed in horses of any age.[3] Radiographically, these cyst-like lesions appear as subchondral radiolucent defects (Figs. 18–2 and 18–3). Joint communication may be present; radiographic confirmation of such communication requires that the x-ray beam strike the area of joint involvement tangentially (see Fig. 18–3). Thus, even if joint communication is present, it may not be identified radiographically. These osseous cyst–like lesions are often bilateral, and if one is identified, the opposite stifle should be radiographed. Occasionally, osseous cyst–like lesions are found in the lateral condyle or the proximal tibia, but these locations are less common sites of occurrence when compared with the medial femoral condyle.

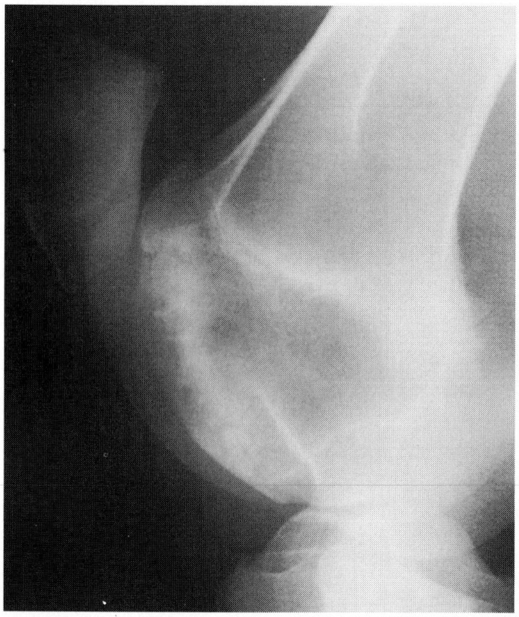

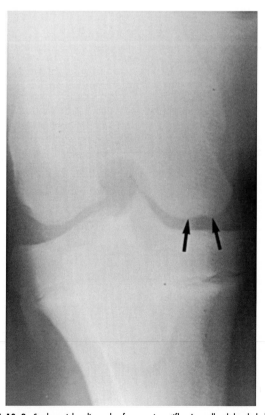

FIGURE 18–1. Stifle of a horse with osteochondrosis of the lateral trochlear ridge of the femur, lateromedial view. The lateral trochlear ridge has an irregular margin, and the subchondral bone is sclerotic.

FIGURE 18–2. Caudocranial radiograph of an equine stifle. A small subchondral defect is present in the medial femoral condyle *(arrows)*. This lesion may be considered as a part of the osseous cyst–like lesion syndrome. It could not be seen in the lateral view.

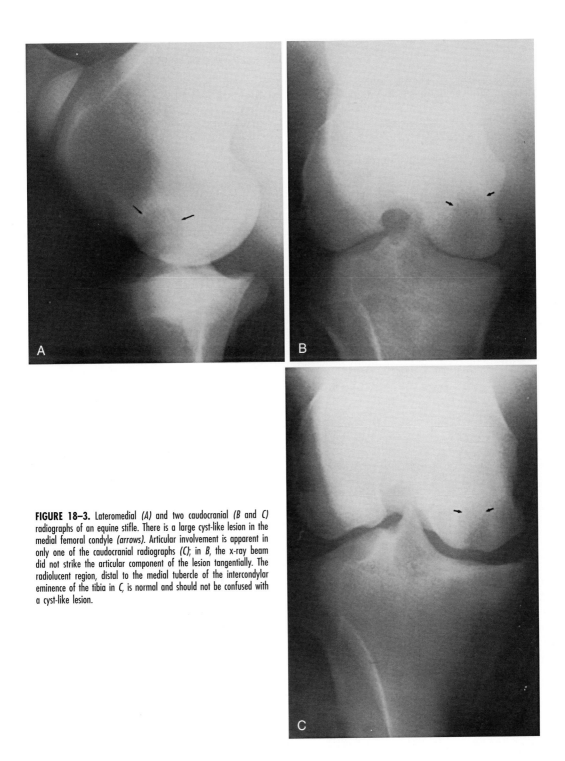

FIGURE 18–3. Lateromedial *(A)* and two caudocranial *(B* and *C)* radiographs of an equine stifle. There is a large cyst-like lesion in the medial femoral condyle *(arrows)*. Articular involvement is apparent in only one of the caudocranial radiographs *(C)*; in *B*, the x-ray beam did not strike the articular component of the lesion tangentially. The radiolucent region, distal to the medial tubercle of the intercondylar eminence of the tibia in *C*, is normal and should not be confused with a cyst-like lesion.

Normal radiographs do not necessarily rule out osteochondrosis. In one study, 40 percent of radiographically normal horses and 78 percent of horses with mild flattening of the subchondral bone had abnormal cartilage on arthroscopic examination.[4]

Sepsis

In foals, a common cause of stifle sepsis is bacteremia due to umbilical infection. The radiographic appearance of stifle osteomyelitis is similar to that of bone infections elsewhere in the body; the resulting bone lesion is aggressive. There is usually soft-tissue swelling, which may reflect cellulitis as well as joint effusion, and osteolytic lesions often occur in the femur, patella, or tibia (Fig. 18–4). If the infection progresses, sclerosis reflecting new bone formation may be seen, and an active periosteal reaction may develop.

Skin laceration or puncture, with subsequent bacterial contamination, is another cause of septic stifle changes in horses. Changes may be limited to the soft tissue, in which instance only soft-tissue swelling is seen. If bone is involved, typical changes of osteomyelitis are seen.

Trauma

Traumatic alterations in the equine stifle should be evaluated in the same manner as in the stifle joint of other animals.[5] Degenerative joint disease may develop as a result of external trauma or wear and tear. Signs are identical to those seen in degenerative joint disease in other joints, including periarticular osteophyte formation (Fig. 18–5), decrease in the size of

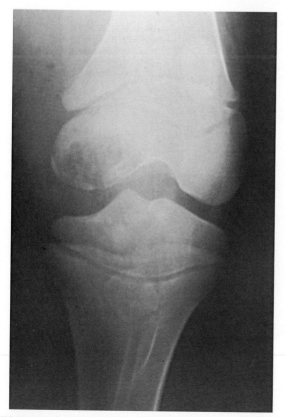

FIGURE 18–4. Caudocranial radiograph of the stifle of a foal with septic arthritis and femoral osteomyelitis. There is an aggressive, primarily osteolytic lesion in the medial femoral condyle. In addition, there is gas in the soft tissues medial to the medial femoral condyle. This radiographic appearance in the equine stifle is virtually diagnostic for bacterial osteomyelitis.

articular spaces, and subchondral osteolytic defects due to synovial hyperplasia. Care must be taken in the evaluation of articular space size because this determination is influenced by the geometric relationship of the x-ray beam, the articular space, and the cassette.

Distal Patellar Changes

Fragmentation, enthesophyte formation, subchondral irregularity, and radiolucency of the distal patella all have been reported in adult horses with stifle lameness (Fig. 18–6).[6] One of the potential causes of these changes is instability of and stress on the distal patella caused by medial patellar desmotomy.[7]

Tumoral Calcinosis

Tumoral calcinosis (calcinosis circumscripta) may appear clinically as a hard nodule on the lateral aspect of the stifle.[8] Radiographically the nodule contains punctate areas of mineralization. The cause of tumoral calcinosis is unknown; affected horses usually are not lame.

THE TARSUS

Radiographic Technique

For routine examination of the tarsus, four radiographic projections should be made: lateromedial, dorsoplantar, dorsolateral-plantaromedial oblique, and dorsomedial-plantarolateral oblique. Oblique projections are recommended routinely because of the complex nature of the tarsus and the tendency for some abnormalities to remain undetected in dorsoplantar or lateromedial projections.

In young foals, physes are visible in the distal tibia and tuber calcanei. In addition, the lateral malleolus appears as a separate structure; it fuses with the tibia at approximately 100 days of age.[9] In some foals, the first and second tarsal bones appear as separate structures after birth; in other horses, fusion may take place before birth. One author estimates that the first and second tarsal bones are radiographically separate in approximately 20 percent of 6-month-old foals.[9]

The use of a grid for tarsal radiography is not necessary. It is important that the horse bear weight on the joint when the radiographs are made.

Radiographic Abnormalities

Osteochondrosis and Osseous Cyst–Like Lesions

There are at least three distinct manifestations of osteochondrosis and osseous cyst–like lesions in the tarsus. First, osteochondrosis may affect the cranial aspect of the intermediate ridge of the tibial cochlea.[10] In this instance, a cleavage line may be seen in the cranial aspect of the intermediate ridge, which reflects formation of a large osteochondral fragment. This fragment may be seen in the lateromedial projection but is more clearly seen in the dorsomedial-plantarolateral projection (Fig. 18–7). Genetic factors may play a role in the development of this manifestation of osteochondrosis.[11]

Second, osteochondrosis may develop on the lateral or medial trochlear ridge of the talus, resulting in a radiolucent defect involving the margin of the affected talus (Fig. 18–8).[11] Third, osseous cyst–like lesions may be found in the distal

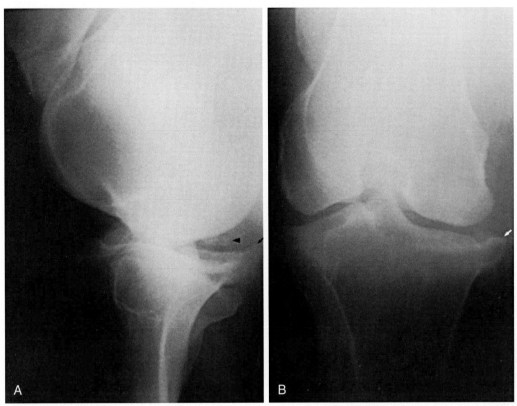

FIGURE 18–5. The stifle of a horse with degenerative joint disease, lateromedial *(A)* and caudocranial *(B)* views. There is a large periarticular osteophyte on the medial tibial condyle *(arrow)* and mineralization of the medial meniscus *(arrowhead).*

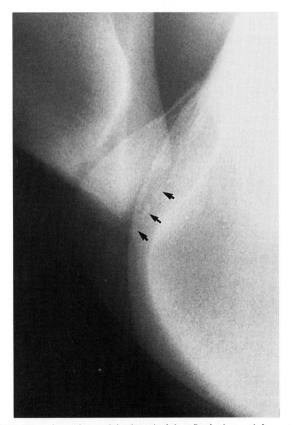

FIGURE 18–6. Close-up lateromedial radiograph of the stifle of a horse with fragmentation and radiolucency of the distal patella *(arrows)* following medial patellar desmotomy.

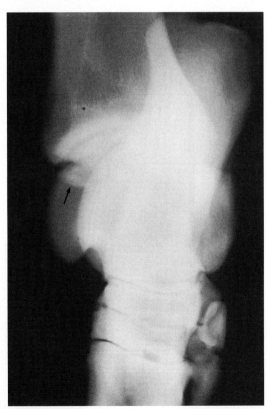

FIGURE 18–7. The tarsus of a horse with osteochondrosis of the tibial intermediate ridge, dorsomedial-plantarolateral view. There is an osteochondral fragment of the distal tibia *(arrow).* Osteophytes are present on the dorsolateral aspects of the distal intertarsal and tarsometatarsal articulations, which are indicative of degenerative joint disease.

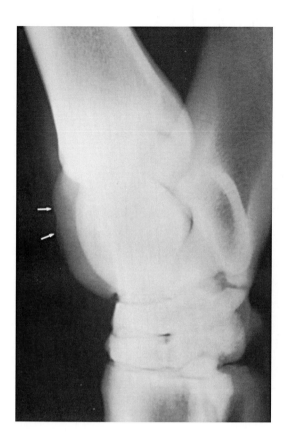

FIGURE 18–8. The tarsus of a horse with osteochondrosis of the medial trochlear ridge of the talus (arrows), lateromedial view. The dorsal margin of the medial trochlear ridge is irregular. Note the normal "beak-like" bone projection on the distal margin of the medial ridge of the talus.

FIGURE 18–9. Lateromedial (A) and dorsoplantar (B) radiographs of the tarsus of a foal with a compression fracture of the third tarsal bone.

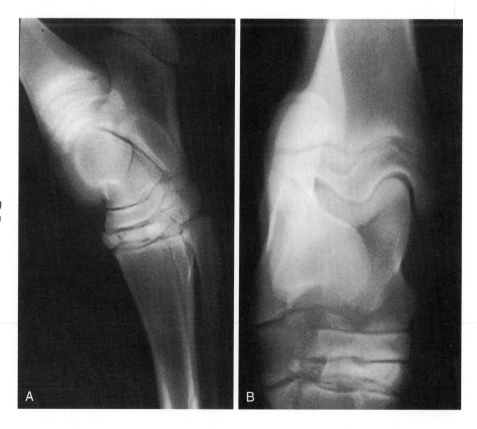

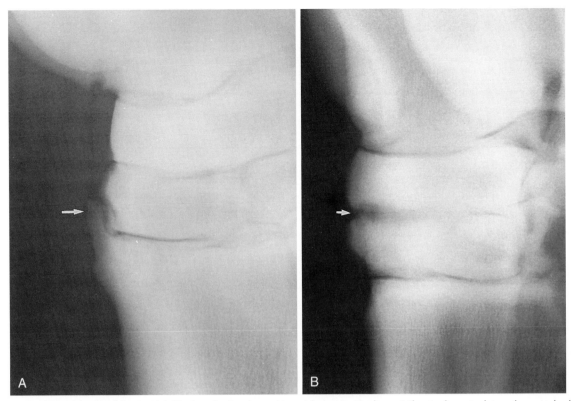

FIGURE 18–10. Lateral *(A)* and dorsolateral-plantaromedial *(B)* radiographs of two horses with tarsal degenerative joint disease. *A,* There is a large osteophyte on the proximodorsal aspect of the third metatarsal bone *(arrow)*. *B,* There is irregularity and radiolucency of the distal intertarsal joint *(arrow)*.

tibia, the proximal aspect of the third metatarsus, the talus, or the calcaneus. All three manifestations of osteochondrosis, osseous cyst–like lesions, or both are often bilateral, and if identified, radiographs of the contralateral limb should be made.

Another condition that has been described as a form of osteochondrosis is compression of the third tarsal bone in foals. This condition has also been described as aseptic or avascular necrosis of the third tarsal bone. The exact cause of this condition is unknown. Nevertheless, an extensive compression-type fracture of the third tarsal bone is occasionally observed in foals (Fig. 18–9).[12] Many of these foals also have an associated angular limb deformity, which may be secondary to the fracture or may have been present before fracture and may have contributed to mechanical failure of the third tarsal bone.

Trauma

Whether the result of external trauma or joint wear and tear, degenerative joint disease of the tarsus is common, especially in the distal intertarsal and tarsometatarsal joints. Periarticular osteophyte formation is the most commonly observed radiographic sign of tarsal degenerative joint disease in horses. In instances in which the disease is severe, however, there may be subchondral bone lysis, ankylosis, or both. This feature of degenerative joint disease in the equine tarsus is not commonly seen in other joints.[13, 14] Tarsal joint space narrowing without subchondral bone lysis is difficult to evaluate radiographically because it is not often possible to obtain a radiograph with the x-ray beam parallel to the joint surface. The clinical significance of radiographically detectable changes of tarsal degenerative joint disease is debatable be-

cause there is poor clinical correlation between these changes and lameness.[15]

Periarticular osteophytes are usually best seen in the dorsolateral-plantaromedial oblique projection because the disease begins dorsomedially in many horses. Radiographic changes may frequently be seen in other tarsal projections as well (Fig. 18–10; see also Fig. 18–7).

Other Conditions

Fractures and sepsis of the tarsus are relatively common. Radiographic evaluation of these conditions is straightforward, and radiographic signs are similar to those described elsewhere in this text.

References

1. Pascoe JR, Pool RR, Wheat JD, et al: Osteochondral defects of the lateral trochlear ridge of the distal femur of the horse: Clinical, radiographic and pathologic examination and results of surgical treatment. Vet Surg 13:99, 1984.
2. Peterson H, and Reinland S: Periarticular subchondral bone cysts in horses. *In* Proceedings of the 14th Annual Meeting of the American Association of Equine Practitioners, Philadelphia, 1968, p 245.
3. Stewart B, and Reid CF: Osseous cyst-like lesions of the medial femoral condyle in the horse. J Am Vet Med Assoc 180:254, 1982.
4. Steinheimer DN, McIlwraith CW, Park RD, et al: Comparison of radiographic subchondral bone changes with arthroscopic findings in the equine femoropatellar and femorotibial joints: A retrospective study of 72 joints (50 horses). Vet Radiol Ultrasound 36:478, 1995.
5. Sanders-Shamis M, Bukowiecki CF, and Biller DS: Cruciate and collateral ligament failure in the equine stifle: Seven cases (1975–1985). J Am Vet Med Assoc 193:573, 1988.
6. McIlwraith CW: Osteochondral fragmentation of the distal aspect of the patella in horses. Equine Vet J 22:157, 1990.

7. Squire KRE, Blevins WE, Frederick M, et al: Radiographic changes in an equine patella following medial patellar desmotomy. Vet Radiol *31*:208, 1990.
8. Dodd DC, and Raker CW: Tumoral calcinosis (calcinosis circumscripta) in a horse. J Am Vet Med Assoc *157*:968, 1970.
9. Smallwood JE, Auer JA, Martens RJ, et al: The developing equine tarsus from birth to six months of age. Equine Pract *6*:7, 1984.
10. Stromberg B, and Rejno S: Osteochondrosis in the horse. Acta Radiol [Diagn] (Stockh) *358*:139, 1978.
11. Schougaard H, Romme JF, and Phillipson J: A radiographic survey of tibiotarsal osteochondrosis in a selected population of trotting horses in Denmark and its possible genetic significance. Equine Vet J *22*:288, 1990.
12. Dewes HF: The onset and consequences of tarsal bone fractures in foals. NZ Vet J *30*:129, 1982.
13. McIlwraith CW: Current concepts in equine degenerative joint disease. J Am Vet Med Assoc *180*:239, 1982.
14. Morgan JP: Radiographic diagnosis of bone and joint diseases in the horse. Cornell Vet *58*(suppl):28, 1968.
15. Hartung K, Munzer B, and Keller H: Radiographic evaluation of spavin in young trotters. Vet Radiol *24*:153, 1983.

STUDY QUESTIONS

1. The most common location of osseous cyst–like lesions in the equine stifle is the
   A. Medial femoral condyle.
   B. Lateral femoral condyle.
   C. Intermediate ridge of the tibia.
   D. Patella.
   E. None of the above.

2. Approximately _____ percent of radiographically normal horses may have arthroscopic evidence of abnormal cartilage in the stifle joint.
   A. 5 percent.
   B. 15 percent.
   C. 40 percent.
   D. 75 percent.
   E. 90 percent.

3. The most common cause of stifle joint infection in foals is
   A. Kicked by dam.
   B. Intra-articular injections.
   C. Secondary to mastitis.
   D. Secondary to umbilical infection.
   E. Secondary to fistulous withers.

4. Which of the following is *not* a typical manifestation of osteochondrosis of the equine tarsus?

   A. Fragmentation (separation) of the intermediate ridge of the tibia.
   B. Radiolucent defect on the lateral or medial ridge of the tibia.
   C. Osseous cyst–like lesion of the distal tibia.
   D. Failure of the lateral malleolus to unite with the tibia.

5. Which view of the tarsus will project the calcaneus in the most unobstructed fashion?
   A. Lateromedial.
   B. Dorsoplantar.
   C. Dorsolateral-plantaromedial.
   D. Dorsomedial-plantarolateral.

6. The sustantaculum tali is part of which bone?
   A. Calcaneous.
   B. Talus.
   C. Tibia.
   D. Femur.

7. The relationship between radiographic severity of degenerative joint disease of the equine tarsus and clinical lameness is strong. (True or False)

8. Joint space width in the equine tarsus is relatively easy to assess accurately with the use of radiography. (True or False)

(Answers appear on page 637.)

Chapter 19

The Carpus

J. Gregg Boring

The equine carpus is composed of seven to nine cuboidal bones arranged in two rows, opposed proximally by the radius (antebrachiocarpal joint) and distally by the three metacarpal bones (carpometacarpal joint). The intercarpal joint (middle carpal or midcarpal joint) joins the proximal and distal rows of carpal bones.

The antebrachiocarpal, middle carpal, and carpometacarpal joints all are synovial joints. The middle and carpometacarpal joints communicate between the third and the fourth carpal bones; the antebrachiocarpal joint is separate.[1, 2] Collectively, there are approximately 26 side-to-side and proximal-to-distal bone articulations. The irregularly curved surfaces are compounded by superimposition of the various sizes, shapes,

and positions of the individual carpal bones. This anatomic complexity necessitates the use of multiple radiographic views to examine the carpal region adequately.

RADIOGRAPHIC EXAMINATION

Five standard views have been suggested for radiographic evaluation of the carpus:[3] the dorsopalmar (DPa), lateromedial (LM), flexed lateromedial (FLM), dorsolateral-palmaromedial oblique (DL-PaMO), and dorsomedial-palmarolateral oblique (DM-PaLO) views (Fig. 19–1). The exact positioning

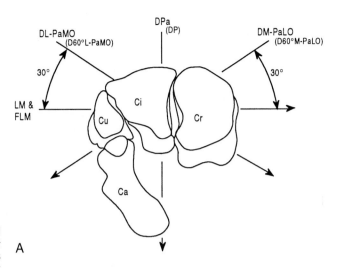

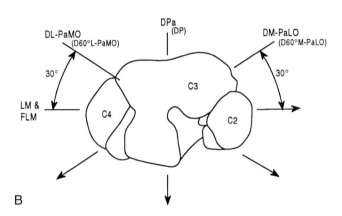

FIGURE 19–1. Five standard radiographic projections. Diagram of the proximal *(A)* and distal *(B)* rows of equine carpal bones. Directional terms describing the point of entrance to the point of exit of the primary x-ray beam are designated. The terminology shown in parentheses describes the angulation of the x-ray beam. DL-PaMO, dorsolateral-palmaromedial oblique; DPa, dorsopalmar; DM-PaLO, dorsomedial-palmerolateral oblique; Ca, accessory carpal; Cu, ulnar carpal; Ci, intermediate carpal; Cr, radial carpal; LM, lateromedial view; FLM, flexed lateromedial view.

used to produce the oblique views is described by identifying the degree of obliquity from the dorsal aspect of the carpus. Therefore, the oblique views are more appropriately the dorsal 60-degree lateral–palmaromedial oblique (D60°L-PaMO) and the dorsal 60-degree medial–palmarolateral oblique (D60°M-PaLO).

In addition to the five standard views, oblique views of the dorsal surface of the carpus are of value for more complete evaluation of some carpal fractures (Fig. 19–2).[4] These dorsal-surface views are designated as dorsoproximal-dorsodistal obliques (DPr-DDiO).[5] The direction of the x-ray beam may be chosen to project the dorsal aspect of either the distal radius or the distal row of carpal bones. The proximal row of carpal bones may also be evaluated by positioning the x-ray beam at an intermediate degree of angulation between those shown (see Fig. 19–2). Generally, views of the dorsal surface of the carpus are made when there is intracapsular soft-tissue swelling or when radiographic abnormalities explaining the clinical signs, or joint distention, are not seen in the five standard projections of the carpus.

RADIOGRAPHIC INTERPRETATION

For standardization, it is recommended that carpal radiographs be placed on the illuminator in a standard fashion. The order recommended, from the viewer's left to right, is the DPa, LM, FLM, obliques, and special dorsal-surface projections.

Soft-Tissue Swelling

Soft-tissue swelling may be intracapsular, extracapsular, or both. Each of the three carpal joints has a distinct joint capsule with specific origins and attachments (Fig. 19–3), and there is communication between the middle and the carpometacarpal joints.[6] The LM and D65°L-PaMO views are best for identifying intracapsular distention (Fig. 19–4A and B). Intracapsular distention is seen with fracture, secondary joint disease, septic arthritis, and serous arthritis. A radiographic diagnosis of serous arthritis (carpitis) is infrequently made and should be considered after bony changes have been ruled out. Extracapsular swelling is typically diffuse and ill-defined over the dorsum of the carpus (see Fig. 19–4C). This swelling often extends from the distal radius to the proximal portion of the third metacarpus, with the maximum degree of swelling not occurring at the level of a joint.[6] Extracapsular swelling can be produced by bursitis, tenosynovitis, and cellulitis.

Fractures

Carpal fractures are subjectively described as being a chip, a corner, or a slab. Chip fractures are the most common type and are usually seen as a small periarticular osseous body. A corner fracture is larger than a chip fracture, involves a more significant amount of subchondral bone, and tends to appear square or rectangular (Fig. 19–5B). Slab fractures extend

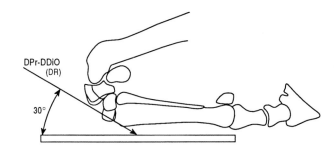

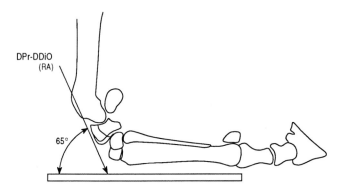

FIGURE 19–2. Dorsoproximal-dorsodistal oblique (DPr-DDiO) projections of the equine carpus. These views are used to project the dorsal aspects of the equine carpal bones and the distal end of the radius. DR, view to project distal row; RA, view to project distal radius.

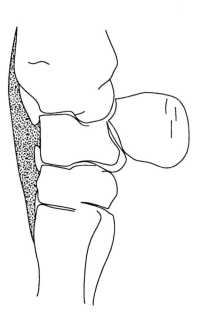

FIGURE 19–3. The origins and attachments of the joint capsule of the carpus. The middle carpal (intercarpal) and carpometacarpal joints communicate between the third and the fourth carpal bones, but the antebrachiocarpal joint cavity remains separate.[1] (From O'Brien TR, Morgan JP, Park RD, et al: Radiography in equine carpal lameness. Cornell Vet *61:*666, 1971; with permission.)

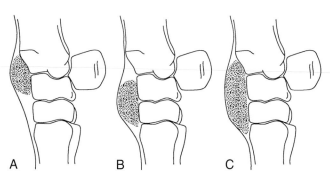

FIGURE 19–4. Intracapsular and extracapsular soft-tissue swelling. Intracapsular swelling of the antebrachiocarpal *(A),* middle, and carpometacarpal joints *(B).* Extracapsular swelling *(C)* is seen with cellulitis, tenosynovitis, and bursitis. (From O'Brien TR, Morgan JP, Park RD, et al: Radiography in equine carpal lameness. Cornell Vet *61:*666, 1971; with permission.)

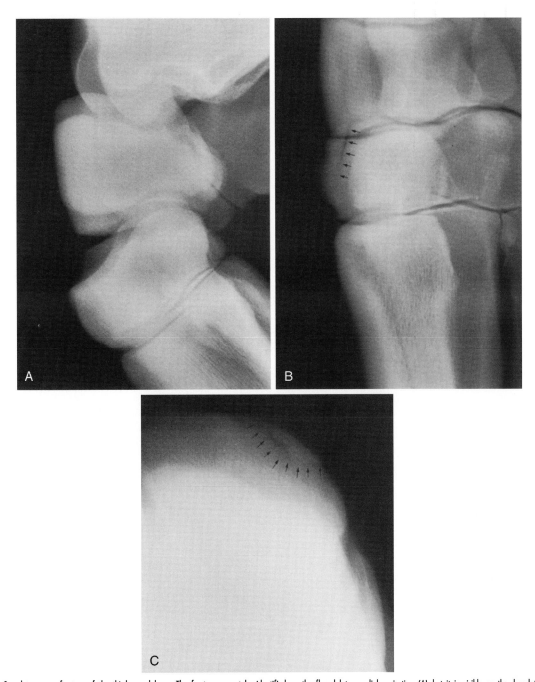

FIGURE 19–5. Complete corner fracture of the third carpal bone. The fracture cannot be identified on the flexed lateromedial projection *(A)*, but it is visible on the dorsolateral-palmaromedial oblique (DL-PaMO) projection *(B; arrows)*. The fracture appears to be incomplete, with the proximal end involving the articular cartilage. *C,* Dorsoproximal-dorsodistal oblique (DPr-DDiO) view exhibits the fracture to be complete. The DL-PaMO and DPr-DDiO views together identify this finding as a corner fracture *(arrows)* in contrast with a slab fracture, which would extend through the entire thickness of the bone, interrupting both articular surfaces.

from one subchondral surface to another, involving two joint spaces, for example, the middle carpal and carpometacarpal surfaces for a third carpal bone slab fracture.

Radiographs must be interpreted to determine whether a fracture is acute or chronic. An acute fracture appears as a discrete body, with the point of its origin being sharply marginated. A chronic fracture appears more rounded and less opaque, with resorption of bone at its origin (Fig. 19–6D). A fracture seen on any projection must be evaluated on the other views, especially on DPr-DDiO projections, to determine the fragment size, the presence of additional fractures, and the degree of subchondral bony changes.

Fractures are the most common injury in mature performance horses. Thoroughbreds have almost twice the incidence of carpal fractures as do Quarter horses.[7] The most common sites of carpal fractures, in descending order of incidence, are the radial carpal, the third carpal (see Fig. 19–5), the distal end of the radius (Fig. 19–7), and the intermediate carpal bone (Fig. 19–8). Fractures of the radial carpal bone account for more carpal fractures than all other carpal bones combined.[7] The dorsodistal corner of the radial carpal bone is the most typical site (see Fig. 19–6).

The FLM and D60°L-PaMO projections are particularly valuable in isolating these radial carpal fractures; the former

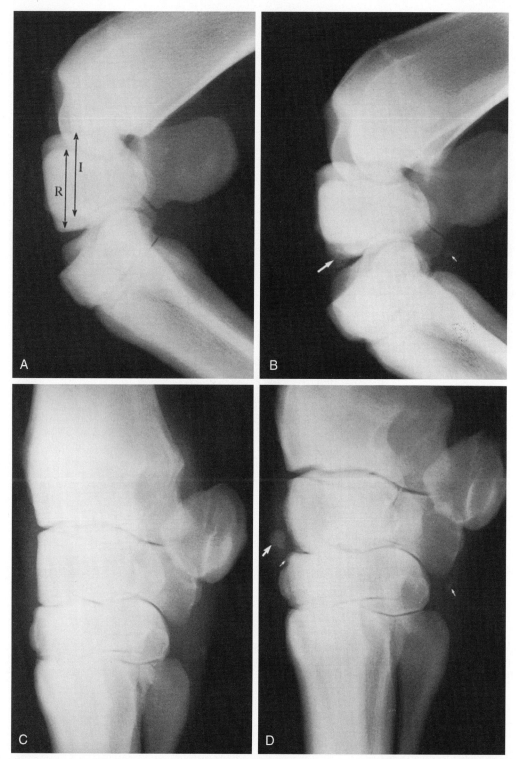

FIGURE 19–6. Chronic fracture of the distal radial carpal bone. *A,* Flexed lateromedial view (FLM) of a normal carpus. Note the distal shift of the radial carpal bone separating the dorsoproximal and dorsodistal corners of the radial (R) and intermediate (I) carpal bones. *B,* A rounded (chronic) corner fracture is seen on the distal radial carpal bone *(large arrow),* and a small fragment *(small arrow)* has become displaced to the palmar aspect of the middle carpal joint. Eighty-nine percent of all carpal fractures have been reported to be visible with this view.[8] *C,* Normal carpus in the dorsolateral-palmaromedial oblique (DL-PaMO) view. This view is necessary for evaluating completely fractures of the distomedial radius, radial, and third carpal bones. *D,* Note the small periarticular osteophyte *(small dorsal arrow)* on the third carpal bone not visible on the FLM view. This osteophyte is indicative of secondary joint disease. Secondary joint disease was initiated by a long-standing radial carpal bone fracture *(large arrow).* A small piece of the chip fracture is located in the palmar aspect of the joint *(small palmar arrow).*

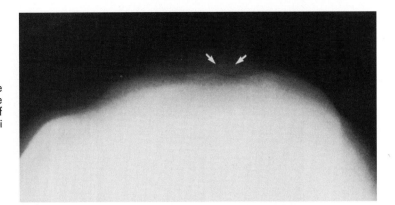

FIGURE 19–7. Dorsoproximal-dorsodistal oblique (DPr-DDiO) projection of the distal end of the radius. Standard views exhibited only intracapsular soft-tissue swelling of the antebrachiocarpal joint. This projection highlights the dorsal aspect of the distal radius. A small bone fragment can be seen under the extensor carpi radialis tendon (arrows).

alone was shown in one study to isolate 89 percent (127 of 143) of all carpal fractures.[8] The FLM projection separates the proximal and distal borders of the radial and intermediate carpal bones by shifting the radial carpal bone distally as a result of the action of the cranial aspect of the radial trochlea in the flexed position (Fig. 19–9).[1]

Fractures of the third carpal bone with minimal displacement of the fracture fragment are the most difficult to evaluate in the five standard projections.[4] Small cortical fractures from the distal radius are also difficult to see on standard radiographic projections. By projecting the dorsal surface of the carpus radiographically (see Fig. 19–2), the dorsal aspects of the distal radius and third carpal bone may be evaluated. Fractures of the third carpal bone may appear to be simple fractures on standard views. On DPr-DDiO views, however, they are sometimes recognized as comminuted. The radiographic projection of the dorsal surface of the carpus also often reveals that fractures suspected of being incomplete or nondisplaced are actually complete or displaced.[4] The degree of subchondral sclerosis of carpal bones may also be evaluated.

In horses with carpal fractures, it is important to evaluate comminution, thickness of fracture, and extent of secondary fracture lines. The presurgical assessment of a third carpal bone slab fracture should also include the degree of reduction produced by flexing the carpus (FLM projection) and the best plane for screw placement (DPr-DDiO projection).

Postsurgical radiographic examinations are useful for assessing the degree of bony union, the stability of the surgical implants, and the alignment of the fracture fragment(s). Severe soft-tissue swelling preoperatively and postoperatively prevents complete carpal flexion and may limit the radiographic evaluation.

Angular Limb Deformities

Angular limb deformities in foals probably have a multifactorial origin; radiographic diagnosis should be correlated with the foal's morphologic and geometric appearance.[9, 10] Angular deformities involving the carpus are usually present at birth or begin to manifest within the first 2 weeks of life.[10] Most foals have some angular deformity at birth but are normal by 2 weeks of age.[11] Radiographic examinations are indicated for those foals that remain angulated after 2 weeks of age. In these foals, early treatment is necessary to prevent uneven axial compression of the growth plates, which perpetuates the existing angular deformity.[10]

Joint instability may be related to flaccid or damaged periarticular structures, such as collateral ligaments. Instability may also result from disturbances in growth of the distal radial physis, imbalance in longitudinal growth from the radial epiphysis, or defects in endochondral ossification of the cuboidal bones of the carpus. Direct external trauma to the physis, epiphysis, or carpal bones also may cause angular deformities at the carpus. These conditions may occur alone or in combination.

Radiographic analysis of carpal deformities should include an initial review of survey radiographs for soft-tissue and osseous abnormalities. A bisecting line should be drawn through the medullary cavity of the radius and third metacarpal bone, forming a pivot point where the lines intersect. The pivot point is usually centered at the region of osseous abnormality (Fig. 19–10A). The degree of angular deformity may be measured, which is important for evaluation of treatment effectiveness.

Joint instability from damaged or lax soft-tissue structures usually places the pivot point at the level of the distal articular cartilage of the radius with no radiographic abnormalities

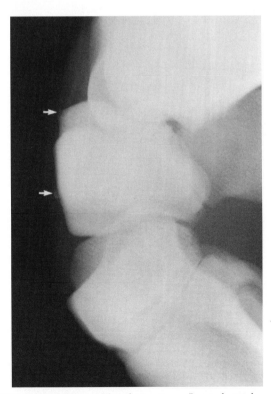

FIGURE 19–8. Intermediate carpal bone fracture. Two small, acute fracture fragments are marginally displaced at the proximal and distal corners of the intermediate carpal bone (arrows). These small chips were vaguely visible on lateral views and could not be specifically associated with either the radial or intermediate carpal bones.

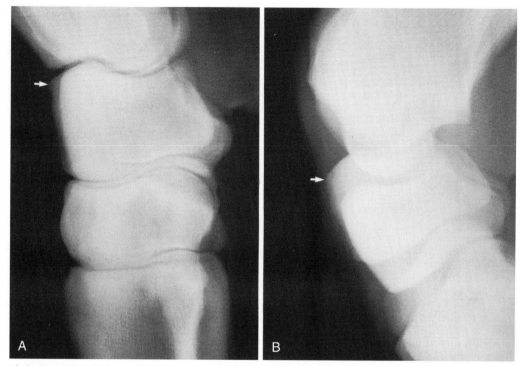

FIGURE 19–9. A nondisplaced proximal intermediate carpal bone fracture may be difficult to identify. *A,* There is a periarticular irregularity seen on the lateromedial projection *(arrow). B,* The fracture is clearly identified *(arrow)* on the flexed lateromedial view at the proximal border of the intermediate carpal bone.

of the carpal bones. Growth imbalances of the metaphysis have a pivot point directly or slightly proximal to the physeal growth plate, with metaphyseal flaring and sclerosis and an irregular wave pattern to the physeal plate (see Fig. 19–10*B*). Growth imbalances of the metaphysis have a pivot point between the joint space and the physis. Ossification defects of the cartilaginous precursors of the cuboidal (carpal) bones have a pivot point in the row of bones where the lesion exists (see Fig. 19–10*A*). Direct trauma may involve the growth centers, with a pivot point corresponding to the area involved. Locations of pivot points are not always reliable; therefore, secondary osseous and soft-tissue alterations should be included in the evaluation.[9, 10, 12] The metacarpophalangeal joint should also be radiographed (DPa and LM) when there is an angular limb deformity. This is done to determine secondary growth imbalances and if the physes of the third metacarpus and proximal aspect of the proximal phalanx are open.

Septic Arthritis

Acute septic arthritis produces intracapsular distention and severe lameness. Contrary to popular belief, intra-articular gas produced by organisms is rare. In the acute phase, radiographic signs other than swelling are not seen unless the joint infection is an extension of osteomyelitis (Fig. 19–11*A* and *C*). Widening of the joint space is usually a result of a lack of full weight bearing on the limb. In subacute and chronic stages, cartilage and bone changes occur, producing an irregular bone margin and joint surface and narrowing of the joint space. These latter findings result from subchondral bone and cartilage destruction. Clinical history and signs help determine whether the origin of septic arthritis is due to hematogenous spread, a penetrating wound, iatrogenic

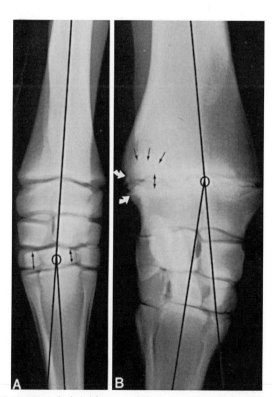

FIGURE 19–10. Angular limb deformities in foals. *A,* Dissecting lines through the radius and third metacarpal bones intersect and form a pivot point over the third carpal bone. An 8-degree angular deformity is present because of a hypoplastic (ossification defect of the cartilaginous precursor) third carpal bone *(short arrow)* on the lateral aspect. *B,* Bisecting lines form a pivot point at the growth plate of the distal radius. Note the prominent bone flaring *(white arrows)* at the metaphyseal and epiphyseal margins. Metaphyseal sclerosis *(single-pointed arrows)* and the irregular wave pattern to the physis *(double-pointed arrow)* indicate growth imbalances of the metaphysis and the epiphysis.

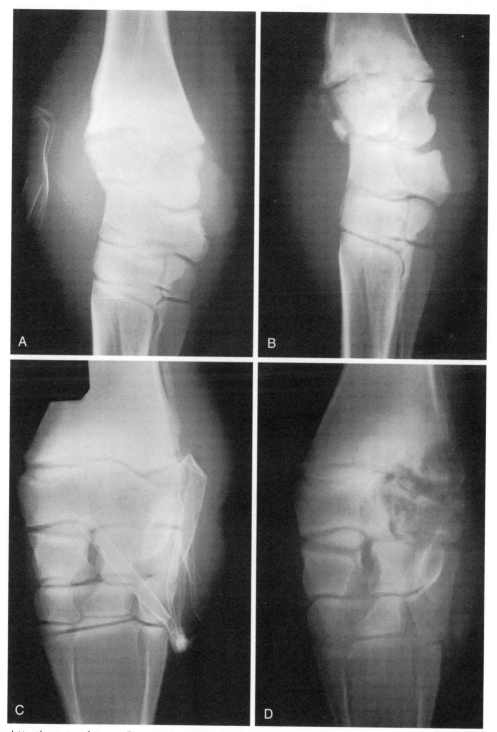

FIGURE 19–11. Septic arthritis with extensive soft-tissue swelling on initial examination *(A and C)*. Initial radiographs demonstrate a dome-like soft-tissue swelling adjacent to the radial physis and epiphysis (a drain tube is visible). Some gas is seen on the dorsopalmar view with periosteal reaction. Repeat radiographs after 10 days *(B and D)* delineate aggressive bone destruction of the metaphysis, physis, and epiphysis, with breakdown of the subchondral bone compatible with extension into the antebrachiocarpal joint. A dome-like soft-tissue swelling is adjacent to the antebrachiocarpal joint, but extracapsular swelling is also evident.

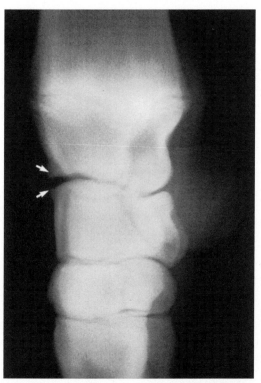

FIGURE 19–12. Periarticular osteophytes *(arrows)* indicate secondary joint disease. The degree of osteophyte formation may not correlate with the severity of the clinical signs.

Secondary Joint Disease

Secondary joint disease is joint degeneration and may involve articular cartilage, bone, or both. This joint disease is termed *secondary* because the primary abnormality is related to growth abnormalities (conformation), damaged articular cartilage, weak or damaged supporting soft-tissue structures, steroid injections, and other traumatic or developmental disorders.

Joints with the greatest range of motion are most commonly and severely involved. For this reason, the antebrachiocarpal and middle carpal joints are the most commonly and severely involved carpal joints.

The radiographic signs of secondary joint disease are capsular distention (see Fig. 19–4), periarticular osteophytes (Fig. 19–12), narrowing of joint spaces, irregular subchondral bone, and subchondral sclerosis. A significant number of productive or destructive changes must occur before radiographic signs are visible. Therefore, the earliest visible radiographic changes should be considered significant with any clinically lame horse. Narrowing of joint spaces without other signs of secondary joint disease is usually a result of cartilage degeneration or a positioning artifact.

Miscellaneous Disorders

Aseptic soft-tissue injuries may produce extracapsular swelling. A thorough clinical examination must be done, but diagnostic ultrasonography is often required for a more definitive diagnosis. Chronic or severe injury produces extracapsular swelling, and focal areas of increased soft-tissue opacity may result from dystrophic calcification (Fig. 19–13).

Some lucent regions in the carpus are normally seen and should not be diagnosed as a clinical problem. The more common examples are seen at the lateral aspect of the distal

causes, or extension from a septic process adjacent to the joint (see Fig. 19-11B and D).[13] In acute septic arthritis, cytopathologic evaluation of joint fluid is necessary for prompt diagnosis and treatment.

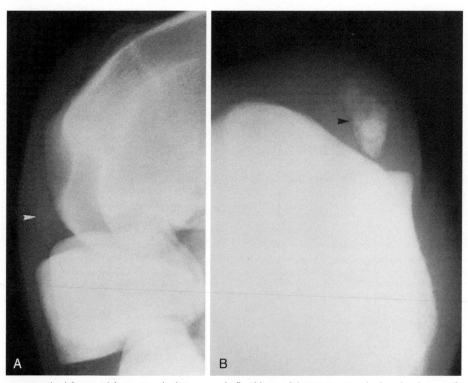

FIGURE 19–13. Chronic tenosynovitis with calcification. Calcification *(arrowheads)* is seen on the flexed lateromedial (FLM) view *(A)* and is located in the groove for the common digital extensor tendon on the dorsoproximal-dorsodistal oblique (DPr-DDiO) view *(B)*, which is obliqued because of poor positioning.

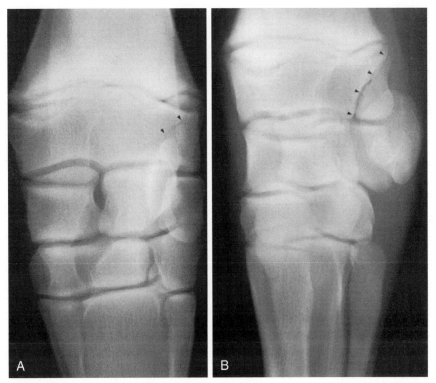

FIGURE 19–14. Distal radial and ulnar epiphyses of a young foal. The distal ulnar physis *(arrows)* is evident on the dorsopalmar (DPa) *(A)* and dorsal 60-degree lateral–palmaromedial oblique (D60°L-PaMO) *(B)* views. The distal ulnar and radial epiphyses fuse at about 3 or 4 months of age to form the lateral styloid process of the distal radius. The distal ulnar epiphysis should not be confused with a large fracture fragment.

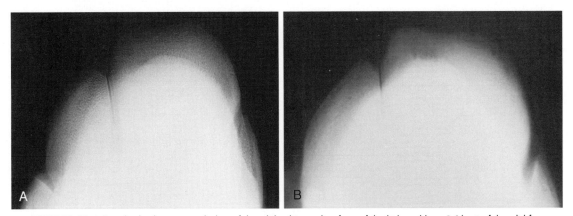

FIGURE 19–15. *A,* Normal trabecular pattern to the bone of the radial and intermediate fossae of the third carpal bone. *B,* Sclerosis of the radial fossa.

radial epiphysis and the palmar region of the ulnar, second, or fourth carpal bones. These radiographic findings are incidental and considered developmental variations.

In the foal, the lateral aspect of the distal radial epiphysis has a physis between it and the distal ulnar epiphysis (styloid process), which appears as a lucent line (Fig. 19–14). Fusion occurs at 3 or 4 months of age, but it may be incomplete, resulting in an oval lucency in the mature horse.

Subchondral sclerosis is an important radiographic finding seen in high-performance horses.[14, 15] A loss of normal trabecular pattern in the subchondral bone is seen as an increased bone opacity resulting from thickening of the trabeculae and loss of the intertrabecular spaces. This finding is commonly seen in the third carpal bone but may also be identified in the radial carpal bone.[16] Third carpal bone sclerosis is more frequently identified in the radial fossa and is best evaluated on the DPr-DDiO projection (Fig. 19–15). This finding is associated with varying degrees of lameness and may only be· diagnosed radiographically. It has been associated with focal subchondral lucent defects and is considered a precursor to a slab or corner fracture.

References

1. Smallwood JE, and Shively M: Radiographic and xerographic anatomy of the equine carpus. Equine Pract 1:22, 1979.
2. Getty R (Ed): Sisson and Grossman's The Anatomy of Domestic Animals. Philadelphia, WB Saunders, 1975.
3. Morgan JP, Silverman S, and Zontine WJ: Techniques of Veterinary Radiography. Davis, CA, Veterinary Radiology Associates, 1975.
4. O'Brien TR: Radiographic diagnosis of "hidden" lesions of the third carpal bone. In Proceedings of the 23rd Annual Meeting of the American Association of Equine Practitioners, Vancouver, BC, 1977, pp 343–354.
5. Smallwood JE, Shively MJ, Rendano VT, et al: A standardized nomenclature for radiographic projections used in veterinary medicine. Vet Radiol 26:2, 1985.
6. O'Brien TR, Morgan JP, Park RD, et al: Radiography in equine carpal lameness. Cornell Vet 61:666, 1971.
7. Thrall DE, Lebel JL, and O'Brien TR: A five-year survey of the incidence and location of equine carpal chip fractures. J Am Vet Med Assoc 158:1366, 1971.
8. Park RD, Morgan JP, and O'Brien TR: Chip fractures in the carpus of the horse: A radiographic study of their incidence and location. J Am Vet Med Assoc 157:1305, 1970.
9. Pharr JW, and Fretz PB: Radiographic findings in foals with angular limb deformities. J Am Vet Med Assoc 179:812, 1981.
10. Fretz PB: Angular limb deformities in foals. Vet Clin North Am [Large Animal Pract] 2:125, 1980.
11. Adams OR: Lameness in Horses, 3rd Ed. Philadelphia, Lea & Febiger, 1974.
12. Guffy MM, and Coffman JR: The variability of angular deformity of the carpus of foals. In Proceedings of the 15th Annual Meeting of the American Association of Equine Practitioners, Montreal, 1970, pp 437–458.
13. Morgan JP: Radiographic diagnosis of bone and joint diseases in the horse. Cornell Vet 58:28, 1968.
14. O'Brien TR, De Haan CE, and Arthur RS: Third carpal bone lesions of the racing Thoroughbred. In Proceedings of the 31st Annual Meeting of the American Association of Equine Practitioners, Toronto, 1985, pp 515–524.
15. De Haan CE, O'Brien TR, and Koblik PD: A radiographic investigation of third carpal bone injury in 42 racing Thoroughbreds. Vet Radiol 28:88, 1987.
16. Young A, O'Brien TR, and Pool RR: Exercise-related sclerosis in the third carpal bone of the racing Thoroughbred. In Proceedings of the 34th Annual Meeting of the American Association of Equine Practitioners, San Diego, 1988, pp 339–346.

STUDY QUESTIONS

1. A standard radiographic examination of the carpus should consist of how many views? Name them.

2. What are the two conditions that define the need to make dorsoproximal-dorsodistal oblique projections of the carpus?

3. How does one decide whether to make the dorsoproximal-dorsodistal oblique projection of the distal radius or distal row of carpal bones?

4. A dorsal 45-degree lateral–palmaromedial oblique compared to a dorsal 60-degree lateral–palmaromedial oblique is:
   A. Closer to the lateromedial projection.
   B. Closer to the dorsopalmar projection.

5. What are the three general types of carpal bone fractures identified radiographically?

6. What bone of the carpus has the highest incidence of fracture?

7. Why should a carpal radiographic examination be done on a foal with angular limb deformity?

8. Why is a radiographic examination of the metacarpophalangeal area needed when there is an angular limb deformity originating in the distal radius growth plate?

9. A horse was referred for surgery of a slab fracture of the third carpal bone, and lateromedial and dorsal 60-degree lateral–palmaromedial oblique radiographs accompanied the horse. You advise the owner that another radiographic examination is required. The owner questions the need for another examination only 2 days after the first examination. How would you explain your need for another examination?

10. On the flexed lateromedial view, how can the intermediate and radial carpal bones be differentiated?

(Answers appear on pages 637 and 638.)

Chapter 20

The Metacarpus and Metatarsus

Stephen K. Kneller

ANATOMIC CONSIDERATIONS

Third Metacarpus and Metatarsus—the Cannon Bone

Radiographically, the third metacarpus and metatarsus (MC III and MT III) are basically the same (Fig. 20–1). The midportion of the dorsal cortex is thicker than the remaining cortex, thinning gradually toward the ends of the bone. This varying cortical thickness is often mistaken for a disease process. The palmaroplantar cortex is more uniform in thickness and is interrupted at the junction of the proximal and middle one third by the nutrient foramen. In contrast to the nutrient foramina of smaller bones, those in MC III and MT III are more similar to channels, which may be mistaken for lesions on lateral and oblique views, especially in the hindlimb (Fig. 20–2).

The palmaroplantar cortex is flattened proximally, often resulting in visualization of both medial and lateral aspects on a lateral view. There is no visible proximal physis at birth. The distal epiphysis is within the metacarpophalangeal (metatarsophalangeal) joint and is one of the first sites to become abnormal in metabolic bone disease, although its appearance varies in the normal animal at different ages.

On the lateral view, the metacarpus and metatarsus differ from each other at the distal end (see Fig. 20–1). The metacarpus is relatively straight, whereas the distal end of the metatarsus usually curves slightly, giving the dorsal border a slightly convex appearance.

Second and Fourth Metacarpi and Metatarsi—the Splint Bones

The second and fourth metacarpi (MC II, MC IV) and metatarsi (MT II, MT IV) are small bones that articulate with the carpus or tarsus and taper distally. The size and shape are variable among animals and between limbs.[1] There is a variable degree of natural outward curvature. The distal end is usually in the form of a slight bulbous enlargement of variable size and shape, but the margins are smooth and distinct.

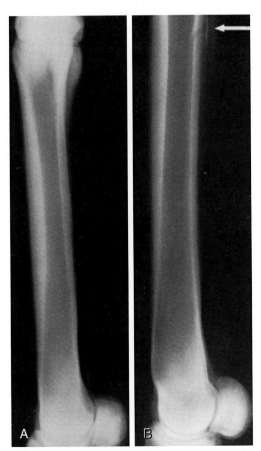

FIGURE 20–1. Normal lateral radiographs of the metacarpus *(A)* and the metatarsus *(B)*. Note that the metacarpus is straight, whereas the metatarsus curves slightly at the distal end. The dorsal cortex in both bones is thicker, especially at the midportion. The large nutrient foramen is evident in the metatarsus *(arrow)*.

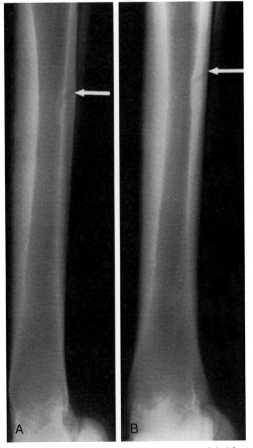

FIGURE 20–2. Lateral *(A)* and dorsomedial-plantarolateral *(B)* views of the left metatarsus of a 1-year-old Thoroughbred colt. The nutrient foramen appears as a channel through the plantar cortex of third metatarsus *(arrows)*.

In the forelimb, the medial splint bone (MC II) is usually longer than the lateral (MC IV), although MC IV may be the same length or longer than MC II. In the hindlimb, when compared with MT II, MT IV is relatively massive and irregular at the proximal aspect, often extending proximal to MT III.

The proximal epiphysis of the splint bones, apparently present in the fetus, is fused at birth. The distal epiphysis is cartilaginous and, therefore, is not visible radiographically at birth. As it ossifies, the distal epiphysis is separated from the body of the bone by cartilage until fusion occurs. Care should be taken to avoid mistaking this normal structure for a fracture (Fig. 20–3).

Mach Bands—False Fracture Lines

A visual phenomenon in radiography that causes some confusion is edge enhancement, or mach bands.[2] This phenomenon is especially evident in radiographs of equine metacarpi and metatarsi. Simply stated, as one bone edge crosses another on a radiograph, a radiolucent line may appear. This line may be often seen on the palmaroplantar aspect of the equine metacarpus and metatarsus, resulting in erroneous diagnoses of cortical fracture of MC III or MT III as well as fractures of the smaller metacarpal and metatarsal bones (Fig. 20–4). To guard against making erroneous diagnoses, the anatomic contour of each bone must be followed carefully,

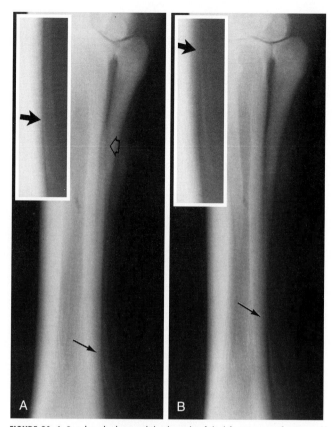

FIGURE 20–4. Dorsolateral-palmaromedial radiographs of the left metacarpus of a 2-year-old Standardbred gelding with a soft-tissue injury over the fourth metacarpus (MC IV), 10 cm distal to the carpus. *A,* There is a radiolucent line in MC IV at the site of injury *(open arrow);* in a slightly different oblique view *(B),* this line cannot be seen. The radiolucent line in *A* is due to overlapping margins of the third metacarpus (MC III) with MC IV, which may be confirmed by tracing the margins away from the point in question. Also, note the radiolucent line across the distal end of MC IV in *A (solid arrow in inset),* which moves proximally in *B (solid arrow in inset)* as the point of overlap moves proximally. The midportion of the palmar cortex of MC III is also affected by this phenomenon. The black lines causing this confusion are called *mach bands* and should not be mistaken for fracture lines.

with additional radiographs obtained for clarification as needed.

CHARACTERIZATION OF LESIONS

Soft-Tissue Enlargement and Mineralization

Abnormal size and shape of the soft tissues in the metacarpal and metatarsal areas may be evident on radiographs as (1) enlargements over the dorsal surface, with early metacarpal periostitis; (2) generalized enlargements along the palmaroplantar surface, with suspensory desmitis and flexor tendon abnormalities; and (3) localized areas along the small metacarpal or metatarsal bones, usually proximally, with interosseous ligament damage. Because there is normally minimal soft tissue in these areas, such soft-tissue abnormalities should also be evident on visual inspection and palpation of the horse.

The purpose of radiographically evaluating the soft tissues is threefold. First, in a busy practice, there is a temptation to perform a quick physical examination and proceed with radiographic examination. Finding soft-tissue enlargements radiographically should stimulate a more thorough physical examination of the area in question. Second, although thor-

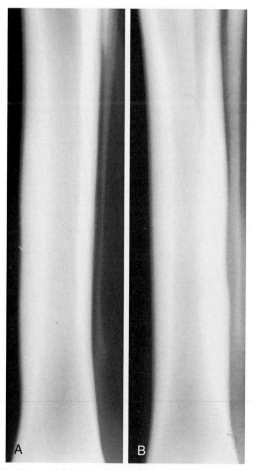

FIGURE 20–3. Dorsomedial-plantarolateral *(A)* and dorsolateral-plantaromedial *(B)* radiographs of the left pelvic limb of a 4-month-old Quarter horse filly in which the second metatarsus *(A)* and fourth metatarsus *(B)* can be seen. The distal epiphyses have not fused to the diaphyses.

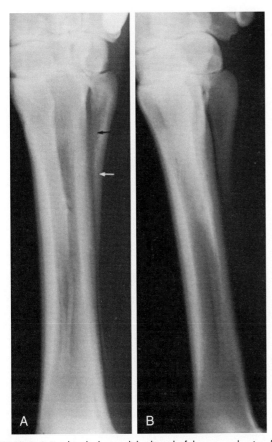

FIGURE 20–5. A, Dorsolateral-palmaromedial radiograph of the metacarpal region of an 11-year-old Morgan mare in which the fourth metacarpus (MC IV) can be seen. The space between the third metacarpus (MC III) and MC IV is not clearly seen, suggesting mineralization of the interosseous ligament (arrows). B, Same view at a different angle. There is a clear separation of MC III and MC IV with no abnormal mineralization.

Mineral opacity between the small metacarpal or metatarsal bones and MC III or MT III is a common finding as a sequela to trauma to the interosseous ligament (splint disease). This opacity may be actual mineralization of the interosseous ligament or an associated periosteal reaction. As in any dystrophic mineralization, this radiographic sign is not evident until some time after the injury. Accurate positioning is imperative when evaluation of the mineralization of the interosseous ligament is attempted because overlap of the bones may produce a similar appearance (Fig. 20–5). In some horses, because of the bone contour, multiple views at slightly different angles must be made to separate the bones completely throughout the length of overlap. When this mineralization is evident, the animal has had damage in the interosseous ligament. Splint disease is discussed more thoroughly in the following section.

Periosteal Response

On high-quality radiographs, periosteal surfaces of the metacarpus and metatarsus should be smooth and well defined. Because of the geometry of the bones, the dorsal surface of MC III or MT III may appear indistinct on radiographs unless a high-intensity illuminator (hot light) is used. Periosteal reaction is a healing response, and its appearance depends on the stage of healing. If the inciting cause is removed, the periosteal response becomes mature and smooth over time.

The dorsal surface of MC III may develop a periosteal reaction because of microfractures; this is commonly referred to as metacarpal periostitis or bucked shins (Fig. 20–6). Care should be taken to evaluate the cortex for fracture lines (see section on cortical bone abnormalities).

ough study of the radiographs is paramount, finding a soft-tissue abnormality should lead to an in-depth review of the underlying bony structures to evaluate the extent of the lesion and to characterize it further. The third purpose is correlation of abnormalities, evaluating the association or lack of association of bony lesions with soft-tissue enlargements in size, shape, and proximity as well as relative activity. For example, in many horses, tendons and ligaments may be delineated because of the loose, fat-laden adventitia interposed between them. In such horses, a low degree of inflammation may sometimes be appreciated as a loss of visualization of these margins on high-quality radiographs.

Soft-tissue mineralization may be identified, especially in the suspensory ligament and flexor tendon areas. Surface debris and medication should be removed to avoid confusion. Mineralization within the soft tissues is usually dystrophic owing to injury of some duration. The injury may be from work-related stress, resulting in damaged or torn structures, or it may be caused by drug injections.

Penetrating foreign objects may also be present in soft tissues. Therefore, it is important to be familiar with the normal appearance of soft tissue because only then may foreign objects having an opacity similar to adjacent soft tissue be recognized as a disturbance of the normal size, shape, and opacity relationships.

Mineralization in the skin and subcutaneous tissues may result from surface injuries and must be differentiated from deeper mineralization. In the hindlimb, the chestnut may contain mineral and be mistaken for disease.

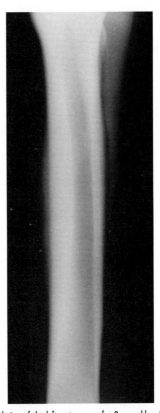

FIGURE 20–6. Lateral view of the left metacarpus of a 2-year-old racing Quarter horse. There is a layer of periosteal new bone on the dorsal aspect of the midportion of the third metacarpus. The right third metacarpus had similar changes.

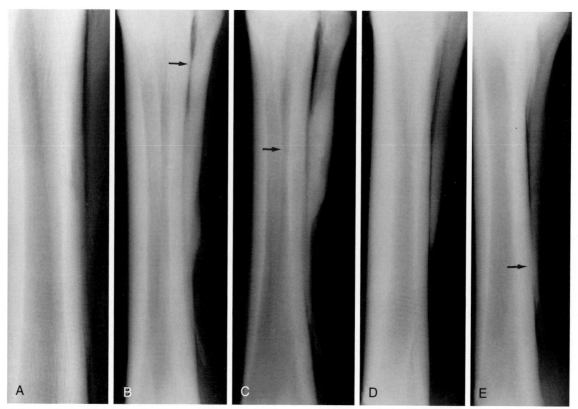

FIGURE 20–7. Dorsomedial-palmarolateral radiographs of the metacarpal region of several horses with different appearances of damaged interosseous ligaments (*splint lesions*). *A,* A 13-year-old Thoroughbred gelding (hunter-jumper) with a recent interosseous injury. Slight periosteal response and a small amount of cortical bone lysis are evident. This is the typical appearance of a 2- to 3-week-old lesion. *B,* A 3-year-old Standardbred gelding. The periosteal response is more organized but still active. It involves approximately the entire attachment area of the interosseous ligament with a separate site of reaction proximally *(arrow). C,* A 2-year-old Standardbred gelding. As in *B,* this lesion is chronic, but it appears active and most likely is at least 6 weeks old. The periosteal reaction is large and opaque over a localized area, but it has not become smooth. The large mass may produce abnormal pressure on surrounding soft tissues. The nutrient foramen *(arrow)* should not be confused with a lesion. *D,* A 2-year-old Thoroughbred filly. The lesion on the midportion of the second metacarpus (MC II) is inactive. This is typical of a 3- to 6-week-old lesion that has been protected with rest. Such a lesion would be expected to become solid with no enlargement. *E,* A 5-year-old Standardbred gelding. The lesion is near the distal end of MC II *(arrow).* It is opaque and smooth, blending together with the cortex of the third metacarpus (MC III) and MC II as a chronic inactive lesion. Lameness may result from concussion of MC II and the interosseous ligament, exaggerated by the distal fusion of MC II to MC III. The appearance of the proximal end is caused by overlap of MC II, MC III, and the fourth metacarpus.

Another relatively common location for periosteal response is between MC (MT) II and MC III, with lesions between MC (MT) III and MC IV occurring less frequently. These lesions are usually associated with the proximal one half of the splint bones and are secondary to interosseous ligament damage (splint disease) (Fig. 20–7). The periosteal response is variable in size; initially the response is ill defined and irregular and gradually becomes smooth, opaque, and smaller as it matures, fusing the small bones to the larger bones. A large, irregular periosteal response may mimic a fracture, yet a fracture may be masked by the callus formation.

Indistinct margins or small amounts of active periosteal reaction may be seen on the distal ends of the small metacarpal or metatarsal bones owing to irritation from suspensory ligament disease (Fig. 20–8).

Cortical Bone Abnormalities

Cortical lysis in the metacarpal and metatarsal bones is usually associated with localized trauma. Injury to the periosteum of MC III or MT III may cause death of the outer one third of the bone, with a resulting sequestrum (Fig. 20–9). This is related to the thick cortex of these bones and the inability of the endosteal blood supply to maintain viability of the dorsal cortex following periosteal disruption.

Following damage to the interosseous ligament, multiple small lytic lesions may be seen along the opposing surfaces of the metacarpal and, less often, metatarsal bones, presumably because of disruption of fibrous attachments and resultant inflammation.

Metacarpal and metatarsal fractures are common, especially in racing horses. The most common fracture site in these regions is the distal one half of MC II and IV and MT II and IV. As mentioned previously, care must be taken to avoid mistaking cartilaginous plates and mach bands as fractures. Fractures may also occur in the proximal one half of MC II and IV and MT II and IV, and these fractures may be mistaken for typical "splints."

Aside from complete fractures of MC III and MT III, which are obvious, incomplete fractures may be difficult to diagnose. They do, however, occur in specific locations. These incomplete stress fractures are usually seen in racing horses. The lesion most readily diagnosed is the sagittal distal condylar fracture (Fig. 20–10). This fracture frequently affects MC III, extending proximally from the metacarpophalangeal joint; it may or may not be significantly displaced. Often, this fracture may be seen only on the dorsopalmar or slightly oblique view, and it may be easily missed on underexposed radiographs.

Stress fractures may also be found in the dorsal cortex, especially associated with metacarpal periostitis (Fig. 20–11). These fractures occur most often on the dorsomedial aspect near the junction of the middle and distal one third of the

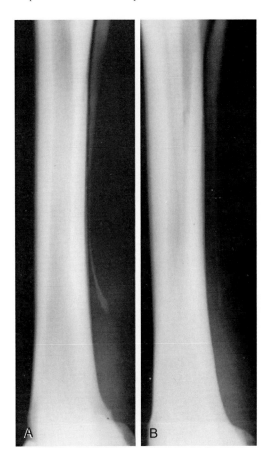

FIGURE 20–8. Dorsomedial-plantarolateral view of the second metatarsus (MT II) *(A)* and dorsolateral-plantaromedial view of the fourth metatarsus (MT IV) *(B)* in an 8-year-old Standardbred gelding. Soft-tissue enlargement is present on the plantar surface of the metatarsal area. MT II is deviated sharply at the distal end, and MT IV is separated from the third metatarsus. Both MT II and MT IV have indistinct margins on the distal ends consistent with periosteal irritation.

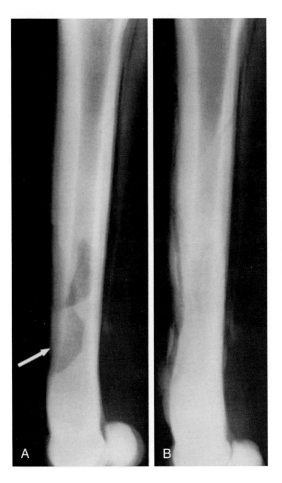

FIGURE 20–9. *A,* Lateral view of the right metatarsal region of a 3-year-old Quarter horse mare 10 days after the limb was severely injured, exposing a large portion of the third metatarsus (MT III). The large radiolucent areas overlying MT III are due to missing portions of soft tissue. A faint, dark line is present within the dorsal cortex of MT III *(arrow)*, indicative of fracture or impending sequestration. *B,* A lateral view, 3 weeks later. The sequestered bone can now be seen to extend proximally. Periosteal response is present around the lesion.

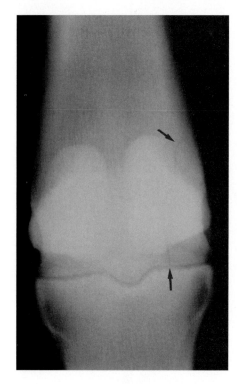

FIGURE 20–10. Dorsopalmar radiograph of the left front limb of a 4-year-old Thoroughbred stallion. A sagittal fracture is present in the lateral distal condyle of the third metacarpus (arrows). This lesion was not visible on lateral or oblique views.

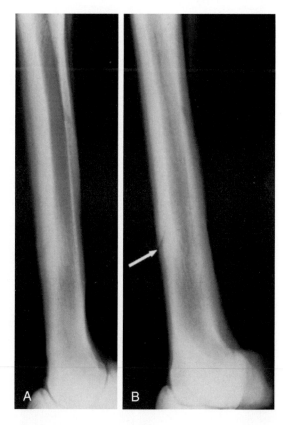

FIGURE 20–11. Lateral (A) and dorsolateral-palmaromedial (B) views of the left metacarpal region of a 6-year-old Thoroughbred gelding that became lame immediately after a race 2 weeks before the radiographs were made. The stress fracture (arrow) evident in B is barely visible in A.

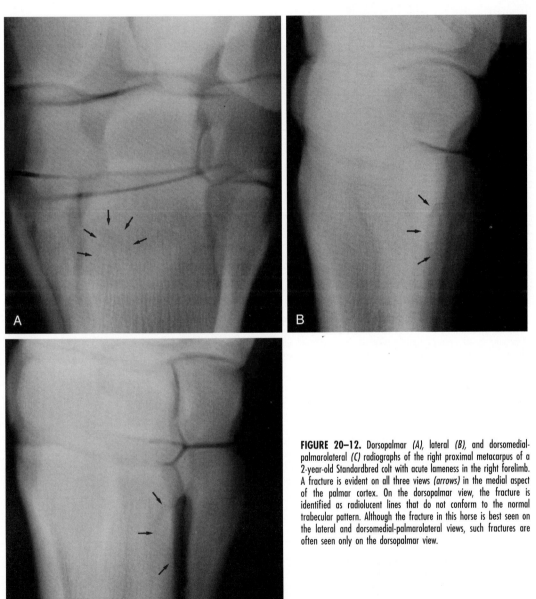

FIGURE 20–12. Dorsopalmar *(A),* lateral *(B),* and dorsomedial-palmarolateral *(C)* radiographs of the right proximal metacarpus of a 2-year-old Standardbred colt with acute lameness in the right forelimb. A fracture is evident on all three views *(arrows)* in the medial aspect of the palmar cortex. On the dorsopalmar view, the fracture is identified as radiolucent lines that do not conform to the normal trabecular pattern. Although the fracture in this horse is best seen on the lateral and dorsomedial-palmarolateral views, such fractures are often seen only on the dorsopalmar view.

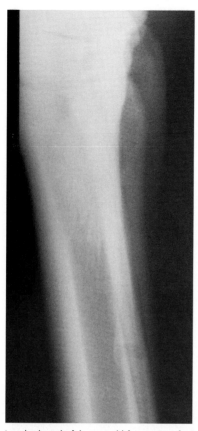

FIGURE 20–13. Lateral radiograph of the proximal left metacarpus of a 3-year-old Standardbred with lameness in the left forelimb. The proximal portion of the medullary cavity contains an irregular region of increased opacity originating from the palmar cortex (compare with Fig. 20–14). This opacity results from endosteal bone response owing to injury of the palmar cortex. A vertical fracture line was seen on the dorsopalmar view.

bone. Because of their shape, these lesions have been called *saucer fractures*.

Fractures also occur in the palmaroplantar cortex. The most common site is approximately 2 to 3 cm from the proximal articular surface, although they may occur in the midportion of the bone. Associated lesions have been reported as avulsion fractures, stress fractures, and stress response, sometimes linked with disease of the suspensory

ligament.[3–5, 7] Some appear radiographically only on the dorsopalmar (dorsoplantar) view as a thin crescent-shaped or linear-shaped region of decreased opacity. Other appearances include an irregular trabecular pattern or slight increased opacity in the proximal portion of MT III or MC III (Fig. 20–12). Typically, these abnormalities are medial to the midsagittal plane. In lateral and oblique views, fractures or increased opacity may be seen adjacent to the palmaroplantar cortex (Fig. 20–13; see Fig. 20–12). Overexposed or underexposed radiographs may lead to misinterpretation of this condition. Additionally, because of the large number of overlying bone margins, fractures in this area may be difficult to see. Scintigraphy has aided in proving the presence of fractures that are difficult to see radiographically.[6, 8]

Abnormal shape of MC III and MT III results from growth disturbance and is most often seen at the distal end of the bone. This shape change may be seen as a single, localized problem, or it may be seen in conjunction with more proximal limb abnormalities.

Although there is considerable variety in the size and shape of the small metacarpal and metatarsal bones, abaxial deviation of the distal ends is often associated with suspensory desmitis, presumably from outward pressure exerted by the enlarged ligaments (see Fig. 20–8). If this outward curving is noted, the suspensory ligaments should be evaluated for inflammation and enlargement, but apparent deviation should not be considered diagnostic for suspensory desmitis.

References

1. Getty R: Sisson and Grossman's The Anatomy of the Domestic Animals, 5th Ed. Philadelphia, WB Saunders, 1975.
2. Lane EJ, Proto AV, and Phillips TW: Mach bands and density perception. Radiology *121*:9, 1976.
3. Bramlage LE, Gabel AA, and Hackett RP: Avulsion of the origin of the suspensory ligament in the horse. J Am Vet Med Assoc *176*:1004, 1980.
4. Lloyd KCK, Koblik P, Reagle C, et al: Incomplete palmar fracture of the proximal extremity of the third metacarpal bone in horses: Ten cases (1981–1986). J Am Vet Med Assoc *192*:798, 1988.
5. Dyson S: Proximal suspensory desmitis: Clinical, ultrasonographic, and radiographic features. Equine Vet J *23*:25, 1991.
6. Devous MD, and Twardock AR: Techniques and applications of nuclear medicine in the diagnosis of equine lameness. J Am Vet Med Assoc *184*:318, 1984.
7. Pleasant RS, Baker GH, Muhlbauer MC, et al: Stress reactions and stress fractures of the proximal palmar aspect of the third metacarpal bone in horses: 58 cases (1980–1990). J Am Vet Med Assoc *201*:1918, 1992.
8. Edwards RB, Ducharme NG, Fubini SL, et al: Scintigraphy for diagnosis of avulsions of the origin of the suspensory ligament in horses: 51 cases (1980–1993). J Am Vet Med Assoc *207*:608, 1995.

STUDY QUESTIONS

1. The cortical thickness of the metacarpal/metatarsal bones of the horse is normally uniform on dorsal and palmar/plantar aspects; thus, a thicker dorsal cortex is indicative of disease. (True or False)

2. On a lateral view, the distal end of the metacarpus of the horse is relatively straight, whereas the distal end of the metatarsus is curved. (True or False)

3. The length of small metacarpal/metatarsal bones (MC/MT II and IV) is typically uniform on an individual horse. (True or False)

4. The multiple linear bone edges on the palmar/plantar aspect of the equine metacarpal/metatarsal region results

in mach bands, which may be misdiagnosed as fracture lines. (True or False)

5. Metacarpal periostitis ("bucked shins") usually causes periosteal response on the dorsal aspect of the metacarpal diaphysis and may be associated with visible cortical fractures. (True or False)

6. Although *splint bones* is a name given to the small metacarpal/metatarsal bones (MC/MT II and IV), *splint lesions* is a name for damage of the interosseous ligament between these bones and the cannon (MC/MT III). (True or False)

7. Small cortical bone (stress) fractures may be difficult to

demonstrate or recognize. Because of this, it is helpful to recognize typical locations. In MC/MT III, what three sites are most common?

8. On the palmar/plantar aspect of the limb in the metacarpal/metatarsal region, erroneous diagnosis of fracture may occur without careful attention to specific bone margins. The false appearance of fracture lines is due to what visual phenomenon?

9. What normal structure near the mid-diaphysis of MC/MT III may be mistaken for a fracture or lytic lesion?

10. Indistinct periosteal margins and flaring of the distal ends of the small metacarpal or metatarsal bones may be caused by enlargement of what soft-tissue structure?

(Answers appear on page 638.)

Chapter 21

The Metacarpophalangeal (Metatarsophalangeal) Articulation

Ron D. Sande

The anatomic structures of the metacarpophalangeal (MCP) and metatarsophalangeal (MTP) articulations are so similar that it is difficult to differentiate the right from the left or the forelimb from the hindlimb on radiographs. The MCP articulation is most often involved with pathologic change, perhaps owing to the support function of the forelimb and the characteristic difference in weight bearing and concussion.

The MCP or MTP articulations are hinge joints formed by the distal end of the metacarpus (metatarsus) and the proximal end of the proximal phalanx. The articular surface of the proximal phalanx is concave and bears a sagittal groove or depression corresponding to the sagittal ridge at the distal end of the third metacarpus or metatarsus (MC III or MT III). This ridge and groove divide the bearing surface into two unequal parts. The largest surface is on the medial side, where axial loading is greatest. The sagittal ridge is received into a similar depression at the palmar* surface created by the proximal sesamoids and the intersesamoidean ligament. There are two radii of articulation of the joint. The dorsal radius serves the weight-bearing portion, and the palmar radius conforms to the articulation with the proximal sesamoids.[1] The junction of these radii of articulation may be confused with pathologic flattening of the articular surface.

The joint capsule attachments are at the proximal end of the proximal phalanx and are immediately periarticular with no redundant capsule or cul-de-sacs. The capsule attaches to the distal end of MC III or MT III at the periarticular margins. Dorsally, there is a cul-de-sac that extends proximally and forms a pouch that allows for full flexion of the joint. There is a bursa interposed between the extensor tendons and the dorsal joint pouch. The palmar joint capsule extends proximal to the sesamoids between the suspensory ligament and MC III or MT III.[1]

Ligaments associated with the MCP and MTP articulations are important to their function and stability and, when injured, give rise to significant pathologic change (see Figs. 22–10 to 22–12). *Lateral* and *medial collateral ligaments* arise from the fossae on either side of the distal end of MC III and

MT III and attach to the roughened area on the medial and lateral aspects of the proximal phalanx distal to the articular margin. The *suspensory* (interosseous) *ligament* branches to form attachments to the abaxial surfaces of the proximal sesamoids. The *annular ligament* and the *collateral sesamoidean ligament* have fibers perpendicular to the axis of the suspensory ligament and ultimately have some insertion at the distal ends of second and fourth metacarpus or metatarsus (MC or MT II and IV). The *intersesamoidean ligament* connects the proximal sesamoids and fills the space between them. This ligament forms one part of the MCP or MTP articulation. *Distal sesamoidean ligaments* are best remembered as superficial, middle, and deep. The superficial ligament attaches distally to the proximal palmar surface of the middle phalanx. The middle ligament attaches to the palmar surface of the proximal phalanx. The deep, or cruciate, sesamoidean ligaments originate from the basilar border of each sesamoid and attach to the opposite eminence on the proximal palmar border of the proximal phalanx.[1]

RADIOGRAPHIC EXAMINATION

The intent of the examination should be to visualize the articular and periarticular skeletal structures and the adjoining soft tissues. The examination should include the proximal interphalangeal joint and the distal ends of the metacarpi or metatarsi. Identification markers recorded in the emulsion are essential in radiographic examination of the MCP or MTP articulation; right versus left, and forelimb versus hindlimb should also be designated. If oblique views are obtained, it is important to designate the projection. Markers should be placed to the lateral surface of all views, with the exception of the lateromedial view, when markers should be placed dorsally.[2]

Survey radiographic examination should include a lateromedial, a dorsopalmar, and two oblique projections (dorsal 45-degree–lateral-palmaromedial and dorsal 45-degree–medial-palmarolateral) with the limb bearing weight if possible. The lateromedial projection should be made with the primary beam centered at the articulation and directed paral-

---

Palmar(o) is used throughout this chapter with the understanding that *plantar(o)* should be substituted if reference is being made to the hindlimb.

lel to an imaginary line connecting the collateral fossae at the distal MC III or MT III. Because the plane of the joint is at an angle to the bearing surface of the hoof (i.e., the ground), the primary beam may be directed from dorsal proximal to palmar distal at approximately 30 to 40 degrees, that is, dorsal 35-degree–proximal-palmarodistal oblique. This should result in the projection of the proximal sesamoids over the distal MC III or MT III and the joint space projected with maximum width.[3, 4]

The dorsal 45-degree–lateral-palmaromedial and dorsal 45-degree–medial-palmarolateral oblique projections should be a routine part of the survey examination. Special projections may be derived according to the information gained from survey radiographs. The lateromedial projection during flexion is performed while the foot is held off the ground as if the sole of the hoof were being inspected. Alternate positions include variations in the degree of flexion and flexed oblique views. These projections may provide better visualization of subarticular surfaces at the dorsal aspect of distal MC III or MT III, the proximal part of the proximal phalanx, and the dorsal or articular margins of the proximal sesamoid bones.[4]

The dorsodistal-palmaroproximal projection is made while the limb is not bearing weight; this study yields a tangential image of the articular margin of the distal metacarpus or metatarsus. The foot is elevated on a block, and the limb is extended. The primary beam direction is approximately 125 degrees to the axis of the metacarpus or metatarsus.[5] The degree of flexion and the angle of the primary beam determine the tangent of the joint surface that is visualized.

The palmaroproximal-palmarodistal projection is used to visualize the palmar articular surface of MC III or MT III and the proximal sesamoids. Positioning of the patient requires that the x-ray tube be placed close to the abdominal wall. The limb is positioned as far caudal as possible, and the foot is placed on a supporting tunnel containing a cassette.[4] Some magnification results from the use of this projection.

The abaxial surfaces of the proximal sesamoids may be examined by placing a cassette medial or lateral to the joint. The x-ray beam is then directed in a palmaroproximolateral-dorsodistomedial or palmaroproximomedial-dorsodistolateral direction.[6]

Contrast arthrography of the MCP or MTP joint is sometimes useful (see Fig. 21–2). Five to 10 mL of water-soluble contrast medium containing 300 to 400 mg/mL of iodine is adequate. Injection of contrast medium should follow arthrocentesis and withdrawal of an equal volume of synovial fluid. Injection is made into the lateral pouch of the joint, proximal to the lateral sesamoids and dorsal to the suspensory ligament. The joint should be vigorously flexed, extended, and massaged before radiography to distribute the contrast medium throughout the joint.[4]

RADIOGRAPHIC INTERPRETATION OF DISEASES OF THE METACARPOPHALANGEAL (METATARSOPHALANGEAL) ARTICULATION

Joint disease in the horse is often associated with repeated trauma, and as with any species, the changes may be characteristic of the joint and of the function required of the horse. A study of race track injuries in horses has provided an overview of pathologic findings and pathogenesis of MCP or MTP joint disease.[7] Lameness and distention of a joint are clinical signs that typically precede the request for radiographic examination. The earliest signs of joint disease may remain obscure on radiographs because wear lines in the articular cartilages and synovial hypertrophy are usually not

recognized. Radiographs of the contralateral joint may be made for comparison, and although pathologic change is often bilateral, it is usually in different stages of development.

Joint Effusion

Joint effusion, sometimes called *osselets*, is usually a result of trauma, with degenerative changes in the joint capsule. Radiographic signs include soft-tissue swelling and joint distention. Dystrophic calcification of the periarticular soft tissues may also be present.[8]

Villonodular Synovitis

Villonodular synovitis is characterized by a firm, nonfluctuating swelling at the dorsal aspect of the joint. The villonodular masses arise from enlargement of the proximal fibrous tabs of the joint capsule and are associated with trauma. The condition is usually diagnosed by clinical signs, history, and palpation. Radiographic signs include mild to severe erosion of the distal MC III or MT III at a point just distal to the dorsal joint capsule attachment.[9–11] Periarticular bony proliferation may be present (Fig. 21–1). With the use of arthrography, a radiolucent, space-occupying mass can usually be identified in the dorsal cul-de-sac of the joint (Fig. 21–2).

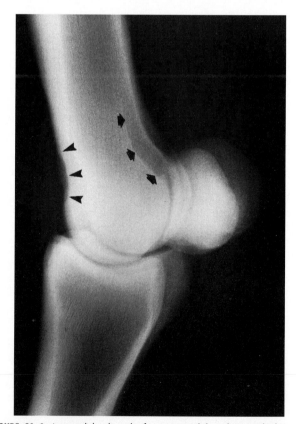

FIGURE 21–1. Lateromedial radiograph of a metacarpophalangeal joint with changes of villonodular synovitis. Swelling is present dorsal to the joint. There is erosion of bone at the dorsoproximal joint capsule attachment *(arrowheads)* and early evidence of supracondylar lysis at the palmar cortex *(arrows)*. Bony proliferation is visible at the proximodorsal periarticular border of the proximal phalanx.

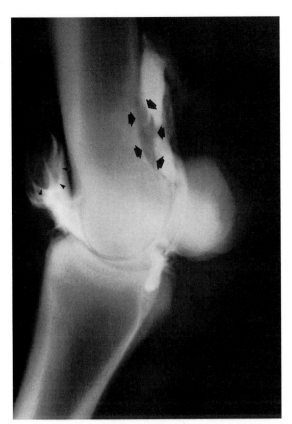

FIGURE 21-2. Positive-contrast arthrogram (same horse as in Fig. 21–1). There are two radiolucent, space-occupying masses in the dorsoproximal joint space *(arrowheads)*. A space-occupying mass at the palmar surface fills the area of supracondylar lysis *(arrows)*.

Supracondylar Lysis

In MC III or MT III, supracondylar lysis is similar to the villonodular sign except that it occurs at the palmar surface of the bone.[7] Changes are caused by chronic proliferative synovitis. Radiographic signs are joint distention and lysis of bone at the palmar cortex of MC III or MT III, distal to the joint capsule attachment (see Fig. 21–1). Arthrography may be difficult to perform because of the presence of hypertrophied synovium and diminished synovial joint space. Contrast medium permeates an undulating, irregular mass filling defect. The concavity formed in the bone is usually readily apparent (see Fig. 21–2).

Degenerative Joint Disease

Degenerative joint disease is a nonspecific term describing deterioration of articular and periarticular structures. The pathologic events culminate in degenerative hypertrophic osteoarthritis regardless of the causes or biochemical alterations.

The first stages include cartilage degeneration and formation of wear lines that are characteristic of hinge joints. These lines are grooves in the articular surface that are oriented parallel to the direction of joint motion. Blisters form in the surface, and subsequent wear results in narrowing of the joint space. If reduction in the width of a joint space is confirmed on two radiographic views, there is little doubt that cartilage thickness has been reduced. Progressive loss of joint width is a subjective finding and must be carefully assessed with clinical signs to determine its significance (Fig. 21–3).

Radiographic signs of degenerative joint disease are soft-tissue swelling, narrowed joint space, and bone remodeling with lysis or proliferation. These findings may occur in any combination. Joint capsule thickening may be suspected but is probably not visualized, even on high detail radiographs. Soft-tissue swelling results from hypertrophy and proliferation of other periarticular tissues.

In chronic arthritis, there is sclerosis or eburnation of subchondral bone with loss of trabecular architecture as a result of erosion and loss of the articular cartilage. Constant stress and tension or trauma at the joint capsule attachments result in enthesophyte formation (Fig. 21–4). Similar but not identical are the bony osteophytes that form at the joint margin in response to damage to the articular surface.

Cortisone Arthropathy

The changes associated with cortisone arthropathy involve articular and periarticular structures and have variable degrees of degeneration and proliferation. Repeated steroid injections result in localized demineralization of bone and decreased trabecular detail. Chronic changes include mineralization in the periarticular soft tissues, probably associated with deposition of some steroid within those structures. A differential diagnosis of steroid-induced arthritis should be considered in the presence of degenerative change or collapse of subchondral bone with mineralization in periarticular soft tissue (Fig. 21–5).

Osteochondrosis

Osteochondrosis may be found in the distal aspect of MC III or MT III.[12–14] The radiographic findings are well-demarcated,

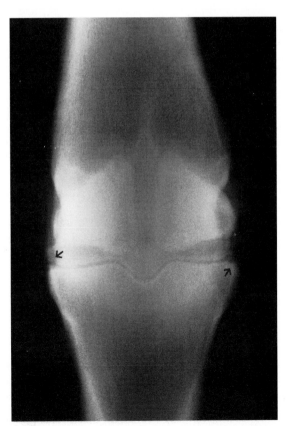

FIGURE 21-3. Dorsopalmar radiograph with changes of chronic degenerative joint disease. There is narrowing of the joint space and formation of osteophytes at the joint margins *(arrows)*.

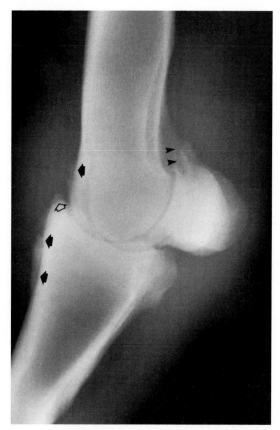

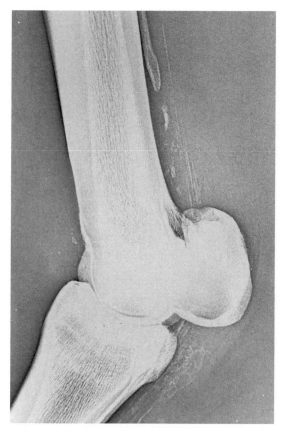

FIGURE 21–4. Lateromedial radiograph of a horse with chronic degenerative joint disease, sesamoiditis, and desmitis. There is generalized soft-tissue swelling and joint distention. Chronic osteochondral fractures are present at the apices of the proximal sesamoids *(arrowheads).* Degenerative bony proliferation is present at the dorsoproximal surface of the proximal phalanx and at the joint capsule attachment on the dorsodistal surface of the third metacarpus *(solid arrows).* A periarticular osteophyte is evident on the dorsal rim of the proximal phalanx *(open arrow).* Other changes include supracondylar lysis, remodeling of bony trabeculae in the proximal sesamoids, and bony proliferation at the attachments of the deep sesamoidean ligaments at the proximal palmar aspect of the proximal phalanx.

FIGURE 21–5. Xeroradiograph of a horse with cortisone arthropathy. There is narrowing of the joint space. Coarse bone trabeculae are indicative of demineralization of bone. Mineralization in periarticular soft tissues is typical of cortisone arthropathy.

oval radiolucencies that may extend several centimeters deep to the articular margins. A lateromedial radiograph of the joint may better indicate the depth of the lesion in the condyle. The shape of the defect may be a shallow concavity, a deep concavity, crescentic, oval, or circular.[15] The changes are found at the junction of the radii of articulation between the MCP or the MTP joint and the metacarposesamoidean or metatarsosesamoidean articular surface (Fig. 21–6). These lesions have been called *traumatic osteochondrosis,* an indication of the controversy regarding their cause.[7] Arthrographically, there may be cavitation of the joint surface, although advanced degenerative subchondral bony changes may be found, and the cartilage may be intact, yet dimpled, at the joint surface.

Osteochondral fragments of the palmar aspect of the joint have been given three classifications.[16] Type I fragments occur at the proximal end of the phalanx, just medial or lateral to the sagittal groove, and type II fragments have origin from the palmar eminence of the proximal phalanx. Type III has origin from the basilar margin of the sesamoid and is discussed later as a basilar fracture. Type I or II fragments have the highest incidence in Standardbreds. These were originally reported as avulsion fractures.[17, 18] Because of the anatomic origin and symmetry of the lesion and breed predilection, it has been reported that these fragments are the result of osteochondrosis (Figs. 21–7 and 21–8). These fragments are

the subject of much interest and some controversy. Studies have been reported regarding radiography,[19–21] etiology,[22] heritability,[23, 24] effect of patient size,[25] epidemiology,[26–27] surgical treatment,[28, 29] and prognosis.[21]

Osteochondrosis of the sagittal ridge of MC III or MT III is usually diagnosed in young horses and occurs with variable radiographic expression (Fig. 21–9). Radiographic signs may

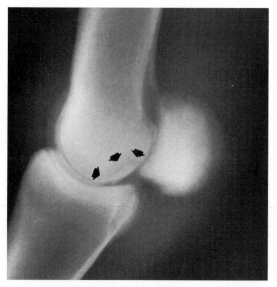

FIGURE 21–6. Lateromedial radiograph of a horse with distal metacarpal osteochondrosis. An opaque osteochondral fragment is present within a deep concavity of radiolucency *(arrows).*

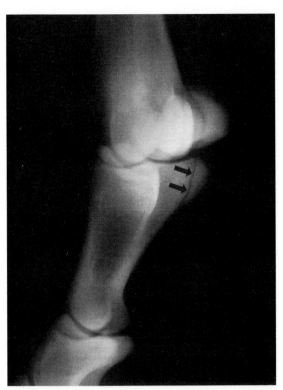

FIGURE 21–7. Dorsal 45-degree medial-palmarolateral radiograph of the metacarpophalangeal joint with a type II fragment *(arrows)* originating from the medial palmar eminence of the proximal phalanx.

vary from flattening to large excavations of subchondral bone of the sagittal ridge. Lesions are best visualized on flexed lateral projections of the MCP or MTP joint. Fragments, containing bone, may be found in close association to the bone defect.[21, 30]

Septic Arthritis

Septic arthritis may be associated with hematogenous distribution of microorganisms, as occurs with omphalophlebitis or by direct contamination because of trauma or nonsterile technique. Radiographic signs of early septic arthritis are periarticular soft-tissue swelling and distention of the joint. Progression of the disease results in malalignment, subluxation, or collapse of the joint. Bony changes consist of subchondral bone lysis and periosteal proliferation at the joint margins (Fig. 21–10). The cartilage space may appear increased at areas of subchondral bone lysis. Diminished joint space is evidence of the loss of articular cartilage that precedes subchondral bony change.

The radiographic sign of an increase in the apparent joint space must be critically analyzed. Incomplete ossification of the cartilage model is present in young, developing animals and progressively diminishes with skeletal maturity. Increased thickness of the articular cartilage has not been documented in animals. Excessive fluid or soft tissue in the joint space, as occurs with immune-mediated arthritis, results in a wider joint space. These diseases have not been documented in the horse, but the author has observed horses in which these signs were consistent with that diagnosis.

Nonseptic inflammatory joint diseases have varied causes and may be difficult to classify. Radiographic signs are distention of the joint and displacement of periarticular soft tissues.

If the condition is chronic, bony excrescences at the joint margins or periarticular osteophytes may be found.

Slab Fractures

Fractures in the distal condyle of MC III or MT III may be difficult to visualize radiographically. The radiographic signs include uneven joint surface, interruption of the metaphyseal cortex, and presence of a radiolucent fracture line extending from the joint surface to the cortex. These fractures usually occur at the lateral side of the joint (Fig. 21–11) and may be completely displaced, completely nondisplaced, or incomplete. Prognosis following surgical treatment varies.[29, 31]

Fractures of the proximal phalanx may communicate. Fracture location and severity must be considered relative to surgical repair and prognosis.[32]

Periarticular Chip Fractures

Chip fractures are more common in horses that have raced, and they occur about equally in the forelimbs. They may arise from the medial or lateral eminences at the proximodorsal periarticular rim of the proximal phalanx but occur more frequently at the medial side.[33] Acute chip fractures may have sharp borders and geometric configurations. Chronic chip fractures have smooth, rounded borders. The latter are usually attached to the joint capsule or to the joint margin as an exostosis (Fig. 21–12). Free joint bodies may displace or move about within the joint.

Osteochondral fragments arising from the plantarolateral eminences of the proximal phalanx (see Fig. 21–12, *open arrow*) have been reported as fractures.[7, 17, 18, 22, 34] These frag-

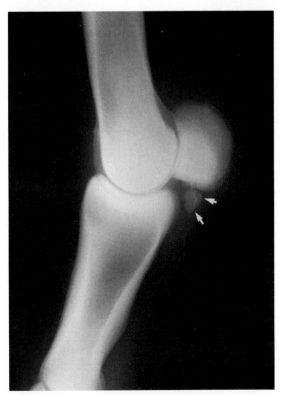

FIGURE 21–8. Lateromedial radiograph of a metacarpophalangeal joint with a type III fracture *(arrows)* originating from the basilar margin of a proximal sesamoid.

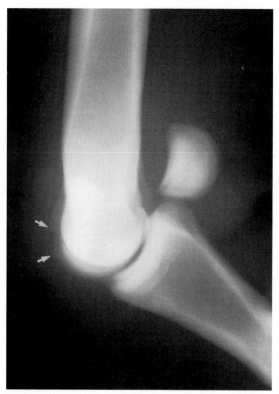

FIGURE 21–9. Lateromedial radiograph of a flexed metacarpophalangeal joint with osteochondrosis of the sagittal ridge of the third metacarpus. Excavation of subchondral bone can be seen between the *arrows*. A periarticular fragment is present at the dorsoproximal margin of the proximal phalanx.

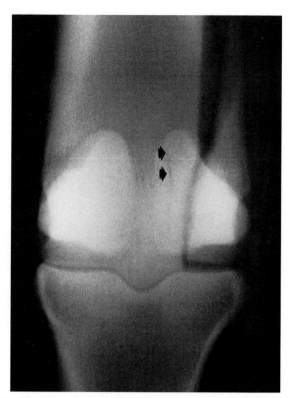

FIGURE 21–11. Dorsopalmar radiograph of a horse with a slab fracture of the lateral condyle of the third metacarpus. Some fracture lines may be difficult to visualize *(arrows)*. Marked displacement of a fragment such as this is often not present.

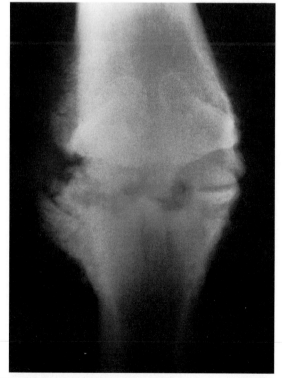

FIGURE 21–10. Dorsopalmar radiograph of a horse with chronic septic arthritis. Generalized soft-tissue swelling is present. The joint space has collapsed, and there is severe erosion of subchondral bone of the opposing joint surfaces. Bony proliferation is evident on all periarticular surfaces. The palisading nature of the periosteal reaction is typical of osteomyelitis.

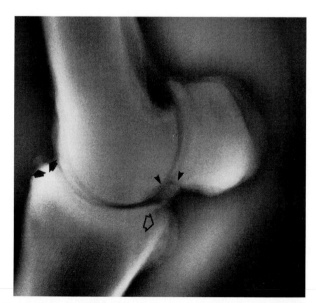

FIGURE 21–12. Lateromedial radiograph of a horse with chronic degenerative joint disease. An osteochondral (chip) fracture is present at the dorsal periarticular rim of the proximal phalanx *(solid arrows)*. A basilar osteochondral fracture of the proximal sesamoid is evident *(arrowheads)*. There is bony proliferation at the attachment of the deep sesamoidean ligaments at the palmaroproximal border of the proximal phalanx *(open arrow)*. Villonodular erosion of bone and supracondylar lysis are apparent.

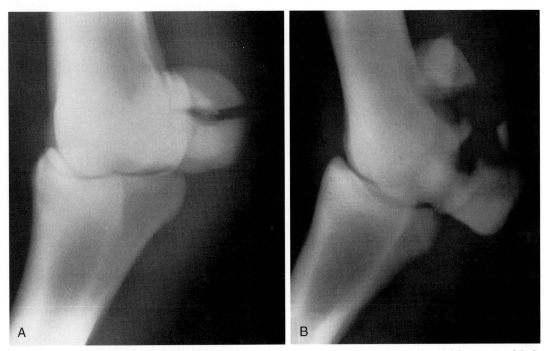

FIGURE 21–13. *A,* A dorsal 45-degree medial-palmarolateral radiograph. Fractures through the medial sesamoid are apparent. The joint is extended, but separation of the fragments is minimal. The suspensory ligament remains intact. *B,* Lateral radiograph of a horse with fractures of the medial and lateral proximal sesamoids. The joint is hyperextended, and there is marked separation of the fragments. The suspensory ligament has separated.

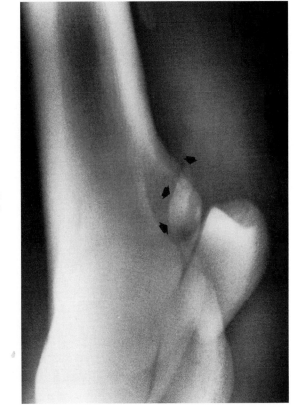

FIGURE 21–14. Palmaroproximolateral-dorsodistomedial radiograph of a horse with a periarticular fracture of the medial proximal sesamoid *(arrows).* The fracture originates at an articular surface and emerges at the abaxial surface of the sesamoid.

ments have been discussed previously and are considered by some as being a manifestation of osteochondrosis.[16, 19–28, 35, 36]

Fractures of the Proximal Sesamoids

Proximal sesamoid fractures are consistently of three types: apical, midbody, or basilar.[29] Some may be found as osteochondral fragments separated from the sesamoid apex (apical fractures; see Fig. 21–4) or base (basilar fractures, type III[16]; see Figs. 21–8 and 21–12). Fractures through the body of the sesamoid may have a narrow cleavage line, indicating that the suspensory apparatus remains intact (Fig. 21–13A). Wide separation of sesamoid fragments usually indicates bilateral sesamoid fractures and separation of the fibers of the suspensory ligament (see Fig. 21–13B). Hyperextension of the MCP or MTP joint is apparent if stress is applied to the joint or if the limb is bearing weight.

Abaxial fractures are detected with the use of special radiographic projections. These fractures result from avulsion of bone by a portion of the attachment of the branches of the suspensory ligament on the medial or lateral aspect of the respective proximal sesamoid (Fig. 21–14). A review of the clinical aspects of apical[37] and basilar[38] sesamoid fractures is available.

Sesamoiditis

Sesamoiditis is indicated radiographically by bony proliferation on nonarticular surfaces of the proximal sesamoids.[39] Linear or cystic lysis may appear to penetrate the sesamoid from the abaxial surface (Fig. 21–15). Sesamoiditis is usually

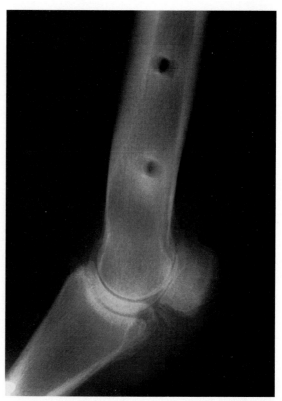

FIGURE 21–16. Lateromedial radiograph of distal third metacarpus, the metacarpophalangeal joint, and the proximal phalanx of a horse that recently had a "walking cast" support removed from the leg. There is some bone sclerosis around transverse pin tracts, but the remaining bone has advanced osteopenia. There is generalized remodeling of bone, and the cortices are thin. Osseous trabeculae are coarse and irregular with no organized pattern. The sesamoids have a sponge-like appearance, and avulsion of bone has occurred along the basilar margins.

associated with degenerative change in the suspensory ligament and degenerative remodeling or fracture at the distal ends of the minor metacarpals (see Fig. 21–15).

Disuse Atrophy of Bone

Disuse atrophy occurs more rapidly in the proximal sesamoid bones but may be recognized in the tubular bones as a reduction in bone opacity. Trabeculae within the bone become large and coarse. This change occurs as a result of altered stress or axial weight bearing and does not signify primary pathologic change in the fetlock (Fig. 21–16).

References

1. Getty R: Sisson and Grossman's The Anatomy of the Domestic Animals, 5th Ed. Philadelphia, WB Saunders, 1975, pp 357–360.
2. Rendano VT: Equine radiology: The fetlock. Mod Vet Pract 58:871, 1977.
3. Allan GS: Radiography of the equine fetlock. Equine Pract 1:40, 1979.
4. Morgan JP: Techniques of Veterinary Radiography, 5th Ed. Ames, Iowa State University Press, 1993.
5. Hornof WJ, and O'Brien TR: Radiographic evaluation of the palmar aspect of the equine metacarpal condyles: A new projection. Vet Radiol 21:161, 1980.
6. Palmer SE: Radiography of the abaxial surface of the proximal sesamoid bones of the horse. J Am Vet Med Assoc 181:264, 1982.
7. Pool RR, and Meagher DM: Pathologic findings and pathogenesis of racetrack injuries. Vet Clin North Am [Equine Pract] 6:1, 1990.
8. Gillette EL, Thrall DE, and Lebel JL: Carlson's Veterinary Radiology, 3rd Ed. Philadelphia, Lea & Febiger, 1977, p 435.
9. Barclay WP, White KK, and Williams A: Equine villonodular synovitis: A case survey. Cornell Vet 70:72, 1979.

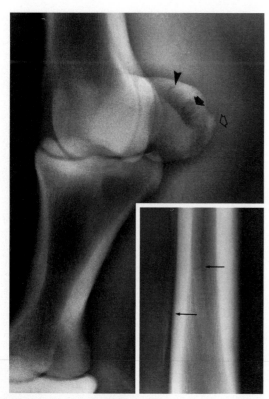

FIGURE 21–15. Dorsal 45-degree medial-palmarolateral oblique view of a horse with chronic sesamoiditis, desmitis, and fractures of the second and fourth metacarpi (MC II and IV); the medial proximal sesamoid is projected. Degenerative remodeling is present with tunneling *(arrowhead)*, cystic change *(solid arrow)*, and an abaxial fracture *(open arrow)*. Inset, There are fractures at the distal ends of MC II and MC IV *(arrows)*.

10. Nickels FA, Grant BD, and Lincoln SD: Villonodular synovitis of the equine metacarpophalangeal joint. J Am Vet Med Assoc 168:1043, 1976.

11. van Veenendaal JC, and Moffat RE: Soft-tissue masses in the fetlock joint of horses. Aust Vet J 56:533, 1980.

12. Petterson H, and Reiland S: Periarticular subchondral "bone cysts" in horses. Clin Orthop 62:95, 1969.

13. Hornof WJ, O'Brien TR, and Pool RR: Osteochondritis dissecans of the distal metacarpus in the adult racing thoroughbred horse. Vet Radiol 22:98, 1981.

14. Edwards GB: Interpreting radiographs: 2. The fetlock joint and pastern. Equine Vet J 16:4, 1984.

15. O'Brien TR, Hornof WJ, and Meagher DM: Radiographic detection and characterization of palmar lesions in the equine fetlock joint. J Am Vet Med Assoc 178:231, 1981.

16. Foerner JJ, Barclay WP, Phillips TN, et al: Osteochondral fragments of the palmar/plantar aspect of the fetlock joint. In Proceedings of the 33rd Annual Meeting of the American Association of Equine Practitioners, 1987, p 739.

17. Birkeland R: Chip fractures of the first phalanx in the metatarsal phalangeal joint of the horse. Acta Radiol 319(suppl):73, 1972.

18. Petterson H, and Ryden G: Avulsion fractures of the caudoproximal extremity of the first phalanx. Equine Vet J 14:333, 1982.

19. Sandgren B: Bony fragments in the tarsocrural and metacarpo- or metatarsophalangeal joints in the Standardbred horse—a radiographic survey. Equine Vet J 6(suppl):66, 1988.

20. Carlsten J, Sandgren B, and Dalin G: Development of osteochondrosis in the tarsocrural joint and osteochondral fragments in the fetlock joints of Standardbred trotters: I. A radiological survey. Equine Vet J 16(suppl):42, 1993.

21. Grøndahl AM, and Engeland A: Influence of radiographically detectable orthopedic changes on racing performance in Standardbred trotters. J Am Vet Med Assoc 206:1013, 1995.

22. Dalin G, Sandgren B, and Carlsten J: Plantar osteochondral fragments in the fetlock joints of Standardbreds: Result of osteochondrosis or trauma? Equine Vet J 16(suppl):62, 1993.

23. Grøndahl AM, and Dolvik NI: Heritability estimations of osteochondrosis in the tibiotarsal joint and of bony fragments in the palmar/plantar portion of the metacarpo and metatarsophalangeal joints of horses. J Am Vet Med Assoc 203:101, 1993.

24. Philipsson J, Andréasson E, Sandgren B, et al: Osteochondrosis in the tarsocrural joint and osteochondral fragments in the fetlock joints in Standardbred trotters: II. Heritability. Equine Vet J 16(suppl):38, 1993.

25. Sandgren B, Dalin G, Carlsten J, et al: Development of osteochondrosis in the tarsocrural joint and osteochondral fragments in the fetlock joints of Standardbred trotters: II. Body measurements and clinical findings. Equine Vet J 16(suppl):48, 1993.

26. Grøndahl AM: The incidence of bony fragments and osteochondrosis in the metacarpo- and metatarsophalangeal joints of Standardbred trotters: A radiographic study. Equine Vet Sci 12:81, 1992.

27. Sandgren B, Dalin G, and Carlsten J: Osteochondrosis in the tarsocrural joint and osteochondral fragments in the fetlock joints in Standardbred trotters: I. Epidemiology. Equine Vet J 16(suppl):31, 1993.

28. Fortier LA, Foerner JJ, and Nixon AJ: Arthroscopic removal of axial osteochondral fragments of the plantar/palmar proximal aspect of the proximal phalanx in horses: 119 cases (1988–1992). J Am Vet Med Assoc 206:71, 1995.

29. Copelan RW, and Bramlage LR: Surgery of the fetlock joint. Vet Clin North Am [Large Anim Pract] 5:221, 1983.

30. Yovich JV, McIlwraith CW, and Stashak TS: Osteochondritis dissecans of the sagittal ridge of the third metacarpal and metatarsal bones in horses. J Am Vet Med Assoc 186:1186, 1985.

31. Rick MC, O'Brien TR, Pool RR, et al: Condylar fractures of the third metacarpal bone and third metatarsal bone in 75 horses: Radiographic features, treatments, and outcome. J Am Vet Med Assoc 183:287, 1983.

32. Holcombe SJ, Schneider RK, Bramlage LR, et al: Lag screw fixation of noncomminuted sagittal fractures of the proximal phalanx in racehorses: 59 cases (1973–1991). J Am Vet Med Assoc 206:1195, 1995.

33. Yovich JV, and McIlwraith CW: Arthroscopic surgery for osteochondral fractures of the proximal phalanx of the metacarpophalangeal and metatarsophalangeal (fetlock) joints in horses. J Am Vet Med Assoc 188:273, 1986.

34. Nixon AJ, and Pool RR: Histologic appearance of axial osteochondral fragments from the proximoplantar/proximopalmar aspect of the proximal phalanx in horses. J Am Vet Med Assoc 207:1076, 1995.

35. Barclay WP, Foerner JJ, and Phillips TN: Lameness attributable to osteochondral fragmentation of the plantar aspect of the proximal phalanx in horses: 19 cases (1981–1985). J Am Vet Med Assoc 191:855, 1987.

36. Grøndahl AM: Incidence and development of ununited proximoplantar tuberosity of the proximal phalanx in Standardbred trotters. Vet Radiol Ultrasound 33:18, 1992.

37. Spurlock GH, and Gabel AA: Apical fractures of the proximal sesamoid bones in 109 Standardbred horses. J Am Vet Med Assoc 183:76, 1983.

38. Parente EJ, Richardson DW, and Spencer P: Basal sesamoidean fractures in horses: 57 cases (1980–1991). J Am Vet Med Assoc 202:1293, 1993.

39. Blevins WE, and Widmer WR: Radiology in racetrack practice. Vet Clin North Am [Equine Pract] 6:31, 1990.

STUDY QUESTIONS

1. Survey radiographic examination of the metacarpophalangeal joints and the metatarsophalangeal joints:
   A. Requires only left and right markers because the hindlimb and the forelimb are distinctly different.
   B. Should include four orthogonal projections, flexed lateral projections, and skyline projections.
   C. Should be centered over the diaphysis of the third metacarpus and the exposure made with the limb not supporting weight.
   D. Should be made before making special projections or contrast studies of the joint.

2. Villonodular synovitis of the metacarpophalangeal or metatarsophalangeal joint is:
   A. Usually the result of low-grade infection.
   B. A sequela to osteochondrosis and some nutritional disturbances.
   C. The result of repetitive or single-event trauma.
   D. Usually occurs with degenerative joint disease and cartilage degradation.

3. Lateromedial projection of the left metacarpophalangeal joint of a 2-year-old Thoroughbred filly, presented with forelimb lameness and swelling at the metacarpophalangeal joints (Fig. 21–17). Give the radiographic findings, diagnosis, and suggestions for additional radiographic examination.

4. Fractures that communicate with the metacarpophalangeal or metatarsophalangeal joint:

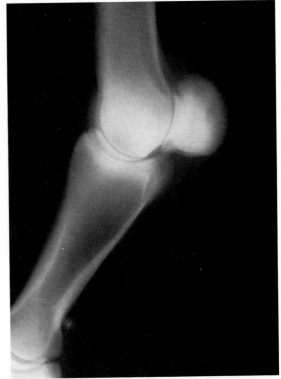

FIGURE 21–17

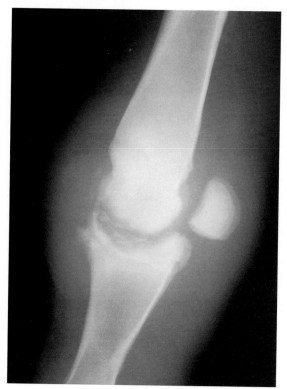

FIGURE 21-18

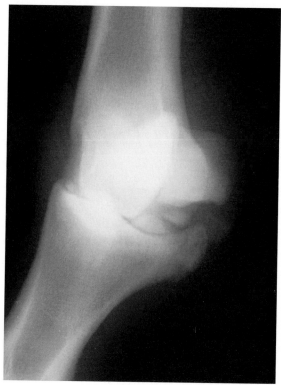

FIGURE 21-19

A. Are most common at the medial condyle of the right metacarpus in young racing Thoroughbreds.
B. May involve any of the bony components of the fetlock joint.
C. Are usually exercise limiting but not prohibiting.
D. Result in crippling lameness.

5. Supracondylar lysis of the metatarsus or metacarpus is:
   A. Similar to villonodular synovitis except that it occurs at the plantar (palmar) surface of the bone.
   B. Diagnosed most easily with the use of contrast arthrography.
   C. Is commonly seen as a sequela to cortisone injections.
   D. Is a common sequela to septic arthritis.

6. A 6-month-old Appaloosa filly was presented with an open, draining wound dorsal to the fetlock (Fig. 21-18). List the radiographic findings and diagnosis.

7. Degenerative joint disease of the metacarpophalangeal or metatarsophalangeal joint:
   A. Can best be diagnosed by radiographic signs of periarticular bone proliferation and subchondral bone remodeling.
   B. Is most often a sequela to septic arthritis.
   C. Is a nonspecific term for progressive deterioration of all tissue components of the joint.
   D. Is a specific joint disease resulting from repetitive trauma.

8. Osteochondrosis of the metacarpophalangeal or metatarsophalangeal joint:
   A. Is diagnosed more frequently in the proximal sesamoids.
   B. Has rather clearly defined heritability.
   C. Is often diagnosed in Standardbreds at the proximal palmar/plantar margin of the proximal phalanx.
   D. Has been mistakenly diagnosed as traumatic avulsion of apophyses and fractures of the sagittal ridge of the third metacarpus.

9. A dorsomedial-plantarolateral projection of the left metatarsophalangeal joint of a 2-year-old Standardbred gelding was obtained (Fig. 21-19). Describe the radiographic findings and give your diagnosis.

10. Diseases of the proximal sesamoids, referred to as *sesamoiditis:*
    A. Acquire the name because, with the exception of fractures, the majority of the diseases result in inflammation and irritation of the periosteum.
    B. Are often associated with changes in the suspensory ligament and tissues removed from the fetlock joint.
    C. Are inflammatory diseases of the bone that lead to degenerative joint disease.
    D. Result in separation of the bone because of progressive weakening and avulsion of the supporting ligamentous structures.

(Answers appear on page 638.)

Chapter 22

The Phalanges

Sandra V. McNeel • Elizabeth A. Riedesel

TECHNICAL FACTORS

The *significance* of many radiographic abnormalities of the equine phalanges is difficult to ascertain unless pertinent facts obtained from the patient's clinical history and physical examination are correlated with the radiographic findings. Diagnostic nerve blocks are used to localize the lesion more specifically, especially in the horse with multiple abnormalities identified during the physical examination.[1]

Patient Preparation

Dirt, skin lesions, and iodine-containing medications can all produce opacities that complicate radiographic interpretation. Consequently the patient should be examined closely to be sure that all such material has been removed from the hair coat. Shoes and any additional pads used in corrective shoeing should be removed to obtain optimal radiographs of the distal phalanx and navicular bone. The sole and sulci of the frog should be thoroughly cleaned with a hoof pick. The sulci may then be filled with a material of soft-tissue opacity (such as Play-Doh, Rainbow Crafts, Cincinnati, OH) to the level of the solar surface (Fig. 22–1). Packing the central and collateral sulci eliminates the radiolucent linear opacities seen when the air-filled sulci become superimposed on the distal phalanx in the dorsal 65-degree–proximal-palmarodistal* view (Fig. 22–2).

---

*Palmar(o) is used throughout this chapter with the understanding that *plantar(o)* should be substituted if reference is being made to the rear digit.

Recommended Views

The equine foot is structured such that certain anatomic areas can be imaged as a group. These groupings and the projections needed to evaluate them optimally are listed in Table 22–1. Excellent, complete descriptions of patient positioning[2-5] and examples of normal radiographic anatomy[4-7] are available, and the reader is referred to these sources for additional information. Normal radiographic anatomy is also presented in Chapter 47.

NORMAL RADIOGRAPHIC ANATOMY (INCLUDING VARIATIONS)

Osseous Structures

The foot axis (as seen on the lateromedial view of the digit) is the angle described by an imaginary line that divides the middle phalanx into dorsal and palmar halves. This line should also divide both proximal and distal phalanges into dorsal and palmar halves. When the line is carried through the distal phalanx, it should create an angle of 45 to 50 degrees (front) or 50 to 55 degrees (hind) with the bony solar margin.[4] Figure 22–3 illustrates the normal axis of a foredigit. Variations in the angle occur with conformational differences in individual horses.[8]

A nutrient foramen occurs as an inconsistent radiographic finding in the proximal phalanx of approximately 85 percent of Thoroughbreds and Standardbreds.[9] When present, it is seen as a radiolucent line running obliquely through the dorsal aspect of the mid-diaphyseal cortex (see Fig. 22–3). These foramina should not be mistaken for fractures. Variations may also occur in the appearance of trabeculae in the medullary cavity of the proximal phalanx (Fig. 22–4). A prominent radiolucent center in the medullary cavity surrounded by a ring-like radiopacity is illustrated in Figure

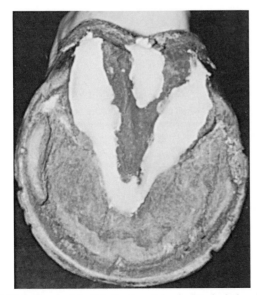

FIGURE 22–1. The sole of the foot after the central and collateral sulci have been filled (packed) with a pliable material of similar radiopacity as the sole (Play-Doh).

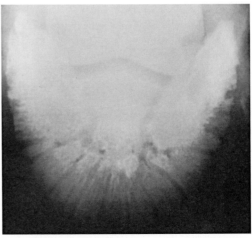

FIGURE 22–2. Dorsal 65-degree–proximal-palmarodistal view of a normal distal phalanx with the sulci packed. Note the good definition of vascular channels without superimposed air artifacts.

Table 22-1
VIEWS FOR EQUINE PHALANX EVALUATION

Examination	Structures Evaluated	Views
Pastern	Proximal phalanx Proximal interphalangeal joint Middle phalanx	Dorsal 45°–proximal-palmarodistal oblique Lateromedial Dorsal 35°–lateral-palmaromedial oblique Dorsal 35°–medial-palmarolateral oblique
Distal phalanx	Distal phalanx Distal interphalangeal joint	Dorsopalmar with horizontal beam and/or dorsal 45°–proximal-palmarodistal oblique with horse standing on cassette Dorsal 65°–proximal-palmarodistal oblique with horse standing on cassette Lateromedial, with foot on block so as to include solar margin of distal phalanx and soft tissues of sole on the radiograph Two oblique views: dorsal 65°–proximal 45°–lateral-palmarodistomedial and dorsal 65°–proximal 45°–medial-palmarodistolateral. Obliques are especially useful when distal phalanx fracture is suspected

22–4B; this is a normal variation in trabeculation and does not indicate cyst formation.

If the lateromedial view is slightly oblique, two normal structures become more prominent and can be misinterpreted as pathologic. The first is the V-shaped attachment of the oblique sesamoidean ligament along the palmar cortex of the proximal phalanx. The second is the eminence for attachment of the collateral ligament of the distal interphalangeal joint along the dorsum of the middle phalanx (see Fig. 22–16).

The radiographic appearance of the normal distal phalanx varies in several respects.[10-12] The most obvious difference is the distribution of vascular channels. Although the pattern of vascular channel formation is unique to individual animals, the major channels identified at the solar margin should communicate with the solar canal. Figure 22–5 demonstrates some of the variations in the number of vascular channels, their distribution, and the patterns of radiation

from the solar canal. A smoothly rounded notch in the toe of the distal phalanx may be seen in the normal horse. This notch is referred to as the *crena marginis solearis* or, more commonly, the *crena* or toe notch.

The shape of the extensor process of the distal phalanx may also differ among individual animals (Fig. 22–6).[10] The margin of the normal process, however, is smooth, regardless of its shape. The palmar processes of the distal phalanx become more extensively ossified with age. The morphologic development of the palmar process has been described in the foal (3 to 32 weeks of age).[13] Compare the palmar processes of the three horses (5 months old, 8 years old, and 15 years old) in Figure 22–7.

Soft Tissue

Knowledge of the attachment sites of the joint capsules, tendons, and ligaments of the foot is imperative for accurate

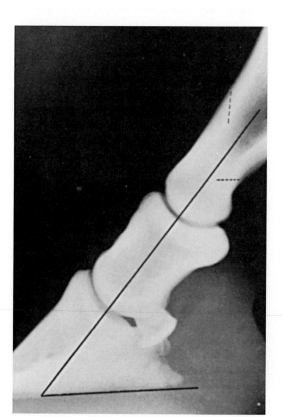

FIGURE 22–3. Normal lateromedial view of a front digit. The axis of the foot, measured through the plane of the middle phalanx and solar margin of the distal phalanx, is 47 degrees. *Dashed lines* represent the location of small nutrient foramina that are variably present in the normal horse.

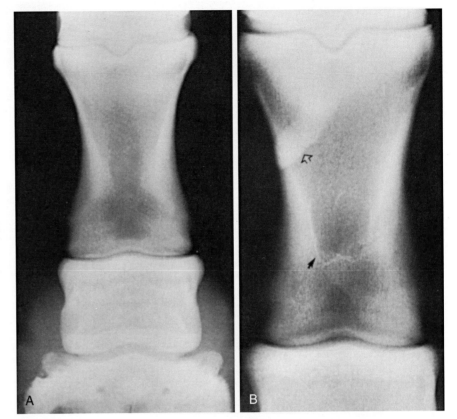

FIGURE 22–4. Dorsopalmar view of two normal equine proximal phalanges. *A*, Note the normal thickness of the lateral and medial cortices of the proximal phalanx at the junction of the middle and distal one third of the bone. The radiolucent medullary cavity is seen between the thickest parts of the cortex. The widest joint space is usually the distal interphalangeal joint, with the joint spaces becoming progressively more narrow toward the metacarpophalangeal joint. *B*, A thin rim of opaque trabeculation surrounds the central medullary cavity of the proximal phalanx *(solid arrow)*. The ergot is elongated in this animal and is seen because of its summation with the proximal phalanx *(open arrow)*.

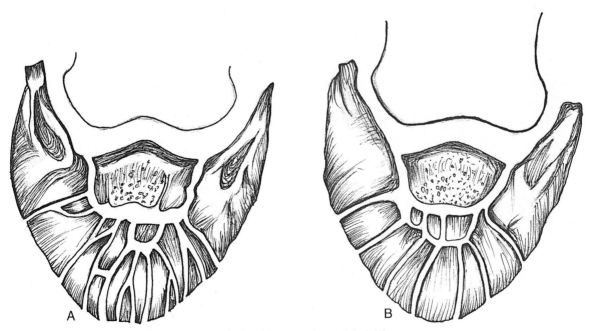

FIGURE 22–5. *A* and *B,* Two variations in the pattern of vascular channel formation in the normal distal phalanx.

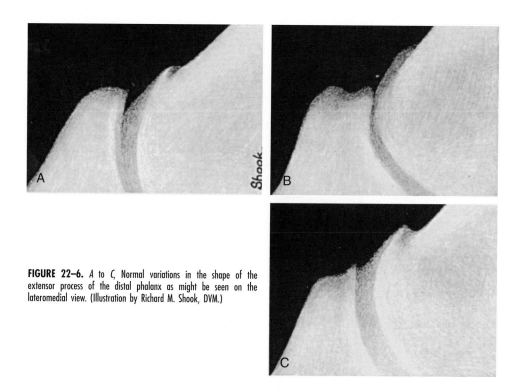

FIGURE 22–6. *A* to *C*, Normal variations in the shape of the extensor process of the distal phalanx as might be seen on the lateromedial view. (Illustration by Richard M. Shook, DVM.)

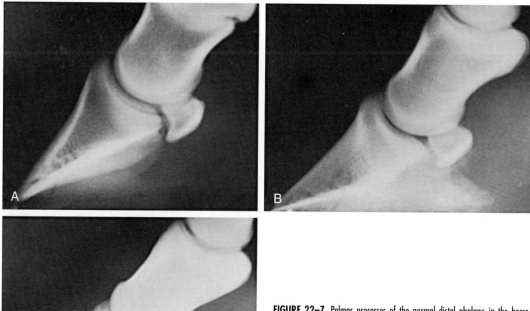

FIGURE 22–7. Palmar processes of the normal distal phalanx in the horse become more extensively ossified with age. *A*, Lateromedial view of a 5-month-old foal. *B*, Lateromedial view of an 8-year-old Standardbred. *C*, Lateromedial view of a 15-year-old Arabian cross-breed.

interpretation of the osseous changes seen in radiographs of the phalanges. Figures 22–8 through 22–10 illustrate the attachment sites of these major structures. Additional information on soft-tissue attachments is available.[14] The ergot may create a radiopacity when superimposed on the proximal phalanx in the dorsopalmar view (see Fig. 22–4B). In the lateromedial view, the ergot opacity can be seen along the palmar surface of the skin.

Articular Cartilage

In the properly positioned dorsal 45-degree–proximal-palmarodistal view of the normal foot, the metacarpophalangeal, proximal interphalangeal, and distal interphalangeal joints can be visualized. The metacarpophalangeal joint is usually the narrowest of these articulations, the proximal interphalangeal joint is slightly wider, and the distal interpha-

langeal joint is the widest of the three joint spaces (see Fig. 22–4A). If the horse is not bearing weight evenly on the leg, the asymmetric loading forces can cause the appearance of narrowing of the loaded side and widening of the nonloaded side of the joint (see Fig. 22–24F). This artifact can be recognized because it similarly affects all three joints, as seen on the dorsopalmar view.

ROENTGEN SIGNS OF THE PROXIMAL AND MIDDLE PHALANGES

Number

Rare congenital anomalies may cause an abnormal number of digits or phalanges to be present. Polydactylism in the horse is often associated with a complete supernumerary

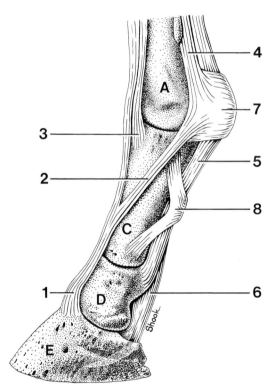

FIGURE 22–8. Lateral view of the tendon and ligament attachments of the thoracic digit (superficial tissues). (Illustration by Richard A. Shook, DVM.)

The following anatomic key is designed for Figures 22–8 through 22–10.

A. Third metacarpal bone.
B. Proximal sesamoid bone.
C. Proximal phalanx.
D. Middle phalanx.
E. Distal phalanx.
F. Distal sesamoid (navicular) bone.
  1. Common digital extensor tendon.
  2. Extensor branch of the interosseous (suspensory) ligament.
  3. ateral digital extensor tendon.
  4. Interosseous (suspensory) ligament.
  5. Superficial digital flexor tendon.
  6. Deep digital flexor tendon.
  7. Superficial transverse metacarpal ligament (palmar annular ligament).
  8. Proximal digital annular ligament.
  9. Superficial (straight) sesamoidean ligament.
  10. Middle (oblique) sesamoidean ligament.
  11. Deep (cruciate) sesamoidean ligament.

12. Metacarpophalangeal joint capsule (blended with fibers from the common digital extensor tendon).
13. Distal palmar recess of the metacarpophalangeal joint.
14. Dorsal recess of the proximal interphalangeal joint capsule.
15. Palmar recess of the proximal interphalangeal joint.
16. Proximal interphalangeal joint capsule (blended with fibers from the common digital extensor tendon).
17. Dorsal recess of the distal interphalangeal joint.
18. Palmar recess of the distal interphalangeal joint.
19. Collateral sesamoidean ligament.
20. Distal sesamoidean impar ligament.
21. Podotrochlear bursa.
22. Medial collateral ligament of the metacarpophalangeal joint.
23. Lateral collateral ligament of the proximal interphalangeal joint.
24. Medial collateral ligament of the distal interphalangeal joint.

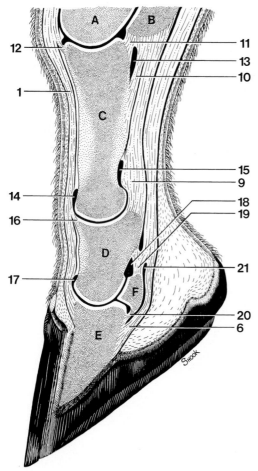

FIGURE 22–9. Tendon, ligament, and joint capsule attachments of the thoracic limb digit, sagittal section. (See *Anatomic Key* in legend for Fig. 22–8.) (Illustration by Richard A. Shook, DVM.)

metacarpophalangeal joint in addition to the phalanges of the digit.

Contour (Margination)—Periosteal Bone Proliferation

The underlying cause of periosteal new bone growth may be determined by evaluating the extent and the specific location of the lesion. In the instance of a focal area of periosteal reaction, consider whether the lesion is at a site of attachment for a tendon, ligament, or joint capsule. Previous sprain or strain injuries of tendons or ligaments and stretching of joint capsules as a result of intracapsular hemorrhage or joint effusion stimulate periosteal new bone growth, referred to as *enthesophyte formation*, at the fibro-osseous junction (Fig. 22–11). Focal periosteal proliferation that is not located at an attachment site may be due to previous direct trauma or to inflammation or infection of overlying soft tissues.

Diffuse periosteal new bone formation that involves multiple phalanges in one limb is suggestive of extensive infection, especially if accompanied by inflammation. Diffuse, symmetric periosteal proliferation involving multiple phalanges of all four limbs indicates a systemic process, such as hypertrophic osteopathy. The osseous lesions of this uncommon disorder are a sequela to chronic pulmonary (or, rarely, abdominal) space-occupying masses. Intrathoracic lesions that have been reported to cause hypertrophic osteopathy in the horse include tuberculosis, pulmonary abscesses, pulmonary neoplasms, ovarian neoplasia with pulmonary metastasis, rib fracture with adhesions, and pulmonary infarction.[15]

The smoothness of the margin and the radiopacity of the added periosteal bone may also be useful in determining the relative aggressiveness and chronicity of the lesion.

Four expressions of periosteal proliferation commonly occur in the equine proximal and middle phalanges (Fig. 22–12). The first is a smoothly margined and mildly opaque bone formation (see Fig. 22–12B), which is indicative of recent subperiosteal hemorrhage owing to trauma or elevation of the periosteum by exudate secondary to spread of infection from adjacent bone or soft tissue. The second is a smooth-margined, opaque bone formation suggestive of inactive, remodeled trauma (see Fig. 22–12C). The third is an irregular-margined, mildly opaque bone formation (see Fig. 22–12D). In this instance, recent or active periosteal damage because of direct trauma, avulsion injury of soft-tissue attachments, or infection (acute periostitis) is likely. Finally, an irregular-margined, opaque bone formation (see Fig. 22–12E) is indicative of chronic periostitis owing to infection or chronic strain on soft-tissue attachments or rarely to hypertrophic osteopathy.

Radiopacity

When alteration of bone radiopacity is identified, the location of the abnormality may help determine the underlying cause. Therefore, in the following discussion, the location and change in bone opacity are considered as an integrated unit.

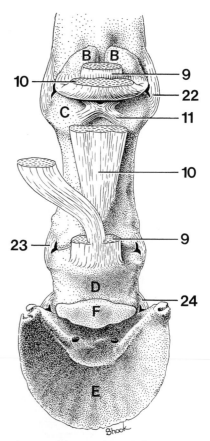

FIGURE 22–10. Palmar view of the sesamoidean and collateral ligament attachments of the digit. (See *Anatomic Key* in legend for Fig. 22–8.) (Illustration by Richard A. Shook, DVM.)

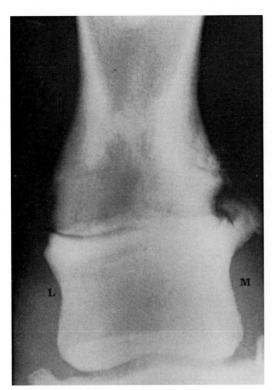

FIGURE 22–11. Dorsopalmar view in which there are large enthesophytes at the attachments of the medial collateral ligament. In addition, collapse of the medial portion of the proximal interphalangeal joint with subchondral sclerosis of the opposed surfaces of the proximal and middle phalanges is seen. Osteoarthritis is secondary to trauma. L, lateral; M, medial.

Increased Opacity, Subchondral Location

This finding is indicative of sclerosis caused by degenerative joint disease initiated by chronic instability, previous trauma, or poor conformation. A narrowed joint space, periarticular osteophytes, and enthesophytes may also be seen in advanced degenerative joint disease (see Fig. 22–11).

Increased Opacity, Periosteal Location

This alteration is usually seen with trauma, inflammation, or infection, as described previously.

Decreased Opacity of All Parts of the Phalanges

If radiographic exposure factors are correct, diffuse decrease in bone opacity may be due to disuse. Resorption of small trabeculae, as occurs with disuse, can cause the proximal sesamoid bones and phalanges to appear abnormally coarse, in addition to being of decreased opacity. Rarely does a calcium or phosphorus nutritional imbalance lead to sufficient demineralization of the appendicular skeleton to be identified radiographically.

Focal Decreased Opacity

Osteochondrosis occurs as a solitary radiolucent defect located in the subchondral bone, which often is surrounded by a radiopaque rim or diffuse sclerosis. Figure 22–13 illustrates two examples of such a defect, one with and one without accompanying secondary joint disease. When osteochondrosis occurs in the proximal and middle phalanges, the lesions are usually found in the distal portion of the proximal phalanx and less commonly in the distal subchondral bone of

the middle phalanx. These lesions are generally associated with joint effusion or lameness in horses of training age, that is, younger than 3 years of age. One report indicated a higher incidence of occurrence in the pelvic limb in a group of Quarter horses,[16] although either the thoracic or the pelvic limb may be affected.

Osteochondrosis defects in the distal part of the proximal phalanx frequently lead to extensive degenerative joint disease in the proximal interphalangeal joint (see Fig. 22–13B). In these instances, surgical arthrodesis may be warranted to allow return to useful function.[17–19] In one series of 13 horses in which solitary lesions of phalangeal osteochondrosis were treated by conservative management, lameness disappeared in seven horses over a period of 1 month to 2.5 years.[20] In four of these animals, the osteochondrosis defect could not be identified radiographically 1.5 to 2.5 years after the initial diagnosis. The extreme variation in outcome of phalangeal osteochondrosis may be associated with the size of the defect, the extent of associated articular cartilage fragmentation, and degenerative joint disease.

A solitary radiolucent defect in the body of the phalanx may be due to cortical bone necrosis and sequestrum formation (Fig. 22–14) or, rarely, to a congenital defect, such as monostotic fibrous dysplasia (nonossifying fibroma).[21] The latter anomaly can be distinguished by its thin-walled, cyst-like architecture, which may occupy the entire diaphyseal portion of the bone. Pathologic fracture through the thinned cortex of the phalanx may cause acute, severe lameness.

Multiple Radiolucent Subchondral Bone Defects

These changes are seen in septic arthritis (Fig. 22–15), osteochondrosis, some instances of degenerative joint disease, and steroid arthropathy.[4, 22–25] The origin of joint sepsis may be a penetrating puncture wound, extension from an adjacent infectious site (e.g., soft-tissue abscess or epiphyseal osteomyelitis), a hematogenous route, or iatrogenic (after arthrocen-

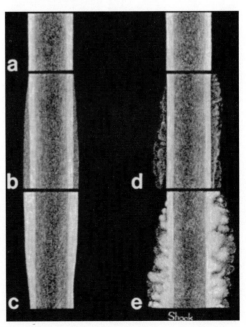

FIGURE 22–12. Variable appearance of contour and opacity of periosteal bone proliferation: A, Normal cortex. B, Smooth margin, mildly opaque periosteal bone formation. C, Smooth margin, opaque bone formation. D, Irregular margin, mildly opaque bone formation. E, Irregular margin, opaque bone formation. Note the loss of distinction between periosteal new bone and original cortex in C and E. (Illustration by Richard A. Shook, DVM.)

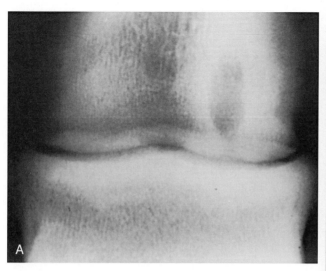

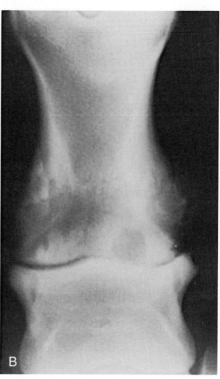

FIGURE 22–13. Dorsopalmar view of solitary, radiolucent subchondral bone defects (osteochondrosis) of the proximal phalanx. *A,* Elliptic defect with surrounding zone of sclerosis, without osteoarthrosis, in a 1-year-old Thoroughbred. *B,* Spheric defect surrounded by sclerotic subchondral bone. Collapse of contiguous joint space and periarticular osteophyte formation indicate the presence of osteoarthrosis in a 6-year-old Quarter horse that had been lame for 1 month.

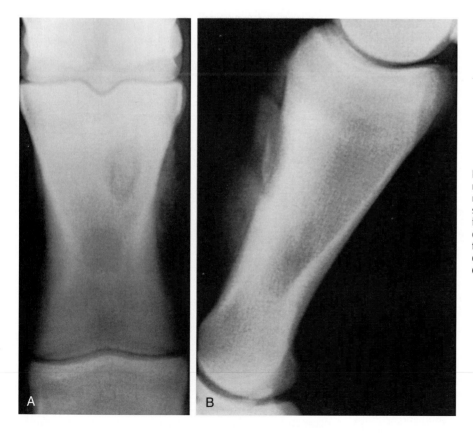

FIGURE 22–14. Sequestrum formation involving the proximal phalanx. *A,* In the dorsopalmar view, there is an ovoid radiolucent defect in the proximal part of the phalanx that surrounds a smaller oval opacity. Active periosteal new bone formation is also evident. *B,* In the lateromedial view, the cortical sequestrum, the defect in the underlying cortex, and the adjacent periosteal proliferation are visible. Sequestration of bone may be caused by trauma-induced avascular necrosis or by bacterial osteomyelitis.

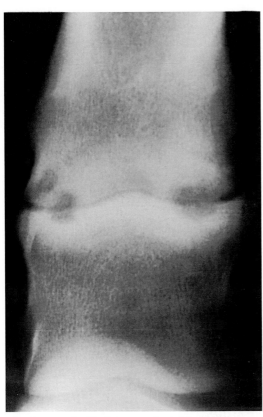

FIGURE 22–15. Decreased width of the proximal interphalangeal joint space with large, multiple, indistinctly margined subchondral bone defects. The radiographic signs in this foal are due to septic arthritis with erosion of articular cartilage leading to osteomyelitis of the subchondral epiphyseal bone. The absence of the periosteal reaction, which usually accompanies lysis owing to osteomyelitis, suggests a fulminating infection.

tesis or intra-articular corticosteroid therapy). The osseous defects represent osteomyelitis and necrosis at the subchondral bone and cartilage junction.[24] The adjacent joint space is often concomitantly narrowed owing to destruction of articular cartilage.

The pathogenesis of articular cartilage loss in degenerative joint disease is multifactorial, and its description is found elsewhere.[25–27] Multiple *punctate* radiolucent subchondral defects may be seen in combination with periarticular osteophytes, uneven narrowing of the joint space, and sclerosis in some horses with severe chronic degenerative joint disease.

Decreased Opacity Adjacent to the Physis

In the proximal or middle phalanx, this is a rare radiographic sign. Physeal growth disturbances usually affect the larger long bones. Septic embolization from bacteremia can produce sites of necrosis at multiple physes.

PROXIMAL PHALANX FRACTURE

Fractures of the proximal phalanx occur in different parts of the bone, depending on the type of stress applied. The most common fracture types are chip fracture at the proximal dorsal surface and spiral or longitudinal fracture of the body (diaphysis).[19, 28] Osteochondral fragments of the palmar or plantar proximal tuberosity are described in Chapter 21.

The most common fracture involving the proximal phalanx is the chip fracture of the proximal dorsomedial edge (Figs.

22–16 and 22–17).[28] Overextension of the metacarpophalangeal joint, as occurs with fatigue in racing horses, allows impaction of the dorsal edge of the proximal phalanx with the dorsal surface of the third metacarpus (MC III). The medial proximal margin of the proximal phalanx is larger in area than the lateral margin and therefore contacts MC III first during extension. The greater percentage of weight borne on the thoracic limbs results in a higher incidence of these fractures at the metacarpophalangeal joint. The size of the fragment, the amount of articular surface included, the presence or absence of degenerative joint disease, and any previous treatment with intra-articular corticosteroids are all taken into consideration (along with clinical signs of lameness or swelling and economic factors) when determining whether surgical excision of the fragment is warranted.[29, 30]

Three types of sagittal fractures occur in the proximal phalanx, each with distinct management needs and prognosis.[31, 32] First, incomplete fractures begin at the proximal articular surface and extend a variable distance (usually not more than 25% of the length of the bone) distally within the body. These are commonly found in the hindlimb of Standardbreds. Second, complete nondisplaced sagittal fractures extend from the proximal articular surface of the proximal phalanx to the proximal interphalangeal joint. These usually occur in the forelimbs of Thoroughbreds and hindlimbs of Standardbreds. Third, complete displaced simple fractures are due to the rotary force applied down through the midsagittal ridge of the third metatarsus (MT III) as the horse makes a sharp turn with the foot bearing full weight. Thus, a combination of twisting and axial compression occurs simultaneously. The rotating midsagittal ridge of MT III acts as a wedge driving

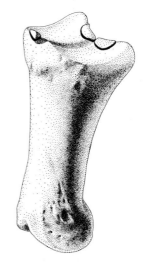
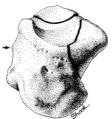

FIGURE 22–16. Dorsomedial view of the common sites of chip or avulsion fracture involving the proximal or middle phalanx. The most common fracture is chip fracture of the dorsomedial proximal tuberosity of the proximal phalanx. Avulsion fracture of the palmar (plantar) process of the proximal phalanx may involve the weight-bearing articular surface. Torsion while the digit is under maximal axial compression may cause fragmentation of the palmar or plantar processes of the middle phalanx. The *arrow* indicates the normal eminence for attachment of the collateral ligament of the distal interphalangeal joint. (Illustration by Richard A. Shook, DVM.)

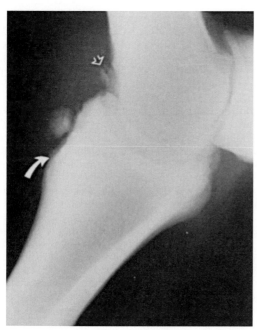

FIGURE 22–17. Lateromedial view of the metacarpophalangeal joint. Small chip fragments from the dorsoproximal edge of the proximal phalanx are evident *(open arrow)*. There is also periosteal proliferation and sclerosis *(curved arrow)* with avulsion fragmentation or dystrophic calcification of the insertion of the lateral digital extensor tendon.

into the more stationary proximal phalanx. Oblique projections are often necessary to evaluate completely the extent and direction of fracture planes, especially if internal fixation is contemplated. Careful evaluation of the radiograph may be required for identification of the incomplete spiral or longitudinal fracture (Fig. 22–18).

MIDDLE PHALANX FRACTURE

Fractures of the middle phalanx occur more frequently in the pelvic limb of middle-aged horses.[4] These fractures are also more common in horses that perform activities during which the bone is subject to extreme torque and compressive forces, for example, barrel racing, calf roping, and cutting. Types of fractures that occur in the middle phalanx include chip fracture (rare), fracture of a single caudal eminence (unusual), fracture of both lateral and medial caudal eminences (frequent), or comminuted fractures (most common) (Fig. 22–19).

Comminuted fractures most frequently involve the proximal interphalangeal joint but may also extend into the distal interphalangeal joint. If both joints are affected, the prognosis is considerably worse. In one study, a 50 percent survival rate and 10 percent chance of return to athletic function were reported in horses with biarticular involvement. Horses with a simple caudal eminence fracture involving only one articulation had an excellent prognosis for pasture soundness and greater than 30 percent chance of return to athletic function.[33] Because it is critical to identify accurately the number and direction of fracture planes and the extent of articular involvement, careful study of all four radiographic projections (see pastern examination, Table 22–1) should be used to gain a thorough understanding of the fracture configuration.[34]

ROENTGEN SIGNS OF INTERPHALANGEAL JOINT ABNORMALITIES

Alignment

Alteration in the relative position of the phalanges may occur owing to congenital, developmental, or traumatic causes.

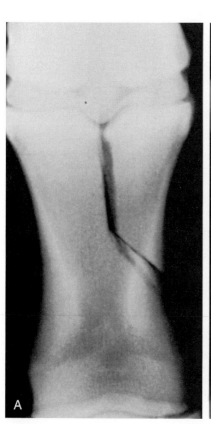
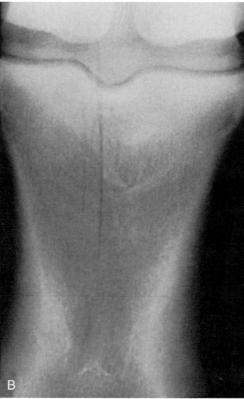

FIGURE 22–18. Complete *(A)* and incomplete *(B)* longitudinal fracture of the proximal phalanx. The plane of the primary x-ray beam must be parallel to the fracture plane to identify this lesion when no fragment displacement is present.

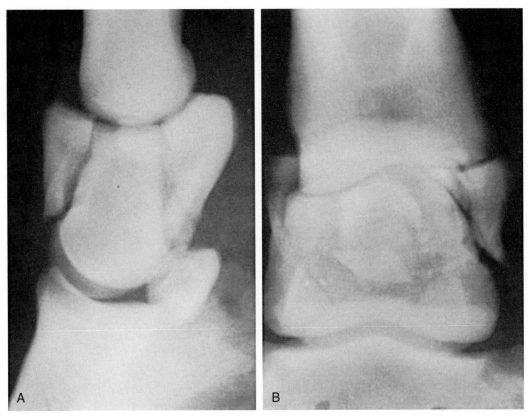

FIGURE 22–19. *A and B,* Comminuted, multiple fractures of the middle phalanx. In the lateromedial view *(A),* the palmar fracture extends into the distal interphalangeal joint in the area of the navicular bone.

Radiographs demonstrate the most common changes in alignment as dorsal or palmar subluxation of the affected joint.

Flexural Deformity of the Distal Interphalangeal Joint

The clinical appearance of an almost vertical hoof wall indicates an underlying increased flexion of the distal phalanx with respect to the middle phalanx (Fig. 22–20). This deformity may be either congenital or acquired. Factors that may lead to congenital deformities include genetic influences and teratogenic insults, such as pregnant mares ingesting locoweed, being fed goitrogenic diets, or experiencing influenza during embryonic developmental stages of gestation.[4, 35] The acquired form is frequently related to pain, which initiates a flexion withdrawal response; lack of exercise; or poor nutritional management in the growing foal. Both overfeeding and imbalanced diets have been cited as potentiating factors.[36] The exact manner in which these various influences interact to produce flexural deformities is unknown, but several theories suggest a difference in the rate of bone growth versus tendon and ligament lengthening.[36, 37] These theories all imply a faster rate of lengthening for bone than for the flexor tendon–check ligament unit.

It has been theorized that the deformity is caused by a rapid increase in length of MC III or MT III at its distal physis. Bone growth rate then occurs more rapidly than the rate at which the inferior check ligament (accessory ligament of the deep digital flexor tendon) can passively lengthen. Increasing tension on this tendon-ligament unit leads to flexion of the distal interphalangeal joint, with the foal assuming a "toe dancer" stance. Secondary changes that occur if the deformity persists include shortening of the joint capsules and suspen-

sory ligaments of the navicular bone and pododermatitis resulting from abnormal wearing of the hoof wall at the toe.[38, 39]

Flexural Deformity of the Proximal Interphalangeal Joint

This abnormal alignment is uncommon and may be either congenital or acquired (Fig. 22–21). Visually, there is bulge in the dorsal pastern contour that has been referred to as *dorsal subluxation.*[40, 41] Thoroughbred race horses have developed this malalignment following injury to the soft-tissue support structures of the metacarpophalangeal joint.[40] Dorsal subluxation has also occurred after corrective desmotomy of the suspensory ligament for treatment of flexural deformities of the metacarpophalangeal joint.[40] A number of young horses have been observed with this deformity in the hindleg. The flexion is prominent when the horse is non–weight-bearing, but with full weight the alignment is reduced, often accompanied by a clicking sound.[41, 42] A combination of deep digital flexor tendon contracture and concomitant superficial digital flexor tendon laxity has been postulated as the cause for this hindlimb deformity.[41]

Hyperextension of the Proximal Interphalangeal Joint

This is an unusual appearance that occurs with rupture of both the straight sesamoidean ligament and the superficial digital flexor tendon. It may also be seen in combination with overextension of the distal interphalangeal and metacarpophalangeal joints as a congenital deformity in foals.

Hyperextension of the Distal Interphalangeal Joint

This malalignment may occur in newborn foals as a congenital abnormality affecting all three joints of the foot, or it may

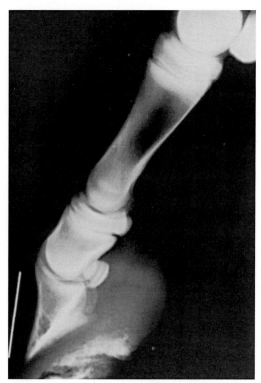

FIGURE 22–20. Flexural deformity of the distal interphalangeal joint in a 4-month-old foal. The dorsal surface of the distal phalanx remains parallel to the dorsal hoof wall *(white line),* but both of these structures assume an abnormally vertical position.

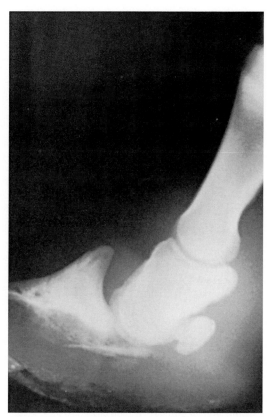

FIGURE 22–22. Luxation of the distal interphalangeal joint secondary to osteomyelitis and pathologic fracture of the flexor surface of the distal phalanx. Dorsal displacement of the distal phalanx is due to avulsion of the deep digital flexor tendon insertion and the subsequent unreciprocated pull of the common digital extensor tendon. The distal sesamoidean impar ligament is also ruptured, allowing proximal displacement of the navicular bone.

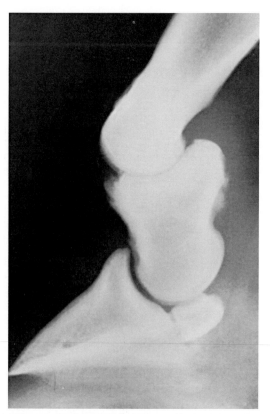

FIGURE 22–21. Dorsal subluxation of the proximal interphalangeal joint. Enthesophytes of the dorsal joint capsule and superficial digital flexor tendon insertion indicate the chronicity of this injury.

be seen in adults owing to an acquired lesion affecting only the distal interphalangeal joint. In the foal, the flexor tendons may be weak at birth, thus providing inadequate support for the digit and allowing the metacarpophalangeal joint to contact the ground. Weakened flexor tendons may also be seen secondary to poor nutrition, secondary to slow or incomplete recovery from a systemic disease, or after prolonged periods of external support (splinting or casting) of the leg.[31] Acquired overextension is seen with rupture of the deep digital flexor tendon or avulsion of its insertion (Fig. 22–22). This lesion occurs with traumatic laceration of the tendon or extension of infection from a deep sole abscess to the palmar surface of the distal phalanx.

Pericapsular Soft Tissues

Roentgen signs include alteration of thickness or opacity of the tissues surrounding the joints. To visualize these changes, technical factors must allow definition of soft tissue as well as bone. Use of a relatively higher kVp and lower mAs produces a radiograph with longer scale of contrast and better resolution of soft tissues.

Increased pericapsular soft-tissue thickness may be seen with intracapsular fluid accumulation, extracapsular inflammation (cellulitis), or fibrosis. If radiographic signs of soft-tissue enlargement are strictly confined to the region of the joint, intracapsular fluid accumulation is the likely cause. If the enlargement extends proximally and distally beyond the sites of joint capsule attachment, extracapsular fluid or fibrosis is present, which obscures evaluation of intracapsular changes.

Increased opacity within pericapsular soft tissues is usually due to dystrophic mineralization. Lesions that commonly become mineralized include chronic sprain or strain of supporting ligaments (see Fig. 22–17), pericapsular deposition of corticosteroids, or focal necrosis secondary to neurectomy (Fig. 22–23). Ossification of the collateral cartilages of the third phalanx should not be mistaken for dystrophic mineralization of soft tissue (see under Ossification of Collateral Cartilages [Sidebones]).

Decreased opacity within the soft tissues is associated with the presence of air or gas in the subcutis or fascial planes of tendons and ligaments. Soft-tissue gas commonly follows diagnostic nerve block, open skin wound, or rarely a gas-producing organism.

Joint Space Width and Subchondral Bone Opacity

Joint space width and subchondral bone opacity are two important roentgen signs of joint disease that are considered together because the appearance of the subchondral bone affects the visualization of the joint space. Figure 22–24 illustrates normal and abnormal appearances of bone and joint space in a stylized proximal interphalangeal joint. In the normal proximal interphalangeal joint (see Fig. 22–24A), the subchondral bone is smooth, broader, and more opaque in the middle phalanx than in the proximal phalanx. The zone of soft-tissue opacity between the adjacent bones is commonly referred to as the *joint space*, although it is actually produced by the opposing articular cartilages of the proximal and middle phalanges. In a radiograph of a normal horse

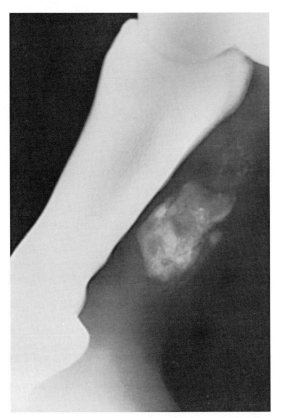

FIGURE 22–23. Dystrophic calcification in the palmar soft tissues secondary to previous neurectomy.

obtained during weight bearing, this zone should be of uniform width across the entire surface of the joint.

Increased Width, No Change in Subchondral Bone

The most common cause of this radiographic appearance is the lame horse that is non–weight-bearing at the time of radiography (see Fig. 22–24B). Lack of axial weight compression allows slight distraction of the adjacent bones, to the limit allowed by the joint capsule and supporting collateral ligaments. This roentgen sign may also be seen in early septic arthritis, when increased synovial fluid accumulation and exudate are present in the joint cavity but before osseous changes occur.[43] Generally, in animals evaluated for suspected joint disease, the process has progressed beyond this stage.

Increased Width, Decreased Opacity, and Irregular Contour of Subchondral Bone

This appearance indicates an aggressive process that is eroding both articular cartilage and subchondral bone (see Fig. 22–24C). These signs occur most frequently in septic arthritis that has extended to osteomyelitis. Increased joint width suggests production of large amounts of exudate or cellular debris.

Decreased Width, Subchondral Bone Uniform in Opacity, With or Without Sclerosis

This abnormality may affect the entire width of the joint evenly, or it may occur in only part of the joint (see Fig. 22–24D). Pathologic narrowing of the joint space is caused by loss of articular cartilage because of injury or conformational defect and subsequent abnormal wear of cartilage surfaces. Artifactual narrowing of the entire joint space may be produced by angulation of the primary x-ray beam such that the beam and joint surface are no longer parallel.

Decreased Width, Irregular Contour, and Nonuniform Opacity of Subchondral Bone

This combination of abnormalities may be seen in the septic joint after erosion of articular cartilage with extension of infection to the subchondral bone (see Fig. 22–15) or in chronic osteoarthrosis owing to instability, in which cystic degenerative changes are occurring in the subchondral bone (see Fig. 22–24E). Sclerosis of adjacent portions of the proximal or middle phalanx occurs with advancing chronicity of the lesion. The radiolucent defects seen in the subchondral bone owing to inflammation are usually multiple and small and have poorly defined margins when compared with lesions produced by osteochondrosis (see Fig. 22–13).

Increased Width on One Side of Joint Only, No Subchondral Bone Changes

If the metacarpophalangeal joint and both interphalangeal joints show similar widening, the patient is probably not bearing weight evenly on the foot (see Fig. 22–24F). Asymmetric weight distribution causes the unloaded side of the joint to be wider than the loaded side of the joint. This is a common radiographic artifact.

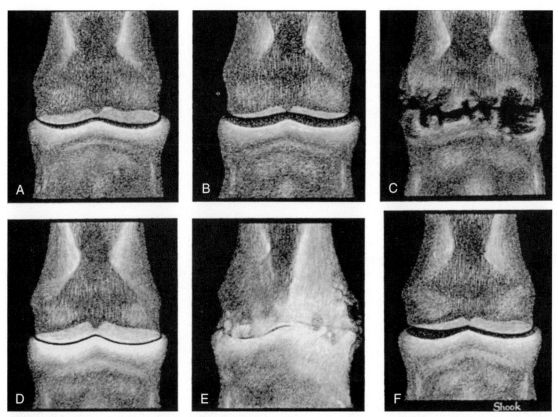

FIGURE 22–24. Common changes in joint space width, subchondral bone opacity, or both, seen in the proximal interphalangeal joint. *A,* Normal joint space and subchondral bone. *B,* Widened joint space, no subchondral bone changes—non–weight-bearing at time of radiography or increased intra-articular fluid volume. *C,* Widened joint space, lysis of subchondral bone—active septic arthritis. *D,* Uniformly narrowed joint space, no subchondral bone changes—artifact caused by angulation of the primary x-ray beam or degenerative wearing and loss of articular cartilage. *E,* Narrowed joint space, irregular opacity and contour of subchondral bone—chronic low-grade septic arthritis or chronic osteoarthritis owing to trauma-related instability or poor conformation. *F,* Widened joint space on the lateral or medial side, no subchondral bone changes—asymmetric weight distribution on the foot (a common artifact). (Illustration by Richard A. Shook, DVM.)

Periarticular Bone Margins

New bone formation often occurs in the interphalangeal area in association with chronic joint diseases. One pattern of bone proliferation is a sharply margined lipping of the periarticular surface in response to instability of the joint. This appearance is seen frequently in the proximal interphalangeal joint, in which remodeling of the opposing bones creates a flatter, broader articular surface, with spiculated osteophytes along the edge of the middle phalanx (Fig. 22–25). Instability may be primary (congenital malformation of articular surfaces and poor conformation) or secondary (trauma owing to overuse, laceration of supporting ligaments, sequelae after intra-articular fracture, or large osteochondrosis defect). Another common type of new bone formation is the enthesophyte (bone spur), which forms at the attachment site of the joint capsule or collateral ligaments (see Figs. 22–11 and 22–21). As previously stated, these areas of new bone growth indicate ossification of the fibro-osseous attachment or focal stimulation of underlying periosteum.[27]

ROENTGEN SIGNS IN THE DISTAL PHALANX

Number

A supernumerary distal phalanx may be seen in polydactylism, as previously described. Agenesis of the distal phalanx has also been reported.[44] Abnormalities of this magnitude are uncommon.

Position

The normal orientation of the distal phalanx to the hoof is maintained by the interdigitating leaves of the laminar corium and the horn-like lamellae of the hoof wall. The laminar corium is attached to the dorsal surface of the distal phalanx by a modified periosteum, which contains a tightly meshed network of blood vessels.[45]

Palmar deviation (rotation) of the toe of the distal phalanx is a common occurrence in laminitis. The earliest radiographically detectable sign of laminitis has been described as an increased thickness (>20 mm) of the soft tissues dorsal to the distal phalanx as seen on the lateral view (Fig. 22–26).[12] This thickening of laminar tissues occurs without palmar deviation and can be seen as early as 48 to 72 hours after the onset of laminitis.[46]

Numerous causes for acute laminitis have been proposed, including vasoconstriction of the digital vessels, microthrombosis, perivascular edema, and arteriovenous shunting at the coronary band.[47-51] Mechanistic causes may vary with the inciting cause and amount of time during the developmental stages of acute laminitis. The resulting necrosis or ischemia of the laminae and lamellae of the foot, however, results in loss of support for the dorsal surface of the distal phalanx. With loss of the laminar or lamellar junction, the weight of the horse, the leverage force placed at the toe (as the hoof breaks over in midstride), and the pulling force of the deep digital flexor tendon combine to force the toe mechanically away from the hoof wall (Fig. 22–27).[4, 50]

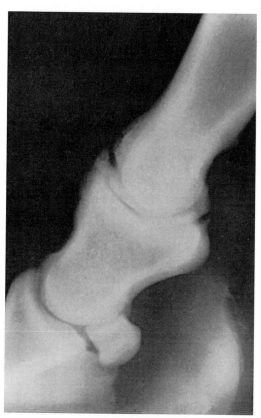

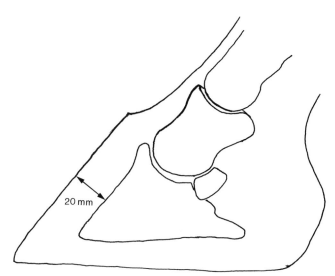

FIGURE 22–26. The earliest radiographic sign that may be seen with laminitis is thickening of the soft tissues dorsal to the distal phalanx, that is, when this measurement *(black arrow)* is greater than 20 mm.[46] The normal mean (±SD) for dorsal hoof wall soft-tissue thickness in Thoroughbreds has been reported to be 14.3 (±1.0) mm at the region indicated by the black arrow.[12]

FIGURE 22–25. Osteoarthrosis of the proximal interphalangeal joint. The contours of the opposing surfaces of the proximal and middle phalanx are flattened. The articular surfaces are also broader as a result of remodeling and new bone formation at the periarticular margins. These periarticular osteophytes are often sharply spiculated in the mildly unstable joint.

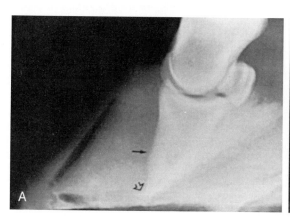

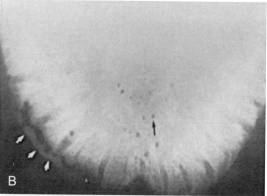

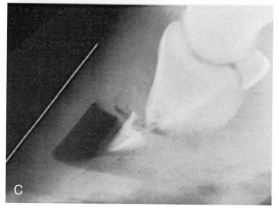

FIGURE 22–27. *A,* Severe palmar deviation-rotation of the distal phalanx owing to laminitis. Gas is seen between the hoof wall and the soft tissues of the corium. Indistinct dorsal surface *(solid arrow)* and angulation ("ski-tip" appearance) of the toe of the distal phalanx *(open arrow)* are additional changes seen in chronic laminitis. *B,* Pathologic type VI fracture of the distal phalanx secondary to laminitis. A thin bone segment is separated from the solar margin *(white arrows).* Punctate radiolucent defects *(black arrow)* are enlarged vascular channels viewed end-on. *C,* Fracture of the toe with concurrent palmar deviation-rotation and a large accumulation of gas between the hoof wall and the laminar corium.

Linear radiolucency at the laminar or lamellar junction is another radiographic abnormality that may be seen with acute laminitis. This is seen as a single linear lucency on the lateral view or as a series of parallel linear lucencies in the dorsal 65-degree–proximal-palmarodistal oblique view of the third phalanx. This linear radiolucency has been attributed to air dissecting between the hoof wall and the laminar corium when necrosis has eroded through to the coronary band or white zone of the sole or to nitrogen that moves from the blood into the partial vacuum created by the displacement of the toe and the adjacent lamina.[52]

Chronic laminitis may be characterized by the following radiographic changes in the distal phalanx: palmar deviation of the toe, indistinct dorsal surface, increased number of vascular channels directed to the dorsal surface, pathologic fracture of the toe, and remodeled shape of the toe to an elongated "ski-tip" appearance. These changes are demonstrated in Figure 22–27. The degree of distal phalanx deviation has been used as a prognostic sign in the evaluation of horses with laminitis. In a series of 91 horses, the degree of rotation was inversely correlated with return to athletic performance. Horses with less than 5.5 degrees of deviation had a favorable prognosis for return to athletic work, horses with 6.8 to 11.5 degrees of deviation had a guarded prognosis, and horses with more than 11.5 degrees of deviation were not useful as performance animals, but some could be salvaged for breeding.[53] In a more recent study, however, the degree of rotation or distal displacement of the distal phalanx did not correlate with outcome, and lameness severity was a more accurate predictor.[54] Thus, additional factors such as degree of lameness and rapidity of response to therapy should also be considered when evaluating prognosis.[55]

Dorsal displacement of the distal phalanx is uncommon, occurring secondary to stretching or rupture of the deep digital flexor tendon. The phalanx maintains its orientation to the hoof wall so that the toe of the hoof is also elevated from the ground (see Fig. 22–22).

Contour

Alterations in contour are those changes that affect the normal shape of the margins of the distal phalanx. The location of the radiographic abnormality may provide a clue to the cause of the lesion.

Indistinct, Domed Dorsal Margin

This sign, seen on the lateromedial view, indicates chronic strain on the modified periosteum, resulting in minimal periosteal proliferation (see Fig. 22–27A). When these changes are chronic, the normal straight dorsal surface of the distal phalanx becomes rounded. This appearance is one of the radiographic signs of previous chronic laminitis or other focal inflammation.

Indistinct, Irregular Solar Margin

Diffuse roughening of the solar border, creating a ragged, lacy appearance when viewed on the lateromedial or dorsal 65-degree–proximal-palmarodistal oblique projection, may be an indication of chronic bruising and mild inflammatory response (pedal osteitis). Because there is considerable variation in the appearance of the solar surface of the normal distal phalanx, however, this radiographic sign may be misleading. A positive response to hoof testers; an increased number and diameter of vascular channels, seen concomitantly with demineralization of the toe; and thinning of the sole of the foot increase the probability of pedal osteitis as a current cause of lameness. It should be noted that once pedal osteitis becomes inactive, there is frequently little change in the appearance of the roughened contour of the solar margin. Thus, clinical signs must be considered to determine whether a radiographically irregular margin of the distal phalanx is an indicator of current or previous pathology.

Irregular Extensor Process

A defect at the base of the extensor process or fragment proximal to the process indicates fracture or incomplete ossification of this structure. Fractures may occur owing to abnormal strain on the common digital extensor tendon or to overextension of the distal interphalangeal joint. Because this abnormality can be bilateral, incomplete development from separate centers of ossification must be considered as another possible cause. Small bone opacities adjacent to the process are not considered significant if the horse is clinically sound. When the articular surface is involved, the defect is more important and may lead to secondary osteoarthritis of the distal interphalangeal joint (Fig. 22–28).[56]

Irregular Fragmentation at the Toe

Solar margin fractures have been added to the standard classification of distal phalanx fractures as type VI.[57] Table 22–2 lists descriptions of each fracture type. Type VI fractures may be traumatic or pathologic in origin. Pathologic type VI fractures occur secondary to pedal osteitis, laminitis, or osteomyelitis, and the associated roentgen signs of the latter lesions accompany the fragments seen at the solar margin. Bone fragments are usually thin and may be overlooked if exposure factors are not optimal or if the foot is not properly cleaned before radiographic examination.

Table 22–2
CLASSIFICATION OF DISTAL PHALANX FRACTURES

Type	Description	Prognosis
I	Nonarticular fracture of palmar or plantar process	Good outcome with corrective shoeing and 3–12 mo rest
II	Articular fracture extending from the distal interphalangeal joint to the solar margin	Guarded
III	Midsagittal articular fracture that divides the phalanx into equal parts	Guarded
IV	Extensor process fracture	Guarded for large fragments with articular involvement
V	Comminuted fracture of body or fracture owing to foreign object penetration or osteomyelitis	Insufficient data to determine
VI	Solar margin fracture	Good outcome if not complicated by laminitis or severe pedal osteitis

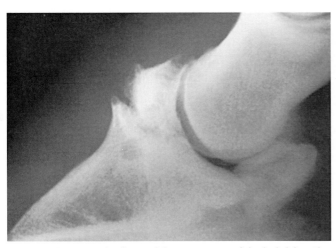

FIGURE 22–28. Long-standing fracture of the extensor process of the distal phalanx. The fracture extends into the articular surface of the distal interphalangeal joint and has led to degenerative osteoarthrosis.

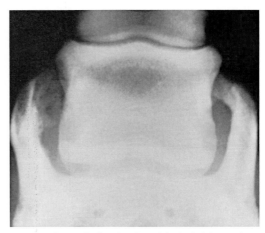

FIGURE 22–29. Ossification of collateral cartilage of the distal phalanx. Uniform ossification is seen in both the lateral and the medial collateral cartilage. Such advanced changes usually do not cause lameness if the foot is broad at the heel.

Ossification of Collateral Cartilages (Sidebones)

This is a common finding in radiographs of the distal part of the digit, especially in draft breed horses. When the proximal edge of the ossified collateral cartilage extends beyond the proximal margin of the navicular bone, sidebone formation is considered present[11] (Fig. 22–29). Even an extensive degree of ossification may not be clinically significant, especially in older horses, horses with a broad foot, and horses that have no pain on manipulation of the heel area.

Asymmetric calcification of the collateral cartilages may indicate increased stress on the ossified portion (Fig. 22–30). Careful physical examination is warranted in such an instance to determine if localized disease is present within the foot. The appearance of the navicular bone should also be closely evaluated in the previous example because collateral cartilage ossification may accompany a more significant degenerative lesion in the navicular bone.[56]

A radiolucent linear defect or gap in the ossified cartilage usually indicates the junction between a separate, peripheral ossification center and that part of the cartilage that is ossifying from the palmar process of the phalanx. In a study of Finnish trotters, almost all radiolucent gaps between separate ossification centers were located in the middle or distal part of the ossified cartilage.[58] Fracture of the ossified collateral

cartilage is unusual. Response to digital pressure applied at the coronary band in the area of the suspect fracture helps to differentiate a fracture from an incomplete pattern of ossification.

Radiopacity

Abnormal opacity identified in the distal phalanx is most often radiolucent. The shape and number of abnormal opacities commonly found are subsequently described.

Solitary Linear Decreased Opacity

Traumatic fracture is the most common cause of this sign. Osteomyelitis and improper shoeing have also been suggested as possible causes for fracture of the distal phalanx. Because the hoof wall restricts displacement of a bone fragment, diagnosis of the fracture depends on visualization of the fracture line. If the plane of the primary x-ray beam is not parallel to the fracture plane, the superimposed parts of the bone obscure the fracture line, and diagnosis may be missed.

Therefore, four views of the distal phalanx are recommended when a fracture is suspected: (1) dorsal 65-degree–proximal-palmarodistal oblique with the horse standing on

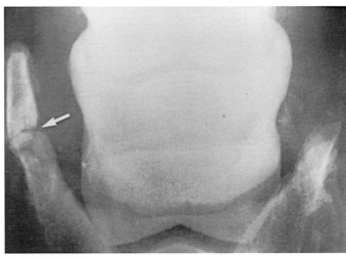

FIGURE 22–30. Asymmetric ossification of the collateral cartilage of the distal phalanx may indicate abnormal stress on the affected side of the foot and warrants close examination of the heel and navicular bone for additional abnormalities. The radiolucent defect *(arrow)* is a cartilage remnant between two separate centers of ossification, not a fracture.

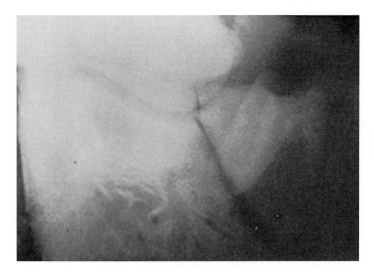

FIGURE 22–31. Type II fracture of the distal phalanx. Dorsal 65-degree–proximal 45-degree–lateral-palmarodistomedial view. This projection is often necessary to determine whether the fracture extends into the distal interphalangeal joint, as it does in this horse.

the cassette, (2) lateromedial, (3) dorsal 65-degree–proximal 45-degree–lateral-palmarodistomedial oblique, and (4) dorsal 65-degree–proximal 45-degree–medial-palmarodistolateral oblique (see Table 22–2 for fracture description classification).[32, 57]

Type II fractures were found most often in one report of 65 horses.[59] The lesions usually involved the lateral aspect of the left front distal phalanx or the medial aspect of the right front distal phalanx (Fig. 22–31).[59, 60] In that series, of fractures in racehorses, the forelimb that bore the most weight in turns was at greatest risk (horses were raced counterclockwise). Another report of 274 horses found that type VI was the most frequently identified type of fracture.[57]

The progression of healing of a distal phalanx fracture is difficult to determine radiographically owing to the minimal amount of external osseous callus produced by this bone.

The periosteum of the distal phalanx is poorly developed and does not respond aggressively to the stimulation of direct trauma. Treatment by corrective shoeing and stall rest has led to healing in 3 to 19 months, with young horses and nonarticular fractures showing the most rapid and complete progression to bony union.

Palmar process ossicles have been identified radiographically in the forelimbs of foals aged 3 to 32 weeks.[61] Although it has been suggested that these ossicles may be separate centers of ossification, the appearance in the majority of foals studied was consistent with fracture healing.[13, 61] Radiographically, these are seen as triangular-to-oblong fragments. Radiography is an insensitive method for identifying all foals affected with these fractures, however. Lameness directly attributed to these fractures is uncommon. Foals through 12 weeks of age have a lucent line between the proximal and

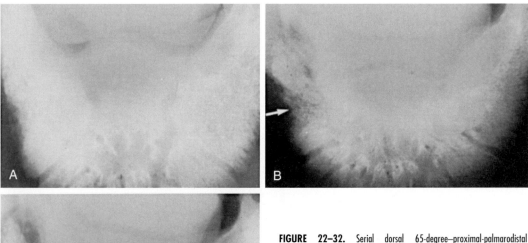

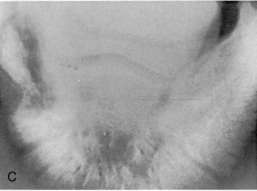

FIGURE 22–32. Serial dorsal 65-degree–proximal-palmarodistal projections of the palmar processes of the distal phalanx in an acutely lame 5-year-old Thoroughbred. *A,* Initial examination shows minimal radiographic abnormality. *B,* Six days later, a radiolucent defect *(arrow)* is evident in the medial palmar process with loss of trabecular bone detail (compare with lateral palmar process). *C,* Nine days later, more extensive lysis of bone has occurred, with separation of a sequestered fragment. The radiographic diagnosis is osteomyelitis with sequestrum formation.

distal angles of the palmar process. This line is normal and should not be mistaken for a fracture.

Multiple Linear Decreased Opacities

This appearance is usually due to increased size and number of vascular channels (hypervascularity) secondary to inflammation from laminitis (see Fig. 22–27) or chronic bruising of the sole and distal phalanx (pedal osteitis).

Solitary Rounded Decreased Opacity

If the defect is sharply defined with a distinct margin between it and the rest of the phalanx, the lesion may be a bone cyst; a remnant of an old, currently inactive infection; osteochondrosis; or, rarely, a congenital vascular malformation or keratoma.[56, 62–64] If the margin of the defect is indistinct and tends to fade into the surrounding bone, an infectious lesion, such as an abscess and osteomyelitis with sequestration, should be considered.[63] Figure 22–32 illustrates serial radiographs that were made of the distal phalanx of a horse with a draining tract over a period of 15 days. These images illustrate the degree and rapidity of osseous destruction that may occur with osteomyelitis. Repeat or follow-up radiographs may be useful in the work-up of the persistently lame horse in which no radiographic changes were initially noted.

RADIOGRAPHIC INTERPRETATION

Use of the roentgen sign approach may assist greatly in understanding and interpreting radiographic abnormalities in the equine phalanges. Many of the osseous or joint changes discussed in this text, however, do not completely remodel when the initial stimulus that created them is removed or the disease process reaches an inactive state. Therefore, determining the current significance of lesions seen on radiographs can be difficult, especially in the acutely lame horse with radiographic evidence of previous disease. Additionally, in some instances of acute lameness, pathologic changes occurring in the bone have not progressed to the severity that makes them radiographically detectable. Nuclear imaging techniques appear to offer significant advantages over radiography in these situations. The radionuclide bone scan is a sensitive test for early bone injury because it reflects changes in skeletal mineral metabolism and physiology rather than in bone density (g/cm^3) and structure. Bone scans have also been used to determine the degree of activity of radiographically identified lesions.[65] Although nuclear scintigraphic examination is not practical for the private practitioner, many university teaching hospitals and some private veterinary referral centers have the capability to perform these studies, and referral for this examination is possible.

References

1. Nyrop KA, Coffman JR, DeBowes RM, et al: The role of diagnostic nerve blocks in the equine lameness examination. Comp Contin Ed Vet Pract 5:S669, 1983.
2. Morgan P, and Silverman S: Techniques of Veterinary Radiography, 3rd Ed. Davis, CA, Veterinary Radiology Associates, 1982.
3. Morgan JP, Neves J, and Baker T: Equine Radiography. Ames, Iowa State University Press, 1991.
4. Stashak TS: Adams' Lameness in Horses. Philadelphia, Lea & Febiger, 1987.
5. Ticer JW: Radiographic Positioning and Technique in Veterinary Practice. Philadelphia, WB Saunders, 1984.
6. Schebitz H, and Wilkens H: Atlas of Radiographic Anatomy of the Horse. Philadelphia, WB Saunders, 1978.
7. Smallwood JE, and Holliday SD: Xeroradiographic anatomy of the equine digit and metacarpophalangeal region. Vet Radiol 28:166, 1987.
8. Bushe T, Turner TA, Poulos P, et al: The effect of hoof angle on coffin, pastern, and fetlock joint angles. Proc Am Assoc Equine Pract 33:729, 1987.
9. Kneller SK, and Losonsky JM: Variable locations of nutrient foramina of the proximal phalanx in forelimbs of Thoroughbreds. J Am Vet Med Assoc 197:736, 1990.
10. Rendano VT, and Grant B: The equine third phalanx: Its radiographic appearance. J Am Vet Radiol Soc 19:125, 1978.
11. Butler FA, Colles CM, Dyson SJ, et al: Clinical Radiology of the Horse. London, Blackwell Scientific Publications, 1993.
12. Linford RL, O'Brien TR, and Trout DR: Qualitative and morphometric radiographic findings in the distal phalanx and digital soft tissues of sound Thoroughbred racehorses. Am J Vet Res 54:38, 1993.
13. Kaneps AJ, Stover SM, and O'Brien TR: Radiographic characteristics of the forelimb distal phalanx and microscopic morphology of the lateral palmar process in foals 3–32 weeks old. Vet Radiol Ultrasound 36:179, 1995.
14. Weaver JCB, Stover SM, and O'Brien TR: Radiographic anatomy of soft tissue attachments in the equine metacarpophalangeal and proximal phalangeal region. Equine Vet J 24:310, 1992.
15. Messer NT, and Powers BE: Hypertrophic osteopathy associated with pulmonary infarction in a horse. Comp Contin Ed Vet Pract 5:S636, 1983.
16. Trotter GW, McIlwraith CW, Norrdin RW, et al: Degenerative joint disease with osteochondrosis of the proximal interphalangeal joint in young horses. J Am Vet Med Assoc 180:1312, 1982.
17. Trotter GW, and McIlwraith CW: Osteochondritis dissecans and subchondral cystic lesions and their relationship to osteochondrosis in the horse. Equine Vet Sci 5:157, 1981.
18. Trotter GW, and McIlwraith CW: Osteochondrosis in horses: Pathogenesis and clinical syndromes. In Proceedings of the 27th Annual Convention of the American Association of Equine Practitioners, New Orleans, 1981, pp 141–160.
19. McIlwraith CW, and Goodman NL: Conditions of the interphalangeal joints. Vet Clin North Am [Equine Pract] 5:161, 1989.
20. Pettersson H, and Reiland S: Periarticular subchondral bone cysts in horses. Clin Orthop 62:95, 1969.
21. Attenburrow DP, and Heyse-Moore GH: Non-ossifying fibroma in phalanx of a Thoroughbred yearling. Equine Vet J 14:59, 1982.
22. Hackett RP: Intra-articular use of corticosteroids in the horse. J Am Vet Med Assoc 181:292, 1982.
23. Pool RR, Wheat JD, and Ferraro GL: Corticosteroid therapy in common joint and tendon injuries of the horse: I. Effects on joints. In Proceedings of the 26th Annual Convention of the American Association of Equine Practitioners, Anaheim, CA, 1980, pp 397–406.
24. Firth EC: Current concepts of infectious polyarthritis in foals. Equine Vet J 15:5, 1983.
25. McIlwraith CW: Idiopathic synovitis, traumatic arthritis and degenerative joint disease. In Proceedings of the 27th Annual Convention of the American Association of Equine Practitioners, New Orleans, 1981, pp 125–139.
26. McIlwraith CW: Pathobiology and diagnosis of equine joint disease. In Proceedings of the 27th Annual Convention of the American Association of Equine Practitioners, New Orleans, 1981, pp 115–123.
27. Pool RR, and Meagher DM: Pathologic findings and pathogenesis of racetrack injuries. Vet Clin North Am [Equine Pract] 6:1, 1990.
28. Kawcak CE, and McIlwraith CW: Proximodorsal first phalanx osteochondral chip fragmentation in 336 horses. Equine Vet J 26:392, 1994.
29. Yovich JV, and McIlwraith CW: Arthroscopic surgery for osteochondral fractures of the proximal phalanx of the metacarpophalangeal and metatarsophalangeal joints in horses. J Am Vet Med Assoc 188:273, 1986.
30. Speirs VC: Assessment of the economic value of orthopedic surgery in Thoroughbred racehorses. Vet Clin North Am [Large Anim Pract] 5:391, 1983.
31. Foerner JJ, and McIlwraith CW: Orthopedic surgery in the racehorse. Vet Clin North Am [Equine Pract] 6:147, 1990.
32. Gabel AA, and Bukowiecki CF: Fractures of the phalanges. Vet Clin North Am [Large Anim Pract] 5:233, 1983.
33. Colahan PT, Wheat JD, and Meagher DM: Treatment of middle phalangeal fractures in the horse. J Am Vet Med Assoc 178:1182, 1981.
34. Doran RE, White NA, and Allen D: Use of a bone plate for treatment of middle phalangeal fractures in horses: Seven cases (1979–1984). J Am Vet Med Assoc 191:575, 1987.
35. McIlwraith CW, and James LF: Limb deformities in foals associated with ingestion of locoweed by mares. J Am Vet Med Assoc 181:255, 1982.
36. Owen JM: Abnormal flexion of the corono-pedal joint or "contracted tendons" in unweaned foals. Equine Vet J 7:40, 1975.
37. Fackelman GE: Equine flexural deformities of developmental origin. In Proceedings of the 26th Annual Convention of the American Association of Equine Practitioners, Anaheim, CA, 1980, pp 97–105.
38. Fackelman, GE: Tendon surgery. Vet Clin North Am [Large Anim Pract] 5:381, 1983.
39. Fackelman GE, Auer JA, Orsini J, et al: Surgical treatment of severe flexural deformity of the distal interphalangeal joint in young horses. J Am Vet Med Assoc 182:949, 1983.

40. Grant BD: The pastern joint. *In* Mansmann RA, and McAllister EG (Eds): Equine Medicine and Surgery, 3rd Ed. Santa Barbara, CA, American Veterinary Publications, 1982, p 1056.

41. Shiroma JT, Engel HN, Wagner PC, et al: Dorsal subluxation of the proximal interphalangeal joint in the pelvic limb of three horses. J Am Vet Med Assoc *195*:777, 1989.

42. Wagner PC, and Watrous BJ: Equine Pediatric Orthopedics—A Practitioner Monograph. Santa Barbara, CA, Veterinary Practice Publishing, 1991.

43. Barber SM: Subluxation and sepsis of the distal interphalangeal joint of a horse. J Am Vet Med Assoc *181*:491, 1982.

44. Taylor TS, and Morris EL: Agenesis of the distal phalanx in a mule. Vet Radiol *24*:63, 1983.

45. Kainer RA: Clinical anatomy of the equine foot. Vet Clin North Am [Equine Pract] *5*:1, 1989.

46. O'Brien TR, and Baker TW: Distal extremity examination: How to perform the radiographic examination and interpret the radiographs. *In* Proceedings of the 32nd Annual Convention of the American Association of Equine Practitioners, Nashville, 1986, pp 553–566.

47. Ackerman N, Garner HE, Coffman JR, et al: Angiographic appearance of the normal equine foot and alterations in chronic laminitis. J Am Vet Med Assoc *166*:58, 1975.

48. Colles CM, Garner HE, and Coffman JR: The blood supply of the horse's foot. *In* Proceedings of the 25th Annual Convention of the American Association of Equine Practitioners, Miami, 1979, pp 385–389.

49. Hood DM, and Stephens KA: Physiopathology of equine laminitis. Comp Contin Ed Vet Pract *3*:S454, 1981.

50. Coffman JR, Johnson JH, Finocchio EJ, et al: Biomechanics of pedal rotation in equine laminitis. J Am Vet Med Assoc *156*:219, 1970.

51. Goetz TE: Anatomic, hoof and shoeing considerations for the treatment of laminitis in horses. J Am Vet Med Assoc *190*:1323, 1987.

52. O'Brien TR: Personal communication. Davis, University of California, Davis, 1996.

53. Stick JA, Jann HW, Scott EA, et al: Pedal bone rotation as a prognostic sign in laminitis of horses. J Am Vet Med Assoc *180*:251, 1982.

54. Hunt RJ: A retrospective evaluation of laminitis in horses. Equine Vet J *25*:61, 1993.

55. Baxter GM: Acute laminitis. Vet Clin North Am [Equine Pract] *10*:627, 1994.

56. Reid CF: Radiography and the purchase examination in the horse. Vet Clin North Am [Large Anim Pract] *2*:151, 1980.

57. Honnas CH, O'Brien TR, and Linford RL: Distal phalanx fractures in horses: A survey of 274 horses with radiographic assessment of healing in 36 horses. Vet Radiol *29*:98, 1989.

58. Ruohoniemi M, Tulamo R-M, and Hackzell M: Radiographic evaluation of ossification of the collateral cartilages of the third phalanx in Finnhorses. Equine Vet J *25*:453, 1993.

59. Scott EA, McDole M, and Shires MH: A review of third phalanx fractures in the horse: 65 cases. J Am Vet Med Assoc *174*:1337, 1979.

60. Scott EA, McDole M, Shires MH, et al: Fractures of the third phalanx (P₃) in the horse at Michigan State University, 1964–1979. *In* Proceedings of the 25th Annual Convention of the American Association of Equine Practitioners, Miami, 1979, pp 439–449.

61. Kaneps AF, O'Brien TR, Feddem RF, et al: Characterization of osseous bodies of the distal phalanx of foals. Equine Vet J *25*:285, 1993.

62. Vershooten F, and De Moor A: Subchondral cystic and related lesions affecting the equine pedal bone and stifle. Equine Vet J *14*:47, 1982.

63. Baird AN, Seahorn TL, and Morris EL: Equine distal phalangeal sequestration. Vet Radiol *31*:210, 1990.

64. Lloyd KCK, Peterson PR, Wheat JD, et al: Keratomas in horses: Seven cases (1975–1986). J Am Vet Med Assoc *193*:967, 1988.

65. Chambers MD, Martinelli MJ, Baker GJ, et al: Nuclear medicine for diagnosis of lameness in horses. J Am Vet Med Assoc *206*:792, 1995.

STUDY QUESTIONS

1. A 7-year-old Quarter horse mare, retired from racing, presented with a history of intermittent lameness of the right front leg when exercised. There is pain in the proximal interphalangeal joint. Radiographs of this region show multiple, small radiolucent subchondral bone defects in the distal first phalanx, accompanied by a narrowed joint space and mature periarticular osteophytes. The radiographic changes are most likely those of:
   A. Severe chronic degenerative joint disease.
   B. Osteochondrosis.
   C. Acute, active septic osteoarthritis.

2. A focal area of solid, ovoid calcification is identified in the soft tissues palmar and slightly proximal to the proximal border of the navicular bone on the lateromedial view of the foot of a 10-year-old Quarter horse gelding. What additional radiographic projection would provide the best image to determine whether this calcification is within the collateral cartilage of the distal phalanx or the deep digital flexor tendon?

3. What are three common radiographic signs seen with chronic laminitis?

4. A 10-year-old Arabian cross-breed mare is presented with lameness and swelling along the lateral aspect of the left front pastern. The owner reports the duration of both the lameness and the swelling to be about 10 days. Radiographs of the region show a smooth-surfaced periosteal opacity arising from the lateral cortex of the proximal phalanx. What factors should be considered to determine the significance of the radiographic findings?

5. A 4-year-old Thoroughbred stallion in race training develops an acute lameness in the left front foot. On a dorsal 65-degree–proximal-palmarodistal oblique view of the distal phalanx, a linear radiolucency is noted extending from the solar margin at the lateral quarter into the body of the bone. What are your rule-outs, and what additional information (or radiographic projections) would be useful in making the diagnosis?

6. What steps should be taken before radiography of the distal phalanx to achieve the best-quality images?

7. A 12-year-old Arabian gelding is presented for a precompetition physical examination (horse does competitive trail riding). The horse has not competed for 2 years because of problems with "tying-up syndrome." During the past 2 years, the horse has been used for riding lessons, with no reported lameness. On physical examination, the horse is mildly lame in both front feet at the trot. The horse is sore through the quarters and toes of both front feet with hoof testers. Figure 22–33 A to C are the lateral and dorsal 65-degree–proximal-palmarodistal oblique views of the right front foot (radiographs of the contralateral foot appeared similar). Identify the abnormal radiographic signs, and make your diagnosis.

8. A 17-year-old Quarter horse stallion has been lame for 5 days, with frequent periods of laying down. The horse is not responding to symptomatic treatment for laminitis. On physical examination, the horse is lame on both front feet but more on the left. There is soft-tissue swelling around the left coronary band. Identify the radiographic abnormalities in Figure 22–34 A and B, and make your diagnosis.

9. A 2-month-old Belgian/Percheron filly has a severe right hindleg lameness of 1 week's duration. She touches only the heels to the ground, with no weight on the toe. A plantar digital nerve block done to aid working with the foot relieved the lameness. A sole abscess was found at

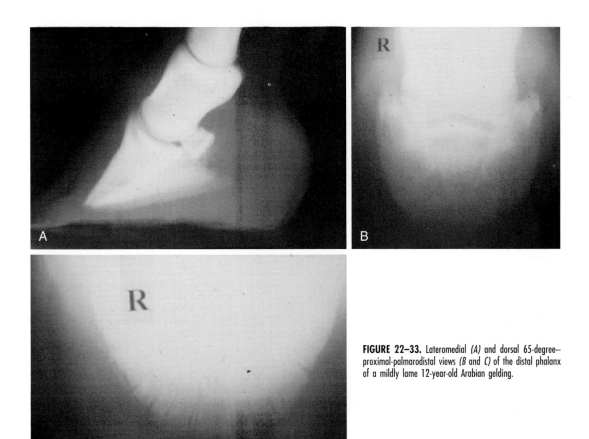

FIGURE 22–33. Lateromedial *(A)* and dorsal 65-degree–proximal-palmarodistal views *(B and C)* of the distal phalanx of a mildly lame 12-year-old Arabian gelding.

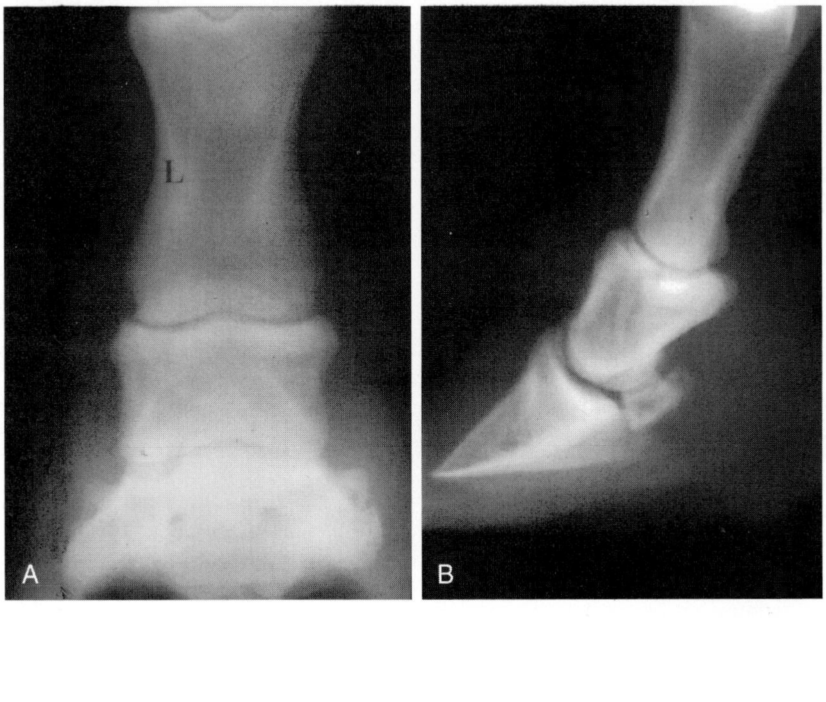

FIGURE 22–34. Lateromedial *(A)* and dorsopalmar *(B)* views of the left front foot of a 17-year-old Quarter horse stallion, lame for 5 days.

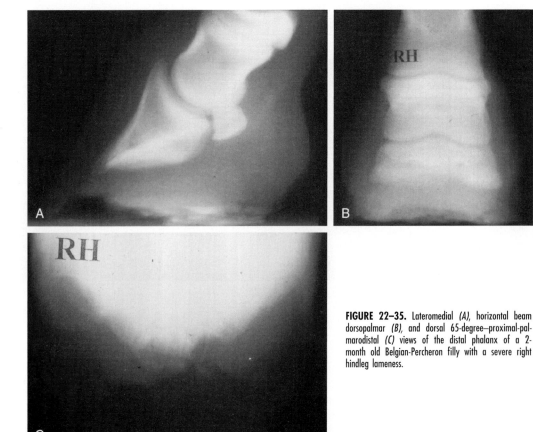

FIGURE 22–35. Lateromedial *(A)*, horizontal beam dorsopalmar *(B)*, and dorsal 65-degree–proximal-palmarodistal *(C)* views of the distal phalanx of a 2-month old Belgian-Percheron filly with a severe right hindleg lameness.

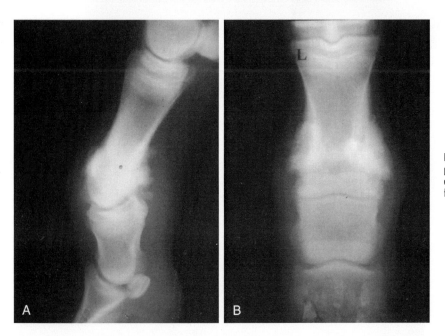

FIGURE 22–36. Lateromedial *(A)* and dorsal *(B)* 45-degree–proximal-palmarodistal oblique view of the left front phalanges of a 4-month-old Quarter horse colt with enlargement distal to the fetlock, but no lameness.

the toe. It was opened for drainage and appeared to dissect into both medial and lateral sole areas. The foot was soaked and packed. Three days later, the filly was somewhat better but still lame. Radiographs were made at this time (Fig. 22–35 *A* to *C*). Describe the radiographic changes, and make your diagnosis.

10. A 4-month-old Quarter horse colt was presented for

evaluation of chronic enlargement of the left forefoot distal to the fetlock without lameness. Physically, there was a nonpainful swelling circumferentially around the left front pastern and a firm prominence along the dorsal surface of the joint. Describe the radiographic abnormalities in Figure 22–36 *A* and *B*, and make your diagnosis.

(Answers appear on pages 638 to 640.)

Chapter 23

The Navicular Bone

Robert L. Toal

ANATOMY

The normal radiographic anatomy of the navicular bone is shown in Chapter 47. The navicular bone is shuttle shaped and has two surfaces (articular and flexor), two borders (proximal and distal), and two extremities (medial and lateral) (Fig. 23–1).[1] The articular surface conforms with the condyles of the middle phalanx, whereas the distal border just dorsal to the impar ligament has a small articular surface that articulates with the distal phalanx. The distal articular surface of the navicular bone and the articular surface of the distal phalanx are usually parallel but can be convergent.[2] The flexor surface has a prominent central ridge. The deep digital flexor tendon, protected by a bursa, passes over the flexor surface. The navicular bone is held in position by three strong ligaments. The paired suspensory navicular ligament originates from the dorsolateral aspects of the proximal phalanx and attaches to the proximal navicular border and extremities. The distal sesamoidean, or impar, ligament originates on the distal navicular border and inserts on the distal phalanx with the deep digital flexor tendon. Blood vessels and sensory nerves traverse these ligaments and ramify into the navicular bone and synovial membrane via both borders (see Fig. 22–9).[3] There is no evidence of an anatomic communication between the distal interphalangeal joint and the navicular bursa.[4]

INDICATIONS FOR RADIOGRAPHY

Indications for navicular radiography include the assessment of bony changes in navicular syndrome, identification of significant bone abnormalities during prepurchase examination, assessment of bone or bursal involvement in foot wounds or abscesses, evaluation of suspected trauma, and collection of information about the morphologic progression or remission of navicular bone abnormalities.

PREPARATION FOR RADIOGRAPHIC EVALUATION

Accurate radiographic evaluation of the navicular bone depends on a radiograph that is properly positioned and prop-

erly exposed and on a foot that is free of distracting artifacts. Proper preparation for navicular radiography is similar to that for the distal phalanx discussed in Chapter 22.

Positioning aids, such as a reinforced cassette, grooved wooden blocks, and a cassette tunnel, assist in radiographic evaluation of the navicular bone (Fig. 23–2). Use of a grid for angular dorsoproximal-palmarodistal views is optional. A grid improves radiographic detail by reducing film fog from scatter radiation. Because the grid is fragile, its use is limited to techniques during which the foot does not bear weight directly on the grid.

RADIOGRAPHIC VIEWS

The location of the navicular bone and its complex shape require that multiple views be made for complete radiographic evaluation. Commonly used radiographic views include the angular dorsoproximal-palmarodistal views, the lateromedial view, and the palmaroproximal-palmarodistal view.[2]

Dorsoproximal-Palmarodistal Views

Angular dorsoproximal-palmarodistal views of the navicular bone may be made by two different hoof-positioning techniques.[5–7] In one method (high coronary stand-on route), the foot rests directly on a reinforced cassette, cassette tunnel, or grooved wooden block. The x-ray beam is centered just proximal to the coronary band and angled 45 or 65 degrees proximally from horizontal. In the other method (upright pedal route), the hoof rests on the toe in tiptoe fashion with the dorsal hoof wall positioned either 80 or 90 degrees from horizontal; the x-ray beam is directed horizontally (Fig. 23–3).

Stand-on techniques are technically easier but result in slightly more magnification of the navicular bone when compared with the upright pedal route.[6] Magnification can be

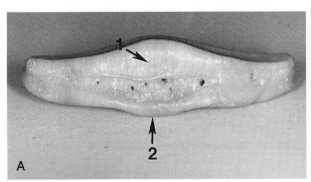
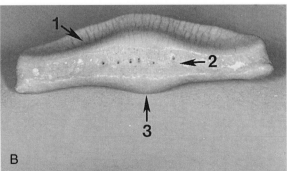

FIGURE 23–1. Gross photographs of the navicular bone. *A,* En face view of the distal border. Note (1) the small articular surface with the distal phalanx and (2) the projection off the distal border where the impar ligament attaches. *B,* En face view of the proximal border. Note (1) the articular surface with the middle phalanx, (2) the proximal border itself where the suspensory navicular ligament attaches, and (3) the navicular ridge. The view in *B* is analogous to that obtained in a palmaroproximal-palmarodistal radiograph.

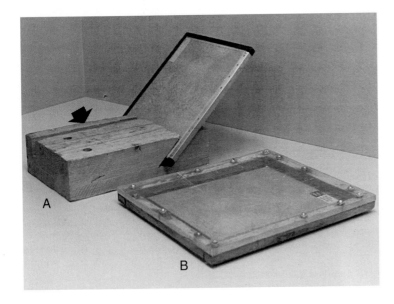

FIGURE 23–2. Types of positioning aids for navicular radiography. *A*, A wooden block for angular dorsoproximal-palmarodistal views. The longitudinally oriented slot *(arrow)* is used for lateral views. The grooves are of sufficient width to allow combined insertion of a grid and cassette. *B*, A cassette tunnel covered with Plexiglas protects the cassette (and grid) during dorsoproximal-palmarodistal views.

minimized on the high coronary stand-on route with the use of a grooved wooden block. A cassette and grid are placed in a precut groove behind the hoof as it rests on the block. Owing to the position of the cassette, less magnification of the navicular bone occurs when compared with other stand-on techniques (see Fig. 23–3B).

Both of these dorsoproximal-palmarodistal views project the navicular bone behind the middle phalanx. The two navicular extremities and the medulla are readily seen. Visualization of the navicular borders varies, however, because the proximal and distal navicular borders are not parallel (they diverge in a palmar direction), and thus a true geometric projection of these two borders cannot be obtained in a single dorsoproximal-palmarodistal radiograph. By varying the x-ray beam angulation incident on the navicular bone in

the high coronary route or by altering the position of the hoof in the upright pedal route, an accurate projection of either the proximal or the distal navicular border can be obtained.

An undistorted projection of the proximal navicular border is achieved with the use of the 45-degree high coronary stand-on route or the 90-degree upright pedal route. Unfortunately, the distal navicular border is not well visualized by these routes because it is projected below the level of the distal interphalangeal joint. Because only the proximal navicular border can be accurately evaluated in these two projections, they are not routinely used (see Fig. 23–3A and C).

A 65-degree high coronary stand-on route or an 80-degree upright pedal route projects the distal navicular border proximal to the distal interphalangeal joint and superimposes the entire navicular bone behind the middle phalanx. The distal navicular border is well-visualized, and although the proximal border is slightly distorted, it is readily identified. Either one of these two positioning methods is recommended for the angular dorsoproximal-palmarodistal projection because, when done properly, the entire navicular bone is seen (see Fig. 23–3B and D).

Lateromedial View

In the lateral view, it is important to use the best possible positioning technique to project both navicular extremities superimposed. If some degree of angulation occurs, this factor must be recognized and taken into account during interpretation. The foot is placed on a wooden block so the x-ray tube can be positioned low enough to center the beam on the lateral axis of the navicular bone. A wooden block also elevates the hoof, allowing the cassette to straddle it proximally and distally. Thus, the entire hoof can be included on the radiograph.

Palmaroproximal-Palmarodistal View

The palmaroproximal-palmarodistal view (Fig. 23–4) projects the flexor cortex, medulla, and navicular ridge. The concept is to isolate most of the bone between the palmar processes of the distal phalanx. The horse stands on a reinforced cas-

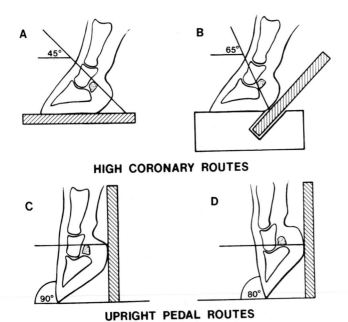

FIGURE 23–3. Angular dorsoproximal-palmarodistal views. High coronary routes (*A*, direct stand-on method; *B*, wooden block technique) and upright pedal routes (*C* and *D*) are illustrated showing beam or hoof angulation relative to the horizontal plane. Only the proximal navicular border is well visualized in *A* and *C*, whereas both proximal and distal borders are clearly projected in *B* and *D*.

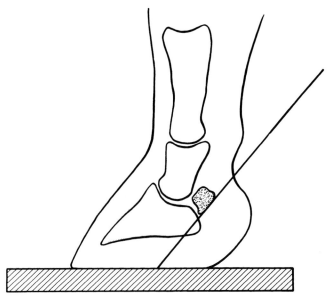

FIGURE 23–4. Palmaroproximal-palmarodistal view. The digit is positioned in extension, with the x-ray beam angled tangentially to the flexor surface.

sette or cassette tunnel. The foot is positioned as far caudal as possible while still bearing weight.[8] Paradoxically, some people prefer that the foot be more slightly forward than in the normal standing position.[8, 9] Regardless of foot location, the primary beam is positioned tangential to the estimated plane of the flexor cortex and is centered between the bulbs of the heel. Too steep of a beam angle with the foot may result in superimposition of the ergot over the navicular bone. Reduced angulation alters the apparent width of the flexor cortex and results in an indistinct interface between cortical and trabecular bone.[8] Oblique palmaroproximal-palmarodistal projections distort the navicular shape and superimpose it behind the palmar processes of the distal phalanx.

Dorsopalmar View

In the dorsopalmar view, the x-ray beam is directed horizontally toward the hoof, which is in a normal weight-bearing position. The foot should be placed on a wooden block. The x-ray beam is centered on the coronary band dorsally while the cassette is palmar. As in the lateromedial view, the wooden block elevates the foot, allowing the cassette to straddle the hoof and the navicular bone. This view is not done routinely but is useful in evaluating the extremities of the navicular bone, particularly when subtle abnormalities are suspected.

NORMAL RADIOGRAPHIC APPEARANCE

In the angular dorsoproximal-palmarodistal views, the navicular bone is of uniform radiopacity. Its spindle shape varies somewhat from horse to horse. The extremities are fairly symmetric and are bluntly pointed. The proximal border is smoothly marginated, although it may appear roughened owing to the summated opacity of the distal end of the middle phalanx over the navicular bone. The distal border has a variable number (four or five on average) of cone-shaped radiolucencies. Their size is variable, possibly being related to degree of work, although their shape should remain somewhat triangular (see Fig. 47–60).

The lateral view offers a clear, unobstructed view of the navicular bone but presents a foreshortened image. Both extremities should be superimposed; a well-defined medullary cavity is visualized. The flexor surface is convex palmarly and is smoothly marginated. In some normal horses, a smoothly marginated dimple of variable depth is seen in the midportion of the sagittal ridge. The proximal and distal borders are smooth, as are the articular surfaces. Some horses may have a mild elongation of the proximal or distal border or both.[2] The joint space between the navicular bone and the distal phalanx is usually parallel, but a convergent joint is sometimes present (see Fig. 47–58).

In the palmaroproximal-palmarodistal view, a well-defined medullary cavity of uniform trabecular pattern with four or five small radiolucent foramina may be seen. The cortex is of homogeneous opacity and is of uniform thickness centrally, with some thinning peripherally. The width of the flexor cortex varies from 2.0 to 3.6 mm because of breed differences and geometric magnification.[2, 8] The flexor surface is smoothly marginated with a prominent central ridge. The sagittal ridge is usually rounded and prominent, but in some horses it may appear flattened normally. A small crescent-shaped radiolucency can be seen within the cortex of the flexor sagittal ridge representing a normal midsagittal synovial fossa. This fossa is occasionally seen as a dimple on the flexor surface on the lateral view. The ends of both extremities are rounded, being variably superimposed over the palmar processes of the distal phalanx. The articular surface is occasionally seen in this view (see Fig. 47–62).

NAVICULAR DISEASE

The term *navicular disease* is used in this discussion despite evidence that navicular origin lameness may be a syndrome of variable etiology. The precise source of pain in navicular lameness remains obscure. Variable response to local analgesia of the medial and lateral palmar digital nerves, the distal interphalangeal joint space, and the navicular bursa is noted. This suggests that sensory nerves innervating the synovial membranes of the collateral sesamoidean ligament, the distal sesamoidean impar ligament, and the navicular bone itself play a separate or combined role in mediating pain in this condition.[4, 10] Navicular disease is primarily a slowly developing intermittent bilateral forelimb lameness[11, 12]; it is occasionally recognized in the hindlimb.[13] Incidence data are skewed by the population characteristics of reporting institutions. In general, navicular disease is most common between 7 and 15 years of age, with a mean age of 9 years at presentation. Males are more involved than females; geldings have a greater risk than stallions; and the highest incidence is in Quarter horses, Thoroughbreds, and Standardbreds.[14, 15]

There are no pathognomonic clinical tests for navicular disease. The diagnosis is based on a characteristic gait, localization of pain to the palmar part of the foot, identification of radiographic signs of navicular degeneration, and elimination of other causes of lameness.[11, 16] When navicular lameness is suspected, both feet should be radiographed because radiographic changes are often bilateral even if clinical signs are not.

The pathophysiology of navicular disease is controversial. Classically, it has been characterized as a navicular bursitis with secondary bone and tendon disease.[5, 11, 16] Thromboembolism of the navicular nutrient arteries has been proposed as another cause, but histopathologic corroboration of this is lacking.[3, 17–22] Other evidence supports the concept that navicular disease is a degenerative arthrosis, albeit with a vascular component.[20, 22–24] Chronic passive venous conges-

Table 23-1
ROENTGEN SIGNS OF NAVICULAR DEGENERATION

Proximal Border and Extremities	Flexor Cortex Changes
Enthesophytes	Cortical erosions
Spurs on extremities	Mineralization of the deep
Remodeling	digital flexor tendon
Distal Border Changes	**Medullary Cavity Changes**
Synovial invaginations	Radiolucent cysts
Small osseous fragments	Sclerosis

tion of the foot has been identified and related to navicular changes of elevated subchondral bone pressure and arterial hyperemia.[20, 25, 26]

Similar confusion exists concerning the significance of radiographic changes in navicular lameness. It has been shown that there is a poor correlation of pathologic and radiographic findings to clinical signs and prognosis.[14, 17, 19, 21, 27] Horses without radiographic abnormalities may have clinical navicular lameness, and horses with pathologic and radiographic changes may be sound.[21, 28] This paradox is explained, in part, by the fact that horses have different pain thresholds, are subjected to wide ranges of physical exercise, and are evaluated in variable stages of disease.[8] Additionally, some pathologic changes may represent insignificant wear lesions or may be located in tissues of soft-tissue opacity and thus are not radiographically discernible.[16, 19] Several authors agree that radiographic signs of navicular disease in an otherwise clinically normal horse are significant and may warrant a cautious prognosis for future soundness.[8, 29] There is no universal agreement, however, as to the clinical significance of all roentgen signs seen in navicular disease.

Roentgen Signs of Navicular Degeneration

Radiographic abnormalities associated with navicular degeneration are varied. Bony abnormalities may occur separately, but usually they occur in combination, unilaterally or bilaterally. Their clinical relevance with respect to presence, ab-

sence, or degree of lameness in a given animal is varied.[27] Additionally, there is no clear association between changes in the radiologic appearance of navicular bones and clinical outcome after treatment.[30] Thus, radiographic changes of navicular degeneration must be interpreted in context with the presenting clinical signs.

The major roentgen signs of navicular degeneration are shown in Table 23–1. Figure 23–5 is a diagram depicting various roentgen signs of navicular degeneration. Radiographic manifestations of navicular degeneration and normal variants are shown in Figures 23–6 through 23–9.

Proximal Border and Navicular Bone Extremities

Dystrophic mineralization at sites of ligamentous or tendon attachment is termed *enthesophytosis*.[22, 31] Mineralization of the suspensory navicular ligament along the proximal border results in a roughened or sawtooth appearance of the bone margin. Pronounced enthesophytes on the extremities of the navicular bone have been termed *spurs*. When enthesophytosis is excessive, the overall shape of the bone is altered. This is termed *remodeling* (see Figs. 23–6B and C and 23–7B).

In general, enthesophytes are manifestations of a degenerative process.[5, 11, 31, 32] They are occasionally seen in nonlame animals, particularly in older, heavily worked animals.[14, 17, 19] Enthesophytes in younger horses and extensive enthesophytes in others should be considered significant, particularly if accompanied by lameness.

Enthesophytes are best seen in angular dorsoproximal-palmarodistal views as new bone formation on the extremities or as bone proliferations along the proximal border (sawtooth border). In the lateral view, excessive remodeling gives the bone an elongated appearance (see Fig. 23–6B). Caution should be exercised because improperly positioned lateral views may artifactually distort the bone profile. Similarly, normal variants exist that resemble remodeling laterally when angular dorsoproximal-palmarodistal images are normal.[22]

Distal Border Changes

The radiolucent invaginations along the distal border of the navicular bone are termed *synovial invaginations*. These are

DORSAL 65° PROXIMAL-   LATEROMEDIAL   PALMAROPROXIMAL-
PALMARODISTAL VIEW   VIEW   PALMARODISTAL VIEW

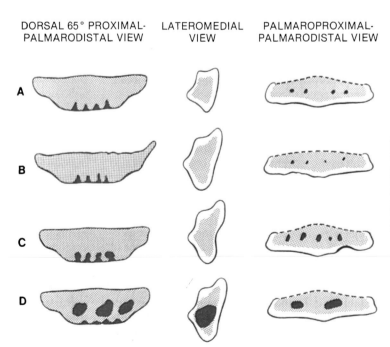

FIGURE 23–5. Radiographic changes seen in navicular degeneration. Dorsal 65-degree–proximal-palmarodistal view: *A,* Normal. *B,* Remodeling—enthesophyte on extremity and sawtooth proximal border. *C,* Lollipop-shaped invaginations on distal border. *D,* Cyst-like lesion formation. Lateromedial view: *A,* Normal. *B,* Elongated navicular profile from remodeling (enthesophyte formation). *C,* Flexor cortical erosion. *D,* Cyst-like lesion formation. Palmaroproximal-palmarodistal view: *A,* Normal. *B,* Flexor cortical erosions. *C,* Enlarged fossae and flexor cortical erosions. *D,* Cyst-like lesion formation. (Modified from Richard Park, Fort Collins, CO; with permission.)

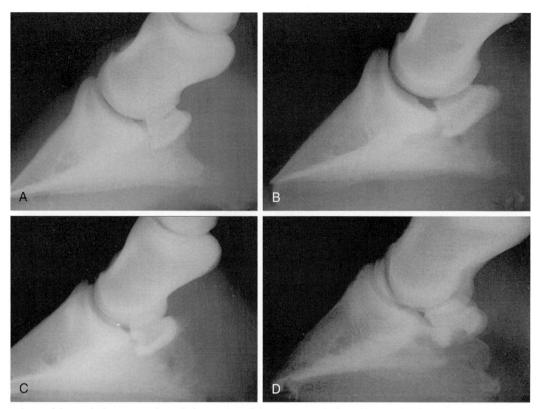

FIGURE 23–6. Lateral views of the navicular bone. *A,* Normal navicular bone. *B,* Proximal elongation as a result of remodeling. *C,* Enthesophyte (spur) on proximal border. *D,* Flexor cortex lysis.

best seen in the dorsal 65-degree–proximal-palmarodistal view. They are normally an inverted cone to popsicle stick in shape. An increase in their size and number are physiologic changes related to type and frequency of work.[2, 3] A change to a lollipop or mushroom shape is considered to signal an abnormal degenerative change (see Fig. 23–7*C*).[22, 23] These abnormal synovial invaginations may be a sign of an arthrosis of the distal interphalangeal joint, albeit a navicular manifestation. The presence of synovial invaginations in the extremities of the navicular bone has been considered abnormal by some, but their presence does not correlate with lameness.[27]

Horses with clinical navicular disease have a high incidence of abnormal synovial invaginations, but their clinical specificity remains uncertain. This is because lollipop-shaped synovial invaginations have been reported in 11 percent of normal horses, and there is no correlation with degree of lameness in confirmed navicular lameness.[27]

Radiolucent changes of the distal border cannot be seen well in lateromedial views. The palmaroproximal-palmarodistal view, however, projects them end-on within the trabecular portion of the bone. Increases in size of visible fossae in this view are abnormal (see Fig. 23–9*A*).[8, 9] The range of

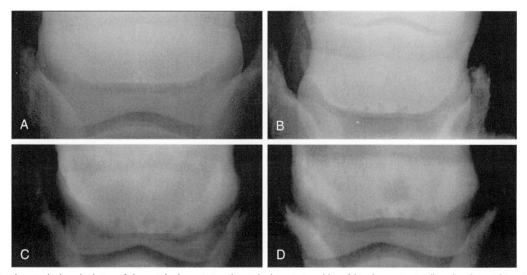

FIGURE 23–7. Dorsal proximal-palmarodistal views of the navicular bone. *A,* Normal navicular bone. *B,* Remodeling of lateral extremity. *C,* Lollipop-shaped synovial invaginations of the distal navicular border. *D,* Cyst-like cavitation over the plane of the navicular medullary cavity. Remember that flexor cortical erosions often falsely mimic medullary cavity cysts on dorsoproximal-palmarodistal views. Thus, the palmaroproximal-palmarodistal view is needed in this situation to determine accurately the location of the lesion.

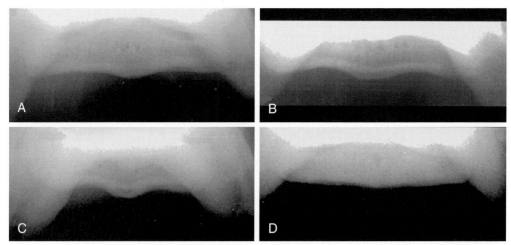

FIGURE 23–8. Normal variations in the appearance of the navicular flexor cortex are shown. The flexor cortex should be smoothly marginated and have an abrupt demarcation from the less opaque medullary spongiosa. *A,* Prominent sagittal ridge. *B,* Blunted sagittal ridge. *C,* Crescent-shaped radiolucency in sagittal ridge. *D,* Altered beam angulation and patient motion result in indistinct interface between the cortex and the medullary spongiosa falsely suggesting navicular sclerosis.

normal shape variation of fossa appearance for this view, however, has not been established. It is the author's opinion, therefore, that distal border radiolucent changes are more consistently evaluated with the use of angular dorsoproximal-palmarodistal views, especially when there is only minimal enlargement.

Mineralization associated with the distal sesamoidean impar ligament is another degenerative change. This has similar significance to enthesophytes involving the proximal border. Occasionally, osseous fragments can be seen associated with the distal border. These can be seen in normal and lame horses alike. Small osseous fragments occasionally indicate chip fractures of the distal border and are discussed further under fractures. Small osseous fragments of the distal border are best seen in the angular dorsoproximal-palmarodistal views.

Flexor Cortex Changes

Gross pathologic involvement of the navicular flexor fibrocartilage is varied. Lesions include yellowish discoloration, cartilage thinning, focal erosions, and cartilage ulcerations, with or without subchondral bone involvement.[5, 19, 23] Some of the abnormalities may be age-related phenomena, but all have been seen in navicular disease to varying degrees.[17, 19]

Bursae, tendon, and cartilage changes are not usually seen radiographically; only subchondral bone defects are routinely detectable. Early lesions are best seen on the palmaroproximal-palmarodistal view, whereas severe defects may be recognized in other views as well. Abnormal roentgen signs consist of cortical thinning with subchondral bone lysis (fuzzy margins of the cortex) and diffuse to localized demineralization within the flexor compact bone (see Fig. 23–9).[8] Flexor cortex erosions are rarely seen in sound horses and have a significant correlation to the presence and degree of lameness.[2, 27] It is not unusual for large flexor cortical erosions to simulate medullary cyst-like lesions in the dorsopalmar view. It is important to localize such cyst-like lesions radiographically. Flexor cortical erosions are often associated with tendinous adhesions, whereas medullary cysts are not.[23, 31] This added information may be important in the overall manage-

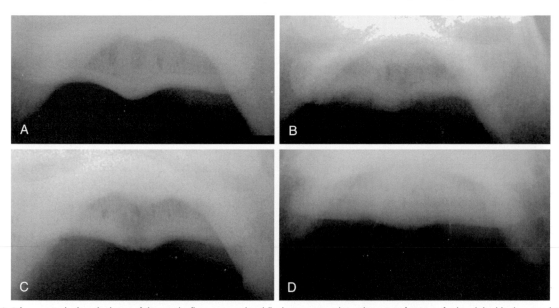

FIGURE 23–9. Palmaroproximal-palmarodistal views of the navicular flexor cortex and medulla showing various abnormalities. *A,* En face view of enlarged distal border synovial invaginations. *B,* Subtle flexor cortex erosions resulting in a loss of the normal smooth flexor contour. *C,* Large focal cortical lysis causing disruption of the flexor cortex over the sagittal ridge. *D,* Extensive subchondral bone sclerosis. This was also seen on other views.

ment of the animal. Navicular variants of a flat sagittal ridge and a crescent lucency within the cortex of the sagittal ridge exist (see Fig. 23–8). These should not be misdiagnosed as navicular degeneration. Studies have shown the crescent-shaped radiolucency either to be a centrally located concavity of the sagittal ridge or to be associated with the formation of a second linear bony ridge dorsal and parallel to the flexor surface.[34, 35] The tiny gap between these two plates of bone is responsible for the radiolucent crescent. Regardless of the explanation, a crescent-shaped radiolucency may be seen normally in the flexor eminence on the palmaroproximal-palmarodistal view in some horses (see Fig. 23–8C).

Well-positioned lateral radiographs depict the flexor cortex in profile axially. Minor dimpling of the navicular ridge in this view may be a normal variant or may be the result of geometric distortion. Abrupt irregular cavitations are abnormal (see Fig. 23–6D). It is recommended that abnormalities of the flexor cortex observed on a lateral radiograph be further evaluated with the use of the palmaroproximal-palmarodistal view.

Dystrophic mineralization of the deep digital flexor tendon may be seen in conjunction with flexor erosions. This finding is reported rarely and indicates severe tendon degeneration, rendering a poor prognosis.[22, 36] Faint visualization of the deep digital flexor tendon on the lateral view is a frequent normal finding. Diseased tendons that are sufficiently mineralized may be seen in both lateral and palmaroproximal-palmarodistal views.

Medullary Cavity Changes

Medullary trabecular disruption in the form of trabecular lysis or cyst-like cavitations is abnormal. These changes are rarely seen in sound horses (see Fig. 23–7D). These radiolucencies may be seen on the angular dorsoproximal-palmarodistal, palmaroproximal-palmarodistal, and occasionally lateral views. They range in size from 0.5 to 1.5 cm and are round to oval. They usually are single but may be multiple. Marginal sclerosis is variable, ranging from complete to none at all.

Lytic lesions located within the middle or distal phalanx may be superimposed over the navicular bone. By evaluating other views or by repeating the dorsoproximal-palmarodistal view at a different angle, it is possible to see if the suspect lesion changes in position or remains associated with the navicular bone. Similarly, lucent artifacts that result from air trapped in the frog by packing material should not be misinterpreted as radiolucent bone lesions. Air pockets usually present as linear radiolucent shadows. When there is doubt, repacking the frog should be done.

Extensive erosions of the flexor cortex can falsely mimic medullary cavity cysts on angular dorsoproximal-palmarodistal views. On a palmaroproximal-palmarodistal view, the suspect lesion can be localized as to whether it originates from the flexor cortex or the medullary cavity (see Fig. 23–9C and D).

Sclerosis of the medullary spongiosa is said to be an early finding in horses lame because of navicular disease.[2, 8, 27] This is seen as a fine trabecular pattern that blends with the subjacent flexor cortex resulting in an indistinct interface between the flexor cortex and the medullary spongiosa.[2, 8] This finding can also be seen in normal horses as a result of a poorly positioned radiograph (see Fig. 23–8D).[2, 27]

Normal Radiographic Findings

It should be realized that many horses with clinical navicular lameness have normal radiographs.[15] These animals may

have disease that better falls into the category of navicular bursitis. Before arriving at this assessment, however, an adequate number of high-quality radiographs should be obtained.

Technetium-99m bone scintigraphy is an extremely valuable adjunct when radiographic findings are equivocal or when the bone is normal, but disease of the navicular bursa is suspected. This is true because nuclear scintigraphy is more sensitive than radiography in identifying early soft-tissue and bone abnormalities, although a scintigram provides primarily physiologic as opposed to anatomic information. Because physiologic alterations associated with navicular degeneration are likely to precede gross anatomic changes, scintigraphy of the navicular bone should be done when clinical signs are compatible with navicular lameness but radiographs are normal.[37]

FRACTURES

Navicular fractures are infrequently reported. Therefore, data are not available to draw firm conclusions about their incidence and pathophysiology. Most navicular fractures are traumatic or pathologic in origin. Both chip and complete fracture types have been described. A diagram of navicular fractures is shown in Figure 23–10.

Care should be taken to avoid misinterpreting artifacts as navicular fractures. The sulci of the frog may cast overlying radiolucent shadows in the dorsoproximal-palmarodistal projection that simulate complete navicular fracture. This situation occurs when the foot is unpacked or when air is trapped in the sulcus by packing material. Sulcal lines typically extend above and below the navicular bone. Complete fractures are confined to the bone and are seen on dorsoproximal-palmarodistal and palmaroproximal-palmarodistal views. Gravel or debris in the foot or a foot with scaly horn may simulate chip fractures. By proper hoof preparation (cleaning, paring, and packing), these artifacts can be elimi-

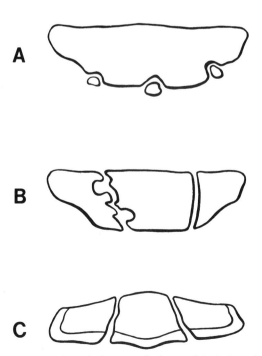

FIGURE 23–10. Types of navicular fractures. *A,* Chip fractures of the distal navicular border, dorsal 65-degree–proximal-palmarodistal projection. *B* and *C,* Complete navicular fractures, dorsal 65-degree–proximal-palmarodistal and palmaroproximal-palmarodistal projections.

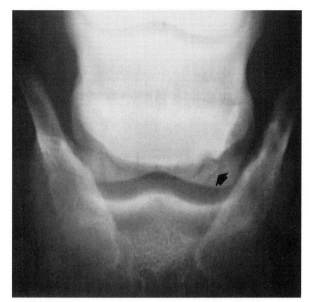

FIGURE 23–11. Chip fracture at the distal navicular border. The small fragment *(arrow)* and the underlying fracture bed can be seen.

nated. Lateral views or dorsoproximal-palmarodistal radiographs taken at different angles help to localize a suspect opacity. When in doubt about navicular fractures, the hoof should be cleaned and repacked before more radiographs are made.

Osseous Fragments of the Distal Border

Small osseous fragments associated with the distal border of the navicular bone and impar ligament are occasionally seen. These osseous bodies have more than one pathogenesis. They may be due to chip fractures, damage to the impar ligament with secondary mineralization, separate centers of ossification within the impar ligament, and synovial osseous metaplasia.[24, 31] When present, osseous bodies may be unilateral or bilateral, involve both the medial and the lateral aspect of the bone, or involve only one side of the bone. Larger fragments are most often found on the medial side of the bone.

Osseous bodies that are true chip fractures may appear as small (0.2 to 1.2 cm), rectangular bone fragments separated from the distal border by a radiolucent zone. A fracture bed within the navicular bone corresponding in size and shape to the fragment is often seen.[38] Dystrophic mineralization of the impar ligament may have a similar appearance, but a fracture bed is not seen.

The presence of osseous bodies does not indicate navicular disease but usually occurs in association with other roentgen signs of navicular disease. They have not been shown to influence clinical signs or prognosis of navicular disease (Fig. 23–11).

Complete Fractures

Complete navicular fractures may occur in normal or diseased navicular bones.[10, 39–45] They are most frequently seen in the forelimb, but hindlimb fractures have been reported.[44] Initiating causes include direct navicular trauma and repeated concussive forces on a pathologic navicular bone in a neurectomized patient. Lameness associated with complete fractures is usually acute but may be chronic and is moderate to severe. In general, long-term prognosis for competitive performance is poor.[38] Postmortem studies of limited numbers of fractured navicular bones show fibrous unions between the fragments.[40] Variable instability is inherent because of the hinge-like motion allowed by the fibrous component.

Usually, one or two vertical or oblique fracture lines may be seen within the body or the body-extremity junction of the navicular bone. A prominent fracture line is usually present. Fracture fragments have irregular-to-smooth margins and are minimally displaced. Occasionally, fragments have mild degenerative changes of bony resorption and sclerosis subjacent to the fracture line (Fig. 23–12A). Healing is thought to be from a noncalcified fibrous union because bony union is not observed radiographically, regardless of fracture duration. The absence of periosteum and progenitor cells, constant fragment motion, and influx of regional synovial fluid are all thought to play a role in navicular fracture healing with fibrous rather than bony union.

Multipartite Sesamoids

Bilaterally symmetric fractures are occasionally seen in minimally lame animals with otherwise normal navicular bones. This finding has fostered the belief that multipartite sesamoids may represent multiple ossification centers that have not fused. Congenital multipartite sesamoids are occasional, incidental findings in other species. Although the navicular bone develops from a single ossification center, aberrant formation is theoretically possible.[1] Radiographic differentiation between a congenitally multipartite navicular bone and a chronic fracture is impossible. Radiographically, multipartite (bipartite or tripartite) sesamoid bones are often bilateral. Individual fragments have smooth, rounded margins with wide radiolucent gaps between them. In addition, multiple ossification centers initially cause no to minimal lameness. If instability is present, however, degenerative changes resulting in lameness may occur.

In some lame horses, a multipartite navicular bone also has changes compatible with advanced navicular degenera-

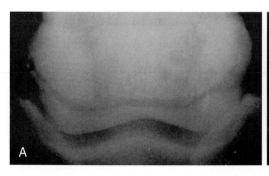
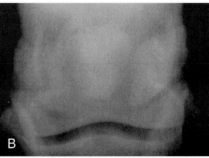

FIGURE 23–12. *A,* Complete navicular bone fractures. *B,* Tripartite navicular bone, which is probably congenital in origin.

tion. This circumstance has two plausible explanations. One is that there has been a pathologic fracture of a primarily diseased bone. Another is that fracture or multiple ossification centers are present initially. The resultant instability causes chronic secondary degenerative changes. Thus, multipartite sesamoid bones seen in conjunction with severe degenerative navicular changes are difficult to classify as either fractured or multipartite (see Fig. 23–12B).

NAVICULAR SEPSIS

Navicular sepsis may result from penetrating puncture wounds or deep lacerations that involve the bursa or the bone itself. Roentgen signs relative to the navicular bone following a puncture wound to the navicular bursa vary. The length of time between the initial injury and the first radiographic evaluation influences the findings.[45]

If a horse presents within 3 weeks of injury and initial radiographs are negative, a fistulogram or radiograph made after insertion of a blunt probe should be considered. This examination aids in establishing if the puncture wound involves the navicular bursa or bone (Fig. 23–13). This information is important because a puncture wound that involves a bone or bursa warrants a more cautious prognosis and more vigorous therapy because osteomyelitis may result. A negative fistulogram does not eliminate the possibility that the navicular bone or bursa was involved in the initial injury because partial tract healing in the deeper areas of the wound could prevent passage of contrast medium during fistulography, resulting in a falsely negative study.

Regardless of whether a fistulogram is done during the initial evaluation, follow-up radiographs should be made within the subsequent 3 to 12 weeks because radiographic evidence of navicular infection may take 6 weeks or longer to become apparent. Also, it has been estimated that 50 percent of horses with initially negative radiographs subsequently develop radiographic signs of bone infection. Once present, navicular osteomyelitis may progress and result in

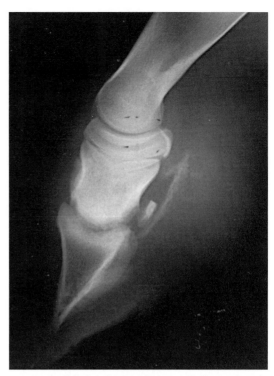

FIGURE 23–14. Lateral forefoot of a young horse 4 weeks after a nail puncture of the navicular bursa. There is septic arthritis of the distal interphalangeal joint, osteolysis and displacement of the navicular bone, and dystrophic mineralization of the deep digital flexor tendon.

serious complications leading to chronic lameness that may eventually necessitate euthanasia.

Of the standard projections to evaluate the navicular bone, the lateral and palmaroproximal-palmarodistal views are more valuable than the angled dorsoproximal-palmarodistal views in detecting and staging osteomyelitis of the navicular bone.

Initial roentgen signs of navicular bone infection appear as focal areas of decreased opacity in the flexor cortical bone with disruption and irregularity of the flexor surface. These lesions are initially located abaxial to the sagittal ridge. The greater the duration of the injury without treatment, the more extensive the disease in terms of depth of the irregularity into the navicular bone and the abaxial extent of it.

More severe chronic findings associated with puncture wounds and navicular osteomyelitis include septic osteomyelitis of the distal interphalangeal joint (Fig. 23–14), secondary joint disease, pathologic fractures of the navicular bone, and subluxation of the distal interphalangeal joint. Rupture of the deep digital flexor tendon or navicular impar ligament causes subluxation of the distal interphalangeal joint. In some horses, degenerative changes similar to those seen in navicular disease have been observed as long-term sequelae.

MISCELLANEOUS CONDITIONS

Another condition that affects the navicular bone is degenerative arthritis. The navicular bone participates in forming the distal interphalangeal joint. The articular border of the navicular bone adjacent to the middle phalanx is normally rounded. Periarticular osteophytes can be seen that result in subtle, pointed, spur-like projections. These have been seen in normal horses as well as in horses lame from navicular

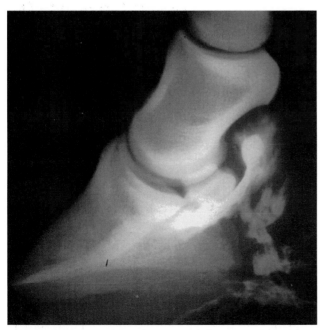

FIGURE 23–13. Fistulogram after a nail puncture wound. There is communication of the tract with the navicular bursa.

disease; thus, their significance is uncertain. Reports of significant pathologic processes involving the articular cartilages in navicular disease are rare.[19] It is believed, however, that some changes seen in navicular degeneration are a form of distal interphalangeal joint arthrosis.[19, 20, 22] Congenital absence of the navicular bone (agenesis) has been reported.[47, 48]

References

1. Getty R: Sisson and Grossman's The Anatomy of the Domestic Animals. Philadelphia, WB Saunders, 1975.
2. Kaser-Hotz B, and Ueltschi G: Radiographic appearance of the navicular bone in sound horses. Vet Radiol Ultrasound 33:9, 1992.
3. Colles CM, and Hickman J: The arterial supply of the navicular bone and its variations in navicular disease. Equine Vet J 9:150, 1977.
4. Bowker RM, Ruckershouser SJ, Kelly BV, et al: Immunocytochemical and dye distribution studies of nerves potentially desensitized by injections into the distal interphalangeal joint of the navicular bursa of horses. J Am Vet Med Assoc 203:1708, 1993.
5. Oxspring GE: The radiology of navicular disease with observations on its pathology. Vet Rec 15:1434, 1935.
6. Campbell JR, and Lee R: Radiological techniques in the diagnosis of navicular disease. Equine Vet J 4:135, 1972.
7. Reid CF: Equine Extremity Radiography in Positioning and Exposure Guide for Veterinary Radiography. Wilmington, DE, DuPont X-Ray Systems, 1978.
8. O'Brien TR, Millman TM, Pool RR, et al: Navicular disease in the Thoroughbred horse: A morphologic investigation relative to a new radiographic projection. J Am Vet Radiol Soc 16:39, 1975.
9. Rose RJ, Taylor BJ, and Steel JD: Navicular disease in the horse: An analysis of seventy cases and assessment of a special radiographic view. J Equine Med Surg 2:492, 1978.
10. Dyson SJ, and Kidd L: A comparison of responses to analgesia of the navicular bursa and intra-articular analgesia of the distal interphalangeal joint in 59 horses. Equine Vet J 25:93, 1993.
11. Stashak TS (Ed): Adam's Lameness in Horses, 4th Ed. Philadelphia, Lea & Febiger, 1987.
12. Rose RJ: The treatment of navicular disease—a review and current concepts. Presented at the 29th Annual Convention of the American Association of Equine Practitioners, Las Vegas, 1983.
13. Valdez H, Adams OR, and Peyton LC: Navicular disease in the hindlimbs of the horse. J Am Vet Med Assoc 172:291, 1978.
14. Ackerman N, Johnson JH, and Dorn CR: Navicular disease in the horse: Risk factors, radiographic changes, and response to therapy. J Am Vet Med Assoc 170:183, 1977.
15. Wright IM: A study of 118 cases of navicular disease: Clinical features. Equine Vet J 25:488, 1993.
16. Pool RR, Meagher DM, and Stover SM: Pathophysiology of navicular syndrome. Vet Clin North Am [Equine Pract] 5:109, 1989.
17. Colles CM: Ischaemic necrosis of the navicular bone and its treatment. Vet Rec 104:133, 1979.
18. Fricker CH, Riek W, and Hugelshofer J: Occlusion of the digital arteries—a model for pathogenesis of navicular disease. Equine Vet J 14:203, 1982.
19. Doige CE, and Hoffer MA: Pathologic changes in the navicular bone and associated structures of the horse. Can J Comp Med 47:387, 1983.
20. Svalastoga E: Navicular disease in the horse—a microangiographic investigation. Nord Vet Med 35:131, 1983.
21. Ostblom L, Lund C, and Melsen F: Histologic study of navicular bone disease. Equine Vet J 14:199, 1982.
22. Poulos PW, and Smith MF: The nature of enlarged "vascular channels" in the navicular bone of the horse. Vet Radiol 2:60, 1988.
23. Svalastoga E, Reimann I, and Nielsen K: Changes of the fibrocartilage in navicular disease in horses. Nord Vet Med 35:373, 1983.
24. Svalastoga E, and Neilsen K: Navicular disease in the horse—the synovial membrane of bursa podotrochlearis. Nord Vet Med 35:28, 1983.
25. Svalastoga E, and Smith M: Navicular disease in the horse—the subchondral bone pressure. Nord Vet Med 35:31, 1983.
26. Colles CM: Concepts of blood flow in the aetiology and treatment of navicular disease. Presented at the 29th Annual Convention of the American Association of Equine Practitioners, Las Vegas, 1983.
27. Wright IM: A study of 118 cases of navicular disease: Radiological features. Equine Vet J 25:493, 1993.
28. Turner T, Kneller S, Badertscher R, et al: Radiographic changes in the navicular bones of normal horses. In Proceedings of the 32nd Annual Meeting of the American Association of Equine Practitioners, 1986, pp 309–314.
29. Huskamp B, and Becker M: Diagnose und prognose der röntgenologischen Veranderungen an den Strahl-beinen der Vordergliedma Ben der Pferde unter besonderer Beruecksichtigung der Ankau fsuntersuchung: Ein Versuch zur Schematisierung der Befunde. Praktische Tierarzt 61:858, 1980.
30. Wright IM: A study of 118 cases of navicular disease: Treatment by navicular suspensory desmotomy. Equine Vet J 25:501, 1993.
31. Poulos P, Brown A, Brown E, et al: On navicular disease in the horse: A roentgenological and patho-anatomic study: II. Osseous bodies associated with the impar ligament. Vet Radiol 30:54, 1989.
32. Turner TA: The anatomic, pathologic, and radiographic aspects of navicular disease. Comp Contin Ed Vet Pract 4:350, 1982.
33. MacGregor C: Radiographic assessment of navicular bones based on changes in the distal nutrient foramina. Equine Vet J 18:203, 1986.
34. Poulos P, and Brown A: On navicular disease in the horse: A roentgenological and patho-anatomic study: I. Evaluation of the flexor central eminence. Vet Radiol 30:50, 1989.
35. Berry C, Pool R, Stover S, et al: A radiographic/morphologic investigation of a radiolucent crescent within the flexor central eminence of the navicular bone in the Thoroughbred. In Proceedings of the American College of Veterinary Radiology Annual Meeting, Chicago, 1990.
36. Turner TA: Dystrophic calcification of the deep digital flexor tendons resulting from navicular disease. Vet Med Small Anim Clin 77:571, 1982.
37. Trout DR, Hornof WJ, and O'Brien TR: Soft-tissue and bone-phase scintigraphy for diagnosis of navicular disease in horses. J Am Vet Med Assoc 198:73, 1991.
38. van De Watering CC, and Morgan JP: Chip fractures as a radiologic finding in navicular disease of the horse. J Am Vet Radiol Soc 16:206, 1975.
39. Lillich JD, Ruggles AJ, Gabel AA, et al: Fracture of the distal sesamoid bone in horses: 17 cases (1982–1992). J Am Vet Med Assoc 207:924, 1995.
40. Vaughan LC: Fracture of the navicular bone in the horse. Vet Rec 73:895, 1961.
41. Arnbjerg J: Spontaneous fracture of the navicular bone in the horse. Nord Vet Med 31:429, 1979.
42. Reeves MJ: Miscellaneous conditions of the equine foot. Vet Clin North Am [Equine Pract] 5:221, 1989.
43. Smythe RH: Fracture of the navicular bone in the horse—comment. Vet Rec 73:1009, 1961.
44. Kaser-Hotz B, Ueltshci G, Hess N, et al: Navicular bone fractures in the pelvic limb in two horses. Vet Radiol Ultrasound 32:283, 1991.
45. Rick MC: Navicular bone fractures. In White NA, Moore JN (Eds): Current Practice of Equine Surgery. Philadelphia, JB Lippincott, 1990, pp 602–605.
46. Richardson GL, and O'Brien T: Puncture wounds into the navicular bursa of the horse: Role of radiographic evaluation. Vet Radiol 26:203, 1985.
47. Reid CF: Radiology panel—film interpretation session notes. In Proceedings of the 22nd Annual Convention of the American Association of Equine Practitioners, Dallas, 1976, p 7.
48. Modransky C, Thatcher C, Welker F, et al: Unilateral phalangeal dysgenesis and navicular bone agenesis in a foal. Equine Vet J 19:347, 1987.

STUDY QUESTIONS

1. The suspensory navicular ligament attaches to which one of the following?
   A. Flexor surface.
   B. Flexor and articular surface.
   C. Proximal border and extremities.
   D. Distal border and flexor surface.
   E. None of the above.

2. The best radiographic projection to obtain a true unobstructed view of the distal border of the navicular bone is the:
   A. Palmaroproximal-palmarodistal.
   B. 65-degree–dorsoproximal-palmarodistal.
   C. 45-degree–dorsoproximal-palmarodistal.
   D. Dorsopalmar view.
   E. None of the above.

3. Which one of the following does not represent a normal manifestation of the flexor cortex of the navicular bone?
   A. Blunt-pointed sagittal ridge.
   B. Flat sagittal ridge.
   C. Crescent-shaped lucency in sagittal ridge.
   D. Cortical erosion of the flexor surface.
   E. Flexor cortex width of 3 mm.

4. Which one of the following is true about synovial invaginations with respect to the navicular bone?
   A. Most prominent on the distal border.
   B. Are seen in sound horses less than 2 percent of the time.
   C. Increased size but triangular shape suggests age or work changes.
   D. Lollipop shape is abnormal.
   E. Are suggestive of navicular sepsis.

5. Medullary cysts seen on angular dorsoproximal-palmarodistal views either can be within the navicular spongiosa or can represent a focal flexor cortical lytic lesion. (True or False)

6. Osseous fragments of the distal border of the navicular bone are due to which one of the following?
   A. Chip fractures.
   B. Impar ligament mineralization.
   C. Separate ossification centers.
   D. Synovial osseous metaplasia.
   E. All of the above.

7. Congenital multipartite sesamoids and complete navicular fractures can always be differentiated radiographically. (True or False)

8. When complete navicular fractures occur, why do they heal with a fibrous rather than an osseous union?

9. After a nail puncture wound to the navicular bursa, if initial radiographs are inconclusive, follow-up radiographs should be done when?
   A. Within 3 to 12 weeks.
   B. Within 12 to 16 weeks.
   C. Within 16 to 20 weeks.
   D. No follow-up films are indicated because a negative initial study was seen.

10. What are proposed pathophysiologic mechanism(s) of navicular disease syndrome?
   A. Infection due to *Haemophilus navicularis*.
   B. Progressive navicular bursitis.
   C. Degenerative arthrosis.
   D. Osteochondrosis.
   E. Ischemic necrosis of the navicular.

(Answers appear on page 640.)

Chapter 24

The Larynx, Pharynx, and Trachea

Stephen K. Kneller

LARYNX AND PHARYNX

Anatomic Considerations

The pharynx, bordered by the base of the tongue and the retropharyngeal wall, is divided into oropharynx and nasopharynx by the soft palate, which extends to the level of the epiglottis. On high-quality lateral radiographs, most of the laryngeal structures can be identified (Fig. 24–1).[1] Laryngeal structures are difficult to see on ventrodorsal views because of other overlying structures. In lateral radiographs, the transverse basihyoid bone is usually obvious because it is projected on-end and may be mistaken for a foreign object.

Radiographs of brachycephalic dogs as well as those of obese animals are more difficult to interpret because of the larger amount of soft tissue and fat (Fig. 24–2). This results in a lower air:tissue ratio, providing less contrast as well as more irregular opacities.

In young animals (2 to 3 months of age), laryngeal structures may not be well defined because they are not sufficiently mineralized. Mineralization in laryngeal cartilaginous structures, including the epiglottis, is recognized as an aging change. Mineralization may be seen in animals as young as 2 to 3 years of age and is expected earlier in large and chondrodystrophic dogs. In one study, 96 of 99 clinically normal dogs of random breeds and random age greater than 1 year had radiographic laryngeal mineralization.[2] The cricoid cartilage is usually the first laryngeal cartilage to become mineralized.

In a routine lateral view with the head in a normal position, the larynx is usually ventral to the first two cervical vertebrae. It is usually just slightly more ventral than the main portion of the cervical trachea. If the radiograph is made with the head extended, the larynx is pulled slightly cranial and is closer to the spine. Additionally, the hyoid bones are at a lesser angle with one another, and the ventrodorsal diameter of the pharynx may be compressed. If the radiograph is made with the head in flexion, the larynx may be as far caudal as C4. In this position, air flow is compromised, decreasing the air:tissue ratio. This makes structures more difficult to see, and overlying skin folds are more likely.

Depending on the phase and depth of respiration during radiography, the tip of the epiglottis may be just dorsal or ventral to the soft palate, or it may be on the ventral floor of the pharynx. This variation may be seen in normal animals; however, in the presence of swallowing disorders, radiographic and fluoroscopic examination should be performed during swallowing to determine if the epiglottis moves normally.

The hyoid bones are relatively well defined and easy to identify in the dog and cat. The key to diagnostic accuracy is simply a familiarity with the normal appearance. These bones

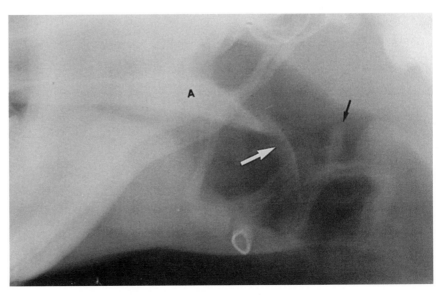

FIGURE 24–1. A normal lateral radiograph of the laryngeal region of a 6-month-old mixed-breed dog. The soft palate (A) separates the nasopharynx from the oropharynx. The epiglottis *(white arrow)* extends from the larynx to the tip of the soft palate. The cranial cornua of the thyroid cartilage *(black arrow)* should not be mistaken for a foreign object. Note the end-on view of the basihyoid bone.

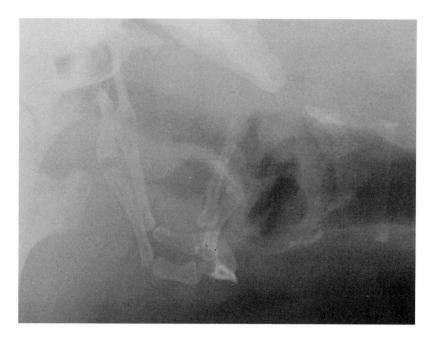

FIGURE 24–2. A normal lateral radiograph of the laryngeal region of an obese 13-year-old German shepherd dog. Notice that nonmineralized structures are more difficult to define owing to compromise of the air space.

have been mistakenly diagnosed as foreign objects. The configuration and relative position of the hyoid bones are rather uniform among small animals; however, the position of the head, tongue, and larynx during radiography causes variation in angles between hyoid bones. Oblique views may cause significant distortion, leading to erroneous diagnosis. Few radiographic abnormalities are evident in the hyoid bones. The most common abnormalities are fractures or dislocation.

Radiographic Signs of Disease

Abnormal Size and Shape

As mentioned previously, the size and shape of the pharynx and larynx vary with breed and degree of obesity. Generalized swelling may be detected if it is severe. This swelling may be erroneously diagnosed, however, in smaller, heavy-bodied, and obese animals. A severely elongated soft palate may be seen radiographically, although direct visual inspec-

tion is a more accurate method of evaluation. Radiographic examination may be an aid in assessing the degree of airway compromise in brachycephalic breeds before corrective surgery of external structures is pursued. Although specific airway diameter cannot be assessed, the relative size of the soft palate, epiglottis, and larynx can be evaluated.

Space-Occupying Lesions Within the Airway

Mass lesions, such as abscesses, polyps, neoplasms, and granulation tissue, may be readily identified with appropriate radiographic technique, accurate positioning, and knowledge of normal anatomy. When small, these lesions appear as variants in the normal shape of structures, and, when large, they may obliterate air-filled cavities. Such mass lesions may be found at any location (Fig. 24–3). Variation in radiographic technique may be necessary to demonstrate such lesions, owing to the variation in overlying tissue opacity between portions of the skull and cervical region. Depending on the shape, physical density, and architecture, foreign

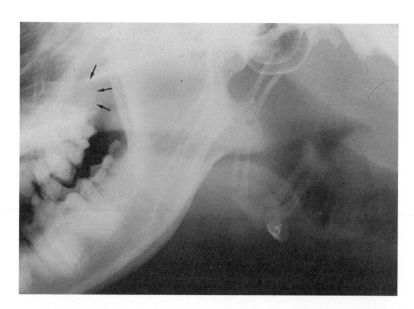

FIGURE 24–3. A lateral radiograph of the pharyngeal region of a 7-year-old Labrador retriever presenting with dyspnea. A neoplastic mass 1 cm in diameter *(arrows)* was found radiographically and confirmed by endoscopic examination and at surgery. Lesions in this area may be easily overlooked, especially on underexposed radiographs. Notice that on this radiograph, the epiglottis is positioned in the ventral pharynx at the base of the tongue region.

objects lodged in the airway may be identified specifically or may appear as space-occupying tissue masses.

Space-Occupying Masses Outside the Airway

Space-occupying masses outside the airway are more difficult to identify because they are not surrounded by gas. These lesions are identified by recognizing displacement or encroachment of the air-tissue interfaces. Although masses may develop at any site, enlargement of specific structures, such as a lymph node and the thyroid gland, should be considered when the cause for such radiographic abnormalities is being determined.

Functional Abnormalities

Functional abnormalities of the larynx are best evaluated by direct visual inspection. Neurogenic disorders result in mild or equivocal radiographic signs.[3] Consistent misplacement of the epiglottis seen on radiographs should prompt visual examination. In the panting dog, the epiglottis lies on the ventral floor of the pharynx.[2] Otherwise, it is in a semierect position, usually with the tip just dorsal or ventral to the soft palate.

TRACHEA

Anatomic Considerations

The trachea is best evaluated on the lateral view; however, the ventrodorsal view is useful to assess displacement of the trachea, principal bronchi, or both. The trachea is a midline structure that may deviate slightly to the right in the cranial mediastinum. This deviation is more exaggerated in short-bodied breeds such as the Boston terrier and should not be mistaken for displacement owing to a mass. On the lateral view, the trachea is nearly parallel to the cervical spine but is slightly closer to the spine in the caudal cervical region than cranial. Because the thoracic vertebrae angle dorsally, there is slight divergence of the trachea from the thoracic spine. The terminal trachea angles slightly ventral at the point of bifurcation into the principal bronchi. The diameter of the trachea is relatively uniform, slightly smaller than the larynx. In normal animals, the trachea does not vary significantly between phases of respiration and remains uniform in diameter.

The trachea is a semirigid tube attached at the larynx and the carina. It is confined in the cervical region but is less constrained in the cranial mediastinum. During radiographic examination in the lateral view, the head and neck should be placed in an erect but not overextended position. Extreme

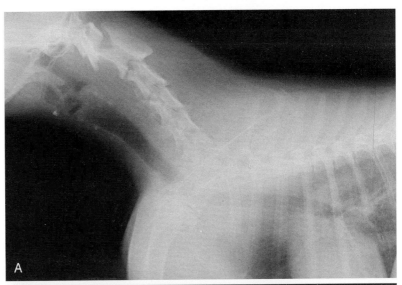

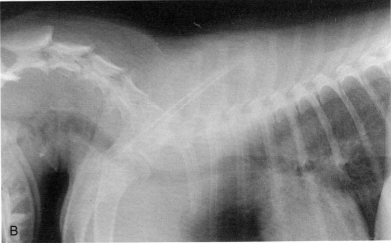

FIGURE 24–4. *A,* Lateral radiograph of a dog with the head and neck correctly positioned. *B,* Lateral radiograph of the same dog with the neck flexed. Notice the variation in tracheal position. This normal variation may be dramatic, leading to misdiagnosis of a mediastinal mass. Notice also, on the flexed view, that the laryngeal region is difficult to interpret.

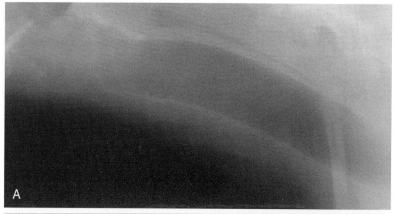

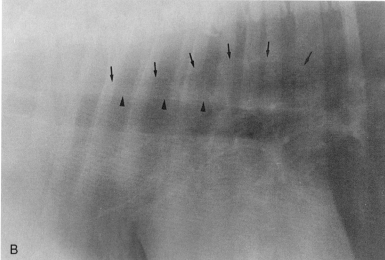

FIGURE 24–5. *A,* Lateral radiograph of a 9-month-old retriever. Because of the gas in the cranial esophagus, the ventral esophageal wall and the dorsal tracheal wall silhouette into one soft-tissue opacity that may be erroneously interpreted as thickening of the tracheal wall. *B,* Lateral thoracic radiograph of an 11-year-old West Highland White terrier. A barely discernible amount of gas is present in the thoracic esophagus *(arrows).* Because of this gas, the ventral esophageal wall is, again, silhouetted against the dorsal tracheal wall *(arrowheads).* Gas is often normally found in this location.

extension of the neck may cause compression and narrowing of the trachea at the thoracic inlet. Conversely, if the neck is flexed, the trachea is likely to bend in the cranial mediastinum, simulating displacement by a cranial mediastinal mass (Fig. 24–4).

Mineralization of the tracheal rings may be seen as an aging process, especially in large and chondrodystrophic dogs, but it is also seen in younger dogs, apparently with no significance. Diseases that stimulate metastatic mineralization may stimulate increased mineralization of the trachea along with other soft tissues.

Radiographic Signs of Disease

As mentioned earlier, displacement of the trachea is a reliable sign of mass lesions in the surrounding soft tissue if positioning artifacts and breed variation are accounted for. A common tracheal displacement is ventral displacement of the larynx and proximal trachea because of thyroid gland enlargement. Lymph node enlargement can be identified by tracheal deviation adjacent to the known location of lymph nodes (see Chapter 28).

In the cervical region, mass lesions must be relatively large to cause tracheal displacement. Unless massive in size, mass lesions that compress the trachea usually involve the trachea rather than simply touch it. Except for tracheobronchial and cranial mediastinal lymph node involvement and gross heart enlargement, compressive masses usually originate from the trachea itself.

Primary tumors of the larynx or trachea are uncommon. In the canine and feline trachea, osteochondroma and carcinomas, respectively, are the most common. Carcinomas are the most common tumor of the canine larynx, whereas lymphosarcoma is the most common feline laryngeal tumor. Tracheal and laryngeal tumors often produce clinical signs consistent with airway obstruction. Most laryngeal and tracheal tumors appear as masses within the lumen of the airway. Neoplastic lesions must be differentiated from polyps or abscesses within the upper airway because these may appear radiographically identical to primary tumors.[4]

Tracheal diameter varies slightly from breed to breed; however, this variation is minimal relative to the size of the animal. English bulldogs are known to have a smaller tracheal diameter than other breeds; however, members of this breed also are more likely to have a pathologically small trachea as a congenital defect.[5] Calculation of the ratio of tracheal diameter to thoracic inlet diameter can be used as a way of assessing tracheal size.[6] In nonbrachycephalic dogs, the mean ratio of tracheal diameter to thoracic inlet diameter was 0.20 ± 0.03 compared with 0.16 ± 0.03 in non-bulldog brachycephalic breeds and 0.13 ± 0.38 in bulldogs. The range in bulldogs was 0.07 to 0.21. The smallest ratio in bulldogs with no clinical signs of respiratory disease was 0.09. The ratio for dogs younger than 1 year of age was slightly smaller than for older dogs. Accurate lateral positioning is necessary for accurate measurements.

Although the common infectious diseases rarely result in detectable thickening of the tracheal wall or narrowing of the lumen, acute dyspnea may occur as the result of in-

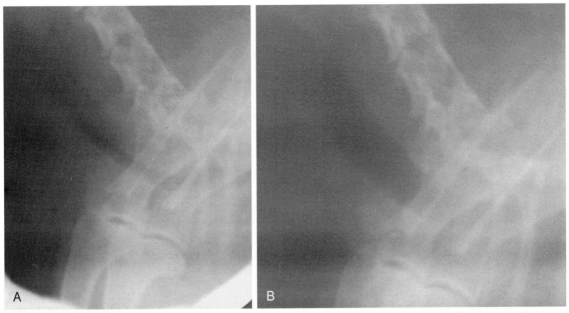

FIGURE 24–6. Inspiration *(A)* and expiration *(B)* radiographs of a 15-year-old Poodle were made during fluoroscopy. The cervical trachea is narrowed on inspiration and is larger than the thoracic trachea on expiration. This finding indicates that the weak trachealis muscle is being pulled into the lumen by negative pressure during inspiration, compromising air flow, and is being forced outward by positive pressure during expiration.

flammatory tracheal disease, with significant decrease in diameter of the tracheal lumen. If the esophagus contains large or small amounts of gas, the esophageal wall may cause a silhouette sign with the dorsal tracheal wall (tracheoesophageal stripe sign), presenting an erroneous appearance of tracheal thickening (Fig. 24–5).

Most tracheal problems are dynamic in nature, resulting in variation in tracheal size in a region related to the phase of

the respiratory cycle (i.e., tracheal collapse). This variation is most often seen in the toy dog breeds because of weakness in the structural rigidity of the trachea. Tracheal collapse, because of its dynamic nature, requires special attention for radiographic documentation.

Dynamic narrowing of the tracheal lumen owing to tracheal instability may occur in the cervical trachea (especially at the thoracic inlet) during inspiration (Fig. 24–6) or in the

FIGURE 24–7. Inspiratory *(A)* and expiratory *(B)* radiographs of an 11-year-old Poodle. The entire thoracic trachea collapses nearly completely during expiration. In many patients, only the caudal trachea collapses, with a characteristic end-expiratory click heard on auscultation.

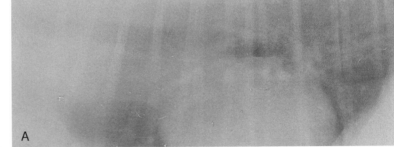

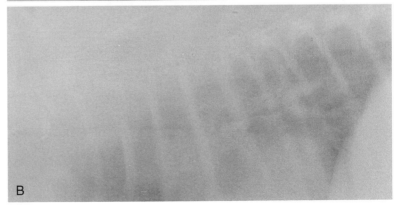

thoracic trachea (especially at the carina) during expiration (Fig. 24–7), or during both. With severe loss of rigidity, the site of collapse may not match with the phase of respiration. At times, the area that collapses may actually "balloon" during the opposite respiratory phase.

Abnormal enlargement of a portion of trachea on inspiration should lead to suspicion of obstruction of air flow cranially. This enlargement may be from disease in the trachea or larynx. It is often seen as a secondary radiographic sign of laryngeal paralysis.[3]

Confusion may occur when tracheal rings or a partial air column can be identified dorsal to the upper margin of the tracheal air column. Although some people believe this is due to overlying structures, tracheography (by injecting contrast medium into the trachea) has proved narrowing of the tracheal lumen in some instances. An explanation of this pattern is redundancy of the trachealis muscle folding into the dorsal trachea, narrowing the actual air space. During fluoroscopic examination, the soft-tissue trachealis muscle sometimes moves in and out of the lumen during respiration. The radiographic pattern may be seen in large dogs with no evidence of respiratory distress, making muscle laxity difficult to blame for the radiographic phenomenon in all dogs. Because the dorsal aspect of the trachea may normally be flattened, a similar pattern may be seen if the trachea is rotated.

To evaluate dynamic tracheal disease fully, lateral radiographs should be made during both inspiration and expiration. Often, suspected abnormalities may be detected in this manner. Abnormalities in the thoracic trachea are exaggerated during coughing. At times, fluoroscopic examination is necessary to demonstrate the dynamic signs.

Narrowing of a region of the trachea has been reported secondary to localized obstruction in the cranial aspect of the trachea in cats.[7] The cause for the localized obstruction may not be radiographically visible, suggesting that discovery of narrowed or collapsed trachea in cats should prompt further investigation by endoscopic examination.

References

1. O'Brien JH, Harvey CE, and Tucker JA: The larynx of the dog: Its normal radiographic anatomy. J Am Vet Radiol Soc 10:38, 1969.
2. Gaskell CJ: The radiographic anatomy of the pharynx and larynx of the dog. J Small Anim Pract 14:89, 1974.
3. Reinke JD, and Suter PF: Laryngeal paralysis in a dog. J Am Vet Med Assoc 172:714, 1978.
4. Carlisle CH, Biery DN, and Thrall DE: Tracheal and laryngeal tumors in the dog and cat: Literature review and 13 additional patients. Vet Radiol 32:229, 1991.
5. Suter PF, Colgrove DJ, and Ewing GO: Congenital hypoplasia of the canine trachea. J Am Anim Hosp Assoc 8:120, 1972.
6. Harvey CE, and Fink EA: Tracheal diameter: Analysis of radiographic measurements in brachycephalic and non-brachycephalic dogs. J Am Anim Hosp Assoc 18:570, 1982.
7. Hendricks JC, and O'Brien JA: Tracheal collapse in two cats. J Am Vet Med Assoc 187:418, 1985.

STUDY QUESTIONS

1. Laryngeal and pharyngeal structures may be difficult to distinguish on high-quality radiographs in which of the following?
   A. Young animals.
   B. Obese animals.
   C. Brachycephalic breeds.
   D. All of the above.

2. Mineralization of laryngeal structures is abnormal if seen in dogs under 5 years of age. (True or False)

3. Except during swallowing, the normal epiglottis is usually seen in radiographs to be flat against the ventral wall of the pharynx. (True or False)

4. Soft-tissue opacity or mass effect lesions within the gas-filled chambers of the larynx or pharynx may be caused by neoplasia, abscess, polyps, or foreign objects. (True or False)

5. The volume of the pharynx may be compromised by outside material, including adipose tissue, abscesses, neoplasia, or enlargement of tissues such as lymph nodes. (True or False)

6. The trachea is a midline structure. Deviation from the midline is abnormal on a ventrodorsal (dorsoventral) view in any patient. (True or False)

7. When radiographing a trachea, to avoid erroneous compression of the tracheal diameter, the patient's neck should be flexed. (True or False)

8. Normal tracheal lumen diameter relative to thoracic inlet diameter is smaller for brachycephalic dogs than for non-brachycephalic dogs. (True or False)

9. If demonstrated radiographically, tracheal collapse tends to occur during inspiration in the cervical region and during expiration within the thorax. (True or False)

10. Normal gas in the esophagus may lead to erroneous diagnosis of tracheal wall thickening. (True or False)

(Answers appear on page 640.)

Chapter 25

The Esophagus

Barbara Jean Watrous

Disorders of the pregastric alimentary tract result in a variety of clinical signs, including regurgitation, dysphagia, abnormal swallowing, and gagging or retching.[1] Other signs include weight loss, failure to gain weight or grow normally, and chronic or recurrent respiratory problems. Aspiration pneumonia, tracheitis, and nasal discharge are frequent complications of esophageal dysfunction. In several systemic neuromuscular diseases, the oropharynx, esophagus, or both may be involved. Indications for evaluation of the upper alimentary tract, therefore, include dysphagia; regurgitation; and recurrent, unexplained respiratory tract infections.

Survey radiographs may allow identification of radiopaque foreign bodies or mass lesions. The survey radiographic examination should include views of the entire esophagus, including the caudal pharynx and cranial abdomen. Views of the skull may be required when oropharyngeal dysphagia is suspected.

Contrast radiographic examination is often necessary to identify lesions or to characterize survey radiographic findings further. Differentiation of functional from morphologic causes of dysphagia may be possible with static contrast studies. Specific evaluation of functional abnormalities, however, may be made only in dynamic fluoroscopic studies. The emphasis in this chapter is on information provided by static survey and contrast radiographic findings.

SURVEY RADIOGRAPHIC FINDINGS

The normal esophagus is a collapsed tube bounded cranially and caudally by functional sphincters. On survey radiographs (Table 25–1), the esophagus is not usually seen because the soft tissues of the cervical esophagus silhouette with surrounding muscles and associated fascia, and the thoracic esophagus is enveloped by the dorsal mediastinum, fascia, and connective tissue.[2]

The absence of abnormal esophageal radiographic findings does not preclude the presence of esophageal disease; such is often encountered with acute esophageal disease. In addition, the presence of indirect signs of esophageal disease should be anticipated. Focal or generalized esophageal dilation may be less apparent when the lumen is fluid filled, creating a positive silhouette sign. The enlarged lumen, however, affects adjacent visible structures. The weight of the dilated esophagus may cause ventral and right lateral tracheal displacement in the cervical and cranial thoracic regions. The cranial and caudal mediastinum widens around the dilated esophagus. Pulmonary interstitial or alveolar infiltrates occur secondary to aspiration. Pleural effusion, pneumothorax or pneumomediastinum, and lobar consolidation are occasionally present secondary to esophageal disease.

The presence of opacity change allows for direct visualization of the normal and abnormal esophagus. Decreased radiopacity, both periesophageal and intraluminal, makes the esophagus visible radiographically. Pneumomediastinum or cervical gas may outline its adventitial surface (Fig. 25–1). Gas may originate from deep skin wounds, tracheal and esophageal rupture, and pulmonary leakage. Perforation of the esophagus may occur from trauma or inflammation; foreign bodies and esophageal surgical procedures are the most common causes. The radiographic signs of an acute perforation are air in the periesophageal tissues of the cervical region and pneumomediastinum. Long-standing perforation of the cervical esophagus leads to cellulitis and abscess formation with persistence of air or with periesophageal mass formation. Mediastinitis and pleuritis result from a chronically perforated thoracic esophagus.

Accumulation of intraluminal gas usually indicates esophageal disease. Occasionally, however, small amounts of swallowed air are seen in the normal esophagus. Common sites for this on the lateral view include the area immediately caudal to the cranial esophageal sphincter (Fig. 25–2), at the

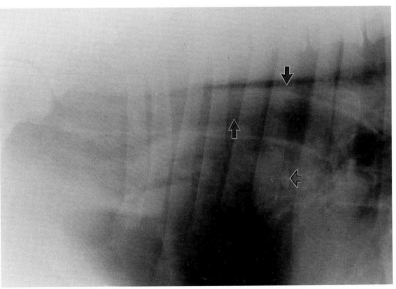

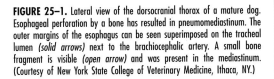
FIGURE 25–1. Lateral view of the dorsocranial thorax of a mature dog. Esophageal perforation by a bone has resulted in pneumomediastinum. The outer margins of the esophagus can be seen superimposed on the tracheal lumen *(solid arrows)* next to the brachiocephalic artery. A small bone fragment is visible *(open arrow)* and was present in the mediastinum. (Courtesy of New York State College of Veterinary Medicine, Ithaca, NY.)

Table 25–1
SURVEY RADIOGRAPHIC FINDINGS

Radiographic Findings	Esophageal Status	Etiologies
Normal	Normal	—
	Abnormal	Neuromuscular disease
		Hiatal hernia
		Foreign body (nonradiopaque)
		Esophagitis
		Early strictures
		Fistulas
Radiolucency		
Regional intraluminal	Normal	Aerophagia
	Abnormal	Foreign bodies (nonradiopaque)
		Gastroesophageal intussusception
		Extraluminal masses
		Esophagitis
		Strictures
		Vascular ring anomalies
		Neoplasia
		Segmental hypomotility
Generalized intraluminal	Normal	General anesthesia
		Central nervous system depression
	Abnormal	Megaesophagus
		Neuromuscular hypomotility
		Hypoadrenocorticism
		Autoimmune myositis
		Autoimmune neuritis
		Myasthenia gravis
		Toxicities
		Neoplasia
		Hypothyroidism
		Trauma
Periesophageal	Normal	Subcutanoeus emphysema
	Abnormal	Perforation
Radiopacity		
Regional intraluminal	Abnormal	Vascular ring anomalies
		Foreign bodies (radiopaque)
		Spirocerca lupi
		Neoplasia
		Gastroesophageal intussusception
		Diverticula
		Periesophageal masses
Generalized intraluminal	Abnormal	Megaesophagus

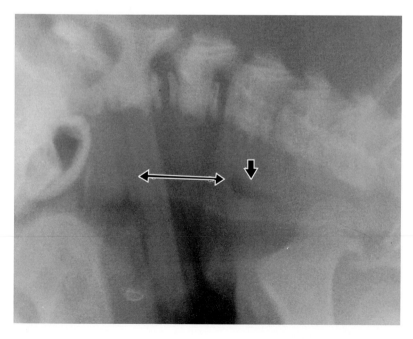

FIGURE 25–2. Lateral view of the neck of a normal 6-week-old puppy that struggled during radiographic examination. Air trapped in the cranial esophagus *(arrow)* just behind the cranial esophageal sphincter *(double-headed arrow)* is commonly seen under these circumstances. (Courtesy of New York State College of Veterinary Medicine, Ithaca, NY.)

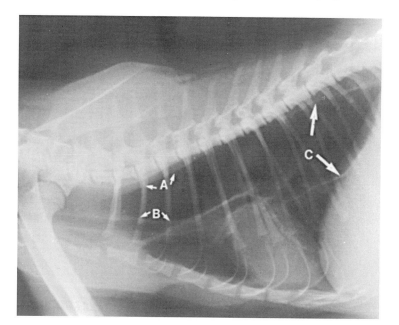

FIGURE 25–3. Lateral view of the thorax of an aged cat with chronic upper airway obstruction. The entire esophagus is visible because it is dilated and air-filled. Hallmarks of esophageal dilation include the sharp interface between the longus colli muscles and the esophageal lumen (A), the tracheal stripe sign with displacement of the trachea ventrally (B), and the paired converging soft-tissue stripes in the dorsocaudal thorax (C). (Courtesy of New York State College of Veterinary Medicine, Ithaca, NY.)

level of the thoracic inlet and dorsal to the heart base. Repeated radiographs should indicate that this focal air accumulation is transient. In the dorsoventral or ventrodorsal view, this gas is often hidden because of superimposition.

Abnormal luminal gas accumulation occurs in most esophageal diseases. Generalized megaesophagus with a gas-filled lumen may be visualized along all or part of its length on survey radiographs. In the lateral view, the cervical portion is apparent beginning just caudal to the cranial esophageal sphincter. When mildly dilated, the esophagus is visible dorsal to the proximal trachea, crossing somewhat lateral to the trachea at the thoracic inlet. As it dilates further, it drapes around the trachea and depresses it ventrally (Fig. 25–3). If the esophagus is fluid filled, the lumen may not be visible because of silhouetting of the soft tissue and fluid (Fig. 25–4A). The thoracic esophagus, when gas filled, may be inadvertently overlooked because of the relative radiolucency of the adjacent lung field. Close scrutiny, however, provides several hallmark findings characteristic of its presence. When

the cranial thoracic esophagus dilates, the dorsal wall abuts against the paired longus colli muscles, which may be seen as a sharp interface from the thoracic inlet to the ventral aspect of T5 or T6. The ventral wall projects lateral and often ventral to the trachea. The draping of the ventral wall over the dorsal tracheal wall results in summation (silhouetting) of the two walls, which creates the *tracheal band* or *tracheal stripe* sign. When gas-distended, the caudal thoracic esophagus is seen as a pair of thin, soft-tissue stripes that converge to a point overlying the diaphragm and cranial abdomen. Absence of the ventral stripe may result from an overlap of the caudal vena cava (see Fig. 25–3).

On the dorsoventral or ventrodorsal view, the dilated, gas-filled cervical esophagus may be hidden by the spine and trachea, although displacement of the trachea to the right may be seen (see Fig. 25–4B). The dilated cranial thoracic esophagus produces a wide cranial mediastinum that is relatively radiolucent. The lateral margins are indented on the left by the descending aorta and on the right by the azygous

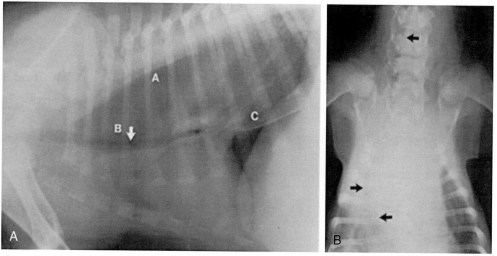

FIGURE 25–4. A, Lateral view of a young dog with megaesophagus. The esophageal lumen is not visible in the cervical region owing to its fluid content. Some hallmark signs (see legend to Fig. 25–3) are apparent in the thoracic region. B, Deviation of the cervical and thoracic portions of the trachea (arrows) by the fluid-filled cranial esophagus may be seen. (Courtesy of New York State College of Veterinary Medicine, Ithaca, NY.)

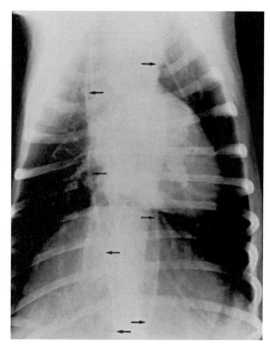

FIGURE 25–5. Dorsoventral view of the thorax of an adult dog with megaesophagus. The lateral walls of the esophagus are seen as thin soft-tissue bands roughly parallel to the spine *(arrows)*. They converge in the caudal thorax. (Courtesy of New York State College of Veterinary Medicine, Ithaca, NY.)

vein. The caudal thoracic esophagus converges to a V at the hiatus of the diaphragm (Fig. 25–5).

Abnormal regional gas accumulation may occur anywhere along the esophagus just cranial to or at the site of localized disease. Gas trapping occurs at the site of acute entrapment of intraluminal foreign bodies, esophagitis, and segmental esophageal hypomotility. Obstruction of the esophageal lumen by vascular ring anomalies (Fig. 25–6), acquired strictures, extraluminal (Fig. 25–7) and intrinsic masses, and chronic foreign bodies may or may not result in air accumulation.

Increased radiopacity associated with esophageal disease may be general or focal. Generalized radiopacity occurs when radiopaque foreign bodies or liquid, food, or foreign material accumulates in the dilated lumen (see Fig. 25–4). The radiopacity is usually heterogeneous because of the entrapment of small gas bubbles in solid or semisolid food. Regional

radiopacity may be a result of lodged radiopaque foreign bodies (Fig. 25–8), localized dilation because of vascular ring anomalies (Fig. 25–9), diverticula or gastroesophageal intussusceptions (Fig. 25–10) and subsequent food or foreign material accumulation (see Fig. 25–9), focal soft-tissue infiltration of the esophageal wall (Fig. 25–11), or dystrophic mineralization (Fig. 25–12). The common locations of various esophageal lesions are listed in Table 25–2.

CONTRAST RADIOGRAPHY

Contrast Media

Many contrast media are available for esophagography, and choosing a specific one should be based on the suspected disease.[3] Barium sulfate cream and paste (Esophotrast, Rhone-Poulenc Rorer Pharmaceuticals Inc., Collegeville, PA; Intropaste, Lafayette Pharmaceutical, Inc., Lafayette, IN; E Z Paste, E Z EM Co., Westbury, NY; Varibar, E Z EM Co.) have been formulated for extreme radiopacity and good adherence to esophageal mucosa. Mucosal irregularities (esophagitis, neoplastic infiltrates) and strictures are readily evaluated with paste or cream. Because of their viscosity, however, they tend to maintain a bolus, failing to disperse well or flow around intraluminal lesions. Admixture with liquid barium suspensions is also poor, resulting in clumping in the gastric lumen when an upper gastrointestinal examination follows an esophagram in which paste was used. Aspiration of paste may lead to asphyxiation; therefore, use of paste is not advised when aspiration is a concern.

Liquid barium sulfate suspensions (e z hd, E Z EM Co.; Liquid Sol-O-Paque, E Z EM Co.; E-Z-Paque, E Z EM Co.) do not adhere well to the mucosa, but a high-density medium (45 to 85 percent w/w) can be used for esophagography because it is relatively safe when aspirated, mixes well with fluid contents, and readily flows around obstructions. Motility problems of the oropharyngeal and esophageal regions should be evaluated first with liquid barium. Barium-coated food may be administered subsequently, particularly in animals with problems in swallowing solids but not liquids. Barium-coated food may best demonstrate early strictures or regional motility disorders.

Oral aqueous iodine solutions (Gastrografin, Bracco Diagnostics, Princeton, NJ; Oral Hypaque Sodium, Nycomed Inc., New York, NY; MD Gastroview, Mallinckrodt Medical Inc., St. Louis, MO) are relatively nontoxic in body cavities. Therefore, their use is indicated when esophageal perforation is

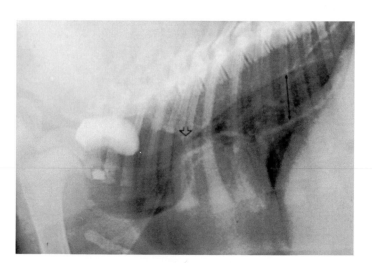

FIGURE 25–6. Lateral view of the thorax of a young dog with a persistent right fourth aortic arch. The characteristic site of obstruction with persistent right fourth aortic arch is just cranial to the tracheal bifurcation *(open arrow)*. An evaluation for possible esophageal dilation caudal to the ring, as was present in this animal *(double-headed arrow)*, must be made. The radiopacities are foreign bodies (stones) within the prestenotic dilated esophageal lumen. Thoracic tracheal depression is evident. Rare causes for other vascular ring anomalies include double aortic arches, aberrant right subclavian artery, and dextroaorta with left subclavian artery. (Courtesy of New York State College of Veterinary Medicine, Ithaca, NY.)

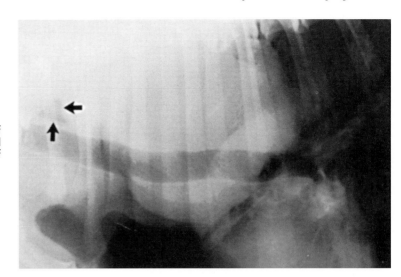

FIGURE 25–7. Lateral view of the dorsocranial thorax of a dog with signs of regurgitation. A thoracic tumor encroached on the esophagus, leading to mild dilation and focal air accumulation at the thoracic inlet *(arrows).* (Courtesy of New York State College of Veterinary Medicine, Ithaca, NY.)

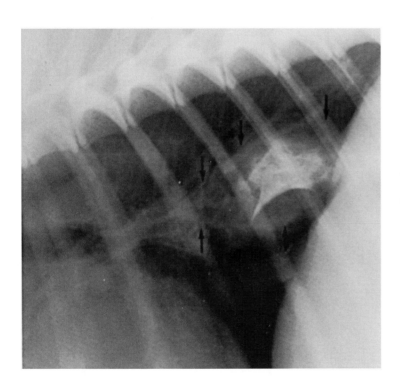

FIGURE 25–8. Lateral view of the dorsocaudal thorax of the dog in Figure 25–7. There is a radiopaque foreign body cranial to the esophageal hiatus. The sharp projection is characteristic of esophageal foreign bodies. A prominent zone of soft tissue *(arrows)* surrounds the bone, indicative of esophageal wall thickening by inflammation. Four common sites of foreign body entrapment are the cranial cervical region, the thoracic inlet, over the base of the heart, and cranial to the hiatus. (Courtesy of New York State College of Veterinary Medicine, Ithaca, NY.)

FIGURE 25–9. Lateral view of the cranial thorax of a young cat with a persistent right fourth aortic arch. There is food accumulation in the dilated segment of the esophagus cranial to the obstruction. The trachea deviates ventrally. (Courtesy of New York State College of Veterinary Medicine, Ithaca, NY.)

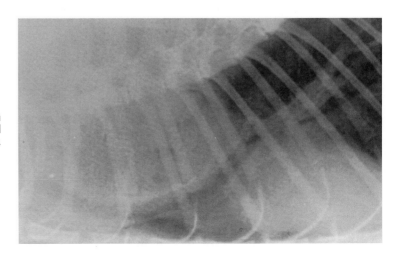

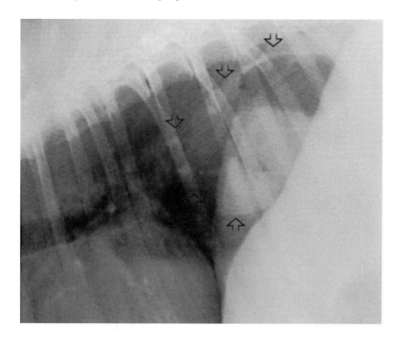

FIGURE 25–10. Lateral view of the caudodorsal thorax of a mature dog with a gastroesophageal intussusception. The radiopacity of the gastric contents may be seen in the caudal thorax superimposed over the left diaphragmatic crus and dorsocaudal lung field *(arrows).* (Courtesy of New York State College of Veterinary Medicine, Ithaca, NY.)

FIGURE 25–11. Lateral view of the caudodorsal thorax of a mature dog. There is an area of soft-tissue opacity between the aorta and caudal vena cava *(arrows).* This is an esophageal leiomyoma. (Courtesy of New York State College of Veterinary Medicine, Ithaca, NY.)

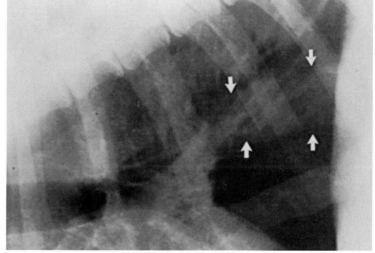

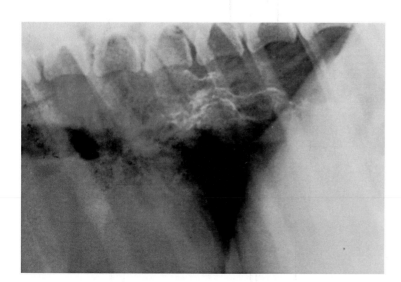

FIGURE 25–12. Survey radiograph of the caudodorsal thorax of a mature dog. There are abnormal linear to amorphous mineral opacities in the dorsal thorax. Differential diagnoses include dystrophic mineralization of the esophagus associated with chronic inflammation or granuloma *(Spirocerca lupi),* neoplasia with mineralization, chronic radiolucent foreign body, and coating of an eroded mucosa by an antacid or enteric-coated agent. (Courtesy of New York State College of Veterinary Medicine, Ithaca, NY.)

Table 25–2
CHARACTERISTIC SITE OF FOCAL ESOPHAGEAL DISEASE

Cervical Region	Cranial Thoracic Region	Caudal Thoracic Region
Achalasia	Vascular ring anomaly	Esophagitis (reflux)
Asynchrony	Esophagitis (reflux)	(patulent caudal esophageal
Chalasia	Stricture	sphincter)
Foreign body	Periesophageal mass	Foreign body
Esophagitis (caustic)	Redundancy	Perforation
Extension of neoplasia	Diverticula	Leiomyoma
Perforation	Foreign body	Gastroesophageal intussusception
Segmental hypomotility	Neoplasia	Hiatal hernia
	Perforation	Esophageal fistula

suspected. These agents are hypertonic and thus, if aspirated, may induce pulmonary edema. In addition, a volume-depleted animal may be further compromised by fluid loss through the gastrointestinal tract from their osmotic effect. If leakage occurs into a fluid-filled pleural space, the resulting dilution may make it difficult to detect the extravasated contrast medium or the site of leakage. Nonionic organic iodide agents (Omnipaque, Mallinckrodt Medical Inc.) are isosmolar and do not create the complications encountered with ionic contrast media. Nonionic agents are more expensive, however. The use of a barium sulfate liquid in the presence of a perforation has instigated some controversy because of the tendency of barium to stimulate a granulomatous reaction on pleural surfaces. The use of barium sulfate is indicated, however, when an oral iodine medium fails to define the problem. Aqueous iodine contrast media are not recommended for routine esophagography because of their poor coating ability.

Technique

Survey radiographs should always be made immediately before an esophagram. This provides for selection of a suitable radiographic technique and for assessment of the status of the esophagus and surrounding tissues. Superimposition of the spine readily obscures even a barium-coated esophageal lumen. Therefore, in addition to the lateral view, either a right or left dorsoventral-lateral oblique position is recommended to rotate the esophagus into a more visible location. On the lateral view, the opacity over the thoracic inlet from the heavy musculature of the brachium can be reduced by moving one thoracic limb cranially and the other caudally.

A fractious animal may be given a nominal dose of phenothiazine tranquilizer (acepromazine maleate, 0.05 mg/lb of body weight subcutaneously or intramuscularly). The esophagus, however, is affected by most central nervous system depressant drugs, and their use is disadvantageous when motility is being evaluated.

Approximately 5 to 20 mL of contrast medium is given to induce several complete swallows for coating the pharynx and esophagus. Oropharyngeal problems are best evaluated by a series of radiographs made in the midst of a swallow and during a pause after the swallow is completed. The esophageal phase should be radiographed after a sufficient pause to ensure complete transport of the last bolus to the stomach.

The normal appearance of the oropharyngeal region after a swallow of contrast medium is coating of the mucosa without significant retention of the contrast medium (Fig. 25–13). A small amount may occasionally remain immediately caudal to the cranial esophageal sphincter. No contrast medium should persist in the piriform recesses or upper airway (nasopharynx, larynx, or trachea) unless laryngotracheal aspiration inadvertently occurs.

The normal canine esophageal mucosa appears as a series of longitudinal folds. The lines are close together through most of its length but may separate slightly at the thoracic inlet as the esophagus passes along the left lateral side of the trachea (Fig. 25–14). The feline esophagus has a similar appearance to the level of the heart base, but the caudal esophagus has obliquely directed folds that correspond to the

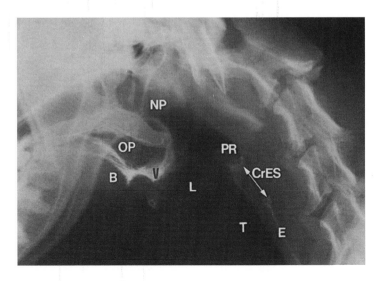

FIGURE 25–13. Normal oropharyngeal contrast medium examination of a mature dog (lateral view). NP, nasopharynx; OP, oropharynx; B, base of tongue; E, esophagus; V, valleculae; L, larynx; T, trachea; PR, piriform recesses; CrES, cranial esophageal sphincter. (Courtesy of New York State College of Veterinary Medicine, Ithaca, NY.)

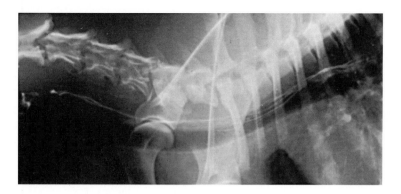

FIGURE 25–14. Normal esophagram (lateral view) of a mature dog using barium sulfate cream. The longitudinal folds often separate at the thoracic inlet.

smooth muscle segment (Fig. 25–15). Oblique views of the dorsoventral or ventrodorsal position eliminate superimposition of the spine for better visualization of the esophagus (Fig. 25–16).

CONTRAST RADIOGRAPHIC FINDINGS

Diseases of the oral stage of swallowing usually involve the tongue. If an abnormality of the oral stage is present, the effect may be on prehension, caudal transport through the oral cavity, or organization of a bolus in the oropharynx by the tongue. Retention of contrast medium in the oral cavity and oropharynx is present radiographically. The subsequent pharyngeal and cricopharyngeal stages are normal (Fig. 25–17).

Pharyngeal stage dysphagia is encountered with neuromuscular disease, inflammatory diseases (Fig. 25–18), and trauma that may be associated with perforation (Fig. 25–19) or fracture of the hyoid apparatus (Fig. 25–20).[4–6] The oral stage is normal, but inadequate pharyngeal peristalsis leads to retention of much of the bolus of contrast medium. Inadequate closure of the pharyngeal egresses (nasopharynx, oral cavity, and larynx) may lead to reflux of contrast medium into these regions.

Cricopharyngeal stage dysphagia may be due to inappropriate opening or nonopening of the cranial esophageal sphincter (cricopharyngeal asynchrony or achalasia) or failure of closure of that sphincter (chalasia). Chalasia is recognized by the persistence of a patent passage between the pharynx and cranial esophagus (Fig. 25–21). Reflux of esophageal contrast medium results in its presence in the pharynx. Pharyngeal paresis often accompanies cricopharyngeal chalasia, which

is an additional cause for pharyngeal retention of contrast medium. Dysfunction of the cranial esophageal sphincter because of asynchrony or achalasia results in interference with transport of the contrast medium. The passage may be visibly distorted, although the pattern of distribution of retained contrast medium is similar to the pattern found in pharyngeal dysphagia (Fig. 25–22). Table 25–3 is a summary of the static contrast radiographic findings in the various oropharyngeal dysphagias.

A diffusely dilated esophagus (megaesophagus) usually produces sufficient diagnostic radiographic signs on survey radiographs to preclude the need for esophagography. On occasion, however, a partially gas-filled and fluid-filled lumen is difficult to detect (see Fig. 25–4A), requiring contrast medium examination. In addition, esophageal dilation may be caused by other than primary neuromuscular abnormalities, for example, neoplasia, inflammation, or hiatal disease. Evaluation of the competency of the cranial esophageal sphincter by examination with contrast medium may be indicated to help establish a prognosis in instances of systemic neuromuscular disease.

Regional dilation without obstruction may occur in primary segmental hypomotility or secondary dysmotility from inflammation, diverticula, and redundancy. Segmental motility disturbances may affect any portion of the esophagus. Reflux esophagitis usually involves the caudal esophagus and may or may not be associated with hiatal herniation (Fig. 25–23), caudal esophageal sphincter chalasia, chronic vomiting, or idiopathic reflux (Fig. 25–24). Diverticula or sacculations of the esophagus are most often encountered cranial to strictures, including those that result from vascular ring anomalies (see Fig. 25–6), but also occur with esophageal or periesophageal inflammation. Esophageal redundancy is an

Text continued on page 284

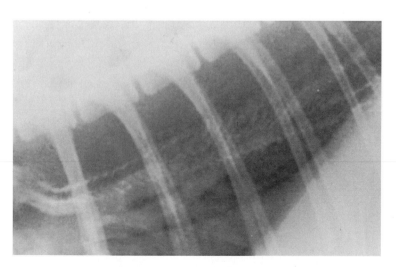

FIGURE 25–15. Normal caudal thoracic esophagram in a mature cat. Note the herringbone mucosal pattern.

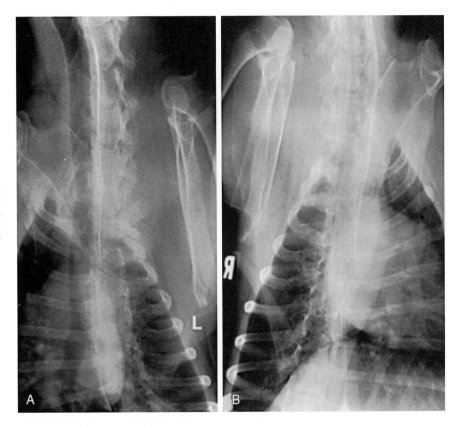

FIGURE 25–16. *A,* Normal esophagram (right dorsoventral oblique view) of a mature dog after administration of a barium sulfate cream. The sternum is to the right of the esophagus and the vertebral column to the left. *B,* Same study as in *A,* left dorsoventral oblique view. The sternum is to the left of the esophagus and the vertebral column to the right.

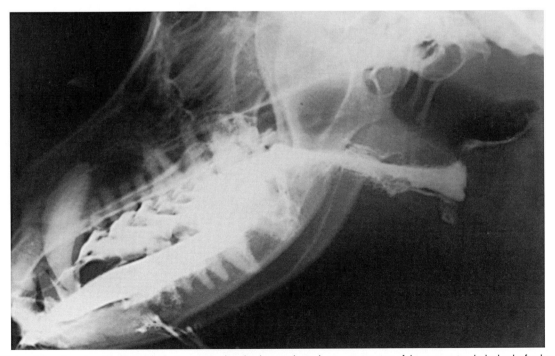

FIGURE 25–17. Lateral view of a mature dog with oral dysphagia owing to a hypoglossal neuropathy. Inadequate stripping action of the tongue against the hard and soft palate prevents caudal transport of ingesta, and there is no resulting bolus formation of contrast medium at the base of the tongue. A small amount of contrast medium has been swallowed, signifying normal pharyngeal and cricopharyngeal function. (Courtesy of New York State College of Veterinary Medicine, Ithaca, NY.)

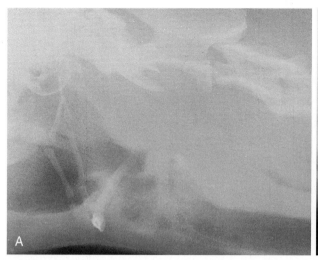
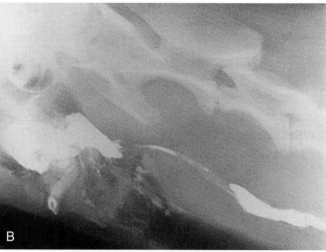

FIGURE 25–18. Pharyngeal-stage dysphagia is a result of inadequate sequential cranial-to-caudal contraction by the pharyngeal muscles. Thus, transport of a bolus through the cranial esophageal sphincter is usually incomplete. Contrast medium is retained in the pharynx and piriform recesses. This dog with chronic laryngitis and pharyngitis has retropharyngeal swelling and inflammation in addition to scarring of the larynx. *A,* Note the short epiglottis and ventrally displaced trachea. Air is retained in the esophagus. *B,* Esophagram; there is pharyngeal retention of contrast medium and laryngotracheal aspiration because of disturbed motility.

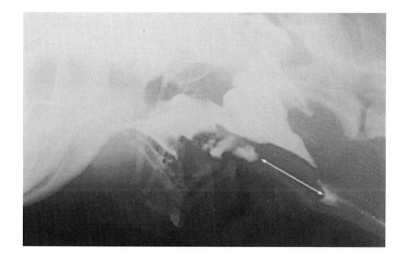

FIGURE 25–19. Pharyngeal laceration secondary to a stick resulted in a retropharyngeal fistula and pharyngeal paresis. There is accumulation of contrast medium in the pharynx, the piriform recesses, and the retropharyngeal abscess. *Double-headed arrow* denotes the cranial esophageal sphincter. (Courtesy of New York State College of Veterinary Medicine, Ithaca, NY.)

FIGURE 25–20. Lateral view of the pharyngeal region of a mature dog. The hyoid apparatus plays an integral role in coordinating laryngeal closure with the oral, pharyngeal, and cricopharyngeal stages of swallowing. Fracture *(arrows)* or dislocation of the hyoid apparatus may disrupt this process, as in this dog. Contrast medium has collected in the oropharynx but cannot be propelled caudally by the pharynx. (Courtesy of New York State College of Veterinary Medicine, Ithaca, NY.)

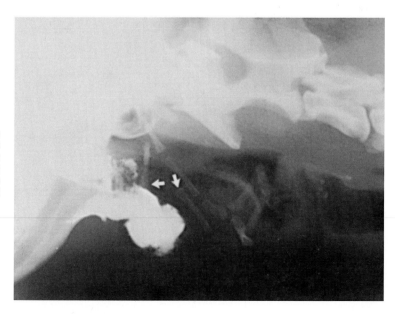

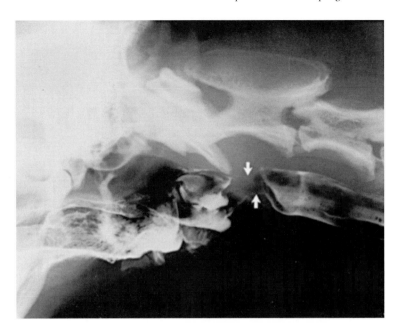

FIGURE 25–21. Lateral view of the pharyngeal region of a mature dog with autoimmune polymyositis. Chalasia *(arrows)* and megaesophagus are present. Contrast medium in the valleculae and piriform recesses may be due to esophagopharyngeal reflux or to pharyngeal paresis. (Courtesy of New York State College of Veterinary Medicine, Ithaca, NY.)

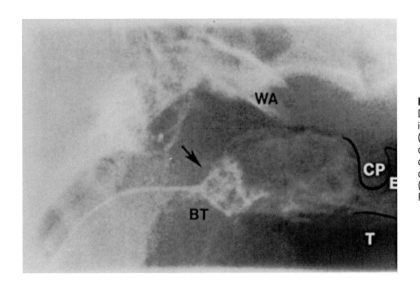

FIGURE 25–22. Lateral esophagram of the pharyngeal region of a dog. During the pharyngeal and cricopharyngeal stages of swallowing, the pharynx is in vigorous contraction *(arrow)* against a closing cranial esophageal sphincter (CP). The floor of this passage is open, allowing air and contrast medium to outline the distorted sphincter. This asynchrony between the pharyngeal and the cricopharyngeal stages occurs more commonly than does true cricopharyngeal achalasia. BT, base of tongue; WA, wings of atlas; E, esophagus; T, trachea. (From Ettinger SJ [Ed]: Textbook of Veterinary Internal Medicine, 2nd Ed. Philadelphia, WB Saunders, 1983; with permission.)

Table 25–3
SUMMARY OF LOCATION OF RETAINED CONTRAST MEDIUM RELATIVE TO TYPE OF OROPHARYNGEAL DYSPHAGIA

		Dysphagia		
Site	Normal	*Oral*	*Pharyngeal*	*Cricopharyngeal*
Oral cavity	+/−	+	−	−
Nasopharynx	−	−	+/−	+/−
Oropharynx	−	+	+/−	+/−
Pharynx	−	−	+	+
Valleculae	+/−	+/−	+	+
Piriform recesses	−	−	+	+
Esophagus	−	−	+/−	+/−
Larynx/trachea	−	−	+	+

+, present; −, absent.

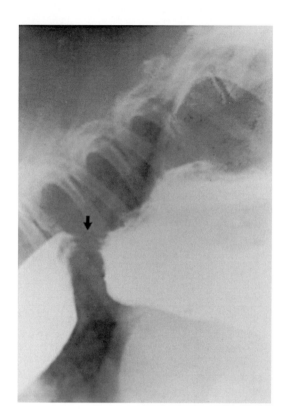

FIGURE 25–23. A hiatal hernia is present. Esophagitis and caudal esophageal dilation result from the gastroesophageal reflux. The caudal esophageal sphincter *(arrow)* is well defined cranial to the diaphragm. (Courtesy of New York State College of Veterinary Medicine, Ithaca, NY.)

FIGURE 25–24. Gastroesophageal reflux is characterized by contrast medium in the caudal esophagus after clearing of this area subsequent to the initial administration of contrast medium. The ventral wall of the esophagus in this dog is thickened *(arrows)* by chronic inflammation, which impairs rapid clearing and further compounds the problem. (Courtesy of New York State College of Veterinary Medicine, Ithaca, NY.)

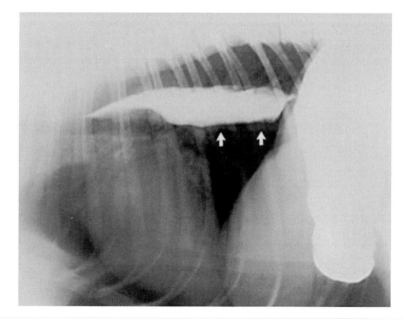

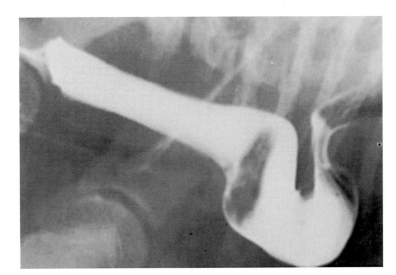

FIGURE 25–25. The cranial thoracic esophagus in this immature bulldog is redundant. The tortuous path may hamper peristalsis. (Courtesy of New York State College of Veterinary Medicine, Ithaca, NY.)

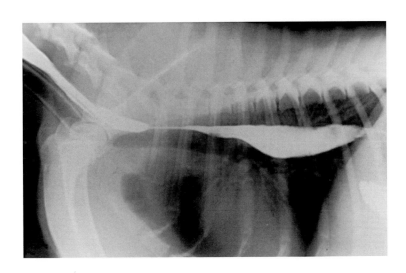

FIGURE 25–26. Lateral esophagram of a young adult dog. There is a cranial thoracic esophageal stricture. The lesion developed after the administration of anesthesia. The extent of the luminal involvement was best demonstrated by placing an esophageal tube while the dog was anesthetized and gradually administering contrast medium to fill the distensible portions of the esophagus. (Courtesy of New York State College of Veterinary Medicine, Ithaca, NY.)

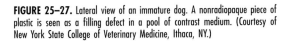

FIGURE 25–27. Lateral view of an immature dog. A nonradiopaque piece of plastic is seen as a filling defect in a pool of contrast medium. (Courtesy of New York State College of Veterinary Medicine, Ithaca, NY.)

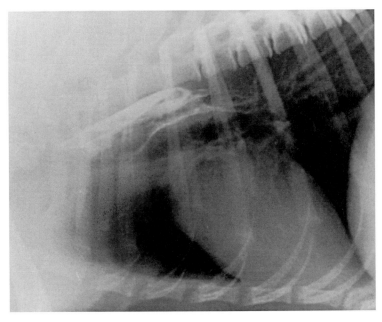

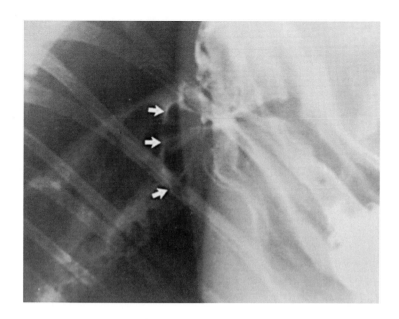

FIGURE 25–28. Gastroesophageal intussusception and related obstruction of the esophagus may be intermittent or persistent. The signs of regurgitation and vomiting were sporadic in this cat. Gastric rugal folds, covered with barium *(arrows)*, project into the dilated caudal esophagus. (Courtesy of New York State College of Veterinary Medicine, Ithaca, NY.)

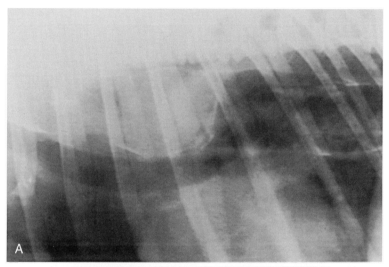

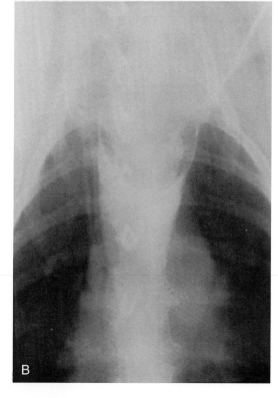

FIGURE 25–29. *A* and *B,* An ovoid soft-tissue filling defect is present within the esophageal lumen of an older dog. A pedunculated tumor was found on endoscopic examination. An esophageal foreign body might have a similar appearance. (Courtesy of New York State College of Veterinary Medicine, Ithaca, NY.)

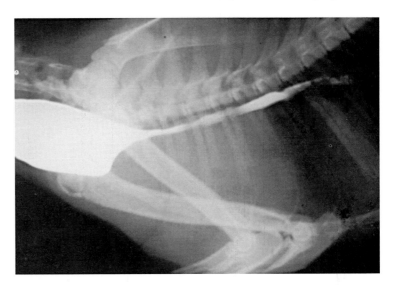

FIGURE 25–30. Lateral esophagram of an immature cat with cranial mediastinal lymphosarcoma. The periesophageal mass causes obstruction of the esophagus owing to restricted expansion capabilities at the thoracic inlet and cranial thorax and to the large mass. (From Ettinger SJ [Ed]: Textbook of Veterinary Internal Medicine, 2nd Ed. Philadelphia, WB Saunders, 1983; with permission.)

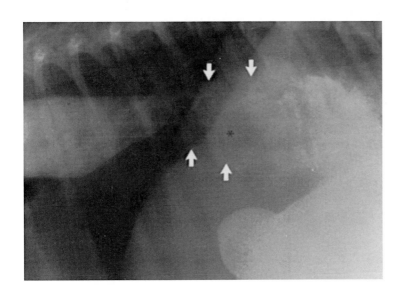

FIGURE 25–31. Lateral esophagram of a puppy. The esophageal lumen is dilated. Contrast medium outlines the dilated abdominal segment, which has a markedly irregular mucosal surface *(arrows)* and a filling defect *(asterisk)*. The diagnosis was granulomatous esophagitis with ulceration. (Courtesy of New York State College of Veterinary Medicine, Ithaca, NY.)

FIGURE 25–32. Lateral esophagram of a young dog. There is simultaneous filling of the right caudal lobe bronchus and the esophagus, indicating a bronchoesophageal fistula. (From Ettinger SJ [Ed]: Textbook of Veterinary Internal Medicine, 2nd Ed. Philadelphia, WB Saunders, 1983; with permission.)

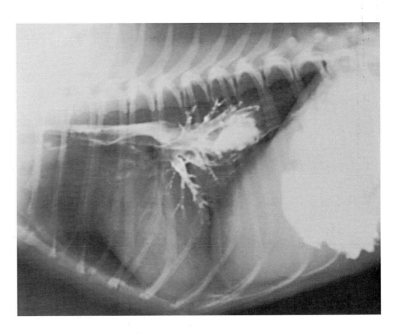

occasional incidental finding, but this disorder may be problematic in young brachycephalic breeds, especially English bulldogs and Shar-peis. Regional dilation may be demonstrated at the site of deviation in the thoracic inlet (Fig. 25–25).

Obstructions eventually lead to dilation of the esophageal lumen cranial to the site but, acutely, may not be apparent on survey radiographs. The source of obstruction may be intrinsic (strictures [Fig. 25–26], foreign bodies [Fig. 25–27], gastroesophageal intussusception [Fig. 25–28], and intraluminal masses [Fig. 25–29]) or extrinsic (periesophageal masses [Fig. 25–30]). Masses often cause the esophagus to deviate around them. The location of the mass determines the rapidity of onset of esophageal obstruction and the degree of dilation given the limited space available in certain sites along the path of the esophagus (i.e., the thoracic inlet). Mural masses may trap small amounts of luminal contrast medium, but they rarely cause obstruction until they are large (Fig. 25–31). Dysphagia is usually the result of regional dysmotility.

Esophageal fistulas may have extravasation of contrast medium along a tract, with dispersion of the contrast medium into the pulmonary parenchyma via an airway (esophagotracheal or esophagobronchial) or directly (esophagopulmonary) (Fig. 25–32). Fistulas should not be mistaken for inadvertent aspiration and subsequent alveolarization of contrast medium during a routine swallow.

An increase in esophageal wall thickness can be identified only in the thoracic region. Confirmation of a thickened wall because of inflammation or neoplasia can be made by using esophagography (see Fig. 25–24). Because the periesophageal fascia and muscle in the cervical region and the liver and stomach in the cranial abdomen silhouette with the adjacent esophageal wall, thickening of these areas can be presumed only by the presence of concurrent changes in the mucosal contour. Infiltration by neoplasia or by inflammatory or granulation tissue usually distorts the mucosal surface, obliterating the longitudinal or oblique folds (see Fig. 25–31).

References

1. O'Brien TR: Esophagus. In O'Brien TR (Ed): Radiographic Diagnosis of Abdominal Disorders in the Dog and Cat: Radiographic Interpretation, Clinical Signs, Pathophysiology. Philadelphia, WB Saunders, 1978, pp 141–203.
2. Kealy JK: The abdomen. In Diagnostic Radiology of the Dog and Cat, 2nd Ed. Philadelphia, WB Saunders, 1987, pp 41–59.
3. Brawner WR, and Bartels JE: Contrast radiography of the digestive tract: Indications, techniques and complications. Vet Clin North Am [Small Anim Pract] 13:599, 1983.
4. Watrous BJ: Clinical presentation and diagnosis of dysphagia. Vet Clin North Am [Small Anim Pract] 13:437, 1983.
5. Watrous BJ: Esophageal disease. In Ettinger SJ (Ed): Textbook of Veterinary Internal Medicine: Diseases of the Dog and Cat. Philadelphia, WB Saunders, 1983, pp 1191–1233.
6. Jones, BD, Jergens AE, and Guilford WG: Disease of the esophagus. In Ettinger SJ (Ed): Textbook of Veterinary Internal Medicine: Diseases of the Dog and Cat, 3rd Ed. Philadelphia, WB Saunders, pp 1255–1277.

STUDY QUESTIONS

1. Increased radiopacity associated with the esophagus may be due to:
   A. Foreign body.
   B. Dystrophic mineralization.
   C. A and B.

2. Accumulation of intraluminal gas always indicates esophageal disease. (True or False)

3. Causes for the presence of gas surrounding, and therefore making visible, the cervical esophagus include:
   A. Pneumomediastinum.
   B. Deep fascial gas.
   C. Esophageal perforation.
   D. All of the above.

4. This survey radiographic examination is of a 10-year-old neutered male domestic shorthaired cat (Fig. 25–33). He was presented for sudden onset of dyspnea. What radiographic signs are present? What are the radiographic conclusions? What may cause the combined radiographic findings?

5. Dilation of the esophagus may cause:
   A. Leftward and ventral deviation of the intrathoracic trachea.
   B. Leftward and dorsal deviation of the intrathoracic trachea.
   C. Rightward and ventral deviation of the intrathoracic trachea.
   D. Rightward and dorsal deviation of the intrathoracic trachea.

6. Focal dilation of the esophagus just cranial to the heart base is often seen with vascular ring anomalies. Name another esophageal disease that may appear similar to vascular ring anomalies.
   A. Nonradiopaque foreign body lodged at the heart base.
   B. Esophageal stricture located at the heart base.
   C. Esophagitis.
   D. Esophageal redundancy.
   E. All of the above.

7. If you suspect esophageal mucosal disease, which contrast medium would be indicated to demonstrate this?
   A. Liquid barium sulfate suspension.
   B. Barium sulfate paste.
   C. Ionic organic iodide contrast medium for oral administration.
   D. Nonionic isosmolar organic iodide contrast medium for oral administration.

8. A megaesophagus is usually well visualized when filled with positive contrast medium. In the dorsoventral or ventrodorsal radiograph, the cranial thoracic esophagus is indented by what two structures?
   A. Aorta and spine.
   B. Cranial vena cava and spine.
   C. Spine and azygous vein.
   D. Aorta and azygous vein.

9. A 4-year-old neutered female mixed-breed dog presented for intractable vomiting and gagging. In survey thoracic radiographs, there was a large heterogeneous

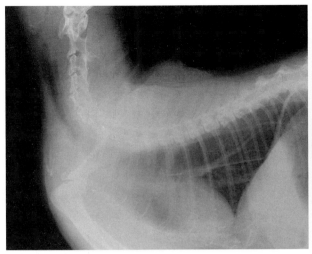

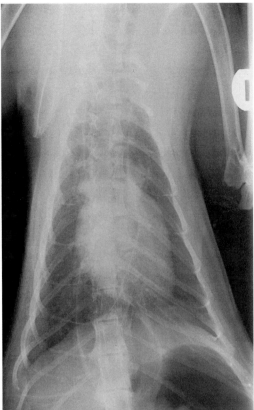

FIGURE 25–33

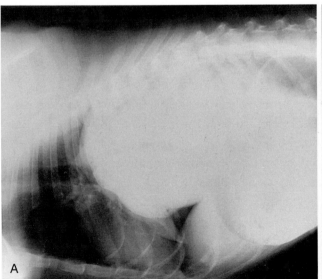

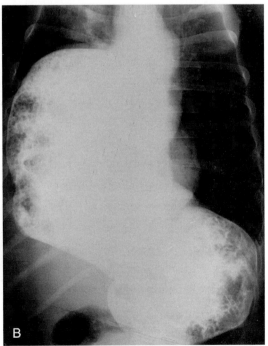

FIGURE 25–34

mass located in the caudal right thoracic region. A barium swallow was performed using liquid barium sulfate suspension (Fig. 25–34). What is your list of radiographic differential diagnoses, in decreasing order of likelihood?

10. Why should survey radiographs of the entire esophagus be obtained before an esophagram?

(Answers appear on page 640.)

Chapter 26

The Thoracic Wall

Charles R. Root • Robert J. Bahr

The thoracic wall consists of skin, fat, subcutaneous muscles, ribs (or sternum ventrally), intercostal muscles, parietal pleura, and the associated vasculature and nerves.[1, 2] Normal thoracic radiographic anatomy is well described.[1, 3–5] The radiographic manifestations of disease of the thoracic wall are rarely pathognomonic. As a result, accurate differentiation may be difficult or impossible. The key to accurate complete radiologic assessment lies in (1) recognition of basic radiographic signs of disease; (2) description of each in terms of abnormal size, shape, position, number, and opacity; (3) application of a working knowledge of the pathogenesis of the major categories of disease; and (4) coupling of the radiographic signs with historical, physical, and laboratory findings. Such a systematic approach, although seldom yielding unequivocal conclusions, may help rule out specific diseases and may result in the suggestion of specific diagnostic tools to further an understanding of the problem.

SPECIAL PROCEDURES

Routine thoracic radiographic examination often yields enough information to permit assessment of the thoracic wall. Using high kVp–low mAs technique, the contrast between the subcutaneous muscles and fat may not be as striking as that produced with low kVp–high mAs techniques. Therefore, supplemental projections with reciprocal adjustments in mAs and kVp may produce relatively better subcutaneous detail. Occasionally, oblique projections, horizontal-beam projections, or a contrast radiographic procedure may be helpful.

The only contrast radiographic procedure of much value is fistulography. Previously, pleurography was useful in some instances, but it has been largely replaced by sonography.[6–9] Fistulography is of potential use in the presence of a chronic draining tract that either has failed to heal or has recurred after treatment. Such a history is highly suggestive of a foreign body. Fistulography should be performed with care if the lesion is suspected to be infected and if the tract potentially communicates with a body cavity. Syringes, organic iodide contrast medium, pediatric Foley catheters, and various catheter adapters are needed for fistulography. The tract is cannulated with the appropriate catheter or catheter adapter (previously filled with contrast medium to avoid introduction of air bubbles). The catheter or catheter adapter must be large enough to seal the tract against significant reflux of contrast medium around the device, or the cuff of the Foley catheter must be inflated for the same purpose. Diluted contrast medium (5 to 10 percent w/v) is then injected. Undiluted contrast medium should not be injected because small or relatively faintly radiopaque filling defects may be obliterated. The volume is variable, but the tract should be filled until mild back-pressure is detected in the syringe or until a *small amount* of contrast medium refluxes around the catheter. Lateral, dorsoventral or ventrodorsal, oblique, and horizontal-beam projections are then made. These radiographs are carefully scrutinized for evidence of filling defects in the contrast medium or of communication of the contrast medium with the intercostal tissues, ribs, sternum, vertebral column, or underlying body cavity.

RADIOGRAPHIC SIGNS

Skin and Subcutaneous Tissue

Focal extracostal opacities (Fig. 26–1) may be caused by mammary nipples, engorged ticks, neoplasms, abscesses, granulomas, scabs, or metallic foreign bodies (such as bullet fragments and shotgun pellets). Only metallic foreign bodies are easily identified radiographically. The others are homogeneous fluid opacities that may not be well demarcated. Oblique or tangential projections may be necessary to assess fully some cutaneous and subcutaneous lesions and most artifacts (such as wet hair or cutaneous debris).

Diffuse extracostal opacities (Fig. 26–2) may be produced by cellulitis, contusion, edema, hypodermoclysis fluid, or neoplasia. Usually the normal subcutaneous fat striations are disturbed, commonly being obliterated but possibly only displaced if the lesion is well delineated and slowly developing (e.g., benign neoplasia).

Focal extracostal lucencies (Fig. 26–3) may be produced by laceration or punctures of skin or subcutaneous tissue by external sharp trauma, by fractured rib ends,[10] by abscesses with gas-forming organisms, by small amounts of gas in subcutaneous injections, and by lipomas. Lipomas are usually better circumscribed and less lucent than the others.

Diffuse extracostal lucencies (Fig. 26–4) may be produced by subcutaneous or intrafascial emphysema[10, 11] or by intermuscular and subcutaneous accumulation of fat because of obesity. The former is more frequently caused by external trauma but may be secondary to pneumomediastinum.

Ribs

Radiographic signs of lesions of the ribs in dogs and cats have been described.[5] Focal costal opacities (Fig. 26–5) may be

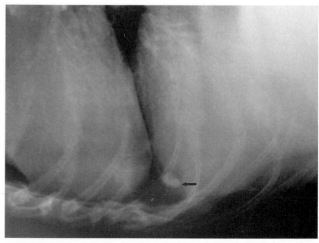

FIGURE 26–1. Left lateral thoracic radiograph of a dog with a nipple *(arrow)* superimposed over the caudoventral thorax. Similar focal extracostal lesions may be produced by engorged ticks, pedunculated tumors, or scabs. See Figure 2–15 for more information.

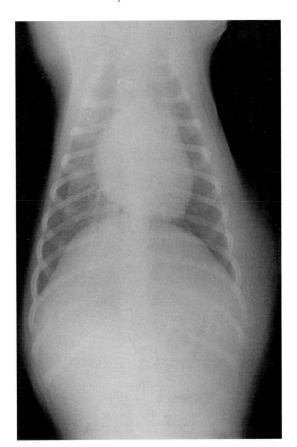

FIGURE 26–2. Dorsoventral thoracic radiograph of a dog with diffuse left subcutaneous swelling caused by hypodermoclysis. A similar radiographic finding may be produced by cellulitis or contusion.

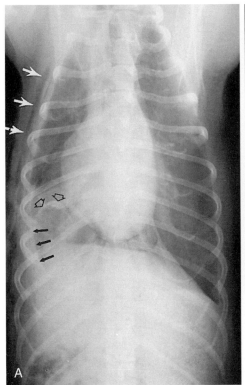

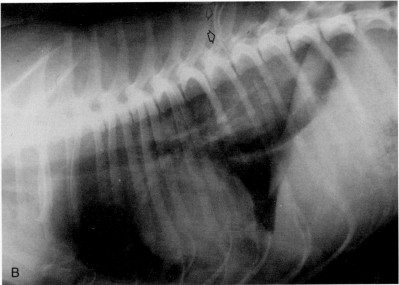

FIGURE 26–3. Ventrodorsal (A) and lateral (B) thoracic radiographs of a dog that had been attacked by another dog. There is focal subcutaneous gas (white arrows) along the right lateral thoracic wall because of penetration. There is also a severely displaced fracture of the right eighth rib (open arrows) and adjacent pleural effusion (black arrows). Abscesses, subcutaneous injections containing small air bubbles, and occasionally fractured ribs (fracture lines) also may produce focal extracostal lucencies. (Courtesy of the Santa Cruz Veterinary Hospital, Santa Cruz, CA.)

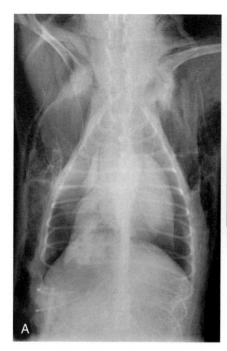

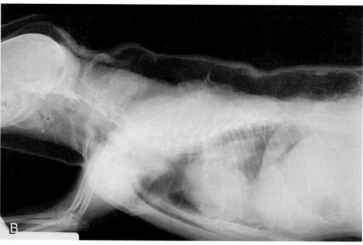

FIGURE 26–4. Dorsoventral *(A)* and lateral *(B)* thoracic radiographs of a dog with diffuse subcutaneous and intrafascial emphysema secondary to penetrating trauma (dogfight) of the caudal right hemithorax (fractured right 8th to 10th ribs with intercostal lacerations, the latter causing severe widening of the right 9th intercostal space). This type of emphysema may be initiated by pneumomediastinum, trauma near the thoracic inlet or axilla, or direct external trauma. In this dog, the trauma established communication with the pleural space, resulting in bilateral pneumothorax. Gas is also visible in the fascial planes of the neck.

caused by neoplasia,[5, 10] bacterial osteomyelitis,[5] fungal osteomyelitis, healing fractures, foreign bodies (e.g., shotgun pellets), and multiple cartilaginous extostoses.[2, 11, 12] The first three may be difficult to differentiate radiographically because they all may involve combinations of bone formation and bone lysis. Although both primary and metastatic rib neoplasia may produce lysis, sclerosis, or both, primary tumors tend to occur near the costochondral junction or within the distal third of the rib, whereas metastatic tumors generally occur in the midportion or proximal half of the rib.[5] Chondrosarcomas are the most common primary neoplasms involving the ribs in dogs; their radiographic signs are similar to, and often difficult to distinguish from, those of osteosarcoma.[13] Radiopaque foreign bodies are uncommon, but be-

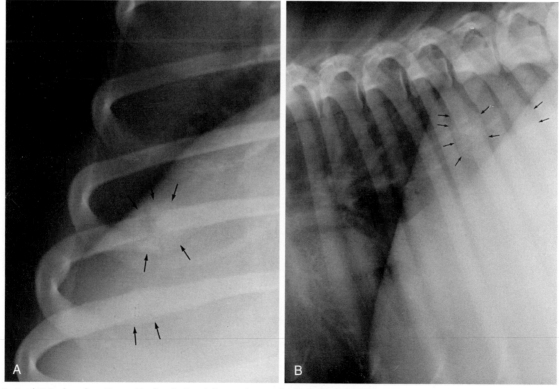

FIGURE 26–5. *A* and *B,* Focal costal opacities resulting from healing rib fractures *(arrows).* This dog had been hit by a car several weeks before these radiographs were made. Notice the exuberant periosteal callus, which produces a focal costal opacity. The more cranial of the two affected ribs also has a central radiolucency representing the remodeling changes associated with early fracture healing. Other lesions that may produce a focal costal opacity include neoplasia and focal inflammation.

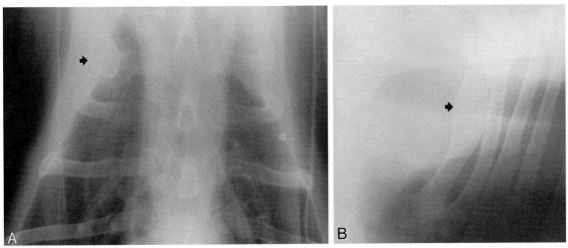

FIGURE 26-6. *A* and *B,* Radiographs of a dog with an old, healed fracture *(arrows)* of the first right rib. Its union is complete, and there is a smooth, focal costal opacity bridging the fracture site.

cause they are usually the result of gunshot wounds, they present little diagnostic confusion. Multiple cartilaginous exostoses (osteochondroma), as the common name implies, involve many sites, including ribs,[2, 5, 11, 12, 14, 15] skull, and long bones. Healed rib fractures[16] generally produce local smooth bony enlargement (Fig. 26–6) at the fracture sites, as a result of exuberant callus formation in response to constant respiratory motion during healing.

Diffuse costal opacities may be caused by exuberant periosteal reaction associated with chronic bacterial osteomyelitis. In patients who have lived in or visited the southwestern United States, coccidioidomycosis[5, 14, 17, 18] may produce a diffuse sclerotic periosteal reaction (Fig. 26–7).

Focal costal lucencies (Fig. 26–8) may be caused by fractures,[14, 19] neoplasia,[5, 13, 14] or osteomyelitis. Of these, fractures

are easiest to diagnose and usually are easily differentiated radiographically from neoplasia and osteomyelitis. Care must be taken not to mistake the natural angulation of the proximal portions of the ribs for nondisplaced fractures; this is especially true in lateral or ventrodorsal radiographs that are slightly obliqued.

Focal intercostal soft-tissue opacities are rare, but suggest neoplasia or focal inflammation. If the opacities are large or solid and substantive, there may be cranial and caudal displacement of the adjacent ribs. Focal intercostal metal opacities are usually the result of gunshot wounds. These findings are often incidental and insignificant.

Focal intercostal lucencies (Fig. 26–9) are most often caused by penetrating trauma. These lesions may or may not penetrate the pleural space and may or may not be associated

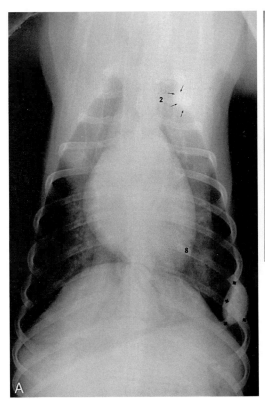

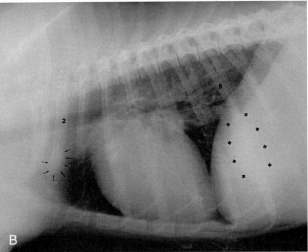

FIGURE 26–7. Dorsoventral *(A)* and right lateral *(B)* thoracic radiographs of a dog with costal coccidioidomycosis. The lesions are sclerotic opacities involving the left second and eighth ribs *(arrows).* (Courtesy of Department of Veterinary Medicine and Surgery, College of Veterinary Medicine, University of Missouri, Columbia, MO.)

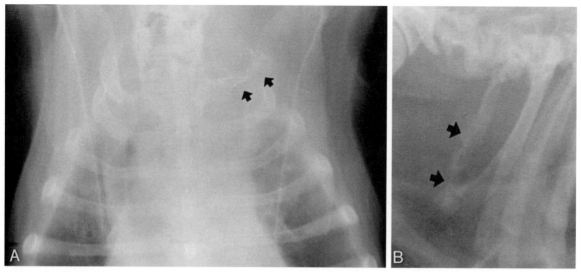

FIGURE 26–8. Ventrodorsal *(A)* and left lateral *(B)* thoracic radiographs of a dog with destruction *(arrows)* of the left first rib caused by a tumor. There is dextrad displacement and lateral extrinsic compression of the trachea secondary to a cranial mediastinal mass. Histopathologic diagnosis was not obtained. Focal costal lucency may be produced by neoplasia or osteomyelitis. (Courtesy of Parkwood Pet Clinic, Woodland Hills, CA.)

with fractures or displacement of ribs. They appear as a radiolucent interruption of normal homogeneous intercostal soft tissue. It is also possible for focal intercostal lucencies to develop after a fracture of a rib that lacerates adjacent lung. In this instance, there usually is pneumothorax, and there may be accompanying focal or diffuse subcutaneous or intrafascial emphysema. Intercostal abscess formation may be a late sequela of external penetration of intercostal tissue. If gas-forming organisms are present, a focal intercostal lucency may develop. Such lucency, in contrast to that seen in acute injury, is well circumscribed and confined rather than angular and poorly localized.

Expansile rib lesions,[11, 13] regardless of their radiographic opacity, potentially cause displacement or divergence of the adjacent ribs. This effect is usually much better seen in the ventrodorsal or dorsoventral projections than in lateral views, and supplemental ventrodorsal oblique projections may be necessary to appreciate fully the expansile nature of the lesion. The ribs, similar to other bony structures, do not react to pathologic insult with an *either/or* response. Often there is both lysis and production of bone. Certain combinations of an increase and decrease in opacity may have differential diagnostic significance. For instance, a focal opacity surrounded by focal lysis may suggest osteomyelitis with seques-

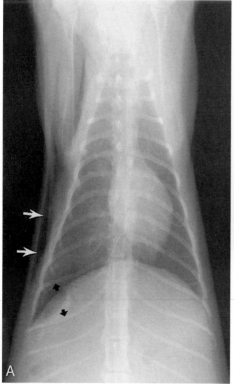

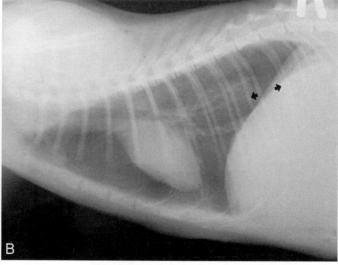

FIGURE 26–9. Dorsoventral *(A)* and right lateral *(B)* thoracic radiographs of a cat with intercostal lacerations *(arrows)*, which have resulted in widening of the right 10th intercostal space. This lesion was the result of a dog bite. Note the long zone of right lateral subcutaneous emphysema *(white arrows)* along the right thoracic wall in *A.* Pneumothorax is also present.

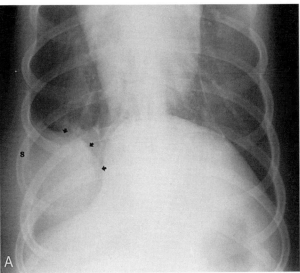

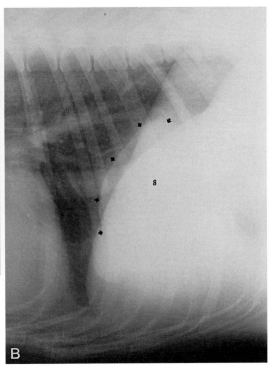

FIGURE 26–10. Dorsoventral (A) and left lateral (B) thoracic radiographs of a dog with an extrapleural mass adjacent to the eighth rib on the right (arrows). The diaphragm is displaced, and there is both external and internal protrusion of the mass (arrows). The broadly based indentation in the region where the internal protrusion joins the thoracic wall in A is characteristic of extrapleural lesions.

tration, whereas reactive bone surrounding a mottled lytic area may represent a neoplastic process or early fracture repair with remodeling changes.

Medial extension of a pathologic process from the thoracic wall, from ribs, or from intercostal tissue often causes broadly based medial displacement of parietal pleura. This pleural displacement often results in displacement of adjacent lung and produces the characteristic *extrapleural sign* (Figs. 26–10 and 26–11).[5, 11, 13, 20] The extrapleural sign is best seen when the primary beam strikes the lesion tangentially. Visualizing the extrapleural sign may require supplemental oblique projections. A characteristic of the extrapleural sign is a broadly based indentation of adjacent lung and medial deviation of the pleural space. Lesions capable of producing the extrapleural sign include any process by which tissue protrudes inward from outside the parietal pleura. Examples are primary costal neoplasia,[11] metastatic costal neoplasia, subpleural hemorrhage,[11] primary pleural neoplasia, metastatic pleural neoplasia, and healing fractures of the ribs. Mesothelioma[21] is a good example of a lesion that should produce the extrapleural sign. Unfortunately, this lesion often produces severe pleural effusion that precludes visualization

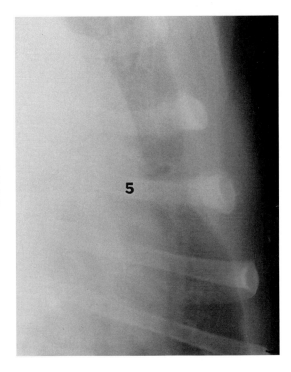

FIGURE 26–11. Dorsoventral thoracic radiograph of a dog with an extrapleural lesion adjacent to the fifth rib on the left. Note the smoothly marginated, broadly based indentation of the lung. The lesion was a subpleural hematoma resulting from trauma. Costal neoplasia is another type of lesion that may produce the extrapleural sign. If this opacity were of pulmonary origin, it would form either a right or an acute angle with the thoracic wall rather than having a tapering junction.

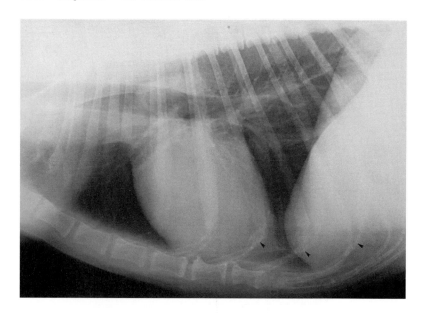

FIGURE 26–12. Left lateral thoracic radiograph of a dog with stippled mineralization *(arrowheads)* of the costal cartilages. This is a normal finding that usually progresses from caudal to cranial as the animal matures.

of the extrapleural sign, unless supplemental radiography immediately follows large-volume thoracocentesis.

Sternum

Stippled mineralization of costal cartilages[19] is probably the most frequent radiographic observation associated with the sternum. This finding (Fig. 26–12) is generally of no clinical significance,[14, 17] is most often a normal aging change, and usually progresses from caudal to cranial as the patient grows older. Pathologic changes in sternebral opacity, shape, or location are rarely observed but can be produced by neoplasia,[2] chronic inflammation,[2, 11] or trauma.[2, 14, 16] If pathologic, such changes should be expected to be accompanied by one or more of the following other radiographic signs: displace-

ment of adjacent costal cartilages, focal or diffuse intercostal opacity, and the extrapleural sign.

Pectus excavatum (Fig. 26–13) and other sternal anomalies (including fewer than normal numbers of sternebrae and sternal dysraphism) have been seen in animals with congenital peritoneopericardial diaphragmatic hernia.[2, 22] Pectus excavatum and peritoneopericardial diaphragmatic hernia are congenital defects that occur at roughly the same time during gestational development, suggesting a more than casual relationship between sternal conformation and the other two lesions. In the lateral projection, radiographic signs of pectus excavatum include dorsal displacement of the caudal sternum and, secondarily, the cardiac silhouette. In dorsoventral or ventrodorsal views, the heart is usually displaced to the left.[14] There may be fewer than eight sternebrae, and the presence of a silhouette sign joining the ventral diaphragm

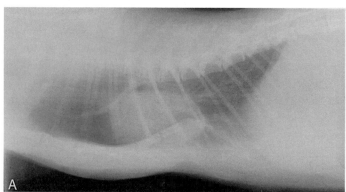

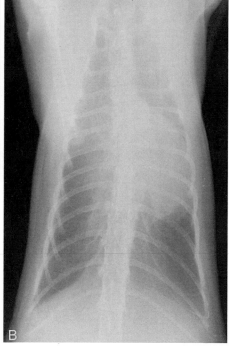

FIGURE 26–13. Left lateral *(A)* and dorsoventral *(B)* thoracic radiographs of a cat with pectus excavatum. The heart is displaced dorsally and to the left by the sternal deformity. This cat does not have a peritoneopericardial diaphragmatic hernia. The number of sternebrae (eight) in this cat is normal.

and the caudal aspect of the cardiac silhouette is highly suggestive of concomitant congenital peritoneopericardial diaphragmatic hernia.[2, 23]

References

1. Allan GS: Thoracic radiology excluding the heart, lungs and great vessels. Aust Vet Pract 10:146, 1980.
2. Suter PF: Thoracic Radiography: A Text Atlas of Thoracic Diseases of the Dog and Cat. Wettswil, Switzerland, Peter F. Suter, 1984.
3. Schebitz H, and Wilkens H: Atlas of Radiographic Anatomy of Dog and Cat, 3rd Ed. Berlin, Paul Parey, 1977.
4. Ticer JW: Radiographic Technique in Veterinary Practice, 2nd Ed. Philadelphia, WB Saunders, 1984.
5. Dennis R: Radiographic diagnosis of rib lesions in dogs and cats. Vet Annual 33:173, 1993.
6. Bhargava AK, Burt JK, Rudy RL, et al: Diagnosis of mediastinal and heart base tumors in dogs using contrast pleurography. J Am Vet Radiol Soc 11:56, 1970.
7. Bhargava AK, Rudy RL, and Diesem CD: Radiographic anatomy of the pleura in dogs as visualized by contrast radiography. J Am Vet Radiol Soc 10:61, 1969.
8. Burt JK: Contrast pleurography. In Ticer JW (Ed): Radiographic Technique in Small Animal Practice. Philadelphia, WB Saunders, 1974.
9. Rudy RL, Bhargava AK, and Roenigk WJ: Contrast pleurography: A new technique for the radiographic visualization of the pleura and its various reflections in dogs. Radiology 91:1034, 1968.
10. Douglas SW, and Williamson HD: Veterinary Radiological Interpretation. Philadelphia, Lea & Febiger, 1970.
11. Myer W: Radiography review: The extrapleural space. J Am Vet Radiol Soc 14:157, 1978.
12. Morgan JP, Carlson WD, and Adams OR: Hereditary multiple exostosis in the horse. J Am Vet Med Assoc 140:1320, 1962.
13. Brodey RS, Misdorp W, Riser WH, et al: Canine skeletal chondrosarcoma: A clinicopathologic study of 35 cases. J Am Vet Med Assoc 165:68, 1974.
14. Kealy JK: Diagnostic Radiology of the Dog and Cat. Philadelphia, WB Saunders, 1979.
15. Pool RR, and Carrig CB: Multiple cartilaginous exostosis in a cat. Vet Pathol 9:350, 1972.
16. Roenigk WJ: Injuries to the thorax. J Am Anim Hosp Assoc 7:266, 1971.
17. Gillette EL, Thrall DE, and Lebel JL: Carlson's Veterinary Radiology, 3rd Ed. Philadelphia, Lea & Febiger, 1977.
18. Morgan JP: Radiology in Veterinary Orthopedics. Philadelphia, Lea & Febiger, 1972.
19. Owens JM: Radiographic Interpretation for the Small Animal Clinician. St. Louis, Ralston Purina, 1982.
20. Lord PF, Suter PF, Chan KF, et al: Pleural, extrapleural, and pulmonary lesions in small animals: A radiographic approach to differential diagnosis. J Am Vet Radiol Soc 13:4, 1972.
21. Thrall DE, and Goldschmidt MH: Mesothelioma in the dog: Six case reports. J Am Vet Radiol Soc 19:107, 1978.
22. Evans SK, and Biery DN: Congenital peritoneopericardial diaphragmatic hernia in the dog and cat: A literature review and 17 additional case histories. Vet Radiol 21:108, 1980.
23. Berry CR, Koblik PD, and Ticer JW: Dorsal peritoneopericardial mesothelial remnant as an aid to the diagnosis of feline congenital peritoneopericardial diaphragmatic hernia. Vet Radiol 31:239, 1990.

STUDY QUESTIONS

1. If properly positioned and exposed routine thoracic radiographs fail to produce sufficient contrast for accurate interpretation of suspected chest wall lesions, which of the following change(s) in radiographic technique for supplemental examination may be helpful:
   A. Lower the kVp and compensatorily raise the mAs.
   B. Raise the kVp and compensatorily lower the mAs.
   C. Raise both the kVp and the mAs.
   D. Lower both the kVp and the mAs.
   E. Increase the focal-film distance.

2. Describe in detail the technique for *fistulography* of a draining chest wall lesion. Include indications, contraindications, patient preparation, supplies, procedure, complications, and potential radiographic signs.

3. List several artifacts that may be confused with lesions of the thoracic wall.

4. How is a subcutaneous lipoma generally differentiated from another focal extracostal lucency? From a benign subcutaneous neoplasm? From a subcutaneous injection (vaccination, medication)? From obesity? From hypodermoclysis fluid? From a subcutaneous or intrafascial abscess? From subcutaneous emphysema?

5. Which of the following lesions is often associated with cranial and caudal diversion of respectively adjacent ribs?
   A. Intercostal mass.
   B. Parietal pleural mass.
   C. Expansile rib lesion.

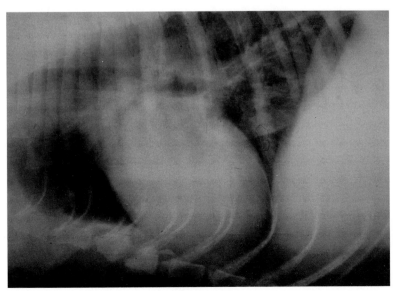

FIGURE 26–14

D. Fractured rib.
E. Subcutaneous abscess.
F. Intercostal muscle laceration or tearing.

6. Which of the following may be expected to produce the *extrapleural sign*?
   A. Intercostal mass.
   B. Parietal pleural mass.
   C. Expansile rib lesion.
   D. Fractured rib.
   E. Subcutaneous abscess.

7. Stippled mineralization of costal cartilages is an abnormal

aging change, is not seen often, and involves the affected ribs randomly. (True or False)

8. Name two congenital defects, one involving the ventral portion of the thoracic wall and one involving the phrenicodiaphragmatic ligament, which may occur concomitantly.

9. Image interpretation (Fig. 26–14): List the major radiographic signs.

(Answers appear on pages 640 to 641.)

Chapter 27

The Diaphragm

Richard D. Park

The diaphragm is the musculocutaneous partition between the thoracic and abdominal cavities. Embryologically the diaphragm is formed by the septum transversum ventrally and by the mesentery of the foregut and two pleuroperitoneal folds dorsally.

The diaphragm provides approximately 50 percent of the mechanical respiratory force for inspiration.[1] The diaphragm also acts as a mechanical partition or barrier between the thorax and abdomen. Lymph vessels from the abdomen penetrate the diaphragm and drain into thoracic lymph nodes and vessels. Thus, inflammatory and neoplastic abdominal diseases may spread to the mediastinum and pleural space. Lymph flow from the thorax to the abdomen does not occur.[2]

The diaphragm consists of a tendinous center and three thin peripheral muscles: the pars lumbalis, the pars costalis, and the pars sternalis. The pars lumbalis consists of the right and left crura, which attach to the cranial ventral border of L4 and the body of L3. This attachment results in these vertebrae occasionally having a concave, indistinct ventral margin that may be mistaken for bone lysis. The pars costalis attaches in an oblique direction to the 13th through 8th ribs, and the pars sternalis attaches to the xyphoid cartilage.[3] The diaphragm is convex and extends into the thorax from its attachments. In doing so, the phrenicocostalis and phrenicolumbalis recesses are created.

There are three openings through the diaphragm: (1) The dorsally located aortic hiatus encloses the aorta, azygous, and hemiazygous veins and the lumbar cistern of the thoracic duct; (2) the centrally located esophageal hiatus encloses the esophagus and vagal nerve trunks; and (3) the caudal vena cava foramen is located at the junction of the muscular and tendinous portions of the diaphragm.

NORMAL RADIOGRAPHIC ANATOMY

Radiographically, only a small portion of the diaphragm can be visualized on any one view. It appears as a thin, convex structure of soft-tissue opacity extending in a cranial and ventral direction. Radiographic visualization of the diaphragm is dependent on adjacent structures being of different opacity. Most of the thoracic surface is visible because of the adjacent gas-filled lungs. Parts of the thoracic surface are not visualized where the lung is not in contact with the diaphragm, that is, the phrenicocostalis and phrenicolumbalis recesses. A large portion of the abdominal surface is not seen because the adjacent liver silhouettes with it. The ventral abdominal diaphragmatic surface is visible on the lateral view when fat is present within the falciform ligament. The dorsal aspect of the left diaphragmatic crus and the gastric wall appear as one linear structure when gas is present in the gastric cardia.

Diaphragmatic structures that may be distinctly visualized radiographically are the right and left crura, the intercrural cleft, and the cupula (body) (Figs. 27–1 to 27–4). Associated structures that may also be seen are the caudal vena cava and the caudal ventral mediastinum. On the lateral view, the right crus of the diaphragm blends with the caudal vena caval border, and the gastric fundus may be seen adjacent to the abdominal surface of the left crus. The intercrural cleft is a shorter, convex, opaque line caudal and ventral to the crura (see Figs. 27–1 and 27–2). The cupula is the most cranial convex portion of the diaphragm on both the lateral and the dorsoventral or ventrodorsal views. Also, on these views, the thoracic surface of the diaphragm may be visualized as one, two, or three convex projections into the thoracic cavity (see Figs. 27–3 and 27–4).

Several normal variations of diaphragmatic position and shape may be seen radiographically. Factors that cause this variable appearance are both real and apparent. Real factors consist of breed, age, obesity, respiration, and gravity. Apparent factors are x-ray beam centering and animal positioning during radiographic examination. When all permutations of these variables are considered, more than 51,000 combinations are possible.[4] Obviously, most of these variables are not radiographically significant; however, some must be recognized and understood. Changes that are most apparent radiographically are the position, shape, and visualization of the cupula and crura. The relative position of the crura is most dependent on position and size of the animal and primary x-ray beam centering.

The most dependent crus is usually displaced cranially

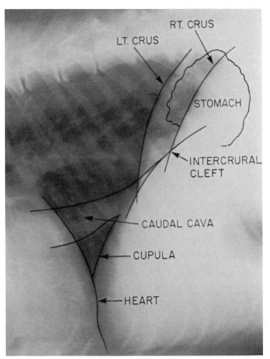

FIGURE 27–1. Left lateral recumbent radiograph of the diaphragmatic region of a normal dog.

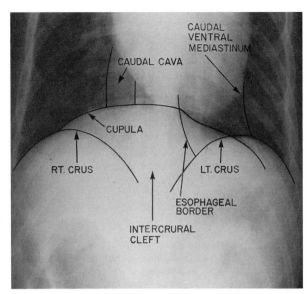

FIGURE 27–3. Ventrodorsal view of the diaphragmatic region of a normal dog with the cupula and both crura projecting into the thorax.

when an animal is in lateral recumbency. In right lateral recumbency, the crura appear to be parallel (see Fig. 27–2); in left lateral recumbency, they sometimes appear to cross (see Fig. 27–1). The crura also appear to be more extensively separated, that is, up to 2.5 vertebral lengths, if the animal is

slightly rotated or if the x-ray beam is centered over the mid or cranial thorax.[4]

The radiographic appearance of the diaphragm in ventrodorsal or dorsoventral projections varies with centering of the x-ray beam. The diaphragm may appear as a single, dome-shaped structure (see Fig. 27–4) or as two or three separate domed structures (see Fig. 27–3). The three structures represent the cupula and two crura. A single, domed diaphragm may be seen on a ventrodorsal or dorsoventral view when the x-ray beam is centered on the midabdomen or midthorax. Two or three separate domed structures are seen when the animal is in the ventrodorsal position and the x-ray beam is centered on the midthorax or on a dorsoventral view with the x-ray beam centered on the midabdomen.[4]

The diaphragmatic position and shape vary with respiration and intra-abdominal pressure. The normal intersection point of the diaphragm and spine is between T11 and T13 but may vary between T9 and L1. The diaphragm changes

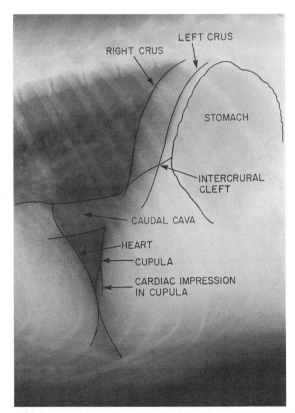

FIGURE 27–2. Right lateral recumbent view of the diaphragmatic region of a normal dog.

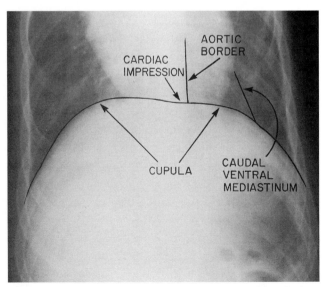

FIGURE 27–4. Dorsoventral view of the diaphragmatic region of a normal dog with only one convex shape projecting into the thorax.

position with normal respiration from one half to two verte-bral lengths. On extreme inspiration, the diaphragm changes position and shape. On a lateral thoracic view made in ex-treme inspiration, the diaphragm is oriented more vertically; the shape changes from convex to straight. The diaphragm is displaced cranially by increased intra-abdominal pressure, which may be produced by obesity, ascites, gastric or intesti-nal distention, abdominal pain, and abdominal masses.

Separate diaphragmatic structures are not seen as distinctly in the cat, probably because of the relatively small thoracic size (Fig. 27–5). On extreme inspiration, particularly if the animal is in respiratory distress, small symmetric muscle projections are noted from the thoracic diaphragmatic surface in the ventrodorsal or dorsoventral view (Fig. 27–6).

RADIOGRAPHIC SIGNS OF DIAPHRAGMATIC DISEASE

The signs associated directly with the diaphragm are not as numerous and specific as those that are found in many other

organs. Radiographic changes observed most frequently with diaphragmatic disease are general or local outline loss of the thoracic diaphragmatic surface and changes in diaphragmatic shape and position (Table 27–1).

The thoracic diaphragmatic surface outline may be obliter-ated or not visualized radiographically if anything of the same opacity, such as organs of soft-tissue opacity and fluid, is adjacent to the surface. Changes in the diaphragm shape occur most frequently on the cupula; they are often normal and are caused by contact with the heart (Fig. 27–7) or the position of the animal during radiographic examination. The shape and position may also appear altered in some large-breed dogs, with the body appearing more convex and ex-tending to a more cranial position in the thorax. This may be the result of a flaccid tendinous membrane or associated with a peritoneopleural hernia, which often produces no clinical signs.

Thoracic masses, or lung disease, adjacent to the dia-phragm; hiatal and small traumatic diaphragmatic hernias; and chronic pleural inflammatory reactions are the most

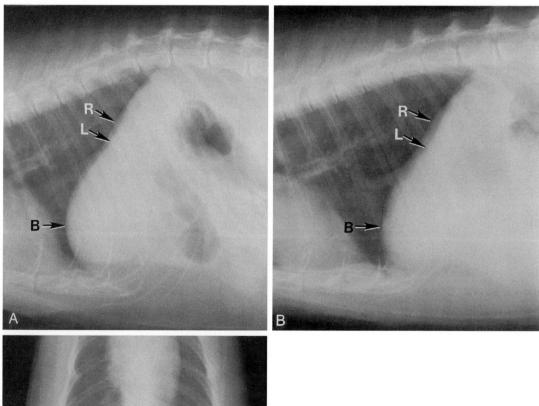

FIGURE 27–5. Radiographs of the diaphragmatic region of a normal cat. *A,* Left lateral recumbent view. *B,* Right lateral recumbent view. *C,* Ventrodorsal view. The right (R) and left (L) diaphragmatic crura are almost superimposed on both recumbent views with little change in position. The body (B) has a convex shape projecting into the thorax. In *C,* the diaphragm projects as a single convex opacity into the caudal thorax *(arrows).*

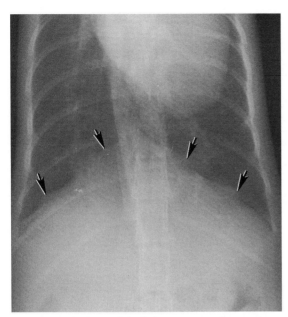

FIGURE 27-6. Ventrodorsal view of the diaphragmatic region of a normal cat on deep inspiration. Small, regularly spaced projections *(arrows)* are evident along the thoracic diaphragmatic surface. This so-called tenting reflects pulling of the diaphragm against its costal attachments.

frequent causes of shape changes. An asymmetric diaphragmatic shape may occur with unilateral tension pneumothorax or hemiparalysis. Suspected hemiparalysis should be confirmed by observing respiration under fluoroscopy.

Positional changes consist of cranial and caudal displacement. Because the position of the diaphragm varies with the respiratory cycle, minor changes are difficult to diagnose and in most instances are not clinically significant. Severe positional changes may be significant and indicative of tho-

racic or abdominal disease. Cranial diaphragmatic displacement is usually associated with abdominal disease (see Table 27–1) or generalized diaphragmatic paralysis, which should be confirmed with fluoroscopic observation. In some instances, pleural fluid between the lungs and diaphragm produces a pseudodiaphragm. This occurrence should not be mistaken for the actual diaphragmatic outline.

Caudal diaphragmatic displacement is usually associated with severe respiratory disease (Fig. 27–8). The caudally positioned diaphragm is an attempt by the animal to increase the level of systemic Po_2, which may be low because of ventilation or perfusion deficiencies in the lungs. Bilateral tension pneumothorax may also cause a caudally displaced diaphragm from increased pleural pressure. In most instances of pneumothorax, however, the caudally displaced diaphragm is probably an attempt to increase respiratory ventilation.

Although many of the general radiographic signs of diaphragmatic disease are not specific, they should be observed and their cause should be determined. In some instances, additional radiographic studies, such as positional views and contrast medium studies, may be indicated to determine the cause of the radiographic signs observed.

DIAPHRAGMATIC DISEASES

The most frequently observed diaphragmatic diseases in the dog and cat are traumatic and congenitally predisposed hernias. Motor or innervation disturbances occur less frequently.

Diaphragmatic Hernias

A diaphragmatic hernia is a protrusion of abdominal viscera through the diaphragm into the thorax. Diaphragmatic hernias that may be recognized radiographically include trau-

Table 27–1
RADIOGRAPHIC SIGNS OF DIAPHRAGMATIC DISEASES

Radiographic Signs	Causes
General loss of thoracic surface outline	Bilateral pleural fluid Generalized pulmonary disease in caudal lung lobes
Localized or partial loss of the thoracic surface outline	Thoracic masses adjacent to the diaphragm Diaphragmatic hernias Focal pulmonary disease in caudal lung lobes
Shape changes	Thoracic masses adjacent to the diaphragm Hiatal hernias Small diaphragmatic hernias Pleural reaction on the diaphragmatic surface Neoplasia Hemiparalysis of the diaphragm Unilateral tension pneumothorax
Position changes Cranial displacement	Obesity Peritoneal fluid Abdominal pain Abdominal masses or organ enlargement; liver enlargement and masses frequently cause cranial displacement Generalized diaphragmatic paralysis Cranial displacement of the cupula caused by a diaphragmatic defect with the peritoneum and pleura intact
Caudal displacement	Severe respiratory distress—ventilation or perfusion problems Tension pneumothorax Caudal displacement of the cupula caused by contact with the heart

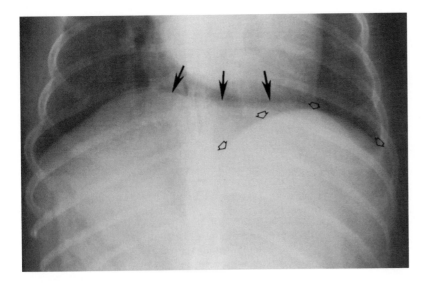

FIGURE 27–7. Ventrodorsal view of the diaphragmatic region of a normal dog. A cardiac impression *(solid arrows)* is present on the diaphragmatic body (cupula). The left diaphragmatic crus *(open arrows)* is distinctly visible. The right crus cannot be visualized as a separate structure.

matic, peritoneopericardial, hiatal, mediastinal, and those secondary to congenital diaphragmatic defects.

Abdominal trauma is the most common cause of diaphragmatic hernias. A high momentary increase in abdominal pressure when the glottis is open produces a high pleuroperitoneal pressure gradient that may result in a diaphragmatic hernia. The high pleuroperitoneal gradient may produce a rent in the muscular portion of the diaphragm or herniate abdominal viscera through congenitally weak or defective areas. Clinical signs that may be observed with diaphragmatic hernias are dyspnea, pain, vomiting, regurgitation, muffled heart sounds, and a weak femoral pulse.[5, 6] Some diaphragmatic hernias may not cause clinical signs and are detected incidentally.

Radiology plays an important role in confirming a diagnosis of diaphragmatic hernia and may provide information about location, extent, contents, and secondary complications associated with the hernia.[7–11] If a diagnosis cannot be confirmed from survey radiographs (Table 27–2), additional imaging procedures may be performed to add further diagnostic information. The radiographic procedures consist of administration of barium sulfate per os, positional radiographic views, removal of pleural fluid and reradiographing the thorax, and peritoneography.

To ascertain the position of the stomach and proximal small bowel, a small amount (20 to 40 mL) of barium sulfate (30 percent w/v) can be given per os and radiographs obtained after 15 to 20 minutes (Fig. 27–9). Positional radiographs made with a horizontal x-ray beam help identify solid organ structures (Fig. 27–10). Thoracocentesis and pleural fluid removal followed by another radiographic examination provide better radiographic visualization of thoracic structures. Positive-contrast peritoneography can be performed by injecting 1 mL/kg of body weight of a tri-iodinated contrast medium into the peritoneal cavity. The animal should then be positioned such that gravity allows the contrast medium to gravitate around the liver and the diaphragm. Incomplete visualization of the abdominal surface of the diaphragm is the most consistent positive-contrast peritoneographic sign of a diaphragmatic hernia (Fig. 27–11).[12, 13] Any or all of these

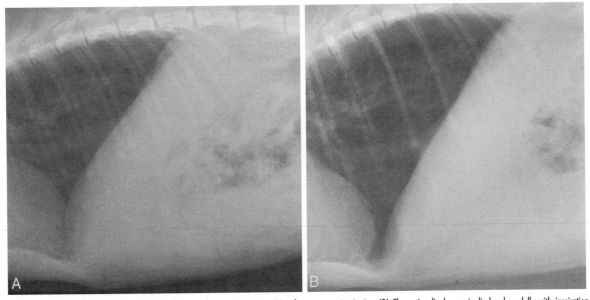

FIGURE 27–8. Lateral views of the diaphragmatic region of a normal cat on expiration *(A)* and on extreme inspiration *(B)*. The entire diaphragm is displaced caudally with inspiration and has a more flat contour when compared with the expiratory radiograph.

Table 27–2
RADIOGRAPHIC SIGNS ASSOCIATED WITH TRAUMATIC DIAPHRAGMATIC HERNIA

Abdominal viscera within the thorax
   Gas-filled or ingesta-filled bowel
   Gas-filled or ingesta-filled stomach
   Identifiable parenchymal organs, such as the liver and
     spleen
Displacement of abdominal structures—cranial
   Liver
   Small bowel
   Stomach
   Spleen
Displacement of thoracic structures—generally displaced away
   from an abnormal opaque area in the thorax
   Heart
   Mediastinum
   Lungs
Partial or complete loss of the thoracic diaphragmatic surface
   outline
   Pleural fluid or mass
   Lung fluid or mass
Cranial displacement or angulation of a diaphragmatic
   segment seen on the lateral view
Pleural fluid

procedures may be used, but the most simple procedures should be used first. Peritoneography with tri-iodinated contrast medium should be used after other diagnostic procedures have failed to provide the needed information.

Ultrasonographic examination of the diaphragm may add diagnostic information in difficult patients, particularly those in which pleural fluid is present and obliterates soft tissue.

The examination is best done transhepatically.[14] Ultrasonographic signs of a diaphragmatic hernia are identification of abdominal structures within the thorax, particularly the liver, and an interruption in the diaphragmatic outline.[14–16] An interruption in the diaphragmatic outline may not be consistently seen with diaphragmatic hernias.[17]

Traumatic Diaphragmatic Hernias

In one study, only one half of the animals presenting with a traumatically induced diaphragmatic hernia had a known history of trauma.[6] Traumatic diaphragmatic hernias usually involve the muscular part of the diaphragm.[6, 18] In one report, it was suggested that there is equal incidence on right and left sides[14]; in another report, it was stated that there was a higher incidence on the right side in the dog.[6] The organs that most frequently herniate through the diaphragm, in order, are the liver, small bowel, stomach, spleen, and omentum.[6, 9, 18–20]

The most consistent radiographic signs of traumatic diaphragmatic hernias are abdominal viscera within the thorax, displacement of abdominal or thoracic organs or both, partial or complete loss of the thoracic diaphragmatic surface outline, asymmetry or altered slope to the diaphragm on the lateral projection,[11] and pleural fluid (Fig. 27–12).

Identification of abdominal structures in the thorax is a conclusive sign of a diaphragmatic hernia. Small bowel is easily identified when it is gas-filled; when fluid-filled, it appears as a tubular structure. The stomach may be filled with gas, fluid, or ingested material. Ingested material usually has a granular appearance and is easily identified radiograph-

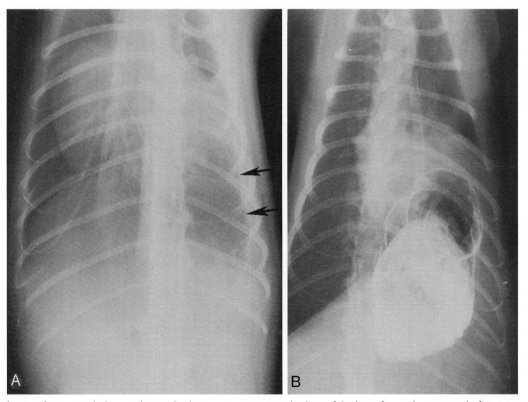

FIGURE 27–9. Confirmation of a traumatic diaphragmatic hernia with a barium gastrogram. *A,* Ventrodorsal view of the thorax of a cat. There is increased soft-tissue opacity in the left caudal thorax with obliteration of the left diaphragmatic outline. There is displacement of the left caudal lung lobe away from the thoracic wall *(arrows)* by pleural fluid. The heart is displaced toward the right thoracic wall, which may be accentuated by the slightly oblique position of the animal. *B,* Following administration of barium sulfate, the stomach is easily identified in the left caudal thorax, thus confirming a left-sided diaphragmatic hernia.

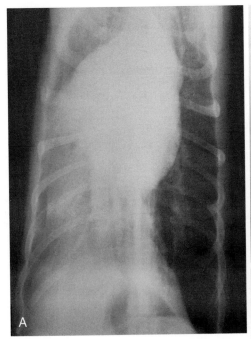

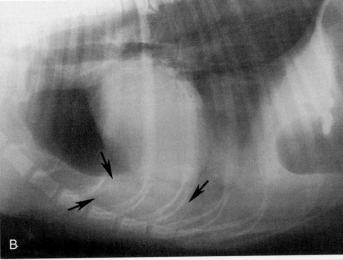

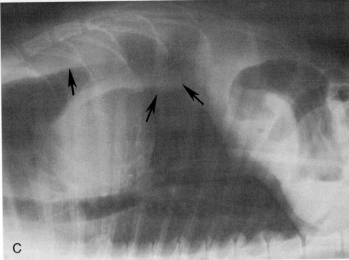

FIGURE 27–10. Ventrodorsal *(A)*; lateral *(B)*; and dorsal recumbent, horizontal-beam lateral *(C)* views of a dog with a traumatic diaphragmatic hernia. *A,* There is an increased soft-tissue opacity in the caudal right thorax with loss of the thoracic diaphragmatic surface outline over the cupula. *B,* The heart is displaced dorsally, and a soft-tissue opacity is seen between the heart and the sternum *(arrows).* The thoracic diaphragmatic outline is indistinct over the cupula. *C,* The soft-tissue opacity *(arrows)* remains in the same position, which indicates that the opacity is a solid structure and not free pleural fluid. This finding is compatible with a diaphragmatic hernia.

ically. In addition, gastric rugal folds may provide a marker for identifying the stomach within the thorax. A herniated, gas-distended stomach may appear as a unilateral left pneumothorax, and the stomach should be decompressed and repositioned immediately by surgical intervention (Fig. 27–13).[6] Such instances are life-threatening because of potential or actual cardiovascular tamponade.

Herniated solid abdominal parenchymal organs are difficult to distinguish from localized pleural fluid, pulmonary opacity, or both. Omentum is the most difficult to detect unless it is herniated in association with other abdominal organs. In such instances, it provides a fat opacity and helps outline other abdominal visceral organs.

In the absence of identifying abdominal organs in the thorax, cranial abdominal organ displacement or absence of abdominal organs from their normal location serves as an excellent radiographic sign for identifying diaphragmatic hernias. The liver, spleen, small bowel, and stomach are organs to assess most closely for displacement. Inclusion of the cranial abdomen on the thoracic radiograph when diaphragmatic hernia is suspected is helpful to evaluate abdominal organ displacement. Barium sulfate may also be administered to identify the stomach and to help detect mild to moderate gastric displacement not observed on survey radiographs.

The heart, mediastinum, and lungs may also be displaced, depending on the amount and position of abdominal organs within the thorax. The heart and lungs are usually displaced cranially and laterally by herniated abdominal viscera, and the mediastinum is usually displaced laterally.

A localized diaphragmatic surface outline loss usually indicates the area through which the diaphragmatic hernia has occurred. Abdominal viscera and pleural fluid adjacent to the thoracic diaphragmatic surface cause the outline loss. This occurrence must be distinguished from the many other thoracic conditions that produce a soft-tissue opacity adjacent to the diaphragm. Occasionally the torn diaphragmatic segment or muscle may be displaced in a cranial direction from the diaphragm, producing an almost horizontal diaphragm outline in one area. When present, this is a reliable radiographic sign of diaphragmatic hernia.

Pleural fluid is consistently present with chronic diaphragmatic hernias or if a herniated abdominal organ, most usually the liver,[20] is strangulated through a small diaphragmatic opening. Pleural fluid is a nonspecific sign of a diaphragmatic hernia and often masks other more important radiographic signs. Thoracocentesis and aspiration of the pleural fluid are often necessary before the hernia can be detected with certainty.

Congenitally Predisposed Diaphragmatic Hernias

Approximately 15 percent of all diaphragmatic hernias are congenitally predisposed.[9] Included in this group are perito-

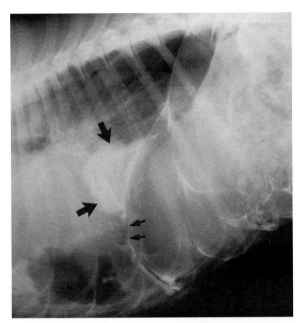

FIGURE 27–11. A lateral abdominal radiograph of a positive-contrast peritoneogram. There is an indistinct outline to the abdominal surface of the diaphragm *(small arrows)*, with contrast medium present within the pleural cavity *(large arrows)*. These are reliable radiographic signs of a diaphragmatic defect and a diaphragmatic hernia.

Table 27–3

RADIOGRAPHIC SIGNS ASSOCIATED WITH PERITONEOPERICARDIAL DIAPHRAGMATIC HERNIAS

Abdominal organs identified in the pericardial sac; gas, ingested material, or structures of soft-tissue opacity may be present

Large, round cardiac silhouette

Convex projection of the caudal cardiac silhouette

Indistinguishable border of the ventral thoracic diaphragmatic surface and the caudal ventral cardiac silhouette

Confluent silhouette between the diaphragm and the heart

Dorsal peritoneopericardial mesothelial remnant between the heart and diaphragm on the lateral view in cats

neopericardial diaphragmatic hernias, hiatal hernias, and diaphragmatic defects. Herniation in association with congenital diaphragmatic defects may occur in an animal of any age after some form of abdominal trauma or transitory increase in intra-abdominal pressure. Defects in diaphragmatic development may be present and never result in a hernia.

Peritoneopericardial Diaphragmatic Hernias

With a peritoneopericardial diaphragmatic hernia, abdominal viscera herniates into the pericardial sac through a congenital hiatus formed between the tendinous portion of the diaphragm and the pericardial sac. They have been reported in litter mates,[21] and it has been suggested that this trait is carried on a simple autosomal recessive gene in cats, with a 1:500 to 1:1500 rate of incidence.[22] The hernia may have been present from birth, or it may be developmental. Mild increases in intra-abdominal pressure may cause abdominal organs to herniate through a congenital hiatus.

Peritoneopericardial hernias may produce clinical signs, or they may be an incidental radiographic finding. These hernias may be present in old or young animals,[5, 23–27] with the liver, stomach, omentum, and small bowel most frequently herniated.

Radiographic signs associated with peritoneopericardial hernias are listed in Table 27–3. Herniated abdominal organs in the pericardial sac are usually caudal, or caudal and lateral to the heart. Gas-filled or ingesta-filled hollow visceral organs are usually not difficult to identify within the pericardial sac. Radiographically, gas within the bowel is in abrupt contrast to the adjacent structures of soft-tissue opacity. As stated previously, ingested material usually has a granular radiographic appearance. Solid parenchymal organs, unless surrounded by omentum, are difficult to distinguish as separate

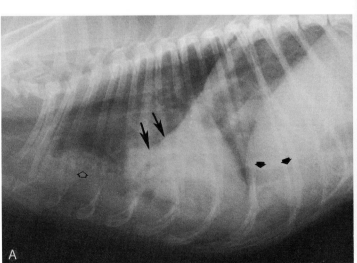

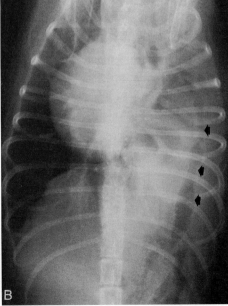

FIGURE 27–12. Lateral *(A)* and ventrodorsal *(B)* views of the thorax of a dog with a traumatic diaphragmatic hernia. Radiographic signs compatible with a diaphragmatic hernia in *A* are gas-filled and ingesta-filled bowel *(open arrow)* within the thorax, cranial displacement of abdominal structures (i.e., small bowel [*small solid arrows*]), and a cranially displaced diaphragmatic segment *(large solid arrows)*. Radiographic signs in *B* are the heart displaced away from the herniated viscera, gas-filled small bowel within the thorax *(arrows)*, cranially displaced abdominal structures (i.e., small bowel, stomach, and liver), and loss of the left diaphragmatic surface outline.

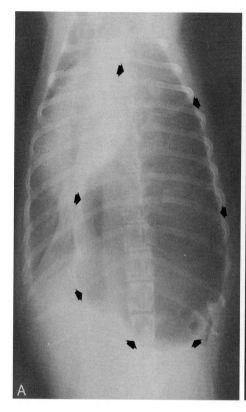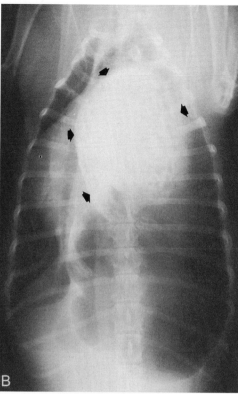

FIGURE 27–13. Ventrodorsal views of the thorax of a dog with a traumatic diaphragmatic hernia without *(A)* and with *(B)* barium in the stomach. *A,* The gas-filled stomach *(arrows)* is herniated into the left hemithorax, simulating a unilateral tension pneumothorax; it displaces the heart and lungs to the right side. The normal gastric and left diaphragmatic outlines are not present. *B,* Barium is present in the cranial part of the stomach *(arrows),* and there is severe gaseous gastric distention.

structures within the pericardium. When abdominal organs are herniated into the pericardial sac, cranial and ventral organ displacement within the abdomen may be seen, but the displacement is usually not as pronounced as that noted with traumatic diaphragmatic hernias.

A large, round cardiac silhouette and a cardiac silhouette with an abnormal convex projection on the caudal border are signs consistent with peritoneopericardial diaphragmatic hernias. These two signs are dependent on the amount of abdominal viscera within the pericardial sac. Large amounts of viscera produce a large, round cardiac silhouette, whereas smaller amounts, such as a portion of the liver or stomach, may produce an abnormal convex caudal cardiac border. A large, round silhouette must be differentiated from pericardial effusion, generalized heart enlargement, or both. An abnormally convex caudal cardiac border must be differentiated from neoplasia, pleural granulomas, or localized pleural fluid.

An indistinguishable outline to the ventral diaphragmatic surface and the caudal ventral cardiac silhouette is produced by the communication between the two structures. This finding must be differentiated from normal contact between the heart and diaphragm, pleural fluid, localized pleuritis, and pleural granulomas.

An apparently confluent silhouette between the heart and diaphragm may appear as a wide caudal mediastinum; depending on the size of the communication, it may or may not be seen radiographically. This confluent silhouette must also be differentiated from other pathologic conditions that have been listed. On the lateral view, identification of the dorsal peritoneopericardial mesothelial remnant between the heart and diaphragm is a consistent radiographic sign of peritoneopericardial hernia in cats (Fig. 27–14).[28] Additional radiographic studies that may be performed to confirm a diagnosis include administration of barium sulfate per os, nonselective angiography,[29] peritoneography, and pericardi-

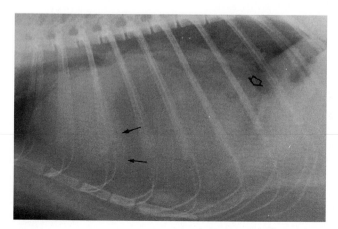

FIGURE 27–14. Lateral view of a feline thorax. The cat has a peritoneopericardial diaphragmatic hernia. The faint outline of a dorsal peritoneopericardial mesothelial remnant is present cranial to the diaphragm *(open arrow).* The liver, omentum, and spleen are herniated into the pericardial sac. The caudal border of the heart is visible *(black solid arrows)* because of fat in the adjacent omentum.

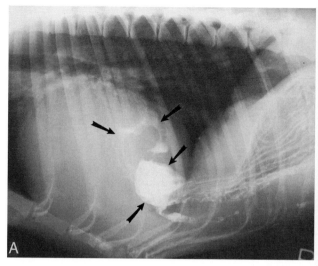
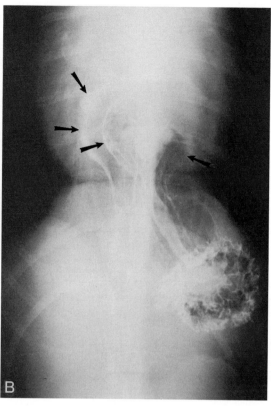

FIGURE 27–15. Lateral *(A)* and ventrodorsal *(B)* views of the thorax of a dog with a peritoneopericardial diaphragmatic hernia. *A,* The pyloric antrum and proximal duodenum are herniated into the caudal aspect of the pericardial sac and are filled with barium *(arrows).* The stomach is angled in an abnormal cranial direction, and there is a convex soft-tissue protrusion on the caudal heart border. *B,* The barium-filled pyloric antrum and proximal duodenum *(arrows)* are within the caudal aspect of the pericardial sac. The pyloric antrum and fundus of the stomach are displaced cranially, and the caudal heart border has an abnormal convex shape.

ography. Barium sulfate may be used to demonstrate gastrointestinal structures within the pericardial sac or cranial ventral displacement of abdominal structures (Fig. 27–15).

Peritoneography with negative-contrast or positive-contrast medium may be used to evaluate for the presence of a peritoneopericardial hernia. For this study, the animal is positioned to allow gravitation of contrast medium from the peritoneum into the pericardial sac or to outline the abdominal surface of the diaphragm. This maneuver may not be successful because of the inability to gravitate contrast medium through a small or obstructed hiatus. Nevertheless, a defect in the outline of the peritoneal surface of the diaphragm may be outlined.[13] Ultrasonography has also been used to diagnose peritoneopericardial diaphragmatic hernias successfully.[14–17]

Hiatal Hernias

Hiatal hernias are produced when a portion of stomach enters the thorax through the esophageal hiatus. These hernias are reported to occur through a congenitally or traumatically enlarged esophageal hiatus; they also may result from contraction of the longitudinal esophageal muscle.[30, 31]

There are two recognized types of hiatal hernias:[32] sliding and paraesophageal. The gastroesophageal sphincter and a portion of the stomach, usually the cardia, are herniated into the thorax with sliding hiatal hernias.[33] Sliding hiatal hernias are usually congenital and seen in younger animals.[32] They are often associated with esophagitis from gastroesophageal reflux. As the name implies, the caudal esophagus and the cardia slide intermittently from the abdomen into the thorax. Because the hernia is dynamic, it may not be seen on any one radiograph; fluoroscopic examination is often necessary to make a diagnosis. Patients with nonsliding hiatal hernias have been reported, with the gastroesophageal sphincter and the gastric cardia displaced through the esophageal hiatus and fixed within the thorax.[34] The number of reported sliding

hiatal hernias in animals is not high.[35–42] The low incidence may be a reflection of the subtle clinical signs and intermittent manifestations on survey radiographs.

A paraesophageal hiatal hernia is produced when the cardia or cardia and fundus of the stomach herniate through, or along side of, the esophageal hiatus and become positioned adjacent to the esophagus. They are usually static and do not slide between the thorax and abdomen, and the gastroesophageal sphincter is in a normal position.[31, 33, 43] The herniated stomach may cause esophageal obstruction from external pressure on the caudal esophagus.

Hiatal hernias have been reported in both the dog and the cat.[34, 37, 39–42] They have been reported associated with other esophageal conditions in Chinese Shar-peis.[42] Clinical signs reported with hiatal hernias include vomiting, regurgitation, excessive salivation, dysphagia, and dyspnea.[34, 41, 42] This condition may be suspected from the clinical signs and survey radiographic findings, but it must be confirmed with an esophagram.

Radiographic signs of a hiatal hernia consist of survey findings and those observed with an esophagram (Table 27–4). The most consistent survey radiographic sign is stomach displacement. The cardia appears to be stretched toward the diaphragm or may extend into the thorax. This displacement produces an abnormal shape to the cardia and fundus remaining in the abdomen. The caudal esophagus may or may not be distended, and a soft-tissue opacity (mass) may be seen adjacent to the left diaphragmatic crus. The size and visibility of this mass depend on the amount of stomach that has actually herniated into the thorax.

A dilated caudal esophagus is usually best detected and evaluated with an esophagram. An esophagram is also helpful to differentiate the type of hiatal hernia. The caudal esophageal sphincter and a portion of the cardia are seen cranial to the diaphragm with a sliding hiatal hernia.[44] The caudal esophageal sphincter can be identified as a concentric, smooth 1- to 2-cm narrowing in the caudal esophagus (Fig.

Table 27–4
RADIOGRAPHIC SIGNS ASSOCIATED WITH SLIDING HIATAL HERNIAS

Survey Radiographs

Soft-tissue mass adjacent to the left diaphragmatic crus
Loss of thoracic surface outline on the left diaphragmatic crus
Cranial displacement of the gastric cardia produces an
   abnormal gastric shape
Dilated esophagus
Pneumonia

Esophagram

Dilated esophagus
Hypomotile esophagus
Gastroesophageal sphincter within the thorax represented by a
   circumferentially narrowed area of the esophagus
Gastric cardia within the thorax
Gastroesophageal reflux

Table 27–5
RADIOGRAPHIC SIGNS ASSOCIATED WITH GASTROESOPHAGEAL INTUSSUSCEPTIONS

Survey Radiographs

Soft-tissue mass adjacent to the diaphragm
Cranial displacement of the stomach with or without the spleen
   or duodenum
Dilated esophagus

Esophagram

Intraluminal filling defect in the caudal esophagus
Barium outline of rugal folds
No barium within the stomach

27–16). Displacement and narrowing of the caudal esophagus by the cardia and fundus are seen with paraesophageal hiatal hernias, along with barium opacification of the herniated stomach (Fig. 27–17).

Gastroesophageal Intussusception

Gastroesophageal intussusceptions occur when the stomach, with or without the spleen, duodenum, pancreas, and omentum, invaginates through the esophageal hiatus into the caudal esophagus.[31, 33, 45, 46] They occur mostly in male and German shepherd dogs and animals with a pre-existing dilated esophagus.[46] Gastroesophageal intussusceptions usually produce an esophageal obstruction, which results in rapid deterioration of the animal's condition with a high mortality rate; therefore, a timely diagnosis is essential.[46]

On survey radiographs, a large soft-tissue mass is seen adjacent to the diaphragm, usually accompanied by a dilated esophagus. With an esophagram, gastroesophageal intussusceptions produce a large intraluminal filling defect within the

caudal esophagus, rugal folds may be outlined with barium, and barium usually does not enter the stomach (Table 27–5 and Fig. 27–18).

Diaphragmatic Defects

Congenital diaphragmatic defects in the dog and cat have been reported rarely.[47-50] The defects are created when the septum transversum or the pleural peritoneal folds do not develop and fuse to form a complete diaphragm. The diaphragmatic defect allows abdominal viscera to enter the thoracic cavity and may produce clinical signs consistent with a traumatic diaphragmatic hernia.

In humans, diaphragmatic defects have a familial incidence with a multifactorial mode of inheritance.[51] Congenital defects in dogs have been reported in the muscular diaphragm, dorsolateral in position,[47] and in the membranous diaphragm associated with umbilical hernias.[48-50]

The radiographic signs of congenital diaphragmatic defects are the same as those listed for traumatic diaphragmatic hernias. With membranous defects, however, the liver is displaced cranially, while remaining in the caudal ventral thorax, often confined to the mediastinum (Fig. 27–19).

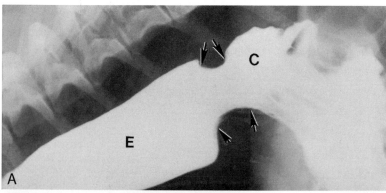
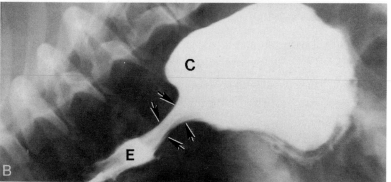

FIGURE 27–16. Lateral views of barium esophagram in a patient with a sliding hiatal hernia. *A,* Contrast medium distends the caudal esophagus (E), the gastroesophageal sphincter *(arrows),* and the cardia (C). The gastroesophageal sphincter and gastric cardia are displaced cranial to the diaphragm through the esophageal hiatus. *B,* The esophagus (E) and gastroesophageal sphincter *(arrows)* are outlined but are not distended with barium; most of the barium has passed into the stomach. The gastroesophageal sphincter and gastric cardia (C) are herniated through the esophageal hiatus and are cranial to the diaphragm.

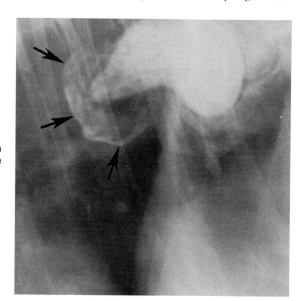

FIGURE 27–17. Lateral view of the thorax. Barium is outlining a paraesophageal hiatal hernia. The barium outlines the gastric cardia *(arrows)*, which is cranial to the diaphragm. The cardia has herniated through the esophageal hiatus adjacent to the caudal esophagus, which is not opacified.

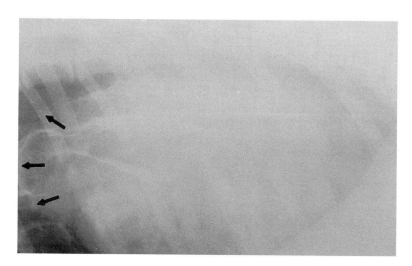

FIGURE 27–18. Lateral radiograph of the caudodorsal aspect of the thorax of a dog with a gastroesophageal intussusception. Barium outlines its cranial aspect *(arrows)*. The large soft-tissue mass in the caudal dorsal thorax is the stomach intussuscepted into the caudal esophageal lumen. Note the barium coating of the gastric rugae; this feature is characteristic of gastroesophageal intussusception.

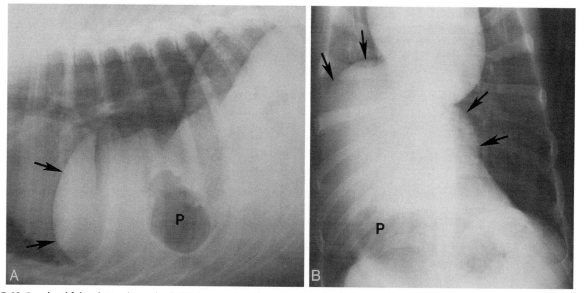

FIGURE 27–19. Recumbent left lateral *(A)* and ventrodorsal *(B)* radiographs of the thorax of a dog with a diaphragmatic defect. The defect was in the cupula, with the pleura and peritoneum intact. The liver *(arrows)* and gas-filled pyloric antrum (P) are within the thorax. The stomach and liver are displaced cranially.

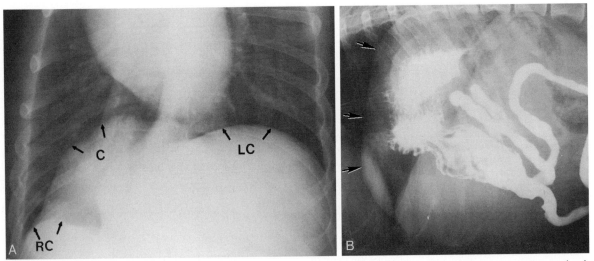

FIGURE 27–20. Ventrodorsal *(A)* and lateral *(B)* radiographs of the cranial abdomen. There is hemiparalysis of the left diaphragm. *A*, The left diaphragmatic crus (LC) is cranial to the right crus (RC). The cupula (C) and right crus are in a normal inspiratory position. *B*, The cranial position of the left diaphragmatic crus *(arrows)* causes the gastric cardia and fundus to be displaced cranially.

Motor Disturbances of the Diaphragm

The diaphragm is the principal muscle of respiration and is innervated by the phrenic nerve. Motor disturbances in most instances are clinically asymptomatic and have not been well documented in animals.

Motor disturbances of the diaphragm consist of unilateral paralysis, bilateral paralysis, and diaphragmatic flutter.[1] Diaphragmatic paralysis may be produced by pneumonia, trauma, myopathies, and neuropathies, or the cause may be unidentified.[1] Diaphragmatic paralysis may be suspected from survey radiographs that show cranial displacement of one or both diaphragmatic crura (Fig. 27–20). Confirmation of paralysis is best achieved with fluoroscopy. Unequal movement between the crura is seen with unilateral paralysis. With bilateral paralysis, minimal or no diaphragmatic movement or a paradoxic cranial displacement of the flaccid diaphragm may occur during inspiration.[52] Bilateral paralysis may be more difficult to confirm with fluoroscopy because diaphragmatic movement is sometimes produced by compensatory abdominal muscle contraction during respiration.

Diaphragmatic flutter is most often associated with contractions of the diaphragm synchronous with the heart beat. The condition is usually transient in nature and can be diagnosed easily with fluoroscopy by observing contractions of the diaphragm in synchrony with the heart beat.[53]

Muscular Dystrophy

Muscular dystrophy caused by dystrophin deficiency has been reported in dogs[54] and cats.[55, 56] In cats, an irregular scalloped appearance of the diaphragm, particularly along the ventral margin, was a consistent finding observed on radiographs after 7 months of age.[55] The scalloped margin noted best on the lateral view should not be confused with the normal scalloping observed on the ventrodorsal view in cats on maximum inspiration (see Fig 27–6). Muscular hypertrophy produced with feline muscular dystrophy has also been reported to cause a megaesophagus from extraluminal hiatal obstruction. Definitive laboratory tests, such as immunofluorescence or immunoblot tests, are necessary to establish the diagnosis in such patients.

References

1. Shim C: Motor disturbances of the diaphragm. Clin Chest Med *1*:125, 1980.
2. Rivero O, and del Castillo H: Lymphatics of the diaphragm in the dog. Acta Radiol [Diagn] (Stockh) *17*:663, 1976.
3. Miller ME, Christensen GC, and Evans HE: Anatomy of the Dog. Philadelphia, WB Saunders, 1964.
4. Grandage J: The radiology of the dog's diaphragm. J Small Anim Pract *15*:1, 1974.
5. Schulman J: Peritoneopericardial diaphragmatic hernia in a dog. Mod Vet Pract *60*:306, 1979.
6. Garson HL, Dodman NH, and Baker GJ: Diaphragmatic hernia: Analysis of fifty-six cases in dogs and cats. J Small Anim Pract *21*:469, 1980.
7. Farrow CS: Radiographic diagnosis of diaphragmatic hernia. Mod Vet Pract *64*:979, 1983.
8. Silverman S, and Ackerman N: Radiographic evaluation of abdominal hernias. Mod Vet Pract *58*:781, 1977.
9. Wilson GP III, and Hayes HM Jr: Diaphragmatic hernia in the dog and cat: A 25-year overview. Semin Vet Med Surg *1*:318, 1986.
10. Levine SH: Diaphragmatic hernia. Vet Clin North Am [Small Anim Pract] *17*:411, 1987.
11. Stokhof AA, Wolvekamp WTC, Hellebrekers LJ, et al: Traumatic diaphragmatic hernia in the dog and cat. Tijdschrift Diergeneesk *111*(Suppl 1):62S, 1986.
12. Rendano VT: Positive contrast peritoneography: An aid in the radiographic diagnosis of diaphragmatic hernia. J Am Vet Radiol Soc *20*:67, 1979.
13. Stickle RL: Positive-contrast celiography (peritoneography) for the diagnosis of diaphragmatic hernia in dogs and cats. J Am Vet Med Assoc *185*:295, 1984.
14. Lamb CR, Mason GD, and Wallace MK: Ultrasonographic diagnosis of peritoneopericardial diaphragmatic hernia in a Persian cat. Vet Rec *125*:186, 1989.
15. Hay WH, Woodfield JA, and Moon MA: Clinical, echocardiographic, and radiographic findings of peritoneopericardial diaphragmatic hernia in two dogs. J Am Vet Med Assoc *195*:1245, 1989.
16. Hashimoto A, Kudo T, and Sawashima I: Diagnostic ultrasonography of noncardiac intrathoracic disorders in small animals. Research Bulletin of the Faculty of Agriculture, Gifu University *55*:235, 1990.
17. Hodges RD, Tucker RL, and Brace JJ: Radiographic diagnosis [peritoneopericardial diaphragmatic herniation in a dog]. Vet Radiol Ultrasound *34*:249, 1993.
18. Carb A: Diaphragmatic hernia in the dog and cat. Vet Clin North Am [Small Anim Pract] *5*:477, 1975.
19. Wilson GP, Newton CD, and Burt JK: A review of 116 diaphragmatic hernias in dogs and cats. J Am Vet Med Assoc *159*:1142, 1971.
20. Boudrieau RJ, and Muir WW: Pathophysiology of traumatic diaphragmatic hernia in dogs. Comp Contin Ed Vet Pract *9*:379, 1987.
21. Feldman DB, Bree MM, and Cohen BJ: Congenital diaphragmatic hernia in neonatal dogs. J Am Vet Med Assoc *153*:942, 1968.
22. Saperstein G, Harris S, and Leipold HW: Congenital defects in domestic cats. Feline Pract *6*:18, 1976.
23. Bjorck GR, and Tigerschiold A: Peritoneopericardial diaphragmatic hernia in a dog. J Small Anim Pract *11*:585, 1970.
24. Gourley IM, Popp JA, and Park RD: Myelolipomas of the liver in a domestic cat. J Am Vet Med Assoc *158*:2053, 1971.

25. Rendano VT, and Parker RB: Polycystic kidneys and peritoneopericardial diaphragmatic hernia in the cat: A case report. J Small Anim Pract 17:479, 1976.
26. Weitz J, Tilley LP, and Moldoff D: Pericardiodiaphragmatic hernia in a dog. J Am Vet Med Assoc 173:1336, 1978.
27. Evans SM, and Biery DN: Congenital peritoneopericardial diaphragmatic hernia in the dog and cat. Vet Radiol 21:108, 1980.
28. Berry CR, Koblik PD, and Ticer JW: Dorsal peritoneopericardial mesothelial remnant as an aid to the diagnosis of feline congenital peritoneopericardial diaphragmatic hernia. Vet Radiol 31:239, 1990.
29. Willard MD, and Aronson E: Peritoneopericardial diaphragmatic hernia in a cat. J Am Vet Med Assoc 178:481, 1981.
30. Edwards MH: Selective vagotomy of the canine oesophagus—a model for the treatment of hiatal hernia. Thorax 31:185, 1976.
31. Teunissen GHB, Happ RP, Van Toorenburg J, et al: Esophageal hiatal hernia: Case report of a dog and a cheetah. Tijdschr Diergeneesk 103:742, 1978.
32. Ellison GW, Lewis DD, Phillips L, et al: Esophageal hiatal hernia in small animals: Literature review. J Am Anim Hosp Assoc 20:783, 1984.
33. Ellis FH Jr: Controversies regarding the management of hiatus hernia. Am J Surg 139:782, 1980.
34. Prymak C, Saunders HM, and Washabau RJ: Hiatal hernia repair by restoration and stabilization of normal anatomy: An evaluation in four dogs and one cat. Vet Surg 18:386, 1989.
35. Rogers WA, and Donovan EF: Peptic esophagitis in a dog. J Am Vet Med Assoc 163:462, 1973.
36. Gaskell CJ, Gibbs C, and Pearson H: Sliding hiatus hernia with reflex oesophagitis in two dogs. J Small Anim Pract 15:503, 1974.
37. Alexander JW, Hoffer RE, MacDonald JM, et al: Hiatal hernia in the dog: A case report and review of the literature. J Am Anim Hosp Assoc 11:793, 1975.
38. Iwasaki M, DeMartin BW, DeAlvarenga J, et al: Congenital hiatal hernia in a dog. Mod Vet Pract 58:1018, 1977.
39. Robotham GR: Congenital hiatal hernia in a cat. Feline Pract 9:37, 1979.
40. Peterson SL: Esophageal hiatal hernia in a cat. J Am Vet Med Assoc 183:325, 1983.
41. Bright RM, Sackman JE, NeNovo D, et al: Hiatal hernia in the dog and cat: A retrospective study of 16 cases. J Small Anim Pract 31:244, 1990.
42. Stickle R, Sparschu G, Love N, et al: Radiographic evaluation of esophageal function in Chinese Shar Pei pups. J Am Vet Med Assoc 201:81, 1992.
43. Miles KG, Pope ER, and Jergens AE: Paraesophageal hiatal hernia and pyloric obstruction in a dog. J Am Vet Med Assoc 193:1437, 1988.
44. Steiner GM: Gastro-oesophageal reflux, hiatus hernia, and the radiologist with special reference to children. Br J Radiol 50:164, 1977.
45. Pollock S, and Rhodes WH: Gastroesophageal intussusception in an Afghan hound. J Am Vet Radiol Soc 11:5, 1970.
46. Leib MS, and Blass CE: Gastroesophageal intussusception in the dog: A review of the literature and a case report. J Am Anim Hosp Assoc 20:783, 1984.
47. Bath GF: Congenital diaphragmatic hiatus in a dog: Case report. J S Afr Vet Assoc 47:55, 1976.
48. Nicholson C: Defective diaphragm associated with umbilical hernia. Vet Rec 98:433, 1976.
49. Sawyer SL: Defective diaphragm associated with umbilical hernia. Vet Rec 98:490, 1976.
50. Swift BJ: Defective diaphragm associated with umbilical hernia. Vet Rec 98:511, 1976.
51. Wolff G: Familial congenital diaphragmatic defect: Review and conclusions. Hum Genet 54:1, 1980.
52. Greene CE, Basinger RR, and Whitfield JB: Surgical management of bilateral diaphragmatic paralysis in a dog. J Am Vet Med Assoc 193:1542, 1988.
53. Mainwaring CJ: Post-traumatic contraction of the diaphragm synchronous with the heartbeat in a dog. J Small Anim Pract 29:299, 1988.
54. Cooper BJ, Winand NJ, Stedman H, et al: The homologue of the Duchenne locus is defective in X-linked muscular dystrophy of dogs. Nature 334:154, 1988.
55. Berry CR, Gaschen FP, and Ackerman H: Radiographic and ultrasonographic features of hypertrophic feline muscular dystrophy in two cats. Vet Radiol Ultrasound 33:357, 1992.
56. Gaschen FP, and Swendrowske MA: Hypertrophic feline muscular dystrophy: A unique clinical expression of dystrophin deficiency. Feline Pract 22:23, 1994.

STUDY QUESTIONS

1. What two factors relating to physical alignment during the radiographic examination affect the appearance of the diaphragm on a dorsoventral or ventrodorsal radiograph?

2. On a recumbent lateral radiograph of the thorax, which diaphragmatic crus is displaced cranially?

3. The thoracic surface of the diaphragm is easily visualized radiographically because of the adjacent air-filled lungs. What conditions obliterate or cause the diaphragmatic surface not to be visible radiographically?

4. Identifying abdominal structures within the thorax is pathognomonic for diagnosing a diaphragmatic hernia. What two other radiographic signs are most credible for identifying diaphragmatic hernias?

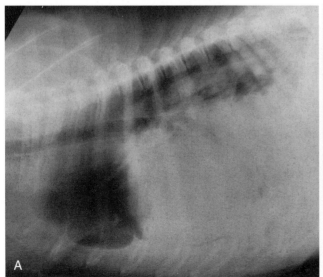

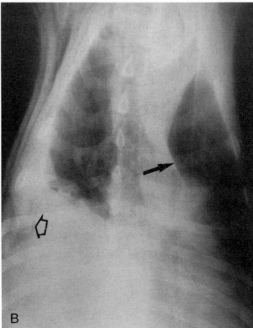

FIGURE 27–21

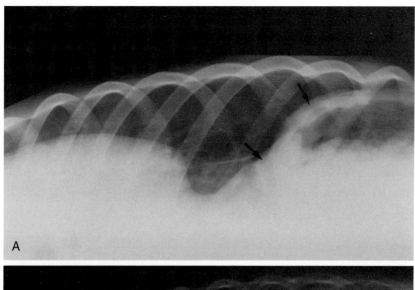

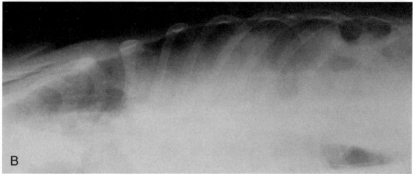

FIGURE 27-22

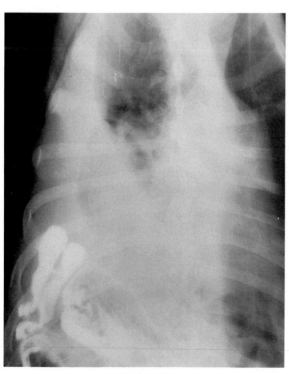

FIGURE 27-23

5. In cats with a peritoneopericardial diaphragmatic hernia, what structure is commonly identified on the lateral thoracic view?

6. What are the most reliable radiographic signs observed on the lateral thoracic radiograph for suspecting a hiatal hernia?

7. What radiographic sign is a consistent finding with muscular dystrophy in cats?

8. What radiographic signs can be identified on the lateral and ventrodorsal thoracic radiographs (Fig. 27–21A and B), and what is your specific or differential diagnosis?

9. What other diagnostic imaging modalities or techniques could be used to help determine a specific diagnosis (referring to Fig. 27–21)?

10. What radiographic signs are present on the lateral decubitus views (Fig. 27–22A and B) and the upper gastrointestinal study (Fig. 27–23) that would confirm the diagnosis of a traumatic diaphragmatic hernia in the right caudal thorax?

(Answers appear on pages 641 to 642.)

Chapter 28

The Mediastinum

Donald E. Thrall

NORMAL ANATOMY

The mediastinum is the two layers of mediastinal pleura and the space between them. The two mediastinal pleural layers are part of the right and left pleural sacs. Each pleural sac is composed of mediastinal, diaphragmatic, costal, and pulmonary pleura (Fig. 28–1). These pleural components are continuous. When speaking of the mediastinum or mediastinal disease, one is usually referring to some abnormality involving the space between the two layers of mediastinal pleura rather than a primary abnormality of a mediastinal pleural layer.

The mediastinum extends from the thoracic inlet to the diaphragm and is primarily located in the median plane of the thorax, essentially dividing the thoracic cavity into right and left halves (Fig. 28–2). The mediastinum may be subdivided into a cranial portion cranial to the heart, a middle portion at the level of and containing the heart, and a caudal portion caudal to the heart. The mediastinum may also be divided into dorsal and ventral portions by a dorsal plane through the tracheal bifurcation. Organs present in the mediastinum are listed in Table 28–1.

There is controversy regarding whether the mediastinal pleura is fenestrated. Some sources suggest that it is,[1]

whereas others suggest it is not.[2] Regardless of whether the mediastinal pleura is fenestrated or just extremely fragile, it is common for pleural space disease to be bilateral (i.e., not contained to one pleural cavity by the mediastinum). For example, in one study of induced pneumothorax in dogs, 22 of 24 dogs having air injected into one pleural space quickly developed bilateral pneumothorax.[3] Unilateral pleural space disease or pleural space disease with asymmetric distribution may occur if (1) the mediastinum is not fenestrated or the mediastinal pleura remains intact, (2) existing fenestrations have been closed by inflammatory disease, or (3) the pleural space contents are too large or viscid to pass through any existing fenestrations.

The mediastinum, in contrast to the pleural space, is not a closed cavity. The mediastinum communicates cranially with the fascial planes of the neck via the thoracic inlet. Caudally the mediastinum communicates with the retroperitoneal space through the aortic hiatus. These communications provide the means for the spread of mediastinal disease to the neck and abdomen and vice versa.

Of the mediastinal organs listed in Table 28–1, only the heart, trachea, caudal vena cava, aorta, and, in young animals, thymus are visible in normal thoracic radiographs. Oc-

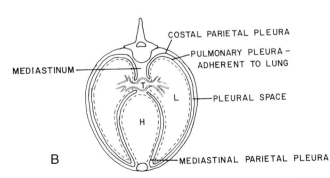

FIGURE 28–1. Drawings of the thorax in dorsal (A) and transverse (B) planes illustrating the relationship of the pleural layers. A, Note the continuity of the costal, mediastinal, and diaphragmatic parts of the parietal pleura. (Lungs have not been included in A.) B, Note how the mediastinal pleura is reflected onto the lung as pulmonary pleura. Note also that the pleural space is not continuous with the mediastinum. T, trachea; L, lung; H, heart.

Table 28–1
MEDIASTINAL ORGANS

Organ	Cranial Mediastinum	Middle Mediastinum	Caudal Mediastinum
Cranial vena cava	x		
Thymus	x		
Sternal lymph nodes	x		
Aortic arch	x		
Brachiocephalic artery	x		
Left subclavian artery	x		
Mediastinal lymph nodes	x		
Trachea	x	x	
Right and left vagosympathetic trunk	x	x	
Dorsal intercostal arteries and veins	x	x	x
Internal thoracic arteries and veins	x	x	x
Esophagus	x	x	x
Thoracic duct	x	x	x
Right and left sympathetic trunks	x	x	x
Right and left phrenic nerves	x	x	x
Descending aorta		x	x
Bronchoesophageal arteries and veins		x	x
Azygous vein		x	x
Heart		x	
Tracheobronchial lymph nodes		x	
Main pulmonary artery		x	
Main pulmonary veins		x	
Principal bronchi		x	
Caudal vena cava			x
Right and left vagus nerves			x

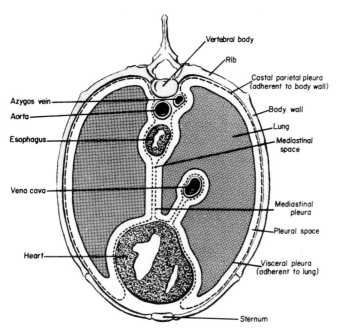

FIGURE 28–2. Cross-section of the canine thorax in a transverse plane. The mediastinum divides the thorax into right and left halves. Note that the mediastinum (mediastinal space) does not communicate with the pleural space. (From Thrall DE, and Losonsky JM: Dyspnea in the cat: II. Radiographic aspects of intrathoracic causes involving the mediastinum. Feline Pract 8:47, 1978; with permission.)

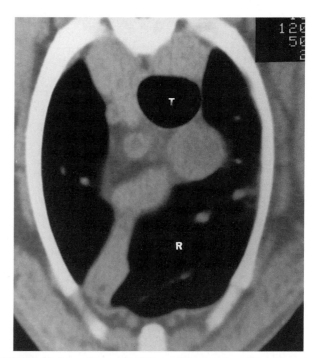

FIGURE 28–4. Computed tomographic (CT) image of the canine thorax. This transverse plane image is at the level of the second thoracic vertebra. Note the greater thickness of the mediastinum dorsally in comparison to ventrally. This greater thickness accounts for the opacity seen ventral to the trachea in lateral thoracic radiographs (see Fig. 28–3). Note the vessels ventral to the trachea (T). There is insufficient fat for these vessels to be seen in radiographs, but the superior inherent contrast of CT allows them to be seen. Note also the cranioventral mediastinal reflection; the ventral mediastinum is being pushed to the left by the right cranial lung lobe (R).

casionally the normal esophagus may be seen (see Chapter 25). Other mediastinal organs are not seen because (1) they are not large enough to absorb a sufficient number of x-rays, (2) there is insufficient fat in the mediastinum to provide contrast, or (3) they are in contact with other mediastinal structures of the same radiopacity and cannot be seen because of the silhouette sign. An example of silhouetting of mediastinal structures is the appearance of the cranial mediastinum in a lateral thoracic radiograph. A distinct opacity is usually visible in the cranial mediastinum ventral to the trachea, but individual organs cannot be discerned (Fig. 28–3). The opacity is due to the absorption of x-rays by cranial mediastinal organs, that is, the left subclavian artery, brachiocephalic trunk, cranial vena cava, mediastinal lymph nodes,

and possibly the thymus. These organs are not seen individually, however, because they are in contact with each other and there is usually little fat in the cranial mediastinum. Thus, the margin of these vessels in the cranial mediastinum is obliterated. On the lateral projection, the cranial mediastinum is more radiopaque just ventral to the trachea than just dorsal to the sternum because of the greater thickness of the mediastinum ventral to the trachea (Fig. 28–4; see Fig. 28–3).

In ventrodorsal or dorsoventral thoracic radiographs, most

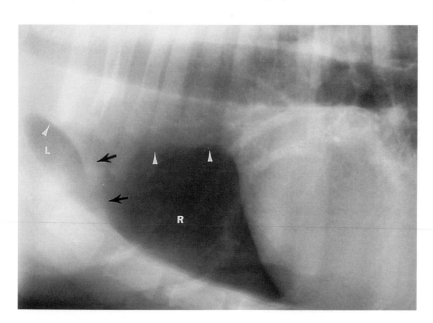

FIGURE 28–3. Left lateral radiograph of the thorax of a normal dog. The opacity ventral to the trachea (*white arrowheads indicate ventral margin of opacity*) is part of the cranial mediastinum. Although there are several different organs in this part of the mediastinum (e.g., left subclavian artery, brachiocephalic trunk, and cranial vena cava), they cannot be discerned because they are in contact with each other and there is insufficient surrounding fat to provide contrast. The mediastinum extends dorsally from the vertebrae ventrally to the sternebrae, but it is most radiopaque immediately ventral to the trachea because its thickness is greatest in this location (see Fig. 28–4). Note also the cranioventral mediastinal reflection (*black arrows*) between the cranial portion of the left cranial lobe (L) and the right cranial lobe (R), which appears as a curving line of soft-tissue opacity that extends from the end of the first rib in a caudoventral direction to the second sternebra (see Fig. 28–4).

of the cranial mediastinum is superimposed on the spine, and the width of the mediastinum is usually less than approximately two times the width of the spine (Fig. 28–5). In obese patients, the cranial mediastinum may be widened by fat accumulation, and the resultant opacity can be confused with a mediastinal mass (Fig. 28–6).

There are three mediastinal reflections, two of which are frequently identified in normal thoracic radiographs: (1) the cranioventral mediastinal reflection, (2) the caudoventral mediastinal reflection, and (3) the vena caval mediastinal reflection or the plica vena cava.

On a ventrodorsal or dorsoventral radiograph, the cranioventral mediastinal reflection appears as a curving radiopaque line, with the concave surface on the patient's right, extending from approximately T1 or T2 to the region of the main pulmonary artery (see Figs. 28–4 and 28–5). This reflection is caused by extension of the right cranial lobe across the midline pushing the mediastinum to the left (see Fig. 28–4). The thickness of the cranioventral mediastinal reflection is affected by the amount of fat it contains. On the lateral view, the cranioventral mediastinal reflection and the margin of the right cranial lobe may frequently be identified immediately cranial to the heart (see Fig. 28–3). The cranioventral mediastinal reflection is not visible in every thoracic radiograph. The thymus lies in the cranioventral mediastinal reflection, and the thymus can frequently be identified in ventrodorsal or dorsoventral radiographs of young animals. The thymus is not as readily seen on lateral views of the

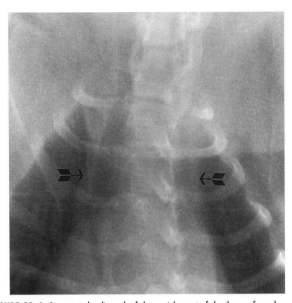

FIGURE 28–6. Dorsoventral radiograph of the cranial aspect of the thorax of an obese dog. The cranial mediastinum contains a large amount of fat and appears wider than twice the diameter of the thoracic spine (arrows). Care should be taken to avoid misinterpreting a wide mediastinum in an obese animal as an abnormal mediastinal mass.

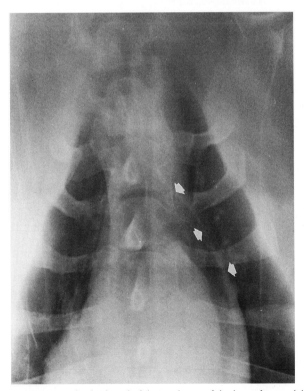

FIGURE 28–5. Ventrodorsal radiograph of the cranial aspect of the thorax of a normal dog. The cranial mediastinum is superimposed on the cranial aspect of the thoracic spine; it is relatively indistinct. As an approximation, the width of the normal cranial mediastinum in ventrodorsal or dorsoventral radiographs should not be greater than twice the diameter of the cranial thoracic spine. Note the mediastinal reflection between the right cranial lobe and the cranial part of the left cranial lobe (arrows); it appears as a curving line of soft-tissue opacity that extends from the C7–T1 junction in a left caudolateral direction to the cardiac silhouette in the region of the main pulmonary artery. See Figure 28–3 for the appearance of this reflection in the lateral view and Figure 28–4 for an illustration of the right lung pushing the mediastinum to the left.

thorax (Fig. 28–7). In lateral projections of the thorax made before the thymus involutes, however, the thymus may silhouette with and obscure the cranial margin of the heart.

The caudoventral mediastinal reflection is seen only on ventrodorsal or dorsoventral radiographs; it cannot be seen in lateral projections. It is created by extension of the accessory lobe (a lobe of the right lung) across the midline, which subsequently pushes the mediastinum to the left. The caudoventral mediastinal reflection appears as a relatively straight radiopaque line in the caudal left hemithorax, extending from the region of the cardiac apex in a caudolateral direction toward the gastric fundus (Fig. 28–8). The caudoventral mediastinal reflection has been incorrectly identified radiographically as the sternopericardiac ligament (also called the *cardiophrenic* or *phrenicopericardiac ligament*), but the sternopericardiac ligament, which is a continuation of the apex of the fibrous pericardium, is not visible radiographically.[4] The thickness of the caudoventral mediastinal reflection depends on the amount of fat it contains (Fig. 28–9). The caudoventral mediastinal reflection is not visible on every ventrodorsal or dorsoventral thoracic radiograph.

The caudal vena caval mediastinal reflection, or plica vena cava, is not visible as a distinct structure in radiographs of the thorax, but its presence as an extension of the mediastinum to the right should be understood (see Fig. 28–2).

PATHOLOGIC MEDIASTINAL CONDITIONS

There are four general classifications of pathologic mediastinal conditions: (1) mediastinal shift, (2) mediastinal masses, (3) mediastinal fluid, and (4) pneumomediastinum.

Mediastinal Shift

A mediastinal shift occurs as a result of unilateral decrease in lung volume (ipsilateral shift), a unilateral increase in lung volume (contralateral shift), or the presence of an intrathoracic mass (contralateral shift). Mediastinal shifts are not

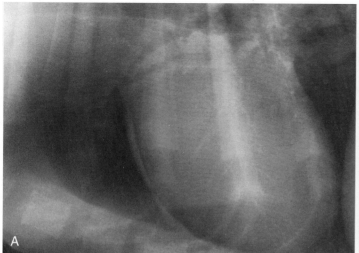

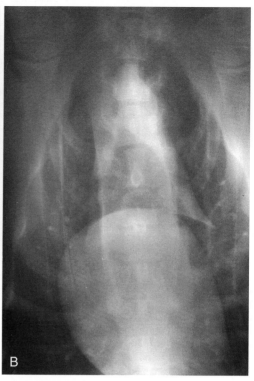

FIGURE 28–7. Lateral *(A)* and ventrodorsal *(B)* radiographs of the thorax of a young dog made before involution of the thymus. In the ventrodorsal view *(B)*, the thymus appears as a sail-shaped area of soft-tissue opacity cranial and to the left of the cardiac base. In the lateral view, the thymus produces a linear region of soft-tissue opacity just cranial to the heart. The thymus may not always be visible in the lateral view in dogs in which it is seen in the ventrodorsal projection.

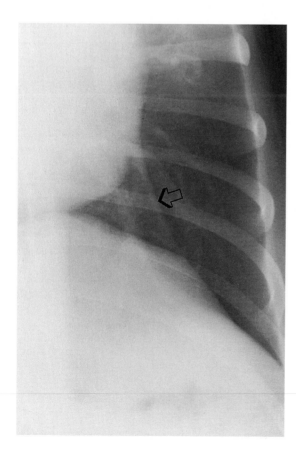

FIGURE 28–8. Ventrodorsal radiograph of the caudal thorax of a normal dog. The caudoventral mediastinal reflection appears as a line of soft-tissue opacity that extends from the region of the cardiac apex in a left caudolateral direction to the diaphragm *(arrow)*.

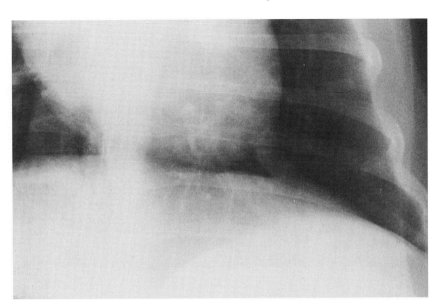

FIGURE 28–9. Ventrodorsal radiograph of the caudal aspect of the thorax of an obese dog. Fat has accumulated in the caudoventral mediastinum, resulting in increased thickness. Compare its appearance in this radiograph with that in Figure 28–8.

readily apparent on lateral radiographs. Therefore, the mediastinal position must be carefully assessed on ventrodorsal or dorsoventral radiographs. The mediastinal position may be evaluated by noting the position of visible mediastinal organs, such as the trachea, heart, aorta, and caudal vena cava, or the previously described mediastinal reflections (Fig. 28–10). Improper patient positioning, such as rotation of the sternum

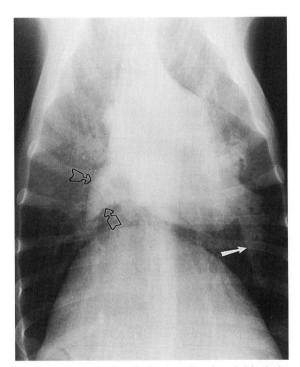

FIGURE 28–10. Ventrodorsal radiograph of a dog with mediastinal shift. The heart and caudoventral mediastinal reflection *(solid white arrow)* are displaced to the left because of decreased volume of the left caudal lung lobe. The right middle lobe is collapsed *(open black arrows)*, and there is alveolar disease in the left caudal lobe. The caudoventral mediastinal reflection does not appear as a radiopaque line as seen in Figure 28–8. Because of the increased opacity within the left caudal lobe, the lobe is silhouetting with the reflection. The caudoventral mediastinal reflection, however, is in contact with the medial portion of the left caudal lobe. Therefore, because the medial margin of the left caudal lobe may be identified as a result of the alveolar disease, the location of the caudoventral mediastinal reflection may be inferred from this information.

to the right or left, may create a false impression of a mediastinal shift.

Mediastinal Masses

Mediastinal mass lesions are common, and the radiographic appearance of many mediastinal masses is similar. The ventrodorsal or dorsoventral projections are more useful than the lateral view in deciding whether an abnormal mass is located in the mediastinum versus the lung. Mediastinal location of a radiographically detectable intrathoracic mass should be considered if (1) the mass lies on or adjacent to the midline (Fig. 28–11), (2) the mass is in a position consistent with one of the three previously described mediastinal reflections (see Fig. 28–7), or (3) the mass deviates a mediastinal structure. Lung masses should not be confused with a mass of mediastinal origin because they usually lie in a position lateral to the mediastinum (Fig. 28–12).

Cranial mediastinal masses often cause elevation of the trachea. Elevation of the trachea, however, may also be produced when there is a large volume of fluid in the pleural space but no mediastinal mass is present (Fig. 28–13). With a large-volume pleural effusion, tracheal elevation results from displacement of lungs as they float in the pleural fluid.[5] Tracheal elevation is not seen when only a small volume of fluid is present in the pleural space unless a mediastinal mass is also present. If pleural effusion is present, definitive identification of a concurrent mediastinal mass may not be possible unless the mass results in compression of the trachea; pleural fluid alone does not result in tracheal compression. If pleural fluid obscures the mediastinum and a mediastinal mass is being considered, removing the fluid and repeating the radiographs may be helpful. Additional radiographs made with a horizontally directed x-ray beam may also be helpful. These horizontal-beam radiographs take advantage of gravity, which causes pleural fluid to migrate away from the area of the suspected mediastinal mass. Ultrasonographic examination is also of value in assessing the cranioventral mediastinum for the presence of a mass.[6] The location of a mass lesion within the mediastinum is helpful in formulating a differential diagnosis. Causes of mediastinal masses are listed in Table 28–2.

Mediastinal lymphadenopathy is one of the most common

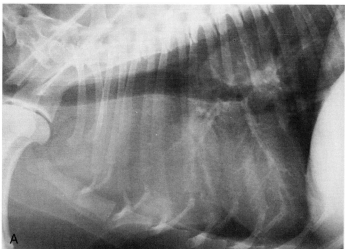

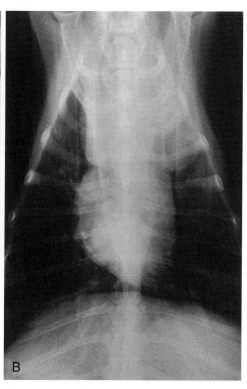

FIGURE 28–11. Lateral (A) and ventrodorsal (B) radiographs of the thorax of a dog with lymphosarcoma. A, A large mass is visible cranial to the heart. Although its position is consistent with mediastinal mass, and there is dorsal displacement of the trachea, this exact position of the mass cannot be determined from the lateral view. B, The mass is centered on the midline, suggesting a mediastinal location. Diagnosis was thymic lymphosarcoma.

causes of a mediastinal mass. The major groupings of lymph nodes in the mediastinum are discussed in the following paragraphs.[7, 8]

The *cranial mediastinal lymph nodes* vary in number and size. Most of them lie along the cranial vena cava and brachiocephalic, left subclavian, and costocervical arteries and are therefore located in the cranial mediastinum, just ventral to the trachea. Afferent lymphatics come from the muscles of the neck, thorax and abdomen, scapula, last six cervical vertebrae, thoracic vertebrae, ribs, trachea, esophagus, thyroid, thymus, mediastinum, costal pleura, heart, and aorta. The cranial mediastinal lymph nodes also receive efferent lymphatics from the intercostal, sternal, middle, and caudal deep

cervical, tracheobronchial, and pulmonary lymph nodes. Efferent channels from the tracheobronchial lymph nodes drain into either the thoracic duct or the left tracheal trunk or both. Enlargement of the cranial mediastinal lymph nodes results in a visible mass in the cranial mediastinum that often elevates the trachea. Enlarged cranial mediastinal lymph nodes may be visible on both lateral and ventrodorsal (dorsoventral) projections (Fig. 28–14). Radiographic identification of enlarged mediastinal lymph nodes in dogs with lymphosarcoma has been identified as a negative prognostic factor.[9]

The *sternal lymph node* is usually represented by a single node on each side in the dog and a single node in the cat. In the dog, there is occasionally only a single median node. The

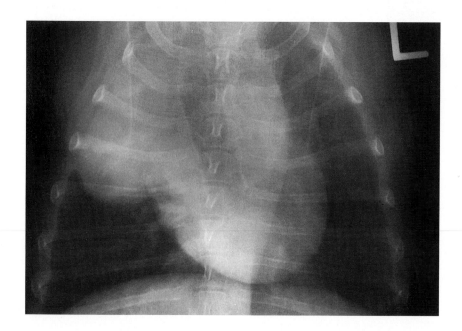

FIGURE 28–12. Ventrodorsal radiograph of the thorax of a dog. There is a large mass in the right cranial hemithorax. The probability of such a mass being in the mediastinum is low because (1) the mass is located lateral to the mediastinum, (2) it is not in a position of one of the mediastinal reflections, and (3) no normal mediastinal organs are displaced (the trachea is normally on the right in the cranial thorax). Diagnosis was primary lung tumor, right cranial lung lobe.

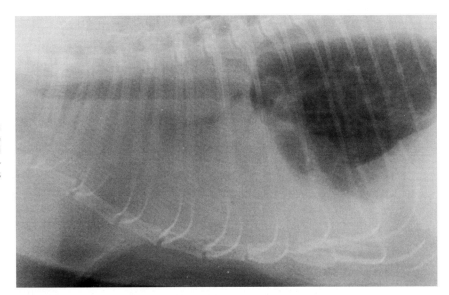

FIGURE 28–13. Lateral radiograph of the thorax of a cat with pleural effusion. The trachea is displaced dorsally, but the presence of a mediastinal mass cannot be confirmed because (1) pleural fluid may be accompanied by tracheal elevation when no mediastinal mass is present, (2) a mass cannot be seen, and (3) there is no compression of the trachea.

sternal node lies in the ventral mediastinum, immediately cranial to the transversus thoracis muscle and medial to the second costal cartilage or second interchondral space, cranioventral to the internal thoracic blood vessels. The afferent lymphatics of the sternal node lie under the transversus thoracis in the fat between this muscle and the dorsal surfaces of the sternal ends of the costal cartilages. They arise in the abdominal wall and perforate the diaphragm near the middle of the costal arch. Afferent vessels receive tributaries from the ribs, sternum, serous membranes, thymus, adjacent muscles, and mammary glands. Clinical evidence of mammary tumor metastasis to the sternal node is uncommon. Diseases of the peritoneal cavity, however, such as pancreatitis or carcinomatosis, may result in clinical and radiographic evidence of sternal lymphadenopathy. Sternal lymphadenopathy appears as an isolated soft-tissue opacity dorsal to the region of the second sternebra and is best seen on the lateral

Table 28–2
CAUSES OF MEDIASTINAL MASSES

Cause of Mass	Mediastinal Location
Lymphosarcoma—cat	Cranioventral
Lymphosarcoma—dog	Perihilar, cranioventral
Inflammatory lymphadenopathy	Perihilar, cranioventral
Neoplastic lymphadenopathy—metastatic	Perihilar, cranioventral
Periesophageal vascular ring	Craniodorsal*
Neurogenic tumor	Dorsal
Paraspinal tumor	Dorsal
Mediastinal abscess—usually secondary to esophageal perforation	Cranioventral, caudoventral, caudal
Generalized megaesophagus	Dorsal
Spirocerca lupi	Caudodorsal
Mediastinal diaphragmatic hernia	Caudoventral
Ectopic thyroid or parathyroid tumor	Cranioventral, perihilar
Thymoma	Cranioventral
Heart-base tumor	Craniodorsal, perihilar
Hiatal hernia	Caudodorsal
Diaphragmatic eventration	Caudodorsal
Hematoma	Variable

*Severe esophagomegaly may appear cranioventrally.

projection, although occasionally there is a sufficiently large mass for the enlargement to be seen on the ventrodorsal view (Figs. 28–15 and 28–16).

The *tracheobronchial lymph nodes* are known as the right, left, and middle tracheobronchial lymph nodes. The right and left nodes lie on the lateral side of their respective bronchus and also contact the trachea. The right node is ventral to the azygous vein, the left ventral to the aorta. The middle tracheobronchial lymph node is the largest of the group. It is in the form of a V and lies in the angle formed by the origin of the primary bronchi from the trachea. Afferent vessels to the tracheobronchial lymph nodes come from the lungs and bronchi primarily, but they also come from the thoracic parts of the aorta, esophagus, trachea, heart, mediastinum, and diaphragm. Enlargement of the tracheobronchial lymph nodes is commonly seen with generalized lymphoreticular neoplasms or inflammatory lung disease and results in visualization of a soft-tissue opacity in the region of the tracheal bifurcation on the lateral view (see Fig. 28–15). Enlargement of the tracheobronchial lymph nodes is usually more apparent on the lateral than on the ventrodorsal or dorsoventral projection. Lateral divergence or separation of the principal bronchi may be apparent on the ventrodorsal view (Fig. 28–17; see also Fig. 28–15). The ease with which enlarged tracheobronchial lymph nodes are seen on the lateral view depends on their size and the amount of adjacent lung opacity. Tracheobronchial lymph nodes are unlikely to be seen unless they create a mass approaching 4 to 6 cm in diameter. In instances in which the lymphadenopathy exists with lung disease, the opacity from the lung disease may make the enlarged tracheobronchial lymph nodes more difficult to identify because of the silhouette sign (Fig. 28–18). On the lateral view, enlarged tracheobronchial lymph nodes may result in elevation or depression of the tracheal bifurcation; in some dogs, no change in position of the tracheal bifurcation results from tracheobronchial lymphadenopathy. Enlarged tracheobronchial lymph nodes that result in elevation of the tracheal bifurcation may be confused radiographically with an enlarged left atrium.

Mediastinal Fluid

Free mediastinal fluid is usually of soft-tissue opacity; therefore, it may appear radiographically as a mediastinal mass or

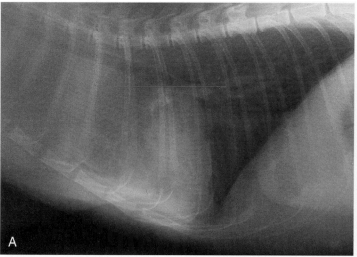

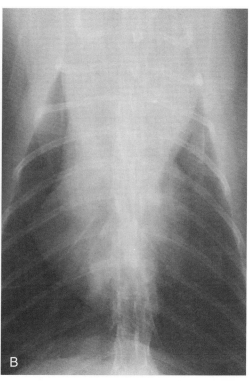

FIGURE 28-14. Lateral *(A)* and ventrodorsal *(B)* thoracic radiographs of a cat with enlargement of the cranial mediastinal lymph nodes. There is a large, homogeneous soft-tissue mass in the cranioventral mediastinum. The mass is elevating the trachea and displacing the cranial lung lobes laterally and caudally. In cats, it is virtually impossible to distinguish between enlargement of the cranial mediastinal lymph nodes and the thymus. Diagnosis was cranial mediastinal lymphosarcoma.

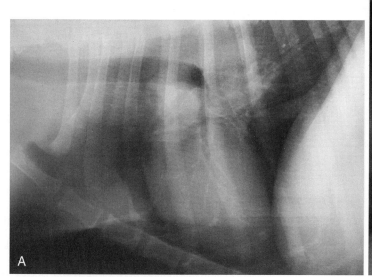

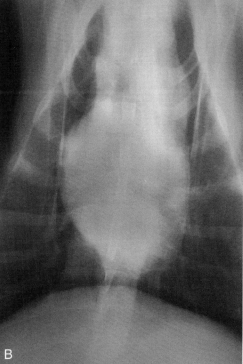

FIGURE 28-15. Lateral *(A)* and ventrodorsal *(B)* thoracic radiographs of a 9-year-old Dalmatian with a history of generalized peripheral lymphadenopathy. In the lateral radiograph, there is a region of soft-tissue opacity just dorsal to the second and third sternebrae owing to enlargement of the sternal lymph node. There is also an ill-defined region of increased opacity around the tracheal bifurcation caused by tracheobronchial lymphadenopathy. The enlarged tracheobronchial lymph nodes have also caused elevation of the trachea just cranial to the bifurcation. In the ventrodorsal view, the enlarged sternal lymph nodes have resulted in widening of the cranioventral mediastinal reflection, and the enlarged tracheobronchial nodes have produced lateral displacement of the principal bronchi (see Fig. 28-17). Diagnosis was lymphosarcoma.

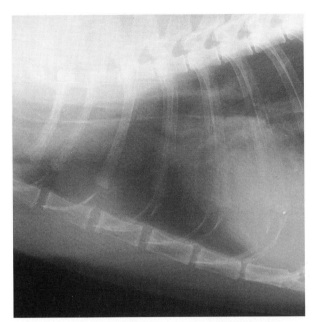

FIGURE 28–16. Lateral thoracic radiograph of a cat with lymphosarcoma. There is a well-defined region of increased opacity dorsal to the third and fourth sternebrae. This opacity represents an enlarged sternal lymph node. Additionally, gas is present ventral to the trachea, which is consistent with pneumomediastinum; this most likely occurred secondary to tracheal puncture when blood was being collected from the jugular vein.

as cardiomegaly if it collects around the heart, or both (Fig. 28–19). If mediastinal fluid is a radiographic consideration, its presence may be detected by horizontal-beam radiography (unless it is trapped or loculated) or ultrasonography. The more common causes of mediastinal fluid include feline infectious peritonitis, trauma, coagulopathy, and esophageal perforation. Mediastinal fluid may also accumulate secondary to an underlying mass.

Pneumomediastinum

Pneumomediastinum is free gas in the mediastinum. Mediastinal gas provides excellent radiographic contrast, thereby

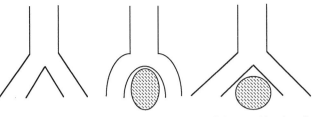

FIGURE 28–17. Illustration of the appearance of the shape of the principal bronchi in the caudal lobes in a ventrodorsal radiograph in the normal state *(left)* and when there is a mass present between them *(middle and right)*. The presence of a mass, such as an enlarged left atrium and a regional lymph node, between the principal bronchi may result in the principal bronchi assuming a curved appearance *(middle)* or being displaced laterally *(right)* or both.

resulting in enhanced visualization of mediastinal organs (Fig. 28–20). If only a small amount of mediastinal gas is present, the only apparent abnormality may be patchy regions of radiolucency in the cranial mediastinum (see Figs. 28–13 and 28–16). The size of the mediastinum is not greatly increased when pneumomediastinum is present. Therefore, pneumomediastinum is not readily seen on ventrodorsal or dorsoventral radiographs (Fig. 28–21). Pneumomediastinum may progress to pneumothorax if mediastinal pressure results in tearing of mediastinal pleura, thus establishing communication between the mediastinum and the pleural space. Dyspnea is usually not seen with pneumomediastinum unless it progresses to pneumothorax. Pneumothorax does not progress to pneumomediastinum. Because of the communication of the mediastinum with the neck and retroperitoneal space, pneumomediastinum may result in subcutaneous emphysema or pneumoretroperitoneum (Fig. 28–22; see Fig. 28–21). Alternatively, gas in the retroperitoneal space or fascial planes of the neck may freely diffuse into the mediastinum.

There are six causes of pneumomediastinum, listed in decreasing order of likelihood:

1. Air escaping into the lung interstitium from sites of alveolar rupture can diffuse in a retrograde direction in loose connective tissue adjacent to bronchi and vessels into the mediastinum.[10] This situation occurs commonly after trauma and also occurs after iatrogenic pulmonary hyperinflation during anesthesia or resuscitation.[11] Pneumothorax is not

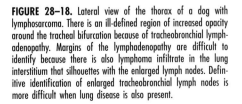

FIGURE 28–18. Lateral view of the thorax of a dog with lymphosarcoma. There is an ill-defined region of increased opacity around the tracheal bifurcation because of tracheobronchial lymphadenopathy. Margins of the lymphadenopathy are difficult to identify because there is also lymphoma infiltrate in the lung interstitium that silhouettes with the enlarged lymph nodes. Definitive identification of enlarged tracheobronchial lymph nodes is more difficult when lung disease is also present.

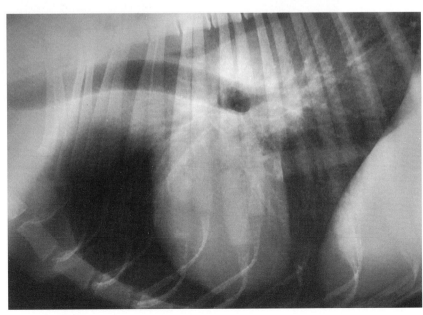

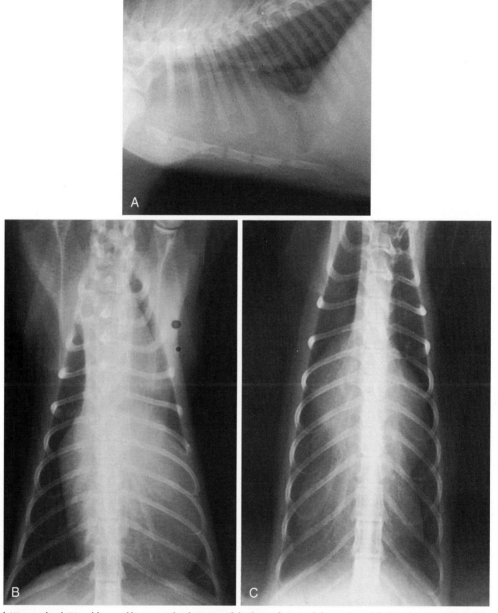

FIGURE 28–19. Lateral *(A)*, ventrodorsal *(B)*, and horizontal-beam ventrodorsal *(C)* views of the thorax of a cat with free mediastinal fluid. *A,* The cardiac silhouette is obscured by homogeneous opacification of the ventral thorax. *B,* The cranial mediastinum is wide, and the cardiac silhouette is enlarged with an unusual, rectangular-appearing right margin. *C,* The heart is clearly seen in the middle of the thorax, and the caudal mediastinum is increased in width owing to caudal gravitation of the free mediastinal fluid. Diagnosis was feline infectious peritonitis. (From Thrall DE, and Losonsky JM: Dyspnea in the cat: II. Radiographic aspects of intrathoracic causes involving the mediastinum. Feline Pract *8:*47, 1978; with permission.)

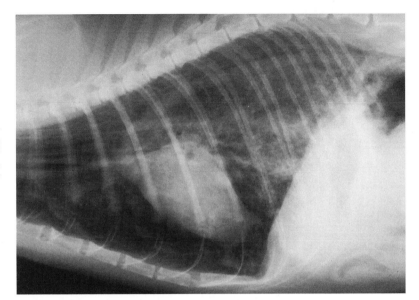

FIGURE 28–20. Lateral view of the thorax of a cat with pneumomediastinum. There is enhanced visualization of the esophagus, adventitial surface of the trachea, cranial vena cava, azygous vein, and major branches of the aortic arch because of contrast provided by free mediastinal gas. The lung is also opacified caudally. (Courtesy of Dr. Mary Mahaffey, University of Georgia, Athens, GA.)

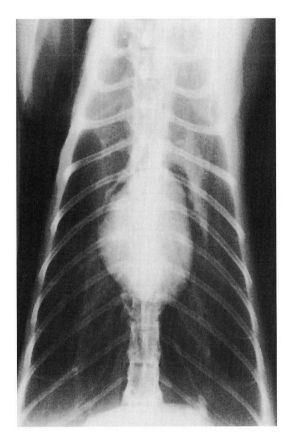

FIGURE 28–21. Ventrodorsal view of a cat with pneumomediastinum. Note the inability to identify the mediastinal gas. The opacity craniolateral to the cardiac base on the cat's left side is probably the thymus, which was displaced laterally by the emphysematous mediastinum. There is gas between the right scapula and the thoracic wall.

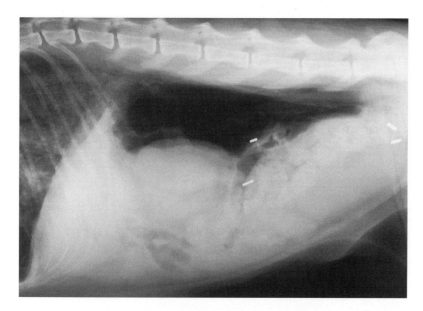

FIGURE 28–22. Abdominal radiograph of the same cat as in Figure 28–20. There is a large amount of gas in the retroperitoneal space as a result of dissection of mediastinal gas caudally through the aortic hiatus. (Courtesy of Dr. Mary Mahaffey, University of Georgia, Athens, GA.)

present when pneumomediastinum results from this mechanism unless the pulmonary pleura becomes torn or the mediastinal air accumulation results in perforation of mediastinal pleura.

2. Caudal extension of gas in neck fascial planes into the mediastinum may occur. Gas in the neck is a common sequela to neck or oral cavity trauma; it also may result from tracheal or esophageal rupture.

3. A hole in the wall of the trachea may occur as a result of trauma or erosion associated with neoplasia or inflammatory disease. If the hole is intrathoracic, air enters the mediastinum directly. If the hole is in the neck, air may dissect along the trachea through the thoracic inlet into the mediastinum. Pneumomediastinum is often observed following jugular venipuncture if the needle inadvertently penetrates the trachea. In cattle and horses, pneumomediastinum is frequently seen following transtracheal aspiration procedures.

4. An esophageal perforation may occur as a result of trauma, inflammation, or neoplasia.

5. Cranial extension of gas from the retroperitoneal space into the mediastinum may occur.

6. A gas-producing organism in the mediastinum is extremely unlikely.

References

1. Schummer A, Nickel R, and Sack W: The Viscera of the Domestic Mammals, 2nd Ed. New York, Springer-Verlag, 1979.
2. Evans HE: The respiratory system. *In* Evans HE (Ed): Miller's Anatomy of the Dog, 3rd Ed. Philadelphia, WB Saunders, 1993, pp 463–493.
3. Kern DA, Carrig CB, and Martin RA: Radiographic evaluation of induced pneumothorax in the dog. Vet Radiol Ultrasound 35:411, 1994.
4. Burk RL: Radiographic definition of the phrenicopericardial ligament. J Am Vet Radiol Soc 17:216, 1976.
5. Snyder PS, Sato T, and Atkins CE: The utility of thoracic radiographic measurement for the detection of cardiomegaly in cats with pleural effusion. Vet Radiol 31:89, 1990.
6. Konde LJ, and Spaulding KA: Sonographic evaluation of the cranial mediastinum in small animals. Vet Radiol 32:178, 1991.
7. Bezuidenhout AJ: The lymphatic system. *In* Evans HE (Ed): Miller's Anatomy of the Dog, 3rd Ed. Philadelphia, WB Saunders, 1993, pp 717–757.
8. Tompkins MB: Lymphoid system. *In* Husdon LC, Hamilton WP (Eds): Atlas of Feline Anatomy for Veterinarians. Philadelphia, WB Saunders, 1993, pp 113–126.
9. Starrak GS, Berry CR, Page RL, et al: Correlation between thoracic radiographic changes and remission/survival in 270 dogs with lymphosarcoma. Vet Radiol Ultrasound, in press.
10. Macklin CC: Transport of air along sheaths of pulmonic blood vessels from alveoli to mediastinum: Clinical implications. Arch Intern Med 64:913, 1939.
11. Brown DC, and Holt D: Subcutaneous emphysema, pneumothorax, pneumomediastinum, and pneumopericardium associated with positive-pressure ventilation in a cat. J Am Vet Med Assoc 206:997, 1995.

STUDY QUESTIONS

1. Which one of the following statements is false?
    A. The mediastinum is a closed space.
    B. The mediastinal pleura is an ineffective barrier to spread of disease from one pleural cavity to another.
    C. The cranial mediastinum appears most opaque in lateral radiographs just ventral to the trachea because its thickness is greatest at this level.
    D. In normal dogs, the width of the mediastinum in ventrodorsal radiographs should be less than approximately two times the thickness of the spine.

2. Which two of the following mediastinal reflections are visible in most normal canine thoracic radiographs?
    A. Cranioventral.
    B. Caudoventral.
    C. Caval.
    D. Plica vena cava.

3. Why is it easier to determine if an intrathoracic mass is located in the mediastinum from ventrodorsal or dorsoventral radiographs rather than from lateral radiographs?

4. Based on the following lateral and ventrodorsal feline thoracic radiographs (Fig. 28–23), list as many roentgen signs as you can which indicate that the opacity seen in the cranial thorax is a mediastinal mass.

5. Based on the following lateral canine thoracic radiograph (Fig. 28–24), the most likely diagnosis is:
    A. Diaphragmatic hernia.

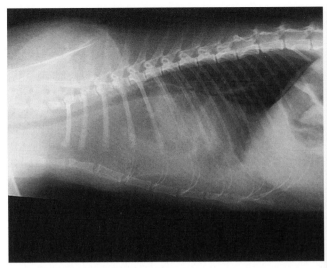

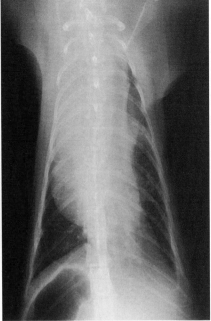

FIGURE 28–23

B. Pleural effusion.
C. Pneumomediastinum.
D. Cranial mediastinal lymphadenopathy.

6. A dog with a ruptured bowel is given barium. The barium extravasates into the peritoneal cavity. Immediate abdominal surgery is successful in repairing the rupture. A thoracic radiograph is made 2 days later because of a cough. Which mediastinal lymph node would be the most likely to have evidence of the previous barium extravasation, and what would the radiographic changes be?

7. Name two imaging techniques that can be used to differentiate between mediastinal fluid and a mediastinal mass.

8. What is the most common cause of pneumomediastinum?

9. Pneumothorax readily progresses to pneumomediastinum. (True or False)

10. Enlargement of the tracheobronchial lymph nodes may cause elevation of the tracheal bifurcation, depression

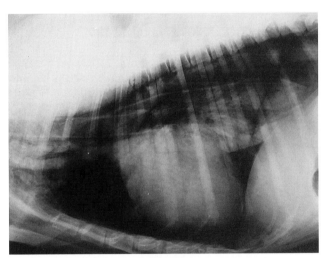

FIGURE 28–24

of the tracheal bifurcation, or no change in tracheal bifurcation position. (True or False)

(Answers appear on page 642.)

Chapter 29

The Pleural Space

Donald E. Thrall

PLEURAL ANATOMY

There are two types of pleura, pulmonary and parietal. Pulmonary pleura, also called *visceral pleura*, covers the lung parenchyma. Parietal pleura is subdivided into three parts; costal parietal pleura lines the inside of the thoracic cage, diaphragmatic parietal pleura covers the diaphragm, and mediastinal parietal pleura forms the boundaries of the mediastinal space.

The left and right pleural sacs are distinct entities, each having continuous costal, diaphragmatic, mediastinal, and pulmonary parts (Fig. 29–1). The pleural space is a potential space between parietal and pulmonary pleural layers and between pulmonary pleural layers in interlobar fissures; it normally contains only a small volume of fluid, which serves as a lubricant.

NORMAL RADIOGRAPHIC APPEARANCE AND PLEURAL THICKENING

Normal pleura is usually not visible radiographically. Pulmonary pleura outside of interlobar fissures cannot be seen because it silhouettes with adjacent soft tissue. Pulmonary pleura within intralobar fissures is surrounded by intrapulmonary air, which provides contrast, but the pleura is so thin that it generally does not absorb a sufficient number of x-rays to produce a detectable radiographic opacity.

Opaque, thin pleural lines are sometimes noted between lobes. Thickened pleura may assume this appearance. Occasionally, however, the x-ray beam strikes normal pleura in an interlobar fissure exactly tangentially, resulting in absorption of a sufficient number of x-rays for the pleura to be

seen. It is impossible to determine radiographically whether isolated, thin pleural lines are normal or whether they represent evidence of slight pleural thickening. In either instance, such a finding is usually of no clinical significance.

When pleural thickening is advanced, more prominent pleural lines may be seen between lung lobes (Fig. 29–2). Thickened pulmonary pleura is not seen radiographically because thickened pleura on the lung surface silhouettes with adjacent soft tissue. In pleural thickening and with pleural effusion, the specific interlobar fissures seen radiographically depend on which fissures are struck tangentially by the x-ray beam. This varies with changes in positioning of the patient.

PLEURAL EFFUSION

Fluid in the pleural space is termed *pleural effusion*. The fluid can be an exudate, transudate, or modified transudate, depending on its cause (Table 29–1). When pleural effusion is present, radiographically detectable changes result. The nature of these changes depends on the volume of fluid, the relationship of the animal to the x-ray beam, the distribution of the fluid, and whether the fluid is free or loculated.

Free Pleural Effusion

The typical radiographic changes associated with free pleural effusion are the same, regardless of fluid type, because neither the distribution of free pleural fluid nor its opacity is related to the cause. Free pleural fluid distributes itself according to gravity and the ability of the lung to expand, that is, lung compliance. Thus, the appearance of pleural effusion

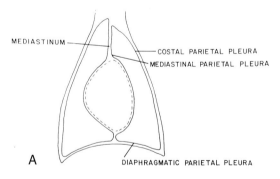

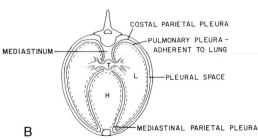

FIGURE 29–1. Drawings of the thorax in dorsal *(A)* and transverse *(B)* planes illustrating the relationship of the pleural layers. *A,* Note the continuity of the costal, mediastinal, and diaphragmatic parts of the parietal pleura. (Lungs have not been included in *A.*) *B,* Note how the mediastinal pleura is reflected onto the lung as pulmonary pleura. Note also that the pleural space is not continuous with the mediastinum. T, trachea; L, lung; H, heart.

MEDIASTINUM — COSTAL PARIETAL PLEURA
— MEDIASTINAL PARIETAL PLEURA

DIAPHRAGMATIC PARIETAL PLEURA

A

COSTAL PARIETAL PLEURA
PULMONARY PLEURA – ADHERENT TO LUNG

MEDIASTINUM

PLEURAL SPACE

MEDIASTINAL PARIETAL PLEURA

B

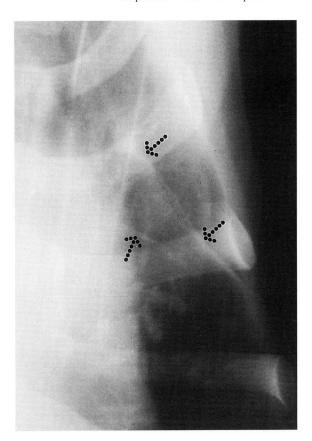

FIGURE 29–2. Ventrodorsal thoracic radiograph of a dog in which interlobar fissures *(arrows)* are visible. These fissures are thicker than normal and may be due to either pleural thickening or a small pleural effusion. In this dog, pleural effusion was not identified when the thorax was radiographed using a horizontally directed x-ray beam, indicating that the interlobar fissures were visible because of either trapped fluid or, more likely, pleural thickening.

in lateral, ventrodorsal, and dorsoventral radiographs made with a vertically directed x-ray beam is different.[1] Roentgen signs of free pleural fluid are listed in Table 29–2.

Interlobar Fissures

The thickness and number of interlobar fissures seen with pleural fluid depend on the amount of fluid and the relative position of the patient and the x-ray beam (Fig. 29–3). Approximately 100 mL of fluid must be present in the pleural space of a medium-sized dog before widened interlobar fissures are visible.[2] Visualization of widened interlobar fissures owing to accumulated fluid results from the x-ray beam striking the fluid-containing fissure tangentially. Some fluid-containing fissures may not be seen because their relationship to the x-ray beam is not tangential.

With small effusions, interlobar fissures are most likely to

be seen on ventrodorsal rather than dorsoventral radiographs. This is because when the patient is in ventral recumbency, small effusions collect dorsal to the sternum and do not enter fissures or increase overall thoracic radiopacity to a sufficient degree to be seen.[2] In lateral radiographs, small effusions usually result in visualization of fissures. As the volume of fluid increases, the number of interlobar fissures seen as well as their thickness increases (Figs. 29–4 and 29–5).

Horizontal-Beam Radiography

It may not be possible to identify small effusions on survey radiographs if the x-ray beam fails to strike a fluid accumulation tangentially. To enhance fluid detection, a horizontally directed x-ray beam may be used to ensure a tangential relationship between the x-ray beam and the fluid collection. If free pleural fluid is present, it gravitates into the dependent portion of the dependent hemithorax where the x-ray beam

Table 29–1
CAUSES OF PLEURAL FLUID

Cause	Fluid Type
Congestive heart failure	M
Pyothorax	E
Malignancy	M
Pneumonia	M, E
Trauma	M
Coagulation defect	M
Hypoproteinemia	T
Mediastinitis	M, E
Chylothorax	M
Diaphragmatic hernia	M

M, modified transudate; E, exudate; T, transudate.

Table 29–2
ROENTGEN SIGNS OF FREE PLEURAL FLUID

Visualization of widened interlobar fissures; fissure is of soft-tissue opacity
Retraction of pleural surface of lung away from pleural surface of thoracic wall; space between lung and thoracic wall is of soft-tissue opacity
Increased soft-tissue opacity dorsal to sternum on lateral radiographs; opacity frequently has scalloped margins
Blunting of costophrenic sulci in ventrodorsal radiographs
Decreased visualization of the heart in dorsoventral radiographs
Obscured diaphragmatic outline in dorsoventral and lateral radiographs

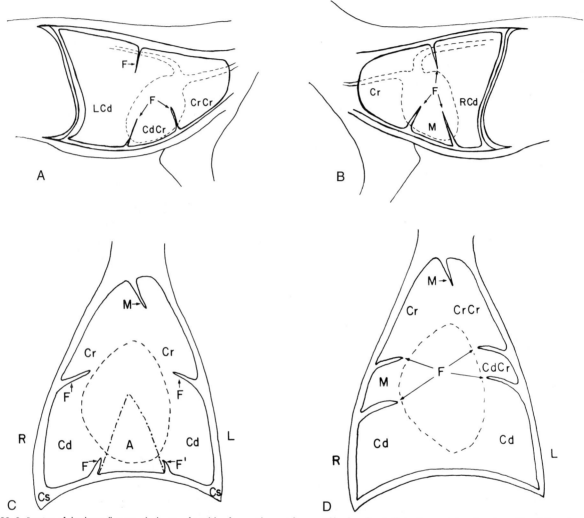

FIGURE 29–3. Drawings of the thorax illustrating the location of interlobar fissures. The exact fissures visible when pleural effusion is present depend on the position of the patient, the volume of fluid, and whether the x-ray beam strikes the fissure tangentially. Only fluid-filled fissures struck tangentially are seen. *A,* Fissures of the lateral aspect of the left lung (looking medial to lateral). These fissures are more likely to be seen when the patient is in left lateral recumbency. *B,* Fissures of the lateral aspect of the right lung (looking medial to lateral). These fissures are more likely to be seen when the patient is in right lateral recumbency. *C,* Fissures on the dorsal aspect of the lungs. These fissures are more likely to be seen when the patient is in dorsal recumbency. Note that the costophrenic sulcus becomes rounded when patients with pleural effusion are in dorsal recumbency. *D,* Fissures on the ventral aspect of the lungs. These fissures are more likely to be seen when the patient is in ventral recumbency. F, interlobar fissure; F', mediastinal reflection between the left caudal lobe and the accessory lobe (pleural fluid may accumulate adjacent to this reflection); CrCr, cranial part of left cranial lobe; CdCr, caudal part of left cranial lobe; Cd, caudal lobe; Cr, right cranial lobe; Md, right middle lobe; A, accessory lobe; Cs, costophrenic sulcus; M, mediastinal reflection; L, left; R, right.

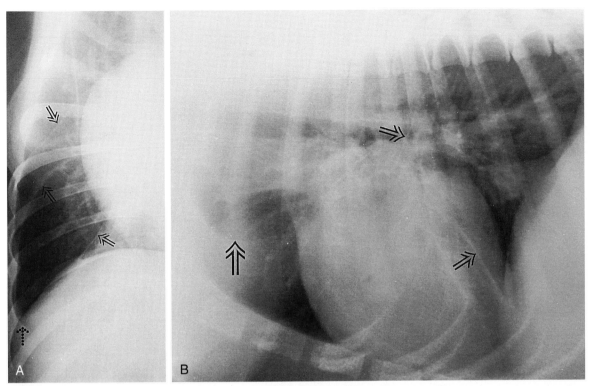

FIGURE 29–4. Ventrodorsal *(A)* and left lateral *(B)* thoracic radiographs of a dog with a moderate pleural effusion. *A,* Numerous interlobar fissures are seen *(double open arrows)*; some have more fluid within than others. The costophrenic sulcus is blunt *(dotted black arrow)*. *B,* Fewer interlobar fissures are also visible in the lateral radiograph *(small double arrows)*. The cranial part of the left cranial lobe has been displaced dorsally *(large double arrow)* by surrounding fluid. (Courtesy of the University of Georgia.)

intersects it tangentially (Fig. 29–6). A sharply demarcated, straight fluid line is not seen in patients with pleural fluid when radiographed with a horizontal x-ray beam because the configuration of the fluid is altered by the adjacent lung, which retracts because of elastic recoil. Sharp fluid lines are seen in horizontal-beam radiographs only when there is a free fluid–free air interface. Horizontal-beam radiographs may be useful in distinguishing between pleural fluid and an intrathoracic mass as a cause of an intrathoracic opacity (Figs. 29–7 and 29–8).

Retraction of Lung Margin

Pleural fluid results in retraction of the pulmonary pleural surface of the lung away from the parietal pleural surface of the thoracic wall or diaphragm. The magnitude of this separation depends on the volume of fluid present and the compliance of the lung. With normal lungs or with lungs of uniformly decreased compliance, retraction of the lungs away from the thoracic wall is uniform, and the degree of collapse is a function of fluid volume. When only a portion of the total lung volume has decreased compliance, that part of the lung retracts less than normal lung. Thus, when nonuniform retraction of lung is seen in patients with pleural effusion, underlying pulmonary disease that has altered lung compliance should be considered.

Retraction of lung from the thoracic wall can be seen on lateral, dorsoventral, and ventrodorsal radiographs (see Fig. 29–5). With pleural effusion, there is fluid surrounding the lung, but the fluid is most apparent radiographically when the x-ray beam is tangential to the fluid (Fig. 29–9). Therefore, there is typically more pleural fluid present than one would predict based on the severity of the radiographic changes.

Retrosternal Opacification

In lateral radiographs, free pleural fluid often results in an increased radiopacity dorsal to the sternum (see Figs. 29–5C and 29–7). This finding is the result of fluid having collected in the ventral thorax, probably layered against the ventral mediastinum in the nondependent hemithorax. If the patient has a unilateral effusion and the fluid is in the dependent hemithorax, this opacity may not be present because there is no fluid in the nondependent hemithorax to layer against the mediastinum. The margin of the retrosternal opacity created by pleural effusion usually appears scalloped because of adjacent, partially collapsed lung, which alters the configuration of the fluid.

Blunting of Costophrenic Sulci

Whether or not the costophrenic sulci become blunted by pleural fluid depends on the position of the patient during radiographic examination. In sternal recumbency, fluid gravitates ventrally, and the costophrenic sulci typically appear normal. In dorsal recumbency, fluid gravitates into the dorsal portion of the thorax resulting in blunting of costophrenic sulci.

There are other differences between dorsoventral and ventrodorsal radiographs when free pleural fluid is present.[1] In dorsoventral radiographs, the fluid that has gravitated ventrally silhouettes with the heart and ventral part of the diaphragm. In ventrodorsal radiographs, pleural fluid does not as readily obscure the heart and diaphragm because the fluid is distributed over a larger area in the dorsal thorax, where it does not contact the heart or dome of the diaphragm (Fig. 29–10; see also Fig. 29–5). Fluid does not tend to obscure the heart as readily in ventrodorsal radiographs because the

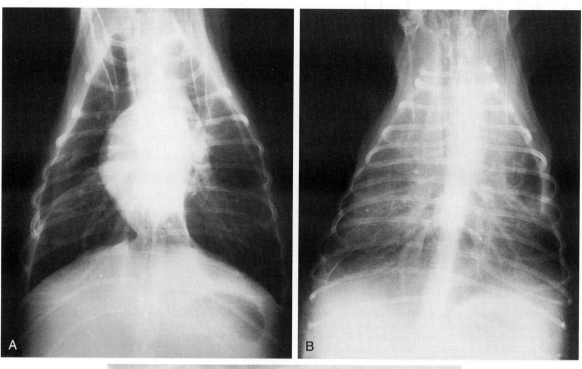

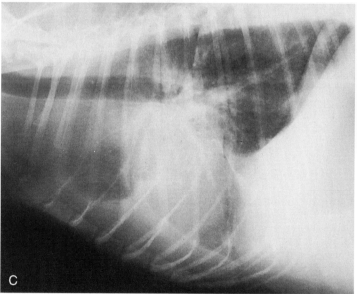

FIGURE 29–5. Ventrodorsal *(A)*, dorsoventral *(B)*, and left lateral *(C)* views of the thorax of a dog with a large volume of fluid in the pleural space. *A,* There are numerous interlobar fissures, and the right caudal lobe is separated from the thoracic wall by an area of soft-tissue opacity. The cardiac silhouette is visible. Note the appearance of the costal cartilages; they should not be mistaken for interlobar fissures. The concave aspect of costal cartilages faces cranially, whereas the concave aspect of interlobar fissures faces caudally. *B,* Interlobar fissures and lung displacement away from the thoracic wall are again evident. The cardiac silhouette is not visible, the diaphragm is obscured, and the overall radiopacity of the thorax is increased (see Fig. 25–10 for explanation). *C,* There are interlobar fissures, the cardiac silhouette is partially obscured by surrounding fluid, and the overall radiopacity of the thorax is increased. In addition, there is an area of radiopacity just dorsal to the sternum, the margins of which are scalloped owing to fluid accumulation in the ventral thorax.

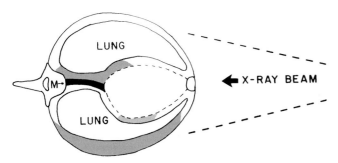

FIGURE 29-6. The demonstration of pleural fluid by horizontal-beam radiography. Fluid is represented by the gray stippled areas. Fluid in the nondependent hemithorax layers against the mediastinum (assuming the mediastinum is complete). This fluid (nondependent side) is not radiographically detectable. Fluid in the dependent hemithorax gravitates to the area between the lung and the thoracic wall where the horizontally directed x-ray beam strikes it tangentially. M, mediastinum.

fluid is located dorsally, above the heart, and does not silhouette with it (see Fig. 29–10).

Atypical Distribution of Free Pleural Fluid

An atypical distribution of free pleural fluid most often results from parts of the lung having different compliance. When a portion of a lung has decreased compliance, fluid present in the pleural space tends to accumulate around it because it is less expansile (more collapsed) than other parts of the lung. Thus, atypical fluid distribution may be a clue to an underlying pulmonary lesion (see Fig. 29–13). These atypical collections result in an intrathoracic radiopacity that is usually irregularly marginated and shaped when compared with opacities typically seen with pleural effusion. These collections may be confused with thoracic wall or pulmonary lesions.

Free pleural fluid is usually equally distributed between the right and left pleural spaces. In some patients, however, there is an asymmetric fluid distribution. Causes of unilateral pleural effusion or an effusion more voluminous in one pleu-

ral space include a difference in compliance between lungs, the closing of mediastinal fenestrations from inflammation or a mass, and an anatomically complete mediastinum. In extensive, unilateral effusion, it may be difficult to identify whether the resultant opacity is caused by a pathologic process in the pleural space, the thoracic wall, or the lung.

Pitfalls in Pleural Fluid Diagnosis

Sometimes an erroneous radiographic diagnosis of pleural fluid is made. Thickened pleura may have an appearance identical to pleural fluid (see Fig. 29–2). A distinction may be made by using a horizontally directed x-ray beam.

Mineralized costal cartilages are sometimes confused with pleural effusion. Their position is similar, but the concave surface of costal cartilages is directed cranially, whereas the concave surface of fluid-filled fissures is directed caudally (see Fig. 29–5C).

Thoracic wall deformities, such as those seen in chondrodystrophoid breeds, may result in increased radiopacity at the margin of the lung field. Without knowledge of this fact, the opacity may be incorrectly misinterpreted as retraction of the lung from the thoracic wall because of pleural fluid (Fig. 29–11).

Significance of Pleural Fluid

Pleural fluid may result from a primary pleural disorder, such as pleural neoplasm, but most often it is a sign of disease elsewhere. It is usually impossible to determine the cause of pleural effusion from radiographs. When pleural fluid is present, structures are obscured, and extremely large lesions can go unidentified.

When pleural fluid is identified, careful scrutiny of the radiograph is necessary. Occasionally, subtle radiographic findings such as a rib lesion or asymmetric distribution of free fluid are noted, which can be of great help in the evaluation of the patient. In patients with a large pleural effusion, the indiscriminate approach of using a horizontally directed

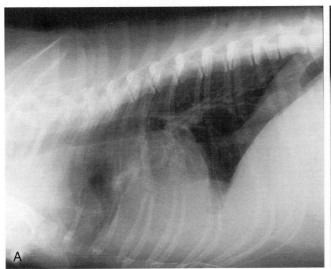
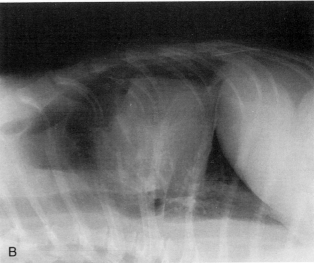

FIGURE 29-7. Right lateral *(A)* and horizontal-beam lateral (dog in dorsal recumbency) *(B)* views of a dog with pleural effusion. *A,* There is an opacity dorsal to the sternum, which is consistent with fluid but may also be a mass. In the ventrodorsal view (not shown), there was only minimal evidence of pleural effusion. To clarify the significance of the opacity, the horizontal-beam view was made. *B,* The fluid has gravitated dorsally and can be seen adjacent to the spine as a soft-tissue opacity separating the lung from the thoracic wall. Also, there is no longer an opacity adjacent to the sternum. Thus, the opacity seen in *A* dorsal to the sternum was fluid. Note that there is not a sharp horizontal *fluid line.* Horizontal fluid lines are seen in horizontal-beam radiographs only when there is a gas-fluid interface. In *B,* the contour of the fluid is conforming to the shape of the partially collapsed lung.

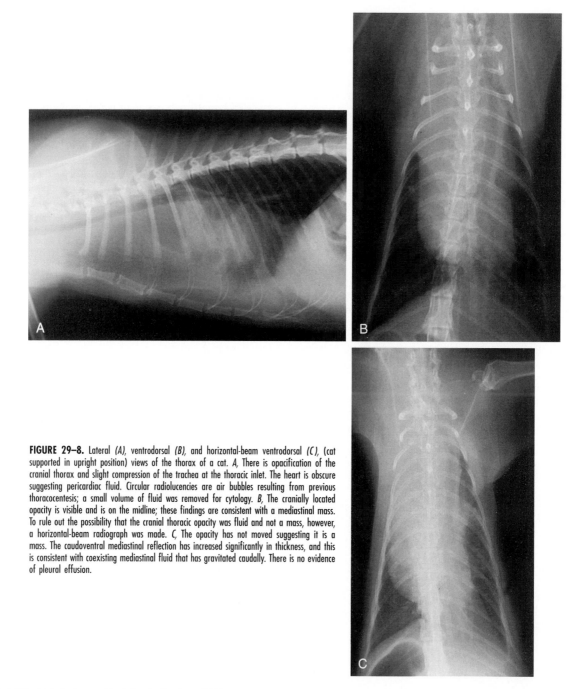

FIGURE 29–8. Lateral *(A)*, ventrodorsal *(B)*, and horizontal-beam ventrodorsal *(C)*, (cat supported in upright position) views of the thorax of a cat. *A,* There is opacification of the cranial thorax and slight compression of the trachea at the thoracic inlet. The heart is obscure suggesting pericardiac fluid. Circular radiolucencies are air bubbles resulting from previous thoracocentesis; a small volume of fluid was removed for cytology. *B,* The cranially located opacity is visible and is on the midline; these findings are consistent with a mediastinal mass. To rule out the possibility that the cranial thoracic opacity was fluid and not a mass, however, a horizontal-beam radiograph was made. *C,* The opacity has not moved suggesting it is a mass. The caudoventral mediastinal reflection has increased significantly in thickness, and this is consistent with coexisting mediastinal fluid that has gravitated caudally. There is no evidence of pleural effusion.

X-RAY BEAM

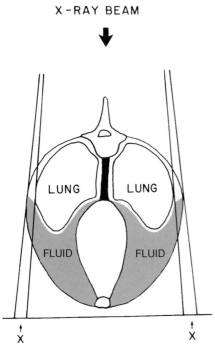

FIGURE 29–9. Principle of lung retraction owing to pleural effusion. This patient with a large pleural effusion is radiographed in ventral recumbency. Fluid, therefore, has gravitated ventrally, resulting in dorsal displacement of lung. There has been extensive dorsal displacement of ventral lung, but this is not apparent radiographically because the fluid collected ventral to the lung has not been struck tangentially by the x-ray beam. The only lung retraction that is apparent is in the regions indicated by *x* because here fluid between the lung and thoracic wall is struck tangentially by the x-ray beam. In the region between the x's, thoracic radiopacity is increased, the heart is obscured, and pulmonary vessels in the partially collapsed lung are visible (compare with Fig. 29–5*B*).

x-ray beam with various patient positions to search for other lesions is unrewarding and should not be done. Making additional radiographs after some of the fluid has been removed may provide important information.

All pleural effusions are clinically significant, and it is important to attempt to reach a definitive diagnosis. In small

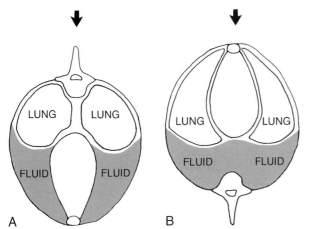

FIGURE 29–10. Effect of dorsal versus ventral recumbency on the radiographic appearance of pleural effusion. *A,* The patient is in ventral recumbency, and fluid gravitates ventrally. The fluid is in contact with the heart, thus obscuring the heart from view. When the patient is placed in dorsal recumbency *(B),* the fluid gravitates dorsally and is not in contact with the heart; thus, the cardiac silhouette is visible. The absolute depth of the fluid is greater when the patient is in ventral recumbency *(A)* because the ventral part of the thoracic cavity is narrower, and the fluid rises to a higher level. Thus, overall thoracic radiopacity is greater when the patient is in ventral recumbency.

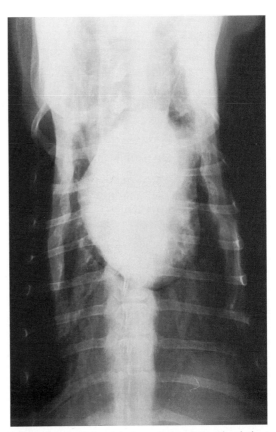

FIGURE 29–11. Ventrodorsal view of the thorax of a normal Basset hound. The sternum is displaced slightly to the left. There is an area of soft-tissue opacity adjacent to the thoracic wall on the dog's left side and an area of radiolucency adjacent to the thoracic wall on the right side. These are artifacts created by the irregular thoracic wall configuration in this chondrodystrophic dog. The opacity on the left side is due to the prominent costochondral region; rotation of the patient resulted in its being located at the periphery of the thorax. The location and appearance of this opacity may result in its being confused with pleural effusion; however, interlobar fissures are not seen. On the right side, the opacity created by the costochondral deformity is located closer to the midline because of patient rotation. Lateral to this opacity is normal lung, which appears radiolucent because of the sharp contrast provided by the costochondral opacity. The radiolucency of this lung may be confused with pneumothorax. A horizontal-beam radiograph of the thorax in this dog was normal (i.e., no pleural effusion or pneumothorax).

effusions, there may be no abnormal clinical signs, whereas large effusions usually result in dyspnea. It should not be assumed, however, that small effusions are less significant than large ones. Thoracocentesis with appropriate fluid analysis should be done when pleural fluid is identified.[3]

Simultaneous Pleural and Peritoneal Effusion

Occasionally, simultaneous pleural and peritoneal effusions are detected. In one study, 32 out of 48 dogs with simultaneous peritoneal and pleural effusion had either neoplastic or cardiovascular disease. Simultaneous pleural and peritoneal effusion is an indicator of severe disease with poor prognosis.[4]

PNEUMOTHORAX

Gas in the pleural space is termed *pneumothorax.* Air can enter the pleural space from the outside or from the lung or mediastinum (Table 29–3). The character of the changes resulting from gas in the pleural space depends on the volume of gas and the relative position of the patient and x-

Table 29–3
CAUSES OF PNEUMOTHORAX

Trauma
Lung rupture
Chest wall rent
Extension of pneumomediastinum
Rupture of cavitary lung mass

Table 29–4
ROENTGEN SIGNS OF PNEUMOTHORAX

Retraction of pleural surface of lung away from pleural surface of
    thoracic wall; space between lung and thoracic wall is radiolucent
Lung markings do not extend all the way to thoracic wall
Lung has increased opacity because of collapse
Appearance of dorsal displacement of the heart on the lateral view

ray beam. Roentgen signs of pneumothorax are listed in Table 29–4.

Retraction of the lung from the thoracic wall can be seen on lateral, ventrodorsal, and dorsoventral radiographs. In a small pneumothorax, this separation is small and may appear as a fine radiolucent line (Fig. 29–12). As in pleural effusion, air surrounds the lung but is most apparent radiographically when the air is struck tangentially by the x-ray beam (see Fig. 29–12). Visualization of gas-containing interlobar fissures is not common with pneumothorax because gas cannot enter the fissures of the collapsed lung.

Pneumothorax results in lung collapse because of the lung elasticity and the increase in pleural space pressure. As lung volume decreases, it contains less air and becomes more radiopaque (Fig. 29–13). The degree of increased opacity is directly related to the degree of collapse, and the increased

opacity may interfere with evaluation of the lung. The pulmonary collapse is also responsible for the lack of visible lung markings extending to the periphery of the thoracic cavity, a common radiographic sign of pneumothorax.

If the pneumothorax is open, that is, with no valve at the site of gas entrance, gas may continue to enter the pleural space until pleural pressure equals atmospheric pressure. At this point, the lung is maximally collapsed but still maintains roughly the shape of a normal lung because of its elasticity.

Separation of the heart from the sternum is commonly seen in lateral radiographs of patients with pneumothorax (see Fig. 29–12). The heart appears elevated from the floor of the thorax, but actually it is displaced into the dependent hemithorax owing to lack of underlying inflated lung to support the heart in its normal midline position. As the heart falls into the dependent hemithorax, it slides dorsally creating

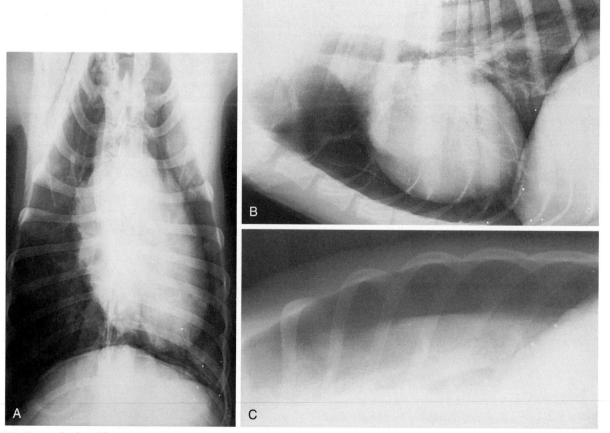

FIGURE 29–12. Ventrodorsal (A), left lateral (B), and right lateral recumbent horizontal-beam (C) radiographs of a dog with pneumothorax. A, The heart is shifted to the left, but evidence of pneumothorax is not seen because the air has risen and accumulated ventral to the sternum where it is not struck tangentially by the x-ray beam. There is a linear region of gas medial to the right scapula and an area of hemorrhage in the left caudal lobe. B, There is a thin radiolucent line between the diaphragm and a caudal lobe caused by gas in the pleural space. The heart is separated from the sternum, and there is a radiolucent area between the sternum and the heart. There are opaque interlobar fissures extending caudoventrally from the carina and superimposed on the cardiac apex region owing to concurrent pleural effusion. C, The extent of pneumothorax is readily apparent. By placing the patient in right lateral recumbency and by using a horizontally directed x-ray beam, air in the left hemithorax was struck tangentially by the x-ray beam. The mAs was decreased by 50 percent to facilitate air visualization by rendering the lung more radiopaque.

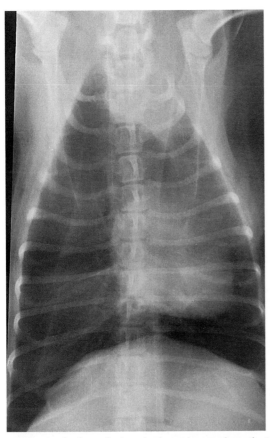

FIGURE 29–13. Ventrodorsal view of a dog with a large right pneumothorax. The right lung is partially collapsed and therefore is of increased radiopacity. The radiolucent area lateral to the right lung is due to gas in the pleural space. The heart has shifted to the left. There is a region of homogeneously increased opacity in the left cranial hemithorax that is due to either lung consolidation or a focal region of pleural effusion. If the opacity is due to pleural effusion, it signifies abnormal lung compliance in the adjacent lung. Altered lung compliance is a common cause of asymmetric pleural effusion.

suggested that pneumothorax is easier to detect in dorsoventral radiographs than in ventrodorsal radiographs.[8]

In most animals, pneumothorax is bilateral, and this relates either to a bilateral source of pleural air or to movement of air across the mediastinum. Results from a study of induced pneumothorax suggest that air can readily move across the mediastinum because bilateral pneumothorax was observed in 22 of 24 dogs in which a unilateral pleural space injection of air occurred.[7] Unilateral pneumothorax, however, can occur for the same reasons as unilateral pleural effusion. There is some controversy regarding the appearance of unilateral pneumothorax in lateral radiographs depending on whether the affected side is dependent or nondependent. Unilateral pleural space air may be more apparent if the affected side is nondependent because the air collects around the dorsocaudal portion of the caudal lobe. In this situation, the air collection is struck tangentially by the x-ray beam. If the affected side is dependent, the air may appear to collect against the mediastinum and is struck en face by the x-ray beam (Fig. 29–15). It has also been stated, however, that unilateral pneumothorax is more apparent when the affected pleural cavity is dependent.[7]

Tension Pneumothorax

Tension pneumothorax occurs when pleural space pressure exceeds atmospheric pressure during both phases of respiration. Tension pneumothorax results from a check-valve mechanism at the origin of pleural space gas. In tension pneumothorax, the increased pleural pressure causes the lung to collapse to a greater degree than its maximal collapse in an open pneumothorax. Thus, it may no longer maintain the shape of a lung but may assume the appearance of a relatively amorphous opacity, often compressed against the midline. With unilateral tension pneumothorax, the increased pleural space pressure tends to cause a contralateral mediastinal shift. Tension pneumothorax may also result in caudal displacement of the diaphragm to the degree that its

the appearance of elevation when seen on a lateral radiograph (Fig. 29–14). Although pneumothorax is the most common cause of the appearance of elevation of the cardiac silhouette on the lateral view, this radiographic sign has also been seen with decreased heart size, as a normal finding in dogs with extremely deep thoracic cavities, and in patients with hyperinflated lungs.

As with pleural effusion, diagnosis of pneumothorax may not be possible from survey radiographs. The likelihood of diagnosing pneumothorax is increased by using a horizontally directed x-ray beam and placing the patient in a position such that the x-ray beam is tangent to the area of air accumulation, such as in lateral recumbency. Decreasing the mAs by 50 percent enhances visualization of the air in the horizontal-beam radiograph by rendering the lung more opaque (see Fig. 29–12C). Justification for use of horizontal-beam radiography to detect pneumothorax should be based on the suspected underlying cause. For example, a pneumothorax resulting from lung disease is a potentially serious event,[5, 6] whereas a small pneumothorax occurring after trauma with no associated clinical signs may not be significant.

Some attention has been given to identifying the best radiographic view to use to detect pneumothorax. In one study of induced pneumothorax, the vertical-beam left lateral recumbent and the horizontal-beam ventrodorsal views were the most effective for detection of pneumothorax. The right lateral view was most sensitive for detection of differences in the *amount* of air in the pleural space.[7] It has also been

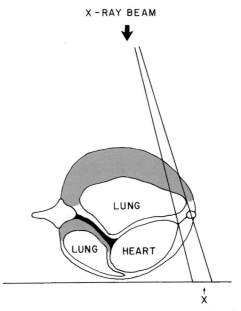

FIGURE 29–14. Principle of separation of the heart from the sternum in lateral radiographs with pneumothorax. When the patient is placed in lateral recumbency, the lack of a fully inflated lung in the dependent hemithorax allows the heart to gravitate. As the heart falls into the dependent hemithorax, it slides dorsally because of the shape of the thoracic wall, thus creating a space between the heart and the sternum. As x-rays pass through this space, the heart appears separated from the sternum on the lateral view by the distance x.

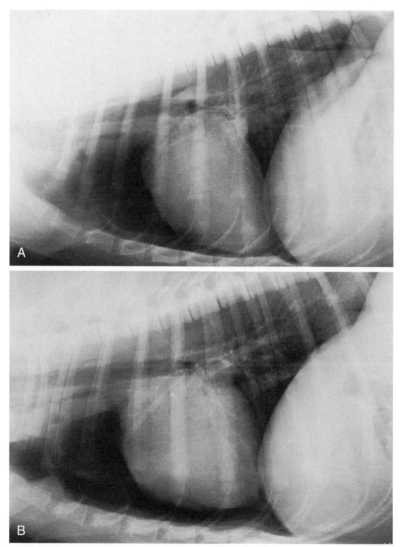

FIGURE 25–15. Right (A) and left (B) lateral thoracic radiographs of a dog with a large left and a small right pneumothorax. A, The large pneumothorax is nondependent and collects around the left caudal lobe, resulting in clear visualization of collapse of the lobe. There is a small area of radiolucency ventral to the heart owing to a slight shift in cardiac position to the right. Note the lack of heart displacement because of the almost fully inflated dependent right lung, which supports the heart on or near the midline. There is a traumatic lung bulla in the right caudal lobe. Pneumomediastinum is also present. B, The large pneumothorax is now dependent. Rather than being located between the lung and the thoracic wall, where it can be struck tangentially by the x-ray beam, air is layered against the dependent side of the mediastinum. There is increased separation between the heart and the sternum owing to atelectasis of the dependent left lung, which permits the heart to fall into the dependent hemithorax. Pneumomediastinum is also present.

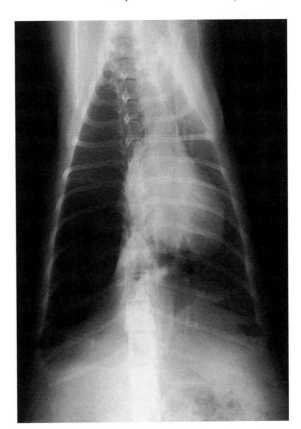

FIGURE 29–16. Ventrodorsal view of the thorax of a cat with tension pneumothorax. The increased pleural space pressure has displaced the diaphragm caudally to the extent that its costal attachments appear as tent-like projections from its thoracic surface. Additionally the heart is shifted to the left by the increased right pleural space pressure.

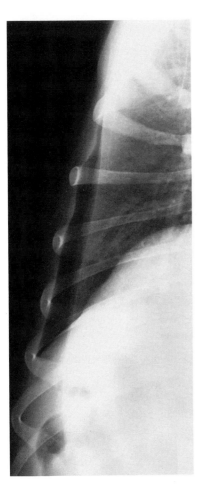

FIGURE 29–17. Ventrodorsal view of the thorax of a dog in which a skin-fold artifact is visible. These artifacts may easily be confused with pneumothorax. The skin fold itself has the appearance of a lung margin, with adjacent radiolucency that may be due to gas in the pleural space. No lung markings are visible in the region lateral to the lung. The correct assessment of skin-fold artifact is made by noting that the caudal extent of the lung margin extends beyond the limits of the thoracic cavity. Additionally, no air is seen between the lung and the diaphragm.

costal attachments become visible (Fig. 29–16). It is important to recognize tension pneumothorax because it is a potentially fatal condition requiring immediate thoracocentesis.

Pitfalls in Pneumothorax Diagnosis

Skin folds can result in an extremely radiolucent area superimposed over the lateral aspect of the thorax on ventrodorsal views. In many patients, it may not be possible to identify lung markings in the radiolucent area. In these instances, the correct diagnosis of skin-fold artifact is usually made by noting that the opacity of the fold extends beyond the limits of the thorax (Fig. 29–17).

In chondrodystrophoid breeds, the costochondral region often appears opaque. If the dog's sternum is rotated slightly to one side for the ventrodorsal or dorsoventral view during radiographic examination, the area peripheral to the opacity appears radiolucent and can be convincing evidence for pneumothorax. Lung markings may be difficult to identify in this radiolucent region, and it may be necessary to resort to the use of horizontal-beam radiography (see Fig. 29–11).

References

1. Groves TF, and Ticer JW: Pleural fluid movement: Its effect on appearance of ventrodorsal and dorsoventral radiographic projections. Vet Radiol 24:99, 1983.
2. Lord PF, Suter PF, Chan KF, et al: Pleural, extrapleural and pulmonary lesions in small animals: A radiographic approach to differential diagnosis. J Am Vet Radiol Soc 13:4, 1972.
3. Bauer T, and Woodfield JA: Mediastinal, pleural, and extrapleural diseases. In Ettinger SJ, Feldman EC (Eds): Textbook of Veterinary Internal Medicine, 4th Ed. Philadelphia, WB Saunders, 1995, pp 812–842.
4. Steyn PF, and Wittum TE: Radiographic, epidemiologic, and clinical aspects of simultaneous pleural and peritoneal effusions in dogs and cats: 48 cases (1982–1991). J Am Vet Med Assoc 202:307, 1993.
5. Yoshioka M: Management of spontaneous pneumothorax in 12 dogs. J Am Anim Hosp Assoc 18:57, 1982.
6. Schaer M, Gamble D, and Spencer C: Spontaneous pneumothorax associated with bacterial pneumonia in the dog—two case reports. J Am Anim Hosp Assoc 17:783, 1981.
7. Kern DA, Carrig CB, and Martin RA: Radiographic evaluation of induced pneumothorax in the dog. Vet Radiol Ultrasound 35:411, 1995.
8. Aronson E, and Reed AL: Radiology corner—pneumothorax: Ventrodorsal or dorsoventral view. Does it make a difference? Vet Radiol Ultrasound 36:109, 1995.

STUDY QUESTIONS

1. For interlobar fissures to be visualized radiographically when pleural effusion is present, the x-ray beam must strike the fissures:
   A. Tangentially.
   B. Perpendicularly.
   C. At maximal inspiration.
   D. At maximal expiration.

2. Small pleural effusions are typically seen more clearly in dorsoventral rather than ventrodorsal radiographs. (True or False)

3. When a horizontal x-ray beam is used to radiograph the thorax of a patient with pleural effusion, a straight fluid line is typically seen. (True or False)

4. List at least three roentgen signs of pleural effusion present in Figure 29–18.

5. Was the dog in Figure 29–18 in dorsal or sternal recumbency when the radiograph was made?

6. The finding of simultaneous pleural and peritoneal effusion:
   A. Is usually the result of overzealous fluid administration.
   B. Has no particular significance.
   C. Is typically associated with a poor prognosis.
   D. Is usually due to a diaphragmatic hernia.

7. Visualization of interlobar fissures is more common with pleural effusion than with pneumothorax. (True or False)

8. List three radiographic signs that would suggest that a pneumothorax is a tension pneumothorax.

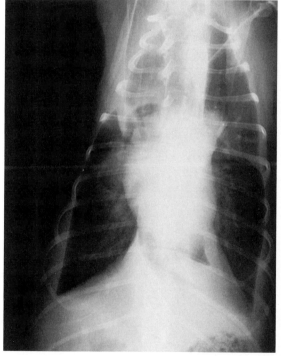

FIGURE 29–18

9. List two reasons for a false radiographic diagnosis of pneumothorax.

10. Describe how costal cartilages can be distinguished from a fluid-containing interlobar fissure.

(Answers appear on page 642.)

Chapter 30

The Heart and Great Vessels

Charles R. Root • *Robert J. Bahr*

Recommended routine radiographic projections for evaluation of the heart vary.[1-4] Some clinicians prefer dorsoventral over ventrodorsal projections, and others recommend right lateral rather than left lateral views. Most seem to offer logical justification for their preferences, depending on suspected clinical diagnoses and the organs or structures of interest. The dorsoventral projection is often recommended over the ventrodorsal view for assessment of the cardiac silhouette,[3, 5, 7] whereas the ventrodorsal projection is often recommended for the lung.[5, 6] In cats, the size and shape of the heart appear to be more variable with patients in dorsal recumbency than when they are sternal.[7] The comparative differences in radiographic appearances of the canine heart in dorsal versus ventral recumbency also have been reported.[8] In the authors' opinion, the left lateral projection results in less distortion in position of the cardiac silhouette than does right lateral dependency, although this point is subject to debate.[1-2]

Short exposure times are vital if blurring because of patient motion is to be avoided.[1, 2, 9] Obliquity of the thorax, especially in the ventrodorsal or dorsoventral projection, should be avoided. Accurate assessment of cardiac chamber size in the ventrodorsal or dorsoventral view is not possible if the degree of obliquity results in the tips of the dorsal spinous processes of the thoracic vertebrae having been projected outside the boundaries of their respective thoracic vertebral bodies.[10]

SPECIAL PROCEDURES

Critical radiographic assessment of diseases of the heart and great vessels is best accomplished using echocardiography or rapid-sequence contrast radiographic examination of the various cardiac chambers (angiocardiography) or portions of one or more of the great vessels (angiography). Such special radiographic procedures are rarely employed in practice owing to the expense of the equipment and the infrequent indications for use. A simple cassette changer for use in private practice has been described.[11] Several conditions can be evaluated by nonselective intravenous angiocardiography.[12] Survey[1, 2, 4, 5, 12, 13] and contrast[1-3, 12] radiographic signs of acquired and congenital cardiovascular diseases have been published.[1-3]

NORMAL RADIOGRAPHIC ANATOMY

Normal cardiovascular radiographic anatomy has been described.[1, 2, 4, 5, 13, 14] Several points are worthy of discussion, however. The external and internal boundaries of the individual chambers of the heart cannot be directly visualized on survey radiographs. Rather, their external margins merge with those of adjacent chambers because they are all contained within the pericardial sac and surrounded by a small amount of fluid. The coronary arteries cannot be seen, although pulmonary vessels superimposed on the cardiac silhouette in the lateral projection are sometimes mistaken for these arteries (see Fig. 2–14). Similarly the junctions of the left atrium and left ventricle may often only be inferred radiographically, as can the point at which the right ventricle and atrium join. The internal features of the cardiac chambers are completely invisible radiographically unless contrasted by an opaque medium during angiocardiography. Echocardiography is now accepted as the method of choice for assessment of cardiac anatomic and pathologic features.

RADIOGRAPHIC SIGNS

Individual Cardiac Chamber Enlargement

The major radiographic signs of left ventricular failure, right ventricular failure, common congenital heart diseases, and common acquired heart diseases are summarized in Table 30–1. Survey radiographic signs of individual cardiac cham-

Table 30–1
SUMMARY OF RADIOGRAPHIC SIGNS OF DISEASES OF THE HEART, GREAT VESSELS, AND PULMONARY PARENCHYMAL VASCULATURE

Defect	Left Atrium	LV	Right Atrium	RV	CVC	Aorta	MPA	ART	VNS
LHF	+	+	−	−	−	−	−	−	+
RHF	−	−	+/−	+	+/−	−	−	+/−	−
PDA	+	+	−	−	−	+	+	+	
PS	−	−	+/−	+	+/−	−	+	−/↓	+
AS	−	+	−	−	−	+	−	−	−
VSD	+/−	+/−	−	+/−	−	−	−	+/−	+/−
TET	−	+*	+/−	+	+/−	−	+	−/↓	−
EIS	+/−	+/−	−	+	−	−	+/−	+/−	+/−
MI	+	+/−	−	−	−	−	−	−	+/−
HWD	−	−	+/−	+	+/−	−	+/−	↑	−

LV, left ventricle; RV, right ventricle; CVC, caudal vena cava; MPA, main pulmonary artery; ART, parenchymal pulmonary arteries; VNS, parenchymal pulmonary veins; LHF, left-sided heart failure; RHF, right-sided heart failure; PDA, patent ductus arteriosus; PS, pulmonic stenosis; AS, aortic stenosis; VSD, ventricular septal defect; TET, tetralogy of Fallot; EIS, Eisenmenger's complex; MI, mitral insufficiency; HWD, heartworm disease; +, abnormal; −, normal; +/−, may be either normal or abnormal; ↑, enhanced or increased in size; ↓, diminished or reduced in size.
*This is often a false impression, created by levad cardiac apex shift owing to severe right ventricular enlargement.

ber enlargement have been described and illustrated.[2, 15] In humans, simultaneous enlargement of two or more cardiac chambers appears to diminish the accuracy of radiographic assessment of cardiac disease[16]; the same is probably true in animals. Unfortunately, there are no reliable radiographic measurement techniques that can be used to assess cardiomegaly. Although measurement techniques have been reported,[17] their routine clinical application is equivocal[2, 5, 18] and inaccurate for several reasons. First, the range of patient sizes is great, and there is considerable breed and individual variation in normal thoracic conformation. Second, it is impossible to correlate radiographic exposure routinely with respiration, heart cycle, and precise positioning of the thorax. Therefore, assessment of cardiac size is subjective at best. There are certain radiographic signs, however, that seem to correlate well with specific cardiac lesions, especially when considered in light of clinical history, physical findings, and other radiographic observations.[3]

Left Atrium

The left atrium is situated immediately ventral to the left main stem bronchus. Therefore, left atrial enlargement causes dorsal deviation of the left main stem bronchus as viewed in the lateral projection (Fig. 30–1). Furthermore, in the same view, there is an increase in height of the caudodorsal border of the heart, often obliterating the left atrioventricular junction (loss of the caudal waist). Viewed dorsally, the normal left atrium is roughly between the left and right main stem bronchi. Therefore, in the ventrodorsal or dorsoventral projection, left atrial enlargement causes the left and right main stem bronchi to diverge (see Fig. 30–1). Distention or enlargement of the left atrial appendage (auricle) is less often recognized radiographically. Occasionally, it is recognized in the ventrodorsal or dorsoventral projection and produces focal bulging of the left cardiac border between the main pulmonary artery and the apex of the heart (Fig. 30–2).

Left Ventricle

Because the left ventricle is relatively thick walled, hypertrophy causes little distortion of its contour in the lateral projection; rather, it tends to elongate, causing dorsal dis-

placement of the trachea (Fig. 30–3).[2] This dorsal displacement involves the entire intrathoracic portion of the trachea, from the thoracic inlet to the carina, resulting in a decrease in the angle between the trachea and the thoracic vertebrae. Pleural effusion may cause similar tracheal displacement, at least in cats, even in the absence of significant cardiomegaly.[19] Therefore, when the cardiac silhouette is obscured by the presence of pleural fluid, the tracheovertebral angle is probably not a reliable sign of left ventricular elongation. The caudal margin of the left ventricular wall may become convex. In the ventrodorsal or dorsoventral projection, there is rounding and left displacement of the normally straight left side of the cardiac silhouette (see Fig. 30–3), and the apex of the heart may become further rounded at its point of contact with the diaphragm.

Right Atrium

In the ventrodorsal or dorsoventral view, assessment of right atrial enlargement is difficult. In the lateral projection, enlargement of the right atrium occasionally may cause dorsal bowing of the terminal portion of the trachea (Fig. 30–4). This finding may cause the caudal trachea (over the cranial portion of the heart base) to assume a distinct hook shape. It should be noted that the carina remains in its normal location unless there is concomitant left atrial or ventricular enlargement. In other words, in instances of selective right atrial enlargement, a line drawn from the middle of the tracheal lumen at the thoracic inlet through the midportion of the carina should duplicate the normal angle of the trachea with the vertebral column.

Considerable variation also exists in the appearance of the junction of the cranial border of the heart with the ventral border of the cranial vena cava in the lateral projection. This region may become either accentuated or obliterated as a result of right auricular enlargement; whatever changes occur are somewhat dependent on breed variation in normal thoracic conformation.

Right Ventricle

Rounding and enlargement of the right ventricle cause increased cardiosternal contact in the lateral projection and bulging of the right ventricular component of the cardiac

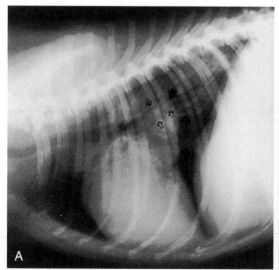
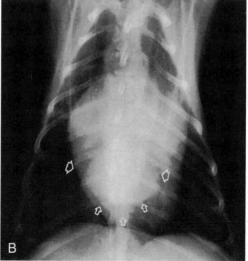

FIGURE 30–1. Right lateral *(A)* and dorsoventral *(B)* thoracic radiographs of a dog with left atrial enlargement owing to mitral insufficiency. *A,* The enlarged left atrium is clearly seen *(solid arrow)*, and there is dorsal deviation of the left main stem bronchus *(open arrows)*. *B,* There is divergence of the left and right caudal lobar bronchi, both caudal lobar bronchi *(open arrowheads)* bowing around the enlarged left atrium *(small open arrows)*, and the caudal portion of the base of the heart is increased in opacity *(small open arrows)*. (Courtesy of Grand Avenue Pet Hospital, Santa Ana, CA.)

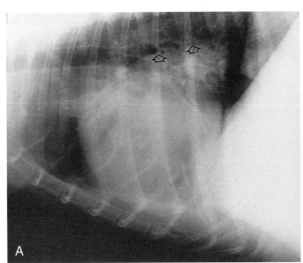

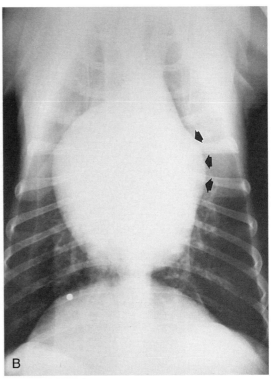

FIGURE 30–2. Left lateral *(A)* and ventrodorsal *(B)* thoracic radiographs of a dog with enlargement of the left atrium and auricle owing to mitral insufficiency. Notice the bulging auricle *(solid arrows)* along the left side of the cardiac silhouette in the ventrodorsal view and elevation of the left main stem bronchus *(open arrows)* in the lateral projection.

silhouette in the ventrodorsal or dorsoventral view (Fig. 30–5). The latter lesion has been described as the *reversed D* sign. In some instances, presumably because of hypertrophy rather than dilation of the right ventricular wall, the apex of the heart is elevated from the sternum (Fig. 30–6) in the lateral projection. In most instances, right ventricular enlargement has little obvious effect on the positions of the structures at the base of the heart.

Changes in the Great Vessels

There are several notable pathologic alterations in the radiographic appearances of the aorta, the caudal vena cava, and

the main pulmonary artery.[2] Some of these changes are quite specific, whereas others may have several possible causes.

Caudal Vena Cava

The caudal vena cava is variable in diameter, depending on the stage of the cardiac cycle and various disease states. Therefore, there is no specific ratio of measurements between the width of the caudal vena cava and any other thoracic structure. Because of its normal variation in size, it is not a sensitive indicator of the existence of cardiac disease. If it is persistently large, right-sided congestive heart failure should

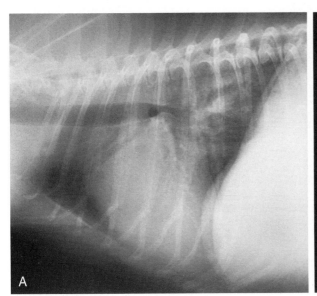

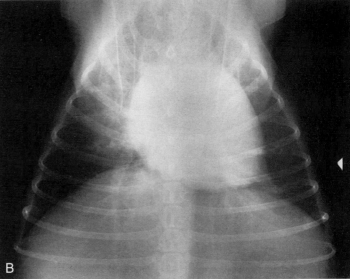

FIGURE 30–3. Right lateral *(A)* and dorsoventral *(B)* thoracic radiographs of a dog with enlargement of the left ventricle owing to mitral insufficiency. *A,* There is elongation of the heart, resulting in dorsal displacement of the entire intrathoracic portion of the trachea. Left atrial enlargement is also present. *B,* The left side of the cardiac silhouette is more rounded than normal and is displaced to the left. In addition, the cardiac apex is more rounded at its point of contact with the diaphragm.

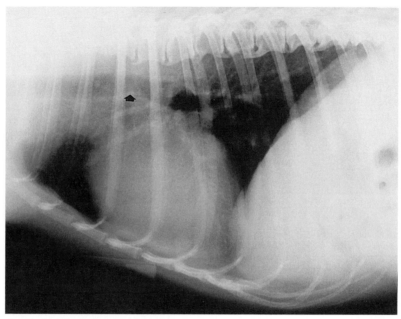

FIGURE 30–4. Left lateral thoracic radiograph of a dog with enlargement of the right atrium. Notice that the caudal portion of the intrathoracic trachea is deviated (bowed) dorsally *(arrow)*. The carina is not elevated, ruling out left atrial or ventricular enlargement.

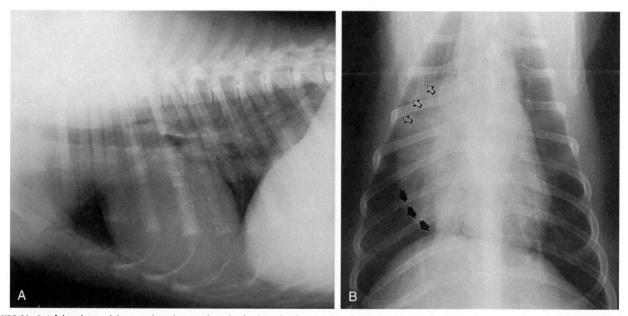

FIGURE 30–5. Left lateral *(A)* and dorsoventral *(B)* thoracic radiographs of a dog with right ventricular enlargement. In the lateral projection, there is extensive cardiosternal contact, whereas in the dorsoventral projection, the right ventricle is rounded and bulges more than normal *(arrows)* into the right hemithorax. The latter observation has been referred to as the *reversed D* sign. Right atrial enlargement is also evident in the dorsoventral view as the prominent bulge in the 10- to 11-o'clock position *(open arrows)*.

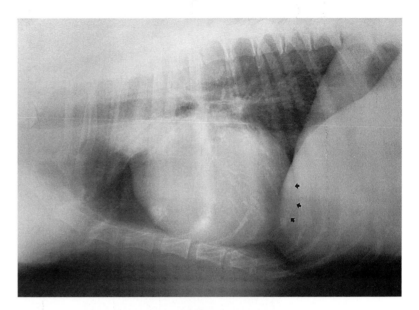

FIGURE 30–6. Left lateral thoracic radiograph of a dog with marked rounding of the right ventricle. Notice that the apex *(arrows)* of the heart no longer contacts the ventral floor of the thorax. This radiographic sign is suggestive of hypertrophy, rather than dilation, of the right ventricle.

be considered. If it is small in both projections or in repeated radiographs, hypovolemia should be considered.

Aorta

The aortic arch may be segmentally enlarged, as might occur as the result of patent ductus arteriosus (Fig. 30–7). The entire aortic arch may also be dilated. In this instance, the result is widening of the caudal portion of the cranial mediastinum (Fig. 30–8) or a bulge on the cranial aspect of the heart on the lateral view. In aged cats, the aortic arch may be elongated and thereby appear somewhat redundant; this is often accompanied by an exaggerated, horizontal alignment of the heart (increased sternal contact), occurring in 28 to 40 percent of cats 10 to 15 years of age and older. In the ventrodorsal or dorsoventral projection, the aorta may be seen bulging into the left hemithorax at the junction of the left caudal aspect of the cranial mediastinum with the left cranial aspect of the heart. The exact cause for these aging changes has not been conclusively documented.[20]

Main Pulmonary Artery

Enlargement of the main pulmonary artery appears in the ventrodorsal or dorsoventral view as a bulge on the left cranial part of the cardiac silhouette in the 12:30- to 2-o'clock position (Fig. 30–9), the so-called pulmonary knob sign.

Heart Failure

Left-Sided Heart Failure

The left atrium is enlarged, often causing dorsal deviation of the left main stem bronchus. The left ventricle is elongated, causing dorsal displacement of the base of the heart (elevation of the trachea results in decreased angle of the trachea with respect to the thoracic portion of the vertebral column). In early left-sided congestive heart failure (Fig. 30–10), there is regional hilar, perihilar, and central lobar unstructured interstitial pulmonary infiltrate (interstitial edema). The pulmonary veins may be dilated. As pulmonary edema progresses (Fig. 30–11), alveolar infiltrate (air bronchogram sign) appears. This alveolar edema may begin in the hilum and

progress (with increasing severity) into the peripheral portions of the lung fields, but more generalized edema formation also occurs. With alveolar pulmonary edema, the pulmonary vessels disappear owing to the presence of the alveolized infiltrate (silhouette sign).

Right-Sided Heart Failure

Except for right-sided heart failure resulting from heartworm disease, congenital pulmonic stenosis, tricuspid dysplasias, primary degenerative tricuspid insufficiency, and some types of feline cardiomyopathy, the right ventricle rarely fails without pre-existing left ventricular failure. Hypertrophy usually precedes dilation, sometimes resulting in elevation of the cardiac apex from the floor of the thoracic cavity in the left lateral projection. When right-sided heart failure is advanced, the dilated right ventricle contacts the sternum over a greater than normal distance (increased cardiosternal contact) in the lateral projection. In the ventrodorsal or dorsoventral projection, the right ventricle bulges into the right hemithorax, creating the *reversed D* sign. The vena cava may be dilated, but this is a radiographic sign that must be interpreted with caution because the size of the vena cava is somewhat dependent on the stage of the heart cycle. To be significant, enlargement of the vena cava must be seen in both projections and must be consistent in repeated radiographic examinations. Secondary to failure of the right ventricle, there may be pleural effusion (which obscures the heart or diaphragm, or both, owing to the silhouette sign) (Figs. 30–12 and 30–13), hepatomegaly, splenomegaly, renal enlargement, thickened small bowel wall, ascites, or combinations of the foregoing radiographic signs.

Congenital Cardiovascular Lesions

Patent Ductus Arteriosus

Although other congenital vascular lesions may mimic the clinical signs of patent ductus arteriosus,[21] the radiographic signs are reliable. There is segmental enlargement of the descending aortic arch, causing a rounding of the junction between the heart and cranial vena cava in the lateral view and elongation of the cardiac silhouette in the dorsoventral projection, resulting in a distinct bulge along the left side of

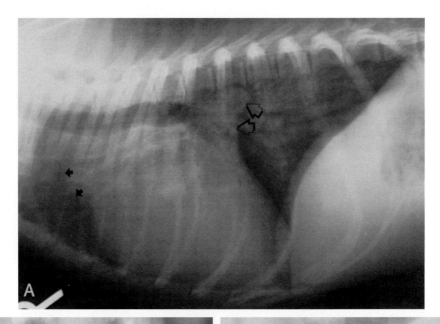

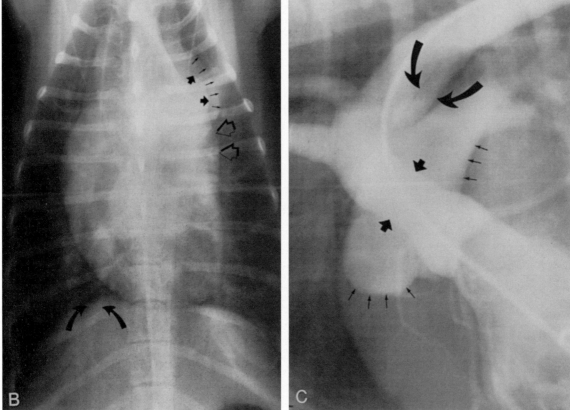

FIGURE 30–7. Right lateral (A) and dorsoventral (B) thoracic radiographs of an 8-month-old female miniature longhaired Dachshund with patent ductus arteriosus. In the dorsoventral projection (B), aneurysmal dilation of the proximal descending aorta (small, thin arrows) is making the cardiac silhouette appear elongated and creates a distinct bulge. A second distinct bulge (large, solid arrows) just craniolateral to the descending aorta is caused by dilation of the main pulmonary artery segment. A third distinct bulge (large open arrows) along the left cardiac border is caused by enlargement and protrusion of the left auricle. Note the enlarged right caudal lobe pulmonary vein (curved arrows) and its adjacent artery, caused by pulmonary overcirculation. In the lateral projection (A), the hugely dilated left atrium (large open arrows) and the filling of the region of the junction of the right ventricle and the cranial vena cava (small solid arrows) caused by aortic and main pulmonary artery segment dilation make the heart base appear wider and the entire cardiac silhouette appear elongated. In a selective left ventricular angiocardiogram (C) (different patient), the dilated main pulmonary artery segment (small thin arrows) and the ascending aorta (solid arrowheads) are accentuated by positive-contrast medium, and the patent ductus arteriosus (curved arrows) lies between the descending aorta and the main pulmonary artery segment and is opacified because of the left-to-right shunting of blood.

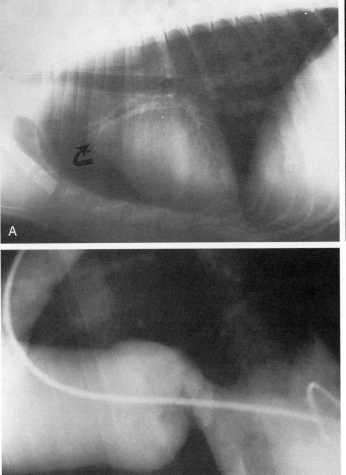

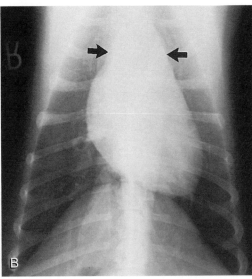

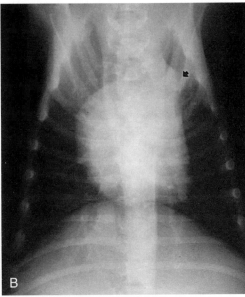

FIGURE 30–8. Right lateral *(A)* and dorsoventral *(B)* thoracic radiographs of an 11-month-old female Rottweiler with aortic stenosis. The left ventricle is not enlarged in either projection, in contrast with some other patients with this defect. The caudal portion of the cranial mediastinum is widened in the dorsoventral projection *(arrows)*, and there is a bulge in the region of the junction of the right ventricle with the cranial vena cava in the lateral view *(curved arrow)*. These radiographic signs are produced by poststenotic dilation of the root of the aorta. *C*, Note the narrow subvalvular region and dilation of the aorta distal to the aortic sinus in the angiocardiogram. The aorta should be no wider than the sinus; enlargement of the aorta distal to the sinus is due to turbulent flow.

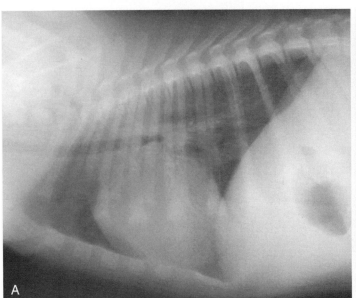

FIGURE 30–9. Left lateral *(A)* and ventrodorsal *(B)* thoracic radiographs of a dog with pulmonic stenosis. There is right ventricular enlargement in both projections, and there is bulging of the main pulmonary artery *(arrow)* in the ventrodorsal projection. The latter radiographic sign is due to poststenotic dilation caused by turbulent flow.

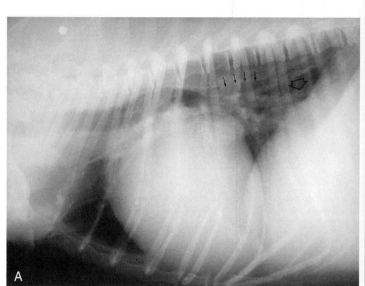
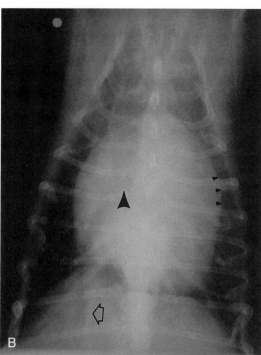

FIGURE 30–10. Right lateral *(A)* and dorsoventral *(B)* thoracic radiographs of an 11-year-old Dachshund with severe, apparently generalized, cardiomegaly and early left-sided heart failure. Note the left ventricular enlargement, indicated by the blunted cardiac apex and tracheal elevation; the left atrial/auricle enlargement, indicated by the dorsal selective deviation of the left caudal lobe stem bronchus *(small, thin arrows)* and prominent bulge in the left cardiac border at the 3-o'clock position *(small arrowheads)*; and the slightly dilated pulmonary veins *(open arrows)*. These veins are not seen as easily as expected, especially in the dorsoventral view, because of a slight, hazy increase in unstructured interstitial pulmonary opacity in the perihilar region bilaterally, caused by interstitial pulmonary edema. The trachea and bifurcation *(large arrowhead)* of the caudal lobe stem bronchi are displaced to the right of midline owing to the severe left heart enlargement, especially so by the left atrial enlargement, which is also causing the left caudal lobe stem bronchus to be less visible in the dorsoventral view. This rightward mediastinal shift makes the right side of the heart appear larger than normal, although for more accurate evaluation of right heart size, ultrasound examination is necessary.

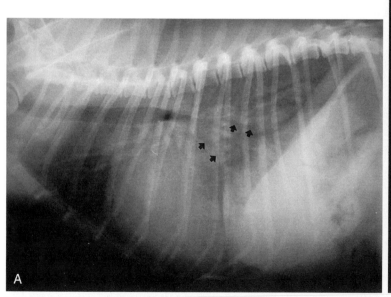
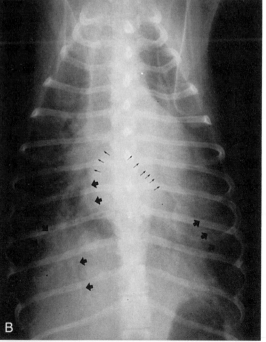

FIGURE 30–11. Right lateral *(A)* and dorsoventral *(B)* thoracic radiographs of an 11-year-old Chihuahua with severe left-sided heart enlargement and advanced left-sided heart failure. The caudal and left heart borders are largely obscured by silhouette sign caused by alveolar pulmonary edema in the perihilar and middle lung regions, evident by the fluid opacity in these lung fields with air bronchogram signs *(larger arrows)*. Silhouette sign also obscures portions of the cupula of the diaphragm and makes all pulmonary vasculature in these regions invisible. The left ventricular enlargement is evident because of the tracheal elevation, and divergence of the caudal lobe stem bronchi *(small thin arrows)* in the dorsoventral view indicates left atrial enlargement, which is also responsible for the rightward displacement of the trachea. Note the absence of radiographic signs (e.g., persistent enlargement of the caudal vena cava, hydrothorax, hepatomegaly, ascites) of right-sided heart failure.

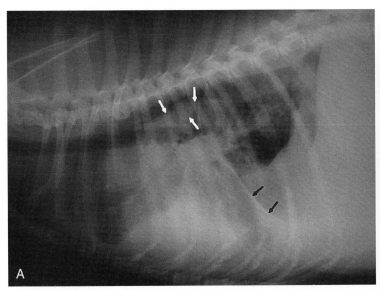

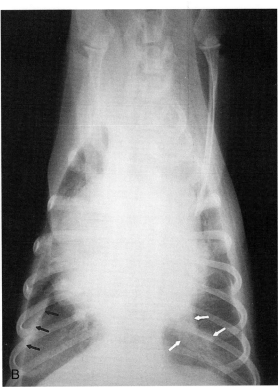

FIGURE 30–12. Left lateral *(A)* and ventrodorsal *(B)* thoracic radiographs of a 6-year-old neutered male Samoyed that had been treated 4 years previously for dirofilariasis. Current history included progressive exercise intolerance and dyspnea. There is severe cardiomegaly (especially right ventricular enlargement), tortuous dilation of the visible portions of the pulmonary arteries *(white arrows)*, hydrothorax *(black arrows)*, and probable ascites. These radiographic signs are compatible with progressive cardiovascular disease secondary to lesions initiated by dirofilariasis, leading to right-sided heart failure. (Courtesy of Animal Medical Clinic of Bothell, Bothell, WA.)

the cranial portion of the cardiac silhouette (see Fig. 30–7). This radiographic sign is theoretically caused by local aortic mural weakness adjacent to the patent ductus arteriosus.[2] Probably because of turbulence and pulmonary hypertension secondary to the effects of overcirculation, the main pulmonary artery segment creates a second distinct bulge just lateral to the aortic dilation in the ventrodorsal or dorsoventral projection. The left ventricle is usually enlarged, as is the left atrium, because of pulmonary overcirculation and distortion of the mitral annulus with secondary mitral insufficiency. In some patients, left atrial enlargement results in protrusion of the left auricle beyond the left cardiac border, creating a third distinct bulge along the left side of the cardiac silhouette in the dorsoventral projection (see Fig. 30–7). Furthermore, the pulmonary vascular pattern is enhanced because of pulmonary overcirculation and hypertension. Frequently the earliest radiographic signs of patent ductus arteriosus are dilation of the preductal aortic arch (on dorsoventral or ventrodorsal projections) and pulmonary overcirculation. The long-term radiographic signs and pathologic effects of patent ductus arteriosus have been described.[22] These include severe enlargement of the left ventricle, marked left atrial enlargement, prominence of the pulmonary vascular pattern and, eventually, left-sided heart failure.[23, 24]

Pulmonic Stenosis

The main pulmonary artery is dilated. Turbulent blood flow creates nonlaminar vector forces that result in dilation of the affected segment of the pulmonary artery or right ventricular outflow tract through a mechanism that is poorly understood.[2] This poststenotic dilation results in distinct bulging of the left craniolateral aspect of the cardiac silhouette in the ventrodorsal or dorsoventral projection (see Fig. 30–9). The pulmonary vascular pattern is usually normal, but in rare instances, the lungs appear hypovascular. In both projections,

the right ventricle is usually enlarged. In the lateral view, the margin between the heart and cranial vena cava sometimes becomes rounded because of a combination of right atrial enlargement and pulmonary artery dilation. The long-term effects of pulmonic stenosis vary considerably (possibly including dyspnea, exercise intolerance, and radiographic signs of right-sided heart failure[23]), according to the degree of right ventricular outflow obstruction.[25]

Aortic Stenosis

There is widening of the caudal aspect of the cranial mediastinum to accommodate poststenotic dilation of the aortic arch. This widening is usually obvious in both lateral and ventrodorsal or dorsoventral projections (see Fig. 30–8). In the lateral projection, the widening distorts the junction between the heart and the cranial vena cava and is caused by poststenotic dilation of the ascending aorta and aortic arch. Also, there is usually elongation of the left ventricle owing to hypertrophy because the heart has had to work against a partially obstructed left ventricular outflow tract. Pulmonary changes are generally absent, unless left ventricular enlargement has caused stretching of the mitral annulus leading to mitral insufficiency and secondary pulmonary edema or venous engorgement. Affected animals often have minimal signs of circulatory disturbance before maturity, but weakness and collapse after exercise may develop in otherwise apparently healthy young adults, often followed by sudden death, probably as a result of myocardial ischemia, which can cause ventricular dysrhythmias.[26]

Ventricular Septal Defect

Radiographic signs depend on the size of the defect and the direction and severity of the shunting of blood. There is

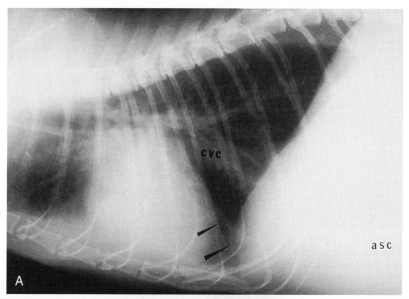

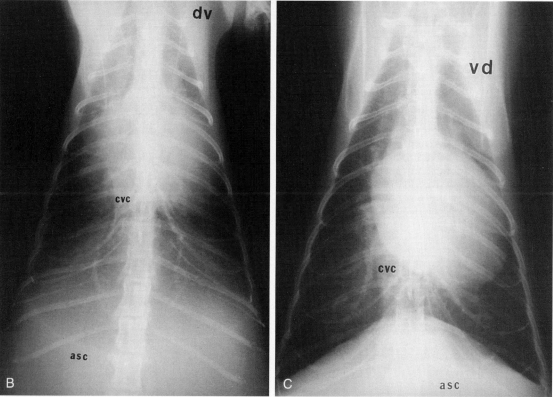

FIGURE 30–13. Right lateral *(A)*, dorsoventral *(B)*, and ventrodorsal *(C)* thoracic radiographs of a 4-year-old, domestic shorthaired cat with right-sided heart failure caused by hypertrophic cardiomyopathy. Note the total loss of visualization of the cardiac borders in the dorsoventral view owing to the silhouette sign caused by moderate, bilateral hydrothorax or pleural effusion. This might be mistaken for a hugely enlarged heart in this view unless pleural fissure lines *(arrowheads)* are noted in the dorsoventral and lateral views, indicating the presence of free pleural fluid. In the ventrodorsal view, the enlarged heart can be seen clearly because of the gravitational shifting of the pleural fluid into the dorsal, paravertebral recesses of the thorax when the patient is turned on his back for ventrodorsal positioning. The apex of the heart has shifted completely into the left hemithorax in the ventrodorsal view, partially owing to fluid-compression atelectasis of the left lung, making the left side of the heart look larger than it really is and de-emphasizing much of the right heart enlargement. In addition to hydrothorax, other radiographic signs of right-sided heart failure seen in this cat include persistent enlargement of the caudal vena cava (cvc) and ascites (asc) (total loss of abdominal serosal detail and abdominal distention) in all three views. Note the relatively normal lungs (radiolucent pulmonary parenchyma with clearly seen pulmonary vessels) in the perihilar region, indicating lack of pulmonary edema (left-sided heart failure).

usually slight biventricular enlargement and left atrial enlargement (Fig. 30–14). The lung fields may be hypervascular but usually not to the same extent as with patent ductus arteriosus.

Tetralogy of Fallot

Tetralogy of Fallot is a complex anomaly that is classically described as the existence of four lesions: pulmonic stenosis, right ventricular hypertrophy, ventricular septal defect, and overriding aorta. Actually, this disorder may be thought of as two primary lesions, each with a secondary lesion. Pulmonary stenosis leads to right ventricular enlargement, and overriding aorta automatically creates a high ventricular septal defect. Radiographically, there may be no abnormalities, but in most instances, there is right ventricular enlargement and the false impression of left ventricular enlargement owing to left displacement of the cardiac apex. Hypovascular lung fields are usually present (Fig. 30–15). Poststenotic dilation of the main pulmonary artery segment may be apparent as enlargement of this structure.

Eisenmenger's Complex

The simplest form of Eisenmenger's complex is morphologically described as consisting of overriding aorta, high ventricular septal defect, and right ventricular hypertrophy.[27] Radiographically, as in tetralogy of Fallot, the right ventricle may be enlarged. The lung markings may not be abnormal, but, in contrast with the findings expected in tetralogy of Fallot, pulmonary hypervascularity is sometimes seen because there is left-to-right shunting. This condition is rare. It can occur in much more complicated forms (in combination with other circulatory anomalies) and is difficult to recognize by survey radiography alone.

Situs Inversus

Situs inversus is an extremely rare congenital malformation in which the thoracic and abdominal viscera are reversed, as mirror images of their normal location. It is usually associated with sinusitis and bronchitis, in which instance the condition is known as *Kartagener's syndrome.*[28, 29] Radiographically (Fig. 30–16), the cardiac apex is on the right, the caudal vena cava

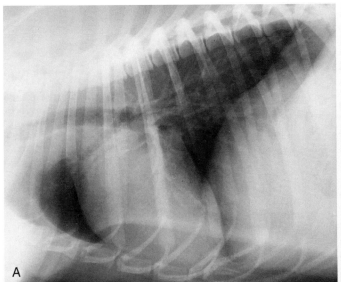

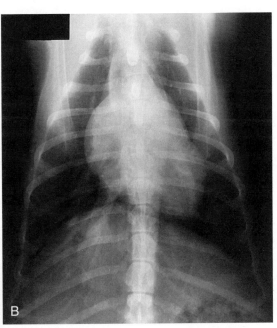

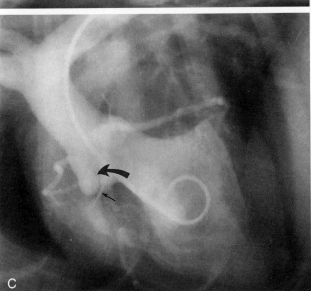

FIGURE 30–14. Right lateral *(A)* and dorsoventral *(B)* thoracic radiographs of a dog with a ventricular septal defect. There is mild biventricular enlargement, and the pulmonary vascular pattern is slightly more prominent than normal. *C,* Ventriculogram. Contrast medium was injected into the left ventricle; there is simultaneous opacification of the right ventricle and main pulmonary artery by contrast medium shunting across a septal defect *(small arrow).* Aortic valvular dysplasia is also present *(curved arrow).*

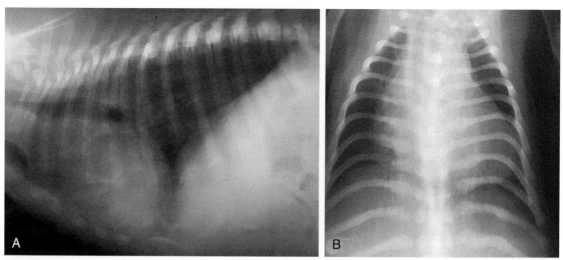

FIGURE 30-15. Right lateral *(A)* and dorsoventral *(B)* thoracic radiographs of a dog with tetralogy of Fallot. There is severe right ventricular enlargement with displacement of the apex to the left, making the left ventricle falsely appear enlarged. The pulmonary vascular pattern is markedly diminished.

is on the left, the accessory lobe of the lungs originates on the left, the pylorus and fundus of the stomach are reversed, the right kidney is more caudad than the left, the liver lobes are reversed, and so forth. Other than the associated respiratory problems, this condition has little significance (beyond humbling those veterinarians who are critical of their technical assistants for allegedly mismarking radiographs).

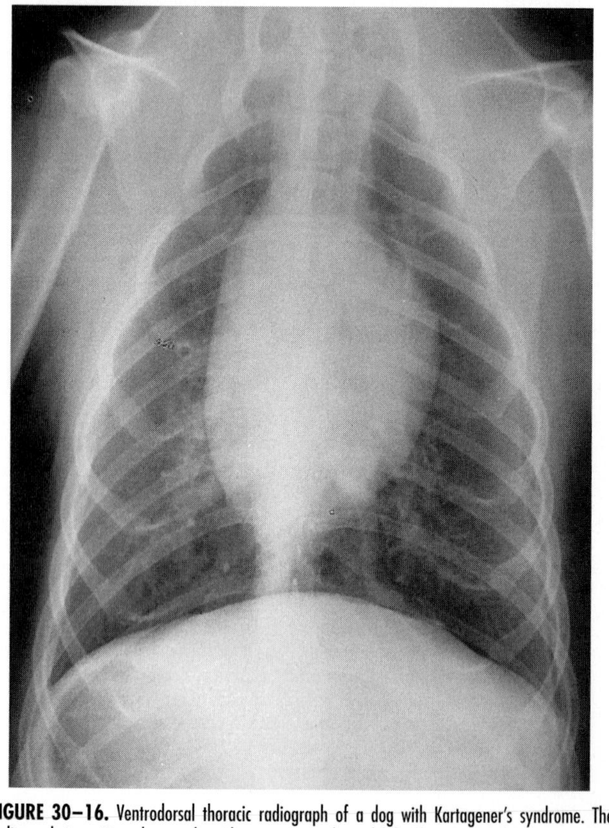

FIGURE 30-16. Ventrodorsal thoracic radiograph of a dog with Kartagener's syndrome. The radiograph is positioned correctly with respect to right and left. There is complete mirror-image positioning of the thoracic and abdominal viscera. The apex of the heart is on the right, the caudal vena cava is on the left, the trachea is on the right, the ventral portion of the caudal mediastinum is on the right, and so forth. Notice also that the bronchial pattern is prominent. Precise labeling of radiographs is needed if this condition is to be diagnosed.

Kartagener's syndrome is one of several possible congenital diseases resulting in malorientation of the thoracic and abdominal viscera.[2]

Acquired Cardiovascular Lesions

Mitral Insufficiency

Insufficiency of the mitral valve produces left atrial enlargement, which, as previously discussed, often causes dorsal deviation of the left main stem bronchus and bowing and lateral divergence of the left and right main stem bronchi (Fig. 30-17). Additionally, by the time the patient is examined clinically, the left ventricle is usually also enlarged, causing dorsal elevation of the axis of the trachea and possible rounding of the normally straight caudal and left borders of the cardiac silhouette. As left-sided heart failure occurs, the pulmonary veins become distended and possibly tortuous, and pulmonary edema occurs, causing interstitial, then alveolar, infiltrate.

Tricuspid Insufficiency

Although much less common as a single lesion than mitral insufficiency, tricuspid insufficiency occasionally exists without other cardiac lesions. Often, however, tricuspid insufficiency is secondary to distortion of the right atrioventricular annulus as a result of mitral insufficiency. Radiographic signs of this disorder, without concomitant left-sided changes,[2] include right atrial enlargement and possible secondary right ventricular enlargement. The right atrium is enlarged, possibly causing dorsal bowing of the trachea over the cranial aspect of the base of the heart. In addition, the right ventricle is enlarged, causing greater than normal sternal contact or elevation of the apex of the heart from the caudoventral floor of the thorax in the lateral projection, or both. In the ventrodorsal or dorsoventral projection, the right ventricle is rounded, bulging into the right hemithorax and causing the *reversed-D* sign. If there is right-sided heart failure, there may be hepatomegaly, splenomegaly, ascites, or pleural effusion.

Heartworm Disease

Heartworm disease is probably the most common cause of acquired cor pulmonale in dogs. The adult parasites most

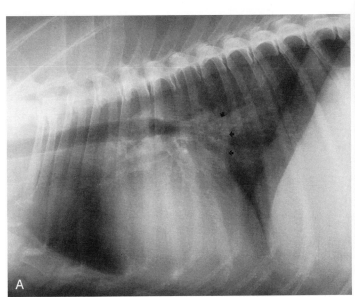
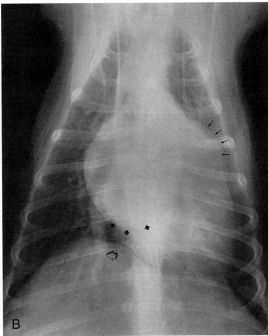

FIGURE 30–17. Right lateral *(A)* and dorsoventral *(B)* thoracic radiographs of a dog with mitral insufficiency. There is left atrial *(large solid arrowheads in A and B)* and left ventricular enlargement, and the left auricle *(small solid arrows in B)* protrudes prominently along the left border of the cardiac silhouette. The trachea is elevated, and the left ventricular contour is rounded in both projections. An enlarged and tortuous right caudal lobar vein may be seen *(open arrow in B)*. Pulmonary edema is not present.

commonly reside in the right ventricle or the pulmonary arteries, occupying space in the lumina, causing physical obstruction of the outflow tract, and destroying normal laminar blood flow in the pulmonary arteries. Typically, as the disease progresses, the vascular intima becomes roughened, irregular, and hypertrophic, further compromising laminar flow. The pulmonary arteries dilate and become tortuous. Perivascular fibrosis follows pulmonary hypertension, and the disease becomes self-perpetuating to the extent that progressive cardiovascular changes may occur even after the parasites are no longer present (see Fig. 30–12). Typical radiographic signs[2, 3, 5] of heartworm disease (Fig. 30–18) include right ventricular enlargement, dilation of the main pulmonary artery at the cranial left border of the ventrodorsal or dorsoventral cardiac silhouette, dilation and tortuosity of the lobar arteries, truncation or pruning of pulmonary arteries, and interstitial or alveolar parenchymal infiltrate. Generally the diameter of the left and right caudal lobar pulmonary arteries should not exceed the width of the ninth rib at the points of intersection of the rib with the corresponding artery in the dorsoventral projection. Also, the cranial lobar arteries should be about the same size as the respective lobar veins, and the diameter of each vessel should not exceed the smallest diameter of the right fourth rib in the left lateral recumbent projection. If right-sided heart failure occurs, the radiographic signs may include ascites, hydrothorax, splenomegaly, or hepatomegaly. Occasionally, adult heartworms may obstruct the caudal vena cava, producing dramatic clinical signs of central hypovolemia and caudal congestion.

Cardiomyopathy

Dilatory cardiomyopathy in cats (rare now that the role of taurine has been defined)[2, 30, 31] (Fig. 30–19) and dogs (Fig. 30–20) usually produces generalized cardiomegaly,[2, 5] al-

though in some patients left atrial and ventricular enlargement may predominate, particularly in Doberman pinschers, which often appear to have only left atrial enlargement on radiographs. If this is the situation, there is usually increase in the size of the pulmonary veins (pulmonary congestion)[32] and various radiographic signs of heart failure. In cats, right ventricular enlargement predominates (in dilatory cardiomyopathy), whereas in dogs left-sided and right-sided failure often occur simultaneously. Therefore, there may be ascites, hepatomegaly, splenomegaly, and pleural effusion associated with right ventricular failure in dilatory cardiomyopathy in cats. In dogs, dilatory cardiomyopathy is often associated with pulmonary edema secondary to left ventricular failure in addition to radiographic signs of right-sided heart failure (distention of the caudal vena cava, hepatomegaly, and pleural effusion, the last-mentioned possibly obscuring the cardiac silhouette). These clinical observations are consistent with the pathologic findings in this syndrome in dogs.[33]

Hypertrophic cardiomyopathy in the cat (Fig. 30–21) produces primarily left atrial enlargement[2, 34] but usually causes little external change in the ventricles. Severe enlargement of the left atrium results in the characteristic valentine heart shape. Occasionally, ventricular enlargement may be obvious in hypertrophic cardiomyopathy (see Fig. 30–13), mimicking that seen in dilatory cardiomyopathy. Secondarily, there may be extracardiac radiographic signs of heart failure, such as ascites, pleural effusion (right-sided heart failure), or pulmonary edema (left-sided heart failure). Assessment of cardiomyopathy has been greatly improved by the use of diagnostic ultrasonography. This technique is now the imaging method of choice for clinical assessment of cardiomegaly.

Pericardial Effusion

As described earlier, the epicardial edges of the heart are normally not visualized because of the presence of a small

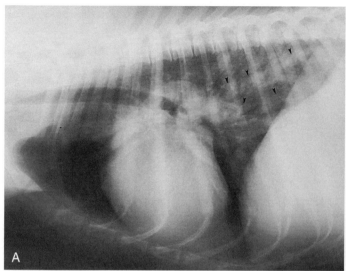

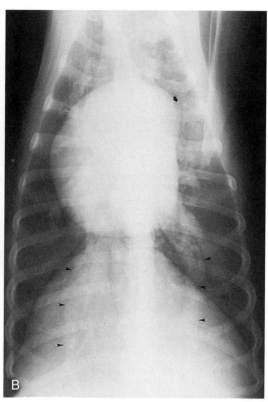

FIGURE 30–18. Left lateral *(A)* and dorsoventral *(B)* thoracic radiographs of a dog with heartworm disease. There is right ventricular enlargement in both projections. The main pulmonary artery *(wide arrowhead)* is distended in the dorsoventral projection, and the left and right caudal lobar pulmonary arteries *(arrowheads)* are dilated and tortuous in both projections. The right cranial lobar pulmonary artery is also enlarged.

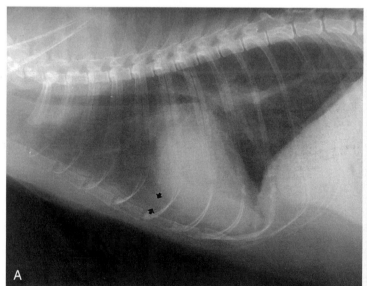

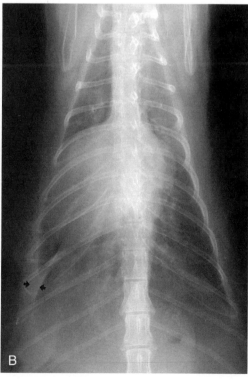

FIGURE 30–19. Left lateral *(A)* and dorsoventral *(B)* thoracic radiographs of a cat with dilatory cardiomyopathy. There is generalized cardiomegaly in both projections. The heart is shifted to the right. Pulmonary vessels are enlarged, and there is pleural effusion *(arrows).*

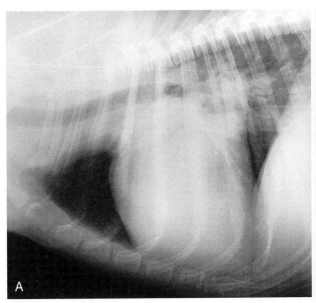

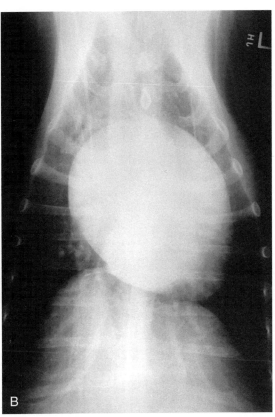

FIGURE 30–20. Left lateral *(A)* and dorsoventral *(B)* thoracic radiographs of a dog with dilatory cardiomyopathy. There is generalized cardiomegaly, and the cardiac silhouette (in addition to being generally enlarged) is somewhat angular in shape.

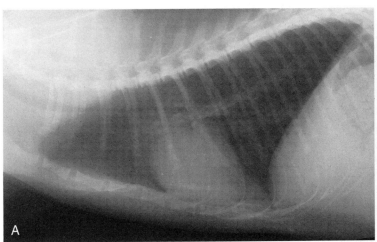

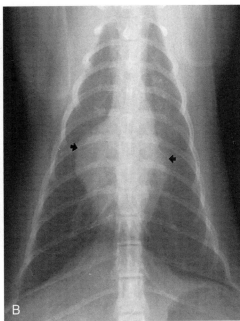

FIGURE 30–21. Right lateral *(A)* and dorsoventral *(B)* thoracic radiographs of a cat with hypertrophic cardiomyopathy. There is little enlargement of the ventricles, but there is an appearance of biatrial enlargement *(arrows in B)* in the dorsoventral projection. Severe left atrial enlargement accounts for the apparent biatrial enlargement.

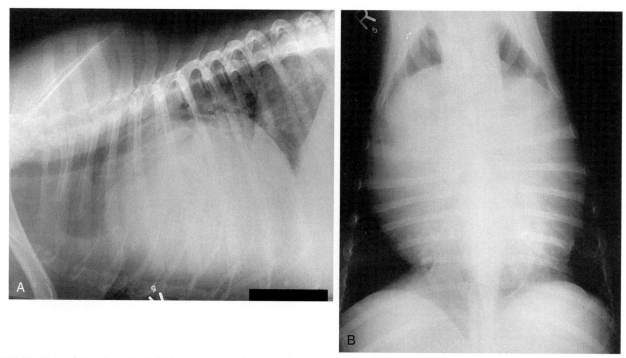

FIGURE 30–22. Lateral (A) and ventrodorsal (B) thoracic radiographs of a 5-year-old male mixed-breed dog with pericardial effusion owing to a right atrial neoplasm. In the ventrodorsal projection, the cardiac silhouette is markedly enlarged and globoid. The edge of the pericardium is distinct in this view because it underwent little motion during the radiographic exposure; it is partially obliterated in the lateral projection owing to free pleural fluid secondary to right-sided heart failure.

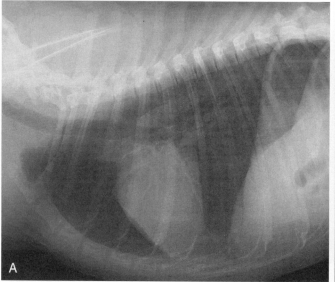

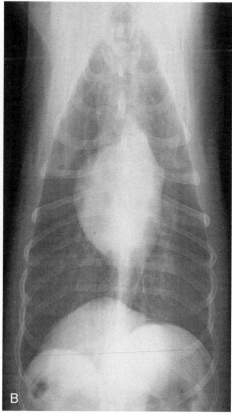

FIGURE 30–23. Lateral (A) and dorsoventral (B) thoracic radiographs of a dog with microcardia owing to hypoadrenocorticism. The heart is markedly smaller than expected relative to the size of the thoracic cavity. Acute hypovolemia produces similar radiographic signs. (Courtesy of the Santa Cruz Veterinary Hospital, Santa Cruz, CA.)

amount of free fluid in the pericardial sac. This fluid, between the pericardial sac and the epicardium, silhouettes with the inside of the pericardial sac and the outside of the heart. Distention of the pericardial sac with large amounts of fluid causes the cardiac silhouette to be enlarged and globoid (Fig. 30–22). In the ventrodorsal or dorsoventral projection, the edge of the pericardial sac may touch the costal margins bilaterally. Furthermore, the edge of the distended pericardial sac is often quite distinct because it undergoes little, if any, motion during systole and diastole. If the efficiency of the cardiac cycle is disrupted by the presence of the pericardial fluid, radiographic signs of congestive heart failure may also be present in the thorax, abdomen, or both. The causes of hydropericardium may be neoplastic, inflammatory, congenital, hemorrhagic,[35] or idiopathic. Among the possible neoplastic causes for hydropericardium are heart base tumors (chemodectomas) and metastatic or primary hemangiosarcomas. Of course, chemodectomas and other neoplasms at the base of the heart do not necessarily involve the pericardial sac. Pericardiocentesis and pneumopericardiography[2, 36] have been recommended to aid in differential diagnosis of pericardial diseases. Diagnostic ultrasonography is now the method of choice for imaging such lesions.

Cardiac Neoplasia

Neoplasms of the heart, whether primary or metastatic, are extremely rare and afford few reliable radiographic signs.[2] Cardiac hemangiosarcomas most commonly involve the right atrium and may produce selective enlargement of that chamber, although this radiographic sign may be obscured by secondary hemopericardium resulting from hemorrhage into the pericardial sac. Metastatic or primary lesions in the myocardium may produce focal irregularity of the border of the cardiac silhouette. Ultrasonography is a more reliable imaging modality for detection and assessment of cardiac neoplasms than is any form of radiographic examination.[37]

Microcardia

Decrease in size of the cardiac silhouette may be absolute or relative.[2] If relative, the thorax has been overinflated by one of several possible conditions, such as emphysema or simple hyperventilation. If absolute, the causes include hypovolemia (due to blood loss, shock, or severe dehydration), atrophic myopathies, and hypoadrenocorticism (due to Addison's disease). The pathogenesis of hypovolemia in Addison's disease is apparently equivocal. Microcardia caused by hypoadrenocorticism has been induced experimentally in dogs.[38] Hypovolemia appears to be the major reason for the decrease in size of the heart in the more acute form of the disease. In the chronically afflicted patient, however, decrease in cardiac size appears to be caused, at least in part, by electrolyte imbalance, which theoretically results in decrease in myocardial mass owing to chronically weak contractions (disuse atrophy). The radiographic sign associated with *microcardia* (Fig. 30–23) is, as the term suggests, the appearance of a smaller than normal cardiac silhouette relative to the size of the thoracic cavity. There are no objective measurements that can be made for assistance in borderline or equivocal situations, but the heart should generally occupy space in the thorax between the fifth and ninth ribs in the lateral projection exposed at maximum inspiration. It should not be widely separated from the diaphragm and the sternum, and its height should be sufficient to create an angle of approximately 10 to 15 degrees between the trachea and the cranial thoracic vertebral column in the dog. In the cat, this angulation may be less obvious and more difficult to measure than

in the dog because of the natural lordosis that exists in the feline cranial thoracic spine.

References

1. Kealy JK: Diagnostic Radiology of the Dog and Cat. Philadelphia, WB Saunders, 1979.
2. Suter PF: Thoracic Radiography: A Text Atlas of Thoracic Diseases of the Dog and Cat. Wettswil, Switzerland, Peter F. Suter, 1984.
3. Watters JW: Radiographic signs of cardiovascular disease. Comp Contin Ed Vet Pract 1:766, 1979.
4. Ticer JW: Radiographic Technique in Veterinary Practice, 2nd Ed. Philadelphia, WB Saunders, 1984.
5. Owens JM: Radiographic Interpretation for the Small Animal Clinician. St Louis, Ralston Purina, 1982.
6. Carlisle CH, and Thrall DE: A comparison of normal feline thoracic radiographs made in dorsal versus ventral recumbency. Vet Radiol 23:3, 1982.
7. Toal RL, Losonsky JM, Coulter DB, et al: Influence of cardiac cycle on the radiographic appearance of the feline heart. Vet Radiol 26:63, 1985.
8. Ruehl WW, and Thrall DE: The effect of dorsal versus ventral recumbency on the radiographic appearance of the canine thorax. Vet Radiol 22:10, 1981.
9. Roenigk WJ: Injuries to the thorax. J Am Anim Hosp Assoc 7:266, 1971.
10. Holmes RA, Smith FG, Lewis RE, et al: The effects of rotation on the radiographic appearance of the canine cardiac silhouette in dorsal recumbency. Vet Radiol 26:98, 1985.
11. Patterson DF, and Botts RP: A simple cassette changer. Small Anim Clinician 1:1, 1960.
12. Stickle RL, and Anderson LK: Diagnosis of common congenital heart anomalies in the dog using survey and nonselective contrast radiography. Vet Radiol 28:6, 1987.
13. Myer CW, and Bonagura JD: Survey radiography of the heart. Vet Clin North Am [Small Anim Pract] 12:213, 1982.
14. Reed JR, Thomas WP, and Suter PF: Pneumopericardiography in the normal dog. Vet Radiol 24:112, 1983.
15. Schnelling C: Radiology of the heart. In Miller M, Tilley L (Eds): Manual of Canine and Feline Cardiology, 2nd Ed. Philadelphia, WB Saunders, 1994.
16. Chikos PM, Figley MM, and Fisher L: Visual assessment of total heart volume and specific chamber size from standard chest radiographs. Am J Roentgenol 128:375, 1977.
17. Hamlin RL: Analysis of the cardiac silhouette in dorsoventral radiographs from dogs with heart disease. J Am Vet Med Assoc 153:1446, 1968.
18. Suter PF, and Lord PF: A critical evaluation of the findings in canine cardiovascular disease. J Am Vet Med Assoc 158:358, 1970.
19. Snyder PS, Sato T, and Atkins CE: The utility of thoracic radiographic measurement for the detection of cardiomegaly in cats with pleural effusion. Vet Radiol 31:89, 1990.
20. Moon ML, Keene BW, Lessard P, et al: Age related changes in the feline cardiac silhouette. Vet Radiol Ultrasound 34:5, 1993.
21. Malik R, Bellenger CR, Hunt GB, et al: Aberrant branch of the bronchoesophageal artery mimicking patent ductus arteriosus in a dog. J Am Anim Hosp Assoc 30:162, 1994.
22. Weirich WE, Blevins WE, and Rebar AH: Late consequences of patent ductus arteriosus in the dog: A report of six cases. J Am Anim Hosp Assoc 14:40, 1978.
23. Darke PGG: Congenital heart disease in dogs and cats. J Small Anim Pract 30:599, 1989.
24. Patterson DF, Pyle RL, Buchanan JW, et al: Hereditary patent ductus arteriosus and its sequelae in the dog. Circ Res 29:1, 1971.
25. Fingland RB, Bonagura JD, and Myer CW: Pulmonic stenosis in the dog: 29 cases. J Am Vet Med Assoc 189:218, 1986.
26. Pyle RL: Congenital heart disease. In Ettinger SJ (Ed): Textbook of Veterinary Internal Medicine, 2nd Ed. Philadelphia, WB Saunders, 1983.
27. Feldman EC, Nimmo-Wilkie JS, and Pharr JW: Eisenmenger's syndrome in the dog: Case reports. J Am Anim Hosp Assoc 17:477, 1981.
28. Carrig CB, Suter PF, Ewing GO, et al: Primary dextrocardia with situs inversus, associated with sinusitis and bronchitis in a dog. J Am Vet Med Assoc 164:1127, 1974.
29. Stowater JL: Kartagener's syndrome in a dog. J Am Vet Radiol Soc 17:174, 1976.
30. Liu S-K: Acquired cardiac lesions leading to congestive heart failure in the cat. Am J Vet Res 31:2071, 1970.
31. Liu S-K, Tashjian RJ, and Patnaik AK: Congestive heart failure in the cat. J Am Vet Med Assoc 156:1319, 1970.
32. Jacobs GJ: Reviewing the various types of primary cardiomyopathy in dogs. Vet Med 91:524, 1996.
33. Van Vleet JF, Ferrans VJ, and Weirich WE: Pathologic alterations in congestive cardiomyopathy of dogs. Am J Vet Res 42:416, 1981.
34. Lord PF, Wood A, Tilley LP, et al: Radiographic and hemodynamic evaluation of cardiomyopathy and thromboembolism in the cat. J Am Vet Med Assoc 164:154, 1974.

35. Gibbs C, Gaskell CJ, Darke PGG, et al: Idiopathic pericardial haemorrhage in dogs: A review of fourteen cases. J Small Anim Pract 23:483, 1982.
36. Thomas WP, Reed JR, and Gomez JA: Diagnostic pneumopericardiography in dogs with spontaneous pericardial effusion. Vet Radiol 25:2, 1984.

37. Thomas WP, Sisson D, Bauer TG, et al: Detection of cardiac masses in dogs by two-dimensional echocardiography. Vet Radiol 25:65, 1984.
38. Rendano VT, and Alexander JE: Heart size changes in experimentally-induced adrenal insufficiency in the dog: A radiographic study. J Am Vet Radiol Soc 17:57, 1976.

STUDY QUESTIONS

1. Why is it not possible to assess cardiovascular disease accurately by physically measuring structures seen on thoracic radiographs?

2. Which of the following are generally accepted as reliable radiographic signs of left atrial enlargement?
   A. Dorsal deviation of the left main stem bronchus in the lateral projection.
   B. Ventral displacement of the caudal vena cava in the lateral projection.
   C. Divergence of the left and right main stem bronchi in the dorsoventral or ventrodorsal projection.
   D. Widening of the arch of the aorta in either projection.
   E. Medial displacement of the right main stem bronchus in the ventrodorsal or dorsoventral projection.

3. Under which circumstances is decrease in the angle between the vertebral column and the trachea (in the lateral radiograph) an unreliable radiographic sign of left ventricular enlargement?

4. Which radiographic sign(s) may help differentiate between right ventricular dilation and right ventricular hypertrophy?

5. Which of the following radiographic signs are generally associated with left-sided heart failure?
   A. Increased cardiosternal contact in the lateral projection.
   B. Elevation of the left main stem bronchus in the lateral projection.
   C. Hepatomegaly.
   D. Ascites.
   E. Alveolar pulmonary infiltrate in the hilar and intermediate zones of the lung fields.
   F. Elevation of the axis of the trachea in the lateral projection.
   G. Free pleural fluid.

6. Which of the following radiographic signs are generally associated with right-sided heart failure?
   A. Increased cardiosternal contact in the lateral projection.
   B. Elevation of the left main stem bronchus in the lateral projection.
   C. Hepatomegaly.
   D. Ascites.
   E. Alveolar pulmonary infiltrate in the hilar and intermediate zones of the lung fields.

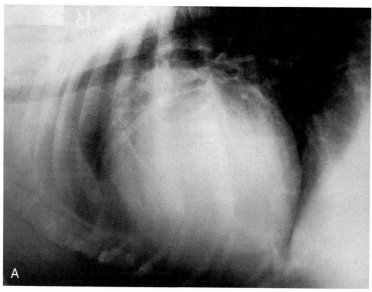

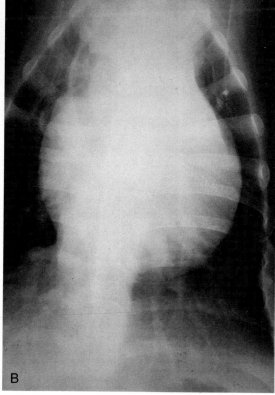

FIGURE 30–24. Left lateral *(A)* and ventrodorsal *(B)* thoracic radiographs of a 9-year-old neutered male Golden retriever with progressive lethargy and exercise intolerance.

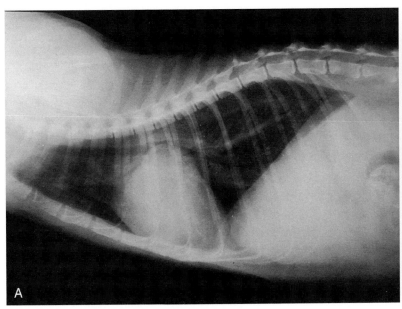

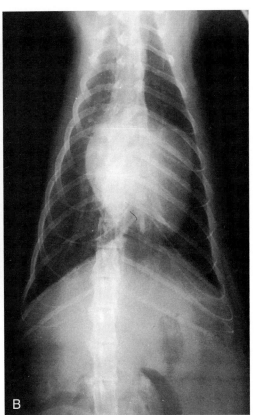

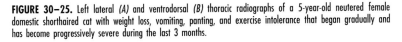

FIGURE 30–25. Left lateral *(A)* and ventrodorsal *(B)* thoracic radiographs of a 5-year-old neutered female domestic shorthaired cat with weight loss, vomiting, panting, and exercise intolerance that began gradually and has become progressively severe during the last 3 months.

F. Elevation of the axis of the trachea in the lateral projection.

G. Free pleural fluid.

7. List the survey radiographic signs generally associated with patent ductus arteriosus. With aortic stenosis. With pulmonic stenosis.

8. List the survey radiographic signs generally associated with heartworm disease. With mitral insufficiency.

9. Radiographic interpretation (Fig. 30–24): List the major radiographic signs.

10. Radiographic interpretation (Fig. 30–25): List the major radiographic signs.

(Answers appear on pages 642 to 643.)

Chapter 31

The Pulmonary Vasculature

John M. Losonsky

Diseases of the cardiovascular and pulmonary systems may result in similar clinical signs.[1] Thoracic radiographs may assist in differentiating pulmonary from cardiac diseases. An important component in evaluating both cardiovascular and pulmonary disease is assessment of the pulmonary vasculature. An attempt should be made to differentiate pulmonary arteries from veins because this provides important information pertaining to circulatory dynamics.

ANATOMY OF THE PULMONARY VASCULATURE

The pulmonary trunk arises from the pulmonary fibrous ring at the conus arteriosus.[2] After coursing 3 or 4 cm, the trunk divides into left and right pulmonary arteries. The left pulmonary artery divides into two or more branches. One of two smaller branches enters the cranial portion of the left cranial lobe (cranial lobar artery of the left cranial lobe). The larger branch subdivides and enters the caudal portion of the left cranial lobe (caudal lobar artery of the left cranial lobe) and the left caudal lobe (left caudal lobar artery).

The right pulmonary artery leaves the pulmonary trunk at almost a right angle and courses to the right. The first branch is the right cranial lobar artery. The vessel then divides into the right middle lobar, accessory lobar, and right caudal lobar arteries.

Commonly, there is one main vein from each lung lobe,

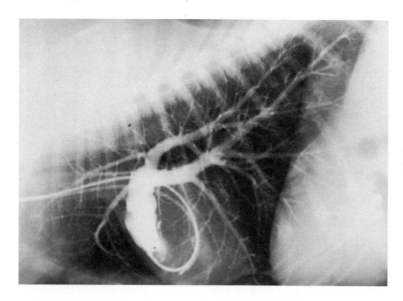

FIGURE 31–1. Lateral pulmonary angiogram of a 2-year-old male mixed-breed dog. The distribution of pulmonary arteries is normal.

but there can be two from the right cranial lobe.[2] The right middle lobar and right cranial lobar veins merge, as do the right caudal lobar and accessory lobar veins, before entering the left atrium. All lobar pulmonary veins from the left lung enter individually into the left atrium.

RADIOGRAPHIC ANATOMY OF THE PULMONARY VASCULATURE

If radiographs are of diagnostic quality, the pulmonary vasculature of the central (hilar) and middle thirds of the lung may be evaluated. In larger dogs, pulmonary vasculature may be seen in the peripheral one third of the lung.

The large left and right pulmonary arteries may be seen on the lateral view from their origin cranial to the tracheal bifurcation (Fig. 31–1). The left pulmonary artery lies dorsal

to the trachea, whereas the right pulmonary artery is ventral to the trachea. On ventrodorsal or dorsoventral radiographs, the left and right pulmonary arteries may be seen extending caudolaterally from the midcardiac region.

Large pulmonary veins may be seen on the dorsoventral view coursing medially to the caudal cardiac region as they merge near the left atrium. Pulmonary arteries and veins are better visualized on a dorsoventral radiograph as opposed to a ventrodorsal radiograph because of a greater degree of lung inflation on the dorsoventral view as well as the more perpendicular relationship of these vessels relative to the primary x-ray beam.[3]

When an artery, bronchus, and vein to a corresponding lobe are seen on a lateral radiograph, the artery is dorsal to the bronchus, and the vein is ventral.[2, 4] The right cranial lobar artery, bronchus, and vein are routinely visible and can serve as reference vessels for evaluation of the pulmonary circulation (Fig. 31–2). The right cranial lobar artery is most

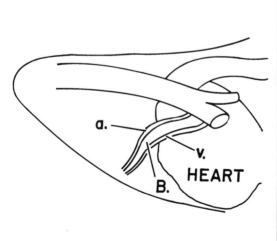

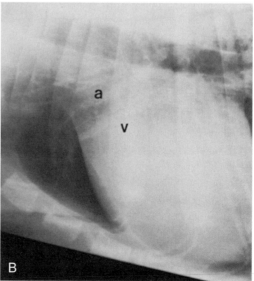

FIGURE 31–2. *A,* Illustration of a lateral canine thoracic radiograph. The location of the right cranial lobar artery (a), vein (v), and bronchus (B) is specified. *B,* Left lateral recumbent view of the thorax of a normal 6-month-old male St. Bernard. Note the right cranial lobar artery (a) and vein (v). The right cranial lobar bronchus is located between the artery and the vein. In this dog, the bronchial wall is visible because it is mineralized. Note that it does not occupy the entire space between the artery and the vein. When the bronchial wall is not mineralized, one should not assume it occupies the entire space between the artery and the vein. (From Thrall DE, and Losonsky JM: A method for evaluating canine pulmonary circulatory dynamics from survey radiographs. J Am Anim Hosp Assoc *12:*457, 1976; with permission.)

commonly visualized when the animal is radiographed in left lateral recumbency (Fig. 31–3), a position in which the right cranial lobe is inflated to a greater extent, resulting in greater separation between these vessels. The right cranial lobar vessels are also located slightly ventral to the opacity produced by the craniodorsal mediastinum, just ventral to the trachea, whereas the paired left cranial lobar vessels are usually superimposed on the mediastinum. In right lateral radiographs, the paired artery and vein supplying the cranial lobes are usually superimposed, making their assessment difficult and prone to error. The paired artery and vein to remaining lobes are not usually seen on lateral views.

When a lobar artery, vein, and bronchus are seen on a dorsoventral radiograph, the artery is lateral to the vein with the bronchus located between the two vessels.[2, 4] The paired arteries and veins of the left and right caudal lung lobes can be identified more frequently on a dorsoventral view than on a ventrodorsal view (Fig. 31–4).[3] Paired arteries and veins are seen less frequently in the remaining lung lobes, although cranial lobe vessels are occasionally seen.

It has been stated that pulmonary arteries are more opaque, are better delineated, have a greater number of branches, and curve cranially and laterally relative to pulmonary veins.[1, 4] The guidelines presented here, however, are more reliable ways to distinguish between pulmonary arteries and veins. Both pulmonary arteries and veins should taper as they course to the periphery of the lung.

ROENTGEN SIGNS OF THE PULMONARY VASCULATURE

Geometric Changes

Size

On the left lateral recumbent radiograph, the right cranial lobar artery and vein should be approximately equal in size. The relative size of these two vessels should be compared, and the size of each should be compared with the right fourth rib just ventral to the spine.[5] The diameter of each

Table 31–1

DISEASES THAT MAY INCREASE THE SIZE OF PULMONARY ARTERIES AND PULMONARY VEINS

Left-to-right shunts
    Patent ductus arteriosus
    Ventricular septal defect
    Atrial septal defect
    Peripheral arteriovenous fistula
Iatrogenic fluid overload
Cardiomyopathy (volume overload)
Mitral insufficiency and heartworm disease

vessel should not exceed the smallest diameter of the right fourth rib.

On the dorsoventral radiograph, the size of caudal lobar arteries and veins should be compared with each other and to the diameter of the ninth rib at the point of intersection of the ninth rib and the corresponding vessel. The artery and vein of each caudal lobe should be similar in size. The diameter of the artery and vein caudal to the ninth rib should not exceed the diameter of that rib.

Table 31–1 is a list of some common diseases in which there can be an increase in size of pulmonary arteries and veins.[5] History, physical examination, electrocardiography, survey thoracic radiographs, angiocardiography, echocardiography, and clinical pathology results can be used to differentiate these conditions. The radiographic changes depend on the severity and duration of the disease (Fig. 31–5). Associated cardiac abnormalities are described in Chapter 30.

Pulmonary arterial enlargement may occur with diseases listed in Table 31–2.[5–9] Heartworm disease in the dog is the most common cause of pulmonary arterial enlargement. In heartworm disease, vessel enlargement occurs because of lesions in the tunica intima and tunica media, or thromboembolic disease, or both. Thoracic radiographic abnormalities seen in spontaneous dirofilariasis are well documented.[10–13] The percentage of dogs with right heart enlargement, main pulmonary artery enlargement, and right cranial lobar pulmonary artery enlargement has been reported.[14] The percentage of right cranial lobar pulmonary artery enlargement was

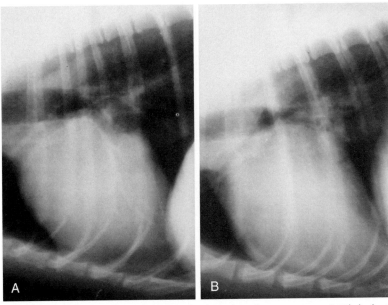

FIGURE 31–3. Lateral views of the thorax of a 12-year-old male Beagle. *A,* With the dog in left lateral recumbency on inspiration. *B,* With the dog in right lateral recumbency on expiration. Note the better visualization of the right cranial lobar vessels in *A.*

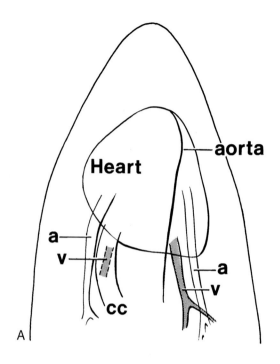

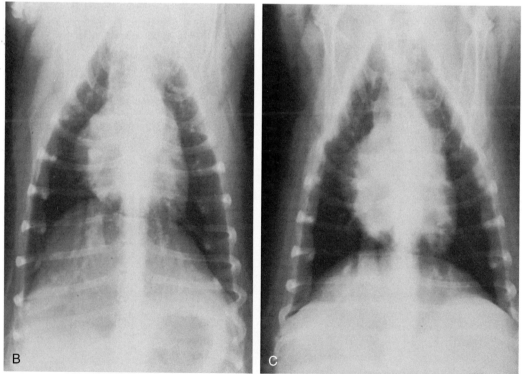

FIGURE 31–4. *A,* Illustration of a dorsoventral canine thoracic radiograph. The location of pulmonary arteries and pulmonary veins to caudal lung lobes is illustrated. a, artery; v, vein; cc, caudal vena cava. Dorsoventral *(B)* and ventrodorsal *(C)* views of a 12-year-old female Dachshund. Note that the caudal lobar arteries and veins are better seen in *B* (sternal recumbency) than in *C.*

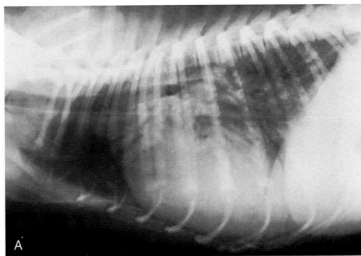

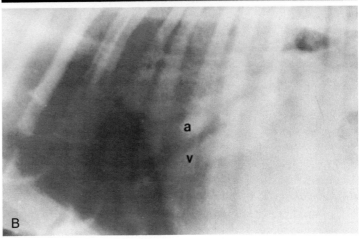

FIGURE 31–5. *A,* Lateral view of the thorax of a 6-month-old male Cocker spaniel with a continuous heart murmur. Note the increase in size of the right cranial lobar artery and vein owing to pulmonary overcirculation associated with a left-to-right shunt. There is also heart enlargement. Note the increased opacity in the caudal lobes owing to hypervascularity. The diagnosis, confirmed angiographically, was patent ductus arteriosus. *B,* A close-up view in which the right cranial lobar artery (a) and right cranial lobar vein (v) are visible. The vein appears larger than the artery. More severe pulmonary vein enlargement, in reference to pulmonary arteries, is common in patent ductus arteriosus because the thin-walled veins are more easily distended. (From Thrall DE, and Losonsky JM: A method for evaluating canine pulmonary circulatory dynamics from survey radiographs. J Am Anim Hosp Assoc *12:*457, 1976; with permission.)

only 47 percent (Fig. 31–6). In that study, caudal lobar pulmonary arteries were not measured because the animals were in dorsal recumbency as opposed to sternal recumbency. In the author's experience, the lobar arteries that enlarge most frequently in spontaneous heartworm disease are the caudal lobar arteries, with a predilection for enlargement of the right more than the left (Fig. 31–7). Experimentally the right caudal lobar artery was the first to enlarge and

Table 31–2
DISEASES THAT MAY INCREASE THE SIZE OF PULMONARY ARTERIES

Tunica intimal proliferation or tunica media
    Hypertrophy
    Dirofilariasis
    Angiostrongyliasis
    Aelurostrongylus (feline)
Thromboembolic disease or primary thromboses
    Dirofilariasis
    Disseminated intravascular coagulation
    Trauma
    Secondary to cardiac diseases
    Angiostrongyliasis
    Renal disease—amyloidosis, glomerulonephritis
    Systemic venous thrombosis
    Septicemia
    Pancreatitis
    Hyperadrenocorticism
Severe chronic lung disease

did so most frequently. The left caudal lobar artery was the next most frequently enlarged vessel.[13, 15–17] It is common in canine heartworm disease to see main pulmonary artery enlargement in association with peripheral pulmonary arterial enlargement (see Fig. 31–7).[14]

In feline heartworm disease, it is *unusual* to see main pulmonary artery enlargement on survey radiographs.[18] With angiography, however, it is possible to see the main pulmonary artery is enlarged in most cats with heartworm disease; the main pulmonary is positioned such that it is not visible in survey radiographs. Parenchymal pulmonary arteries are also enlarged in feline heartworm disease (Fig. 31–8).[19] It has been reported that enlargement of the central and peripheral portions of caudal lobar arteries on the ventrodorsal view, with normal-sized caudal pulmonary veins, represents the earliest radiographic change seen in spontaneous feline heartworm disease. If the diameter of the caudal lobar artery at the seventh intercostal space is 5 mm or larger, 4 mm or larger at the ninth intercostal space, as seen on the ventrodorsal view, this was considered consistent with feline heartworm disease.[19] In experimental infection of cats with third-stage heartworm larvae, most cats had peripheral caudal pulmonary arterial enlargement by 5 months postinfection, but at 9 months postinfection, there was resolution of the peripheral pulmonary arterial enlargement in greater than 50 percent of the cats.[20] Another important aspect of that study was persistent bronchial-interstitial lung opacification, appearing similar to feline allergic lung disease, after vascular changes had resolved.[20] Thus, heartworm disease

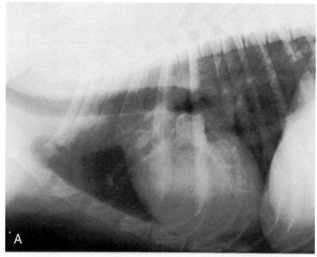

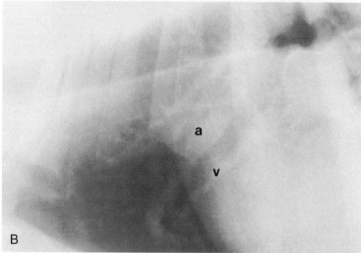

FIGURE 31–6. *A,* Lateral view of the thorax of a 7-year-old male English setter. Note the enlarged right cranial lobar artery relative to the right cranial lobar vein. Diagnosis was heartworm disease. *B,* A close-up view illustrates the size differential between the artery (a) and the vein (v).

should be considered in cats with radiographic evidence of bronchial-interstitial lung opacification even though cardiovascular evidence of heartworm disease is not present.[20]

Other changes with canine heartworm disease that may be used to differentiate it from other diseases are pulmonary artery tortuosity (Fig. 31–9; see also Fig. 31–7), loss of normal tapering (pruning) (see Figs. 31–7 through 31–9), and foci of increased lung opacity along the course of the caudal lobar arteries on the lateral view (Fig. 31–10).[12, 13] The foci of increased opacity in the caudal lobes were present 6 months after experimental infection with L_3 larvae and were still evident 12 months after treatment (Fig. 31–11). These lesions represent peripheral pulmonary arteries with dilation, diverticulations, and tortuosity.[13] Fibrous connective tissue and chronic inflammatory cells may also persist in the arterial wall and perivascular tissue.

Heartworm disease is also the most common cause of thromboembolic disease in that there is arterial occlusion by worm emboli or clots (Fig. 31–12).[12] Pulmonary emboli in heartworm disease have been described as round, irregular, semiopaque pulmonary infiltrates with hazy borders.[11] Pulmonary infarction in heartworm disease is rare.[15, 21]

Pulmonary thrombosis or thromboembolism owing to causes other than dirofilariasis may be associated with normal to reduced lung volume with lobar hyperlucency, re-

duced size of peripheral lung vessels in affected areas, pleural effusion, right ventricular enlargement, and absence of consolidations, atelectasis, or edema commensurate with the severity of the clinical signs.[16] In another report, the radiographic changes included alveolar disease, hyperlucency of a lung lobe or lung region (hypovascular), and pleural effusion, especially with infarction or cardiac disease.[6] In those instances with hyperlucency of a lung lobe or lung region, the major artery (11 instances) or major vein (14 instances) could not be identified or was abruptly attenuated. It is

Table 31–3

DISEASES THAT MAY INCREASE THE SIZE OF PULMONARY VEINS

Cardiac

Volume overload
  Mitral insufficiency
  Early left-to-right shunts—
    thinner wall of vein dilated
    more easily
    Patent ductus arteriosus
    Ventricular septal defect
Primary myocardial disease
  Myocardial failure

Dilatory cardiomyopathy
Diastolic compliance failure
  Hypertrophic
    cardiomyopathy
  Restrictive cardiomyopathy

Noncardiac

Left atrial obstruction
  Neoplasm
  Thrombosis

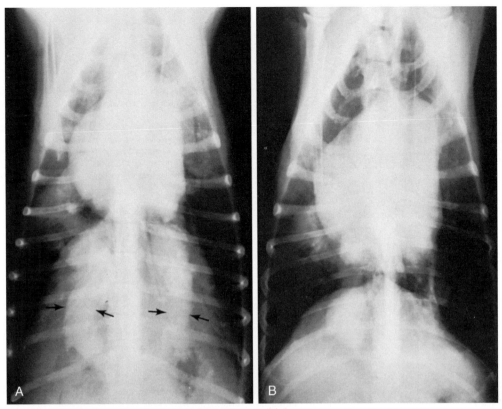

FIGURE 31–7. Dorsoventral (A) and ventrodorsal (B) radiographs of a 4-year-old male German shepherd with heartworm disease. The right and left caudal lobar pulmonary arteries are severely enlarged (arrows), lack the normal uniform tapering (pruning), and are blunted (truncated) at their most distal aspect. Both views show main pulmonary artery enlargement. There is severe tortuosity of the right caudal lobar artery. Note the enhanced visualization of these vessels in the dorsoventral view (A).

important to remember, however, that many patients with pulmonary thromboembolism do not have radiographic changes highly suggestive of arterial occlusion, and definitive diagnosis may require nuclear perfusion scintigraphy or pulmonary angiography.

Table 31–3 outlines the differential diagnoses for pulmonary venous enlargement (Fig. 31–13).[5, 22] Most causes are associated with cardiac disease. Pulmonary venous enlargement is seen most commonly in mitral insufficiency in dogs, dilatory cardiomyopathy in Doberman pinschers, and hypertrophic cardiomyopathy in cats. The incidence of these disease entities has been reported.[23, 24] The radiographic changes associated with cardiac disease are described in Chapter 30.

Table 31–4 is a list of diseases associated with a decrease in size of pulmonary arteries and pulmonary veins.[1] The lung field appears hyperlucent, which results from the pulmonary arteries and veins contributing less soft-tissue opacity to the lung parenchyma because of their reduction in size (Fig. 31–14).

Table 31–4
DISEASES THAT MAY DECREASE THE SIZE OF PULMONARY ARTERIES AND VEINS

Right-to-left shunts
   Tetralogy of Fallot
   Ventricular septal defect with pulmonic stenosis
   Atrial septal defect with pulmonic stenosis
Severe pulmonic stenosis
Hypovolemia
   Shock
   Dehydration
Adrenocortical hypofunction

Shape

Shape changes are most commonly seen in dogs with heartworm disease. With dirofilariasis, in addition to an increase in size of the pulmonary arteries, there may be vascular

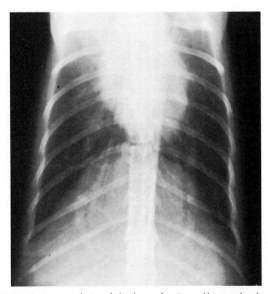

FIGURE 31–8. Dorsoventral view of the thorax of a 3-year-old castrated male domestic shorthaired cat. Note the increase in the size of the caudal lobar arteries and abrupt tapering of the distal portions of the caudal lobar arteries. Enlargement of the main pulmonary artery is not seen; this is common in feline heartworm disease. Six adult heartworms were found at necropsy.

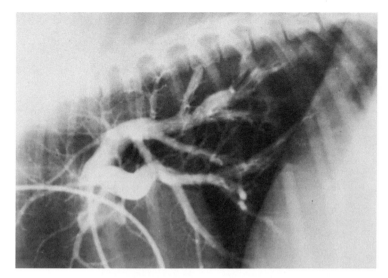

FIGURE 31–9. Lateral pulmonary arteriogram of a mixed-breed dog 12 months after experimental infection with third-stage heartworm larvae. Note the tortuosity of the pulmonary arteries, linear filling defects (adult heartworms), nonuniform arterial tapering, and saccular dilations of the smaller intralobar arteries. Contrast medium was not seen more distally in the caudal lobar arteries on subsequent radiographic examinations, indicative of pulmonary arterial obstruction. (From Rawlings CA, Lewis RE, and McCall JW: Development and resolution of pulmonary arteriographic lesions in heartworm disease. J Am Anim Hosp Assoc 16:17, 1980; with permission.)

FIGURE 31–10. Close-up lateral radiograph of the dorsocaudal lung field of a 4-year-old mixed-breed, neutered female dog. Note the increased dorsocaudal lung opacity. This increased opacity is due to caudal lobar pulmonary arterial enlargement, saccular diverticulations of small arteries, and associated lung disease. The dorsoventral view may be used to confirm that this opacity represents abnormal caudal lobar arteries.

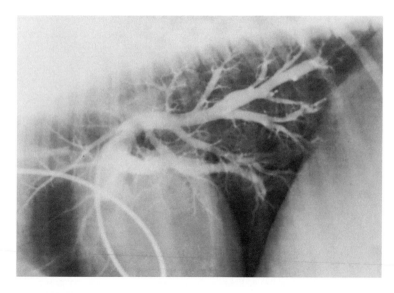

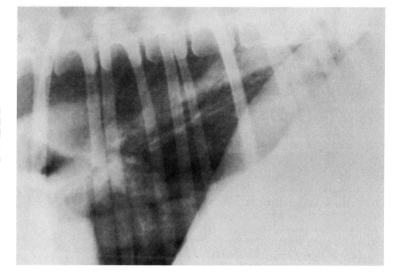

FIGURE 31–11. Lateral pulmonary arteriogram of a mixed-breed male dog 12 months after treatment of heartworm disease. Slight arterial enlargement, saccular dilations of the intralobar arteries, and minimal tortuosity remain. (From Rawlings CA, Lewis RE, and McCall JW: Development and resolution of pulmonary arteriographic lesions in heartworm disease. J Am Anim Hosp Assoc 16:17, 1980; with permission.)

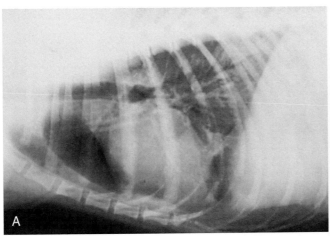

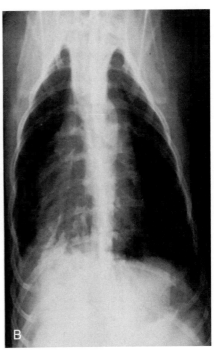

FIGURE 31-12. Lateral (A) and dorsoventral (B) radiographs of a 3-year-old male Siberian husky 1 week after heartworm treatment. The dog was depressed, febrile, and dyspneic. There is alveolar lung disease and decreased volume of the right caudal lung lobe. The heart is displaced slightly to the right owing to the decrease in lung volume. Pleural effusion is present. These radiographic changes represent thromboembolic disease secondary to heartworm therapy.

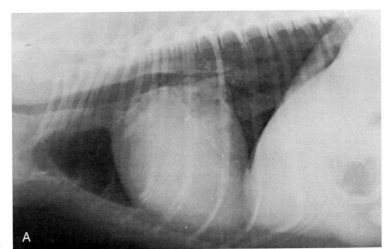

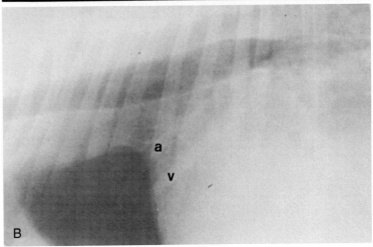

FIGURE 31-13. A, Lateral view of the thorax of an 8-year-old male Poodle. Note the slight pulmonary venous distention—the right cranial lobar vein is larger than the right cranial lobar artery. There is left atrial enlargement. Diagnosis was mitral insufficiency and dysfunction. B, A close-up view of A shows the large right cranial lobar pulmonary vein (v) relative to the artery (a).

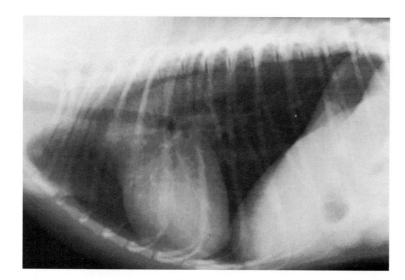

FIGURE 31–14. Lateral view of the thorax of a 9-month-old, neutered female Poodle. Note the lack of opacity in the lung lobes owing to hypovascularity. Tetralogy of Fallot was confirmed at necropsy.

FIGURE 31–15. *A,* Lateral view of the thorax of a 6-year-old male Doberman pinscher. Note the enlargement of the right cranial lobar vein in comparison with the artery. There is loss of margination of the vasculature and increased lung parenchymal opacity owing to heart failure with pulmonary edema. *B,* A close-up view shows the enlarged cranial lobar pulmonary vein *(arrows)* with loss of distinct margination. Diagnosis was dilatory cardiomyopathy with left-sided heart failure.

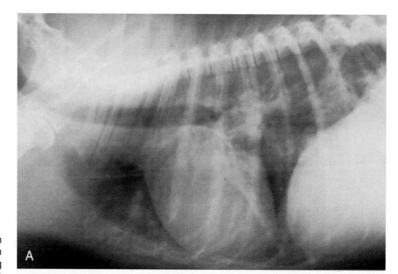

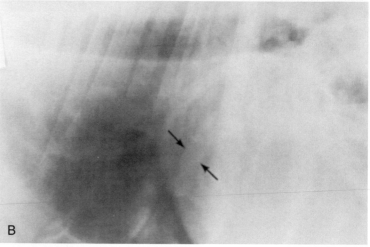

tortuosity (see Figs. 31–7, 31–9, and 31–11), nonuniform tapering from the midportion of the artery distally (see Figs. 31–7 and 31–8), and dilation of smaller arterial branches. These changes may be seen on survey thoracic radiographs, but they are best documented by pulmonary angiography. On survey radiographs of 200 dogs with spontaneous heartworm disease, only 16.5 percent were identified as having tortuous arteries (author's unpublished data). In that study, radiographs of dogs in left lateral recumbency and dorsal recumbency were evaluated. In radiographs made with the animal in ventral recumbency, the caudal lobar arteries are better visualized (see Fig. 31–7).[3] Shape changes with heartworm disease are seen early in the disease and often involve caudal lobar arteries, although they may also be seen in the remaining peripheral arteries.[12–14, 17] Rapid peripheral arterial tapering and focal saccular dilations may occur with any disease that produces pulmonary arterial thrombosis or thromboembolism, but the incidence of occurrence is greater in heartworm disease.

Margination

Loss of pulmonary vessel margins can be focal, multifocal, diffuse, symmetric, or asymmetric (Fig. 31–15). Soft-tissue opaque material (fluid, cells, or debris) in the interstitium or alveoli adjacent to a pulmonary vessel silhouettes with the vessel and obscures its margins.

Radiopacity Changes

The pulmonary arteries and veins are the most prominent structures of the lungs.[1] Therefore, these vessels contribute more opacity to the normal lung parenchyma than any other structures. It is difficult to describe what normal lung opacity should be. Incorrect technical exposures present problems in that underexposed radiographs may create artificial lung opacities, whereas overexposed radiographs may mask increases in lung opacity. Phase of respiration may also alter the opacity of the lung parenchyma. Radiographs made during expiration increase the background lung opacity, whereas those made during inspiration result in less background opacity. Often, there is more lung opacity in older animals because of interstitial fibrosis.[25]

All diseases that produce an increase in size of pulmonary arteries, pulmonary veins, or both increase the opacity of the lung (see Figs. 31–5, 31–10, and 31–15). Abnormalities that result in a decrease in size of pulmonary arteries and veins (see Table 31–4) also decrease lung opacity (see Fig. 31–14). Lobar or sublobar hyperlucency owing to the reduced size of lung vessels (hypoperfusion) has been reported in pulmonary thromboembolism.[9] In another report, loss of visualization of a lobar artery or vein in a lung lobe with pulmonary thrombosis or embolism was mentioned.[6]

Functional Changes

Functional changes involving the pulmonary vasculature may be documented by pulmonary angiography or nuclear scintigraphy. Pulmonary thromboembolic disease occurs when the pulmonary arterial blood flow to a portion of the lung is interrupted by thrombosis or embolism.[26] The occlusion of a pulmonary artery may result in ischemia, hemor-

rhage, or infarction.[6] Loss of surfactant in the occluded lung may result in atelectasis and edema, but hemorrhage, edema, and infarction may have identical radiographic patterns.[6] Pulmonary infarction implies parenchymal necrosis resulting from pulmonary vascular obstruction.[26] Pulmonary infarction is unusual in dogs and cats because of their abundant bronchial arterial supply and the lack of fibrous intralobar septa.

Thromboembolic or primary thrombotic causes listed in Table 31–2 are capable of producing functional pulmonary arterial occlusive diseases. The pulmonary angiogram may show intraluminal filling defects in the artery with compromised blood flow, or total obstruction may be revealed (see Fig. 31–9). Pulmonary thromboembolism occurs most frequently in canine heartworm disease (see Fig. 31–12).

References

1. Ettinger SJ, and Suter PF: Radiographic examination. *In* Canine Cardiology. Philadelphia, WB Saunders, 1970, pp 40–101.
2. Evans HE, and Christensen GC: The respiratory apparatus. *In* Miller's Anatomy of the Dog. Philadelphia, WB Saunders, 1979, p 541.
3. Ruehl WW, and Thrall DE: The effect of dorsal versus ventral recumbency on the radiographic appearance of the canine thorax. Vet Radiol 22:10, 1981.
4. Suter PF: Principles of respiratory function and disease: Normal radiographic anatomy as a basis for a systemic interpretation of diseases of the thorax. *In* Scientific Presentations and Seminar Synopses: 41st Annual Meeting of the American Animal Hospital Association, San Francisco, 1974, pp 707–715.
5. Thrall DE, and Losonsky JM: A method for evaluating canine pulmonary circulatory dynamics from survey radiographs. J Am Anim Hosp Assoc 12:457, 1976.
6. Fluckiger MA, and Gomez JA: Radiographic findings in dogs with spontaneous pulmonary thrombosis or embolism (PTE). Vet Radiol 25:124, 1984.
7. Losonsky JM, Thrall DE, and Prestwood AK: Radiographic evaluation of pulmonary abnormalities after *Aelurostrongylus* inoculation in cats. Am J Vet Res 44:478, 1983.
8. Prestwood AK, Green CE, Mahaffey EA, et al: Experimental canine angiostrongylosis: I. Pathological manifestations. J Am Anim Hosp Assoc 17:491, 1981.
9. Suter PF: Miscellaneous diseases of the thorax. *In* Ettinger SJ (Ed): Textbook of Veterinary Internal Medicine: Diseases of the Dog and Cat. Philadelphia, WB Saunders, 1983, pp 887–890.
10. Ettinger SJ, and Suter PF: Cor pulmonale. *In* Canine Cardiology. Philadelphia, WB Saunders, 1970, pp 425–428.
11. Jackson WF: Radiographic examination of the heartworm-infected patient. J Am Vet Med Assoc 154:380, 1969.
12. Rawlings CA, Lewis RE, and McCall JW: Development and resolution of pulmonary arteriographic lesions in heartworm disease. J Am Anim Hosp Assoc 16:17, 1980.
13. Rawlings CA, Losonsky JM, Lewis RE, et al: Development and resolution of radiographic lesions in canine heartworm disease. J Am Vet Med Assoc 178:1172, 1981.
14. Losonsky JM, Thrall DE, and Lewis RE: Thoracic radiographic abnormalities in 200 dogs with spontaneous heartworm infestation. Vet Radiol 24:120, 1983.
15. Liu SK, Yarns DA, Carmichael JA, et al: Pulmonary collateral circulation in canine dirofilariasis. Am J Vet Res 30:1723, 1960.
16. Tashjian RJ, Liu SK, Yarns DA, et al: Angiocardiography in canine heartworm disease. J Vet Res 31:415, 1970.
17. Thrall DE, Badertscher RR, Lewis RE, et al: Radiographic changes associated with developing dirofilariasis in experimentally infected dogs. Am J Vet Res 41:81, 1980.
18. Schafer M, Berry CR: Cardiac and pulmonary mensuration in feline heartworm disease. Vet Radiol Ultrasound 36:499, 1995.
19. Donahoe JM, Kneller SK, and Lewis RE: In vivo pulmonary arteriography in cats infected with *Dirofilaria immitis*: Pulmonary arteriography in cats infected with *Dirofilaria immitis*. J Am Vet Radiol Soc 17:147, 1976.
20. Selcer BA, Newell SM, Mensour AE, et al: Radiographic and 2-D echocardiographic findings in 18 cats experimentally exposed to *D. immitis* via mosquito bites. Vet Radiol Ultrasound 37:37, 1996.
21. Thrall DE, Badertscher RR, Lewis RE, et al: Collateral pulmonary circulation in dogs experimentally infected with *Dirofilaria immitis*. Vet Radiol 21:131, 1980.
22. Kittleson M: Concepts and therapeutic strategies in the management of

heart failure. *In* Kirk RW (Ed): Current Veterinary Therapy VIII. Philadelphia, WB Saunders, 1983, pp 279–284.

23. O'Grady MR: Acquired valvular heart disease. *In* Ettinger SJ, Feldman EC (Eds): Textbook of Veterinary Internal Medicine: Diseases of the Dog and Cat, 4th Ed. Philadelphia, WB Saunders, 1995, pp 944–958.

24. Sisson DD, and Thomas WP: Myocardial diseases. *In* Ettinger SJ, Feldman

EC (Eds): Textbook of Veterinary Internal Medicine: Diseases of the Dog and Cat, 4th Ed. Philadelphia, WB Saunders, 1995, pp 996–1017.

25. Reif JS, and Rhodes WH: The lungs of aged dogs: A radiographic-morphologic correlation. J Am Vet Radiol Soc 7:5, 1966.

26. Fraser RG, and Paré JP: Diagnosis of Diseases of the Chest. Philadelphia, WB Saunders, 1970.

STUDY QUESTIONS

1. This 9-year-old, neutered male mixed-breed dog has a cough and is exercise intolerant. The most accurate roentgen sign description of the left lateral recumbent (Fig. 31–16*A*) and dorsoventral (see Fig. 31–16*B*) thoracic views is:
   A. Pulmonary lobar arterial enlargement.
   B. Pulmonary lobar venous enlargement.
   C. Both pulmonary lobar arterial and venous enlargement.
   D. Normal pulmonary lobar vasculature.

2. This 10-year-old, spayed female German shepherd is exercise intolerant. The most accurate assessment of the left lateral recumbent thoracic radiograph (Fig. 31–17) is:
   A. Right cranial lobar pulmonary artery enlargement.
   B. Right cranial lobar pulmonary vein enlargement.
   C. Normal size of right cranial lobar pulmonary artery and vein.
   D. Enlargement of right cranial lobar pulmonary artery and vein.

3. This 6-month-old, male Bloodhound tires easily and has a holosystolic heart murmur most prominent in the cranioventral right thorax. The most accurate assessment of this dorsoventral thoracic radiograph (Fig. 31–18) is:
   A. Enlarged caudal lobar pulmonary arteries.
   B. Enlarged caudal lobar pulmonary veins.
   C. Enlarged caudal lobar pulmonary arteries and veins.

4. The most common cause of pulmonary arterial enlargement is:
   A. Mitral insufficiency.
   B. Pulmonic stenosis.
   C. Heartworm disease.
   D. Patent ductus arteriosus.

5. Pulmonary arteries and veins may be reduced in size with which one of the following?
   A. Heartworm disease.
   B. Severe blood loss (hypovolemia).
   C. *Aelurostrongylus.*

6. Which statement is accurate?
   A. On the lateral thoracic view, the large left pulmonary artery is dorsal to the trachea.
   B. On the lateral thoracic view, the large right pulmonary artery is dorsal to the trachea.

7. On the dorsoventral thoracic view, which statement is correct?
   A. Pulmonary arteries are lateral to pulmonary veins.
   B. Pulmonary veins are lateral to pulmonary arteries.

8. The caudal lobar pulmonary arteries are best visualized on which *one* thoracic radiographic view?
   A. Ventrodorsal thoracic view (patient in dorsal recumbency).

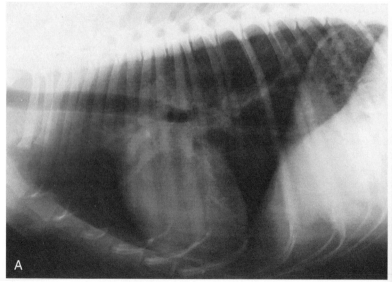

A

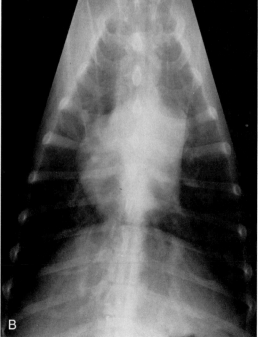

B

FIGURE 31–16

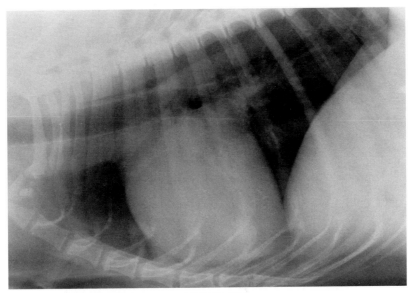

FIGURE 31–17

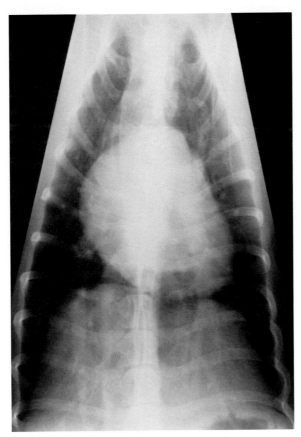

FIGURE 31–18

B. Dorsoventral thoracic view (patient in sternal recumbency).

9. The right cranial lobar pulmonary artery and right cranial lobar pulmonary vein are best visualized and most frequently visualized when the dog or cat is positioned in:
   A. Left lateral recumbency.
   B. Right lateral recumbency.

10. Which *one* of the following disease entities could result in a right cranial lobar pulmonary vein larger in size than the right cranial lobar pulmonary artery?
    A. Pulmonic valvular stenosis.
    B. Pulmonic valvular insufficiency.
    C. Mitral valvular insufficiency.

(Answers appear on page 643.)

Chapter 32

The Canine Lung

Christopher R. Lamb

This chapter describes some of the fundamental aspects of thoracic radiographic technique and normal lung anatomy and some of its variants, and provides guidelines for radiographic diagnosis of lung disease. Although examples of feline lung diseases are not included, the basic principles contained in this chapter pertain to cats as well as dogs.

RADIOGRAPHIC TECHNIQUE

A high-output x-ray machine is important because of the necessity for short exposure times to avoid motion blur associated with breathing. Exposure times of less than 0.05 second generally require at least 200 mAs output. Low-contrast (high kVp–low mAs) techniques are usually advocated for radiography of the thorax because they reduce the relative opacity of the ribs, thereby minimizing interpretive difficulties arising from superimposition of the ribs and intrathoracic structures. In humans, the sensitivity of radiography for pulmonary nodules is higher when high kilovoltages are used.[1] Also, exposure time may be reduced on some machines if a high kVp–low mAs technique is selected.

Thoracic radiographs should be made at the peak of inspiration to maximize the contribution of inhaled air to subject contrast and to ensure consistency (Fig. 32–1). An exception to this rule may be made when a small-volume pneumothorax is suspected, in which instance contrast between the lung and the pleural space may be maximized by obtaining a radiograph at peak expiration.

Methods of positioning dogs for thoracic radiography and the radiographic anatomy of the thorax have been described.[2–4] The author routinely obtains right lateral recumbent and dorsoventral thoracic radiographs of the canine thorax. Rather than advocate specific views, however, the author emphasizes that any particular view provides information principally about the nondependent part of the lung and that there is a corresponding relationship between the view obtained and the location of an observed lesion. For example, a nodule seen on a right lateral recumbent radiograph is usually in the left lung; if a left lateral view is obtained, the lesion may not be visible (Fig. 32–2). This potentially confusing effect is the result of compression of the dependent lung, which expels air and effectively increases lung attenuation and therefore lung opacity. Any difference in attenuation between a soft-tissue nodule and the lung is therefore reduced, often enough to obscure the lung-nodule interface and render the nodule invisible. Conversely, when a nodule is located in the fully aerated, nondependent lung, it has a nodule-lung interface that approximates a soft tissue–gas interface and is therefore readily apparent radiographically. This effect has been discussed in detail elsewhere.[5–8]

When the effect of positioning in dorsal recumbency versus ventral recumbency is considered, an additional effect to be taken into account is geometric distortion because of the diverging primary x-ray beam. This results in magnification of the part of the body closest to the x-ray tube. For this reason, the ventral lung fields are better represented by a ventrodorsal recumbent radiograph than by a dorsoventral

radiograph (Fig. 32–3). Certain other structures, such as the caudal lobe vessels, are seen more clearly on a dorsoventral view.[2, 4]

NORMAL LUNG ANATOMY

Only two components of the canine lung normally contribute to the radiographic image: the large blood vessels and the air. Hence, in an inspiratory radiograph of a normal, healthy dog, the lungs appear as a lucent space through which pulmonary vessels diverge, taper, and branch (Fig. 32–4). Although the position of a bronchus is indicated by the lucent space between two parallel blood vessels, the normal bronchial wall barely contributes to the radiographic image. In certain projections, a normal bronchus may be observed end-on (for example, the right middle lobe bronchus is often seen end-on in a ventrodorsal view), in which instance the wall appears as a distinct but delicate circle flanked by an artery and vein; however, the normal bronchial wall is not visible radiographically when viewed side-on.

Many healthy dogs do have visible bronchial walls because of calcification of the bronchus, which is a clinically insignificant, age-related change that influences the radiographic appearance of the canine lung. Other examples include pleural fibrosis, focal emphysema, interstitial fibrosis, and heterotopic bone formation.[9] The net effect of these changes is a diffuse increase in the lung opacity of old dogs and increased visibility of bronchial walls and pleural surfaces (Fig. 32–5).

Conformation also accounts for some variation in the normal radiographic appearance of the thorax. In brachycephalic or obese dogs, the thoracic wall and mediastinum represent a greater proportion of the total transverse thoracic diameter than in dolichocephalic dogs, so the lung is proportionally smaller, and subject contrast owing to air in the lung is reduced (Fig. 32–6). This effect is in addition to any increase in lung opacity owing to underinflation because of poor conformation of the upper airway, pressure from a distended abdomen, or both, which often occur in brachycephalic dogs.

RADIOLOGY OF LUNG DISEASE

Lung Diseases That Cause Increased Opacity

It is customary to describe the radiographic signs of diffuse lung diseases in terms of four categories that correspond, to some extent, with anatomic divisions of the lung. The four categories of radiographic signs are vascular, bronchial, interstitial, and alveolar.[10] Although this approach (known as pattern recognition) has certain limitations, it is useful because it prompts consideration of each category by the radiologist, thereby acting as a training aid, and because it emphasizes pathoanatomic correlations. Once a radiographic sign is correctly categorized, a preconsidered list of differential diagnoses may be consulted (see Tables 32–1 through 32–6). Hence, pattern recognition encourages logical radiographic interpretation.

One limitation of pattern recognition derives from the fact

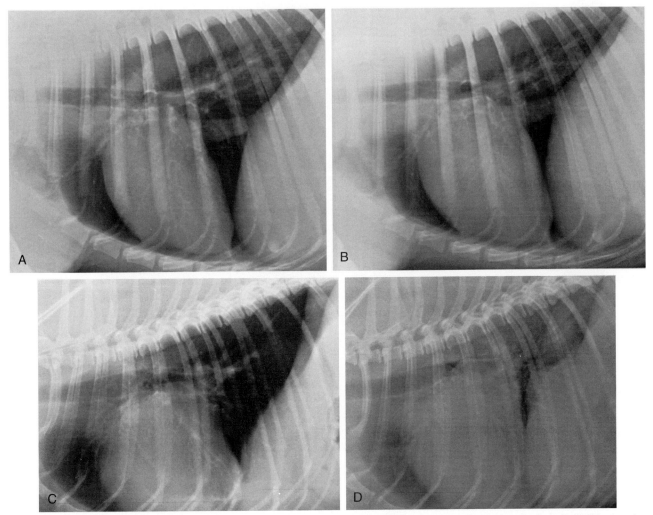

FIGURE 32–1. Examples of the variation in radiographic appearance of the lung in different phases of breathing. *A* and *B*, Recumbent lateral radiographs of a healthy Airedale terrier obtained at peak inspiration *(A)* and peak expiration *(B)*. In expiration, there is cranial displacement of the diaphragm and slightly increased lung opacity. In healthy, deep-chested dogs, these changes are minimal; however, in brachycephalic breeds or dogs with hyperpnea, these differences may be more marked. *C* and *D*, Recumbent lateral radiographs of a hyperpneic Cavalier King Charles spaniel obtained at peak inspiration *(C)* and peak expiration *(D)*. The markedly increased lung opacity in the expiratory radiograph could be misinterpreted as disease, but there is no evidence of pulmonary disease in the inspiratory radiograph. This dog had a cardiac murmur and was radiographed preoperatively as a precaution; the cardiac silhouette is enlarged.

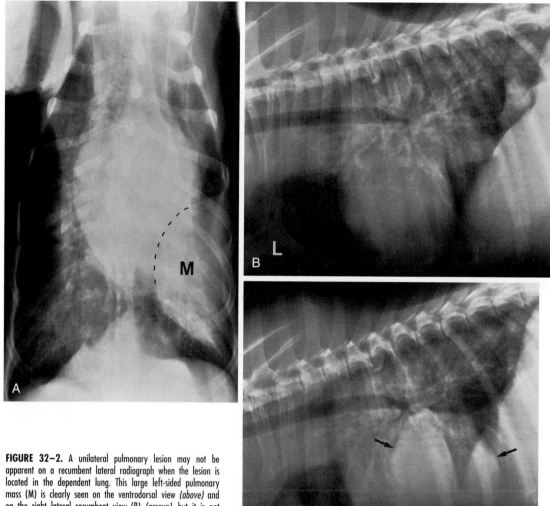

FIGURE 32–2. A unilateral pulmonary lesion may not be apparent on a recumbent lateral radiograph when the lesion is located in the dependent lung. This large left-sided pulmonary mass (M) is clearly seen on the ventrodorsal view *(above)* and on the right lateral recumbent view (R) *(arrows)*, but it is not visible on the left lateral view (L).

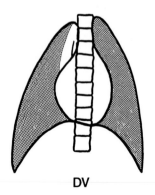
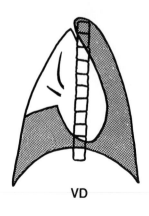

FIGURE 32–3. Lesions in the ventral lung are better seen in ventrodorsal radiographs. The diagram depicts consolidation of the right cranioventral lung as seen in dorsoventral and ventrodorsal radiographs of a large, deep-chested dog. In the dorsoventral view (DV), the lesion is projected close to the midline where it is partially obscured by the heart and spine, whereas in the ventrodorsal view (VD), the lesion is projected away from the midline and is better visualized.

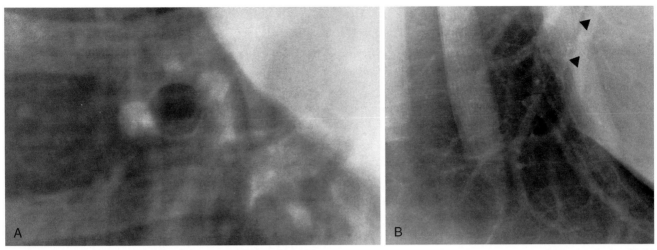

FIGURE 32–4. Close-ups of thoracic radiographs to illustrate the normal appearance of the pulmonary vessels and bronchial wall. *A,* A ventrodorsal view in which the normal right middle lobe artery-bronchus-vein triad can be seen. The bronchus is normally thin walled and has a slightly greater diameter during inspiration than the accompanying blood vessels. *B,* A lateral view in which the cranial lobe vessels are visible. The lucent space between the vessels represents the bronchial lumen; in this dog, the bronchial wall is faintly visible because of calcification *(arrowheads).* In a ventrodorsal or dorsoventral thoracic radiograph, pulmonary arteries are lateral to the corresponding vein, and in a lateral radiograph, pulmonary arteries are dorsal to their respective vein.

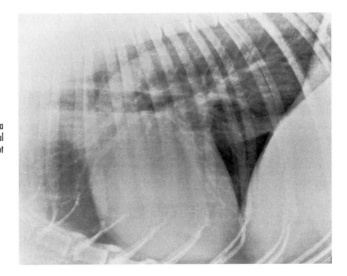

FIGURE 32–5. *Old dog lung.* Left lateral thoracic radiograph of an old retriever in which a mild diffuse increase in lung opacity, owing to a diffuse interstitial pattern and bronchial calcification, can be seen. These signs are typical of age-related pulmonary changes and do not represent clinically significant disease.

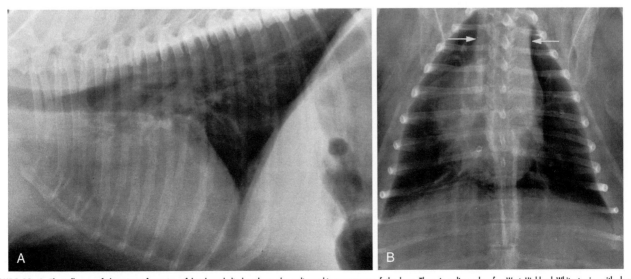

FIGURE 32–6. The influence of thoracic conformation of brachycephalic breeds on the radiographic appearance of the lung. Thoracic radiographs of a West Highland White terrier with dyspnea and exercise intolerance. *A,* In the lateral view, the cranial lung lobes are opaque, and the cranial border of the cardiac silhouette is indistinct. *B,* The cranial lobes are well aerated in the dorsoventral view, but the cranial mediastinum is wide *(arrows)* as a result of fat deposition. The wide mediastinum and relatively narrow cranial lobes account for the appearance of the lateral radiograph, a common finding in brachycephalic or obese dogs.

that the lung can respond in relatively few ways to a wide variety of etiologic factors, so any particular radiographic change is unlikely to be specific for a particular cause. In the instance of interstitial patterns (described subsequently), a wide range of lesions, physiologic factors such as depth of breathing and blood volume, and technical factors may produce radiographic signs that mimic generalized interstitial lung disease. Certain lung diseases may produce mixed radiographic patterns or patterns that change from one type to another over time. Consequently the signalment, history, clinical signs, radiographic techniques used, and sometimes a series of sequential radiographs must all be considered when attempting to diagnose a lung lesion.

Many radiologists routinely ask for information about the signalment and clinical signs when examining radiographs in the belief that this aids interpretation and therefore leads to increased accuracy of diagnosis; however, with respect to thoracic radiographs, there is limited evidence that this is true.[11, 12] An alternative approach involves examination of the radiographs without any knowledge of the patient to avoid distractions and bias. This remains controversial.

Vascular Pattern

Simple visualization of the pulmonary vessels does not constitute a vascular pattern because vessels are normally visible. Changes in vessel diameter, shape, or direction, however, may represent the result of disease. The principal vascular patterns are enlarged vessels and small vessels. Figure 32–7 shows examples of these. A difficulty arises because of the reported wide normal variation in pulmonary vessel size,[13] which prevents the use of measurements for diagnostic guidelines. In extreme instances, recognition of a vascular pattern is relatively straightforward, but within these limits the interpretation of mild changes in expected pulmonary vessel size is subjective. Differences in the relative diameter of artery versus vein are more easily recognized because paired vessels are normally the same size. Artery enlargement may signify pulmonary hypertension, associated with dirofilariasis for example, whereas vein enlargement indicates pulmonary congestion, such as that secondary to mitral regurgitation.

Another effect of changes in pulmonary hemodynamics must be mentioned. If pulmonary blood volume is increased owing to conditions such as venous hypertension and overcirculation, the pulmonary veins may appear enlarged and increased in number in the periphery of the lung, and the overall background opacity of the lung is increased. Conversely, when pulmonary blood volume is decreased owing to causes such as hypovolemia, pulmonary blood vessels appear small and reduced in number, and the lung appears more lucent. Blood in small pulmonary vessels and capillaries is normally an important determinant of lung opacity. This effect must be recognized because increased and decreased pulmonary blood volume can mimic lung infiltration and overinflation, respectively. Further interpretation of abnormalities of the pulmonary vasculature is described in Chapter 31.

Bronchial Pattern

Visualization of the bronchial wall constitutes the bronchial pattern of pulmonary disease. It may result in thickening of the bronchial wall, calcification of the bronchial cartilage, or cellular infiltrate into the peribronchial region.

The critical radiographic sign of a bronchial pattern is a change in the cross-sectional appearance of the bronchus from a thin circle to a thick circle of the same diameter (Fig. 32–8). Increased diameter (with or without thickening of the wall) indicates bronchiectasis. It frequently is simpler to recognize bronchial thickening seen in cross-section than side-on because parallel linear structures on a thoracic radiograph could represent bronchi or vessels. These alternatives may be distinguished by tracing the linear structures peripherally; adjacent arteries and veins diverge in the periphery, whereas bronchial walls converge as the bronchi become progressively smaller.[14] Also, as shown in Figure 32–8, the pattern of branching appears different; vessels produce apparently solitary branches, and bronchi produce paired branches.

Calcification of the bronchial wall causes an increase in opacity but not thickness. It is common in middle-aged and old dogs and is not usually significant.

Thickening of the bronchus is most often associated with chronic inflammation or hypersensitivity. The principal dif-

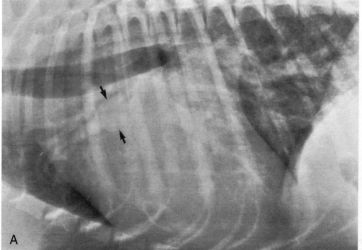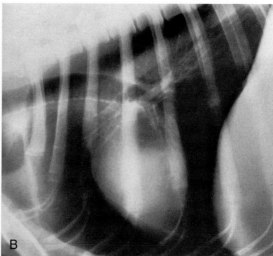

FIGURE 32–7. A, Lateral thoracic radiograph of a young dog with patent ductus arteriosus. The lungs have a diffuse increase in interstitial opacity, most apparent caudally, owing to increased pulmonary blood volume associated with overcirculation. Increased size of blood vessels is sometimes apparent, and in this patient the main pulmonary veins are distended *(arrows)*. B, Lateral thoracic radiograph of a dog with profound hypovolemia. The heart and major pulmonary vessels are small. The lung is hyperlucent because pulmonary blood volume is reduced. Blood in the minor pulmonary vessels and capillaries is normally an important contributor to lung opacity; therefore, in hypovolemia, the lungs appear hyperlucent.

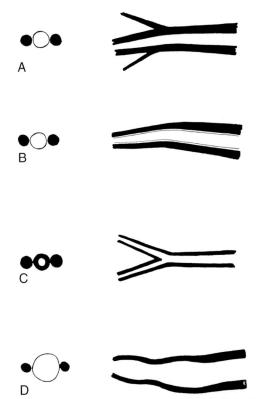

FIGURE 32–8. Variations in the radiographic appearance of the bronchial wall. *A,* In the normal dog, the bronchial wall may be seen end-on as a thin, circular structure between paired vessels but is not visible when viewed side-on. *B,* In many old dogs, calcification of the bronchial cartilage is visible as a thin opaque line paralleling the vessels. *C,* When the bronchial wall is thickened, it appears as a thick ring seen end-on and as a paired branching structure seen side-on. The accompanying blood vessels are normally less apparent radiographically when significant bronchial thickening is present. *D,* Bronchiectasis increases bronchial diameter; a variable bronchial diameter may also be apparent when viewed side-on.

ferential diagnoses for a diffuse bronchial pattern are chronic bronchitis (Fig. 32–9) and pulmonary eosinophilic infiltrates.[15, 16] In some instances, thickening of the peribronchial tissues owing to edema or inflammatory cell infiltrates may

Table 32–1
DIFFERENTIAL DIAGNOSIS OF THE BRONCHIAL PATTERN

Bronchial calcification
Chronic bronchitis
Pulmonary eosinophilic infiltrates
Peribronchial cuffing, e.g., due to edema, bronchopneumonia

mimic a true bronchial pattern. Therefore, peribronchial edema (owing to a variety of acute lung insults) and bronchopneumonia must also be considered (Table 32–1).

Bronchial dilation and loss of the normal tapering and branching space between pulmonary vessel pairs are signs of bronchiectasis (Fig. 32–10).[17] Often, bronchiectasis requires bronchography for confirmation.[18–20]

Interstitial Pattern

Interstitium is the name given to the non–air-containing elements of the lung, excluding the macroscopic blood vessels. The interstitium comprises the alveolar septum, interlobular septum, and microscopic blood vessels. Although detailed classifications of interstitial patterns are available, they may be simply classified as localized or diffuse and nodular or unstructured (Tables 32–2 and 32–3).[21]

Nodular Interstitial Pattern. Pulmonary nodules, clusters of cells that expand and displace the adjacent lung, may be first recognized radiographically when they reach 4 to 5 mm in diameter. Small nodules must be distinguished from pulmonary vessels seen end-on (Fig. 32–11). Pulmonary vessels seen end-on are smaller and less numerous in the periphery of the lung and usually occur close to large vessels. In contrast, lung nodules are not consistently associated with vessels and may be small or large regardless of their location within the lung. Calcification, such as that present in foci of heterotopic bone, enhances visibility of small nodules.

Lung nodules may be solitary or multiple, solid or cavitary (see Table 32–2). The most common solitary nodules in dogs are primary lung tumors, and the most common multiple nodules are pulmonary metastases. The sensitivity of radiography for pulmonary metastasis detection has been estimated as 65 to 97 percent.[7, 22–26] There is evidence that a standard

FIGURE 32–9. Lateral thoracic radiograph of a middle-aged dog with chronic cough attributable to bronchitis. There is a striking bronchial pattern, well seen overlying the heart, as a result of thickening of the bronchial walls.

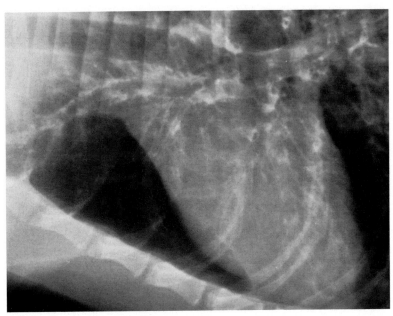

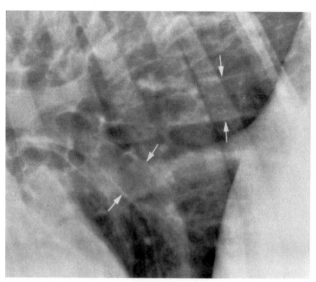

FIGURE 32–10. Close-up of a lateral thoracic radiograph of a 5-year-old female Husky with a history of chronic cough that improved when antibiotics were administered but recurred when medication was discontinued. Endoscopically, there was excessive mucus in the bronchi and evidence of bronchiectasis. This is visible radiographically as loss of the normal tapering of the bronchial walls *(arrows)*. Also the bronchial walls are thickened. Note that the pulmonary vessels are barely visible, a common finding in dogs with severe bronchial disease.

Table 32–2
DIFFERENTIAL DIAGNOSIS OF NODULAR INTERSTITIAL PATTERNS

Noncavitary Nodule

Thoracic wall lesion, e.g., due to skin tumor, tick
Primary lung tumor
Pulmonary metastasis
Granuloma
    Mycotic
    Heartworm associated
    Foreign body
    Eosinophilic (idiopathic)
Fluid-filled bulla
Hematoma
Abscess
Cyst
Mucus-filled bronchus

Cavitary Nodule

Primary lung tumor
Pulmonary metastasis
Mycotic granuloma, e.g., due to blastomycosis
Paragonimiasis
Abscess
Partially fluid-filled lung bulla
Cyst
Bronchiectasis

two-projection thoracic radiographic study (e.g., right lateral and dorsoventral views) is adequate for detection of pulmonary metastasis[26]; however, depending on their position in the lung, lesions can be missed using this approach.[27] Another recommendation, which reflects the importance of detecting metastasis, is to obtain *three* thoracic radiographs (e.g., both left and right lateral and dorsoventral or ventrodorsal views) whenever malignant neoplasia is suspected clinically.

Distinguishing the various causes of pulmonary nodules can be challenging because there is considerable overlap in the appearance of tumors (Fig. 32–12; see Fig. 32–11),[22, 28–31] granulomas (Fig. 32–13),[32–35] and abscesses (Fig. 32–14).[30] The pulmonary lesions of acute paragonimiasis appear radiographically as multiple, 1 to 4 cm in diameter, poorly circum-

scribed nodules; subpleural air-filled cavities and bullae (often septated) develop in chronic infections.[36] Lung cysts and bullae are usually cavitated and thin walled[30, 37] but may be mistaken for solid nodules if fluid filled (Fig. 32–15).[19] Also a fluid-filled or mucus-filled bronchus may be confused with a nodule in some instances (Fig. 32–16).

Unstructured (Hazy) Interstitial Patterns. This category includes a large number of radiographic appearances that share two features: increased lung opacity and obscured, but not obliterated, pulmonary vasculature. The unstructured (hazy) interstitial patterns may include linear (reticular),[38] small nodular (miliary), and reticulonodular components.

A wide variety of causes must be considered when interpretation of a diffuse, hazy interstital pattern is required (see Table 32–3). These include nonpulmonary causes such as

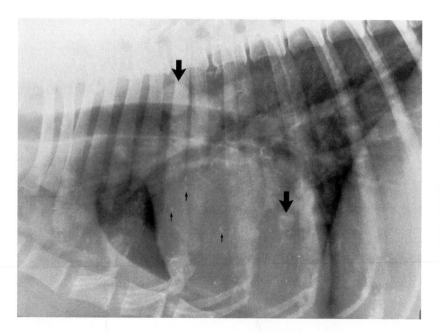

FIGURE 32–11. Lateral thoracic radiograph in which two types of pulmonary nodules are visible. The *large arrows* indicate nodules that are relatively large and spherical and have soft-tissue opacity; these are metastases. The *small arrows* indicate nodules that are small, variably shaped, and more opaque despite their size; these are small foci of heterotopic bone, also known as *pulmonary osseous metaplasia*, which is often found in older dogs. This finding is not clinically significant. If a small pulmonary nodule appears more opaque than a large one, it must be thicker or calcified. Pulmonary vessels viewed end-on are essentially thicker than soft-tissue nodules of the same diameter, so they are more opaque. Heterotopic bone is distinguished from vessels by its variable shape and presence in peripheral parts of the lung where vessels are too small to be seen radiographically.

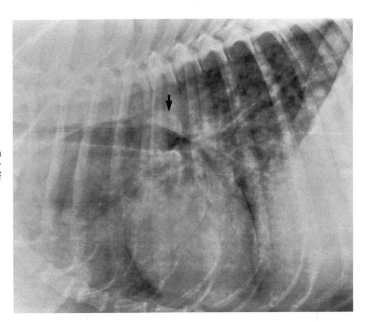

FIGURE 32–12. Lateral thoracic radiograph of a dog with multicentric lymphosarcoma in which diffuse, moderate-to-severe interstitial infiltrate, which includes a small nodular component, can be seen. The caudal trachea appears narrow, probably because of compression by adjacent lymphadenopathy *(arrow)*.

artifact, physiologic variant, and systemic disease. In some patients, knowledge of the history and clinical signs aids interpretation. For example, trauma, near-drowning,[39] and smoke inhalation[40] may produce similar diffuse, hazy interstitial patterns but are readily diagnosed on the basis of the history.

Certain localized, unstructured interstitial patterns may also reflect bronchial disease. For example, bronchial foreign bodies are sometimes diagnosed by the interstitial infiltrate they stimulate around the bronchus rather than by their direct visualization (Fig. 32–17).[41] The right caudal lobe is the most common site of bronchial foreign bodies in dogs. Bronchoesophageal fistula may produce similar signs of localized interstitial infiltrate; diagnosis is based on the results of an esophagram.[42]

Some diseases may produce either nodular or hazy interstitial patterns depending on factors such as duration and severity. Examples include mycotic pneumonia (Fig. 32–18),[32, 35, 43, 44] metastatic neoplasia,[22, 29] and dirofilariasis.[33, 45, 46]

Alveolar Pattern

The alveolar pattern is a radiographic sign of diseases that displace air from the distal air spaces of the lung (and hence it is also referred to as the *air space pattern*). Lung collapse and atelectasis, fluid accumulation, and cellular infiltrates (or combinations of these) may produce alveolar patterns. The radiographic signs of distal air space disease are a relatively homogeneous increase in lung opacity and the air bronchogram.[47] Air bronchograms represent air in the bronchial lumen, surrounded by a relatively homogeneous increase in lung opacity; the bronchial wall itself is not seen (Fig. 32–19). When the bronchus is filled with fluid, cells, or both, the entire affected lobe may appear homogeneous and must be distinguished from a mass.

The distribution of an alveolar pattern may be patchy or diffuse and may change relatively quickly, particularly with fluid accumulations. Changes in the severity and distribution of fluid in the distal air spaces tend to occur more quickly than movements of cellular infiltrates. A time lag between the onset of clinical signs and the radiographic signs of distal air space disease is often observed, and a similar time lag may occur during healing so that in the instance of consolidating bronchopneumonia, the radiographic lesion may persist for several days despite obvious clinical improvement.

The principal differential diagnoses for the alveolar pattern in dogs are summarized in Table 32–4. The two most common causes are pulmonary edema owing to left-sided cardiac decompensation, which typically causes symmetric infiltration of the caudodorsal part of the lung, and bacterial bron-

Table 32–3
DIFFERENTIAL DIAGNOSIS OF UNSTRUCTURED (HAZY) INTERSTITIAL PATTERNS

Diffuse

Artifact
    Underexposure
    End-expiratory exposure
Old dog lung
Lymphosarcoma
Diffuse pulmonary metastasis
Pneumonitis
    Viral—distemper
    Parasitic—*Dirofilaria immitis*
    Metabolic—uremia, pancreatitis, septicemia
    Inhalant—allergy, smoke
    Toxic—paraquat
Disease in transition
    Edema
    Bronchopneumonia
    Hemorrhage

Localized

Partial lung collapse
Contusion
Hemorrhage
Pulmonary embolism
Bronchial foreign body
Disease in transition
    Bronchopneumonia
    Hemorrhage
    Dirofilariasis
    Edema

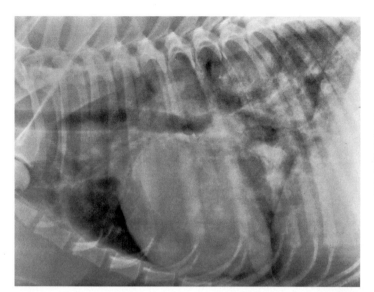

FIGURE 32–13. Lateral thoracic radiograph of an 18-month-old retriever with cough and exercise intolerance. There are several large pulmonary nodules and a moderate interstitial infiltrate, mainly in the dorsal lung fields. The caudal trachea is slightly narrow, compatible with compression by enlarged tracheobronchial lymph nodes. There is enlargement of the right ventricle. Clinicopathologic tests supported heartworm disease, and the pulmonary lesions resolved after treatment with anthelmintics. Final diagnosis was heartworm-associated eosinophilic pneumonitis.

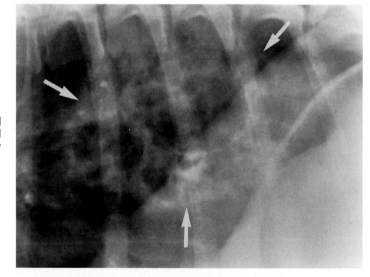

FIGURE 32–14. Close-up of the caudodorsal lung field, in which a poorly marginated cavitated lung mass *(arrows)* can be seen. Primary lung tumor was suspected, and lobectomy was performed. Histologic examination, however, indicated abscess secondary to septic pulmonary infarction.

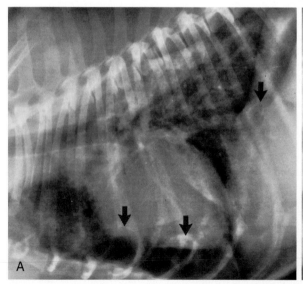
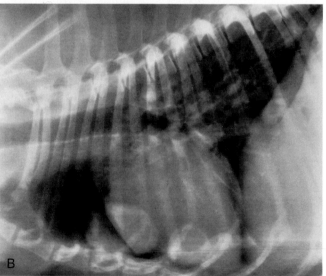

FIGURE 32–15. *A,* Lateral thoracic radiograph of a terrier-cross dog hit by a car about 1 hour previously. The lucent space between the heart and the sternum indicates pneumothorax, and there is a moderate, diffuse interstitial pattern consistent with lung contusion, partial collapse, or both. Close inspection also reveals small gas-filled traumatic lung bullae *(arrows). B,* Repeat radiograph 24 hours later shows resolution of pneumothorax and interstitial pattern. The bullae are partially filled with fluid (probably blood) and now appear as sharply defined, round nodules. At this stage, they may be misinterpreted as other types of pulmonary nodule; however, the history of recent thoracic trauma, the progression from gas-filled to gas and fluid–filled state, and the peripheral location are typical of traumatic lung bullae.

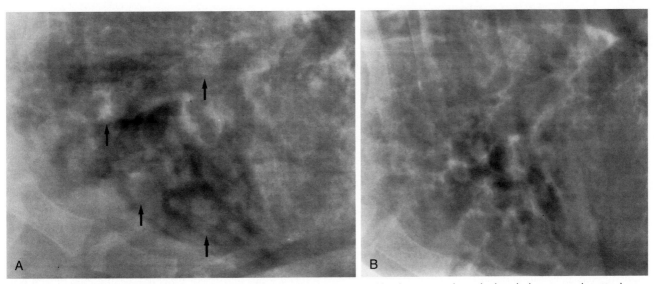

FIGURE 32–16. Close-up of the cranioventral thorax of a dog with chronic recurrent bronchopneumonia and bronchiectasis. *A,* In the initial radiograph, there are several opacities that appear similar to pulmonary nodules *(arrows). B,* In a repeat radiograph of the same area of lung obtained the following day, the nodules have disappeared. Gas-filled, sacculated branching structures consistent with bronchiectasis are now apparent. When interpreting an apparent pulmonary nodule in a dog with chronic airway disease, the possibility that the nodule represents a mucus-filled bronchus should be considered.

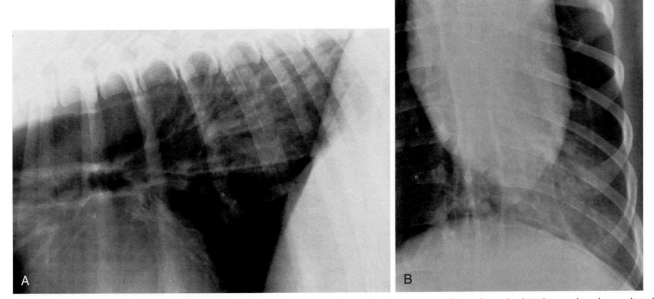

FIGURE 32–17. A 2-year-old male retriever had a chronic persistent cough for several weeks and then developed hemoptysis. Lateral *(A)* and ventrodorsal *(B)* thoracic radiographs were obtained. A marked localized interstitial infiltrate, which obscures the pulmonary vessels, is present in the left caudal lobe. The intensity of the opacity is great and borders on being classified as alveolar in nature. A wheat ear was found lodged in the left caudal lobe bronchus and was removed endoscopically. Opaque bronchial foreign bodies may be visible radiographically but most are nonopaque and are detected only because of the infiltrate that develops around the affected bronchus. When this dog was reradiographed 2 weeks later, the pulmonary infiltrate had resolved. Radiographs were made with the patient under anesthesia; this resulted in the esophagus being dilated and gas filled.

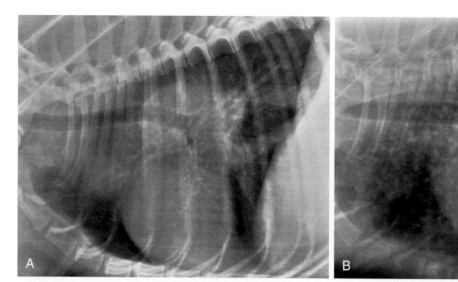

FIGURE 32–18. A, Lateral thoracic radiograph of a dog with cryptococcosis in which a mild diffuse, hazy interstitial pattern and enlarged tracheobronchial lymph nodes can be seen. B, Micronodular interstitial pattern owing to blastomycosis. When so many small nodules are present, the superimposition leads to coalescence of opacities that obscures underlying pulmonary structures.

chopneumonia, which usually has a ventral, often asymmetric, distribution (see Fig. 32–19). Pulmonary hemorrhage may also cause an alveolar pattern. The distribution of pulmonary hemorrhage on radiographs is variable depending on the cause. Hemorrhage associated with trauma is often on the same side as the impact, and thoracic wall lesions, such as rib fractures, may be visible radiographically adjacent to the pulmonary lesion. Hemorrhage secondary to coagulopathy (e.g., coumarin rodenticide toxicity) may have a patchy or generalized distribution.[49] Less common causes of diffuse alveolar patterns include upper airway obstruction,[48] electrocution (Fig. 32–20),[50] uremic pneumonitis,[34] and eosinophilic granulomatosis.[33]

Localized alveolar patterns that correspond to the position of individual lung lobes may occur secondary to collapse or atelectasis. The hallmark of lung lobe collapse is reduced volume of the affected lobe, which may produce a mediastinal shift toward the lesion (Fig. 32–21). In many instances, however, pleural fluid collects around the collapsed lobe, and

a mediastinal shift is not observed.[51] Lung lobe torsion is an uncommon cause of lobar collapse and atelectasis in dogs.[19, 52, 53] Typically an alveolar pattern and reduced lobe volume are observed. Abnormal position of the lobar bronchus may also be apparent.

Mixed radiographic patterns composed of two or more of the four patterns described in this section may be encountered when a disease affects different components of the lung simultaneously or is at different stages of development in different locations in the lung. Neoplasia, dirofilariasis, pulmonary eosinophilic infiltrates, hemorrhage (Fig. 32–22), and smoke inhalation (Fig. 32–23) often produce mixed radiographic patterns.

Hyperlucency

Lung hyperlucency may be recognized when the lung appears less opaque than normal, despite careful selection of exposure factors. In addition to reduced lung opacity, the

Text continued on page 382

Table 32–4
DIFFERENTIAL DIAGNOSIS OF ALVEOLAR PATTERNS

Localized

Bronchopneumonia
Edema
Hemorrhage
Primary lung tumor
Pulmonary metastasis
Lung collapse or atelectasis
   Airway obstruction
   Secondary to pleural effusion
   Compression by adjacent lesion
Dirofilariasis
Pulmonary infarct

Diffuse

Severe bronchopneumonia
Severe edema
Hemorrhage
Near-drowning
Smoke inhalation

Table 32–5
DIFFERENTIAL DIAGNOSIS OF LUNG HYPERLUCENCY

Diffuse

Overexposure
Weight loss
Hypovolemia
Overinflation
   Increased tidal volume
   Upper airway obstruction
   Iatrogenic (anesthesia)
Air trapping
Emphysema

Focal

Bulla
   Congenital
   Acquired
Lobar emphysema
Pulmonary embolism

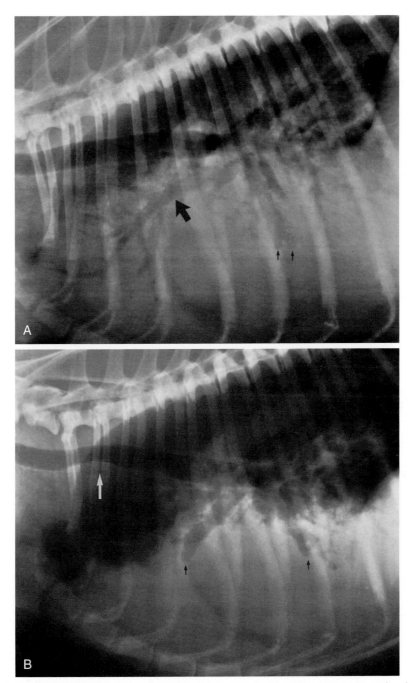

FIGURE 32–19. A 5-year-old Standard Poodle had clinical signs and transtracheal aspirate findings consistent with bronchopneumonia. Treatment with antibiotics, however, produced no sustained improvement. Lateral thoracic radiographs were made with the dog in right lateral recumbency *(A)* and standing with a horizontal x-ray beam *(B)*. In the recumbent lateral radiograph *(A)*, an extensive ventral alveolar pattern and air bronchograms are visible; these are consistent with consolidated bronchopneumonia. The left cranial lobe bronchus *(large arrow)* appears to taper and branch normally, but other bronchi appear dilated and blunt ended *(small arrows)*. This appearance is enhanced in the standing lateral view. Radiographic diagnosis was bronchopneumonia and bronchiectasis. Note the accumulation of mucus in the trachea in the standing lateral view *(white arrow)*.

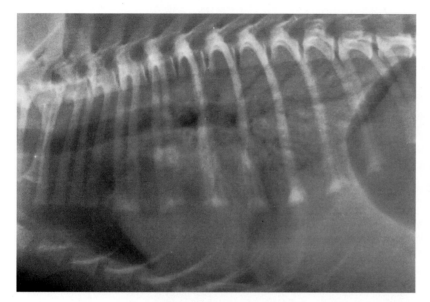

FIGURE 32–20. Lateral thoracic radiograph of a young dog that bit an electric cord. An alveolar pattern with air bronchograms affecting the caudal lobes can be seen. In these instances, electric stimulation of the brain causes a burst of sympathetic nerve discharges, which, in turn, causes acute pulmonary hypertension and pulmonary edema.[50]

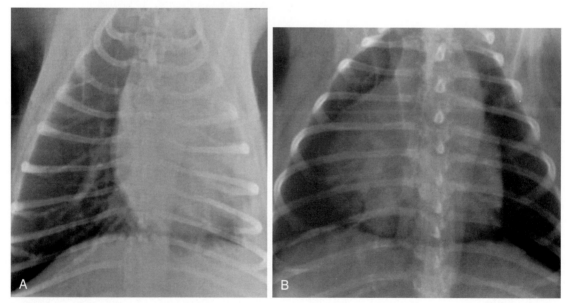

FIGURE 32–21. Example of postural lung collapse in a 5-year-old female Cavalier King Charles spaniel with clinical signs of upper airway obstruction. The pharynx and larynx were examined under anesthesia with the dog in left lateral recumbency. When the thorax was radiographed a few minutes later (dorsoventral, *A*), there was markedly increased opacity of the left lung and mediastinal shift to the left compatible with collapse of the left lung. A repeat dorsoventral radiograph *(B)* of the conscious dog was obtained the following day. The lung has reinflated, and mediastinal structures are in a normal position. No pulmonary lesions are visible. Prolonged lateral recumbency and anesthesia can predispose to postural lung collapse in dogs.

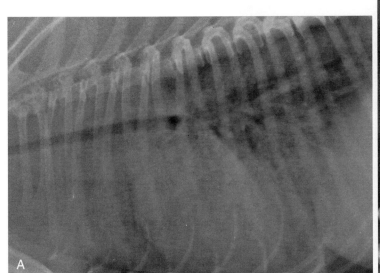
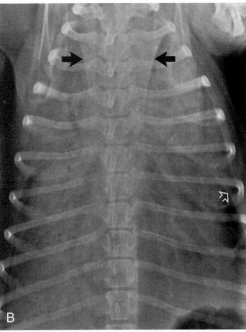

FIGURE 32–22. A 3-year-old female Jack Russell terrier had cough for 2 days then developed pallor, dyspnea, hemoptysis, and melena. In thoracic radiographs (lateral, *A*; dorsoventral, *B*), there is a mixed pulmonary pattern that obscures the cardiac silhouette. The left cranial lobe appears consolidated, and the remainder of the lung has a marked interstitial to alveolar pattern; the pulmonary vessels are most visible in the left caudal lobe indicating that this is the least affected lobe. The tracheal lumen is narrowed as a result of extensive submucosal hemorrhage. Also the cranial mediastinum *(arrows)* and pleural fissures *(open arrow)* appear widened compatible with pleural fluid. The dog died despite treatment. The pathologic diagnosis was pleural, pulmonary, and intestinal hemorrhage compatible with anticoagulant rodenticide toxicity.

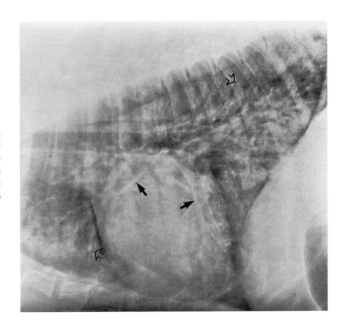

FIGURE 32–23. Lateral thoracic radiograph of a Rottweiler guard dog rescued from a burning warehouse a few hours previously. The dog was in respiratory distress and died a few hours after radiography. This radiograph is an example of a mixed pulmonary pattern with prominent bronchial walls *(closed arrows)*; diffuse, hazy interstitial infiltrate; and peripheral alveolar pattern with air bronchograms *(open arrows)*. These signs are typical of smoke inhalation; the radiographic signs reflect the severe effect of smoke on the bronchial mucosa and surfactant activity that leads to bronchitis, bronchial mucosal and perivascular edema, atelectasis, and alveolar hemorrhage.

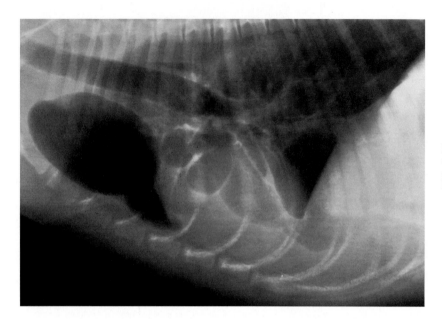

FIGURE 32–24. Lateral thoracic radiograph of a 1-year-old retriever with exercise intolerance and slightly increased respiratory effort. There are several thin-walled, gas-filled bullae in the cranioventral lung field. Final diagnosis was congenital bullous emphysema.

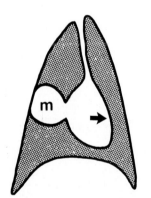
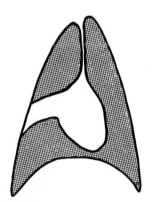
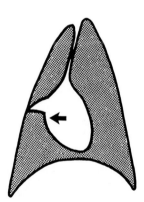

FIGURE 32–25. The principal effect of a lung mass is displacement of adjacent organs, often apparent radiographically as a mediastinal shift away from the lesion. This diagram depicts the effect of a mass (m, *left*), a consolidated right middle lobe that has not changed in volume *(center)*, and a collapsed right middle lobe *(right)*. Note that reduced volume of a lung lobe may produce a mediastinal shift *toward* the lesion, although this effect is often reduced by a redistribution of pleural fluid around the collapsed lobe.[51]

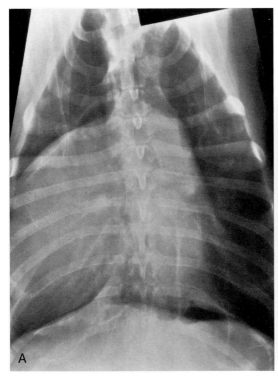

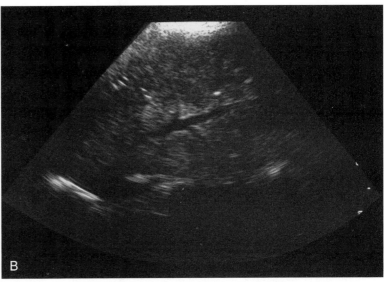

FIGURE 32-26. A 3-year-old female retriever was hit by a car and had a ruptured diaphragm. After surgery to repair this injury, there was persistent pneumothorax and consolidation of the right middle lung lobe. In thoracic radiographs made after referral (ventrodorsal view, *A*), there was an opaque right middle lobe without apparent loss of volume, compatible with consolidation. To define the changes in this lobe better, ultrasonography was performed through an intercostal window *(B)*. The primary bronchus was fluid filled, appearing as an anechoic branching structure (so-called fluid bronchogram). Thoracotomy revealed infarction of the right middle lobe. Although torsion was not present at surgery, torsion secondary to the diaphragmatic rupture was considered to be a likely cause of the infarction. (From Stowater JL, and Lamb CR: Ultrasonography of non-cardiac thoracic diseases in small animals. J Am Vet Med Assoc *195:*514, 1989; with permission.)

FIGURE 32-27. Lateral thoracic radiograph of an old Irish setter presented for lameness evaluation. The radiograph was taken as a routine preanesthetic check, and, unexpectedly, barium was seen in the caudoventral lung. Apparently the dog had a previous upper gastrointestinal study; there was no history of respiratory signs. The location of the barium in this radiograph is typical of aspiration with subsequent translocation to the tracheobronchial lymph nodes *(arrows)*. Most aspirated barium is coughed up within a few minutes; barium uptake by macrophages and migration to regional lymph nodes accounts for a relatively small part of total lung clearance in these patients.

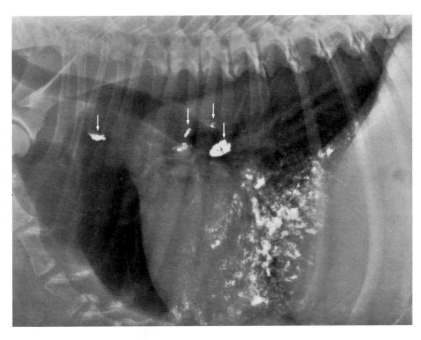

Table 32–6
CALCIFIED LUNG LESIONS

Focal or Multifocal

Bronchial calcification
Heterotopic bone
Granuloma, e.g., due to *Histoplasma*
Osteosarcoma metastasis
Primary lung tumor
Aspirated barium sulfate

Diffuse

Hyperadrenocorticism
Hyperparathyroidism
Chronic uremia
Idiopathic

heart, diaphragm, and ventral aspects of the thoracic vertebrae are sharply defined.

Hyperlucency may be classified as diffuse or focal (Table 32–5). Just as an interstitial infiltrate may be mimicked by underexposure or expiratory exposure, artifactual hyperlucency may be produced by overexposure or overinflation of the lung during anesthesia. Weight loss and hypovolemia also may produce apparent lung hyperlucency by reducing x-ray attenuation in the thoracic wall and lung.

Pathologic causes of lung hyperlucency, such as air trapping or emphysema, may be recognized by concurrent caudal displacement of the diaphragm and the fact that inspiratory and expiratory radiographs appear similar. Causes of focal lung hyperlucency include traumatic lung bulla (see Fig. 32–15), congenital lobar emphysema (Fig. 32–24),[54, 55] and pulmonary thromboembolism.[55]

Pulmonary Mass Lesions

Although the lung nodule was described in the section on interstitial patterns, some additional discussion of mass lesions is required. Lesions that are usefully classified as *masses* are larger than *nodules* and, because of their size, often produce a *mass effect*, that is, displacement of adjacent organs (Fig. 32–25). Unilateral pulmonary masses often cause a mediastinal shift toward the contralateral side. When there is no mass effect and the shape and location of the lesion correspond to a specific lung lobe, consolidation or lobar collapse with local pleural fluid accumulation must also be considered. When these three possibilities cannot be distinguished radiographically, some other imaging study, such as bronchography,[19, 20] ultrasonography (Fig. 32–26),[57] or computed tomography,[58] may be useful.

The differential diagnosis of lung masses is as stated for nodules in Table 32–2. Primary lung neoplasia is the most common cause of a lung mass in dogs.

Calcified Lung Lesions

A variety of lung lesions may calcify.[59, 60] These may be classified as focal or diffuse (Table 32–6). Barium sulfate suspension, which may be deposited in the lung during bronchography or when an upper gastrointestinal contrast study is attempted, may be confused with calcification but is more opaque (Fig. 32–27).

References

1. Kelsey CA, Moseley RD, Mettler FA, et al: Comparison of nodule detection with 70-kVp and 120-kVp chest radiographs. Radiology 143:609, 1982.
2. Ruehl WM, and Thrall DE: The effect of dorsal versus ventral recumbency on the radiographic appearance of the canine thorax. Vet Radiol 22:10, 1981.
3. Spencer CP, Ackerman N, and Burt JK: The canine lateral thoracic radiograph. J Am Vet Radiol Soc 22:262, 1981.
4. Ticer JW: Radiographic Technique in Veterinary Practice, 2nd Ed. Philadelphia, WB Saunders, 1984, pp 275–292.
5. Ahlberg NG, Hoppe F, Kelter U, et al: A computed tomographic study of volume and x-ray attenuation of the lungs of Beagles in various body positions. Vet Radiol 26:43, 1985.
6. Biller DS, and Myer CW: Case examples demonstrating the clinical utility of obtaining both right and left lateral thoracic radiographs in small animals. J Am Anim Hosp Assoc 23:381, 1987.
7. Lang J, Wortman JA, Glickman LT, et al: Sensitivity of radiographic detection of lung metastases in the dog. Vet Radiol 27:74, 1986.
8. Pechman RD: Effect of dependency versus non-dependency on lung lesion visualization. Vet Radiol 28:185, 1987.
9. Reif JS, and Rhodes WH: The lungs of aged dogs: A radiographic-morphologic correlation. J Am Vet Radiol Soc 7:5, 1966.
10. Watters JW: Radiographic signs of pulmonary infiltration. Comp Contin Educ Vet Pract 1:704, 1979.
11. Berbaum KS, Franken EA, Dorfman DD, et al: Influence of clinical history upon detection of nodules and other lesions. Invest Radiol 23:48, 1988.
12. Good BC, Cooperstein LA, DeMarino GB, et al: Does knowledge of the clinical history affect the accuracy of chest radiograph interpretation? Am J Roentgenol 154:709, 1990.
13. Thrall DE, and Losonsky JM: A method for evaluating canine pulmonary circulatory dynamics from survey radiographs. J Am Anim Hosp Assoc 12:457, 1976.
14. Myer CW: Radiography review: The vascular and bronchial patterns of pulmonary disease. Vet Radiol 21:156, 1980.
15. Corcoran BM, Thoday KL, Henfrey JI, et al: Pulmonary infiltration with eosinophils in 14 dogs. J Small Anim Pract 32:494, 1991.
16. Moon M: Pulmonary infiltrates with eosinophilia. J Small Anim Pract 33:19, 1992.
17. Myer CW, and Burt JK: Bronchiectasis in the dog: Its radiographic appearance. J Am Vet Radiol Soc 14:3, 1973.
18. Douglas SW: The interpretation of canine bronchograms. J Am Vet Radiol Soc 15:18, 1974.
19. Walter PA: Non-neoplastic surgical diseases of the lung and pleura. Vet Clin North Am [Small Anim Pract] 17:359, 1987.
20. Webbon PM, and Clarke KW: Bronchography in normal dogs. J Small Anim Pract 18:327, 1977.
21. Myer W: Radiography review: The interstitial pattern of pulmonary disease. Vet Radiol 21:18, 1980.
22. Suter PF, Carrig C, O'Brien TR, et al: Radiographic recognition of primary and metastatic pulmonary neoplasia of dogs and cats. J Am Vet Radiol Soc 15:3, 1974.
23. Tiemessen I: Thoracic metastases of canine mammary gland tumors: A radiographic study. Vet Radiol 30:249, 1989.
24. Holt D, Van Winkle T, Schelling C, et al: Correlation between thoracic radiographs and post mortem findings in dogs with hemangiosarcoma: 77 cases (1984–1989). J Am Vet Med Assoc 200:1535, 1992.
25. Hammer AS, Bailey MQ, and Sagartz JE: Retrospective assessment of thoracic radiographic findings in metastatic canine hemangiosarcoma. Vet Radiol Ultrasound 34:235, 1993.
26. Barthez PY, Hornof WJ, Théon AP, et al: Receiver operating characteristic curve analysis of the performance of various radiographic protocols when screening dogs for pulmonary metastasis. J Am Vet Med Assoc 204:237, 1994.
27. DeHaan CE, Papageorges M, and Kraft SL: Radiographic diagnosis. Vet Radiol Ultrasound 32:75, 1991.
28. Barr FJ, Gibbs C, and Brown PJ: The radiological features of primary lung tumours in the dog: A review of thirty-six cases. J Small Anim Pract 27:493, 1986.
29. Miles KG, Lattimer JC, Jergens AE, et al: A retrospective evaluation of the radiographic evidence of pulmonary metastatic disease on initial presentation in the dog. Vet Radiol 31:79, 1990.
30. Silverman S, Poulos PW, and Suter PF: Cavitary pulmonary lesions in animals. J Am Vet Radiol Soc 17:134, 1976.
31. Shaiken LC, Evans SM, Goldschmidt MH: Radiographic findings in canine malignant histiocytosis. Vet Radiol Ultrasound 32:237, 1991.
32. Ackerman N, and Spencer CP: Radiologic aspects of mycotic diseases. Vet Clin North Am [Small Anim Pract] 12:174, 1982.

33. Calvert CA, Mahaffey MB, Lappin MR, et al: Pulmonary and disseminated eosinophilic granulomatosis in dogs. J Am Anim Hosp Assoc 24:311, 1988.
34. Moon ML, Greenlee PG, and Burk RL: Uremic pneumonitis-like syndrome in ten dogs. J Am Anim Hosp Assoc 22:687, 1986.
35. Walker MA: Thoracic blastomycosis: A review of its radiographic manifestations in 40 dogs. Vet Radiol 22:22, 1981.
36. Pechman RD: The radiographic features of pulmonary paragonimiasis in the dog and cat. J Am Vet Radiol Soc 17:182, 1976.
37. Aron DN, and Kornegay JN: The clinical significance of traumatic lung cysts and associated pulmonary abnormalities in the dog and cat. J Am Anim Hosp Assoc 19:903, 1983.
38. Reif JS, and Rhodes WH: Linear opacities in canine thoracic radiographs. J Am Vet Radiol Soc 9:57, 1968.
39. Farrow CS: Near-drowning in the dog. J Am Vet Radiol Soc 18:6, 1977.
40. Tams TR, and Sherding RG: Smoke inhalation injury. Comp Contin Educ Vet Pract 3:986, 1981.
41. Dobbie GR, Darke PGG, and Head KW: Intrabronchial foreign bodies in dogs. J Small Anim Pract 27:227, 1986.
42. Park RD: Bronchoesophageal fistula in the dog: Literature survey, case presentations, and radiographic manifestations. Comp Contin Educ Vet Pract 6:669, 1984.
43. Burk RL, Corley EA, and Corwin LA: The radiographic appearance of pulmonary histoplasmosis in the dog and cat: A review of 37 case histories. J Am Vet Radiol Soc 19:2, 1978.
44. Millman TM, O'Brien TR, Suter PF, et al: Coccidioidomycosis in the dog: Its radiographic diagnosis. J Am Vet Radiol Soc 20:50, 1979.
45. Ackerman N: Radiographic aspects of heartworm disease. Semin Vet Med Surg 2:15, 1987.
46. Carlisle CH: Canine dirofilariasis: Its radiographic appearance. Vet Radiol 21:123, 1980.
47. Myer W: Radiography review: The alveolar pattern of pulmonary disease. J Am Vet Radiol Soc 20:10, 1979.
48. Kerr LY: Pulmonary edema secondary to upper airway obstruction in the dog: A review of nine cases. J Am Anim Hosp Assoc 25:207, 1989.
49. Berry CR, Gallaway A, Thrall DE, et al: Thoracic radiographic features of anticoagulant rodenticide toxicity in fourteen dogs. Vet Radiol Ultrasound 34:391, 1993.
50. Lord PF: Neurogenic pulmonary edema in the dog. J Am Anim Hosp Assoc 11:778, 1975.
51. Lord PF, and Gomez JA: Lung lobe collapse: Pathophysiology and radiologic significance. Vet Radiol 26:187, 1985.
52. Johnston GR, Feeney DA, O'Brien TD, et al: Recurring lung lobe torsion in three Afghan Hounds. J Am Vet Med Assoc 184:842, 1984.
53. Lord PF, Greiner TP, Greene RW, et al: Lung lobe torsion in the dog. J Am Anim Hosp Assoc 9:473, 1973.
54. Herrtage ME, and Clarke DD: Congenital lobar emphysema in two dogs. J Small Anim Pract 26:453, 1985.
55. Tennant BJ, and Haywood S: Congenital bullous emphysema in a dog: A case report. J Small Anim Pract 28:109, 1987.
56. Fluckiger MA, and Gomez JA: Radiographic findings in dogs with spontaneous pulmonary thrombosis or embolism. Vet Radiol 25:124, 1984.
57. Stowater JL, and Lamb CR: Ultrasonography of non-cardiac thoracic diseases in small animals. J Am Vet Med Assoc 195:514, 1989.
58. Tidwell AS: Diagnostic pulmonary imaging. Prob Vet Med 4:239, 1992.
59. Thrall DE, Goldschmidt MH, Clement RJ, et al: Generalized extensive idiopathic pulmonary ossification in a dog: A case report. Vet Radiol 21:104, 1980.
60. Berry CR, Ackerman N, and Monce K: Pulmonary mineralization in four dogs with Cushing's syndrome. Vet Radiol Ultrasound 35:10, 1994.

STUDY QUESTIONS

1. A large dog has a nodule in the right middle lung lobe. True or false: in a left lateral recumbent radiograph, the nodule is likely to:
   A. Be invisible.
   B. Appear smaller than on a right lateral view.
   C. Be similar in appearance to a right lateral view.

2. List four nonpathologic patient factors that may adversely affect thoracic radiographic quality.

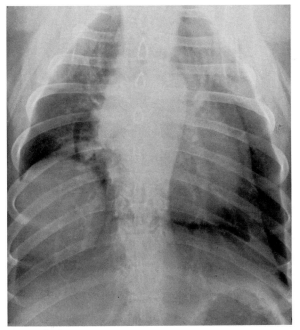

FIGURE 32–28

3. A 5-year-old male Rottweiler was lethargic and had an intermittent cough for 3 weeks. Hematology and serum biochemistry results were within normal ranges. Examine the following dorsoventral thoracic radiograph (Fig. 32–28): Describe the lesion, and list your differential diagnoses.

4. It is normally recommended that thoracic radiographs are exposed at peak inspiration. State an exception to this rule.

5. List three predictable differences in the radiographic appearance of pulmonary nodules and pulmonary blood vessels seen end-on.

6. How might repeating thoracic radiographs within 24 hours aid diagnosis of a pulmonary lesion?

7. Aspiration bronchopneumonia in a dog is likely to be less visible on a dorsoventral thoracic radiograph than a ventrodorsal thoracic radiograph. (True or False)

8. A 9-year-old female German shepherd had a chronic cough and became dyspneic. There was mild pyrexia and neutrophilia. Examine the following thoracic radiographs (Fig. 32–29A and B): Classify the pulmonary pattern. What other relevant radiographic sign is present?

9. Match the following pulmonary lesions with the most appropriate description:
   A. Traumatic pulmonary hemorrhage
   B. Bronchopneumonia

   1. Often produces a mixed radiographic pattern that reflects damage to the bronchi and alveoli

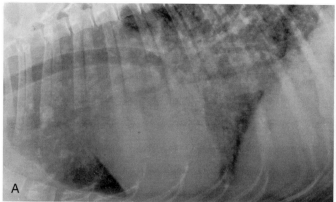

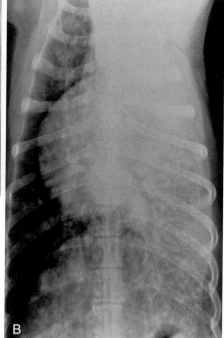

FIGURE 32–29. *A,* Left lateral recumbent. *B,* Dorsoventral.

C. Cardiogenic
   pulmonary edema
D. Smoke inhalation

2. Usually has a bilaterally
   symmetric distribution in
   the caudal lobes
3. Usually affects the ventral
   lung
4. Is often localized and
   asymmetric

10. List five differential diagnoses for pulmonary calcification.

(Answers appear on pages 643 to 644.)

NECK AND THORAX—EQUIDAE

Chapter 33

Larynx, Pharynx, and Proximal Airway

Charles S. Farrow

It is common to evaluate the laryngeal/pharyngeal region radiographically by checking the size, shape, and position of each of its parts against the norm. Using this approach, some patterns emerge in which abnormalities consistently represent a particular disease or disorder, but for the most part diagnoses are based on isolated structural abnormalities. More than structural analysis is required, however, for complete assessment of this anatomic region. Endoscopy has provided valuable functional information. Further, the pharynx, larynx, guttural pouches, and trachea must be conceived of as a functional unit, not merely as individual, unrelated parts. Anatomic abnormalities must be sought and explained in light of observed dysfunction, particularly that which has been witnessed endoscopically. The correlation between radiographic abnormalities and endoscopically observed malfunctions forms the basis for diagnosis in this complex region.

EXAMINATION METHOD

Pharynx and Larynx

The pharynx, larynx, and guttural pouches of the horse are optimally imaged with a single 14 × 17 inch radiograph (Fig.

33–1). The exposure is made with the horse in the standing position, the head held naturally, neither extended nor flexed, with the x-ray beam centered just rostral and slightly dorsal to the mandibular angle. The position of the cassette relative to the right or left side of the head does not influence the appearance of the radiographic image. Likewise, the phase of respiration, either inspiration or expiration, does little to alter regional anatomy.

A ventrodorsal or dorsoventral projection is necessary when evaluating disorders of the guttural pouch in which it is impossible to differentiate right from left and unilateral from bilateral disease. The inherent drawback of this projection is that it requires general anesthesia for optimal radiographic positioning. Oblique projections rarely provide additional information and result in a distorted image.

The position of the horse's head is extremely important. Not only must it be parallel to the cassette and perpendicular to the primary beam, but also it must be in a natural position. If not, the pharynx and guttural pouches appear distorted: elongated and vertically compressed when the head is extended or foreshortened and vertically expanded when flexed. Extension or flexion of the head also causes a reorientation of the soft palate and larynx, in some instances mim-

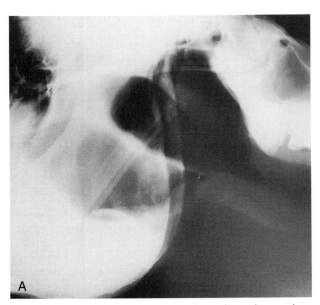
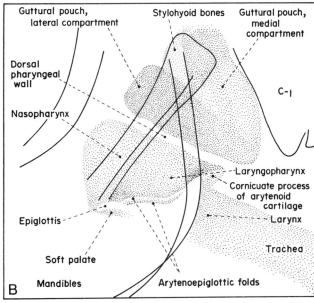

FIGURE 33–1. *A,* Right lateral projection. The normal equine larynx, pharynx, and guttural pouches. *B,* Companion line drawing.

icking disease and in most horses making comparison with radiographic normals difficult and measurement impossible.

Trachea

The cervical trachea requires at least two 14 × 17 or 7 × 17 inch films to be imaged completely, although a single 14 × 17 film images a majority of this organ (Fig. 33–2). The exposures are made with the horse in the standing position. With the exception of obstructive lesions, there is little difference in the relative appearance of inspiratory and expiratory radiographs. A natural head position is not as critical as when the pharyngeal region is being imaged.

Because of the physical and functional relationships of the larynx, pharynx, and guttural pouches, these structures are best imaged collectively on a single film, not as separate images. In so doing, these parts can be visually integrated with their anatomic surroundings: hyoid bones, mandible, cranium, and cranial aspect of the cervical spine.

COMPLEMENTARY EXAMINATIONS

Pharyngography and Esophagography

Pharyngography and esophagography are performed to assess suspected soft palate and epiglottic dysfunction as well as swallowing disorders. This procedure usually differentiates pharyngeal from laryngeal masses and evaluates the ability of the epiglottis to keep ingested material out of the trachea (Fig. 33–3).

Guttural Pouch Opacification

Opacification of one or both guttural pouches with an aqueous iodine solution potentially provides the following information: (1) laterality (right-sided or left-sided involvement), (2) extent (cranial or caudal compartments or both), (3) improved visualization (inner surface), and (4) identification of luminal filling defects (indicative of a mass or mass affect). Additionally, opacification of the guttural pouches establishes

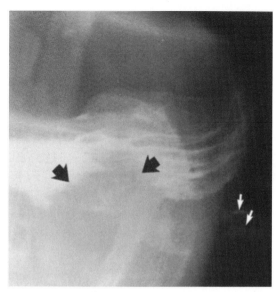

FIGURE 33–3. Laryngogram. There is a large mass ventral to the epiglottis *(large arrows)* and contrast medium within the laryngeal body *(small arrows).*

structural integrity, identifies fistulization, and may be used to verify the location of suitably marked drainage tubes.

APPEARANCE OF LARYNGEAL DISEASE

In terms of what may be specifically identified in a radiographic image, the larynx consists of the epiglottis, the arytenoepiglottic folds, the corniculate process of the arytenoid cartilage, the lateral ventricles, and the body of the larynx. Architectural or spatial alterations to these structures constitute the basis for the radiographic signs of laryngeal disease. These signs include (1) abnormal epiglottic position relative to the soft palate; (2) epiglottic thickening or marginal irregularity; (3) decreased epiglottic size (includes length if measurable); (4) displaced, deformed, indistinct arytenoepiglottic folds or corniculate processes; and (5) laryngeal or paralaryngeal mineralization or gas.[1]

Acute epiglottidis resulting from inflammation or infection typically results in uniform enlargement as observed endoscopically or radiographically.[2] Nasotracheal intubation injury may cause similar changes.[3]

Medium-to-large subepiglottic, epiglottic, and paraepiglottic masses can also be radiographically identified. These lesions, particularly if of the subepiglottic type, may displace the epiglottis in a dorsocaudal direction, effectively increasing the distance between the epiglottis and the soft palate. Unfortunately, it is often not possible to establish the cause of such lesions because of their radiographic similarity. Differential considerations include subepiglottic cyst, granuloma, abscess, and, rarely, tumor (Fig. 33–4).

Inflammation (especially if chronic), postsurgical scarring, and congenital disorders may distort or otherwise alter the appearance of the epiglottic and arytenoid tissues (Figs. 33–5 and 33–6).[4]

Occasionally a primary lesion such as a tumor may occur in one of the arytenoepiglottic folds, causing the proximal part of the larynx to be nearly formless and greatly increased in opacity (Fig. 33–7). Likewise, a paraepiglottic mass or mass affect may distort or obscure the rostral part of the larynx (Fig. 33–8). Paralaryngeal abscessation may occur secondary to laryngeal infection. If fistulation develops, the abscess may

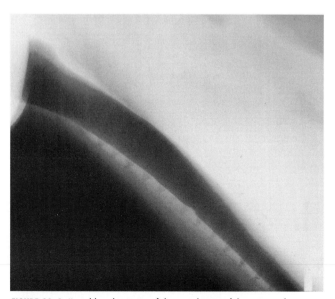

FIGURE 33–2. Normal lateral projection of the cervical region of the equine trachea.

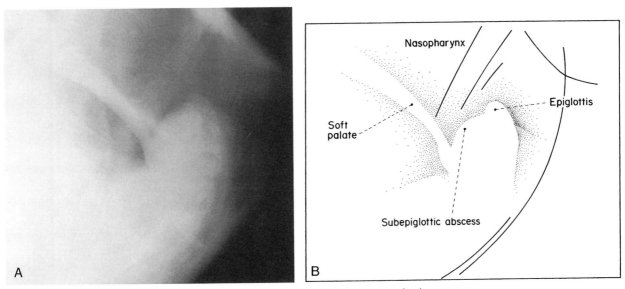

FIGURE 33–4. *A,* Example of a subepiglottic mass, lateral projection. Diagnosis: subepiglottic abscess. *B,* Companion line drawing.

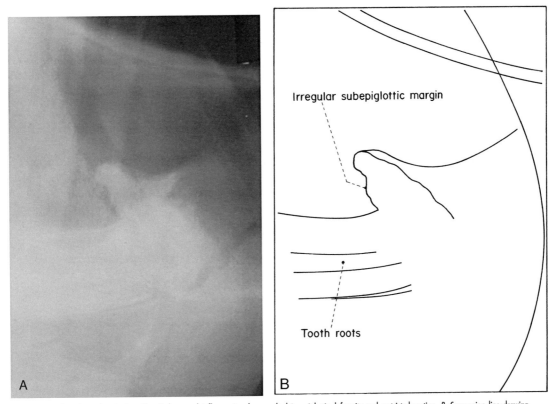

FIGURE 33–5. *A,* Lateral projection. Chronic laryngeal inflammation has resulted in epiglottic deformity and restricted motion. *B,* Companion line drawing.

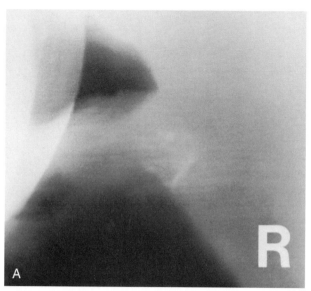
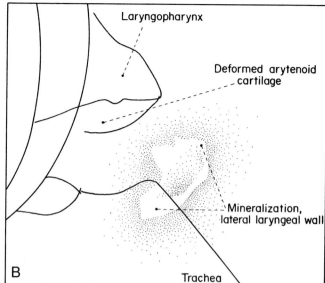

FIGURE 33–6. *A,* Deformity of arytenoid cartilage and associated laryngeal mineralization resulting from surgical failure, lateral projection. *B,* Companion line drawing.

drain into the larynx, its suppurative content being replaced by air, potentially producing a variety of distinctive gas accumulations (Fig. 33–9).[5]

Epiglottic entrapment may or may not be detectable radiographically. Decreased epiglottic size, shape, and positioning relative to the soft palate suggest entrapment; invariable sequential images of the epiglottis do likewise.[6] Epiglottic blunting and dorsal displacement have also been observed in association with entrapment.[7, 8]

Laryngeal mineralization may occur as a function of aging[9] or, alternatively, develop following laryngeal surgery or chronic laryngeal inflammation, arytenoid chrondritis, or arytenoid chondrosis (Fig. 33–10).[10, 11] Such dystrophic calcification may signify altered laryngeal function, especially when associated with enlargement, abnormal margination, or distortion of the arytenoid cartilage. The term *chondroma* is used to describe an arytenoid mass affect.[12]

Potentially, any laryngeal disorder may lead to varying degrees of upper airway obstruction,[13] which may sometimes be inferred radiographically from pharyngeal distention or pulmonary overinflation.

APPEARANCE OF PHARYNGEAL DISEASE

The pharynx, as viewed in a lateral radiographic projection, consists of a large, roughly rectangular, air-filled chamber that is subdivided into three regions: the nasopharynx, which constitutes the major part of the cavity; the laryngopharynx, which is the area immediately dorsal to the arytenoepiglottic folds, and the oropharynx, the area ventral to the caudal aspect of the soft palate, which is typically not visualized because of its similarity to surrounding tissue.

Dorsally the pharynx is bounded by the paired guttural pouches, readily identifiable by their large gas content. The larynx, discussed previously, forms the caudal pharyngeal margin as well as a portion of the ventral border. The soft palate completes the remainder of the ventral pharynx. The rostral aspect of the pharynx is radiographically nonspecific, being a composite image of multiple contiguous and overlapping structures or cavities (see Fig. 33–1). For the purposes of organizational simplicity, the pharyngeal cavity and guttural pouches are considered separately.

Pharyngeal Cavity

Radiographic indications of pharyngeal disease include decreased gas content; alterations in size or contour; and changes in the size, shape, or position of the soft palate. Reduced pharyngeal volume is usually of an extrinsic nature, stemming from disease-induced enlargement of surrounding structures, such as the guttural pouches and retropharyngeal lymph nodes (Fig. 33–11). Gunshot wounds to the throat region may cause extensive pharyngeal and parapharyngeal bleeding as well as injury to the upper airway (Fig. 33–12). Parapharyngeal adenopathy often produces a distinctive con-

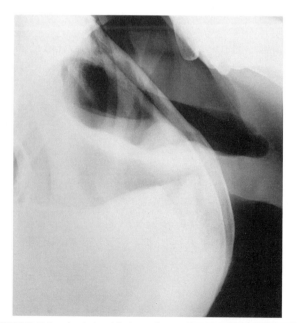

FIGURE 33–7. Lateral projection of the laryngeal region. There is a convexity of the normally concave arytenoepiglottic folds and increased opacity overall (the spherical opacity superimposed on the ventral margin of the guttural pouch field is incidental). Diagnosis: squamous cell carcinoma.

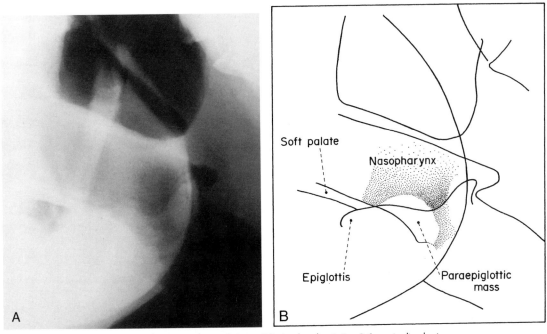

FIGURE 33–8. *A,* Paraepiglottic mass resulting in secondary epiglottic immobilization, lateral projection. *B,* Companion line drawing.

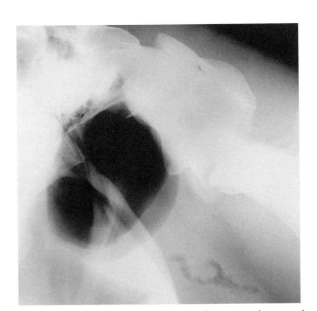

FIGURE 33–9. Lateral projection of the guttural pouches. There is an ovoid gas accumulation dorsal to the larynx. Diagnosis: paralaryngeal abscess.

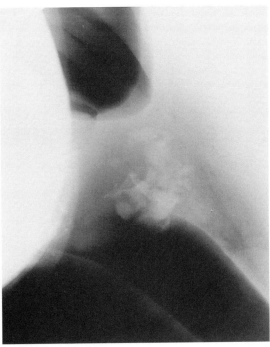

FIGURE 33–10. Lateral projection of the laryngeal region. There are vertically oriented opacities dorsal to the laryngotracheal junction, and mild tracheal stenosis. Diagnosis: dystrophic calcification caused by chronic laryngeal/paralaryngeal inflammation.

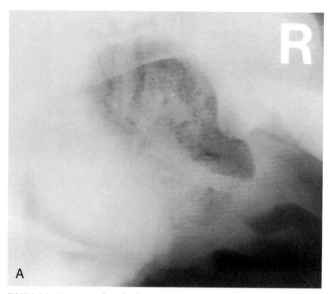

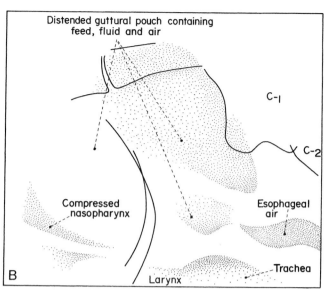

FIGURE 33–11. *A,* Guttural pouch infection resulting in extreme compression of the pharynx, larynx, and trachea, lateral projection. *B,* Companion line drawing.

cavity in the caudoventral margin of one or both guttural pouches (Fig. 33–13). Radiographs made during swallowing may show the tongue filling the majority of the pharynx and thus mimic a pharyngeal mass.[14]

Dorsal displacement of the soft palate is usually associated with organic or functional disorders of the larynx or pharynx (Fig. 33–14). Occasionally, normal horses may have dorsal palatal displacement; however, this is usually only an intermittent finding. When present radiographically, dorsal displacement should be considered abnormal until proved otherwise. Possible laryngeal causes include epiglottic hypoplasia, persistent epiglottic frenulum, epiglottic scarring, and epiglottic entrapment by diseased or malformed arytenoepiglottic folds.

Pharyngeal causes of dorsal palatal displacement include palatal hypoplasia, palatal myositis, ninth and tenth cranial neuropathy, pharyngitis, and secondary causes such as disor-

ders of the guttural pouches and parapharyngeal structures.[15-17] Dorsal displacement of the soft palate, without associated laryngeal disorder, may be linked to airway disease.[18]

Guttural Pouches

The guttural pouches are large, thin-walled, air-filled extensions of the pharynx. Although readily visible because of their air content, their superimposition and close relative proximity afford minimal opportunity for radiographic separation. Oblique projections may be of some use in partially separating the pouches, but only the ventrodorsal view completely eliminates superimposition. Accordingly, assessment of the guttural pouches is usually based on one or more lateral projections.[19]

The radiographic signs of guttural pouch disease include increased air content, decreased air content, fluid level, deformity, intraluminal mass, extraluminal gas or fluid level, pharyngeal compression, and laryngotracheal displacement.

One or both guttural pouches may be distended with gas, fluid, or a combination (Fig. 33–15). With unilateral disease, the abnormal pouch often compresses the adjacent normal pouch to the extent that it becomes invisible radiographically.[20] Severe gaseous distention, also known as tympany, is most frequently seen in foals and young horses; its cause is speculative. The degree of swelling is often so great that the enlarged pouch compresses the pharynx and displaces the larynx and proximal trachea ventrally. This dislocation of the proximal part of the upper airway may severely hamper breathing (Fig. 33–16). Subtotal fluid accumulation in the guttural pouch is usually associated with a distinctive fluid level (Fig. 33–17). It is not possible, however, to distinguish the nature of the fluid. Fortunately the possibilities are few in number, with the two primary considerations being exudate (empyema) and hemorrhage.

Hemorrhage can result from erosion of the internal carotid artery secondary to guttural pouch mycosis,[21] although it may occur secondary to bacterial infection, regional trauma, penetrating foreign body, or gunshot.[22] Exudate may accu-

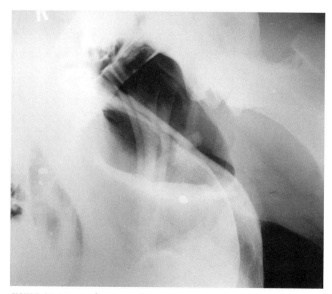

FIGURE 33–12. Lateral projection of the guttural pouches. There is decreased pharyngeal transparency, and multiple bullet fragments. Diagnosis: pharyngeal hemorrhage secondary to gunshot wound.

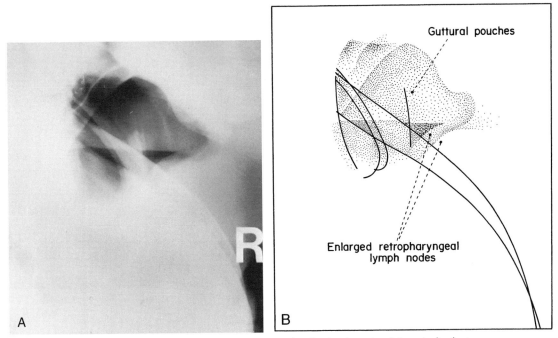

FIGURE 33–13. *A,* Localized adenopathy producing altered contours in the guttural pouches, lateral projection. *B,* Companion line drawing.

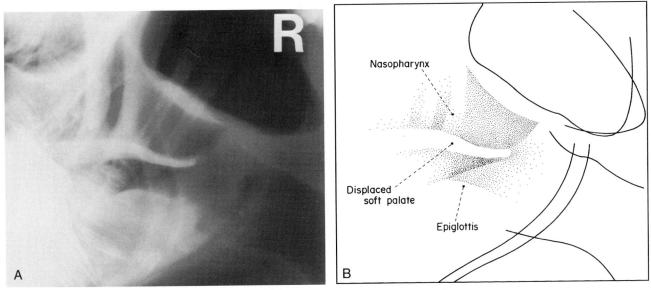

FIGURE 33–14. *A,* Dorsal displacement of the soft palate secondary to palatal hypoplasia, lateral projection. *B,* Companion line drawing.

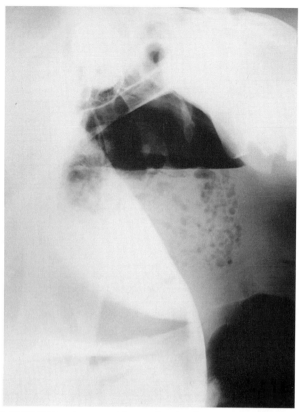

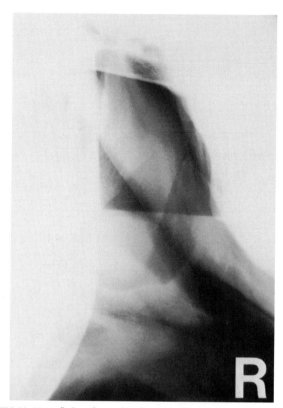

FIGURE 33–15. Lateral projection of the guttural pouches. There is a greatly enlarged guttural pouch filled with a mixture of fluid, air, and floating debris. The pharynx is severely compressed, and the larynx and trachea displaced ventrally, causing nearly complete obstruction of the proximal airway. Diagnosis: necrotic diverticulitis.

FIGURE 33–17. Air-fluid interface resulting from guttural pouch infection, lateral projection.

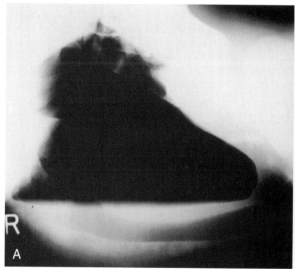

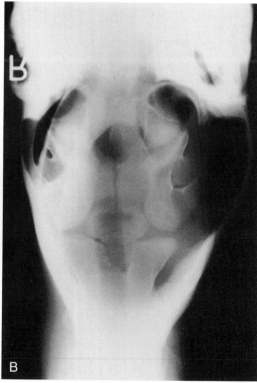

FIGURE 33–16. A and B, Lateral and ventrodorsal projections of the throat region of a young foal. There is gas dissection of the left guttural pouch, with severe tracheal displacement ventrally. Diagnosis: congenital obstruction of the pharyngeal opening to the left guttural pouch.

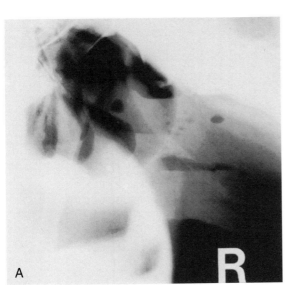

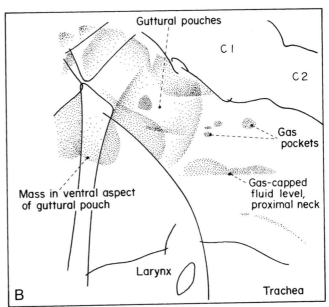

FIGURE 33–18. *A,* Extraluminal gas accumulations and fluid levels developed secondary to chronic guttural pouch infection, fistulation, and extension of the infection into the proximal cervical region, lateral projection. *B,* Companion line drawing.

mulate in the guttural pouch as a result of a ruptured retropharyngeal abscess, regional streptococcal infection, or outflow obstruction secondary to stenosis of the pharyngeal opening.[23] The pouch may also be infected by contaminated instruments, needles, or irrigating solutions. Mycotic infection may extend to the adjacent stylohyoid bone causing bone deposition, destruction, and, in severe instances, pathologic fracture.[24] Most infections are unilateral.[25]

Occasionally, gas or fluid levels are identified in proximity but external to the guttural pouches (Fig. 33–18). Inferentially a guttural pouch origin should be considered, although other gas-containing structures, such as the pharynx, larynx, and trachea, may also leak air after perforation. With regard

to the guttural pouches, it is usually an infection that results in necrosis of the guttural pouch wall and subsequent escape of its gas and infectious content. Fistulas and sinuses sometimes form and often are amenable to sinography. Bacterial gas formation occurs rarely.

Intraluminal masses are identified occasionally if they are of sufficient size and are surrounded by air (Fig. 33–19). Possible causes of such masses include chondroids, inflammatory tissue masses, and blood clots. Tumors may appear similarly; however, they are rare.

Large volumes of luminal fluid may somewhat or entirely obscure one or both guttural pouches. It may be especially difficult to establish the laterality of such lesions because they

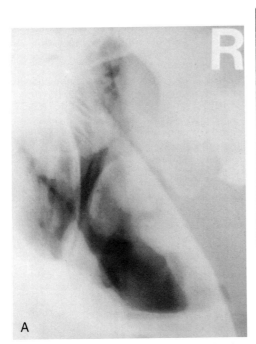

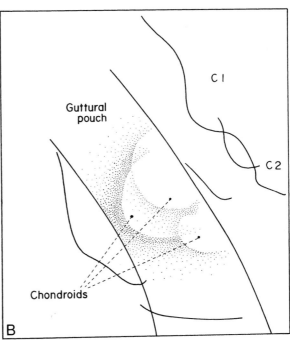

FIGURE 33–19. *A,* Multiple luminal masses (chondroids), lateral projection. *B,* Companion line drawing.

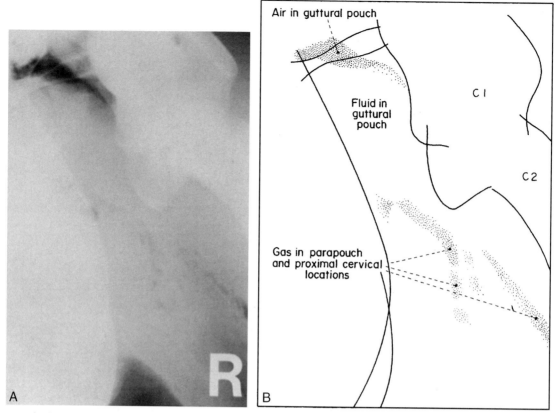

FIGURE 33–20. *A,* Reduced gas content secondary to chronic exudate replacement. Extraluminal and cervical gas is secondary to associated necrosis and gas escape, lateral projection. *B,* Companion line drawing.

frequently compress the uninvolved pouch as well as the pharynx, larynx, and proximal trachea (Fig. 33–20).

TRACHEAL DISEASE

The normal equine cervical trachea may be imaged sufficiently to detect the following structures: the caudal aspect of the larynx, the tracheal lumen, the inner tracheal surface (mucosa), the tracheal rings, and the annular ligaments (by inference the space between tracheal rings) (see Fig. 33–20). The absence or alterations of these normally visible shadows form the radiologic basis for a diagnosis of tracheal disease.

Primary tracheal disorders are only occasionally detected radiographically. Tracheal displacement, however, is common, usually resulting from enlargement of the guttural pouch or cervical part of the esophagus, and may be readily appreciated radiographically (see Figs. 33–11 and 33–15).

The most common indirect indicator of tracheal disease is extratracheal gas. Causes of extraluminal gas include (1) transtracheal aspiration, (2) tracheal fracture after blunt trauma, (3) tracheal perforation caused by penetrating trauma, and (4) tracheal necrosis secondary to tracheal or paratracheal infection or abscess formation (Figs. 33–21 and 33–22); the latter may result in fistula formation.[26–28] Gas may also be seen along the outer margin of the trachea after laryngeal or tracheal surgery and as a complication of wound dehiscence. It is highly unusual for air to reach the tracheal perimeter as a result of a laceration. In the event such a finding is made under these circumstances, it is strongly recommended that upper airway leakage be sought.

Pneumomediastinum is usually the result of tracheal fracture or perforation, the escaping gas dissecting caudally into the mediastinum along the deep fascial planes of the neck (see Fig. 31–21). The origin may, however, be the thoracic trachea or bronchi. Occasionally, air may arise from ruptured alveoli, dissecting in a retrograde fashion along the vascular adventitia into the mediastinum.

Decreased definition of the normally visible tracheal soft tissues may occasionally be seen with infection or trauma; however, the change is subtle. Paratracheal disease or duplication cysts may visually blend with the adjacent trachea, effectively mimicking tracheal disease.[29] The absence of a ventrodorsal view often makes it impossible to make the necessary distinction.

Luminal alterations in the form of tracheal stenosis, collapse, or masses occur occasionally. Most stenotic lesions are the result of tracheotomy-induced scarring related to incorrect surgical technique (Fig. 33–23).[30] Deep cervical lacerations, penetrating foreign bodies, and gunshots may also lead to tracheal scarring and stenosis. Luminal masses are rare, most being tumors or foreign bodies. Tracheal collapse may be congenital or acquired and is often regional in nature. Based on the small number of published reports, it is rare.[31, 32] Tracheal hypoplasia, as in other domestic animals, is associated with a uniformly diminished size, but in contrast to other animals, laryngeal hypoplasia may also be present.[33]

DISEASES OFTEN ASSOCIATED WITH A NORMAL-APPEARING RADIOGRAPH

Pharynx

Pharyngeal lymphoid hyperplasia is radiographically recognizable if the lymphoid plaques are large and project into the

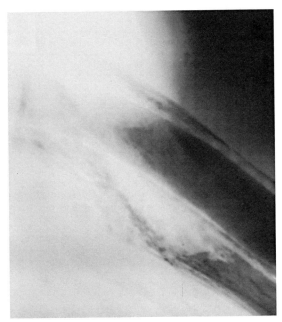

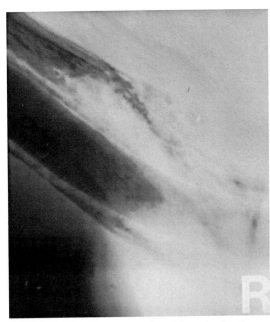

FIGURE 33–21. Extraluminal gas escaping from the cranial cervical trachea 3 hours after transtracheal aspiration, lateral projection.

FIGURE 33–22. Extraluminal gas escaping from the caudal cervical trachea after a penetrating wound, lateral projection.

pharyngeal cavity; otherwise they are indiscernible from the rest of the pharyngeal soft tissues.[34] Likewise, pharyngeal cysts are undetectable unless they are sufficiently large and convex. The same may be said for other pharyngeal masses, such as abscesses or granulomas. Free pharyngeal fluid cannot be detected radiographically.

Larynx

In the horse, there frequently are no radiographic abnormalities associated with epiglottic entrapment (Fig. 33–24). Subsequent endoscopic examinations of the same horses have shown varying degrees of entrapment or, more usually, restricted or limited epiglottic movement. These findings have usually been attributed to a slight inward folding of the arytenoepiglottic folds. Thus, as with any radiographic exami-

nation designed to evaluate altered anatomy, the alteration must be of sufficient magnitude to be recognizable; subtle changes or slight variations from normal are likely to go undetected. For this reason, not only should endoscopy be performed in all horses with suspected epiglottic entrapment, but also it should precede the radiographic examination; the chances of finding a radiographic abnormality are therefore greatly enhanced.

Neither laryngeal hemiplegia nor all but the most extreme epiglottic inflammations can be diagnosed radiographically. Even this type of inflammation may not result in detectable change. All but the largest thyroid tumors are radiographically invisible.[35]

Noisy breathing, with or without distress, is one of the features of hyperkalemic periodic paralysis, a genetic disease of Quarter horses, including young foals. Although endoscopic examination may reveal laryngeal spasm or paralysis,

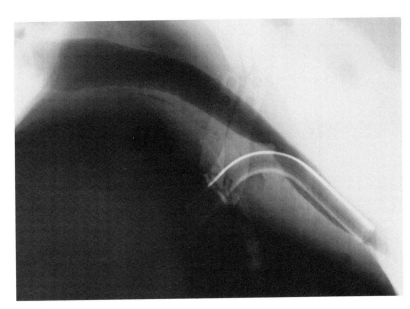

FIGURE 33–23. Lateral projection of the cervical tracheal region. A tracheotomy tube that has caused stenosis at the point of insertion; paratracheal gas indicated leakage.

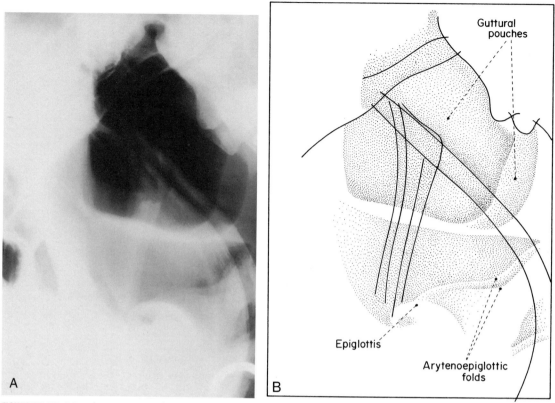

FIGURE 33–24. *A,* Lateral projection. A normal-appearing larynx that, on subsequent endoscopy, showed restricted epiglottic motion. *B,* Companion line drawing.

radiographs are likely to appear normal.[36, 37] Extreme muscular hypertrophy, however, has been known to cause external compression of guttural pouches, with the resulting radiographic appearance of a pharyngeal mass.[38, 39]

Trachea

Tracheitis has not been described radiographically, with or without the use of contrast medium. Tracheal fluid, even in large volumes, is usually not detectable radiographically. Small luminal masses (<1 cm) typically remain unidentified. Tracheograms show only major lesions and rarely identify perforations, including those that produce large volumes of extratracheal air.

References

1. Linford RL, O'Brien TR, Wheat JD, et al: Radiographic assessment of epiglottic length and pharyngeal and laryngeal diameter in the Thoroughbred. Am J Vet Res *44:*1660, 1983.
2. Barclay WP, Phillips TN, and Foerner JJ: Acute epiglottidis in a horse. J Am Vet Med Assoc *181:*925, 1982.
3. Holland M, Snyder JR, Steffey EP, et al: Laryngotracheal injury associated with nasotracheal intubation in the horse. J Am Vet Med Assoc *189:*1447, 1986.
4. Dixon PM, Railton DI, and McGorum BC: Ventral glottic stenosis in 3 horses. Equine Vet J *26:*166, 1994.
5. Farrow CS, and Barber SM: Pharyngeal abscess with laryngeal fistulization in a horse. (What is your diagnosis?) J Am Vet Med Assoc *179:*830, 1981.
6. Ferraro GL: Epiglottic entrapment. *In* White NA, and Moore JN (Eds): Equine Surgery. Philadelphia, JB Lippincott, 1990, p 236.
7. Butler JA, Colles CM, Dyson SJ, et al: Clinical Radiology of the Horse. London, Blackwell Scientific Publications, 1993, pp 347–349.
8. Dik KJ, and Gunsser I: Atlas of Diagnostic Radiology of the Horse. Philadelphia, WB Saunders, 1990, pp 102–103.
9. Orsini PG: Xerographic examination. *In* Beech J (Ed): Equine Respiratory Disorders. Philadelphia, Lea & Febiger, 1991, p 121.
10. Haynes PF, Snider TG, McClure JR, et al: Chronic chondritis of the equine arytenoid cartilage. J Am Vet Med Assoc *177:*1135, 1980.
11. Cahill JI, and Goulden BE: Diseases of the larynx. *In* Colahan PT, Mayhew JG, Merritt AM, et al (Eds): Equine Medicine and Surgery, 4th Ed. Goleta, CA, American Veterinary Publications, 1991, p 411.
12. Dik KJ, and Gunsser I: Atlas of Diagnostic Radiology of the Horse. Philadelphia, WB Saunders, 1990, pp 104–105.
13. Pascoe JR: Pathophysiology of upper airway obstruction. *In* White NA, and Moore JN (Eds): Equine Surgery. Philadelphia, JB Lippincott, 1990, p 213.
14. Honnus CM, Kemper T, and Linford RL: What is your diagnosis? J Am Vet Med Assoc *194:*1769, 1989.
15. Blythe LL, Cardinet GH III, Meaghar DM, et al: Palatal myositis in horses with dorsal displacement of the soft palate. J Am Vet Med Assoc *183:*781, 1983.
16. Haynes PF: Persistent dorsal displacement of the soft palate associated with epiglottic shortening in two horses. J Am Vet Med Assoc *179:*677, 1981.
17. Freeman DE: Dorsal displacement of the soft palate. *In* White NA, and Moore JN (Eds): Equine Surgery. Philadelphia, JB Lippincott, 1990, p 230.
18. Robertson JT: Pharynx and larynx. *In* Beech J (Ed): Equine Respiratory Disorders. Philadelphia, Lea & Febiger, 1991, p 331.
19. Cook WR: The auditory tube diverticulum (guttural pouch) in the horse: Its radiographic examination. J Am Vet Radiol Soc *2:*51, 1973.
20. Barber SM: Diseases of the guttural pouches. *In* Colahan PT, Mayhew JG, Merritt AM, et al (Eds): Equine Medicine and Surgery, 4th Ed. Goleta, CA, American Veterinary Publication, 1991, p 402.
21. Lingard DR, Gosser HS, and Monfart TN: Acute epistaxis associated with guttural pouch mycosis in two horses. J Am Vet Med Assoc *164:*1038, 1974.
22. Bayly WM, and Robertson JT: Epistaxis caused by foreign body penetration of a guttural pouch. J Am Vet Med Assoc *180:*1232, 1982.
23. Freeman DE: Guttural pouches. *In* Beech J (Ed): Equine Respiratory Disorders. Philadelphia, Lea & Febiger, 1991, p 305.
24. Cook WR: The clinical features of guttural pouch mycosis in the horse. Vet Rec *83:*336, 1968.
25. Freeman DE: Guttural pouch empyema. *In* White NA, and Moore JN (Eds): Equine Surgery. Philadelphia, JB Lippincott, 1990, p 240.
26. Farrow CS: Pneumomediastinum in the horse: A complication of transtracheal aspiration. J Am Vet Radiol Soc *17:*192, 1976.
27. Caron JP, and Townsend HGG: Tracheal perforation and widespread subcutaneous emphysema in a horse. Can Vet J *25:*339, 1984.

28. Fubini SL, Todhunter RJ, Vivrette SL, et al: Tracheal rupture in two horses. J Am Vet Med Assoc 187:69, 1985.
29. Peek SF, De LaHunta A, and Hackett RP: Combined esophageal duplication cyst in a Arabian filly. Equine Vet J 27:475, 1995.
30. Freeman DE: Trachea. In Beech J (Ed): Equine Respiratory Disorders. Philadelphia, Lea & Febiger, 1991, p 389.
31. Carig CB, Groenendyk S, and Seawright AA: Dorsoventral flattening of the trachea of a horse and its attempted surgical correction: A case report. J Am Vet Radiol Soc 14:32, 1973.
32. Simmons TR, Peterson M, Parker J, et al: Tracheal collapse due to chrondrodysplasia in a miniature horse foal. Equine Pract 10(10):39, 1988.
33. Dik KJ, and Gunsser I: Atlas of Diagnostic Radiology of the Horse. Philadelphia, WB Saunders, 1990, pp 106–107.
34. Koch C: Disease of the larynx and pharynx of the Horse. Comp Contin Ed Vet Pract 5:S73, 1980.
35. Hillidge CJ, Sanecki RK, Theodorakis MC, et al: Thyroid carcinoma in a horse. J Am Vet Med Assoc 181:711, 1982.
36. Traub Dargatz JL, Ingram JT, Stashak TS, et al: Respiratory stridor associated with polymyopathy suspected to be hyperkinetic periodic paralysis in four Quarter Horse foals. J Am Vet Med Assoc 201:85, 1992.
37. Naylor J: Equine hyperkalemic periodic paralysis. Can Vet J 35:279, 1994.
38. Berry CR: Film reading session; case 5. Vet Radiol Ultrasound 36:332, 1995.
39. Berry CR: Answers for film reading session; case 5. Vet Radiol Ultrasound 36:449, 1995.

STUDY QUESTIONS

1. What are the implications of each of the following errors, potentially made during radiography of the throat?
   A. Head extended.
   B. Head flexed.
   C. Excessively dark image.

2. Radiographically, how can epiglottic dysfunction be evaluated?

3. Which of the following radiographic features characterize pharyngitis?
   A. Increased pharyngeal opacity.
   B. Decreased pharyngeal opacity.
   C. Irregular pharyngeal contours.
   D. Reduced pharyngeal volume.
   E. Increased pharyngeal volume.
   F. Patchy pharyngeal opacities.
   G. None of the above

4. What is *epiglottitis*, and how might it appear radiographically?

5. What are the two most common causes of laryngeal calcification in order of likelihood?

6. What is the major limitation to lateral or oblique projections when attempting to confirm the presence of unilateral guttural pouch disease?

(Answers appear on page 644.)

Chapter 34

The Pleural Space

Ron D. Sande

Examination of the pleural space of the horse is complicated by the large size of the patient. Parallax and magnification are serious problems given the magnitude of pathologic change that is necessary to be seen radiographically.

ANATOMY

The lines of pleural reflection are important landmarks in diagnostic imaging.[1] The parietal pleura is reflected along three major boundaries. The sternal line of reflection is where the costal pleura reflects dorsally to become the visceral pleura of the mediastinum. The vertebral line of reflection is where the costal pleura turns ventrally to form the mediastinal pleura. Perhaps the most important pleural reflection in diagnostic imaging is the diaphragmatic reflection, in which the parietal pleura of the costal surface extends to the surface of the diaphragm and forms the costodiaphragmatic recess or phrenicocostal sinus. This line is the demarcation between the thorax and the abdomen. Externally the anatomic limits may be determined by a line connecting the following points: the 17th intercostal space at the level of

the tuber coxae, the 15th intercostal space at the level of the tuber ischii, the 13th intercostal space at the dorsoventral midpoint, the 11th intercostal space at the level of the point of the shoulder, and a gradually descending line to the point of the elbow. Although it may be difficult to visualize radiographically, this line should be found ventrally at the level of the costochondral junctions caudal to the ninth rib, where it courses caudal and dorsal at a gradually increasing distance from the sternal ends of the ribs to the level of the midshaft of the last rib. It then reflects slightly cranial and dorsal to terminate at the vertebral end of the last intercostal space.

RADIOGRAPHY

Radiographic examination of the equine thorax has become a routine procedure. Advances in technology associated with intensifying screens have effectively increased the capability of mobile radiograph equipment. Despite the sophistication of equipment, it is still difficult to image the cranioventral thorax.

Radiographic examination of the thorax for the purpose of

evaluating the pleural space is performed with the same technique as that used to evaluate other thoracic structures. Horizontal-beam projections are made with the patient standing. The average horse (450 kg) requires at least three and perhaps four 35 cm × 43 cm images on each side for complete examination.[2]

Survey examination for diseases of the pleural space should include at least one right and one left lateral projection of the caudal ventral portion of the thorax. The need for additional projections may be determined based on the preliminary findings and the severity of the disease.

Radiographic Interpretation

Magnification inherent to radiographic examination of the equine thorax results in progressive loss of detail of structures closer to the x-ray tube. Right and left lateral projections permit evaluation of each side of the thorax. Because radiographic detail is better when structures are closer to the film, one may be able to localize lesions in their approximate sagittal plane. A lesion that is near the thoracic wall may have sharp margins in one lateral projection (see Fig. 34–5A), and on the opposite projection it is blurred beyond recognition (see Fig. 34–5B). A lesion located at the midline appears similar or identical, regardless of the projection. Detail of lesions within the pulmonary parenchyma varies according to the sagittal plane in which the lesions exist.

Accumulation of fluid within the pleural space or mediastinum is often a generic finding. Differentiation of transudate, exudate, or blood is impossible without performing a thoracocentesis. Many folds and pockets exist within the mediastinum and pleural sacs. The horse is seldom found in other than a standing position, and, as expected, accumulation of fluid is most often dependent. The earliest sign of fluid in the pleural space is loss of detail in the ventral thorax caudal to the heart (Fig. 34–1). The area cranial to the heart is more difficult to evaluate. Loss of vascular detail within the lung lobes nearest the ventral margins may be the earliest indication of pleural effusion. The volume of fluid required for radiographic detection varies with the size of the patient and the quality of the study. Perhaps no less than 1 or 2 L of fluid in any compartment can be detected in a 450-kg patient. Greater volumes of fluid result in loss of detail progressing dorsally in the thorax, causing a silhouette sign of the respective borders of the diaphragm and the heart. Despite the opinion that fluid moves freely through the mediastinum, it is common to find compartmentalization of the fluid or unilateral fluid; the latter is most often associated with inflammatory conditions and is best studied by using ultrasonography. Fat adjacent to the heart in the mediastinum causes accentuation of the costal border of the lungs in the caudal thorax. This normal finding is often misinterpreted as the accumulation of fluid.

A common error in radiographic interpretation is made when one expects to find a fluid line with pleural effusion. Because of the capillarity and surface tension, a horizontal fluid line is not present unless there is also free gas in the pleural space.

Pneumothorax has multiple causes, although the sources of air are limited to the lung, esophagus, or external body surface. The presence of gas-forming bacteria provides a forum for academic discussion, but radiographic diagnosis is not likely to be made before the death of the patient. It is common to find entrapped gas within an abscess (see Fig. 34–4).

Air in the pleural sacs or mediastinum compartmentalizes rapidly according to the preferred space available. The mass of pulmonary and cardiac tissue in the horse results in dependent displacement of tissue in relation to air. Free air quickly locates dorsally, adjacent to the spine. Sharp visualization of the dorsal lung margins is a reliable sign of air in the pleural spaces. Right and left lateral projections may be necessary to identify the pulmonary margins accurately and to determine the location of the pneumothorax.

ULTRASONOGRAPHY

Ultrasonography may be used for primary examination of the thorax or to augment radiographic findings. Ultrasonography may be used to locate and determine the boundaries of the fluid-filled spaces. Ultrasonographic examination is used to study tissue texture or fluid composition and may be used to guide catheter placement for thoracentesis. The appropriate literature should be consulted for a more complete understanding of this valuable imaging modality.[3–6]

DISEASES OF THE PLEURA AND PLEURAL SPACE

Pleural Effusion

The pathogenesis of pleural effusion is complex, and the causes are many.[7] Pleural effusion may be primary or secondary and may be associated with coexisting diseases. Reports include thoracic metastasis[8–11]; primary neoplasia[12]; abdominal neoplasia[13]; inhaled foreign bodies[14, 15]; primary[16–19] and systemic infection[20]; and secondary to pneumonia, pulmonary abscesses, or trauma.[21] The author's experience also includes pleural effusion associated with esophageal perforation and descending cellulitis and as a sequela to respiratory infections compounded by stress.

Pleural effusion, regardless of cause, is usually detected on physical examination and auscultation. Radiographic examination may be used to substantiate the clinical diagnosis. Radiographic signs vary according to the volume of fluid present; however, negative findings do not preclude the presence of significant disease.[22] Small volumes of fluid result in

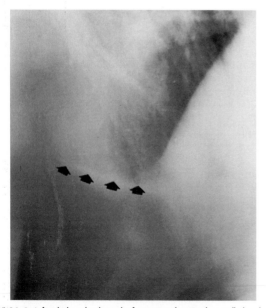

FIGURE 34–1. Left-right lateral radiograph of an equine thorax with a small pleural effusion. The ventral margin of the lung is visible (arrows). There is a silhouette sign of the ventral heart and diaphragm and loss of detail of the distal right middle pulmonary vasculature.

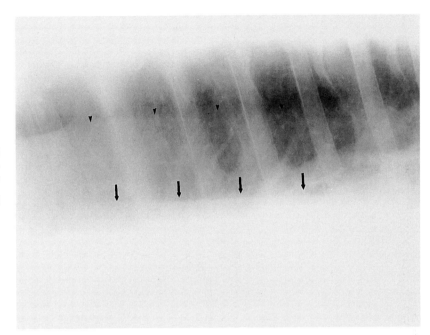

FIGURE 34–2. Left-right lateral radiograph of the dorsocaudal thorax of an adult horse with septic pleuritis. There is increased opacity and loss of detail in the ventral thorax. The opacity from the fluid is so great that the dorsal limit of the fluid *(arrows)* may be confused with the edge of the x-ray beam. Detail of the heart, caudal vena cava, diaphragm, and much of the lung has been obscured. The dorsal margin of the aorta is visible *(arrowheads)*.

increased opacity and loss of detail in the ventrocaudal thorax. The ventral margins of the lung may be outlined, and the vascular detail within the lung may be decreased (see Fig. 34–1). Increased volume of fluid results in progressive silhouetting of the border of the diaphragm, the heart, and the vena cava. These signs are compounded by concomitant collapse of the lungs with an increase in pulmonary opacity and loss of detail owing to excursion of air from the pulmonary parenchyma (Fig. 34–2).

Radiographic evidence of fluid in the pleural space or mediastinum does not provide definitive information that may be of use when differentiating the cause. Despite the radiographic findings, thoracocentesis is necessary. Ultrasonography may be used for locating loculated fluid. Thoracocentesis usually results in pneumothorax. Ultrasonographic examination may be difficult or impossible when air is present in the pleural space. Regarding pleural fluid, prognosis and treatment are often not determined or altered by the radiographic findings.

Pleuritis

Radiographic signs of acute or subacute pleuritis are often not differentiated from those of effusion. The presence of fibrin remains undetected unless it causes restriction of the lung margins. Because the equine lung is not divided by deep fissures, the scalloped borders characteristic of restrictive pleuritis in other species are not typically seen. Accumulation of fibrin may be detected when pleural adhesions and fibrin sheets form and the pleural fluid regresses. The fibrin tags tend to orient vertically within the pleural space or are at least more easily identified when their axes are orthogonal to the vessels and airways within the lung (Fig. 34–3).

More severe chronic fibrinous pleuritis may become compartmentalized, resulting in cavitary pleural disease. Cavitary pleural disease is difficult if not impossible to distinguish from cavitary lung disease. Compartmentalization of pleural fluid often results in confusing images (Fig. 34–4). The inability to perform a dorsoventral or ventrodorsal projection of the

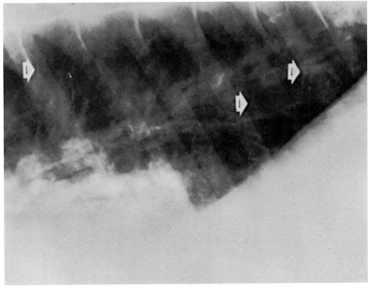

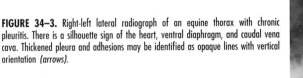

FIGURE 34–3. Right-left lateral radiograph of an equine thorax with chronic pleuritis. There is a silhouette sign of the heart, ventral diaphragm, and caudal vena cava. Thickened pleura and adhesions may be identified as opaque lines with vertical orientation *(arrows)*.

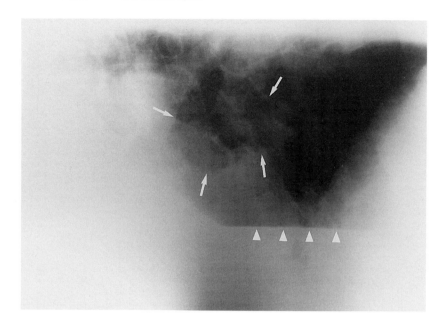

FIGURE 34–4. Left-right lateral thoracic radiograph of the horse in Figure 34–2, made 7 weeks later. Note the cavitary spaces in the lung parenchyma (arrows). Fluid and air, as demonstrated by the interface (arrowheads), are compartmentalized in the pleural space. Similar changes persisted 5 months later.

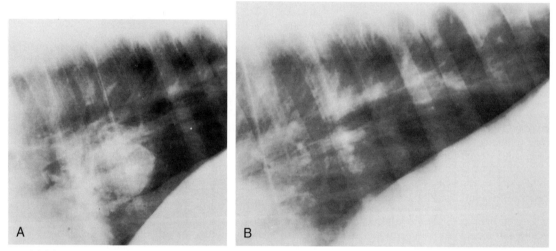

FIGURE 34–5. A, Right-left lateral radiograph of an equine thorax. There is a mass lesion with well-defined margins. Detail of the caudal vena cava and diaphragm is adequate. There is loss of detail in the lung cranial and ventral to the mass. B, Left-right lateral radiograph of the same horse. There is slight loss of detail in the lower left corner of the image. The mass lesion is magnified and superimposed in that area.

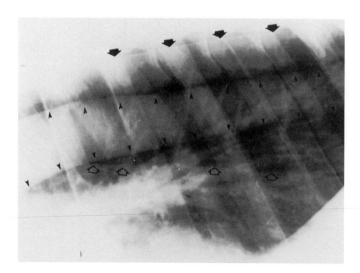

FIGURE 34–6. Right-left lateral radiograph of the thorax of a horse with pneumothorax. Radiographic signs include visible lung border (solid arrows), dorsal margin of the esophagus (open arrows), and increased detail of the margins of the aorta (arrowheads).

equine thorax often limits the radiologist to speculation regarding the location of many lesions.

Pleural and Extrapleural Masses

Differentiation of the causes of pleural and mediastinal masses should be made on the basis of clinical signs, thoracentesis, and biopsy. In the absence of excessive free fluid, a pleural mass may be visualized radiographically. The location of the mass may be determined by the use of opposing projections, as previously described (Fig. 34–5). Tissue masses extending from the pleural surface or in contact with the costal pleura are best examined by using ultrasonography. Radiography is likely to be informative when the lung surface is normal and changes occur deeper in lung tissue or are confined to the mediastinum.[23]

Pneumothorax

The diagnosis of pneumothorax does not identify the actual location of air within the thorax or define the cause. The causes are numerous, and among the more common is jugular venipuncture with subsequent pneumomediastinum progressing to pneumothorax. Free gas in the thorax quickly rises dorsally. In the standing lateral, horizontal-beam projection, air accumulates dorsally. Therefore, the first sign of pneumothorax is visualization of the margins of the lungs. Increased volume of air results in dependent retraction of the lung and decreased opacity in the dorsal thorax (Fig. 34–6). Air within the mediastinum outlines the aorta and does not displace the lung margins.

References

1. Getty R: Sisson and Grossman's The Anatomy of the Domestic Animals. Philadelphia, WB Saunders, 1975.
2. Farrow CS: Radiography of the equine thorax: Anatomy and technic. Vet Radiol 22:62, 1981.
3. Rantanen NW: Ultrasound appearance of normal lung borders and adjacent viscera in the horse. Vet Radiol 22:217, 1981.
4. Rantanen NW, and Ewing RL: Principles of ultrasound application in animals. Vet Radiol 22:196, 1981.
5. Rantanen NW, Gage L, and Paradis MR: Ultrasonography as a diagnostic aid in pleural effusion of horses. Vet Radiol 22:211, 1981.
6. Rantanen NW: Diseases of the thorax. Vet Clin North Am [Equine Pract] 2:49, 1986.
7. Smith BP: Pleuritis and pleural effusion in the horse: A study of 37 cases. J Am Vet Med Assoc 170:208, 1977.
8. Foreman JH, Weidner JP, Parry BW, et al: Pleural effusion secondary to thoracic metastatic mammary adenocarcinoma in a mare. J Am Vet Med Assoc 197:1193, 1990.
9. Morris DD, Acland HM, and Hodge TG: Pleural effusion secondary to metastasis of an ovarian adenocarcinoma in a horse. J Am Vet Med Assoc 187:272, 1985.
10. Rossier Y, Sweeney CR, Heyer G, et al: Pleuroscopic diagnosis of disseminated hemangiosarcoma in a horse. J Am Vet Med Assoc 196:1639, 1990.
11. Meuller PO, Morris DD, Carmichael KP, et al: Antemortem diagnosis of cholangiocellular carcinoma in a horse. J Am Vet Med Assoc 201:899, 1992.
12. Mair TS, Lane JG, and Lucke VM: Clinicopathological features of lymphosarcoma involving the thoracic cavity in the horse. Equine Vet J 17:428, 1985.
13. Harvey KA, Morris DD, Saik JE, et al: Omental fibrosarcoma in a horse. J Am Vet Med Assoc 191:335, 1987.
14. Hultgren BD, Pearson EG, Lassen ED, et al: Pleuritis and pneumonia attributed to a conifer twig in a bronchus of a horse. J Am Vet Med Assoc 189:797, 1986.
15. O'Brien JK: Septic pleuritis associated with an inhaled foreign body in a pony. Vet Rec 119:274, 1986.
16. Benson CE, and Sweeney CR: Isolation of Streptococcus pneumoniae type 3 from equine species. J Clin Microbiol 20:1028, 1984.
17. Sweeney CR, Divers TJ, and Benson CE: Anaerobic bacteria in 21 horses with pleuropneumonia. J Am Vet Med Assoc 187:721, 1985.
18. Rosendal S, Blackwell TE, Lumsden JH, et al: Detection of antibodies to Mycoplasma felis in horses. J Am Vet Med Assoc 188:292, 1986.
19. Hoffman AM, Baird JD, Kloeze HJ, et al: Mycoplasma felis pleuritis in two show-jumper horses. Cornell Vet 82:155, 1992.
20. Mair TS, and Lane JG: Pneumonia, lung abscess, and pleuritis in adult horses: A review of 51 cases. Equine Vet J 21:175, 1989.
21. Collins MB, Hodgson DR, and Hutchins DR: Pleural effusion associated with acute and chronic pleuropneumonia and pleuritis secondary to thoracic wounds in horses: 43 cases (1982–1992). J Am Vet Med Assoc 205:1753, 1994.
22. Prater PE, Patton CS, and Held JP: Pleural effusion resulting from malignant hepatoblastoma in a horse. J Am Vet Med Assoc 194:383, 1989.
23. Reef VB, Boy MG, Reid CF, et al: Comparison between diagnostic ultrasonography and radiography in the evaluation of horses and cattle with thoracic disease: 56 cases (1984–1985). J Am Vet Med Assoc 198:2112, 1991.

STUDY QUESTIONS

1. The pleural cavity of the horse:
   A. Is composed of two potential spaces, each lined by visceral, parietal, diaphragmatic and costal pleura, separated by the mediastinum.
   B. Contains sufficient liquor pleurae to cause blunting of the costophrenic angles on radiographic images.
   C. May be located by finding intercostal spaces 5, 11, and 17 at the level of the shoulder, greater trochanter, and tuber coxae.
   D. Is composed of two distinctly separate spaces, having no communication, that confine a disease to one side.

2. Radiographic examination of the thorax of the horse for evaluation of the pleural space:
   A. Should include ventrodorsal or dorsoventral projections in all horses with thoracic disease.
   B. Should not require a grid when using high kVp and moderate mAs techniques with high-speed screen film combinations.
   C. May require three or four projections in both left and right lateral, horizontal-beam configurations.
   D. Is suitably performed by survey radiography of the caudal, ventral (dependent) pleural space, where fluid will accumulate.

3. Left lateral radiograph of the dorsal, caudal thorax of a 7-year-old Quarter horse gelding with respiratory difficulty after being used as a rodeo horse (Fig. 34–7). What are the significant findings and radiographic diagnosis?

4. Radiographic signs of pleural disease in the horse:
   A. Are first seen as loss of detail in the ventral thorax, cranial to the heart.
   B. Result in loss of detail and obscuration of the aorta, diaphragm, and cardiac margins.
   C. Result in a fluid line, indicating the fluid level in the thorax, on horizontal-beam lateral projections.
   D. May require a fluid or air volume in excess of 2 L for detection by radiography of the thorax.

5. Pneumothorax in the horse is a generic diagnosis usually recognized by the following radiographic sign:

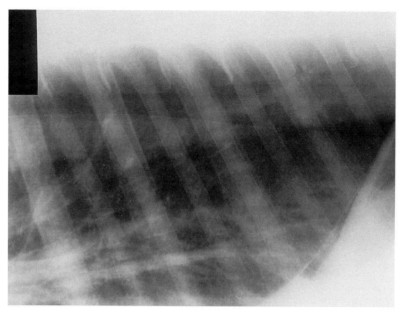

FIGURE 34–7

A. Elevation of the heart and lung margins from the sternum.
B. Clear definition of cardiac margins.
C. Clear definition of the diaphragmatic crura.
D. Clear definition of the dorsal lung margins and aorta.

6. Right lateral projection of the cranial dorsal thorax of a 3-year-old Thoroughbred filly with respiratory distress and elevated temperature following transport between racetracks (Fig. 34–8). What are the significant findings and radiographic assessment?

7. Pleural effusion in the horse:
   A. Results in retraction of lung margins and scalloped lung borders on radiographic images.
   B. Results in progressive obscuration of margins of the heart, diaphragm, and vena cava on radiographic images.
   C. Is characterized by cavitary changes and fluid-air interfaces on radiographic images.
   D. Does not occur as a primary disease and is often associated with radiographic signs of coexisting disease.

8. Diagnostic radiology of the equine thorax, for the study of pleural disease, is better than ultrasonography:
   A. When the disease is in the mediastinum or deep to lung tissue.
   B. When lesions extend from lung margins into the lung parenchyma.

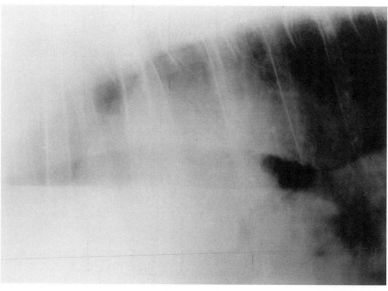

FIGURE 34–8

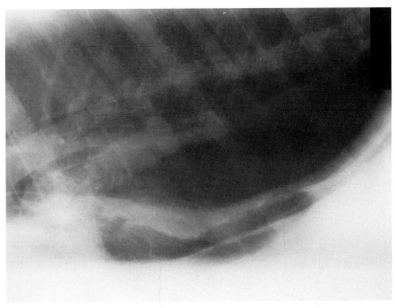

FIGURE 34–9

C. For differentiation of causes of pleural and mediastinal masses.
D. For detection of fibrinous, restrictive pleuritis.

9. Left lateral radiograph of the thorax of a 12-year-old Thoroughbred mare being treated for chronic pleuritis (Fig. 34–9). What are the significant findings and radiographic assessment?

10. Pleural disease in the horse is usually detected first:
    A. By radiography augmented by diagnostic ultrasonography.
    B. By diagnostic ultrasound examination of the thorax.
    C. By auscultation of the thorax.
    D. By radiography of the thorax.

(Answers appear on pages 644 to 645.)

Chapter 35

The Equine Lung

Charles S. Farrow

EXAMINATION METHOD

A foal's thorax may be completely imaged with a 14 inch × 17 inch radiograph (Fig. 35–1A and B). By comparison, four films of this size are needed to image the thorax of an adult horse (Figs. 35–2 through 35–5).

NORMAL APPEARANCE

A standard radiographic examination in an adult horse is composed of four projections: (1) craniodorsal, (2) cranioventral, (3) caudodorsal, and (4) caudoventral. Each requires a different radiographic technique. Cardiovascular assessment is optimized by centering the heart on a single 14 inch × 17 inch film (see Figs. 35–2 to 35–5).

Craniodorsal Projection

The dorsal part of the heart, cranial aorta, and large pulmonary arteries and veins are evident in the craniodorsal

projection. Also seen are the trachea, the tracheal bifurcation, and the continuing bronchi. The lung is visible, but it is difficult to evaluate because of superimposition by the heart and vessels. An accurate assessment of heart size is impossible in this view.

Cranioventral Projection

Most of the heart, aortic origin, cranial mediastinum, and thoracic part of the trachea are visible in the cranioventral projection. The scapulae and one or both humeri usually are visible cranially. The lung is typically overexposed and difficult to see clearly because of the high kilovoltage required to penetrate the thick cardiovascular tissues and the musculature of the partially superimposed proximal forelimbs.

Caudodorsal Projection

The caudodorsal projection provides the largest unobstructed view of the lung. It is important to recognize that normal

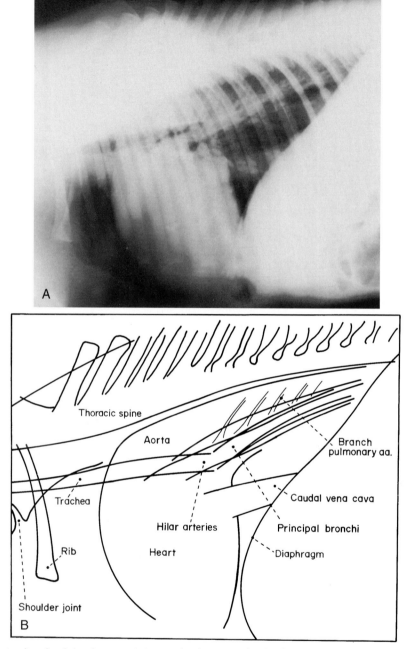

FIGURE 35–1. *A,* Normal foal thoracic radiograph, right lateral projection. *B,* Companion line drawing. Note the relatively large appearance of the heart, a normal finding in foals.

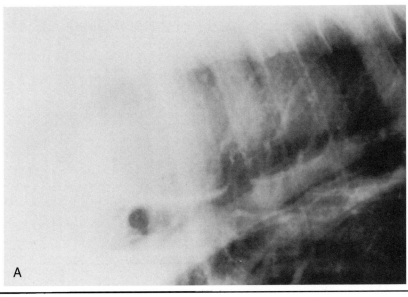

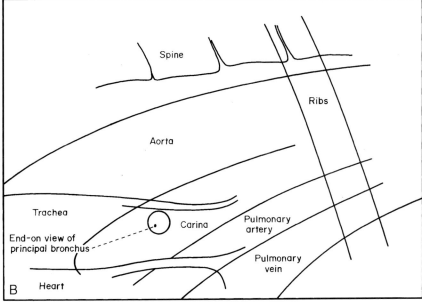

FIGURE 35–2. *A,* Normal adult thoracic radiograph, right lateral projection, dorsocranial aspect. *B,* Companion line drawing.

interstitial lung opacities in the horse are particularly outstanding, especially when compared to dogs and cats. The vascular size and pathways are relatively constant in this region of the lung, making it the ideal for assessing pulmonary circulation. The diaphragm usually appears flattened, or the thoracic side may be slightly convex.

Caudoventral Projection

The caudoventral projection provides for visualization of the caudal part of the heart, the left atrium, and associated pulmonary veins. The caudal vena cava and ventral part of the diaphragm are also visible, which together with the caudal margin of the heart form a characteristically shaped, triangular region in which it is convenient to evaluate lung opacity. Of the four described projections, the caudodorsal and caudoventral views are most apt to reveal any pathologic processes in the lung.

SUPPLEMENTARY PROJECTIONS

Spot Radiographs and Alternate-Side Radiography

Optimal imaging is obtained when a lesion or region of interest is centered radiographically. Thus, once such a lesion has been located in a standard radiographic series, it is often advisable to obtain a radiograph with the lesion centered in the field-of-view to improve image clarity. Clarity may be further enhanced by reducing the distance between the lesion and the film (i.e., obtaining another radiograph with the opposite side of the patient next to the cassette, thereby reducing magnification and improving the sharpness and detail of the image [Fig. 35–6]).

Penetrated View

By using a more penetrating x-ray beam (increased kVp), it is often possible to see additional detail in certain types of lesions, such as a cavitated lung abscess.

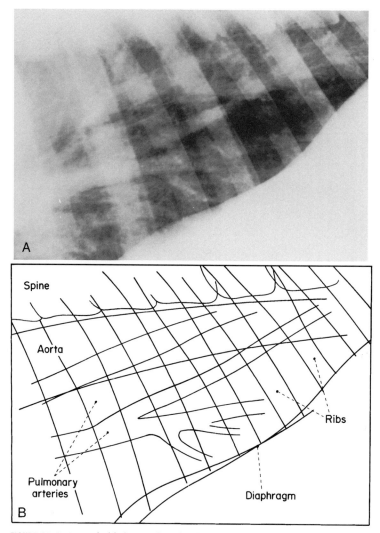

FIGURE 35–3. *A, Normal adult thoracic radiograph, right lateral projection, dorsocaudal aspect. B, Companion line drawing.*

Inspiration-Expiration Comparison Radiographs

In patients with suspected chronic obstructive lung disease, air trapping may be inferred radiographically on the basis of minimal or no difference in lung volume in two sequential radiographs: one on maximal inspiration and one on maximal expiration. This maneuver is especially useful in animals that have otherwise normal radiographic findings. Obviously, care must be taken to be certain that each radiograph was exposed on opposite phases of the respiratory cycle when these sequential examinations are compared.

DIAGNOSTIC LIMITATIONS

The greatest limitation in adult equine thoracic radiography is the inability to view the lung in more than the lateral view. Although alternate-side radiography may be of some help in establishing the laterality of peripherally located lesions, it in no way supplants a ventrodorsal projection.

Because of the enormous size of the horse's thorax (often exceeding 1 m in width), vascular superimposition is marked, especially in the lateral projection. Body fat further degrades the radiographic image owing to scatter and resultant loss of structural definition.

An inability to make postural radiographs, such as decubi-tal and erect projections, prevents the movement of pleural fluid away from potential masses in the ventral aspect of the thorax, particularly those in the cranial mediastinum.

RADIOGRAPHIC OBSERVATIONS

As opposed to a pattern recognition technique for lung assessment (e.g., interstitial versus bronchial versus alveolar opacities), an individual lesion approach as described subsequently can be useful for equine thoracic radiographic interpretation.[1] An individual lesion approach may be employed with any degree of lung involvement: localized, regional, or diffuse. Using this strategy, abnormal pulmonary opacities are placed into one or more of the following broad categories and then related to disorders associated with these types of lesions:[2]

- Pulmonary air loss with replacement (consolidation).
- Pulmonary air loss without replacement (collapse).
- Pulmonary cavitation.
- Spherical lung opacities.
- Linear lung opacities.
- Ring-like lung opacities.
- Nonstructured lung opacities.

The presence of calcification should also be noted.

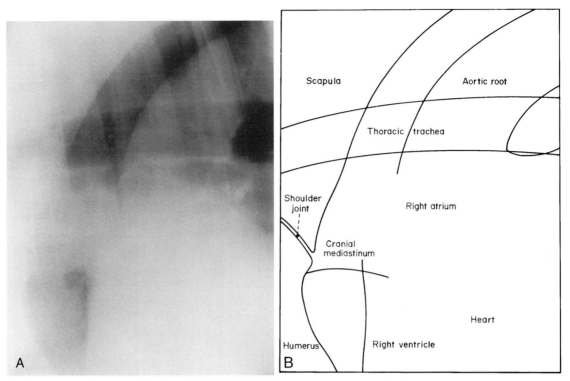

FIGURE 35–4. *A,* Normal adult thoracic radiograph, right lateral projection, ventrocranial aspect. *B,* Companion line drawing.

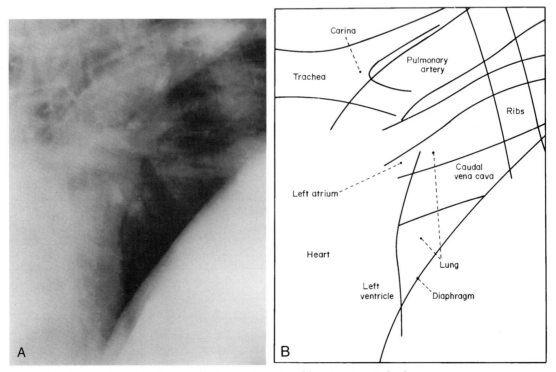

FIGURE 35–5. *A,* Normal adult thoracic radiograph, right lateral projection, ventrocaudal aspect. *B,* Companion line drawing.

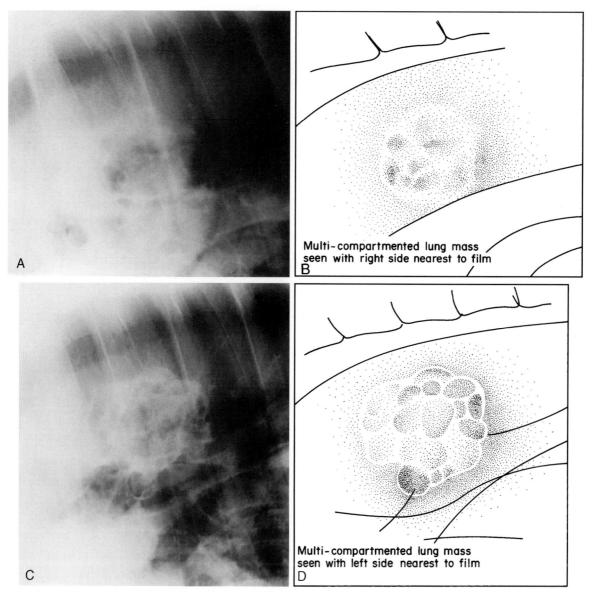

FIGURE 35–6. A, Close-up right lateral thoracic radiograph of central lung region (right side of horse nearest cassette). There is a large, vaguely marginated cavitary lung lesion immediately proximal to the heart base. B, Companion line drawing. C, Close-up left lateral thoracic radiograph of central lung region (left side of horse nearest cassette). The same lung lesion as seen in A is visible, but it is more sharply marginated. The relative improvement in lesion clarity indicates the cavitation is in the left side of the lung. D, Companion line drawing.

Pulmonary Air Loss with Replacement (Consolidation)

Consolidation refers to the replacement of alveolar air by fluid or cells, or both, usually with the maintenance of normal lung volume. The term *pulmonary infiltrate* has also been used in this context but is less precise. The accumulated fluid may be transudative, exudative, or hemorrhagic in nature. Mechanisms of alveolar filling include infection, bleeding, edema, disseminated intravascular coagulation (DIC), near-drowning, smoke inhalation, strangulation, and opportunistic protozoa. The signs of consolidation are as follows.[3]

Lung Opacification

Radiographically the lung should appear dark gray or black. Where air is lost and replaced by liquids or solids, as in pneumonia, the lung becomes light gray or white and is described as opacified. Lung opacification—either partial or complete—is thus the most notable feature of most lung disease. Lung collapse also results in opacification but not to the extent of consolidation. Pleural fluid is more problematic because it may resemble lung opacification, but it usually can be differentiated from the latter by the lack of air bronchograms.

Maintenance of Volume in the Diseased Lobe or Lobes

In addition to a greater degree of opacification, lung consolidation may also be differentiated from collapse by volume maintenance afforded by the fluid that has replaced the air within the diseased alveoli.

Air Bronchogram

Normally, it is not possible to identify medium-sized and small-sized bronchi within the lung because their walls are too thin, and they are filled with air as are the surrounding alveoli; thus, there is little or no discernible contrast between the two lung components. If, however, the individual airway is surrounded by fluid-filled alveoli, it becomes visible as a result of the enhanced contrast afforded to the air-filled bronchus by the contiguous fluid-filled air spaces (Fig. 35–7).

Cardiopulmonary Silhouetting

When consolidated lung is in contact with the heart, and the two structures are projected radiographically, the individual images of the heart and lung are characteristically combined to create a new opacity without evidence of any intervening border. When the line of overlap between the heart and lung is visible, the term *negative silhouette sign* is used, signifying that the lung and heart are superimposed but not in contact. In addition to being helpful in identifying consolidation, the silhouette sign also establishes that the affected lung is in contact with the heart, information that may be surgically useful.

Consolidation of most or all of a single lung lobe with volume preservation is termed *lobar consolidation*. In most instances, this is the result of bacterial pneumonia or, in the context of trauma, pulmonary contusion. Lobar consolidation produces an opaque lobe, typically associated with air bronchograms. Discrete borders are usually formed between the consolidated lobe and the normal adjacent lobes, and there is often cardiopulmonary or diaphragmaticopulmonary silhouetting.

Patchy consolidation (one or more patches of ill-defined opacification) is usually due to infection; sometimes trauma or pulmonary edema; and occasionally immune-mediated pneumonia, DIC, or metastatic tumor. There is no way to differentiate radiographically between these diagnostic possibilities, but in most patients the clinical and laboratory findings point to one of these alternatives as being more likely than the rest.

Cavitation (a hollow area within the lung) occasionally develops within areas of pulmonary consolidation and, in horses, is most often the result of abscessation (see Fig. 35–6). Certain parasites, foreign bodies such as plant awns (foxtails), and some types of primary or metastatic lung tumors may also produce cavitation. Cavitation may be mimicked by sac-

cular bronchiectasis. Cavitary lesions are most often identified because of an associated air-fluid interface—an observation made possible by the communication of the abscess with one or more airways, thus allowing for the drainage of the fluid and subsequent replacement with air. In a lateral projection made with a vertically directed x-ray beam, a fluid line is not seen. Depending on their location, infectious cavitary lesions may rupture to the pleural surface, leading to pneumothorax or pleuropneumonia, or both.

Pulmonary Air Loss Without Replacement (Collapse)

Collapse of one or more lung lobes may be due to a variety of causes but most commonly is caused by external compression resulting from pneumothorax or hydrothorax, combined with the natural tendency of the lung to recoil toward the hilus. Less frequently, lung collapse results from bronchial obstruction, either in the form of a luminal mass or foreign body. The signs of lung collapse are as follows.

Increased Lung Opacity and Decreased Lung Volume

Lung collapse results in an increase in lung opacity but a decrease in volume, in most instances with the maintenance of shape but a proportional diminution in size. A silhouette sign typically results, although with total collapse it may be lost within the normal visual complexity of the hilar region.

When lung collapse occurs, there is usually not only a volume loss on the affected side, but also a compensatory volume increase on the opposite side of the lung. This imbalance in lobar pressures, particularly as it relates to the structures of the mediastinum, results in a shift of the heart toward the side of the lesion. Termed a *cardiac* or *mediastinal shift*, this observation is often invaluable in differentiating consolidation from atelectasis.[4] Unless a ventrodorsal projection is made, however, such an observation is unlikely in a horse.

Spherical Opacities (Lung Nodule, Lung Mass). Spherical lung opacities may be divided according to size: lung nodules measuring roughly less than 0.5 cm in diameter and lung masses measuring roughly 0.5 cm or greater in their

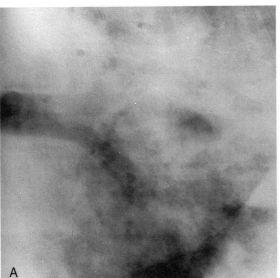
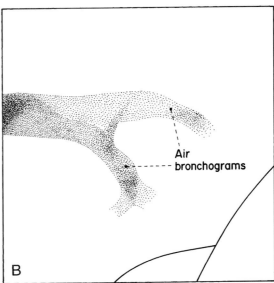

Air bronchograms

FIGURE 35–7. *A,* Close-up lateral thoracic radiograph. There is a large Y-shaped air bronchogram amidst widespread pulmonary consolidation. *B,* Companion line drawing. Diagnosis was pneumonia.

largest dimension. Either may appear sharply or indistinctly marginated, solitary or multiple.

Solitary lung nodules are comparatively rare in horses and are usually indicative of developing abscessation. Focal pneumonia, localized hemorrhage, and infarct are occasionally responsible for a spherical lung opacity. Following the progress of solitary lung lesions with serial radiographic examinations is of great value because the lack of change over a period of months constitutes strong presumptive evidence for a benign tumor or an inactive granuloma.[5]

Multiple small spherical opacities in horses are usually attributable to fungal pneumonia. When calcified, such lesions are most apt to be granulomatous. Some chronic inflammatory lung disease in horses may be associated with ill-defined nodular lung opacities, which apparently arise from the peribronchial tissues; such findings may be mistaken for fungal pneumonia or metastases.

In horses, large circumscribed (mass) lesions are usually abscesses. Less frequently, such a finding represents a primary lung tumor or granuloma. A rapid increase in size favors infectious over neoplastic causes.[6]

Linear Opacities. The term *line shadow* refers to an abnormal linear lung opacity arising from a number of possible disorders. Most commonly, especially if seen in combination with ring shadows, line shadows indicate bronchial or peribronchial disease. It must be remembered, however, that the walls of the large central airways normally cast such shadows, especially in thinner or older horses.

With pneumothorax, the dorsal pleural surfaces are often seen as faint curvilinear opacities diverging from the spinal region in a caudoventral direction toward the diaphragm. No lung vessels are seen between the ventral aspect of the spine and the surface of the partially collapsed lung lobe.

Ring-Shaped Opacities. *Ring shadows* result when large, normal central bronchi or smaller diseased airways are radiographically projected end-on.[7] This end-on view causes the normally thin (and therefore minimally attenuating bronchial wall) to absorb a sufficiently large amount of incident radiation that it becomes highly visible. When viewed slightly askew, such airways may appear eccentrically thickened and be mistaken for bronchial disease. Multiple large ring shadows, other than those normally found in the central lung field, are indicative of bronchiectasis.

Widespread Small Opacities. Thoracic radiographs containing multiple small lung opacities often are difficult to diagnose precisely. Often, it is possible only to render a prioritized differential diagnosis in such situations.[8] Many descriptive terms have been applied to these opacities, the most common being mottling, honeycombing, fine nodular, reticular, and reticulonodular shadows. Such terms may be consolidated into two basic types: *nodular* (to indicate small round shadows) and *reticular* (to describe a net-like pattern of small lines). Disease patterns combining both nodular and reticular elements are referred to as *reticulonodular*.

All of these patterns are due to small lesions in the lung, usually no more than 1 or 2 mm in diameter. Individual lesions of this size, unless calcified, are invisible on a thoracic radiograph. They are seen only because they are superimposed on one another. As such, the abnormal shadows comprising an interstitial lung pattern in a thoracic radiograph typically misrepresent the lesion with respect to both size and shape. Nevertheless, such patterns may, in selected lung disorders, prove diagnostically useful.

Many of these described findings may be mimicked by end-on blood vessels, obesity, emaciation, underpenetration (radiographic image is too light), and patient or respiratory motion.

SPECIFIC LUNG DISEASES

Pneumonia

Equine bacterial pneumonia usually occurs in the ventral half of the lung, often appearing initially as a localized or regional consolidation superimposed on the caudal heart margin.[9] If therapeutically unchecked, many equine pneumonias result in abscessation and pleuritis (Fig. 35–8).[10, 11]

Interstitial pneumonia (alveolitis) occurs in foals as well as adults and is currently theorized to be a distinct disease of unknown cause, occurring in at least two forms.[12] In the foal, the radiographic alterations are often subtle, initially showing as a mild increase in overall lung opacification, sometimes accompanied by prominent bronchi (probably representing peribronchial inflammation). As an aside, the radiographs of pneumonic neonates often appear to have been made during expiration. Although such an appearance may in part be due to expiration, it may also be associated with an elevated respiratory rate and low tidal volume. Further volume loss probably results from luminal obstruction owing to inflammatory secretions.

When thoracic radiographs are made in recumbent foals, postural atelectasis develops almost immediately (assuming the animal was standing previously) and is well advanced if the foal has been recumbent for more than a few hours. Thus, apparent lung opacification in such animals must—at least in part—be attributed to a combination of factors other than disease, including postural atelectasis, hypostatic pulmonary congestion, and reduced ventilation associated with recumbent positioning.

In adult horses 2 years and older, interstitial pneumonia may result in a generalized mild to moderate opacification or a diffuse patchiness, the latter potentially being confused with lung masses such as abscesses, granulomas, or metastases (Figs. 35–9 to 35–11).

Fungal pneumonia also has a range of appearances, a common one being widespread, relatively indistinct spherical opacification (Fig. 35–12). Mixed peribronchial-interstitial patterns have also been observed. *Histoplasma capsulatum* and

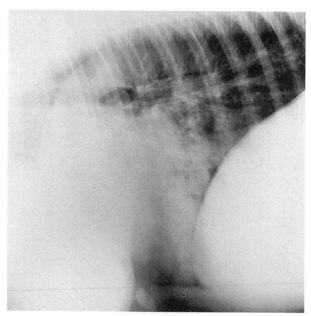

FIGURE 35–8. Lateral thoracic radiograph. There is patchy consolidation beginning at the level of the aorta and extending ventrally where it obliterates the caudal part of the heart. Diagnosis was regional pneumonia with abscessation.

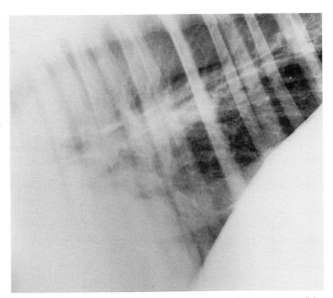

FIGURE 35–9. Lateral thoracic radiograph in which there is a mild increase in overall lung opacity. Diagnosis was mild, diffuse interstitial pneumonia.

Coccidioides immitis are reported most frequently in the southwestern United States, *C. immitis* sometimes appearing as a large solitary lung mass.[13] Some chronic mycotic pneumonia may appear as diffuse ventral consolidation (Fig. 35–13). Viral pneumonia usually does not alter the lung enough to be detected radiographically.

Pulmonary Abscessation

In young horses, and less commonly in adults, pleuropneumonia may lead to abscessation, although abscesses may develop independently.[14] Such lesions may occur deep in the

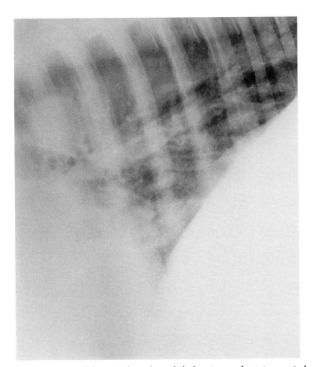

FIGURE 35–10. Lateral thoracic radiograph in which there is a moderate increase in lung opacification and reduced vascular clarity. Diagnosis was moderate, diffuse interstitial pneumonia.

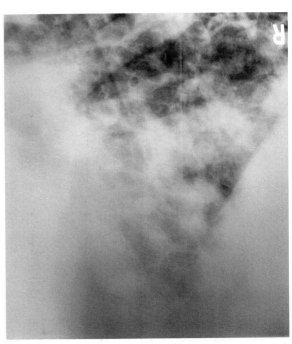

FIGURE 35–11. Lateral thoracic radiograph. There is marked increase in lung opacification obscuring the caudal heart margin and regional vasculature. Although abscesses are suggested radiographically, there were none found at necropsy. Diagnosis was mixed, interstitial consolidative pneumonia.

lung, superficially, immediately beneath the pleural surface, or in the mediastinum. They may be singular or multiple, large or small, and sharply or vaguely marginated. The most characteristic appearance of a pulmonary abscess is that of a baseball-sized opacity located in the caudal third of the lung, often dorsally (Fig. 35–14). Well-marginated pulmonary consolidation may mimic abscessation (Fig. 35–15). Some abscesses communicate with an adjacent bronchus allowing air to enter the abscess cavity, producing a characteristic gas cap (Fig. 35–16).

Pleuropneumonia

In many horses, bacterial pneumonia spreads to the lung surface and into the pleural space.[15] This is termed *pleuropneumonia*.[16] As a result, large volumes of pleural fluid are often produced concealing much of the lung. In such instances, it is often difficult or impossible to distinguish between a viral pleuritis and pleuropneumonia. Fortunately, such a distinction can usually be made using sonography. Where pleural fluid and consolidation or abscessation are seen together, and there is no history of trauma, pleuropneumonia is likely.

Lung Hemorrhage

Injury-Induced Hemorrhage

Blunt or penetrating injury to the lung often produces bleeding, which may be identified in conjunction with other thoracic abnormalities, such as pneumothorax, hemothorax, and rib fractures. The resultant lung consolidation usually resolves in a week or less, often allowing for the differentiation of pulmonary hemorrhage from other forms of consolidation, such as pneumonia, which take longer to disappear.

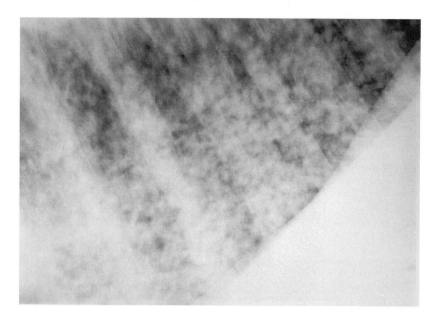

FIGURE 35–12. Close-up lateral thoracic radiograph of caudodorsal lung field. There are diffuse pulmonary nodules. Diagnosis was fungal pneumonia.

Exercise-Induced Hemorrhage

Exercise-induced pulmonary hemorrhage may cause localized, regional, or diffuse parenchymal bleeding, in some instances resulting in sudden death.[17] Often, however, the disorder is not fatal but results in weakness, epistaxis, and radiographically identifiable lesions in the dorsal aspect of the caudal lung lobes. Observed changes range from totally opacified, wedge-shaped regional lesions to nearly transparent, oval-shaped entities, usually located in the caudodorsal part of the lung (Fig. 35–17).[18] Radiologic-pathologic correlation indicates a direct relationship between lesion opacification and severity.[19] Current research is focusing on the relationship between the large cardiac output developed during

racing and the inability of pulmonary capillaries in some horses to withstand the resultant pressure-related stress.[20] Diffuse bleeding disorders such as DIC may resemble pneumonia.[21]

Lung Rupture and the Accumulation of Extrapulmonary Air

Rupture of the lung usually produces some degree of pneumothorax, often associated with pulmonary contusion. Occasionally, there also may be hemothorax. Most such injuries

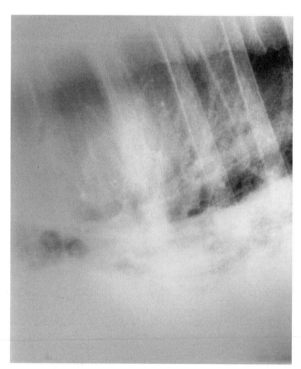

FIGURE 35–13. Close-up lateral thoracic radiograph of the mid-dorsal lung field in which there is consolidation of the ventral half of the lung. Diagnosis was fungal pneumonia.

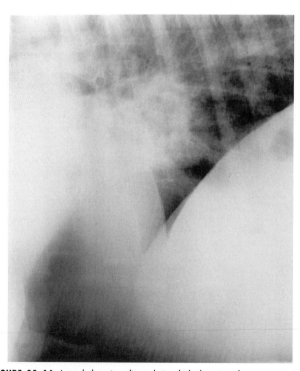

FIGURE 35–14. Lateral thoracic radiograph in which there is a lung mass, partially superimposed on caudal vena cava. Diagnosis was lung abscess.

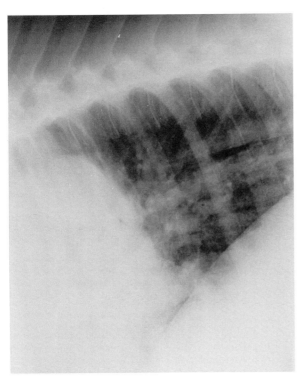

FIGURE 35–15. Lateral thoracic radiograph. There is a well-marginated region of consolidation in the central lung field. Diagnosis was pneumonia, with extensive pulmonary consolidation.

are caused by blunt trauma but may also be incurred by a penetrating thoracic wound (Fig. 35–18).

Pulmonary Hyperemia, Oligemia, and Vascular Deficit

Heart disease, whether congenital or acquired, is the most common cause of altered pulmonary vasculature in the horse. In neonates with persistent fetal intracardiac communications, such as patent foramen ovale, associated pulmonary hypertension results in a diminished vasculature. In

older foals, isolated intracardiac or extracardiac communications typically produce a pulmonary overcirculation. In complex cardiac anomalies in which right-sided outflow obstruction exists, blood may shunt from the right to left sides of the heart causing a reduction in pulmonary blood flow.[22] Congestive heart failure is usually associated with a hyperemic lung, in addition to cardiomegaly and pulmonary edema. Pneumonia may also be associated with regional hyperemia, as is true of most inflammatory conditions. Conversely the pulmonary vasculature often appears small with advanced emphysema and other forms of chronic obstructive lung disease.

Thrombosis, depending on its location and the availability of collateral circulation, may result in a vascular deficit or disappearance of one or more pulmonary vessels, with or without a visible pulmonary infarct. Pulmonary thromboembolism may also be associated with small nodular opacities, although these are extremely difficult to differentiate from end-on vascular projections.[23]

Pulmonary Edema

There are three potential distributions of pulmonary edema: (1) vascular, (2) interstitial, and (3) alveolar, reflecting changes to the lung with increasing pulmonary capillary hydrostatic pressures. Which distribution is present depends on the severity and duration of the inciting condition. Combined patterns are common with pulmonary edema because the excessive circulating blood volume initially enlarges the pulmonary veins and then results in accumulation of fluid in the interstitium (perivascular interstitial tissues) and subsequently the alveoli.[25] Alveolar edema is almost always acute and usually (but not always) bilateral. In the early stages, edema often collects about the hilus—an extremely difficult radiographic determination to make in animals with left atrial enlargement and pulmonary hyperemia and especially difficult in horses, in which only lateral projections are usually available. The causes of pulmonary edema are broadly divided into those due to circulatory causes, such as heart failure or fluid overload, and those that are unrelated to heart disease in which increased capillary permeability is the fundamental disease mechanism. Examples of the latter include aspiration of stomach contents, smoke inhalation,

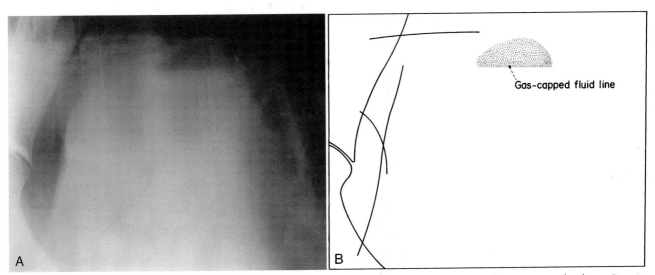

FIGURE 35–16. *A,* Close-up lateral thoracic radiograph centered on the heart. There is a gas-capped fluid line superimposed on the heart base. *B,* Companion line drawing. Diagnosis was communicating lung abscess.

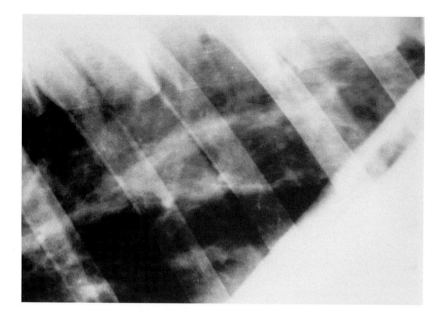

FIGURE 35–17. Close-up lateral thoracic radiograph of caudodorsal lung field in which there is an oval-shaped, ill-defined lung mass adjacent to the dorsal edge of the diaphragm. Diagnosis was exercised-induced pulmonary hemorrhage.

near-drowning, and strangulation. One way of separating cardiac from noncardiac pulmonary edema is the rapidity with which the former may resolve—often in as little as 24 hours with effective therapy.

Noncardiac pulmonary edema has been reported in horses immediately following inhalation anesthesia. Proposed causes included severe alveolar hypoxia related to anesthesia and acute upper airway obstruction during recovery.[26]

Chronic Bronchitis and Bronchiectasis

Chronic bronchial disease is rarely capable of causing enough structural alteration in the bronchi and surrounding connective tissue to be recognized radiographically. When present, bronchial disease is characterized by an outlining or accentuation of the large and middle airways, enhancing their radio-

graphic visibility. Seen on-end, the diseased bronchus resembles a ring, whereas in profile, the effected airway appears as a pair of parallel lines (Fig. 35–19).[27]

Bronchiectasis, generally considered to be an end stage of chronic bronchitis, is characterized by a pronounced accentuation of the large and medium-sized airways, at times accompanied by cylindric or saccular enlargement of one or more bronchi. Because bronchiectatic airways often contain fluid, end-on projections of such bronchi or bronchioles may appear as lung nodules or, in the case of larger airways, lung masses.

Chronic Obstructive Lung Disease

Chronic obstructive lung disease is the most common pulmonary disorder of mature horses throughout most parts of the world. The majority of these disorders are associated with a normal radiograph, whereas the minority have abnormal-appearing lungs. In this latter regard, there are no consistent findings, although the lung and airways are usually diffusely affected—often by linear and ring-shaped opacities or small, poorly defined lung nodules. Functionally, especially in the advanced stages of these disorders, chronic obstructive lung disease may be inferred from the radiographic triad of (1) hyperinflation, (2) hyperlucency, and (3) pulmonary oligemia, particularly if present in both inspiratory and expiratory radiographs. Some of these horses also show a uniform tracheobronchial dilation (see Fig. 35–19).

Allergic Lung Disease

The majority of allergic lungs appear normal radiographically. With long-standing allergic lung disease, there may be excessive *lung markings*, which are believed to represent thickened small airways, many of which are obstructed by abnormal secretions.

Lung Neoplasia

Primary lung tumors are rare in the horse; granular cell tumor (myoblastoma) being the most frequently reported.

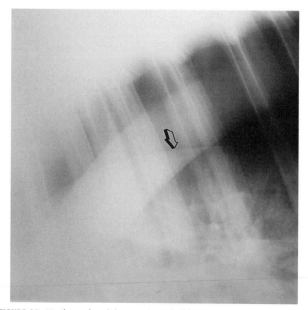

FIGURE 35–18. Close-up lateral thoracic radiograph of the craniodorsal lung field. The surface of collapsed lung *(arrow)* is seen ventral to a large accumulation of pleural air. Diagnosis was pneumothorax and atelectasis.

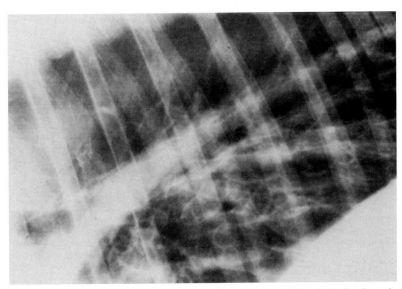

FIGURE 35–19. Close-up lateral thoracic radiograph of the caudodorsal lung field. The large and medium bronchi appear thickened and enlarged as evidenced by numerous line and ring opacities. Diagnosis was emphysema and bronchiectasis.

Secondary lung tumors, or pulmonary metastases, occur occasionally, with one study reporting adenocarcinoma as the most common, arising from primary sites in the thyroid, kidney, ovary, and uterus.

Radiographically, most primary lung tumors appear as a large solitary lung mass, whereas the typical pulmonary metastasis is represented by widespread spherical opacities—usually indistinctly marginated owing to the effects of superimposition.[23] Some metastatic lesions, however, appear as ill-defined nodules and others as patchy consolidation. In contrast to companion animals, widespread spherical opacities in horses are more likely to represent abscessation than cancer.

Mesothelioma affects the pleural surfaces of both the lung and the thoracic cavity and characteristically produces a large volume of pleural fluid, which is usually microscopically di-

agnostic. Radiographically (or sonographically), mesothelioma, and in particular the pleural fluid that it causes, cannot be distinguished from non-neoplastic pleuritis.[28]

Diaphragmatic Hernia

Most diaphragmatic hernias are the result of injury. Radiographic observations are predicated on the following factors: (1) the size and location of the diaphragmatic tear, (2) the extent and location of abdominal content within the thorax, (3) the amount of resultant lung compression, and (4) the volume of fluid produced and accumulated within the thoracic cavity. Cylindric, intrathoracic transparencies strongly suggest herniated intestine (Fig. 35–20). A barium study can also define a herniated stomach or bowel.

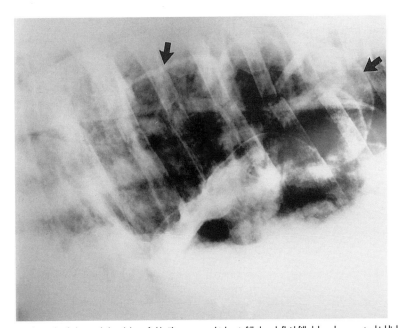

FIGURE 35–20. Close-up lateral thoracic radiograph of the caudodorsal lung field. There are multiple air-filled and fluid-filled bowel segments, highlighted by a large volume of surrounding pleural air *(arrows)*. Ventrally, there is near total opacification, the result of superimposed intestine, liver, atelectasis, and pleural hemorrhage. Diagnosis was diaphragmatic hernia.

References

1. Farrow CS: The perils of pattern recognition. Can Vet J 36:57, 1995.
2. Armstrong P, and Wastie ML: Diagnostic Imaging. Oxford, Blackwell Scientific Publications, 1987.
3. Meyer W: Radiography review: The alveolar pattern of pulmonary disease. J Am Vet Radiol Soc 20:10, 1979.
4. Lord PF, and Gomez JA: Lung lobe collapse. Vet Radiol 26:187, 1985.
5. Reif JS: Solitary pulmonary lesions in small animals. J Am Vet Med Assoc 155:717, 1969.
6. Lillington GA: A Diagnostic Approach to Chest Diseases, 3rd Ed. Baltimore, Williams & Wilkins, 1987.
7. Meyer CW: Radiography review: The vascular and bronchial patterns of pulmonary disease. Vet Radiol 21:156, 1980.
8. Meyer CW: Radiography review: The interstitial pattern of pulmonary disease. Vet Radiol 21:8, 1980.
9. Kangstrom LE: The radiological diagnosis of equine pneumonia. Vet Radiol 9:80, 1968.
10. Raphel CF, and Beech JB: Pleuritis secondary to pneumonia or lung abscessation in 90 horses. J Am Vet Med Assoc 181:808, 1982.
11. Mair TS, and Lane JG: Pneumonia, lung abscesses and pleuritis in adult horses: A review of 51 cases. Equine Vet J 21:175, 1989.
12. Buergelt CD: Interstitial pneumonia in the horse: A fledgling morphological entity with mysterious causes. Equine Vet J 27:4, 1995.
13. Ruoff WW: Fungal pneumonia in horses. In Proceedings of the 34th Annual Convention, American Association of Equine Practitioners, Dec. 4–7, 1988, San Diego, CA, p 423.
14. Lavoie JP, Fiset L, and Laverty S: Review of 40 cases of lung abscesses in foals and adult horses. Equine Vet J 26:348, 1994.
15. Sweeney CR: Causes of pleural effusion in the horse. Equine Vet Ed 4:75, 1992.
16. Farrow CS: Radiographic examination and interpretation. In Beech J (Ed): Equine Respiratory Disorders. Philadelphia, WB Saunders, 1991, pp 89–119.
17. Gunson DE, Sweeney CR, and Soma LR: Sudden death attributable to exercise-induced pulmonary hemorrhage in racehorses: Nine cases (1981–1983). J Am Vet Med Assoc 193:102, 1988.
18. Pascoe JR, O'Brien TR, Wheat JD, et al: Radiographic aspects of exercise-induced pulmonary hemorrhage in racing horses. Vet Radiol 24:85, 1983.
19. O'Callaghan MW, Pascoe JR, O'Brien TR, et al: Exercise-induced pulmonary hemorrhage in the horse: Results of a detailed clinical, post mortem and imaging study: VI. Radiological/pathological correlations. Equine Vet J 19:419, 1987.
20. Wesat JB, and Mathiew-Costello O: Stress failure of pulmonary capillaries as a mechanism for exercise induced pulmonary hemorrhage in the horse. Equine Vet J 26:441, 1994.
21. Morris DD, and Beech J: Disseminated intravascular coagulation in six horses. J Am Vet Med Assoc 183:1067, 1983.
22. Cottrill CM, O'Connor WN, Cudd T, et al: Persistence of fetal circulatory pathways in a newborn foal. Equine Vet J 19:252, 1987.
23. Dik KJ, and Gunser I: Atlas of Diagnostic Radiology of the Horse: Part 3. Diseases of the Head, Neck, and Thorax. Philadelphia, WB Saunders, 1990.
24. Morgan PW, and Goodman LR: Pulmonary edema and adult respiratory distress syndrome. Radiol Clin North Am 29:943, 1991.
25. Staub NC, Nagara H, and Pearce ML: Pulmonary edema in dogs, especially the sequence of fluid accumulation in the lungs. J Appl Physiol 22:227, 1967.
26. Ball MA, and Trim CM: Post anesthesia pulmonary edema in 2 horses. Equine Vet Ed 8:13, 1996.
27. Farrow CS: Radiographic aspects of inflammatory lung disease in the horse. Vet Radiol 22:107, 1989.
28. Mair TS, Hillyer, and Brown PJ: Mesothelioma of the pleural cavity in a horse: Diagnostic features. Equine Vet Ed 4:59, 1992.

STUDY QUESTIONS

1. What is pleuropneumonia? How is it postulated to develop? Is it worse than pneumonia without a pleural component? How difficult is it to diagnose radiographically?

2. Of what use is vascular assessment in the radiographic evaluation of lung disease?

3. A mass with a gas-fluid interface is seen in the dorsal lung field of a 6-year-old horse. What is the most likely diagnosis?

4. What are two significant technical limitations of equine thoracic radiography in relation to canine thoracic radiography?

5. Multiple pulmonary nodules in a horse are less likely to be neoplastic than a similar radiographic finding in a dog. (True or False)

6. Why is a mediastinal shift difficult to identify in equine thoracic radiographs?

7. In which portion of the lung are radiographic changes associated with equine exercise-induced pulmonary hemorrhage most likely to be seen?

8. In which portion of the lung are radiographic changes associated with equine bacterial pneumonia most likely to be seen?

9. Even though it is not possible to obtain ventrodorsal radiographs of the equine thorax, how might one determine if a lung mass is in the right or left lung?

(Answers appear on page 645.)

ABDOMEN—COMPANION ANIMALS

Chapter 36

Abdominal Masses

Charles R. Root

Radiographic differentiation of abdominal masses depends on a good working knowledge of normal radiographic anatomy as well as an appreciation for normal anatomic variations.[1-4] Some abdominal organs, such as the liver, stomach, jejunum, colon, and urinary bladder, are nearly always seen; some, such as the spleen, kidneys, and prostate gland, are typically only partially seen; and some, such as the pancreas, adrenal glands, ovaries, and mesenteric lymph nodes, are seen only if abnormal. When no lesions are detected in the visualized portion of an organ, the remainder of the organ is assumed to be normal *in the context of radiographic differentiation of abdominal masses*. In other words, one must assume normalcy unless there is radiographic evidence to the contrary.

Routine radiography of the abdomen should include ventrodorsal and lateral projections. Right-side dependency allows the tail (distal extremity) of the spleen to gravitate across the midline and thereby be more frequently visualized than with the left side down. Likewise, in left lateral recumbency, the gas-filled pyloric part of the stomach, which may serve as an important landmark, is usually seen. Whether to use a left versus right lateral view routinely is not as important as obtaining supplemental radiographs when needed to alleviate confusion.

Normally visible structures may not be obvious for a variety of reasons, and there may be temptation to perform contrast radiography in such instances. Before resorting to contrast radiography to enhance visualization of poorly delineated abdominal visceral structures, however, one should consider positional radiography. This alternative often yields definitive results quicker and with less manipulation or expense than most contrast radiography. Positional radiography may consist simply of obtaining the opposite lateral, a dorsoventral, or an oblique view, but it also can include horizontal-beam projections, depending on the suspected nature and location of the lesion. In general, positional radiography capitalizes either on the benefits of tangential projections of peripheral lesions or on the effects of gravity on mobile structures or on structures that may contain both fluid and gas.

SPECIAL PROCEDURES

Ultrasonographic assessment of abdominal viscera, when available, has virtually eliminated the need for most special radiographic procedures in differentiation of abdominal masses. When abdominal ultrasonography is not available or if positional radiography is contraindicated or has been unsuccessful, various contrast radiographic procedures may be performed. Special radiographic procedures that have proved helpful in radiographic differential diagnosis of certain abdominal masses include pneumoperitoneography,[1, 2, 5, 6] excretory urography,[7] upper gastrointestinal series,[8] urography,[6] cystography,[7] and celiography.[9]

RADIOGRAPHIC SIGNS

Recognition and assessment of displacement of adjacent abdominal visceral structures are the keys to successful radiographic differentiation of abdominal masses. The effects of abdominal masses on adjacent structures depend on both enlargement and gravity. If the mass is derived from a fixed organ, the effects of gravity and body position are minimal. If the enlarged organ is pendulous, pedunculated, or mobile, however, the combined gravitational and mass effects on adjacent structures may be striking. One should not be surprised by the fact that radiographically demonstrated visceral displacement in dorsal or lateral recumbency may be quite different than that theorized or imagined while the patient is standing or sternal. Visceral displacement may be due to pulsion, traction, or (in hollow viscera only) redundancy. Abdominal masses usually cause displacement of adjacent mobile structures by pulsion. Traction displacement occurs when a structure is pulled from its normal position by some pathologic movement of a structure to which it is attached (e.g., ventral displacement of the caudal pole of the ipsilateral kidney by an ovarian mass, ventral displacement of the duodenum by a mass in the left limb of the pancreas, and ventral displacement of the transverse and ascending portions of the colon by severe colic lymphadenopathy). Redundancy is the third reason a structure appears out of place; the elongated descending colon is probably the most common example, its presence in an atypical location of the caudal abdomen often falsely suggesting enlargement of adjacent structures. Colonic redundancy should be suspected when the colon appears to be displaced and no adjacent mass effect is seen. If adjacent fluid opacity structures are hidden by the presence of ascites, colonic redundancy is not commonly appreciated. This is because, in the presence of ascites, the colon is well seen only if filled with gas; if so, it rises to the highest point in the abdomen where its redundancy is poorly appreciated and, therefore, less confusing.

Several abdominal organs undergo tremendous variation in size under normal circumstances, including the stomach, the urinary bladder, and the uterus. Each of these structures may be pathologically enlarged, and it may be difficult to differentiate radiographically between normal and abnormal enlargement. All other normally visible abdominal organs are enlarged only if abnormal.

The edges of enlarged visceral structures may not be directly visible radiographically. In such instances, enlargement must be inferred by the direction and degree of displacement of adjacent structures. Such displacement may be appreciable even in the presence of diminished abdominal visceral detail.

A discussion of the typical radiographic signs associated with specific enlargements of abdominal organs follows. There are exceptions to the general pattern of visceral displacement, but they are rare. The most common exceptions to typical radiographic signs of abdominal masses are those due to extreme enlargement of the organ in question. Less frequently, redundancy of a hollow viscus may falsely suggest enlargement of an adjacent structure.

Stomach

Enlargement of the stomach (Fig. 36–1), whether postprandial or pathologic, causes caudal displacement of the small bowel, the transverse colon, and the spleen. Splenic displacement in the presence of gastric torsion is variable; in this instance, the spleen may be greatly enlarged because of venous congestion.

Uterus

Uterine enlargement is generally not detected radiographically until it exceeds the diameter of adjacent small bowel.

Further enlargement of the uterine body and horns causes craniodorsal displacement of the small bowel in the lateral projection and mesocranial gathering of the small bowel in the ventrodorsal view (Fig. 36–2). Uterine enlargement often results in tortuous or convoluted homogeneous tubular fluid opacities in the caudoventral abdomen. Further, in the lateral view, there may be separation of the ventral aspect of the colon and the dorsal aspect of the urinary bladder by distention of the body of the uterus. Late pregnancy should be easily distinguished from disease by the presence of fetal skeletal mineralization, a finding that is generally first present at 40 to 45 days of gestation in dogs and cats.

Urinary Bladder

Distention of the urinary bladder (Fig. 36–3) usually produces a homogeneous soft-tissue mass effect in the caudoventral abdomen. In the lateral projection, a full urinary bladder usually causes cranial displacement of small bowel and dorsal displacement of the descending colon. In the ventrodorsal projection, the descending colon may be displaced either to the right or to the left of the urinary bladder. A full urinary bladder may entrap the descending colon to the right of the midline (Fig. 36–4).

Diffuse Hepatomegaly

Generalized enlargement of the liver produces characteristic displacement of the pylorus and pyloric antrum caudally,

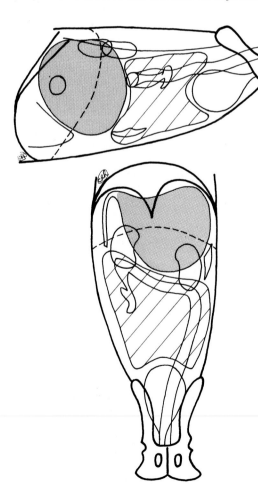

FIGURE 36–1. The radiographic signs of gastric enlargement and the effect of an enlarged stomach on adjacent viscera.

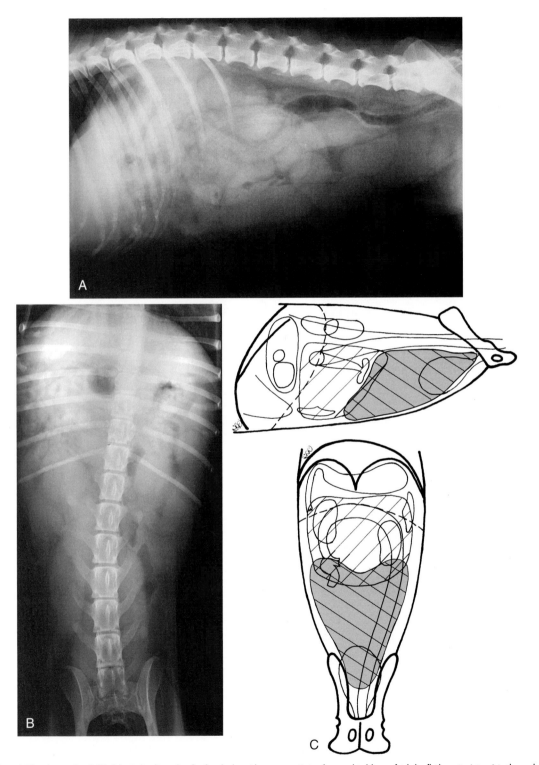

FIGURE 36–2. Lateral *(A)* and ventrodorsal *(B)* abdominal radiographs of a female dog with pyometra. Notice the convoluted loops of tubular fluid opacity (uterus) in the caudoventral abdomen. The small bowel is displaced craniodorsally and in the ventrodorsal view is often displaced medially. The descending colon is often displaced dorsally, as depicted in the associated diagram *(C)*.

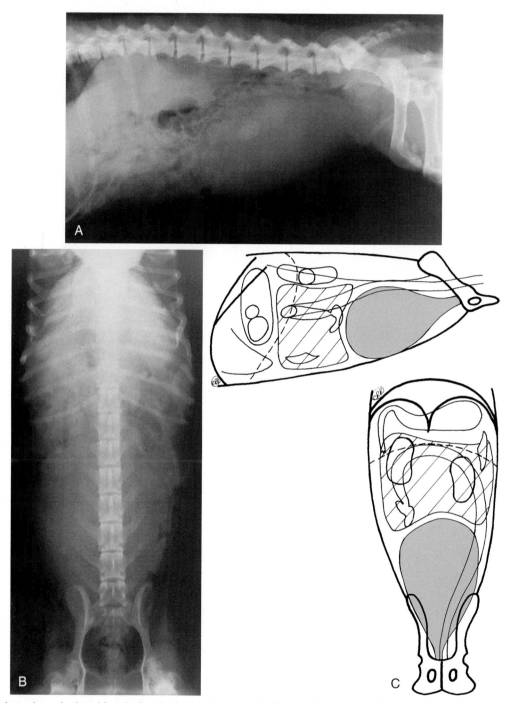

FIGURE 36–3. Lateral (A) and ventrodorsal (B) abdominal radiographs of a dog with a history of dribbling urine. The atonic urinary bladder is distended, displacing the small bowel cranially and the colon dorsally. The line diagrams show the typical visceral displacement (C). (A and B courtesy of the Santa Cruz Veterinary Hospital, Santa Cruz, CA.)

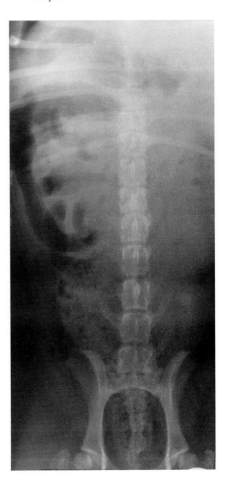

FIGURE 36–4. Ventrodorsal lumbar vertebral radiograph of a dog. Notice that the caudal part of the descending colon is on the right side. This finding is not uncommon, especially when the urinary bladder is full, when the colon is redundant, and when the animal was in left lateral recumbency immediately before being placed on its back for the ventrodorsal radiographic projection. (Courtesy of the Seattle Veterinary Hospital for Surgery, Lynnwood, WA.)

dorsally, and to the left (Fig. 36–5). In the lateral projection, the gastric axis (an imaginary line connecting the fundus, body, and pylorus of the stomach) should be either parallel to the ribs or perpendicular to the spine or somewhere between those two extremes. In the ventrodorsal projection, the gastric axis should be perpendicular to the spine in the dog. Because the pylorus may normally be more caudal in the cat, it can be approximately 30 degrees from perpendicular to the spine in that species, especially in the ventrodorsal projection. In many instances, the enlarged caudoventral edge of the abnormal liver can be seen as it projects beyond the costal margin. When poor abdominal visceral detail prevents direct visualization of the edge of the liver, however, disturbances in the gastric axis are readily apparent if the gastric contents can be seen. Occasionally, a gastrogram may be necessary to characterize generalized hepatomegaly fully.

Focal Lobar Hepatic Masses

Masses developing in the right lateral or right middle lobe of the liver, in the absence of diffuse hepatomegaly, often produce rather specific visceral displacements (Fig. 36–6). There is dorsomedial displacement of the pyloric antrum, pylorus, proximal descending duodenum, and ascending colon. Further, there is caudodorsal displacement of the adjacent small bowel loops and, if the hepatic mass is pedunculated and sufficiently large, craniodorsal displacement of the body of the stomach.

Left lateral or left middle lobar hepatic masses are also quite specific in displacement of adjacent viscera (Fig. 36–7). The head (proximal extremity) of the spleen, the adjacent

small intestine, and the gastric fundus are displaced dorsomedially. The tail of the spleen is variably displaced, but the fundus of the stomach may be strikingly displaced craniodorsally if entrapped by a pedunculated hepatic mass of sufficient size lying to the left.

Central lobar liver masses are rare but usually cause the body of the stomach to be displaced caudodorsally, creating extrinsic indentation of its lesser curvature (Fig. 36–8). Contrast radiography of the stomach may be necessary to appreciate this radiographic sign fully.

Diffuse Splenomegaly

Generalized enlargement of the spleen, if mild, is difficult to verify radiographically. The spleen undergoes considerable nonpathologic variation in size, and there appears to be some overlap of maximal normal and minimal pathologic size. Radiographic assessment of splenic size is subjective, at best. The most acceptable criterion appears to be that a spleen should be considered enlarged if its edges are rounded and if it obviously displaces adjacent viscera (Fig. 36–9).

Splenic Masses

Masses originating in the head of the spleen cause caudodorsal displacement of the adjacent small intestine in the lateral projection. In the ventrodorsal projection, proximal splenic masses cause the small bowel to be displaced caudally and to the right. Also, because the gastrosplenic ligament renders the head of the spleen relatively immobile, masses of the

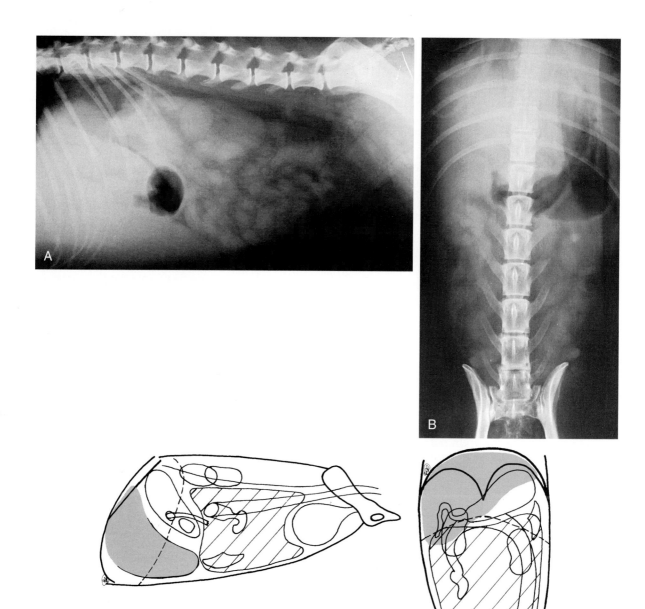

FIGURE 36–5. Lateral (A) and ventrodorsal (B) abdominal radiographs of a dog with generalized hepatic enlargement secondary to diabetes mellitus. There is displacement of the body and pyloric antrum of the stomach caudally, dorsally, and to the left (C). (A and B from Root CR: Abdominal masses: The radiographic differential diagnosis. J Am Vet Radiol Soc 15:26, 1974; with permission.)

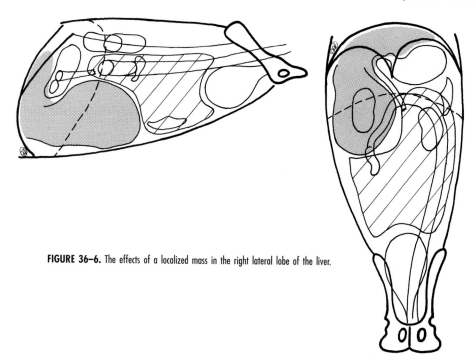

FIGURE 36–6. The effects of a localized mass in the right lateral lobe of the liver.

head of the spleen are often associated with extrinsic cranial displacement of the greater curvature of the stomach, especially in the ventrodorsal view (Fig. 36–10).

Masses that originate in the body or tail of the spleen are the most common cause of a ventral midabdominal mass seen on the lateral view (Fig. 36–11*A*). Distal splenic masses are much less consistent in their displacement of the small bowel than are those of the head of the spleen because the tail and body of the spleen are much more mobile than the head. The small bowel may be displaced in any number of directions or combinations of directions (see Fig. 36–11). Generally, there is dorsal displacement of some portion of the small bowel in the lateral projection. There may also be predominantly caudal or predominantly cranial displacement, however, as well as combinations of cranial and caudal enteric displacement. In the ventrodorsal projection, depending on the location of the splenic mass, the small intestine may be displaced to the left, to the right, caudally, cranially, or peripherally. In fact, subsequent positional radiographs may show considerable variation in enteric visceral displacement. Furthermore, the amount of time a patient is kept in a certain position before radiographs are made may greatly influence the position of the splenic mass.

Splenic Torsion

Splenic torsion may be either secondary to gastric volvulus or independent of other abdominal lesions.[1] In animals in which splenic torsion has existed for several days, only a poorly marginated, generalized, pronounced splenomegaly may be seen (Fig. 36–12).[1] In patients with more recent splenic torsion, it may be possible to identify caudal displacement of the gastric fundus, and the spleen is often dramatically and diffusely enlarged and may be drawn into a C shape as a result of rotation about its own pedicle. If the tail of the spleen is located between the body wall and the right lateral aspect of the enteric viscera, there is often medial displacement of the descending duodenum and ascending colon. Signs of splenic torsion are difficult to identify if the torsion

has resulted in ascites owing to effusion from the splenic capsule.

Mesenteric or Enteric Masses

Circumscribed masses originating in the mesentery and those originating from the bowel wall often produce similar radiographic signs of visceral displacement. Location of such masses is variable and often unstable in serial or positional radiographs. Therefore, visceral displacement is rarely predictable. Masses originating from the root of the mesentery, however, generally produce characteristic peripheral enteric displacement in the ventrodorsal projection and dorsal, cranial, and caudal displacement of the intestine in the lateral projection (Fig. 36–13). They are easily confused with some splenic masses, especially those originating from the tail or body of the spleen. Masses derived from enlargement of the colic lymph node cause ventral and dextrolateral displacement of the ascending colon. Such ventral colonic displacement is best seen with the patient in left lateral recumbency (Fig. 36–14).

Pancreatic Masses

Pancreatic masses are special types of mesenteric masses but may produce specific radiographic signs, depending on the location of the mass within the pancreas. If the mass originates in the left limb of the pancreas (Fig. 36–15), there is almost always lateral displacement of the descending duodenum and extrinsic displacement of the caudodextral wall of the pyloric antrum of the stomach in the ventrodorsal projection. In the lateral projection, the duodenum is usually displaced ventrally. If the mass originates from the right limb of the pancreas, there is usually no extrinsic distortion of the gastric wall, but the adjacent portion of the descending duodenum is displaced ventrally and to the right. Identification of these radiographic signs depends on visualization of

Text continued on page 429

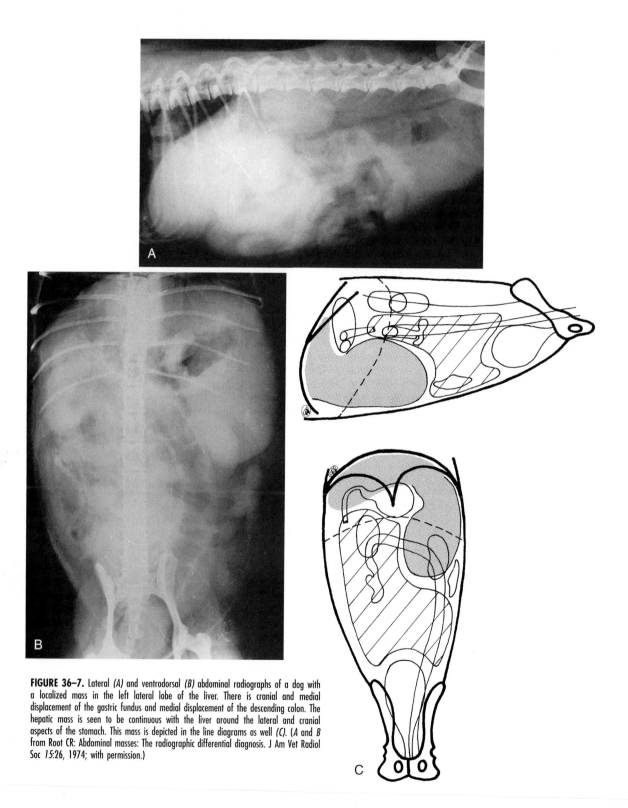

FIGURE 36–7. Lateral *(A)* and ventrodorsal *(B)* abdominal radiographs of a dog with a localized mass in the left lateral lobe of the liver. There is cranial and medial displacement of the gastric fundus and medial displacement of the descending colon. The hepatic mass is seen to be continuous with the liver around the lateral and cranial aspects of the stomach. This mass is depicted in the line diagrams as well *(C)*. *(A* and *B* from Root CR: Abdominal masses: The radiographic differential diagnosis. J Am Vet Radiol Soc *15*:26, 1974; with permission.)

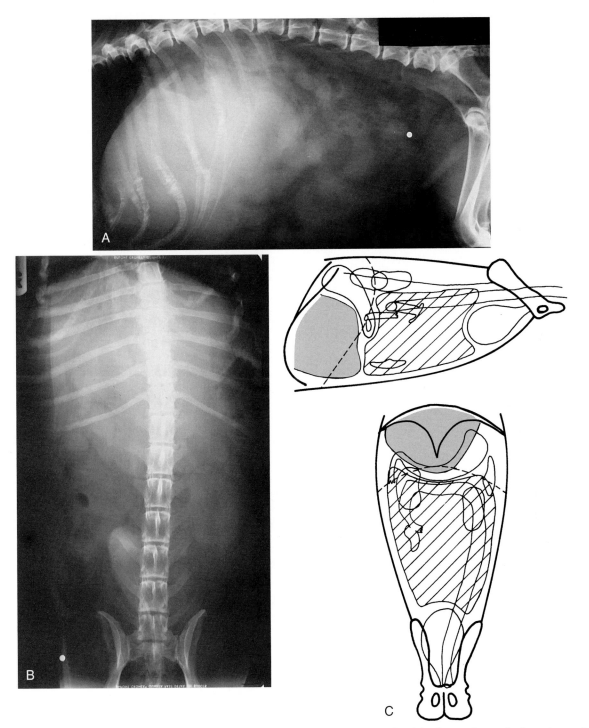

FIGURE 36–8. *A,* Lateral abdominal radiograph of a dog with a large central hepatic mass that displaces the stomach caudally and dorsally. *B,* On the ventrodorsal view, the mass displaces the stomach to the left. Extrinsic indentation of the cranial border of the stomach is best seen in the lateral projection. The line drawings *(C)* illustrate the same effects. (*A* and *B* courtesy of Auburn Valley Animal Clinic, Auburn, WA.)

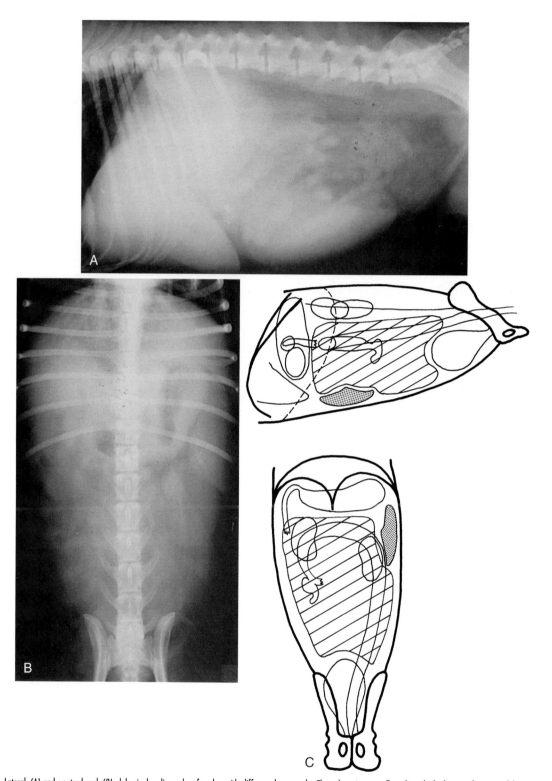

FIGURE 36–9. Lateral *(A)* and ventrodorsal *(B)* abdominal radiographs of a dog with diffuse splenomegaly. The spleen is generally enlarged, displacing adjacent mobile viscera, and its borders are rounded. These radiographic signs are seen in the accompanying line drawings *(C)*. There is also diffuse hepatomegaly. The diagnosis was lymphosarcoma. *(A* and *B* from Root CR: Abdominal masses: The radiographic differential diagnosis. J Am Vet Radiol Soc *15:*26, 1974; with permission.)

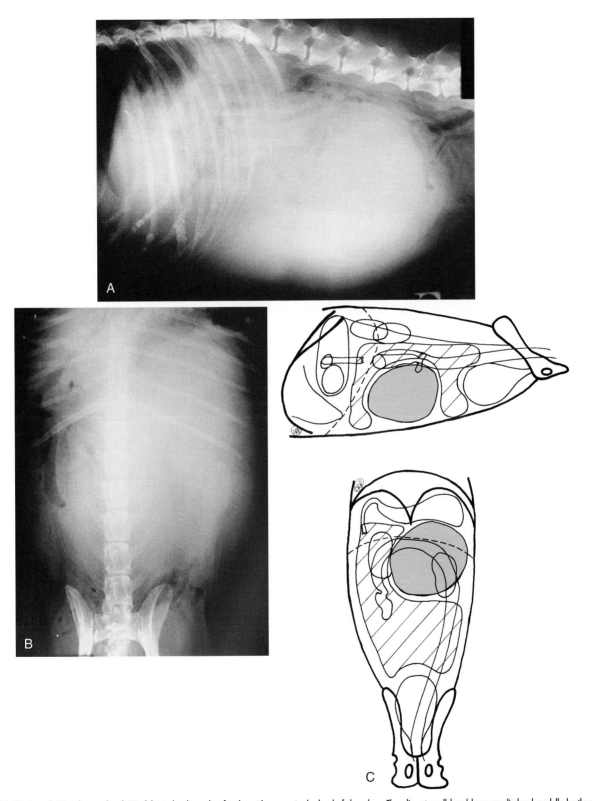

FIGURE 36–10. Lateral *(A)* and ventrodorsal *(B)* abdominal radiographs of a dog with a mass in the head of the spleen. The adjacent small bowel loops are displaced caudally by the mass *(C)*. *(A* and *B* from Root CR: Abdominal masses: The radiographic differential diagnosis. J Am Vet Radiol Soc *15:*26, 1974; with permission.)

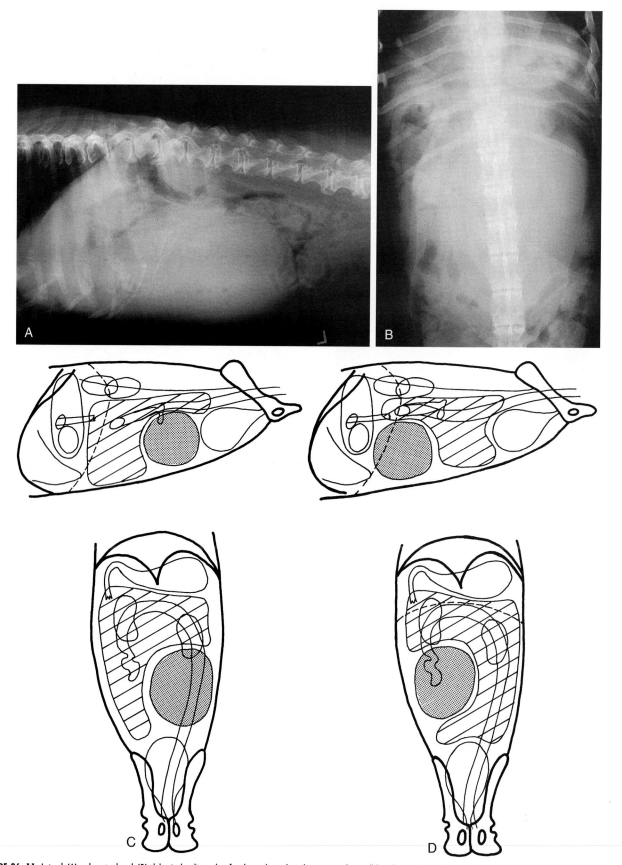

FIGURE 36–11. Lateral (A) and ventrodorsal (B) abdominal radiographs of a dog with a splenic hematoma. The small bowel primarily is displaced caudally. Histopathologic examination is necessary to differentiate benign from malignant splenic masses. C and D, Visceral displacement is variable, depending on the location of the mass within the spleen.

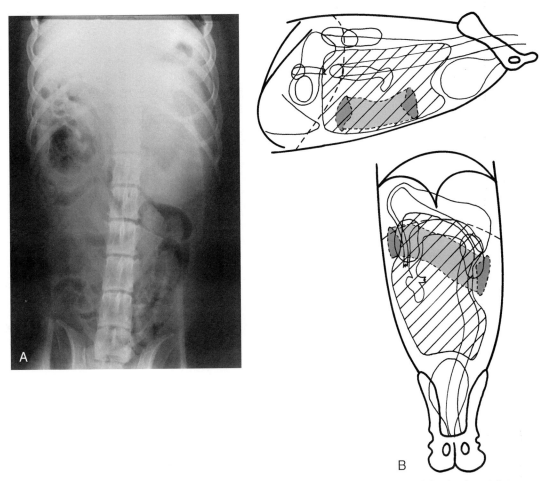

FIGURE 36–12. *A,* Ventrodorsal abdominal radiograph of a dog with torsion of the spleen. Both ends of the spleen are seen end-on, and the spleen has a C shape owing to rotation about its pedicle. *B,* This relationship is diagrammed along with medial displacement of the descending duodenum, which is sometimes seen in torsion of the spleen. This patient had an acute torsion; later the radiographic signs may become more vague after fluid has begun to effuse through the splenic capsule. (*A* courtesy of the Santa Cruz Veterinary Hospital, Santa Cruz, CA.)

the duodenum, sometimes requiring administration of contrast medium.

Kidney Masses

Visualization of the entire contour of the right kidney is rarely possible in survey radiographs because it is embedded in the renal fossa of the caudate lobe of the liver. If its caudal pole is not visible, however, and if there is a homogeneous soft-tissue opacity on the right side of the craniodorsal portion of the abdomen, enlargement of the right kidney should be suspected, and adjacent visceral displacement should be assessed. Enlargement of the right kidney produces medial and ventral displacement of the descending duodenum and ascending colon. There is also usually left and ventral displacement of the adjacent portion of the small intestine (Fig. 36–16).

Direct visualization of the contour of the left kidney is much more reliable than that of the right. Inability to visualize the normal left kidney in either projection may be the first radiographic sign associated with a left renal mass. Left renal masses often produce ventral and medial displacement of the descending colon and adjacent small bowel (Fig. 36–17).

Renal masses, even those of considerable size, remain dorsal in the abdomen. The kidneys are retroperitoneal and, similar to all retroperitoneal structures, are prevented from migrating ventrally by the retroperitoneal fascia. Enlargement of retroperitoneal structures other than the kidneys is rare. In instances of retroperitoneal masses other than renal origin, visualization of the ipsilateral kidney should not be impaired. Renal displacement in such instances depends on the location of the mass. Adrenal masses, masses originating from the epaxial spinal musculature, and masses originating from one of the caudal ribs or one of the lumbar transverse processes (Fig. 36–18) are examples of extrarenal retroperitoneal space-occupying lesions. One note of caution is appropriate: Adrenal pheochromocytoma may invade and replace ipsilateral kidney tissue (Fig. 36–19).[3] Inasmuch as renal masses tend to remain dorsal, progressive enlargement causes ventral displacement of the adjacent mobile visceral structures. Because the kidneys are lateral to the root of the mesentery, renal masses produce medial visceral displacement as they enlarge.

Ovarian Masses

Right ovarian masses are associated with a well-circumscribed homogeneous opacity caudal to the right kidney, separate and distinct from the caudal pole of the kidney. They produce medial, but not ventral, displacement of the descending duodenum and ascending colon. Furthermore, there is ventral deviation of the caudal pole of the right kidney if the ovarian mass is large enough.

Text continued on page 439

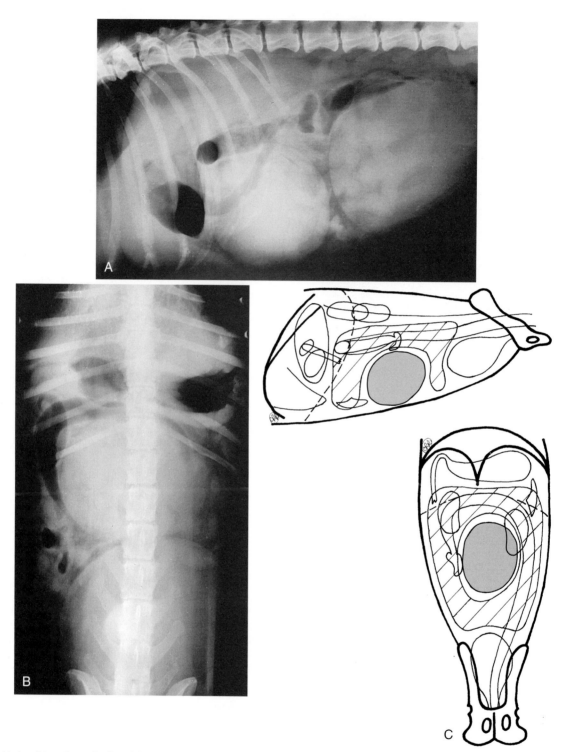

FIGURE 36–13. Lateral *(A)* and ventrodorsal *(B)* abdominal radiographs of a dog with a large cyst in the root of the mesentery. Notice that the small bowel is displaced cranially, caudally, and dorsally in the lateral projection (similar to the displacement that may occur with a splenic mass), but there is peripheral displacement of the bowel in the ventrodorsal projection. *C,* Diagrammatic representation of the typical radiographic signs of a mesenteric mass. *(A* and *B* courtesy of the Animal Medical Center, New York, NY.)

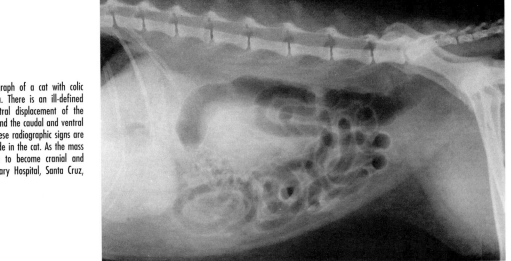

FIGURE 36–14. Lateral abdominal radiograph of a cat with colic lymphadenopathy caused by lymphosarcoma. There is an ill-defined mass in the midabdomen. Notice the ventral displacement of the ascending portion of the colon (feces filled) and the caudal and ventral displacement of the adjacent small bowel. These radiographic signs are typical of enlargement of the colic lymph node in the cat. As the mass enlarges, enteric displacement may change to become cranial and dorsal. (Courtesy of the Santa Cruz Veterinary Hospital, Santa Cruz, CA.)

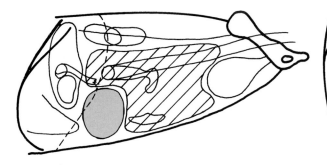

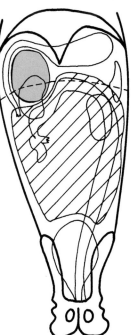

FIGURE 36–15. The radiographic signs that are typical of a mass in the right limb of the pancreas. Notice that the descending duodenum is typically displaced ventrally and laterally by large pancreatic masses.

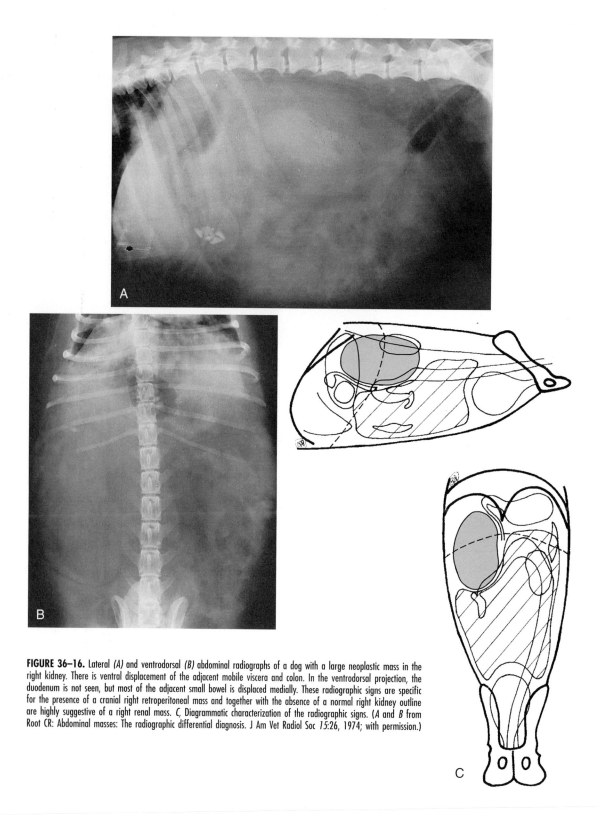

FIGURE 36–16. Lateral *(A)* and ventrodorsal *(B)* abdominal radiographs of a dog with a large neoplastic mass in the right kidney. There is ventral displacement of the adjacent mobile viscera and colon. In the ventrodorsal projection, the duodenum is not seen, but most of the adjacent small bowel is displaced medially. These radiographic signs are specific for the presence of a cranial right retroperitoneal mass and together with the absence of a normal right kidney outline are highly suggestive of a right renal mass. *C,* Diagrammatic characterization of the radiographic signs. (*A* and *B* from Root CR: Abdominal masses: The radiographic differential diagnosis. J Am Vet Radiol Soc *15:*26, 1974; with permission.)

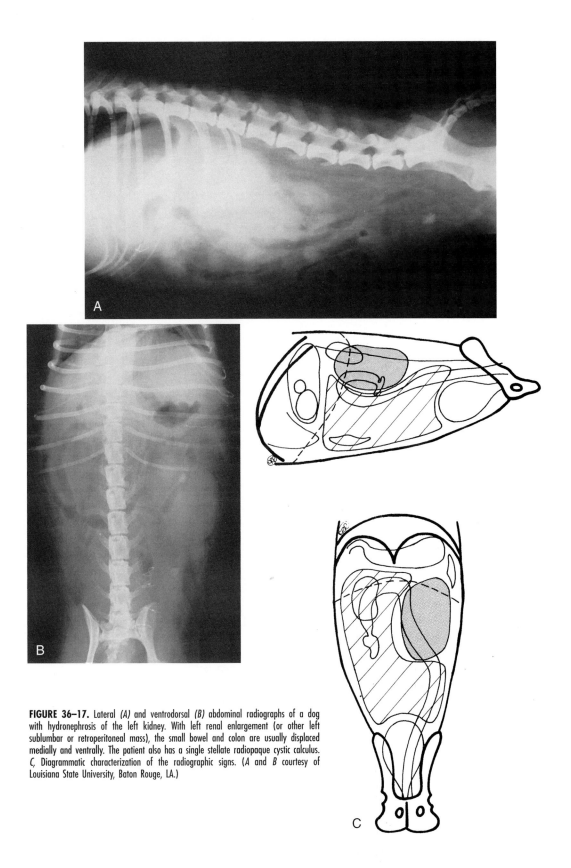

FIGURE 36–17. Lateral *(A)* and ventrodorsal *(B)* abdominal radiographs of a dog with hydronephrosis of the left kidney. With left renal enlargement (or other left sublumbar or retroperitoneal mass), the small bowel and colon are usually displaced medially and ventrally. The patient also has a single stellate radiopaque cystic calculus. *C,* Diagrammatic characterization of the radiographic signs. *(A* and *B* courtesy of Louisiana State University, Baton Rouge, LA.)

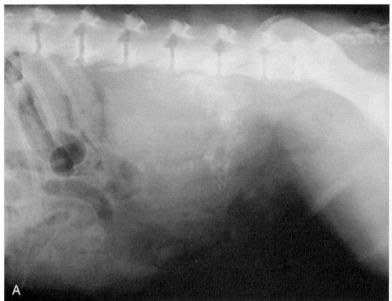

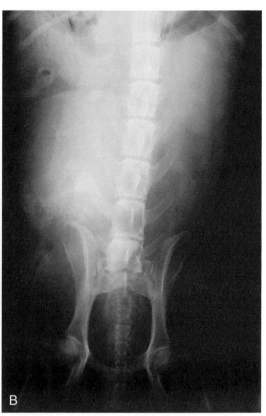

FIGURE 36–18. Lateral *(A)* and ventrodorsal *(B)* abdominal radiographs of a dog with a chondrosarcoma of the transverse process of the right sixth lumbar vertebra. The mass is well circumscribed and contains multiple foci of densely radiopaque material. It does not involve the ipsilateral kidney, but its ventral and medial displacement of adjacent bowel is otherwise typical of a sublumbar or retroperitoneal mass. (Courtesy of Renton Veterinary Hospital, Renton, WA.)

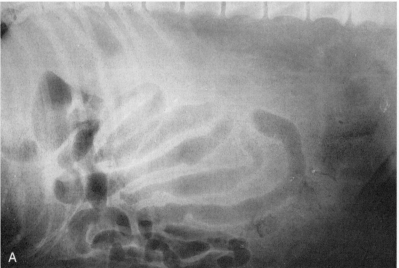

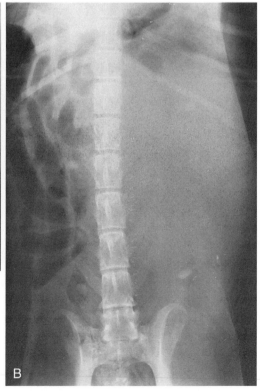

FIGURE 36–19. Lateral *(A)* and ventrodorsal *(B)* abdominal radiographs of a dog with a large mass in the left sublumbar region; notice the typical visceral displacement. The left kidney is not seen, and there is ventral and caudal displacement of the metallic sutures placed during ovariohysterectomy. This lesion proved to be an adrenal pheochromocytoma that had invaded and replaced the left kidney by vascular extension. (From Root CR: Abdominal masses: The radiographic differential diagnosis. J Am Vet Radiol Soc *15*:26, 1974; with permission.)

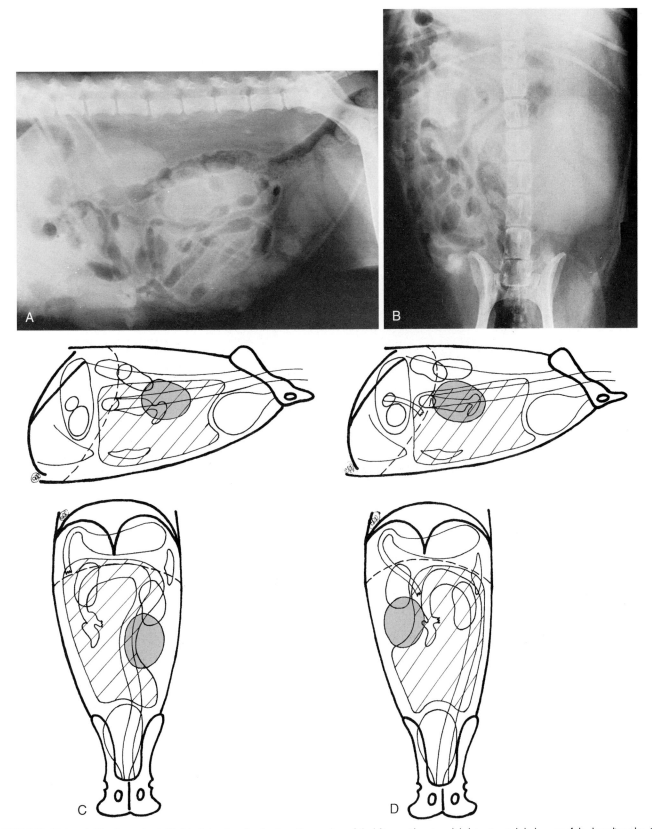

FIGURE 36–20. Lateral *(A)* and ventrodorsal *(B)* abdominal radiographs of a dog with a neoplasm of the left ovary. There is medial, *but not ventral,* displacement of the descending colon. In the lateral projection, the caudal pole of the left kidney is tipped ventrally. The line drawings show the typical radiographic signs of left *(C)* and right *(D)* ovarian masses. *(A* and *B* from Root CR: Abdominal masses: The radiographic differential diagnosis. J Am Vet Radiol Soc *15*:26, 1974; with permission.)

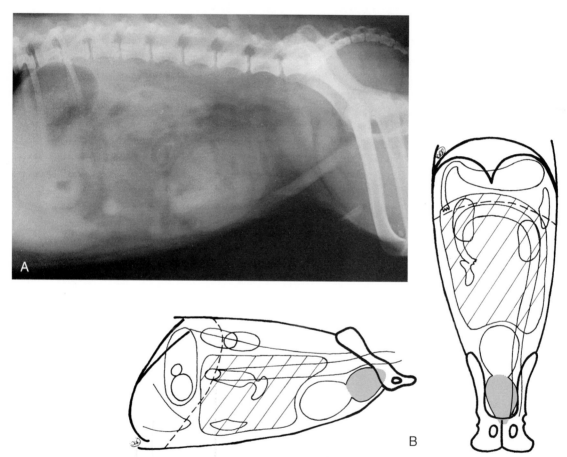

FIGURE 36–21. *A,* Lateral abdominal radiograph of a dog with symmetric prostatomegaly. The ventrodorsal projection is generally noncontributory in this condition. The urinary bladder is displaced cranially, and the prostate gland may be seen at the brim of the pelvis. *B,* Often, there is mild dorsal displacement of the pelvic portion of the descending colon. (*A* from Root CR: Abdominal masses: The radiographic differential diagnosis. J Am Vet Radiol Soc *15:*26, 1974; with permission.)

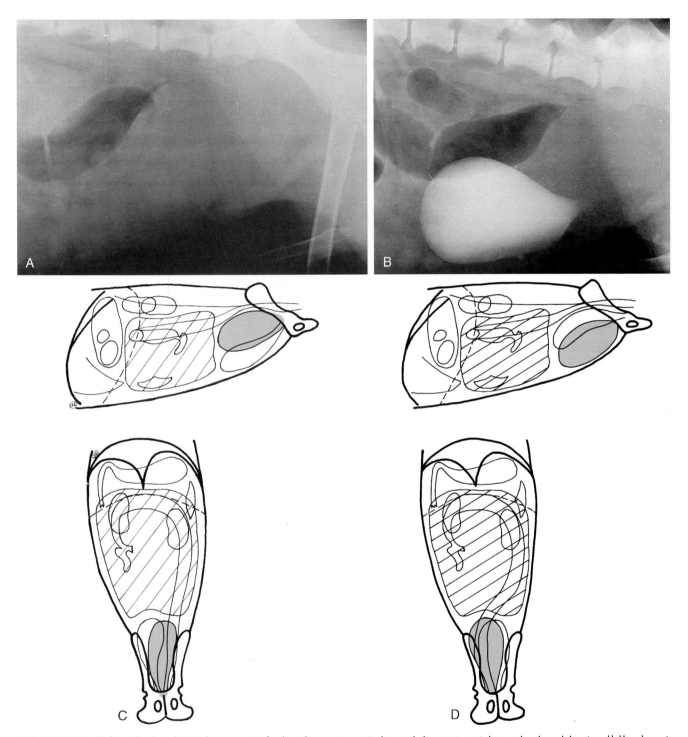

FIGURE 36–22. Lateral abdominal radiograph *(A)* and cystogram *(B)* of a dog with a prostatic cyst. In this animal, the prostatic cyst is between the colon and the urinary bladder, whereas in other dogs, the prostatic cyst may be between the urinary bladder and the ventral body wall *(C and D)*. Cystography or sonography usually must be done to differentiate prostatic cysts from the urinary bladder. The descending colon is usually displaced dorsally. The ventrodorsal projections *(C and D)* generally do not contribute significantly to the evaluation of this lesion. *(A and B from Root CR: Abdominal masses: The radiographic differential diagnosis. J Am Vet Radiol Soc 15:26, 1974; with permission.)*

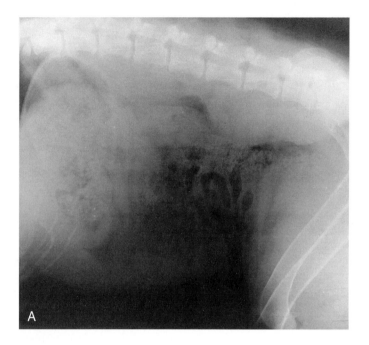

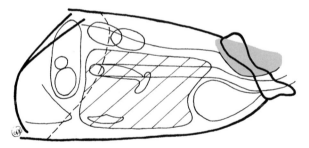

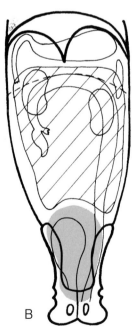

FIGURE 36–23. *A,* Lateral abdominal survey radiograph of a dog with medial iliac lymphadenopathy caused by lymphosarcoma. Notice the ventral displacement of the descending colon. The spleen and liver are also enlarged. *B,* The line drawings represent typical ventral visceral displacement in such lesions. (*A* courtesy of Colorado State University, Fort Collins, CO.)

Left ovarian masses, in addition to producing a space-occupying, soft-tissue mass caudal to the left kidney, usually produce medial, but not ventral, displacement of the descending colon and adjacent small bowel (Fig. 36–20). The caudal pole of the left kidney may be tipped ventrally, depending on the size and location of the mass.

At first consideration, masses originating in the ovaries would seem to be capable of producing visceral displacement identical to that produced by kidneys. *They do not*, and a note of explanation is in order. The ovaries are not retroperitoneal structures. Therefore, as an ovarian mass enlarges, its ovarian ligament stretches, permitting it to gravitate ventrally between the body wall and the descending colon (left ovarian mass) or between the body wall and the descending duodenum and the ascending colon (right ovarian mass). As a result, ovarian masses usually displace adjacent structures medially, *but not ventrally*. Consequently, visceral displacement is best seen in the ventrodorsal view (see Fig. 36–20C and D) and is rarely apparent in the lateral projection. Because the ovarian ligament is attached to the caudal pole of the kidney, a sufficiently pendulous ovary produces ventral deviation of the caudal pole of the ipsilateral kidney in lateral projections.

Prostate Gland

Radiographic signs of diseases of the reproductive system of the male dog[10] and companion animals[11] have been reported. Prostatic diameter, in any direction, should not exceed 70 percent of the height of the pelvic inlet.[12] The prostate gland is normally intrapelvic and is therefore usually not seen radiographically, unless significantly enlarged. If the urinary bladder is distended, however, the normal prostate gland may be cranial to the brim of the pubis. Generalized or symmetric enlargement of the prostate gland produces cranial displacement of the urinary bladder and, possibly, dorsal displacement of the rectum (Fig. 36–21). The ventrodorsal projection is often of little value in assessment of the prostate gland. It should be noted that prostatomegaly (in the absence of distention of the urinary bladder) can displace the colon to either side of the midline. If the prostate gland is painful, the colon may be full of fecal material because the animal may be obstipated.

Eccentric enlargement of the prostate gland, as produced by prostatic cysts or some neoplastic infiltrates, has a variable effect on the adjacent caudal abdominal visceral structures (Fig. 36–22). Depending on the location or site of origin of the prostatic cyst, the urinary bladder may be displaced either cranioventrally or craniodorsally. Contrast radiography is usually necessary to differentiate between the urinary bladder and the prostatic mass in such instances.

Caudal Sublumbar Masses

Masses originating in the caudal sublumbar region are treated separately because their radiographic signs are quite specific (Fig. 36–23). In general, there are few lesions that produce the radiographic signs associated with caudal sublumbar masses. Most such lesions are caused by medial iliac lymphadenopathy, caudal sublumbar muscular masses, or inflammatory granuloma and abscess formation. The descending colon is displaced ventrally in the lateral projection. There is usually a broadly based homogeneous mass in the caudal retroperitoneal space. The ventrodorsal projection is usually noncontributory (see Chapter 37).

References

1. O'Brien TR: Radiographic Diagnosis of Abdominal Disorders in the Dog and Cat. Philadelphia, WB Saunders, 1978.
2. Root CR: Abdominal masses: The radiographic differential diagnosis. J Am Vet Radiol Soc 15:26, 1974.
3. Root CR: Interpretation of abdominal survey radiographs. Vet Clin North Am 4:763, 1974.
4. Schebitz H, and Wilkens H: Atlas of Radiographic Anatomy of Dog and Cat, 3rd Ed. Berlin, Paul Parey, 1977.
5. Ferron RR: Low-cost pocket-sized CO_2 dispenser for medical use. J Am Vet Radiol Soc 17:18, 1976.
6. Ticer JW (Ed): Radiographic Technique in Small Animal Practice, 2nd ed. Philadelphia, WB Saunders, 1984.
7. Root CR: The urinary system. In Ticer JW (Ed): Radiographic Technique in Veterinary Practice, 2nd Ed. Philadelphia, WB Saunders, 1984.
8. Root CR: The gastrointestinal tract. In Ticer JW (Ed): Radiographic Technique in Veterinary Practice, 2nd Ed. Philadelphia, WB Saunders, 1984.
9. Morgan JP: Celiography with iothalamic acid. J Am Vet Med Assoc 145:1095, 1964.
10. Johnston GR, Feeney DA, Rivers B, et al: Diagnostic imaging of the male canine reproductive organs: Methods and limitations. Vet Clin North Am [Small Anim Pract] 21:553, 1991.
11. Root CR, and Spaulding KA: Diagnostic imaging in companion animal theriogenology. Semin Vet Med Surg [Small Anim] 9:7, 1994.
12. Feeney DA, Johnston GR, Klausner JS, et al: Canine prostatic disease—Comparison of radiographic appearance with morphologic and microbiologic findings: 30 cases (1981–1985). J Am Vet Med Assoc 190:1018, 1987.

STUDY QUESTIONS

1. List those structures in the abdomen that are nearly always seen in abdominal radiographs, those that are often only partially seen, and those that are usually seen only if abnormal.

2. Which lateral projection of the abdomen routinely provides better visualization of the spleen? Why?

3. In instances in which differential diagnostic features are lacking in routine radiography, which of the following procedures should be considered as the next step?
   A. Contrast radiography.
   B. Positional radiography.
   C. Exploratory surgery.
   D. Referral.
   E. Ultrasonography.

4. Which of the following contrast radiographic procedures may be helpful in further assessment of a right cranioventral abdominal mass?
   A. Excretory urography.
   B. Cystography.
   C. Upper gastrointestinal series.
   D. Pneumoperitoneography.
   E. Celiography.

5. Name three abdominal structures that may undergo considerable normal variation in size.

6. Caudal, dorsal, and left displacement of the small bowel; dorsomedial displacement of the descending duodenum; and caudal displacement of the transverse colon are suggestive of a mass originating from the:

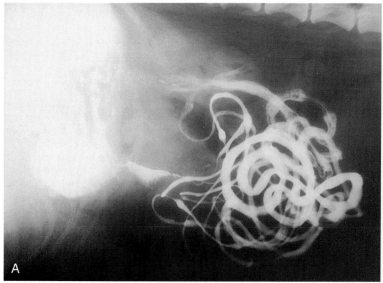

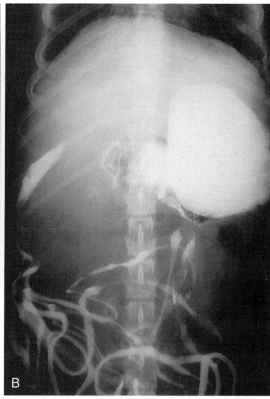

FIGURE 36–24

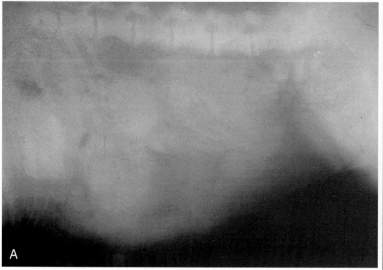

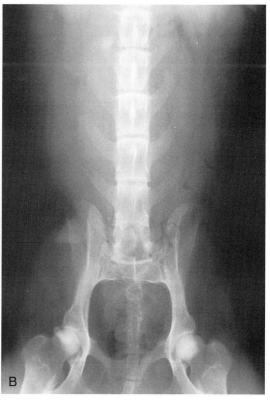

FIGURE 36–25

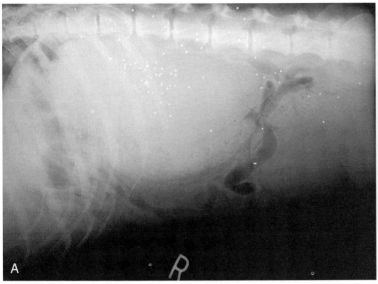

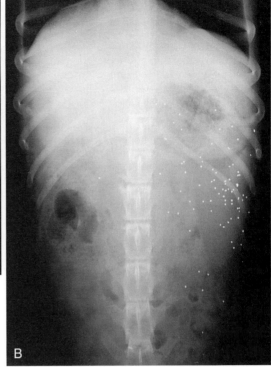

FIGURE 36–26. (Courtesy of South Hill Veterinary Clinic, Puyallup, WA.)

A. Right lateral aspect of the liver.
B. Right kidney.
C. Pancreas.
D. Colic lymph node.
E. Root of the mesentery.

7. Ventral and medial displacement of the descending colon and small bowel are radiographic signs that may be produced by a mass originating from the:
A. Left kidney.
B. Left 13th rib.
C. Left sublumbar muscles.
D. All of the above.
E. All of the above except _____ (specify).

8. The patient is a 7-year-old female German shepherd with progressively severe depression, anorexia, icterus, and vomiting. There is a palpable firm right cranial abdomi-

nal mass. Right lateral (Fig. 36–24A) and ventrodorsal (see Fig. 36–24B) abdominal radiographs were made approximately 30 minutes after oral administration of barium sulfate suspension. List the radiographic signs.

9. Figure 36–25 shows right lateral (A) and ventrodorsal (B) abdominal radiographs of a 4-year-old female Doberman pinscher with a history of acute vaginal hemorrhage. The owner stated that the dog had been bred approximately 30 days before onset of clinical signs, which began after recent vigorous exercise. List the radiographic signs.

10. Figure 36–26 shows right lateral (A) and ventrodorsal (B) abdominal radiographs of a 6-year-old male Weimaraner with a history of anorexia and depression and a large palpable abdominal mass. List the radiographic signs.

(Answers appear on pages 645 to 646.)

Chapter 37

The Peritoneal Space

Mary B. Mahaffey • Don L. Barber

ANATOMY

Limits of the abdominal cavity include (1) the diaphragm cranially; (2) the pelvic inlet caudally; (3) the sublumbar muscles, spine, and crura of the diaphragm dorsally; and (4)

the muscles of the abdominal wall and diaphragm laterally and ventrally. The cranial abdominal cavity is bounded by the caudal rib cage.

The peritoneum is a thin, serous membrane that can be divided into parietal, visceral, and connecting layers, which are all continuous.[1] The parietal peritoneum covers the inner surface of the abdominal cavity and is closely adhered to abdominal musculature. The parietal peritoneum separates extraperitoneal and intraperitoneal spaces. The visceral peritoneum covers the organs of the abdominal cavity either in whole or in part. The connecting peritoneum includes mesenteries, omenta, and intra-abdominal ligaments. The peritoneal space is the space between the parietal and visceral peritoneal layers and is a potential space that normally contains only a small amount of fluid for lubrication.

The space between the dorsal margin of the parietal peritoneum and the abdominal wall is the retroperitoneal space. The retroperitoneal space is extraperitoneal and contains adrenal glands, kidneys, ureters, major blood vessels, and lymph nodes. The retroperitoneal space communicates with the mediastinum cranially and the pelvic canal caudally.[2]

Fat is usually deposited throughout the abdominal cavity and is particularly localized in the falciform ligament, the greater omentum, the mesentery, and the retroperitoneal space.

RADIOGRAPHIC TECHNIQUE

High-quality radiographs are important for radiographic visualization of most peritoneal diseases, especially for recognition of subtle abnormalities. Abdominal preparation is important and is discussed elsewhere.[3] Both overexposure and underexposure can create false results by obscuring or simulating peritoneal diseases. Intra-abdominal contrast and organ visualization are dependent on the difference in opacity between soft-tissue viscera and intra-abdominal fat. This difference in opacity is only slight. Thus, the abdomen is relatively low in inherent contrast, and radiographic exposure techniques that enhance contrast should be used. If possible, the pelvic limbs should be positioned so that the femora are perpendicular to the spine for both lateral and ventrodorsal views. Flexion at the hips can cause superimposition of femoral muscle mass over the caudal abdomen. Pronounced extension at the hips may produce crowding of abdominal viscera and distracting skin folds.

NORMAL RADIOGRAPHIC APPEARANCE

The presence of intra-abdominal fat is important for visceral organ visualization because fat provides an interposed opacity between viscera. Fat in the falciform ligament, greater omentum, mesentery, and retroperitoneal space usually provides adequate interposed opacity between viscera. Without interposed fat, intra-abdominal viscera silhouette to produce a uniform, homogeneous, soft-tissue opacity throughout the abdomen. In mature animals, the amount of fat deposition varies from lean to obese animals (Fig. 37–1). Even thin animals usually have enough fat present to allow organ visualization.

Organ visualization also depends on conformation of the patient. For example, in narrow and deep-chested dog breeds, it may be difficult to visualize intra-abdominal organs on the ventrodorsal radiograph. This may be due, in part, to problems such as overexposure of the thinner caudal abdomen or underexposure of the thicker cranial abdomen. A narrow conformation, however, may also contribute to poor separation of viscera.

The diaphragm is the cranial limit of the abdominal cavity. The cranial surface of the diaphragm is visible because of the interface provided by air in the lungs. The caudal surface of the diaphragm silhouettes with the cranial surface of the liver and is thus not usually visualized. The dorsal limit of the abdominal cavity is defined by the sublumbar musculature and spine. The sublumbar muscles are usually visualized on lateral radiographs owing to the presence of retroperitoneal fat. Cats have a relatively large lumbar muscle mass, which can usually be visualized on lateral and ventrodorsal radiographs (Fig. 37–2). The abdominal wall may be seen because of the contrasting opacity of intraperitoneal fat internally and subcutaneous fat externally. Increasing fat deposition can produce separation and visualization of specific muscle bundles.

ABNORMAL RADIOGRAPHIC FINDINGS

Increased Fluid Opacity

Increased amounts of fluid within the peritoneal cavity cause a loss of the differential opacity interface between soft tissue and fat. Phrases commonly used to describe the loss of differential opacity include *loss of intra-abdominal contrast, decreased visualization of serosal surfaces, increased intra-abdominal soft-tissue opacity,* and *increased intra-abdominal fluid opacity.* Causes for this loss of intra-abdominal contrast include lack of fat, peritoneal effusion, peritonitis, and peritoneal neoplasia. A wet hair coat, or hair coated with ultrasound gel, superimposed over the abdomen may also create irregular opacities that appear to be within the abdomen.

Lack of intra-abdominal fat may be the result of the age of the animal or emaciation. Immature dogs and kittens younger than a few months of age lack sufficient fat to provide intra-abdominal contrast, and thus the abdomen appears as relatively uniform, homogeneous, soft-tissue opacity. The abdomen may also be somewhat pendulous in normal, immature patients. Emaciation causes a similar homogeneous, soft-tissue opacity throughout the abdomen because of a lack of fat (see Fig. 37–1C). In emaciated patients, the abdomen is often tucked up, which can be visualized on radiographs; however, the possibility of coexistent peritonitis cannot be excluded.

Abdominal effusion refers to increased fluid within the abdomen. Intra-abdominal fluid between abdominal viscera provides added overall opacity and silhouettes with viscera, thereby causing a loss of intra-abdominal contrast. Classification of abdominal effusion is broad and includes various types of transudates, exudates, blood, urine, bile, and chyle.[4] In practice, all abdominal fluids are of water or soft-tissue opacity, comparable to the visceral organs.

Peritonitis with edema and inflammation of serosal surfaces and adjacent fat may also cause loss of intra-abdominal contrast. In addition, abdominal effusion is usually present with peritonitis. Peritoneal seeding of neoplastic foci can also cause a loss of intra-abdominal contrast because of the soft-tissue opacity of the nodules as well as possible coexistent effusion.

The radiographic appearance of the aforementioned conditions depends on the cause, severity of the disease, and amount of fluid present. It is a common misconception that accumulation of any amount of intraperitoneal fluid results in complete obliteration of serosal margins. The degree to which serosal margin detail is obscured by fluid is a balance between the amount of fat and fluid present: The more fat present, the more fluid is needed to result in complete obliteration of organ and serosal margins. Thus, organ margins may still be visible when free fluid is present in the intraperitoneal space.

A large volume of abdominal fluid appears as a homogeneous fluid opacity uniformly distributed throughout the ab-

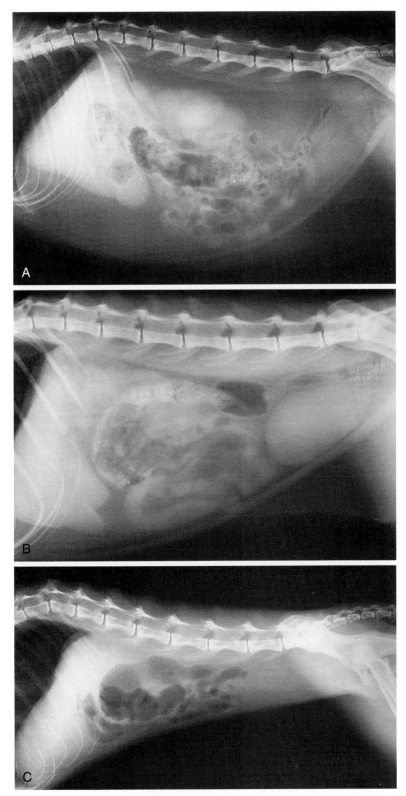

FIGURE 37–1. Lateral views of the abdomen. *A,* Obese cat. Extensive fat deposition in the falciform, omental, mesenteric, and retroperitoneal areas provides interposed opacity between viscera of soft-tissue opacity. *B,* Normal cat. Fat deposition is less than in *A* but is adequate to separate and allow visualization of the viscera. *C,* Emaciated cat. Without interposed fat, viscera silhouette, producing a uniform, homogeneous, soft-tissue opacity throughout the abdomen except for gas in the bowel loops.

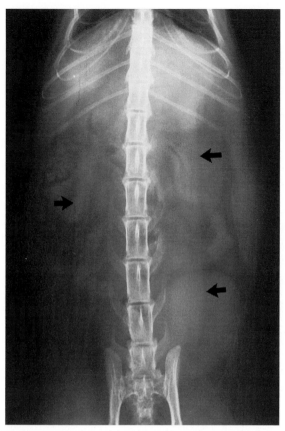

FIGURE 37–2. Ventrodorsal view of the abdomen of a normal cat. Note the margins of the large lumbar muscle mass *(arrows)*.

dominal cavity (Fig. 37–3). The homogeneous appearance is due to total silhouetting of all soft-tissue structures within the abdomen. A large volume of fluid often causes abdominal distention, with outward protrusion of the contour of the abdominal wall. Care must be taken because radiographs of normal immature animals may exhibit similar findings. A large volume of fluid may also displace the diaphragm cranially. If relatively mobile segments of bowel contain gas, they often float to the highest or uppermost area within the ab-

dominal cavity. The presence or absence of coexistent peritonitis cannot be ascertained radiographically.

Smaller amounts of abdominal fluid or peritonitis may produce a mottled, hazy, or irregular fluid opacity on survey radiographs (Fig. 37–4). Individual viscera may be visualized, but there is indistinctness or blurring of the margins of soft-tissue structures. With small amounts of fluid, this appearance may be the result of interdigitation of fluid with folds in the greater omentum and small bowel but without a total silhouette effect.[5] Inflammation of the peritoneum or fat may produce a similar effect. Smaller amounts of effusion may be caused by early fluid accumulation of a generalized process or by more localized diseases.

Manipulation of viscera during laparotomy produces physiologic changes within the abdomen that may appear comparable to peritonitis on radiographs, and these changes may be modified by the amount of induced tissue trauma.[5] Solutions containing water, electrolytes, and relatively low-molecular-weight components are absorbed by the peritoneal membrane within 24 hours.[6] Proteinaceous fluids such as serum, blood, and lymph are absorbed more slowly and may be present for 1 or 2 weeks. These changes can be visualized after laparotomy, and they should not be mistaken for more significant complications. Static or progressive fluid accumulation during this period is abnormal.

One convenient method for assessing the intraperitoneal space for fluid accumulation is to compare the detail and contrast in the intraperitoneal versus the retroperitoneal spaces. Because many diseases resulting in intraperitoneal fluid accumulation do not affect the retroperitoneal space, retroperitoneal detail is often preserved when intraperitoneal fluid has altered the serosal margin of bowel and other intraperitoneal organs (see Fig. 37–4). Normally, detail and contrast in the intraperitoneal and retroperitoneal spaces should be identical. Large volumes of intra-abdominal fluid, however, obscure the retroperitoneal space, even if the fluid is confined to the intraperitoneal space. This phenomenon is due to superimposition by the large fluid volume. Loss of contrast and detail in the retroperitoneal space is an indication of fluid accumulation or, less commonly, inflammation. Fluid accumulation may be confined to the retroperitoneal space, with a normal appearance of the intraperitoneal space (Fig. 37–5). The most common causes of isolated retroperitoneal fluid are hemorrhage and urine leakage. Inflammation and abscessation of the retroperitoneal space may be caused

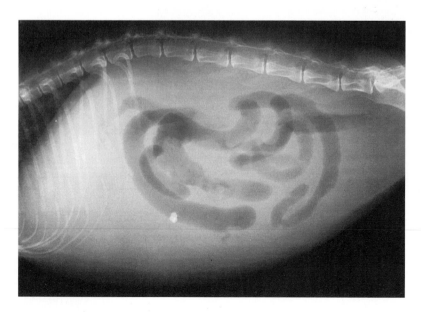

FIGURE 37–3. Lateral view of the abdomen of a cat with a large volume of intraperitoneal fluid. Homogeneous fluid opacity is uniformly distributed throughout a distended abdomen. There is no fluid in the retroperitoneal space, but fascial planes and organs in the retroperitoneal space are not visible because of superimposition of the distended abdomen. Diagnosis was feline infectious peritonitis.

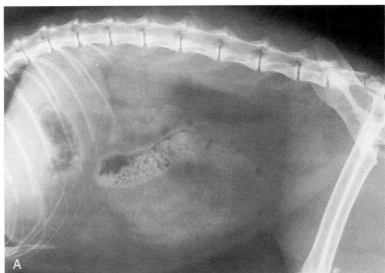

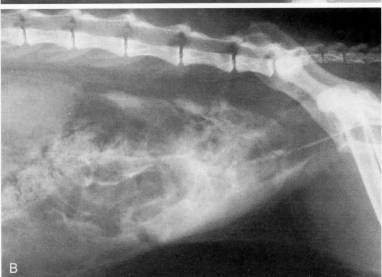

FIGURE 37–4. *A,* Lateral survey radiograph of the abdomen of a cat that had been hit by a car. Mottled, hazy, or irregular fluid opacity within the ventral half of the abdomen produces indistinctness or blurring of the margins of soft-tissue structures. Note that the retroperitoneal space is normal and that a hip is luxated dorsally. *B,* Lateral cystogram of the same cat. There is rupture of the urinary bladder. Note how the fluid interdigitates with bowel loops and mesentery.

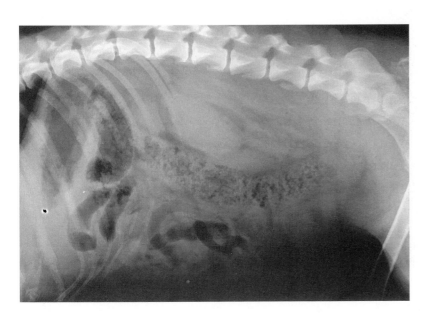

FIGURE 37–5. Lateral view of the abdomen of a dog that had been hit by a car. There is fluid opacity in the retroperitoneal space with blurring of the margin of the lumbar musculature. The streaking is due to interdigitation of the fluid with normal retroperitoneal fat. Note the greater intraperitoneal detail. There is also a sacral fracture with dorsal displacement. Diagnosis was retroperitoneal hemorrhage.

by migrating grass awns, penetrating wounds, foreign bodies, ligatures from ovariohysterectomy, and perforation of the urethra during catheterization.[7, 8]

An ill-defined nodular or granular pattern (Fig. 37–6) may be caused by seeding of the peritoneum with multiple, metastatic neoplastic foci. Examples of tumors associated with such spread include hemangiosarcoma of the spleen and carcinomas of various abdominal organs. The term *carcinomatosis* may be used to describe any cancer disseminated throughout the abdomen, or it may be limited only to carcinomas with this distribution.[9]

Localized radiographic changes of peritoneal disease are most often caused by a small amount of fluid or by localized peritonitis (Fig. 37–7). One of the more common causes of localized peritonitis is acute pancreatitis. The frequency and appearance of radiographic changes caused by acute pancreatitis are variable.[10–12] Changes can usually be localized to the right cranial abdomen, where the right lobe of the pancreas is closely associated with the proximal duodenum and pyloric antrum, or to midline just caudal to the stomach, where the left lobe of the pancreas is located. The major radiographic abnormality is usually an increased, irregular, soft-tissue opacity in the right mid to cranial abdomen, indicating localized peritonitis (Fig. 37–8A). Abscesses, inflammatory masses, and pseudocysts may be sequelae to pancreatitis.[13–15] The proximal descending duodenum may be displaced ventrally or toward the right to produce a broad curvature, and the pylorus of the stomach may be displaced toward the left (see Fig. 37–8B). Less frequently, the transverse colon may be displaced caudally. Bowel loops adjacent to the pancreas, such as the proximal descending duodenum, may contain gas, have loss of tone, and be dilated; spasticity of the duodenum has also been described. Foci of mineralization may occur in areas of fat necrosis.[11] Ultrasonography is of more use than radiography in assessing pancreatitis.

The shape or contour of the abdomen should also be evaluated. Large amounts of abdominal effusion result in a pendulous abdomen. The abdomen may also be pendulous owing to other causes, such as obesity and the muscle weakness of Cushing's syndrome. Emaciation usually causes the abdomen

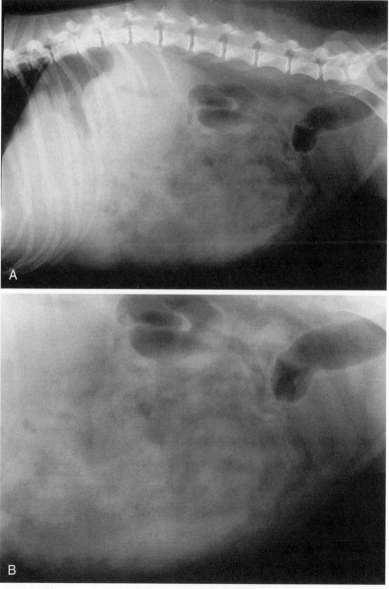

FIGURE 37–6. A, Lateral radiograph of a dog with mottled or irregular fluid opacity within the midventral abdomen that appears as an ill-defined nodular pattern. B, Close-up view. Diagnosis was splenic leiomyosarcoma with peritoneal seeding.

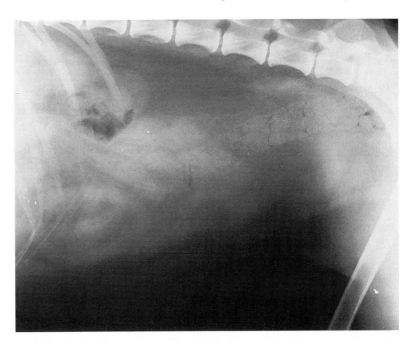

FIGURE 37–7. Lateral view of a dog with subtle changes owing to peritonitis or to a small amount of fluid. The serosal surfaces in the caudoventral abdomen are indistinct. Also note the greater detail in the retroperitoneal in comparison with the intraperitoneal space. Diagnosis was pyometra with small perforation and peritonitis.

to appear tucked up. Trauma of the abdominal wall or localized abdominal pain may produce asymmetric contraction of abdominal muscles.[5]

Intra-abdominal Calcification

Increased mineral opacity, not associated with the gastrointestinal tract, can be seen in various sites within the abdomen. Focal calcified bodies may be found in the peritoneal space (Fig. 37–9). These are thought to be the result of dystrophic calcification of necrotic mesenteric fat and are

not considered clinically significant.[16] Although not common, they are seen more often in cats than dogs. Metastatic calcification of the abdominal vasculature is rare (Fig. 37–10) and is associated with abnormal calcium metabolism primarily in animals with chronic uremia.[16, 17]

Free Abdominal Gas

Although there are many causes of free intraperitoneal gas, the two most common are penetration of the abdominal wall, either by surgery or by penetrating wounds, and perfo-

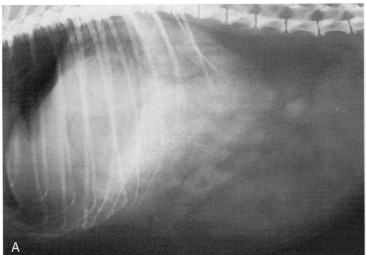

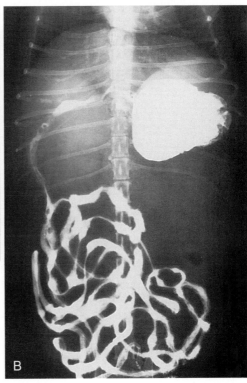

FIGURE 37–8. A, Lateral survey radiograph of a dog with increased, irregular soft-tissue opacity in the mid to cranial abdomen owing to localized peritonitis. B, Ventrodorsal view, upper gastrointestinal tract series. The pylorus is displaced to the left, and the proximal duodenum is broadly curved. Diagnosis was pancreatitis with peripancreatic abscess.

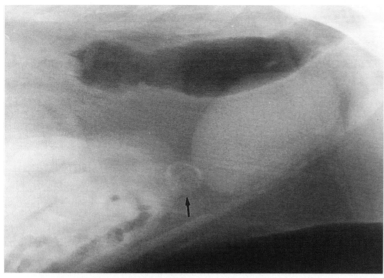

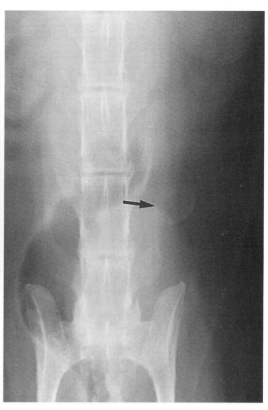

FIGURE 37–9. Close-up lateral and ventrodorsal abdominal radiographs of a cat with a focal calcified body *(arrow)* in the peritoneal space. The calcified body was an incidental finding and thought to be a result of dystrophic calcification of necrotic fat.

ration of the bowel. Not all bowel perforations, however, produce free abdominal gas.[18] Laparotomy is the most common cause of free abdominal gas, and the history is usually known in this instance. Following laparotomy, a moderate amount of gas may persist for days to weeks.[19] Penetrating abdominal wounds are usually diagnosed by physical findings. In patients with a penetrating wound, differentiating whether free abdominal gas is due solely to penetration of the abdomen or concurrent organ rupture is difficult.

A small volume of free abdominal gas is difficult to recognize on conventional radiographs made with a vertically directed x-ray beam because resulting bubbles are small and irregular in shape.[5] Larger gas volumes may coalesce into a larger bubble. This larger bubble may still be difficult to recognize on a radiograph made with a vertical x-ray beam because it is superimposed over other viscera. In addition, this larger bubble may simulate a gas-containing organ, such as the stomach. Such free abdominal gas usually floats to the highest point within the abdomen. In lateral recumbency, this point is usually under the caudal ribs or in the midabdomen. The concurrent presence of abdominal effusion may make recognition of the gas bubble easier because the fluid provides a more uniform, homogeneous soft-tissue background opacity (Fig. 37–11A). A large volume of free abdominal gas is readily detected on survey radiographs because the gas provides contrast to outline serosal surfaces of viscera,

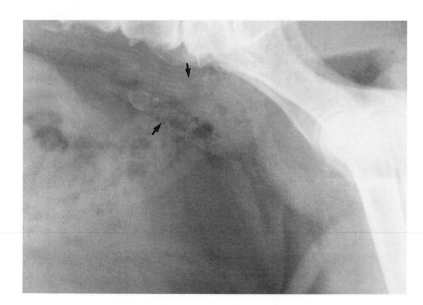

FIGURE 37–10. Close-up lateral view of the caudal abdomen of a 10-year-old dog in chronic renal failure. The external iliac arteries *(arrows)* are visible because of metastatic calcification.

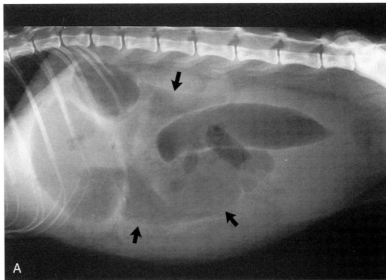

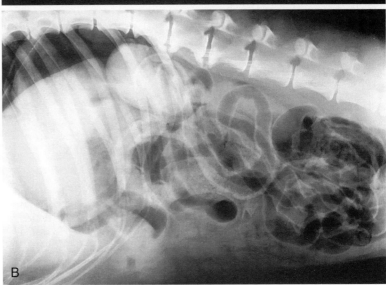

FIGURE 37–11. *A,* Lateral survey radiograph of a cat with abdominal effusion and a moderate amount of free intra-abdominal gas. *Arrows* indicate margins of the gas pocket. *B,* Lateral survey radiograph of the abdomen of a dog immediately after laparotomy. There is a large volume of free abdominal gas that outlines the caudal surface of the right crus of the diaphragm, the cranial pole of the right kidney, the caudal surface of part of the liver, and the serosal surfaces of some bowel loops.

such as bowel loops, the stomach, and the diaphragm (see Fig. 37–11*B*).

Because free gas rises to the highest portion within the abdominal cavity, free gas may be isolated from superimposed structures by using a horizontally directed x-ray beam. With a small volume of gas, it may be preferable to position the patient for 10 minutes before exposure to allow most of the gas to migrate and coalesce at the uppermost portion. The most sensitive projection to detect small volumes of gas is a lateral view, made with a horizontally directed x-ray beam, with the patient in dorsal recumbency and with the cranial portion of the abdomen slightly elevated, so small amounts of gas accumulate between the liver, diaphragm, and ventral abdominal wall (Fig. 37–12*A*).[20] A commonly used projection to document free gas is a ventrodorsal view obtained with the patient in left recumbency with the use of a horizontally directed x-ray beam. Gas usually localizes under the highest portion of the right abdominal wall (see Fig. 37–12*B*), which is usually under the caudal ribs. With larger volumes of gas, the bubble may extend under the diaphragm or along the abdominal wall caudally. Raising or lowering either end of the animal shifts the point of gas accumulation. Exposure factors should be lowered to underexpose the abdomen, and the right abdominal wall should be centered in the x-ray

beam to avoid superimposition of abdominal organs created by divergence of the beam at its periphery. A view with the animal in right recumbency is not recommended because the gas bubble rises to the left side and may be confused with gas within the fundus of the stomach.

Gas may also accumulate in the retroperitoneal space.[8] Retroperitoneal gas is most often the result of extension of pneumomediastinum (see Fig. 28–22) or penetration of the abdominal wall. Retroperitoneal gas is confined to the retroperitoneal space in the dorsal abdomen and is best seen on a lateral radiograph (Fig. 37–13).

Abdominal Wall Abnormalities

Mineralization may occasionally be visualized in the soft tissues surrounding the abdomen. As an example, calcinosis associated with Cushing's syndrome may produce nodular or linear calcification of soft tissues that may be visualized radiographically, most often dorsally and in the ventral abdominal wall.[21] Gas may be seen in the soft tissues surrounding the abdomen from a variety of causes. Abrasions with lacerations often produce a mottled, irregular gas pattern (Fig. 37–14*A*). Tubular or round gas pockets may be

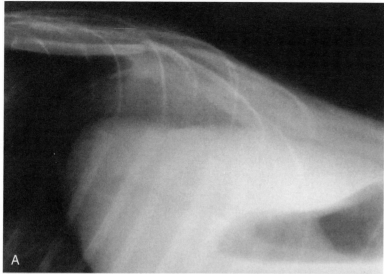

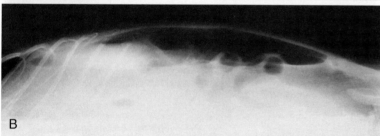

FIGURE 37–12. *A,* Lateral view of the abdomen with the patient in dorsal recumbency with the cranial abdomen slightly elevated and the use of a horizontally directed x-ray beam. Free abdominal gas has accumulated between the diaphragm, liver, and ventral abdominal wall. Diagnosis was ruptured small intestine. *B,* Ventrodorsal view of the abdomen with the patient in left recumbency and the use of a horizontally directed x-ray beam (same as in Fig. 37–11*A*). The free abdominal gas pocket is located under the right abdominal wall and is projected separately from, rather than superimposed over, the abdominal fluid. Diagnosis was ruptured stomach.

contained within herniated bowel loops (Fig. 37–15; see Fig. 37–14*B*). Gas that dissects along fascial planes is most often due to large open wounds or to upper airway perforation or pneumomediastinum. These patterns, however, are not pathognomonic for the cause of the gas accumulation.

ABDOMINAL LYMPH NODES

Abdominal lymph nodes can be divided into two groups: parietal and visceral. Parietal lymph nodes are those that lie in the retroperitoneal space. These lymph nodes receive afferent lymphatics from the spine, adrenal glands, kidneys, caudodorsal abdomen, pelvis, and pelvic limbs. Efferent vessels from these lymph nodes drain into the lumbar trunk, which, in turn, empties into the cisterna chyli. The more cranially located of these lymph nodes may bypass the lumbar trunk and drain directly into the cisterna chyli. Many of the lymph nodes are inconsistently developed and often are absent. The medial iliac lymph nodes, however, the largest lymph nodes of the sublumbar group, are constant. The medial iliac lymph nodes, previously known as the *external iliac lymph nodes*,[1] are located ventral to the vertebra and between the deep circumflex iliac and external iliac arteries.

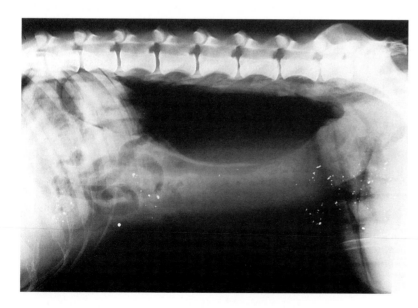

FIGURE 37–13. Lateral view of a dog that had been shot in the caudal abdomen. There is a large volume of gas confined to the retroperitoneal space. There is also gas dissecting along the aorta (ventral to T12) and along the fascial planes of the hindlimb.

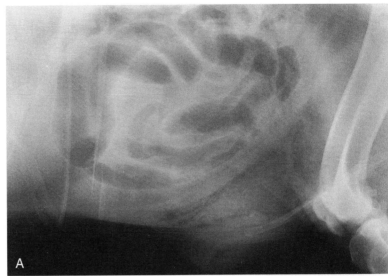

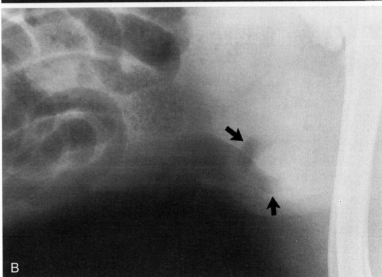

FIGURE 37-14. *A,* Lateral view of the abdomen of a dog that had been hit by a car. Mottled, irregular gas pattern of the soft tissues ventral to the abdominal wall is due to abrasions and lacerations. *B,* Lateral view of the abdomen of a dog with a sharply marginated, tubular gas pocket *(arrows)* ventral to the abdominal wall owing to an inguinal hernia.

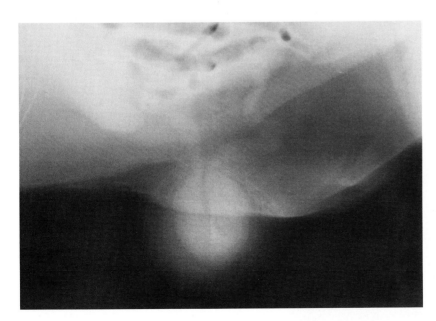

FIGURE 37-15. Lateral view of the ventral abdomen of a dog with an umbilical hernia containing a segment of small bowel. The bowel within the hernia sack is partially obstructed and has become distended.

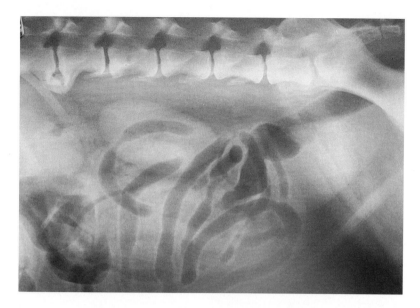

FIGURE 37–16. Lateral view of the abdomen of a normal dog. Note the fat opacity within the retroperitoneal space. Ill-defined nodular soft-tissue opacities in the caudal retroperitoneal space seen ventral to L6 represent end-on projections of the deep circumflex iliac arteries and veins, not lymph nodes. Opacity resulting from superimposition of thigh fascial planes over the retroperitoneal space ventral to L7, as seen in the illustration, is often misdiagnosed as lymphadenopathy. The black dot overlying L4 is a film artifact.

Although some authors state that the medial iliac lymph nodes lie ventral to L5 and L6,[1] it is these authors' experience and that of another author[5] that these lymph nodes are often located ventral to the bodies of L6 and L7. One lymph node is usually present on each side, but occasionally there are two lymph nodes on one or both sides. The medial iliac lymph nodes receive afferent lymphatics from the urogenital tract as well as other structures in the caudal abdomen, pelvis, and pelvic limbs.

The visceral group of abdominal lymph nodes drains the liver, spleen, pancreas, stomach, and intestine. The largest of this group are the cranial mesenteric lymph nodes, which receive afferent lymphatics from the jejunum, ileum, and pancreas. The efferent vessels of the visceral lymph nodes drain into the intestinal trunk, which then empties into the cisterna chyli. Normal abdominal lymph nodes are not seen on survey radiographs because they are not of sufficient size or opacity to be seen as separate structures (Fig. 37–16).

ABNORMALITIES OF THE LYMPH NODES

Abdominal lymph nodes may be seen radiographically only if they are enlarged or mineralized. Abundant retroperitoneal fat present in most dogs also aids in providing contrast between enlarged lymph nodes and surrounding soft-tissue structures. Of the parietal lymph nodes, the medial iliac nodes are usually the only nodes that enlarge to a degree that they may be seen radiographically. Enlarged medial iliac lymph nodes appear as soft-tissue masses in the retroperitoneal space ventral to L6 and L7 (Fig. 37–17). If node enlargement is severe, the lymph nodes may extend more cranially (Fig. 37–18). Frequently, enlarged lymph nodes displace the descending colon and rectum ventrally (Fig. 37–19). One should be cautioned, however, that a ventral course of the colon is not an indication of iliac lymph node enlargement unless a soft-tissue mass is present where the lymph nodes are located. The colon may be normally positioned more ventral than usual without being displaced by a mass. The most common cause of medial iliac lymphadenopathy is neoplasia; however, inflammatory diseases may also cause node enlargement. Neoplastic lymph node involvement may be primary (lymphosarcoma) or metastatic (from caudal abdominal or pelvic neoplasms).[22]

Visceral abdominal lymph nodes are not usually seen on radiographs. They rarely enlarge enough to be seen radio-

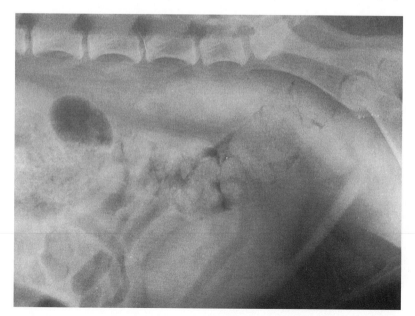

FIGURE 37–17. Lateral view of the abdomen of a dog with lymphosarcoma. The medial iliac lymph nodes are enlarged and appear as a soft-tissue mass with indistinct margins in the retroperitoneal space ventral to L6 and L7.

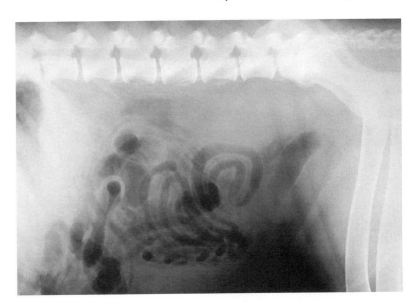

FIGURE 37–18. Lateral view of the abdomen of a dog with lymphosarcoma. Medial iliac lymph node enlargement is severe and appears as a soft-tissue mass in the retroperitoneal space extending caudally from L4 into the pelvic canal.

graphically, they tend to silhouette with surrounding organs, and they are infrequently specifically recognized. Cranial mesenteric lymph nodes may occasionally enlarge sufficiently, however, so as to be seen as an ill-defined central abdominal mass displacing intestine peripherally (Fig. 37–20).

ADRENAL GLANDS

The adrenal glands are located in the retroperitoneal space near the craniomedial border of the kidneys. The left adrenal gland is located more cranially with respect to its corresponding kidney than is the right adrenal gland, which is located near the hilus of the right kidney. The right adrenal gland is bordered dorsally by the psoas minor muscle and the crus of the diaphragm, medially by the caudal vena cava, ventrolaterally by the right kidney, and cranioventrally by the right lateral liver lobe. The left adrenal gland is bordered dorsally by the psoas minor muscle, ventrally by the spleen, laterally by the left kidney, and medially by the aorta.[1] Because of

their small size and soft-tissue opacity, the adrenal glands are not usually seen radiographically.

ABNORMALITIES OF THE ADRENAL GLANDS

Adrenal glands may be seen radiographically only when they are enlarged or mineralized. Radiographically detectable adrenal gland enlargement may be caused by pheochromocytoma,[23] cortical carcinomas, or adenomas.[24, 25] An adrenal mass should be suspected when a soft-tissue or partially mineralized mass is present craniomedial to a kidney; the kidney may be displaced caudolaterally by the mass. Left adrenal masses may displace the fundus of the stomach cranially, the transverse colon caudoventrally, and the left kidney caudally. Masses of the right adrenal gland may be more difficult to detect than those of the left because the right adrenal gland is in close proximity to the liver. Functional adrenal tumors (carcinomas and adenomas) occur with equal frequency in the right or left gland; occasionally, adrenal tumors may occur bilaterally.[25, 26] Of dogs with Cushing's

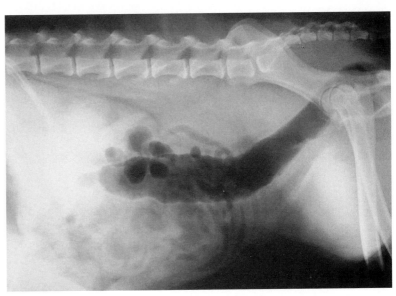

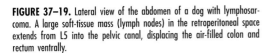

FIGURE 37–19. Lateral view of the abdomen of a dog with lymphosarcoma. A large soft-tissue mass (lymph nodes) in the retroperitoneal space extends from L5 into the pelvic canal, displacing the air-filled colon and rectum ventrally.

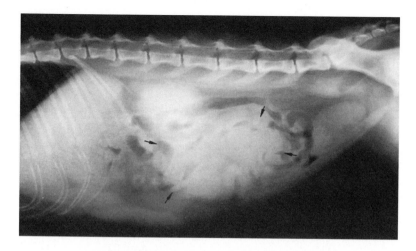

FIGURE 37–20. Lateral view of the abdomen of a cat with mesenteric lymph node enlargement. The enlarged lymph nodes appear as a single, ill-defined soft-tissue mass in the midabdomen *(arrows)*.

syndrome, 10 to 20 percent have functional adrenocortical neoplasms (carcinoma or adenoma).[27, 28]

Computed tomography (CT), ultrasonography, and radiography have been used to image adrenal glands in dogs. Normal and abnormal adrenal glands can be imaged consistently with CT.[29–31] In a study of 41 dogs with functional adrenocortical neoplasms (adenomas and carcinomas), more tumors (72 percent) were found by ultrasound examination than by abdominal radiography (57 percent).[25]

Dystrophic mineralization of adrenal tumors may occur and may be seen radiographically (Fig. 37–21).[24, 25, 32–34] Radiographically visible adrenal calcification in dogs with Cushing's syndrome is highly suggestive of neoplasia. In one study of dogs with functional adrenal tumors, 92 percent of radiographically visible carcinomas and 54 percent of adenomas were calcified.[25] In another study, adrenal calcification was found in 54 percent of carcinomas and 60 percent of adenomas.[24] Carcinomas may invade local tissues, including

the caudal vena cava, and metastasize to the liver, lymph nodes, lungs, and kidneys.[25, 35–37] When adrenal carcinomas are advanced, it may not be possible to determine the origin of the primary mass lesion radiographically. In such an instance, the metastases may be the major radiographic finding, although there may be an ill-defined soft-tissue mass in the craniodorsal abdomen.

Mineralization may occur in non-neoplastic adrenal glands (Fig. 37–22). Radiographically visible adrenal mineralization of unknown cause has been reported in cats.[33, 34] Histologic detection of adrenal calcification was reported in 3.5 percent of dogs, 30 percent of cats, and 50 percent of monkeys in one study[38] and in 25 percent of cats[39] and 1 percent of dogs[40] in two other studies. Calcification occurred in the zona reticularis of the adrenal cortex in the dogs, monkeys, and cats; however, in some cats, calcification affected the entire adrenal cortex and extended into the medulla.[38] Adrenal calcification was not correlated with clinical findings. The

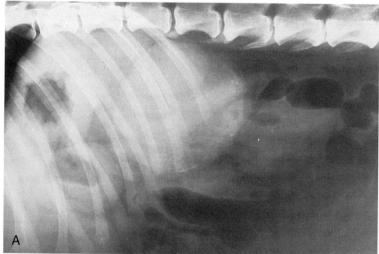

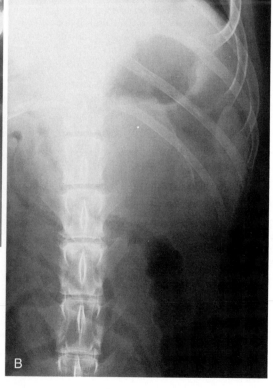

FIGURE 37–21. Lateral *(A)* and ventrodorsal *(B)* abdominal radiographs of a 12-year-old dog. A large, partially mineralized mass is located caudal to the stomach, medial to the spleen, and cranial to the left kidney. The kidney is displaced caudoventrally. The mass is a malignant pheochromocytoma.

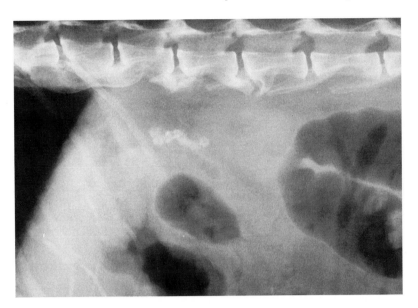

FIGURE 37-22. Lateral radiograph (close-up view) of the abdomen of a 13-year-old cat. Mineral opacities cranial to each kidney are adrenal glands with calcification of the zona reticularis. This finding is clinically insignificant.

cause and pathogenesis of adrenal calcification are unknown. In humans, adrenal calcification has been associated with intra-adrenal hemorrhage, tuberculosis, Addison's disease, tumors (benign and malignant), cysts, Niemann-Pick disease,[41] and Wolman's disease.[42]

It appears that calcification of the adrenal glands in cats is relatively common, but calcification in most animals is not sufficient to be seen radiographically. A normal-sized mineralized adrenal gland in cats and dogs is likely to have no clinical significance.

Adrenal gland dysfunction usually causes secondary changes that are visible radiographically. Radiographic findings of Cushing's syndrome include hepatomegaly, bronchopulmonary mineralization, dystrophic mineralization of the skin and other soft tissues, and adrenal gland enlargement with mineralization, when functional tumors are present.[24, 33, 34] Pulmonary arterial thrombosis has also been reported in dogs with Cushing's syndrome.[43] Esophageal dilation[33] and decreased heart size[44, 45] have been associated with Addison's disease.

References

1. Evans HE, and Christensen GC: Miller's Anatomy of the Dog, 3rd Ed. Philadelphia, WB Saunders, 1993.
2. Johnston DE, and Christie BA: The retroperitoneum in dogs: Anatomy and clinical significance. Comp Contin Ed Vet Pract 12:1027, 1990.
3. Root CR: Interpretation of abdominal survey radiographs. Vet Clin North Am 4:763, 1974.
4. Ettinger SJ, and Barrett KA: Ascites, peritonitis, and other causes of abdominal distention. In Ettinger SJ, and Feldman EC (Eds): Textbook of Veterinary Internal Medicine, 4th Ed. Philadelphia, WB Saunders, 1995.
5. O'Brien TR: The Radiographic Diagnosis of Abdominal Disorders of the Dog and Cat. Philadelphia, WB Saunders, 1978.
6. Boen ST: Peritoneal Dialysis in Clinical Practice. Springfield, Charles C Thomas, 1964.
7. Johnston DE, and Christie BA: The retroperitoneum in dogs: Retroperitoneal infections. Comp Contin Ed Vet Pract 12:1035, 1990.
8. Roush JK, Bjorling DE, and Lord P: Diseases of the retroperitoneal space in the dog and cat. J Am Anim Hosp Assoc 26:47, 1990.
9. Root CR, and Lord PF: Peritoneal carcinomatosis in the dog and cat: Its radiographic appearance. J Am Vet Radiol Soc 12:54, 1971.
10. Gibbs C, Denny HR, Minter HM, et al: Radiological features of inflammatory conditions of the canine pancreas. J Small Anim Pract 13:531, 1972.
11. Kleine LJ, and Hornbuckle WE: Acute pancreatitis: The radiographic findings in 182 dogs. J Am Vet Radiol Soc 19:102, 1978.
12. Suter PF, and Lowe R: Acute pancreatitis in the dog: A clinical study with emphasis on radiographic diagnosis. Acta Radiol (Stockh) 319(suppl):195, 1970.
13. Edwards DF, Bauer MS, Walker MA, et al: Pancreatic masses in seven dogs following acute pancreatitis. J Am Anim Hosp Assoc 26:189, 1990.
14. Salisbury SK, Lantz GC, Nelson RW, et al: Pancreatic abscesses in dogs: Six cases (1978–1986). J Am Vet Med Assoc 193:1104, 1988.
15. Wolfsheimer KJ, Hedlund CS, and Pechman RD: Pancreatic pseudocyst in a dog with chronic pancreatitis. Canine Pract 16:6, 1991.
16. Lamb CR, Kleine LJ, and McMillan MC: Diagnosis of calcification on abdominal radiographs. Vet Radiol 32:211, 1991.
17. Yaphé W, and Forrester SD: Renal secondary hyperparathyroidism, pathophysiology, diagnosis, and treatment. Comp Contin Ed Vet Pract 16:73, 1994.
18. Suter PF, and Olsson SE: The diagnosis of injuries to the intestines, gall bladder and bile ducts in the dog. J Small Anim Pract 11:575, 1970.
19. Probst CW, Stickle, RL, and Bartlett PC: Duration of pneumoperitoneum in the dog. Am J Vet Res 47:176, 1986.
20. Guffy M: A radiological study of hydroperitoneum and pneumoperitoneum in the dog. MS Thesis. Colorado State University, Fort Collins, CO, 1966.
21. Huntley K, Fraser J, Gibbs C, et al: The radiological features of canine Cushing's syndrome: A review of forty-eight cases. J Small Anim Pract 23:369, 1982.
22. Leav I, and Ling GV: Adenocarcinoma of the canine prostate. Cancer 22:1329, 1968.
23. Schaer M: Pheochromocytoma in a dog: A case report. J Am Anim Hosp Assoc 16:583, 1980.
24. Pennick DG, Feldman EC, and Nyland TG: Radiographic features of canine hyperadrenocorticism caused by autonomously functioning adrenocortical tumors: 23 cases (1978–1986). J Am Vet Med Assoc 192:1604, 1988.
25. Reusch CE, and Feldman EC: Canine hyperadrenocorticism due to adrenocortical neoplasia. J Vet Intern Med 5:3, 1991.
26. Ford SL, Feldman EC, and Nelson RW: Hyperadrenocorticism caused by bilateral adrenocortical neoplasia in dogs: Four cases (1983–1988). J Am Vet Med Assoc 202:789, 1993.
27. Meijer JC: Canine hyperadrenocorticism. In Kirk RW (Ed): Current Veterinary Therapy. Philadelphia, WB Saunders, 1980, pp 975–979.
28. Owens JM, and Drucker WD: Hyperadrenocorticism in the dog: Canine Cushing's syndrome. Vet Clin North Am [Small Anim Pract] 7:583, 1977.
29. Voorhout G: X-ray computed tomography, nephrotomography and ultrasonography of the adrenal glands of healthy dogs. Am Res 51:625, 1990.
30. Voorhout G, Stolp R, Rijnberk A, et al: Assessment of survey radiography and comparison with x-ray computed tomography for detection of hyperfunctioning adrenocortical tumors in dogs. J Am Vet Med Assoc 196:1799, 1990.
31. Voorhout G, Stolp R, Lubberink AAME, et al: Computed tomography in the diagnosis of canine hyperadrenocorticism not suppressible by dexamethasone. J Am Vet Med Assoc 192:641, 1988.
32. Huntley K, Frazer J, Gibbs C, et al: The radiological features of canine Cushing's syndrome: A review of forty-eight cases. J Small Anim Pract 23:369, 1982.
33. Ticer JW: Roentgen signs of endocrine disease. Vet Clin North Am 7:465, 1977.
34. Widmer WR, and Guptill L: Imaging techniques for facilitating diagnosis of hyperadrenocorticism in dogs and cats. J Am Vet Med Assoc 206:1857, 1995.

35. Jubb KVF, and Kennedy PC: Pathology of Domestic Animals, 2nd Ed. New York, Academic Press, 1970.
36. Kelly DF, and Darke PGG: Cushing's syndrome in the dog. Vet Rec 98:28, 1976.
37. Siegel ET: Endocrine Disorders of the Dog. Philadelphia, Lea & Febiger, 1977.
38. Ross MA, Gainer JH, and Innes JRM: Dystrophic calcification in the adrenal glands of monkeys, cats, and dogs. Arch Pathol Lab Med 60:655, 1955.
39. Marine D: Calcification of the suprarenal glands of cats. J Exp Med 43:495, 1926.
40. Rajan A, and Mohiyuddeen S: Pathology of the adrenal gland in canines (Canis familiaris). Ind J Anim Sci 44:123, 1974.
41. Bergman SM, and Scouras GC: Incidental bilateral adrenal calcification. Urology 22:665, 1983.
42. Raafat F, Hashemian MP, and Abrishami MA: Wolman's disease: Report of two new cases with a review of the literature. Am J Clin Pathol 59:490, 1973.
43. Burns MG, Kelly AB, Hornof WJ, et al: Pulmonary artery thrombosis in three dogs with hyperadrenocorticism. J Am Vet Med Assoc 178:388, 1981.
44. Rendano VT, and Alexander JE: Heart size changes in experimentally induced adrenal insufficiency in the dog: A radiographic study. J Am Vet Radiol Soc 17:57, 1976.
45. Scott DW: Hyperadrenocorticism (hyperadrenocorticoidism, hyperadrenocorticalism, Cushing's disease, Cushing's syndrome). Vet Clin North Am 9:3, 1979.

STUDY QUESTIONS

1. Figure 37–23 shows lateral (A) and ventrodorsal (B) views of the abdomen of a 1-year-old Rottweiler with a history of lethargy and inappetence. Abdominal distention had been present for 2 weeks. What is the radiographic diagnosis?

2. Figure 37–24 is a lateral abdominal radiograph of a 13-year-old Poodle. The owner noticed a mass in the inguinal region and another near one shoulder. What is the radiographic diagnosis?

3. What is the best radiographic view to detect small quantities of free peritoneal gas using a horizontally directed x-ray beam?
   A. Lateral view, patient standing.
   B. Lateral view, patient in dorsal recumbency.
   C. Ventrodorsal view, patient in left lateral recumbency.
   D. Ventrodorsal view, patient in right lateral recumbency.

4. Which of the following is least likely to result in decreased intra-abdominal contrast?
   A. Peritonitis.
   B. Normal puppy.
   C. Abdominal mass.
   D. Peritoneal metastasis.

5. List three rule-outs for diffuse increase in soft-tissue opacity in the retroperitoneal space.

6. The retroperitoneal space communicates with which of the following?
   A. Mediastinum.
   B. Pelvic canal.
   C. Pleural space.
   D. Peritoneal space.

7. Which of the following structures are not normally identified on survey abdominal radiographs?
   A. Adrenal glands.

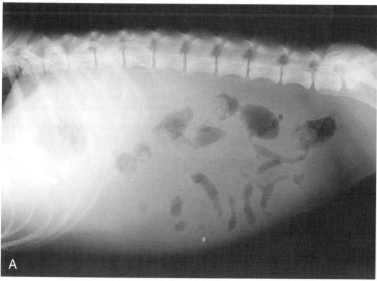

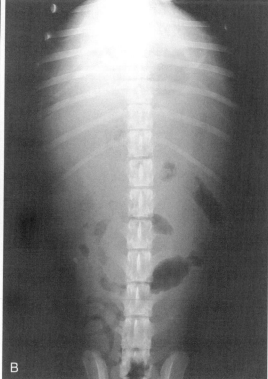

FIGURE 37–23. A and B

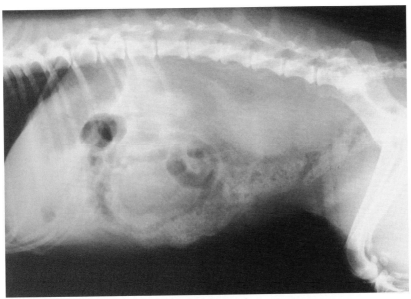

FIGURE 37–24

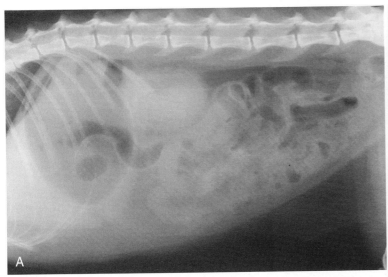

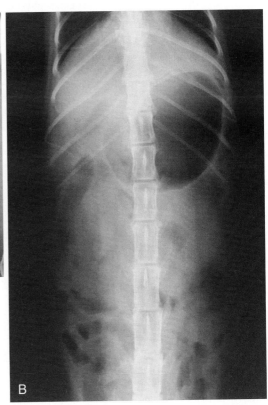

FIGURE 37–25. *A* and *B*

B. Sublumbar lymph nodes.
C. Falciform ligament fat.
D. Caudal surface of the diaphragm.

8. Figure 37–25 shows lateral *(A)* and ventrodorsal *(B)* abdominal radiographs of a 2-year-old cat with vomiting and depression. The owner had seen the cat eat a string 1 week previously. What are the radiographic findings?

9. What is the clinical significance of a normal-sized, mineralized adrenal gland on abdominal radiographs of a cat?

10. Are radiographs more or less sensitive than ultrasound for evaluation of suspected adrenal gland tumors?

(Answers appear on page 646.)

Chapter 38

The Liver and Spleen

Robert D. Pechman, Jr.

Radiographic diagnosis of abnormalities of the liver or spleen depends on recognizing changes in size, shape, position, margination, and radiopacity of these organs. Alterations in size, shape, and margination are common survey radiographic signs of hepatic or splenic disease. Positional changes of these organs are not common, and alterations in radiopacity of the liver and spleen are rare.[1] Abnormalities detected on survey radiographs most often are not specific for any particular disease process; the liver or spleen may appear radiographically normal even when severely abnormal.

Several radiographic procedures have been devised in an attempt to improve the radiographic diagnosis of hepatic or splenic diseases. Portography allows evaluation of the portal venous circulation and detection of portosystemic shunting of blood.[2] Cholangiography and cholecystography are useful in evaluating the biliary system.[3, 4] Angiography may be used to assess the blood supply and structure of these two highly vascular organs.[5]

Alternative imaging techniques have become available that greatly enhance the assessment of hepatic and splenic diseases. Radioisotope scanning of the liver and spleen may be used to evaluate the internal structure of both of these organs or the hepatobiliary system; imaging with ultrasound is particularly effective.[6] Scintigraphic and sonographic imaging techniques are less invasive than radiographic contrast medium examinations.

LIVER

The liver is the largest solid organ in the abdomen and occupies the most cranial aspect of the abdomen. The dimensions of the abdomen are greatest in the region of the liver. Radiographic exposure factors must be adequate to penetrate the liver, yet not so great as to eliminate the slight natural contrast between the liver and surrounding fat. Evaluation of liver size and shape requires evaluation of liver borders and the position of adjacent organs, which may be displaced or altered by an enlarged liver (Fig. 38–1).[1]

The convex cranial margin of the liver is in contact with the diaphragm. The right and left lateral margins of the liver are near the abdominal wall but may be visualized if there is adequate intra-abdominal fat. The ventral border of the liver is usually well defined by the fat in the falciform ligament. The dorsal border of the liver is usually not seen. The concave caudal border of the liver is not directly seen on survey radiographs, but its position can be estimated by its relationship to the right kidney, stomach, and cranial flexure of the duodenum. In lateral radiographs, (1) the dorsocaudal border of the liver is adjacent to the cranial pole of the right kidney, (2) the cranial wall of the stomach defines the caudal margin of the liver in the midabdominal region, and (3) the caudal ventral border of the liver is formed by the left lateral liver lobe. The triangular liver opacity ventral to the pyloric an-

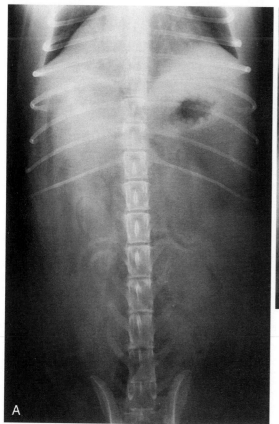

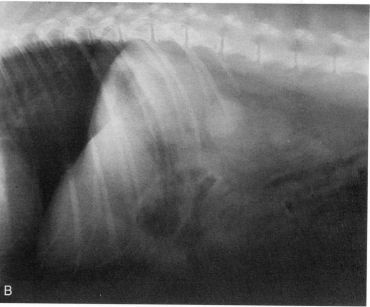

FIGURE 38–1. Ventrodorsal *(A)* and lateral *(B)* radiographs of the abdomen of a normal dog. In the ventrodorsal projection, the stomach is perpendicular to the spine, and the gastric gas shadow identifies the caudal surface of the liver. The gastric gas shadow follows the arch of the ribs in the lateral projection.

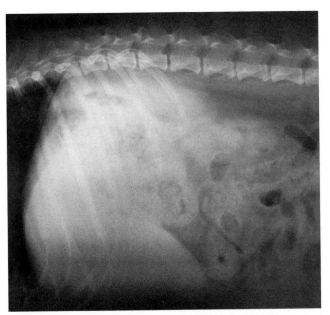

FIGURE 38–2. Generalized hepatomegaly in a dog with Cushing's disease. The liver extends far caudal to the costal arch, and there is dorsal and caudal displacement of the pyloric region of the stomach. The liver margins remain smooth and sharp.

trum is formed by the right medial liver lobe cranially and the left lateral liver lobe caudally.[8]

In ventrodorsal radiographs, the caudal border of the right lateral liver lobe is indicated by the cranial duodenal flexure. The cranial pole of the right kidney defines the caudal border of the caudate liver lobe, and the gastric fundus indicates the caudal border of the left lateral liver lobe. The caudal borders of the right medial, quadrate, and left medial liver lobes are adjacent to the lesser curvature of the stomach.[1, 7, 8]

The apparent shape and position of the liver can be affected by (1) the phase of respiration during which the radiograph is made; (2) the age, breed, and thoracic conformation of the patient; and (3) the position of the patient during radiography.[1, 2] The right liver lobes move cranially during radiography in right lateral recumbency, and the entire liver may move caudally if radiographs are made at peak inspiration. In animals with a deep, narrow thoracic cavity, the liver may be entirely within the portion of the abdomen under the caudal rib cage, whereas the liver may extend slightly beyond the costal arch in animals with a shallow, wide thoracic cavity. The liver is usually larger in young animals than in adults.[2] The liver may be separated from the ventral abdominal wall by a substantial distance because of fat in the falciform ligament; this is particularly true in obese cats. Ligaments that attach the liver to the diaphragm may weaken and stretch in aged or obese dogs, allowing the liver to slide caudoventrally and extend beyond the costal arch.[8] All of these normal variants must be kept in mind when the liver is assessed radiographically.

Alterations in Liver Size

Alterations in liver size may be found in primary liver diseases or secondary to diseases of other organ systems. Survey radiographs may depict increases or decreases in liver size but rarely delineate the cause of the size alteration. Radiographic assessment of liver size is fraught with error and, at best, is inexact and subjective. A quantitative method of evaluating liver size in radiographs of normal dogs has been described,

but the clinical usefulness of this technique remains to be proved.[9]

Hepatomegaly is a reliable radiographic sign of liver disease (Fig. 38–2).[1] Hepatomegaly may be diffuse, with fairly uniform enlargement of all lobes, or it may be focal, with enlargement of only a single lobe. Severe, diffuse hepatomegaly causes a substantial portion of the caudal liver margin to project beyond the costal arch, an obvious increase in size, and, most important, rounding of the caudal liver edges in the lateral radiograph. The stomach is displaced caudodorsally in the lateral projection and caudally and toward the left in the ventrodorsal projection. The right kidney, cranial duodenal flexure, and transverse colon are displaced caudally in the ventrodorsal view.[1, 7] Diffuse hepatomegaly may be caused by inflammatory disease or neoplasia, hepatic venous congestion, fat infiltration, cholestasis, cirrhosis, amyloidosis, or storage diseases.[1, 2]

Focal hepatomegaly is depicted on survey radiographs by displacement of organs adjacent to the affected lobe, and the involved lobe is identified by recognizing which organ or part of an organ is displaced.[10] Right liver lobe enlargement displaces the body and pyloric regions of the stomach dorsally and to the left while the gastric fundus remains in normal position; caudal and left displacement of the gastric fundus with indentation of the lesser curvature of the stomach may be seen with enlargement of the left liver lobes.[7, 10] Focal hepatomegaly, affecting only one or two lobes, may be caused by neoplastic diseases, regenerative nodules of cirrhosis, or localized masses, such as large hepatic abscesses and cysts.[1, 8, 10]

Microhepatia is more difficult to recognize radiographically than is hepatomegaly (Fig. 38–3).[1] Microhepatia may be indicated by cranial displacement of the stomach and decreased distance between the diaphragm and the stomach on the lateral and ventrodorsal projections. Cranioventral slanting

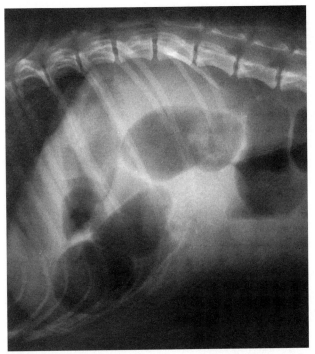

FIGURE 38–3. Microhetatia in a dog with chronic liver disease and hepatic fibrosis. The gas-filled stomach courses cranioventrally, and there is slight cranial displacement of the pyloric region of the stomach. The transverse colon is ventral to the pylorus and is much more cranial than normal. Microhepatica is usually not this dramatic, and caution should be exercised in making the diagnosis.

of the gastric-pyloric axis in the lateral projection and cranial displacement of the right kidney, cranial duodenal flexure, and transverse colon in the ventrodorsal view are additional radiographic signs of microhepatia. Reduced liver size is usually diffuse and may be caused by chronic hepatic disease, fibrosis, hepatic cirrhosis, or congenital anomalies such as congenital portosystemic venous shunts. In dogs with portosystemic shunts, microhepatia is most severe in small breeds with extrahepatic shunts.[11] Reduced liver size may also be seen in normal dogs and cats.[1]

Alterations in Liver Position

Changes in liver position are usually secondary to thoracic diseases or disruption of the diaphragm.[1] The liver may be located more cranially than normal when there is traumatic disruption of the diaphragm and herniation of liver into the thoracic cavity. Congenital peritoneopericardial diaphragmatic hernia, in which a portion of the liver is within the pericardial sac, also results in cranial displacement of the liver (Fig. 38–4). In both instances, the normal diaphragm shadow is incomplete on survey radiographs. Cranial displacement of the liver is indicated by the criteria used to define microhepatica.

Caudal displacement of the liver is usually caused by intrathoracic diseases that displace the diaphragm, and consequently the liver, caudally. Abdominal radiographs made on full inspiration and in patients with a large pleural effusion are commonly characterized by caudal displacement of the liver.[1, 2] Severe overinflation of the lungs, as may occur in chronic obstructive lung disease, also results in caudal displacement of the liver. The radiographic signs of caudal displacement of the liver are those associated with diffuse hepatomegaly—caudal displacement of adjacent organs.

Alterations in Liver Margins

Changes in the normally smooth and fairly pointed liver margins are usually associated with hepatomegaly,[1, 2] but they may be seen in some patients with reduced liver size. The

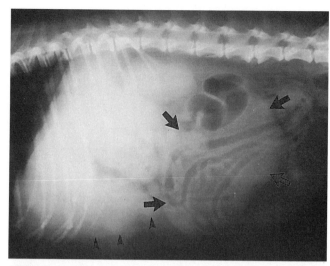

FIGURE 38–5. Nodular liver margins in a dog with splenic hemangiosarcoma and hepatic metastases. The neoplastic mass on the spleen is visible in the midabdomen *(arrows)*. The liver is enlarged, and there is a lumpy appearance of the ventral border *(arrowheads)*. The liver contained numerous metastatic masses that were the cause of the nodular liver margins.

caudal liver margins are often round and blunt in diseases that result in diffuse hepatomegaly, such as right-sided heart failure, hepatic lipidosis, diffuse hepatic neoplasia or inflammation, and amyloidosis.[1, 2, 8]

Liver margins may be round, irregular, and lumpy in patients with hepatic neoplasia, particularly in patients with widespread hepatic metastases, and in patients with cirrhosis with fibrosis and prominent regenerative nodules (Fig. 38–5).[1, 8] Solitary liver masses, such as neoplasms and abscesses near the organ surface, may produce a single lump on the normally smooth liver margin.[1] Liver masses resulting in significant displacement of adjacent organs are discussed in detail in Chapter 36.

Alterations in Liver Radiopacity

The liver is normally of homogeneous soft-tissue opacity; increases or decreases in radiopacity are rare. Increased hepatic radiopacity is caused only by mineralization (Fig. 38–6). Hepatic mineralization, seen as miliary or discrete nodular radiopacities, may occur diffusely or may affect focal areas of one or more lobes.[1] Mineral opacities may be confined to the gallbladder or the biliary or cystic ducts in patients with cholelithiasis.[2, 12, 13] Nodular or miliary parenchymal mineralization may be associated with neoplasia, granulomatous diseases, or mineralized parasitic cysts.[1, 8]

Decreased liver opacity, which also occurs rarely, is due to gas accumulation within the liver. Gas may accumulate in the gallbladder or biliary ducts or within the intrahepatic veins (see Fig. 38–6).[1] Gas within the gallbladder, in the gallbladder wall, or in the pericholecystic liver parenchyma is usually secondary to cholecystitis caused by gas-forming organisms, but it can be due to an open communication with the lumen of the bowel.[1, 8, 14, 15] Gas in the hepatic veins appears as a linear branching pattern of gas opacities,[1] and this may occur secondary to gas embolization during pneumocystography or pneumourethrography.[16] Detection of gas in hepatic vascular structures on survey radiographs is a grave sign.[1]

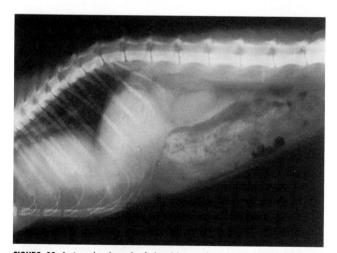

FIGURE 38–4. Lateral radiograph of the abdomen of a cat with a peritoneopericardial diaphragmatic hernia. The cardiac silhouette is greatly enlarged, and the ventral margin of the diaphragm is not visible. The stomach is close to the diaphragm, and there is cranial displacement of the pyloric region of the stomach. The caudoventral margin of the liver, normally ventral to the stomach, is not seen. Radiographic signs of microhepatica are present, but the diagnosis is cranial displacement of the liver owing to a hernia. At surgery, approximately 80 percent of the liver was found in the pericardial sac.

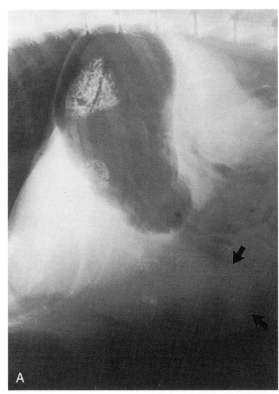
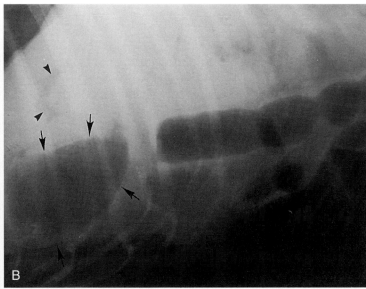

FIGURE 38–6. Alterations in liver opacity. *A,* Increased liver opacity owing to mineralization of *Histoplasma* granulomas. The liver is enlarged, and the caudal edge is noticeably rounded *(arrows)*. *B,* Decreased hepatic opacity is due to gas accumulation within the gallbladder *(arrows)*, gallbladder wall, pericholecystic liver parenchyma, and dilated hepatic biliary duct *(arrowheads)*. This patient had emphysematous cholecystitis caused by *Clostridium.*

Contrast Medium Studies for Evaluation of the Liver

Numerous radiographic contrast medium techniques have been used in dogs and cats in attempts to improve the radiographic diagnosis of liver disease. Techniques such as pneumoperitoneography, cholecystography, cholangiography, and angiography have fallen into disfavor and are not often used. Newer techniques such as nuclear imaging and diagnostic ultrasonography have greatly improved the ability to detect and diagnose liver disease.[6, 8]

Portography is one radiographic procedure that is used occasionally to assess for the presence of portosystemic shunts. Radiographic examination of the portal venous system may be accomplished by several techniques, many of which require equipment not often available in general veterinary practice.[2] Operative portography, however, is a relatively simple technique that may be easily performed without the need for sophisticated imaging equipment or arterial catheterization. Operative portography can be used to evaluate the portal venous circulation for the presence of congenital or acquired portosystemic shunts.[1, 2]

Operative portography is performed by surgically placing a catheter in a jejunal or splenic vein or in the splenic pulp. Aqueous iodinated contrast medium is injected and a radiograph made.[2] A lateral projection is usually adequate for diagnosis, but a ventrodorsal view may be helpful if surgical intervention is contemplated. The portal venous system is usually well defined with operative portography, and portosystemic shunts may be readily identified.

Several congenital and acquired portosystemic shunts have been described.[2] A portopostcaval shunt via the ductus venosus seems to be the most common congenital shunt; acquired portosystemic shunts may involve any of a large number of collateral venous channels (Fig. 38–7).[2]

SPLEEN

The spleen is an elongated, flat, solid organ in the cranial left abdomen, lying just caudal to the stomach. The spleen con-

sists of two main parts: the dorsal extremity (head) and the ventral extremity (tail). The dorsal extremity is less variable in position because of its short gastrosplenic ligament and its location between the gastric fundus and the cranial pole of the left kidney. The ventral extremity is less tightly fixed in position and thus may vary greatly in location.[8, 17]

Radiographically the spleen is an organ of solid, homogeneous soft-tissue opacity that is not consistently visualized in lateral radiographs but is usually seen regularly in ventrodorsal views of the abdomen (Fig. 38–8).[7, 10] The spleen is more likely to be seen in abdominal radiographs made with the animal in right lateral recumbency than in those radiographs made in left lateral recumbency.[7] When seen in the lateral projection, the spleen is near the ventral abdominal wall and just caudal to the liver. In ventrodorsal radiographs, the spleen is a triangular structure of soft-tissue opacity that is slightly caudal and lateral to the gastric fundus.[7, 10] In some animals, particularly cats, the dorsal extremity of the spleen may be seen in the lateral view as a small triangular soft-tissue opacity in the dorsal abdomen just caudal to the gastric fundus.

There are no reliable criteria for the radiographic determination of normal splenic size. Evaluation of splenic size is purely subjective.[10] Radiographically the edges and margins of the normal spleen are smooth and sharp.

Alterations in Spleen Size

Because determination of normal splenic size is subjective, alterations in the size of this organ must be substantial to be recognized. The spleen may increase or decrease in size uniformly and diffusely, or the spleen may enlarge locally, as with a splenic mass (Fig. 38–9).

Diffuse splenic enlargement is often a physiologic response that occurs after the administration of medications. Phenothiazine tranquilizers and barbiturate anesthetics cause diffuse

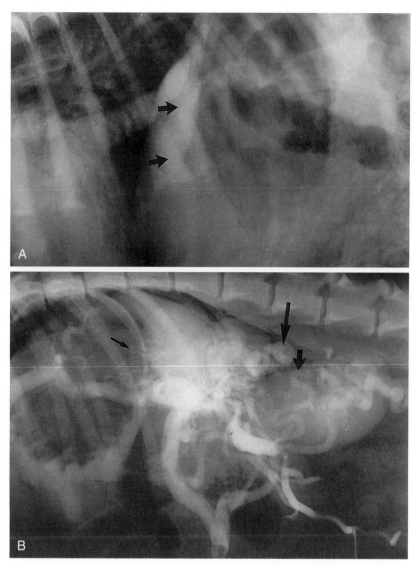

FIGURE 38–7. Contrast portograms in two dogs with portosystemic shunts. *A,* Congenital patent ductus venosus *(arrows)* opacified after injection of contrast medium into the cranial mesenteric artery (cranial mesenteric arterial portography). *B,* Numerous tortuous, collateral venous channels *(arrows)* in a dog with an acquired portosystemic shunt are opacified after injection of contrast medium into a jejunal vein (operative portography).

and often substantial splenic enlargement.[10] Diseases affecting the reticuloendothelial system, such as mastocytosis, lymphosarcoma, and histoplasmosis, also may produce diffuse splenic enlargement.[10, 18, 19] Diffuse splenic enlargement, by itself, is not a reliable sign of disease because the possible causes are numerous, and in many instances enlargement is a normal physiologic reaction. Diffuse splenic enlargement is often seen in patients with splenic torsion or gastric volvulus[18]; splenomegaly is not diagnostic for these conditions but is a supportive radiographic finding.

Primary and metastatic neoplasms are frequent causes of focal splenic enlargement.[10] Subcapsular hematomas also cause focal enlargement of this organ.[18] Splenic masses are recognized by their close association with the spleen in one or both views of the abdomen as well as by the displacement of adjacent organs that they cause.[7, 10] A splenic mass is the most common cause of a midabdominal mass seen on the lateral view. Radiographic diagnosis of splenic masses is discussed in Chapter 36.

Alterations in Spleen Position

Because the spleen is not rigidly fixed, its location can vary greatly, even in normal dogs and cats.[7, 10] Pathologic alter-

ations in spleen position may be seen in patients with traumatic hernias through which the spleen may pass. The dorsal extremity of the spleen is closely attached to the greater curvature of the stomach, so the spleen may be identified in the thorax of some animals with diaphragmatic hernias involving the stomach. Displacement of the stomach, as in gastric volvulus, may also displace the spleen. In patients with splenic torsion, the spleen may be found in an abnormal location, although identification of the spleen may be difficult because of abdominal effusion.[8]

Alterations in Splenic Shape or Margination

Changes in the margins or shape of the spleen are usually the result of splenic masses. The masses distort the normal spleen and produce irregularly lobulated margins. Masses may be neoplastic or may represent large hematomas.[18] Neoplastic masses tend to have lumpy margins with multiple lobulations; hematomas are usually smooth in outline and are spherical.[18] Margins of the spleen may become obscured or obliterated by fluid in the abdomen or around the spleen. This loss of visualization is particularly true in traumatic

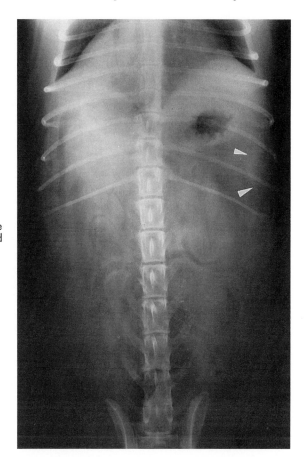

FIGURE 38–8. Ventrodorsal radiograph of the abdomen of a normal dog. The triangular opacity of the normal spleen *(outline and arrows)* is present midway between and slightly lateral to the gastric fundus and the left kidney. The spleen is reliably seen in this location in ventrodorsal radiographs.

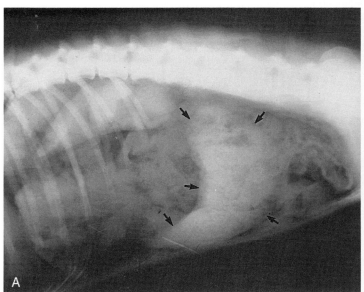

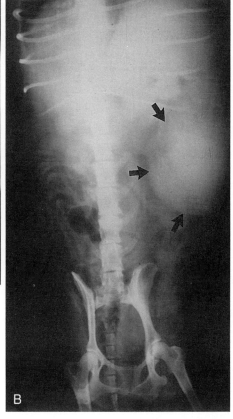

FIGURE 38–9. *A*, The spleen is greatly enlarged in this dog and is clearly seen owing to intra-abdominal gas. The margins of the spleen are smooth *(arrows)*, and no abdominal splenic mass is seen. Splenomegaly is due to the administration of a phenothiazine tranquilizer. *B*, The normal splenic silhouette is not visible in this dog. A large soft-tissue mass *(arrows)* is present where the normal splenic silhouette is expected. A large splenic neoplasm was found at surgery.

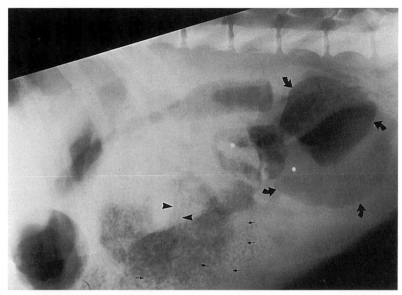

FIGURE 38–10. Alteration in splenic opacity. The spleen contains mottled gas opacities *(small arrows)*, and several veins also contain gas *(arrowheads)* in this dog with splenic torsion. Margins of the spleen are not visible because of intra-abdominal fluid. Free intra-abdominal gas is also present *(curved arrows)*. *Clostridium* was isolated from the spleen after it was removed.

splenic rupture, with hemorrhage initially around the spleen; streaky, hazy areas of increased opacity obscure the normally sharp, clearly defined splenic margins.[8]

Alterations in Radiopacity of the Spleen

Changes in radiopacity of the spleen are rare. Gas accumulation in the splenic pulp may be associated with splenic torsion and subsequent proliferation of gas-forming organisms within the spleen (Fig. 38–10).

References

1. Suter PF: Radiographic diagnosis of liver disease in dogs and cats. Vet Clin North Am [Small Anim Pract] *12*:153, 1982.
2. Suter PF: Portal vein anomalies in the dog: Their angiographic diagnosis. J Am Vet Radiol Soc *16*:84, 1975.
3. Carlisle CH: A comparison of technics for cholecystography in the cat. J Am Vet Radiol Soc *18*:173, 1977.
4. Allan GS, and Dixon RT: Cholecystography in the dog: The choice of contrast media and optimum dose rates. J Am Vet Radiol Soc *16*:98, 1975.
5. Schmidt S, and Suter PF: Angiography of the hepatic and portal venous system of the dog and cat: An investigative method. Vet Radiol *21*:57, 1980.
6. Nyland TG, and Park RD: Hepatic ultrasonography in the dog. Vet Radiol *24*:74, 1983.
7. Root CR: Interpretation of abdominal survey radiographs. Vet Clin North Am *24*:763, 1974.
8. O'Brien TR: The liver. *In* O'Brien TR (Ed): Radiographic Diagnosis of Abdominal Disorders in the Dog and Cat. Philadelphia, WB Saunders, 1978, pp 396–449.
9. Godshalk CP, Kneller SK, Badertscher RR II, et al: Quantitative noninvasive assessment of liver size in clinically normal dogs. Am J Vet Res *51*:1421, 1990.
10. Root CR: Abdominal masses: The radiographic differential diagnosis. J Am Vet Radiol Soc *15*:26, 1974.
11. Bostwick DR, and Twedt DC: Intra and extra hepatic portal venous anomalies. J Am Vet Med Assoc *206*:1811, 1995.
12. Schall WD, Chapman WL Jr, Finco DR, et al: Cholelithiasis in dogs. J Am Vet Med Assoc *163*:469, 1973.
13. Cantwell HD, Blevins WE, Hanika-Rebar C, et al: Radiopaque hepatic and lobar duct choleliths in a dog. J Am Anim Hosp Assoc *19*:373, 1983.
14. Burk RL, and Johnson GF: Emphysematous cholecystitis in the nondiabetic dog: Three case histories. Vet Radiol *21*:242, 1980.
15. Lord PF, Carb A, Halliwell WH, et al: Emphysematous hepatic abscess associated with trauma, necrotic hepatic nodular hyperplasia and adenoma in a dog: A case report. Vet Radiol *23*:46, 1982.
16. Ackerman N, Wingfield WE, and Corley EA: Fatal air embolism associated with pneumourethrography and pneumocystography in a dog. J Am Vet Med Assoc *160*:1616, 1972.
17. Evans HE: The digestive apparatus and abdomen. *In* Evans HE (ed): Miller's Anatomy of the Dog, 3rd Ed. Philadelphia, WB Saunders, 1993, pp 385–462.
18. Couto CG, and Hammer AS: Diseases of the lymph nodes and the spleen. *In* Ettinger SJ, Feldman EC (Eds): Textbook of Veterinary Internal Medicine, 4th Ed. Philadelphia, WB Saunders, 1995, pp 1930–1946.
19. Liska WD, MacEwen EG, Zaki FA, et al: Feline systemic mastocytosis: A review and results of splenectomy in seven cases. J Am Anim Hosp Assoc *15*:589, 1979.

STUDY QUESTIONS

1. The position of the caudal border of the liver can best be estimated by its relationship to the right kidney, stomach, and cranial flexure of the duodenum. (True or False)

2. In this lateral radiograph (Fig. 38–11) of the abdomen of a dog, there is evidence of:
   A. Splenomegaly.
   B. Diffuse hepatomegaly.
   C. A hepatic mass.
   D. Microhepatia.
   E. Lymphosarcoma.

3. In dogs with portosystemic shunts, microhepatia is likely to be most severe in:
   A. Small breeds with intrahepatic shunts.
   B. Large breeds with extrahepatic shunts.
   C. Large breeds with intrahepatic shunts.

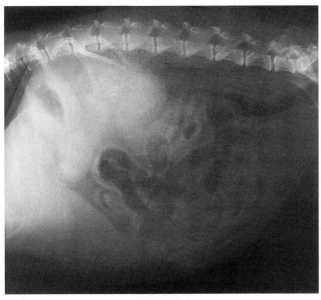

FIGURE 38-11

D. Small breeds with extrahepatic shunts.
E. Dogs with chronic renal disease.

4. Radiopacity of the liver increases as the amount of hepatic fibrosis increases. (True or False)

5. A relatively simple radiographic contrast technique that can easily be used in practice to evaluate the portal venous system is:
A. Operative portography.
B. Cranial mesenteric arteriography.
C. Celiac arteriography.

D. Caudal vena cava venography.
E. Intravenous cholecystography.

6. In a lateral radiograph of the abdomen of a dog (Fig. 38-12), there is radiographic evidence of:
A. A splenic mass.
B. A liver mass.
C. Diffuse hepatomegaly.
D. Hepatic neoplasia.
E. Mesenteric lymphadenopathy.

7. Diffuse and extreme splenic enlargement may be caused by phenothiazine tranquilizers and barbiturate anesthetics. (True or False)

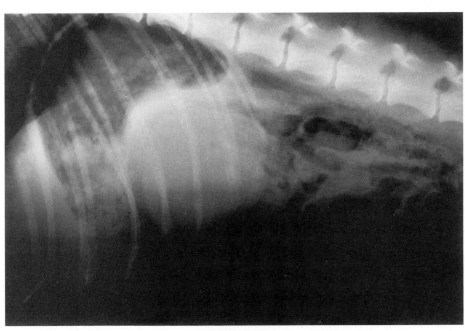

FIGURE 38-12

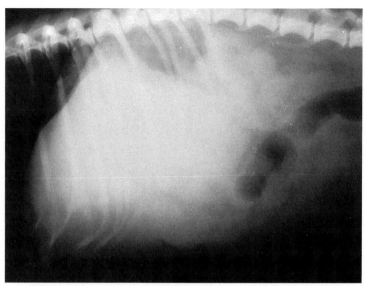

FIGURE 38–13

8. The spleen is more likely to be seen in abdominal radiographs made in left lateral recumbency than in those made in right lateral recumbency. (True or False)

9. In a lateral radiograph of the abdomen of a dog (Fig. 38–13), there is evidence of:
   A. A hepatic mass.
   B. Diffuse hepatomegaly.

C. Diffuse splenomegaly.
D. A splenic mass.
E. Mastocytosis.

10. The presence of a splenic mass in abdominal radiographs is reliable evidence of splenic neoplasia. (True or False)

(Answers appear on page 646.)

Chapter 39

The Kidneys and Ureters

Daniel A. Feeney • Gary R. Johnston

KIDNEYS

Survey radiographs, as well as radiographic procedures with contrast medium, can contribute much information toward the diagnosis of renal and ureteral diseases. The external boundaries of the kidneys can usually be identified on survey radiographs. This identification permits assessment of the size, shape, and radiographic opacity of the kidneys, which may aid in the diagnosis of disease processes. When the kidneys cannot be assessed by survey radiographs, however, or when qualitative functional information is needed, ultrasonography or excretory urography may provide the clinician with much information with minimal patient discomfort.

This chapter specifies the radiographic imaging procedures applicable to the kidneys and places each of these procedures into perspective regarding indications, limitations, contraindications, and pitfalls when applicable. Subsequently the normal radiographic findings based on roentgen signs are described. In addition, the abnormal radiographic findings are described, and at least a partial list of gamuts that should be considered in association with certain roentgen signs is

presented. Cited reference material should be consulted for a more extensive review of the suggested disease processes.

Imaging Procedures

Survey radiographs are the simplest form of radiographic evaluation for small animals. The general indications for the use of survey radiographs to evaluate specific disease processes are outlined in textbooks of general internal medicine or surgery.[1, 2] More specifically, survey radiographs provide information on the external anatomy of the kidney when contrast (both abdominal and retroperitoneal) is adequate to permit their visualization. In addition, it is possible to assess any abnormal opacities near the kidneys, such as air and mineral, which may suggest a pathophysiologic mechanism for the clinical signs of renal disease. Inadequate radiographic contrast, which is generally due to lack of retroperitoneal fat or the presence of peritoneal or retroperitoneal fluid, limits visualization of the kidneys on survey radiographs.

The information available from survey radiographs can be maximized if the patient is properly prepared, such as withholding of food for 24 hours and administration of cleansing enemas at least 1 or 2 hours before radiography. Because the right lateral view permits greater longitudinal separation of the radiographic images of the right and left kidneys, it is the projection most applicable to radiography of the upper urinary tract.[3]

Because of the limitations of survey radiographs, especially when the patient is emaciated or has peritoneal or retroperitoneal fluid, excretory urography is the method of choice to define the anatomic structures and to assess qualitatively the function of the kidneys. It is a relatively simple means of verifying and localizing upper urinary tract disease, and it may be used to assess the reversibility of renal disease. Although excretory urography is not a quantitative measurement of renal function, it may be used to assess the relative function of the kidneys and may be loosely interpreted to assess the pathophysiologic mechanisms of renal failure.[4]

Excretory urography may be used in both azotemic and nonazotemic patients, provided that hydration is adequate. As the degree of renal failure progresses, however, it may be necessary to increase the dose of contrast medium to provide adequate visualization of the kidneys. In any instance, patient hydration should be assessed and determined to be at a normal level before the administration of any contrast medium.[4] It is possible that there may be a temporary decrease in kidney function after excretory urography; an in-depth discussion of this is beyond the scope of this chapter. The clinical significance of this decreased function is considered minimal in the presence of adequate urinary output and patient hydration.

Azotemia is not a contraindication in excretory urography, provided that the patient is adequately hydrated. In other specific disease processes in humans, it has been suspected that excretory urography is contraindicated, but the major underlying factor contributing to the contrast medium–induced problem in these patients appeared to be poor urinary flow secondary to inadequate hydration. For information concerning the specific pathophysiology and management of patients with the unlikely occurrence of contrast medium–induced renal disease or failure, readers are directed to textbooks on renal disease.

The technique of excretory urography is described in detail in Table 39–1. The patient should be prepared as for survey radiographs: Food is withheld, and cleansing enemas are administered.[4–6] Generally, ionic contrast media are used, such as sodium iothalamate and sodium diatrizoate, and are given by bolus intravenous injection. If previous systemic reactions (e.g., shock) have occurred in the patient, however, or the patient is severely compromised medically, nonionic contrast media, such as iopamidol and iohexol, should be considered, or an alternative procedure such as ultrasonography should be sought.[10] The dose of contrast medium for excretory urography is 400 mg iodine per pound of body weight injected via a preplaced cephalic venous or jugular venous catheter.[4–7] Catheter placement should be maintained for at least 15 to 20 minutes after administration of the contrast medium because it provides a readily accessible route in the event of a hypotensive reaction to the contrast medium. There are many suggested filming sequences; however, radiographs obtained immediately and 5, 20, and 40 minutes after injection of contrast medium generally yield the most information.[4, 5, 7]

The interpretative phases of the excretory urogram are the nephrographic and pyelographic phases. Opacification of the

Table 39–1
TECHNIQUE FOR EXCRETORY UROGRAPHY

Routine patient preparation
  24 hours without food; water ad libitum
  Cleansing enema at least 2 hours before radiography
Assess hydration status; proceed only if normal
Obtain survey radiographs
Infuse contrast medium intravenously via the cephalic or jugular vein as rapidly as possible (bolus injection)
  Dose: 400 mg iodine/lb body weight
  Contrast medium: usually sodium iothalamate or sodium diatrizoate, but consider nonionic agents such as iopamidol or iohexol in high-risk patients
Obtain abdominal radiographs in the following sequence:
  Ventrodorsal views at 5–20 seconds, 5 minutes, 20 minutes, and 40 minutes postinjection for general assessment
  Lateral view at 5 minutes postinjection for general assessment
  Oblique views at 3–15 minutes postinjection for ureteral termination in urinary bladder
  Lateral and ventrodorsal views at 30–40 minutes postinjection to observe urinary bladder if retrograde cystography is contraindicated or impossible

Modified from Feeney DA, Barber DL, Johnston, GR, et al: The excretory urogram: Techniques, normal radiographic appearance and misinterpretation. Comp Contin Ed Vet Pract 4:233, 1982; with permission.

functional renal parenchyma is the nephrogram, and opacification of the renal pelves, pelvic recesses, and ureters is the pyelogram. Each phase should be evaluated separately (based on subsequent information in this chapter). The sequence of these phases should then be compared in view of the normal findings yet to be described.

Although procedures in which radiographic contrast media are used provide considerable information relative to urinary tract disease, they may complicate some subsequent determinations for as long as 24 hours. For example, increased urine specific gravity as a result of intravenously administered contrast medium may be erroneously interpreted as adequate renal concentrating ability.[8] In addition, although detailed in vivo studies are not available for all types of urinary pathogens, the influence of contrast media on growth of some urinary tract organisms cannot be ignored.[9] It is recommended, therefore, that samples for culture and renal concentrating ability studies as well as for urine sediment cytologic analysis be obtained before or at least 24 hours after (including several voidings) excretory urography.

Renal ultrasonography is a noninvasive technique in which sound is directed into the tissue and the reflected echoes are reconstructed into two-dimensional images.[10] This procedure requires considerable expertise and sophisticated equipment, but information on renal architecture may be provided without the use of contrast medium. Interpretation of diagnostic ultrasound images is beyond the scope of this book, but the value of ultrasonographic examination for assessment of renal parenchymal and ureteral alterations must not be overlooked.

Normal Radiographic Findings

The normal radiographic findings for both the dog and the cat that may be determined quantitatively are listed in Table 39–2. The most widely used quantification of normal kidney size in the dog and cat is that of renal length, which can usually be assessed on survey radiographs.[1, 3–5, 7, 11–13] In general, the dog kidney is approximately three times the length of the L2 vertebral body as visualized on the ventrodorsal

Table 39–2

QUANTITATIVE APPEARANCE OF NORMAL CANINE AND FELINE EXCRETORY UROGRAMS

Structure	Measurement*	Value†
Kidney	Length	Dog
		$3.00 \pm 0.25 \times L2$
		2.50 to 3.50 × L2
		Cat
		2.4 to 3.0 × L2
		4.0 to 4.5 cm
	Width	Dog
		$2.00 \pm 0.20 \times L2$
		Cat
		3.0 to 3.5 cm
Renal pelvis	Width	Dog
		$0.03 \pm 0.017 \times L2$
		(generally ≤ 2.0 mm)
		Cat
		Not reported
Pelvic recesses	Width	Dog
		$0.02 \pm 0.005 \times L2$
		(generally ≤ 1.0 mm)
		Cat
		Not reported
Proximal ureter	Width	Dog
		$0.07 \pm 0.018 \times L2$
		(generally ≤ 2.5 mm)
		Cat
		Not reported
Distal ureter	Width	Not reported in dogs or cats

*Measurements apply only to the ventrodorsal view.
†L2, the length of the body of the second lumbar vertebral body as visualized on the ventrodorsal view.
Modified from Feeney DA, Barber DL, Johnston GR, et al: The excretory urogram: Techniques, normal radiographic appearance and misinterpretation. Comp Contin Ed Vet Pract 4:233, 1982; with permission.

view. The normal range of kidney size in the dog is from 2.5 to 3.5 times the length of L2.[7, 11] In the cat, the most accepted renal length is that of 2.4 to 3 times the length of the L2 vertebral body,[12] but other values have been suggested.[13] In the authors' experience, however, it is not uncommon for cats older than 10 years of age to have a renal length less than 2.4 times the length of L2. There is no direct association between the apparent small kidney size and laboratory evidence of renal failure when the kidney length is between 2 and 2.4 times the length of L2 in aged cats. Therefore, care must be taken not to overstate prognostic suspicions based on small kidney size in aging cats.

Other quantitative measurements visible only on excretory urograms that may be used to assess the kidneys include measurement of the pyelographic variables, including the width of the pelvic recesses, renal pelvis, and proximal ureter. In general, the renal pelvis and pelvic recesses (sometimes referred to as *pelvic diverticula*) in the dog do not exceed 1 or 2 mm in diameter, and the proximal ureter in the dog does not exceed 2 or 3 mm in diameter. More exact comparisons are given in Table 39–2, which are related to the length of the L2 vertebral body.

The shape of the dog kidney is somewhat elongated, resembling that of a bean, whereas that of the cat is somewhat more rounded, although still somewhat elongated.[1, 4–6] The normal radiographic appearances of the canine and feline kidneys are shown in Figures 39–1 and 39–2. The kidneys in both the dog and the cat are located in the retroperitoneal space[3] and are usually located along the longitudinal axis in association with the last thoracic and first three or four lumbar vertebrae.[1, 6] The right kidney is usually more cranial

than the left, and, as mentioned previously, this separation can be enhanced on the lateral view by using right lateral recumbent positioning.

Renal opacity on survey radiographs is that of homogeneous soft tissue.[1, 3] Visualization of the kidneys on survey radiographs relies on the presence of retroperitoneal fat (perirenal fat) surrounding the kidneys. During excretory urography, the nephrogram is homogeneous, with the exception of the early combined vascular and tubular nephrograms, when the cortex is more radiopaque than the medulla.[4] The pyelogram in the normally functioning kidney is more radiopaque than the nephrogram (see Figs. 39–1 and 39–2).

The dynamic aspects of excretory urography lie in the assessment of nephrographic opacification and fading sequences.[4, 14] The normal nephrogram should be most radiopaque within 10 to 30 seconds after bolus injection of contrast medium. With increasing delay after injection, the nephrographic opacity should decrease progressively; fewer than 25 percent of normal dogs have a detectable nephrographic opacity 2 hours after injection. The pyelogram should be consistently opaque, and the diameter of the ureter should vary with time because of peristalsis (see Figs. 39–1 and 39–2). The degree of nephrographic and pyelographic opacification in combination with the opacification and fading patterns of the nephrogram can be used as a qualitative estimate of renal function.[6, 15] In general, the poorer the renal function, the less opacified are the nephrographic and pyelographic phases of the excretory urogram.

Abnormal Radiographic Findings

Number

Renal aplasia or agenesis may result in the inability to identify one of the kidneys.[1, 2, 16] Unilateral renal agenesis may result in compensatory hypertrophy of the unaffected kidney (Fig. 39–3). There is also the possibility of more than the expected number of kidneys by the phenomenon of renal duplication.[17] The inability to visualize a kidney radiographically may be merely the result of extreme hypoplasia, the consequences of chronic disease, or both.

Size, Shape, and Margination

The combination of these three factors, when applied to the abnormal roentgen appearance of the kidneys, may aid the interpreter in identifying possible gamuts or limiting the possible considerations to a manageable number. These combinations and their differential considerations are discussed subsequently. In many of these differential diagnoses, surgical visualization, microscopic confirmation of the suspected diagnosis, or both are mandatory.

Large, regularly shaped, and smoothly margined kidneys may be encountered in conditions such as compensatory hypertrophy (see Fig. 39–3).[2, 3] In addition, it may also be seen in infiltrative neoplasia, such as lymphosarcoma[1–3]; hydronephrosis, including that caused by the renal parasite *Dioctophyma renale*[1–3, 18]; renal amyloidosis and glomerulonephritis[1, 19]; perirenal pseudocyst[20]; and possibly a large solitary renal cyst.[21] Excretory urography aids in differentiating these possibilities by opacifying the functional renal parenchyma, thus permitting identification of abnormal areas. Characterization of the interface between the normal and abnormal areas is of value in differentiating solitary, well-defined abnormalities, such as a renal cyst, from infiltrative diseases, such as neoplasms.

Large, irregularly shaped kidneys with rough margins must

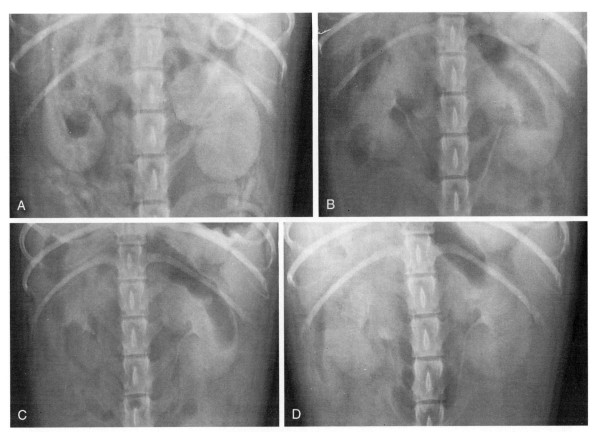

FIGURE 39–1. Ventrodorsal views of a normal dog after intravenous administration of 400 mg iodine per pound body weight in the form of sodium iothalamate. *A,* 10 seconds. *B,* 5 minutes. *C,* 20 minutes. *D,* 40 minutes after injection.

be subdivided into focal abnormalities or multifocal to diffuse renal involvement. If the aforementioned characteristics are focal, major consideration should be given to primary or metastatic renal neoplasms (Fig. 39–4),[3, 4, 6, 22] renal abscess,[3] renal hematoma,[3] and possibly perirenal pseudocyst.[2, 20] If the aforementioned combination of roentgen signs appears to be multifocal or diffuse throughout the kidney, diseases such as polycystic renal disease (Fig. 39–5),[23–26] feline infectious peritonitis,[2, 24, 27] and renal lymphosarcoma[24, 27, 28] should be considered.

If the kidney size is normal, renal shape is regular, and margination is smooth, the presence of renal disease may not be excluded. Diseases such as amyloidosis,[1, 21] glomerulonephritis,[1, 2] and acute pyelonephritis[1] may still be encountered even in the presence of a kidney that appears normal in survey radiographs.

In the kidney that is of normal size but irregular shape with a rough outline, it must be determined whether the process is at one focus or is multifocal to diffuse. Focal variation in renal shape and margination in a normal-sized kidney merits consideration of renal infarct or focal inflammation and renal abscess.[29] Multifocal to diffuse irregularities in shape and margination in the normal-sized kidney are more likely due to chronic pyelonephritis,[2] polycystic renal disease,[30] or both.

The small kidney with regular shape and smooth margins may suggest renal hypoplasia but may also be the result of diseases such as glomerulonephritis, amyloidosis, and familial renal disease of specific dog breeds.[31] Depending on the stage of familial renal disease, it has been suggested that this appearance of the kidney may be encountered in Cocker spaniels[31]; Lhasa apso and Shih tzu dogs[31]; Doberman pinscher[32]

and Samoyed dogs[33]; and possibly in the soft-coated Wheaton terrier,[33] the Norwegian elkhound,[31] and the Standard Poodle.[34] An example of a small, regularly shaped kidney with smooth margins is shown in Figure 39–6 and represents one phase of the disease in the Shih tzu breed.

A small kidney with an irregular shape and rough margins most likely may be attributed to end-stage renal disease and may be from a myriad of causes. When the kidneys are small and renal function is poor, visualization by excretory urographic examination is often limited because it is a combination of glomerular filtration and tubular reabsorption of water that results in concentration of the contrast medium in the renal tubules leading to the increased kidney opacity seen on the radiographic image. In addition, many of these patients have poor body stature owing to their chronic disease, and retroperitoneal fat accumulations are less than optimal. Other diseases that must be considered include amyloidosis,[19] glomerulonephritis and chronic pyelonephritis, and familial renal disease of the Cocker spaniel,[35] Doberman pinscher,[36] Norwegian elkhound,[37] Lhasa apso and Shih tzu dogs,[38] German shepherd,[39] and Standard Poodle.[34] Nonspecific renal dysplasia may manifest as a small, irregularly shaped kidney with rough margins, as may a large infarct or generalized renal ischemia.[40]

Location

Kidneys may maintain relatively normal function while being abnormally located. In animals and humans, ectopic kidneys have been identified in the thorax, intra-abdominal region (not the normal retroperitoneal space), and pelvic ca-

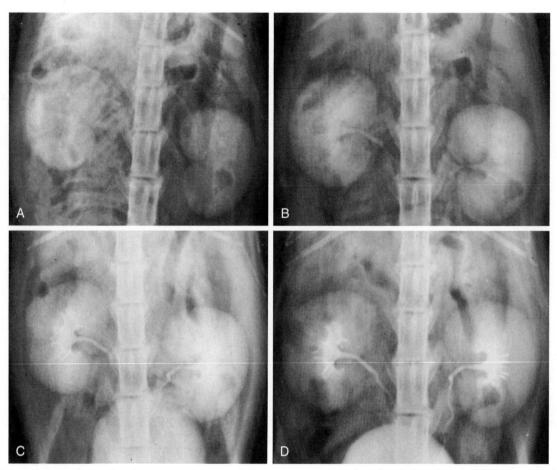

FIGURE 39–2. Ventrodorsal views of a normal cat after intravenous administration of 400 mg iodine per pound of body weight in the form of sodium iothalamate. *A,* 10 seconds. *B,* 5 minutes. *C,* 20 minutes. *D,* 40 minutes after intravenous injection.

nal.[3, 41, 42] Excretory urography and possibly ultrasonography may be of assistance in confirming these unusually located masses as kidneys; excretory urography may aid in the assessment of the functional potential.

In addition to developmental displacement as an ectopic kidney, a kidney may be displaced by an adjacent mass.[3] In particular, adrenal masses may displace either kidney caudally; the right kidney may be displaced caudally by a liver mass, and the left kidney may be displaced caudally by a

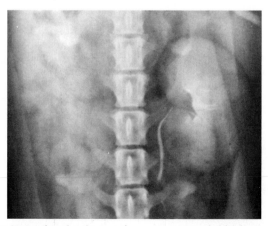

FIGURE 39–3. Radiograph made as part of an excretory urogram. The left kidney is enlarged but is anatomically and functionally normal. The right kidney is not visualized. The left kidney has undergone functional and anatomic compensatory hypertrophy.

mass in the proximal extremity of the spleen. This indirect method of assessing abdominal masses by adjacent organ displacement may be used as an aid in establishing the differential diagnosis.

Radiopacity

On survey radiographs, variations in renal radiopacity (from the expected soft-tissue appearance) may be recognized. The most common opacities recognized include air or mineral. Air may result from vesicoureteral reflux from previous negative-contrast medium procedures involving the lower urinary tract, but it may also be the result of trauma to the perirenal area with leakage of air from intraperitoneal or extra-abdominal sources. Although highly unlikely, gas-forming bacteria may produce air within or around the kidney. Mineral radiopacity may be due to the presence of renal calculi (Fig. 39–7), which are usually magnesium ammonium phosphate in both dogs and cats.[3, 43] Other chemical types of calculi may be encountered with some frequency; however, the radiopacity may vary with the degree of mineralization and is not specific for chemical composition of the calculus. Other mineral opacities within the kidney that must be considered include mineralized cyst,[3] calcified tumors,[3] calcification of the renal parenchyma (nephrocalcinosis),[3, 44] and osseous metaplasia of the renal pelvis in the presence of renal disease.[45, 46] As previously mentioned, loss of retroperitoneal contrast owing to emaciation, the presence of perirenal (retroperitoneal) fluids (i.e., blood or urine), or both may im-

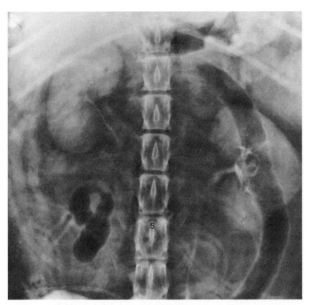

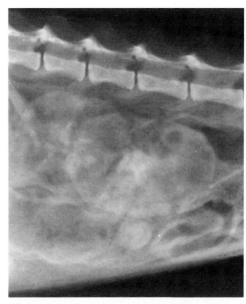

FIGURE 39–4. Ventrodorsal view of a patient 5 minutes after intravenous contrast medium injection for excretory urography. In the midportion of the left kidney, there is a focal area of nephrographic nonopacification with compression and distortion of the renal pelvis and pelvic recesses in the adjacent area. Microscopic diagnosis was renal adenocarcinoma.

FIGURE 39–5. Lateral view of a cat 5 minutes after intravenous contrast medium injection for excretory urography. Kidneys are enlarged, and nephrographic opacification is variable in a random, patchy appearance. Microscopic diagnosis was feline polycystic kidney disease.

pede or preclude visualization of the kidneys. The determination of the need for immediate excretory urographic analysis must be made on the basis of the assessment of the remainder of the body fat stores as well as the clinical history.

Excretory urography causes an increase in the radiographic opacity of the renal parenchyma by the accumulation of contrast medium within the renal tubules and vasculature. The opacity of the renal outflow tract is also increased because of urine that contains concentrated contrast medium. The identifiable structural alterations of the nephrogram[4] and the pyelogram[4] are described in Tables 39–3 and 39–4; Figures 39–3 through 39–6 provide examples of structural nephrographic alteration. Figures 39–8 and 39–9 are examples of two common causes that result in structural alteration of the pyelogram. The use of Tables 39–3 and 39–4 in the separate evaluation of the nephrographic and pyelographic architecture is suggested as a beginning, and common diagnoses (if any occur in both gamut lists) should then be pursued.

Function

The alterations in nephrographic opacification and fading sequences are described in detail in Table 39–5. In general, these changes are classified according to the degree of opacification encountered on the immediate postinjection radiograph as well as the relationship of the subsequently encountered nephrographic opacity in the patient in comparison with the initial opacification.[4, 14] Differential considerations for each of the nephrographic opacification sequences are listed, but those listed are not the only possibilities. Early first (10 to 30 seconds) nephrographic opacification may be delayed in animals with acute and subacute pyelonephritis.[47, 48] Figure 39–10 is an example of an abnormal nephrographic opacity sequence (compare with Fig. 39–1).

Pyelographic alterations associated with changes in renal function generally manifest as poor or undetectable opacification of this phase of the excretory urogram. The opacity of the pyelogram depends on both the filtration of the contrast medium from the blood and the concentration of the contrast medium within the tubules. Loss of either of these capabili-

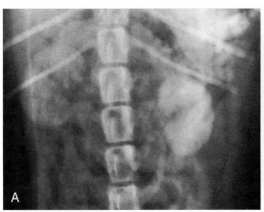

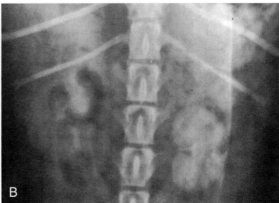

FIGURE 39–6. Ventrodorsal views 10 seconds *(A)* and 5 minutes *(B)* after intravenous contrast medium injection for excretory urography in a 1-year-old Shih tzu. The kidneys are small, nephrographic opacity is poor, and pyelographic opacity is minimal. Microscopic diagnosis was Shih tzu familial renal disease.

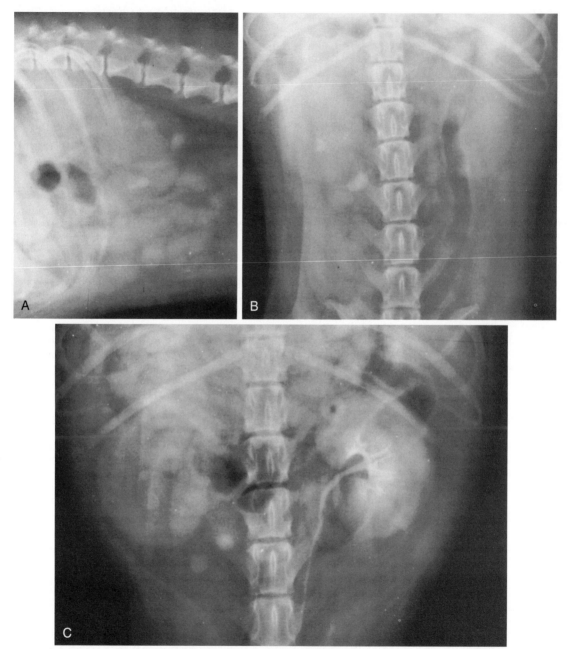

FIGURE 39–7. Lateral *(A)* and ventrodorsal *(B)* radiographs in which there are smoothly marginated, oval, white calcific opacities in the area of the right kidney and ureter. *C,* Ventrodorsal view 5 minutes after intravenous injection of contrast medium for excretory urography. Peripheral opacification of the right nephrogram is identified without accompanying central or pyelographic opacification. Surgical diagnosis was right renal and ureteral calculi with ureteral obstruction and right renal hydronephrosis.

Table 39–3
POSSIBLE STRUCTURAL NEPHROGRAPHIC OPACIFICATION PATTERNS ASSOCIATED WITH CERTAIN RENAL DISEASES*

Opacification Pattern	Renal Disease
Uniform	Normal
	Compensatory hypertrophy
Acute glomerular or tubulointerstitial disease	Perirenal pseudocysts
	Hypoplasia
	Others(?)
Focal, nonuniform	Neoplasm
	Hematuria
	Cyst
	Single infarct
	Hydronephrosis
	Abscess
	Others(?)
Multifocal, nonuniform	Polycystic disease
	Multiple infarcts
	Acute pyelonephritis
	Chronic generalized glomerular or tubulointerstitial disease
	Feline infectious peritonitis
	Infiltrative neoplasia
	Others(?)
Nonopacification	Aplasia/agenesis†
	Renal artery obstruction†
	Nephrectomy or nonfunctional renal parenchyma†
	Insufficient or extravascular contrast medium injection
	Others(?)

*Best identified on radiographs exposed 5 to 20 seconds or 5 minutes after contrast medium injection. Do not overinterpret corticomedullary separation on early postinjection radiographs.

†Only unilateral conditions compatible with life.

ties within the kidneys (assuming adequate dosage and proper route of administration of contrast medium are performed) may result in a less than optimal pyelogram.

Related Abnormal Radiographic Findings

Intra-abdominal Findings Related to Renal Disease

Other organs in the abdomen may be displaced secondary to renal masses.[49] In general, enlargement or a space-occupying mass originating within the left kidney displaces the colon ventrally and the small intestine downward and to the right.[49] Space-occupying masses or enlargement of the right kidney results in displacement of the small intestine (including the duodenum) downward, caudally, and toward the left. In patients with uremia, mineralization of the gastric rugae may occur.[44] Hypoproteinemia secondary to the nephrotic syndrome may result in ascites. Loss of retroperitoneal contrast because of effusion (urine or blood most often from renal trauma) may be noted on survey radiographs and confirmed by excretory urography (Fig. 39–11).

Extra-abdominal Findings Related to Renal Disease

Other tissues, including cutaneous and vascular structures, may undergo calcification secondary to chronic renal disease.[49] Hypertrophic osteopathy may be encountered secondary to renal neoplasms in the absence of pulmonary metastases.[50, 51]

URETERS

Imaging Procedures

The general procedure for interpretation of the kidney should be used to evaluate the ureters. The imaging procedures described for the kidney are equally applicable to the ureter. These techniques are described in the preceding section.

Normal Radiographic Findings

The normal ureters are not visible on survey radiographs. As visualized at excretory urography, there are usually two ureters,[6, 7] and the size of each is usually less than 2 or 3 mm in diameter as these structures exit the kidney. The shape of the ureters is tubular, with segmentation secondary to ureteral peristalsis.[4, 5] The ureters are primarily retroperitoneal[52] but become intraperitoneal as they approach their termination at the bladder trigone.[53, 54] Care should be exercised in the interpretation of the end-on view of the deep circumflex iliac artery as a survey radiographic abnormality related to the ureter.[6] The normal findings for excretory urography relative to the ureter have been described (see Figs. 39–1 and 39–2).[4–7] The function of the ureter is principally assessed relative to the segmentation peristalsis, which can be noted on serial radiographs or at fluoroscopy.[4, 5] In general, if the ureter can be visualized in its entirety from the pelvis of the kidney to the trigone of the bladder, the possibilities of poor ureteral peristalsis, ureteral dilation secondary to partial obstruction, or both must be considered.

Table 39–4
PYELOGRAPHIC APPEARANCE OF SOME COMMON DISEASES OF THE KIDNEY

Pyelonephritis
Acute
  Pelvic dilation
  Proximal ureteral dilation
  Absent or incomplete filling of pelvic recesses
Chronic
  ± Pelvic dilation with irregular borders
  Proximal ureteral dilation
  Short-blunt pelvic recesses

Hydronephrosis
Pelvic dilation
Dilation of pelvic recesses (*note:* recesses may not be distinguishable if pelvic dilation is severe)
Ureteral dilation

Neoplasia
Renal parenchyma
  Distortion, deviation, and/or dilation of renal pelvis
  Distortion or deviation of pelvic recesses
Renal pelvis
  Distortion or dilation of renal pelvis
  Filling defects in renal pelvis

Uroliths and Blood Clots
Filling defects in renal pelvis
Uroliths usually radiolucent compared to contrast medium; blood clots always are radiolucent compared to contrast medium
May be changes as seen in pyelonephritis
± Pelvic dilation

From Feeney DA, Barber DL, and Osborne CA: Advances in canine excretory urography. In 30th Gaines Veterinary Symposium, Gaines Dog Research Center, White Plains, NY, 1981; with permission.

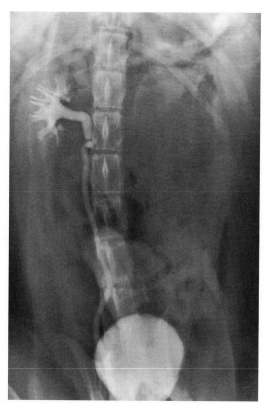

FIGURE 39–8. Ventrodorsal view 40 minutes after intravenous contrast medium injection for excretory urography. The right ureter, renal pelvis, and pelvic recesses are symmetrically enlarged. The left kidney is dramatically enlarged, with only a rim of nephrographic opacification. The central portion of the left kidney is nonopacified, and there is no pyelogram. Necropsy confirmed moderate right and extreme left hydronephrosis secondary to ureteral obstruction by a transitional cell carcinoma of the bladder trigone and proximal urethra.

Abnormal Radiographic Findings

Number

As described previously, agenesis and aplasia of the kidneys and their associated ureters have been reported. Ureteral duplication in the presence of renal duplication in dogs has also been described.[19]

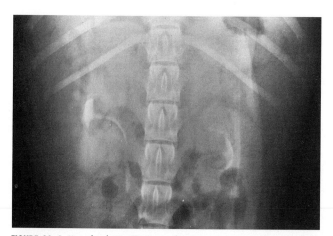

FIGURE 39–9. Ventrodorsal view 20 minutes after intravenous injection of contrast medium for excretory urography. The right and left renal pelves are dilated, but the pelvic recesses cannot be identified. The ureters, particularly the right ureter, are mildly dilated. Radiologic diagnosis was bilateral chronic pyelonephritis.

Table 39–5

POSSIBLE NEPHROGRAPHIC OPACIFICATION SEQUENCES ASSOCIATED WITH CERTAIN RENAL DISEASE PROCESSES

Good initial opacification followed by progressively decreasing opacity:
  Normal
Fair to good initial opacification followed by progressively increasing opacity:
  Systemic hypotension owing to contrast agents
  Acute renal obstruction (including precipitated Tamm-Horsfall mucoprotein in renal tubules)
  Contrast medium-induced renal failure
  Others
Fair to good initial opacification followed by persistent opacity:
  Acute renal tubular necrosis
  Contrast medium–induced renal failure
  Systemic hypotension owing to contrast agents
  Others
Poor initial opacification followed by progressively decreasing opacity:
  Primary polyuric renal failure
  Inadequate contrast medium dose
  Others
Poor initial opacification followed by progressively increasing opacity:
  Acute extrarenal obstruction
  Systemic hypotension existing before contrast medium administration
  Renal ischemia (arterial or venous)
  Others
Poor initial opacification followed by persistent opacity:
  Primary glomerular dysfunction (chronic)
  Severe generalized renal disease

From Feeney DA, Barber DL, and Osborne CA: Functional aspects of the nephrogram in excretory urography: A review. Vet Radiol 23:42, 1982; with permission.

Size, Shape, and Margination

Information pertaining to the size of the ureter, its overall shape, and the mucosal margin characteristics may be combined to assist in the differential diagnosis of ureteral disease. In the following discussion, this triad of roentgen signs is used, and, if possible, differential considerations of disease processes are listed.

A diffusely enlarged ureter with a regular shape and smooth mucosal margins is most likely due to obstruction[4, 6, 55, 56] or to atony induced by infection.[49, 55, 56] Ureteral atony secondary to periureteral inflammation or blunt abdominal trauma has also been described.[6, 52] Ureteral dilation secondary to chronic vesicoureteral reflux is possible but unlikely.[57] A common finding in ectopic ureter is that of diffuse dilation of the abnormal ureter.[6, 53] The cause of this dilation has not been identified, but it is likely to be a combination of obstruction, inflammation, and developmental anomaly.

A focally enlarged ureter with smooth margination is most consistent with a ureterocele or diverticulum (Fig. 39–12).[58–60] In most instances, the ureterocele is a dilation of the submucosal or intramuscular portion of the intravesical ureter as it approaches its point of emptying within the trigone of the urinary bladder. The result is a space-occupying mass within the trigone region that must be differentiated from other bladder or trigonal abnormalities, including neoplasia.

Enlarged ureters of regular shape with roughened or irregular mucosal and mural margins along the entire ureter are suggestive of ureteral fibrosis secondary to chronic inflammation. If the process is focal, the major consideration is primary or metastatic neoplasia; ureteral neoplasia is uncommon.

A small ureter with regular, smooth margins is most likely

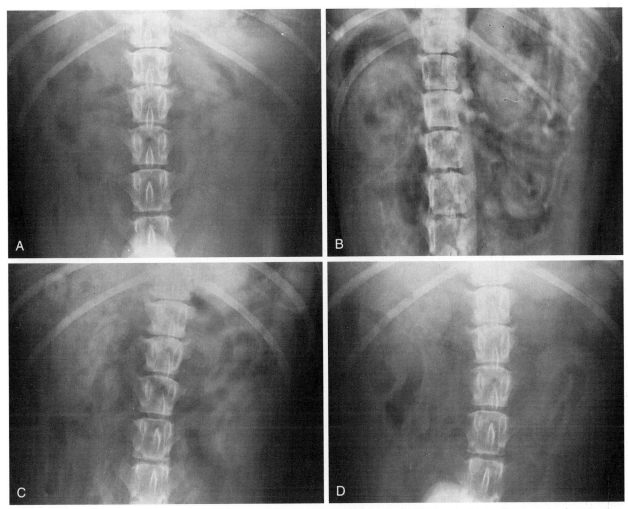

FIGURE 39–10. Ventrodorsal views immediately before *(A)*, 10 seconds after *(B)*, 5 minutes after *(C)*, and 40 minutes after *(D)* intravenous injection of contrast medium for excretory urography. The size of the kidneys is normal, but nephrographic opacification is poor and does not fade with time. Microscopic diagnosis was glomerulonephritis secondary to systemic lupus erythematosus.

due to inadequate contrast medium dose or primary renal oliguria, if the variation involves the entire ureter. If there is a focal decrease in size, compression from an extramural source must be considered. A small, irregularly shaped, rough-margined focal abnormality in a ureter is most likely suggestive of stricture. Stricture may be the result of previous trauma, focal inflammation and secondary fibrosis, or neoplasia.

Location

The abnormal location of the ureter that is most often encountered is ectopic ureter, in which the distal portion of the ureter terminates at a point other than the bladder trigone.[53, 54] The most common site of abnormal ureteral termination is the vagina, followed in relative frequency by the urethra, bladder neck, and uterus. As mentioned in the preceding section, the affected ureter is usually dilated throughout its length; a representative example is shown in Figure 39–13. Another possible cause of abnormal location of the distal portion of the ureter is trauma, usually caused by avulsion of the ureter from the bladder neck. In ureteral avulsion, retroperitoneal effusion may also occur.

Radiopacity

Air in the ureters is most likely associated with vesicoureteral reflux during negative-contrast medium studies of the uri-

nary bladder. Mineralization of the ureter is rare; most mineral opacities in the area of the ureter represent calculi, as shown in Figure 39–7.[4, 6] Loss of retroperitoneal contrast may be an indirect indication of the accumulation of blood or urine or both, one cause of which is ureteral rupture. This loss of retroperitoneal contrast must be interpreted in light of the body fat status in the remainder of the patient. An example of loss of retroperitoneal contrast owing to ureteral rupture and retroperitoneal urine collection is shown in Figure 39–11.

During excretory urography, a reproducible filling defect in the contrast medium column in the ureter may be caused by a calculus,[4, 6] a neoplasm, or a stricture secondary to disease or external compression. Assessment of the margination and opacity of these structures on survey radiographs in combination with the size, shape, and margination of the ureter at excretory urographic examination may help differentiate these considerations. Nonvisualization of a ureteral segment is usually normal because of peristalsis.[4, 5, 7] This segment of the ureter, however, should be visualized at some time in the sequence of radiographs. If the segment is not seen during the sequence, especially in the presence of contrast medium accumulation in the retroperitoneal space or loss of retroperitoneal contrast, ureteral rupture should be considered (see Fig. 39–11).[54] Another consideration in segmental nonvisualization of the ureter is stricture, but there is proximal dilation to provide perspective on the nonvisualized segment.

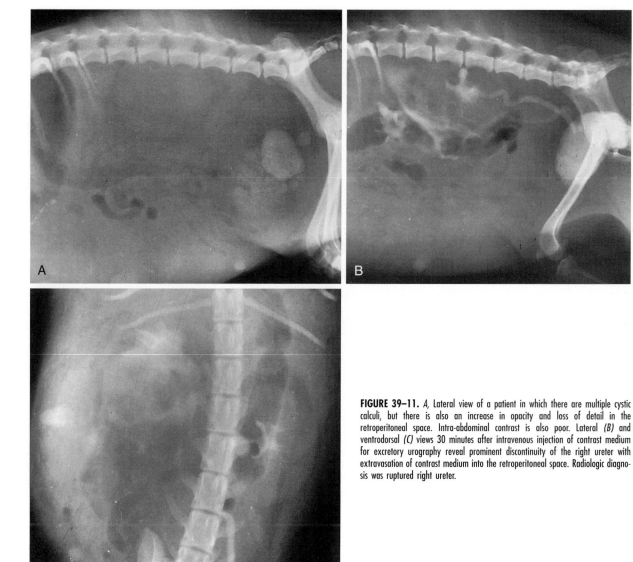

FIGURE 39-11. *A,* Lateral view of a patient in which there are multiple cystic calculi, but there is also an increase in opacity and loss of detail in the retroperitoneal space. Intra-abdominal contrast is also poor. Lateral *(B)* and ventrodorsal *(C)* views 30 minutes after intravenous injection of contrast medium for excretory urography reveal prominent discontinuity of the right ureter with extravasation of contrast medium into the retroperitoneal space. Radiologic diagnosis was ruptured right ureter.

FIGURE 39-12. Lateral *(A)* and ventrodorsal *(B)* views of a patient 40 minutes after intravenous injection of contrast medium for excretory urography. The terminal portion of the left ureter is dilated in its intramural and submucosal path in the urinary bladder and terminates in the proximal urethra. Radiologic diagnosis was ectopic ureter with ureterocele. The radiolucent line in the caudal aspect of the bladder in *B* is the wall of the ureterocele. It is visible because of adjacent contrast medium in the ureteral lumen and in the bladder lumen.

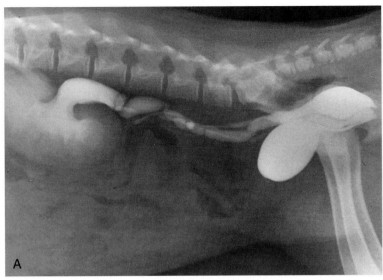

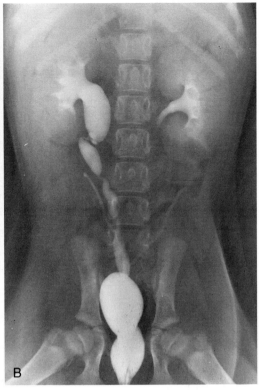

FIGURE 39–13. Lateral (A) and ventrodorsal (B) views of a patient 40 minutes after intravenous injection of contrast medium for excretory urography. The right ureter is extremely dilated, as are the right renal pelvis and pelvic recesses. The right ureter extends dorsal to the bladder trigone and ventral to the vestibule and terminates in the distal urethra. A previous retrograde vaginogram outlined the termination of this ureter as well as the urethral orifice, cervix, and uterine horns. Radiologic diagnosis was ectopic ureter.

Function

Ureteral atony or hypotonia may be induced secondary to intraluminal infection, periureteral inflammation, trauma, or ureteral obstruction (see Figs. 39–8 and 39–13).[4, 6, 48, 52, 55, 56] Differentiation among these possible causes requires complete assessment of the size, shape, and margination of the opacified ureter as well as observation of the site and character of ureteral termination. Comparison with the results of urine cytologic and culture studies is also of value.

Vesicoureteral reflux is the retroflow of urine from the bladder into the ureter either as a low-pressure phenomenon in the presence of incompletely filled bladder or as a high-pressure phenomenon in the presence of a filled bladder or during voiding.[57] Vesicoureteral reflux may be encountered in immature small animals and may be induced during retrograde radiographic procedures. Reflux may also be induced secondary to manual compression of the urinary bladder in an attempt to perform studies such as voiding urethrography. The major significance of vesicoureteral reflux lies in the potential of retroflow of urine contaminated with pathologic organisms from the urinary bladder toward the kidney.

On the basis of the information provided regarding techniques of evaluation, normal radiographic appearance in both survey and contrast radiography, and the differential diagnostic possibilities of the various abnormal findings, the examiner should now be equipped to formulate a differential diagnosis in a given patient. Textbooks of internal medicine should be consulted for the specific nonradiographically oriented tests that may be of value when methods other than exploratory laparotomy or additional radiography are required to make a definitive diagnosis.

References

1. DiBartola SP: Clinical approach and laboratory evaluation of renal disease. *In* Ettinger SJ (Ed): Textbook of Veterinary Internal Medicine, 4th Ed. Philadelphia, WB Saunders, 1995, pp 1706–1719.
2. Osborne CA, Polzin DJ, Feeney DA, et al: The urinary system: Pathophysiology, diagnosis, and therapy. *In* Gourley IA, Vasseur PB (Eds): General Small Animal Surgery. Philadelphia, JB Lippincott, 1985, pp 479–658.
3. Allan G: Radiology in the diagnosis of kidney disease. Aust Vet Pract 12:97, 1982.
4. Feeney DA, Barber DL, and Osborne CA: Advances in canine excretory urography. *In* Proceedings of the 30th Gaines Veterinary Symposium, Gaines Dog Research Center, White Plains, NY, 1981, pp 8–22.
5. Feeney DA, Barber DL, Johnston GR, et al: The excretory urogram: Techniques, normal radiographic appearance, and misinterpretation. Comp Contin Ed Vet Pract 4:233, 1982.
6. Kneller SK: Role of excretory urography in the diagnosis of renal and ureteral disease. Vet Clin North Am 4:843, 1974.
7. Feeney DA, Thrall DE, Barber DL, et al: Normal canine excretory urogram: Effects of dose, time and individual dog variation. Am J Vet Res 40:1596, 1979.
8. Feeney DA, Osborne CA, and Jessen CR: Effects of radiographic contrast media on results of the urinalysis with emphasis on specific gravity. J Am Vet Med Assoc 176:1378, 1980.
9. Ruby AL, Ling GV, and Ackerman N: Effects of sodium diatrizoate on the in vitro growth of three common canine urinary bacterial species. Vet Radiol 24:222, 1983.
10. Feeney DA, Johnston GR, and Walter PA: Imaging the kidney and prostate gland in small animals: Has gray-scale ultrasonography replaced contrast radiography? Probl Vet Med 3:619, 1991.
11. Finco DR, Stiles NS, Kneller SK, et al: Radiologic estimation of kidney size in the dog. J Am Vet Med Assoc 159:995, 1971.
12. Barrett RB, and Kneller SK: Feline kidney measurement. Acta Radiol (Stockh) 319(suppl):279, 1972.
13. Bartels JE: Feline intravenous urography. J Am Anim Hosp Assoc 9:349, 1973.
14. Feeney DA, Barber DL, and Osborne CA: Functional aspects of the nephrogram in excretory urography: A review. Vet Radiol 23:42, 1982.
15. Thrall DE, and Finco DR: Canine excretory urography: Is quantity a function of BUN? J Am Anim Hosp Assoc 12:446, 1976.
16. Robinson GW: Uterus uncornuis and unilateral renal agenesis. J Am Vet Med Assoc 147:516, 1965.
17. O'Hardley P, Carrig PB, and Unshaw R: Renal and urethral duplication in a dog. J Am Vet Med Assoc 174:484, 1979.
18. Senior DF: Parasites of the canine urinary tract. *In* Kirk RW (Ed): Current Veterinary Therapy VII. Philadelphia, WB Saunders, 1980, pp 1141–1143.
19. Barsanti JA, and Crowell W: Renal amyloidosis. *In* Kirk RW (Ed): Current Veterinary Therapy VII. Philadelphia, WB Saunders, 1980, pp 1063–1066.
20. Brace JJ: Perirenal cysts (pseudocysts) in the cat. *In* Kirk RW (Ed): Current Veterinary Therapy VIII. Philadelphia, WB Saunders, 1983, pp 980–981.
21. Stowater JL: Congenital solitary renal cyst in a dog. J Am Anim Hosp Assoc 11:199, 1975.

22. Caywood DD, Osborne CA, and Johnston GR: Neoplasms of the canine and feline urinary tracts. *In* Kirk RW (Ed): Current Veterinary Therapy VII. Philadelphia, WB Saunders, 1980, pp 1203–1212.

23. McKenna SC, and Carpenter JL: Polycystic disease of the kidney and liver in the canine terrier. Vet Pathol 17:436, 1980.

24. Lulich JP, Osborne CA, Walter PA, et al: Feline idiopathic polycystic kidney disease. Comp Contin Ed Vet Pract [Small Anim] 10:1030, 1988.

25. Rendano VT, and Parker RB: Polycystic kidneys and peritoneal pericardial diaphragmatic hernia in a cat. J Small Anim Pract 17:479, 1976.

26. Crowell WA, Hubbell JJ, and Riley JC: Polycystic renal disease in related cats. J Am Vet Med Assoc 175:286, 1979.

27. Walter PA, Johnston GR, Feeney DA, et al: Applications of ultrasonography in the diagnosis of parenchymal kidney disease in cats. J Am Vet Med Assoc 192:92, 1988.

28. Osborne CA, Johnson KH, Kurtz HJ, et al: Renal lymphoma in the dog and cat. J Am Vet Med Assoc 158:2058, 1971.

29. Barber DL: Radiographic evaluation of a focal inflammatory renal lesion. J Am Anim Hosp Assoc 12:451, 1976.

30. Chalifoux A, Phaneuf JB, Oliver N, et al: Glomerular polycystic kidney disease in a dog. Can Vet J 23:365, 1982.

31. Davenport DJ, DiBartola SP, and Chew DJ: Familial renal disease in the dog and cat. Cont Iss Small Anim Pract 4:137, 1986.

32. Witcock BP, and Patterson JM: Familial glomerulonephritis in Doberman pinscher dogs. Can Vet J 20:244, 1979.

33. Bernard MA, and Valli VE: Familial renal disease in Samoyed dogs. Can Vet J 18:181, 1977.

34. DiBartola SP, Chew J, and Boyce JT: Juvenile renal disease in related standard poodles. J Am Vet Med Assoc 183:693, 1983.

35. English PB, and Winter H: Renal cortical hypoplasia in a dog. Aust Vet J 55:181, 1979.

36. Chew DJ, DiBartola SP, Boyce JT, et al: Juvenile renal disease in Doberman pinscher dogs. J Am Vet Med Assoc 182:481, 1983.

37. Finco DR, Kurtz HJ, Low DG, et al: Familial renal disease in Norwegian elkhound dogs. J Am Vet Med Assoc 156:747, 1970.

38. O'Brien TD, Osborne CA, Yano BC, et al: Clinicopathologic manifestations of progressive renal disease in Lhasa Apso and Shih Tzu dogs. J Am Vet Med Assoc 180:658, 1982.

39. Finco DR: Congenital and inherited renal disease. J Am Anim Hosp Assoc 9:301, 1973.

40. Lucke VM, Kelly DF, Darke PG, et al: Chronic renal failure in young dogs—possible renal dysplasia. J Small Anim Pract 21:169, 1980.

41. Wells MJ, Coyne JA, and Prince JL: Ectopic kidney in a cat. Mod Vet Pract 61:693, 1980.

42. Johnson CA: Renal ectopia in a cat. J Am Anim Hosp Assoc 15:599, 1979.

43. Osborne CA, Klausner JS, and Clinton CW: Analysis of canine and feline uroliths. *In* Kirk RW (Ed): Current Veterinary Therapy VIII. Philadelphia, WB Saunders, 1983, pp 1061–1066.

44. Barber DL, and Rowland GN: Radiographically detectable soft-tissue calcification in chronic renal failure. Vet Radiol 20:117, 1979.

45. Hall MA, Osborne CA, and Stevens JB: Hydronephrosis with heteroplastic bone formation in a cat. J Am Vet Med Assoc 160:857, 1972.

46. Miller JB, and Sande RD: Osseous metaplasia in the renal pelvis of a dog with hydronephrosis. Vet Radiol 21:146, 1980.

47. Fuller WJ: Subacute pyelonephritis with a unilaterally non-visualized pyelogram. J Am Anim Hosp Assoc 12:509, 1976.

48. Barber DL, and Finco DR: Radiographic findings in induced bacterial pyelonephritis in dogs. J Am Vet Med Assoc 175:1183, 1979.

49. Root CN: Interpretation of abdominal survey radiographs. Vet Clin North Am 4:763, 1974.

50. Caywood DD, Osborne CA, Stevens JB, et al: Hypertrophic osteoarthropathy associated with a typical nephroblastoma in a dog. J Am Anim Hosp Assoc 16:855, 1980.

51. Nafe LA, Herron AJ, and Burk RL: Hypertrophic osteopathy in a cat associated with renal papillary adenoma. J Am Anim Hosp Assoc 17:659, 1981.

52. Selcer BA: Urinary tract trauma associated with pelvic trauma. J Am Anim Hosp Assoc 18:785, 1982.

53. Faulkner RT, Osborne CA, and Feeney DA: Canine and feline urethral ectopia. *In* Kirk RW (Ed): Current Veterinary Therapy VIII. Philadelphia, WB Saunders, 1983, pp 1043–1048.

54. Owen RR: Canine urethral ectopia. J Small Anim Pract 14:407, 1983.

55. Rose JG, and Gillenwater JY: Effects of obstruction on urethral function. Urology 12:139, 1978.

56. Rose JG, and Gillenwater JY: Effect of chronic ureteral obstruction and infection upon ureteral function. Invest Urol 11:471, 1974.

57. Klausner JS, and Feeney DA: Vesicoureteral reflux. *In* Kirk RW (Ed): Current Veterinary Therapy VIII. Philadelphia, WB Saunders, 1983, pp 1041–1043.

58. Scott RC, Greene RW, and Patnaik AK: Unilateral ureterocele associated with hydronephrosis in a dog. J Am Anim Hosp Assoc 10:126, 1974.

59. Smith CW, and Park RD: Bilateral ectopic ureteroceles in a dog. Canine Pract 1:28, 1974.

60. Stowater JL, and Springer AL: Ureterocele in a dog. Vet Med [Small Anim Pract] 74:1753, 1979.

STUDY QUESTIONS

1. Which of the following diagnostic procedures provides qualitative information on relative renal function?
   A. Survey radiography.
   B. Intravenous urography.
   C. Gray-scale ultrasonography.
   D. Renal biopsy (tissue core).
   E. None of the above.

2. Which of the following must be considered before performing an excretory urogram?
   A. Is there adequate urine production?
   B. Is the patient adequately hydrated?
   C. Is the urinary bladder catheterized?
   D. Is the patient sedated?
   E. A and B.

3. Which of the following tests can potentially be influenced by the presence of radiographic contrast medium in urine?
   A. Sediment cytology.
   B. Specific gravity.
   C. Some bacterial cultures.
   D. Some protein analyses.
   E. All of the above.

4. Which of the following can obscure visualization of the kidneys on either the lateral or ventrodorsal view?
   A. Retroperitoneal fluid.
   B. Lack of retroperitoneal fat.
   C. Infiltrative retroperitoneal mass.
   D. Peritoneal fluid.
   E. A, B, and C.

5. Based on multifocal inhomogeneity of the nephrogram, which of the following conditions would be considered as possible diagnoses?
   A. Glomerulonephritis (glomerulotubular imbalance).
   B. Multifocal metastatic cancer.
   C. Perinephric fluid accumulation (pseudocyst).
   D. Polycystic renal disease.
   E. B and D.

6. Unilateral failure of (or unilateral delay in) renal parenchymal opacification during an excretory urogram may be caused by which of the following?
   A. Poor renal function (e.g., chronic renal disease with azotemia).
   B. Inadequate dose of radiographic contrast medium.
   C. Poor systemic blood pressure owing to contrast medium-induced hypotension.
   D. Ureteral obstruction.
   E. All of the above.

7. Which of the following should be considered if there is unilateral, proportional dilation of the renal pelvis, pelvic recesses, and ureter during an excretory urogram?
   A. Pyelonephritis.
   B. Hydronephrosis.

C. Primary renal parenchymal neoplasia with invasion of the collecting system.
D. All of the above.
E. None of the above.

8. If the observed nephrographic opacity is initially bright but persists with similar intensity on the films made in an excretory urographic series, which of the following should be considered?
A. This is normal.
B. Glomerular dysfunction.
C. Dehydration.
D. Acute extrarenal obstruction.
E. All of the above.

9. An enlarged but smooth and proportionally shaped kidney can be the result of which of the following when viewed by survey radiography?

A. Hydronephrosis.
B. Infiltrative renal disease (e.g., feline infectious peritonitis, amyloidosis).
C. Compensatory hypertrophy.
D. A and B.
E. A, B, and C.

10. Which of the following can cause diffuse, unilateral ureteral dilation when viewed during an excretory urogram?
A. Ectopic ureter.
B. Urinary bladder mass causing obstruction of one ureter at the trigone.
C. Ascending pyelonephritis.
D. A and B.
E. A, B, and C.

(Answers appear on page 647.)

Chapter 40

The Urinary Bladder

Richard D. Park

SURVEY RADIOGRAPHIC EXAMINATION

The urinary bladder is a distensible, round-to-ovoid visceral organ in the caudal abdomen. It serves as a storage reservoir and voiding organ for urine.

A survey radiographic examination of the urinary bladder usually consists of lateral and ventrodorsal views. The lateral view provides better radiographic visualization of the bladder. Good radiographic visualization is limited in the ventrodorsal view by superimposition of the spine and the large bowel. Oblique views may be made to help compensate for poor radiographic visualization on the ventrodorsal view.

Normal Anatomy

The urinary bladder is divided grossly into three parts: the vertex (apex vesicae) cranially, the body (corpus vesicae) in the middle, and the neck (cervix vesicae) caudally (Fig. 40–1).[1–3] Three ligaments formed from peritoneal reflections hold the bladder loosely in position.[3] The middle bladder ligament (ligamentum vesicae medianum) extends along the ventral bladder surface, and two lateral ligaments (ligamenta vesicae laterale) extend along the lateral bladder surfaces. These ligaments often contain large fat deposits, facilitating radiographic visualization of the bladder neck and body. The cranial and dorsal surfaces of the bladder are radiographically visible because of adjacent fat within the omentum and mesentery (Fig. 40–2).

The urinary bladder wall is a musculomembranous structure consisting of mucosal, submucosal, and muscular layers, with the peritoneum closely adherent to the serosal surface providing a separate fourth layer. Neither the thickness of the bladder wall nor the mucosal surface of the bladder can

be assessed on survey radiographs because the adjacent urine has the same radiographic opacity as the bladder wall.

Radiographic visualization of the urinary bladder is compromised by insufficient abdominal fat, inadequate distention, and superimposition opacities. Emaciated or young animals may not have sufficient abdominal fat to provide good tissue contrast adjacent to the urinary bladder. Ingested material in the small bowel, fecal material in the large bowel, muscle tissue from the pelvic limbs, and bone from the spine and pelvis cause superimposition opacities that may obscure

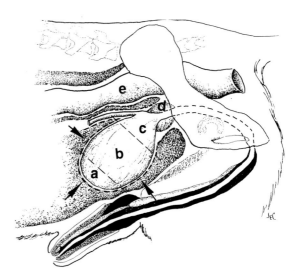

FIGURE 40–1. Lateral view of the abdomen in a normal male dog. a, Vertex. b, Body of the bladder. c, Neck of the urinary bladder. d, Prostate. e, Large bowel. The broken line around the urinary bladder *(arrows)* represents the peritoneal reflection around and adherent to the serosal surface of the urinary bladder.

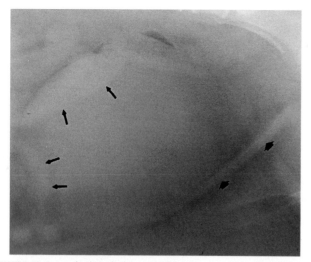

FIGURE 40-2. Lateral radiograph of the caudal abdomen in a normal dog. The bladder neck is well visualized because of fat within the bladder ligaments. The rectus abdominis muscle *(short arrows)* is ventral to the bladder. Bowel is superimposed *(long arrows)* over the cranial and dorsal borders of the bladder.

all or part of the urinary bladder. Focal superimposition opacities may be created by fluid-filled small bowel, nipples, prepuce, and cutaneous masses. Some of these superimposition opacities can be eliminated or minimized by withholding food for 24 hours before the study, giving enemas to clear the large bowel, and pulling the pelvic limbs caudally when the radiograph is made.

Bladder size varies with the amount of urine in the bladder. After voiding, the bladder is small or not visible radiographically. With extreme distention, the cranial bladder border may extend to the umbilicus. Severe distention may occur in a normal bladder if the animal has not had an opportunity to void or will not void because of a strange environment. The urinary bladder in the dog is usually oval, but with distention it becomes more ellipsoid (Fig. 40-3A). The feline urinary bladder is almost always ellipsoid (see Fig. 40-3B).

The bladder is cranial to the pubis, dorsal to the rectus abdominis muscle, caudal to the small bowel and omentum, and ventral to the large bowel. In females, the uterus lies

between the bladder and the rectum. The normal urinary bladder may be partially within the pelvic canal or cranial to the pubis (external to the pelvic canal).[4, 5] The distended urinary bladder is more often located cranial to the pubis but may be within the pelvic canal.[4, 5] The normal urinary bladder in the cat is always intra-abdominal and is located 2 or 3 cm cranial to the pubis. This positioning results from the long bladder neck in the cat,[6] which is not always visible on survey radiographs.

The urinary bladder is a soft-tissue opaque structure. Any opacity greater or less than that of soft tissue detected within the bladder on survey radiographs is abnormal.

Radiographic Signs of Urinary Bladder Disease

Signs of urinary bladder disease on survey radiographs are somewhat limited. In many instances, the signs indicate disease in adjacent structures. Signs that indicate disease of the urinary bladder or of adjacent structures are poor or nonexistent bladder visualization and abnormal bladder position, shape, size, and opacity (Table 40-1).

Inadequate or nonexistent radiographic visualization of the urinary bladder may occur with good or poor serosal detail in the caudal abdomen. If the serosal detail is good and the bladder is not seen, the bladder is either empty or displaced caudally or ventrally. If poor serosal detail is present and the bladder surface is not distinctly seen, free peritoneal fluid or inadequate peritoneal fat may be the cause (Fig. 40-4).

The bladder may be abnormally displaced in various directions.[7] The cause of the displacement may often be determined radiographically by observation of surrounding structures (Fig. 40-5). With severe bladder displacement, such as with hernias, the bladder may not be seen on survey radiographs but may be identified by contrast cystography. A urinary bladder partially within the pelvic canal (Fig. 40-6) may be associated with congenital urinary tract anomalies[8] or, more commonly, a normal variation in position.[4, 5]

It is uncommon to observe a change in shape of the urinary bladder on survey radiographs. Abdominal masses adjacent to the serosal surface of the bladder may distort the bladder shape. Occasionally, tumors originating from the bladder wall protrude from the serosal surface and produce

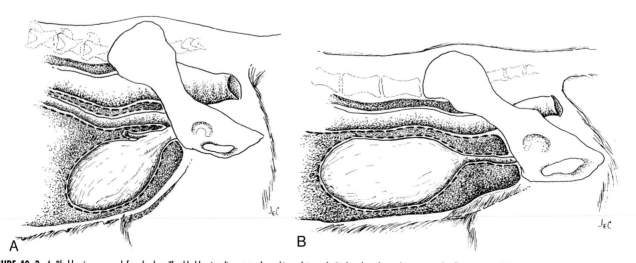

FIGURE 40-3. *A,* Bladder in a normal female dog. The bladder is adjacent to the pubis and is oval. *Broken line* shows the peritoneal reflection around the bladder. *B,* Bladder in a normal cat. The bladder is ellipsoid and has a long neck, which makes the bladder appear to be displaced cranially away from the pubis. *Broken line* shows the peritoneal reflection around the bladder. (From Park RD: Radiology of the urinary bladder and urethra. *In* O'Brien TR [Ed]: Radiographic Diagnosis of Abdominal Disorders in the Dog and Cat. Davis, CA, Covell Park Veterinary Company, 1981, pp 546-547; with permission.)

Table 40–1
URINARY BLADDER: SURVEY RADIOGRAPHIC SIGNS

Radiographic Sign	Gamut of Condition(s) or Disease(s)	Radiographic Sign	Gamut of Condition(s) or Disease(s)
Visualization		***Abnormal Position*** Continued	
Bladder not seen; abdominal serosal outlines are clear	Postvoiding	Caudal displacement	Perineal hernia
	Displaced bladder		Large abdominal mass(es)
	Perineal hernia		Congenital anomalies
	Inguinal hernia		Short urethra
	Pelvic bladder		Ectopic ureters
	Short urethra		Congenital fistulas
	Ectopic ureter		Normal pelvic bladder
	Congenital fistulas	Dorsal displacement	Abdominal mass(es)
	Normal pelvic bladder	***Abnormal Shape***	Mesenchymal neoplasia
Bladder not seen; abdominal serosal outlines are not clearly seen	Ruptured urinary bladder		Adjacent abdominal mass(es)
	Peritoneal fluid		Neoplasia
	Transudate		Abscess or granulomas
	Exudate		Persistent urachal ligament
	Hemorrhage	***Abnormal Size***	
	Emaciated animal	Increased size	Distal urinary obstruction
	Young animal <4 months of age		Urethral obstruction
			Bladder neck obstruction
Abnormal Position			Neurologic deficiencies
Ventral displacement	Abdominal wall hernia	Decreased size	Congenital anomalies
	Inguinal hernia		Ectopic ureters
Cranial displacement	Prostatic disease		Fistulas
	Neoplasia		Diffuse bladder wall disease
	Prostatitis		Cystitis
	Prostatic cyst		Neoplasia
	Hypertrophy		Hemorrhage
Cranioventral displacement	Enlarged uterus	***Opacity Changes***	
	Pyometra	Increased	Calculi
	Pregnancy		Bladder wall mineralization
	Sublumbar mass(es)		Neoplasia
	Large bowel distention		Inflammation
	Uterine stump granuloma or abscess	Decreased	Gas
	Persistent patent urachus or urachal ligament		Iatrogenic
			Emphysematous cystitis

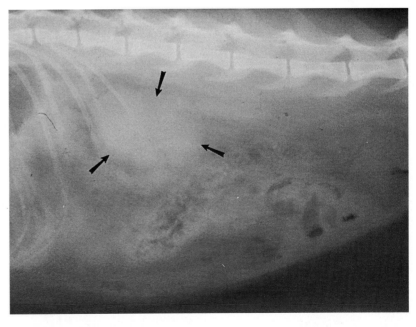

FIGURE 40–4. Lateral radiograph of the abdomen of a cat. The kidneys are easily seen *(arrows)*. The serosal surfaces on the bowel and urinary bladder do not have distinct outlines because of free peritoneal fluid.

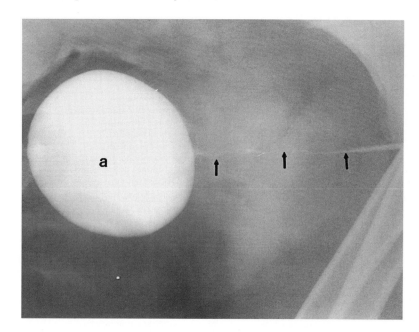

FIGURE 40–5. Positive-contrast cystogram, lateral caudal view, in a male dog. The urinary bladder (a) is displaced cranially from the pubis by a large prostatic mass. The urethra and bladder neck are filled with positive-contrast medium *(arrows)*. Diagnosis was prostatic carcinoma.

a discernible change in bladder shape (Fig. 40–7).[9] A pointed vertex with the bladder appearing elongated may occur with a persistent urachal ligament in the cat.[10]

An abnormally small or large urinary bladder is difficult to diagnose radiographically because of the wide normal variation in bladder size. In most instances, a consistently small or large bladder with associated clinical signs is an indication that a contrast study or ultrasound examination should be performed to determine the cause for the small or large bladder.

Any change in radiographic opacity in the urinary bladder is abnormal and is usually easy to detect. Gas in the bladder may be iatrogenically introduced from catheterization or cystocentesis. Small gas bubbles from iatrogenic causes are usually within the bladder lumen and in the center of the bladder on the recumbent lateral view. Gas in the bladder lumen, in the bladder wall, and occasionally within bladder ligaments occurs with emphysematous cystitis (Fig. 40–8). Em-

physematous cystitis is produced by glucose-fermenting organisms and may be seen in association with diabetes mellitus.[11, 12] Occurrence of emphysematous cystitis without diabetes mellitus also has been reported.[13, 14] Most radiopacities associated with the bladder are calculi. Not all calculi are radiopaque (Table 40–2), however, and thus the absence of radiopacities within the bladder does not rule out the presence of cystic calculi. A horizontal-beam radiograph can be made to diagnose sand-like material within the bladder. This is particularly helpful in cats with feline urologic syndrome.[15] Ultrasonography can also be used to visualize calculi or sand material within the bladder.[16, 17]

CONTRAST CYSTOGRAPHY

Retrograde contrast cystography is a fast, simple, and inexpensive technique that may provide valuable prognostic and

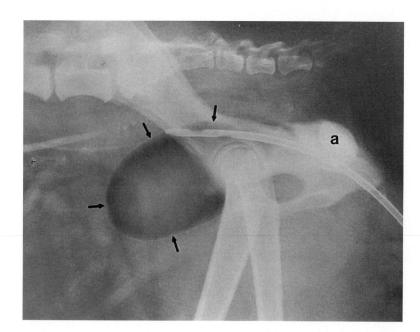

FIGURE 40–6. Lateral radiograph of the caudal abdomen and pelvis after intravenous urography and double-contrast cystography. A radiopaque catheter is present within the bladder, and the bladder is partially within the pelvic canal *(arrows)*. Contrast medium has accumulated in the vagina (a) because of an ectopic ureter.

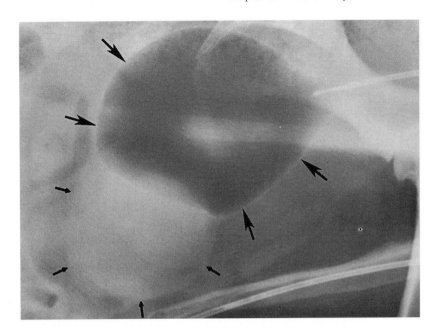

FIGURE 40–7. Oblique view of the abdomen after double-contrast cystography. A mass *(small arrows)* is present on the cranioventral aspect of the gas-filled bladder *(large arrows)*. The mass is a leiomyosarcoma originating from the bladder; it gave the bladder a bilobed appearance on the survey radiograph.

diagnostic information about bladder disease. Indications for contrast cystography are obtained from clinical and radiographic signs. Clinical indications include dysuria, pollakiuria, and intermittent or persistent chronic hematuria. Radiographic signs that indicate the need for contrast cystography include identification of increased or decreased opacity that may be associated with the urinary bladder, evaluation of caudal abdominal masses that may be associated with the urinary bladder, nonvisualization of the bladder after abdominal trauma, and evaluation of the urinary bladder that has an abnormal shape or location.

Voiding cystography is not discussed in this chapter. For more information, the reader is referred to other publications.[18–22] Voiding cystography, coupled with cystometry, is the technique of choice to investigate dynamic bladder diseases such as urinary incontinence and other voiding abnormalities.

Cystography Technique

If possible, food should be withheld for 24 hours and an enema given before a cystographic examination is begun. Fecal material superimposed over the urinary bladder may obliterate important radiographic information.

All catheters and equipment should be sterilized, and the genitalia should be cleaned before the bladder is catheterized. The equipment necessary for bladder catheterization is illustrated in Figure 40–9. To reduce bladder pain and spasm during cystography, 2 to 5 mL of 2 percent lidocaine (Xylocaine) without epinephrine may be injected into the bladder before the procedure is performed.

Complications resulting from catheterization and cystographic procedures occur infrequently and are usually not detrimental to the animal. Iatrogenic trauma, bacterial contamination,[23] or kinked[24] and knotted urethral catheters may

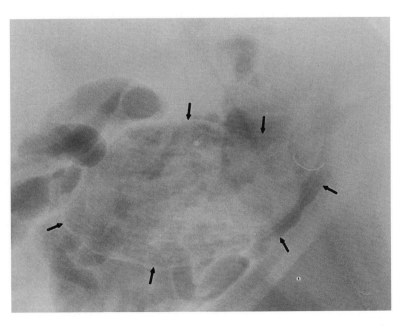

FIGURE 40–8. Lateral view of the abdomen of a dog with gas within the bladder wall, lumen, and bladder ligaments *(arrows)*. Gas in the surrounding bowel loops presents some difficulty in distinguishing gas within the bladder. The animal had cystitis caused by a gas-producing organism but did not have diabetes mellitus.

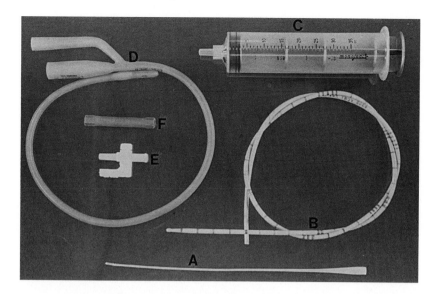

FIGURE 40–9. Equipment for bladder catheterization and cystography: *A*, Tom Cat catheter (Sherwood Medical, St. Louis, MO 63103). *B*, Male urethral catheter. *C*, A large syringe. *D*, A Foley (balloon-type) catheter. *E*, A three-way valve. *F*, A catheter connector for use with the male urethral catheter. (From Park RD: Radiology of the urinary bladder and urethra. *In* O'Brien TR [Ed]: Radiographic Diagnosis of Abdominal Disorders in the Dog and Cat. Davis, CA, Covell Park Veterinary Company, 1981, p 561; with permission.)

occur from improper catheterization techniques. Intramural and subserosal accumulation of contrast medium in the bladder (Fig. 40–10) has been reported after maximal bladder distention with a Foley catheter.[25–28] This complication occurs more frequently in the cat, often with a nondistended bladder and minimal intravesicular pressure. It usually does not result in a clinical problem. Mucosal ulceration, inflammation, and granulomatous reactions may occur, but the changes are usually transitory and produce no serious clinical problems.[29] The most serious complication from negative-contrast cystography is gas embolization into the circulatory system, which may result in death.[30, 31] Fortunately, such complications occur rarely. Also, the likelihood of death from gas embolism may be prevented by the use of nitrous oxide or carbon dioxide instead of room air.

Both negative-contrast and positive-contrast media are used for contrast cystography. Negative-contrast media are room air, carbon dioxide, and nitrous oxide. Positive-contrast media are organic iodides in a 20 percent iodine solution (Table 40–3). Barium should never be used for cystography.[25, 32] The volume of positive-contrast medium used for cystography varies with body weight, species, and pathologic process present in the bladder. An approximation of 10 mL (range of 3.5 to 13.1 mL) of medium per kilogram body weight may be used.[32] The injection should be terminated before the estimated volume has been administered if the bladder feels adequately distended by external palpation, if reflux occurs around the catheter, or if back pressure is felt on the syringe plunger. Moderate bladder distention is recommended because complete distention may obliterate subtle mucosal and bladder wall changes.[33] Four radiographic views of the caudal abdomen (one recumbent lateral, one ventrodorsal, and two recumbent obliques) should be made to examine the contrast medium–filled bladder adequately.

Cystographic Procedures

Retrograde positive-contrast and double-contrast procedures are best for studying the bladder. Positive-contrast cystography is performed by injecting a 20 percent solution of an organic iodide compound into an evacuated bladder via a

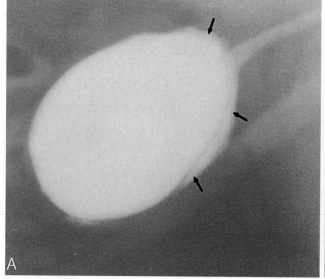

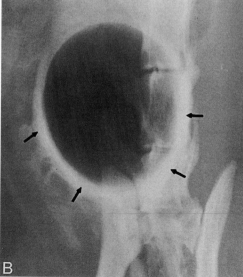

FIGURE 40–10. Positive-contrast *(A)* and double-contrast *(B)* cystograms in which subserosal accumulation of contrast medium may be seen *(arrows)*. This condition usually produces no severe or long-lasting complications. It is caused by a high intraluminal bladder pressure and is predisposed by bladder disease, particularly inflammation.

Table 40-2
RADIOPACITY OF CYSTIC CALCULI ON SURVEY ABDOMINAL RADIOGRAPHS

Calculus Composition	Opacity
Calcium oxalate	Radiopaque
Silica	Radiopaque
Triple phosphate	Radiopaque—small calculi may be nonradiopaque
Cystine	Nonradiopaque, but may have radiopaque stippling
Urate	Nonradiopaque

urethral catheter. The procedure is the method of choice for identifying bladder location and demonstrating bladder tears or ruptures or communications with structures adjacent to the bladder.

A double-contrast cystogram may be performed by injecting a small volume of undiluted positive-contrast medium into an empty bladder. The recommended dose of positive-contrast medium is 0.5 to 1 mL for a cat, 1 to 3 mL for a dog weighing less than 25 lb, and 3 to 6 mL for animals weighing more than 25 lb. Contrast medium injection is followed by bladder distention with negative-contrast medium (Fig. 40–11). Double-contrast cystography is superior for assessing the bladder wall and intraluminal filling defects. The selection of positive-contrast or double-contrast cystography is based on clinical history, clinical signs, radiographic signs, and character of aspirate obtained with bladder catheterization (Fig. 40–12).

Radiographic Signs With Contrast Cystography

Radiographic signs observed with urinary bladder diseases are an irregular mucosal border, intramural thickening, filling defects, and extravasation patterns (Table 40–4). These radiographic changes must be differentiated from artifacts pro-

Table 40-3
ORGANIC IODIDES* AVAILABLE FOR CONTRAST CYSTOGRAPHY

Brand Name	Generic Name	Manufacturer
Conray	60% Meglumine iothalamate	Mallinckrodt
Conray 30	30% Meglumine iothalamate	Mallinckrodt
Conray 400	66.8% Na iothalamate	Mallinckrodt
Hypaque Sodium 20%	20% Na diatrizoate	Nycomed
Hypaque Sodium 25%	25% Na diatrizoate	Nycomed
Hypaque Sodium 50%	50% Na diatrizoate	Nycomed
Hypaque Meglumine 60%	60% Meglumine diatrizoate	Mycomed
Omnipaque†	Iohexol	Nycomed
Renografin-60	52% Meglumine diatrizoate and 8% Na diatrizoate	Bristol-Myers Squibb Co.
Reno-M-60	60% Meglumine diatrizoate	Bristol-Myers Squibb Co.
Renovist‡	35% Na diatrizoate and 34.3% meglumine diatrizoate	Bristol-Myers Squibb Co.
Isovue†	Iopamidol	Bristol-Myers Squibb Co.

*Should be diluted to 20% iodine solution.
†Nonionic contrast medium.
‡Approved for veterinary use by the U.S. Food and Drug Administration.
Mallinckrodt Chemical Works, Diagnostic Products Division, St. Louis, MO.
Nycomed Inc, New York, NY.
Bristol-Myers Squibb Co., Princeton, NJ.

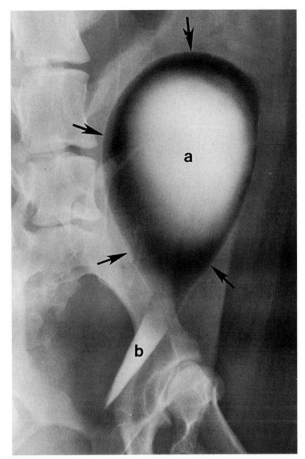

FIGURE 40–11. Oblique radiograph of a normal double-contrast cystogram. The urinary bladder wall (arrows) is clearly seen. The contrast puddle in the dependent portion of the bladder (a) and the contrast medium–filled urethra (b) are easily identified.

duced by factors such as air bubbles and inadequate bladder distention. By noting the number, severity, and distribution of radiographic signs, a specific diagnosis can usually be postulated. If a specific diagnosis cannot be made, the bladder condition, whether normal or abnormal, can be demonstrated. If nonspecific radiographic signs are present or further confirmation is necessary, additional diagnostic tests may be made.

Mucosal Changes

The urinary bladder has a transitional epithelium, which appears smooth on a normal-contrast cystogram. The transitional bladder epithelium is capable of metaplastic, neoplastic, and non-neoplastic proliferation.[35] Mucosal proliferation appears as an irregular outline along the inside bladder surface and may be accentuated with inadequate bladder distention. The distribution of mucosal irregularity is usually focal, but it may be diffuse; it may vary in severity from a slightly irregular brush-type surface to a severe cobblestone appearance (Fig. 40–13). Ulcers may be present with mucosal proliferation. On a double-contrast cystogram, ulcers can be identified if contrast medium adheres to the ulcerated surface. Mild mucosal irregularity may be obliterated on a cystogram if the bladder is completely distended.[33]

Intramural Changes (Bladder Wall Thickening)

A normal bladder has a wall approximately 1 mm thick regardless of the degree of distention.[29] Intramural changes

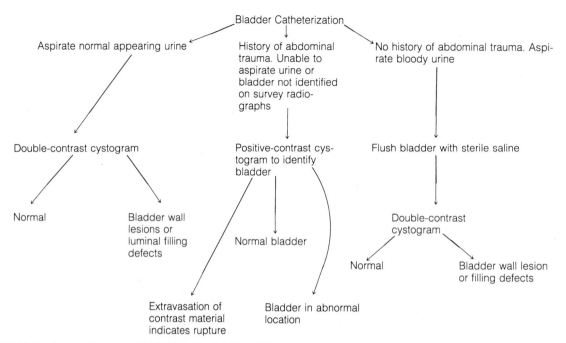

FIGURE 40–12. Selection of cystographic procedure. (Modified from Park RD: Radiology of the urinary bladder and urethra. *In* O'Brien TR [Ed]: Radiographic Diagnosis of Abdominal Disorders in the Dog and Cat. Davis, CA, Covell Park Veterinary Company, 1981, p 564; with permission.)

Table 40–4

RADIOGRAPHIC SIGNS OF PATHOLOGIC PROCESSES OF THE BLADDER

Disease	Mucosal Changes		Intramural Thickening		Filling Defect		Contrast Extravasation	
	Focal	Diffuse	Focal	Diffuse	Attached	Free	Smooth	Irregular
Chronic cystitis	Cranioventral	Occasional	Cranioventral	Occasional (cytoxan-induced cystitis)	Blood clots	Blood clots Calculi	—	—
Polypoid cystitis	Cranioventral	—	Cranioventral	—	Cranioventral	Blood clots	—	—
Acute cystitis	—	—	—	—	—	Occasional blood clots	—	—
Cystic calculi	Cranioventral from cystitis	—	Cranioventral from cystitis	—	—	Calculi and occasional blood clots		
Neoplasia	Any location within bladder	Occasional	Any location within bladder	Occasional	Sessile, occasionally pedunculated	Blood clots	—	—
Bladder contusion	Any location	Large areas of bladder often involved	Any location	Large areas of bladder often involved	Bladder wall hematoma	Blood clots	—	—
Bladder rupture or perforation	—	—	—	—	—	Blood clots	—	Most extravasate is into peritoneal cavity
Traumatic diverticula	—	—	—	—	—	Blood clots	Any location	
Urachal diverticula	Cranioventral associated with cystitis	—	Cranioventral associated with cystitis	—	—	—	Cranioventral	—

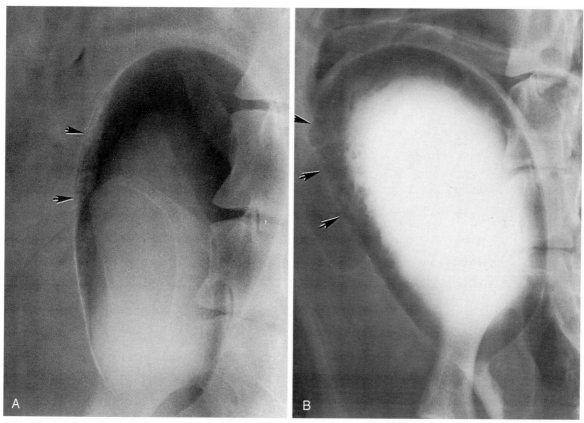

FIGURE 40–13. *A,* Oblique radiograph of the bladder during double-contrast cystography. There is mild mucosal irregularity along the right ventral bladder *(arrows)* caused by chronic bacterial cystitis. *B,* Oblique radiograph of the bladder during double-contrast cystography. Severe mucosal irregularity and mild bladder wall thickening are present along the ventral right bladder *(arrows).*

are demonstrated best with double-contrast cystography and consist of increased bladder wall thickness that is usually focal but may be diffuse (Fig. 40–14). Mild bladder wall thickening may not be demonstrated if the bladder is completely distended.[33] Bladder wall thickening may be caused by cellular infiltration or fibrous tissue proliferation. Cellular

infiltration may result from inflammation, hemorrhage from trauma, or neoplasia. Intramural bladder thickening causes decreased bladder distensibility, which may be symmetric with diffuse intramural bladder disease or asymmetric with focal intramural bladder disease.

Filling Defects

A bladder filling defect is anything occupying space within the bladder lumen that alters normal filling; such a defect occupies space normally filled with contrast medium on a cystogram. All filling defects appear radiolucent when surrounded with positive-contrast medium. The size, shape, number, border contour, position within the bladder, and attachment to the bladder wall should be examined with all bladder filling defects. Observing these filling defect characteristics helps differentiate the nature of the filling defect and ultimately may prove helpful in arriving at a diagnosis (Table 40–5).

Filling defects may be categorized as free or attached. Free luminal filling defects may be caused by air bubbles, calculi, sebaceous or mucous plugs,[34] or blood clots (Fig. 40–15). They are best demonstrated with double-contrast cystography and are seen within the dependent contrast puddle, which is in the center of the bladder on a recumbent lateral view. Attached filling defects may be caused by neoplasia (Fig. 40–16), inflammatory polyps, blood clots, iatrogenic hematomas, and ureteroceles (Fig. 40–17).[36] Mucosal irregularity and ulcers are frequently present on the surface of large attached filling defects. Bladder wall infiltration may be diagnosed as a thickened bladder wall adjacent to the filling defect.[37] Although a specific diagnosis cannot always be made

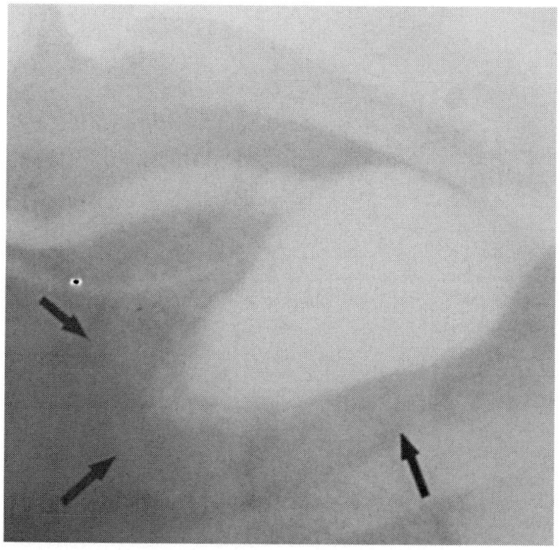

FIGURE 40–14. Lateral radiograph of the urinary bladder filled with positive-contrast medium during intravenous urography. Diffuse bladder wall thickening is present as the result of cytoxan-induced cystitis. The serosal surface *(arrows)* is outlined by fat. Bladder distensibility is decreased by the severe intramural changes. One ureter is distended as a result of obstruction at the ureterovesical junction.

Table 40-5
BLADDER FILLING DEFECTS

Lesion	Shape	Attachment	Border/Contour	Bladder Wall Infiltration (Thickening)
Calculi	Round to slightly irregular	Free in lumen; center of contrast puddle	Indistinct	Variable; usually cranioventral if associated with cystitis
Sebaceous or mucous plug	Round or irregular	Free in lumen; center of contrast puddle	Smooth or irregular, distinct or indistinct	Variable; associated with cystitis
Polyp	Pedunculated or convex	Stalk or sessile	Smooth or irregular, often with ulceration	Variable; bladder wall may be thick at attachment site
Epithelial neoplasia	Irregular or convex	Sessile	Irregular, often with ulceration	Bladder wall often thick or infiltrated at base of attachment
Mesenchymal neoplasia	Convex	Sessile	Usually smooth	Originates within the bladder wall
Blood clots	Irregular	Variable; may be free luminal	Irregular and indistinct	Thickened bladder wall from primary disease process
Bladder wall hematoma	Convex	Sessile	Smooth to slightly irregular	Originates within bladder wall
Ureterocele	Convex to round	Sessile	Smooth	Originates within trigone region of the bladder wall

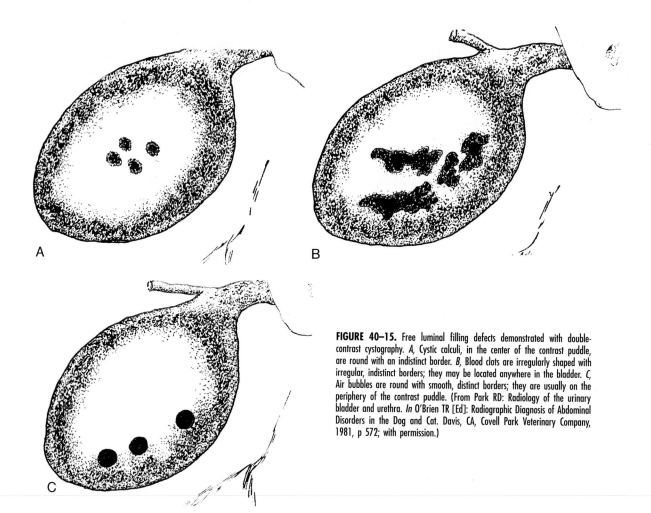

FIGURE 40-15. Free luminal filling defects demonstrated with double-contrast cystography. *A,* Cystic calculi, in the center of the contrast puddle, are round with an indistinct border. *B,* Blood clots are irregularly shaped with irregular, indistinct borders; they may be located anywhere in the bladder. *C,* Air bubbles are round with smooth, distinct borders; they are usually on the periphery of the contrast puddle. (From Park RD: Radiology of the urinary bladder and urethra. *In* O'Brien TR [Ed]: Radiographic Diagnosis of Abdominal Disorders in the Dog and Cat. Davis, CA, Covell Park Veterinary Company, 1981, p 572; with permission.)

FIGURE 40–16. *A,* Double-contrast cystogram. A large neoplastic mass *(arrows)* protrudes into the bladder lumen. There is minimal bladder wall infiltration. Contrast medium coats the ulcerated surface of the neoplasm. *B,* Positive-contrast cystogram. A large neoplastic lesion (transitional cell carcinoma) is present on the right side of the bladder *(arrows).* The neoplasm causes a large filling defect with an irregular surface.

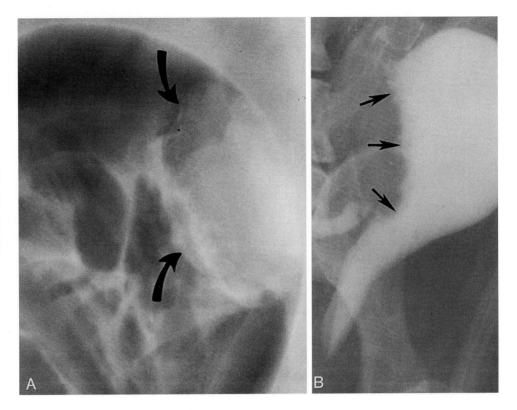

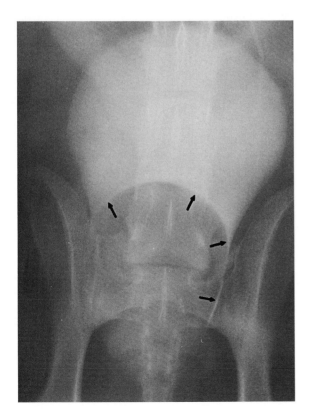

FIGURE 40–17. Ventrodorsal radiograph of the bladder filled with contrast medium during intravenous urography. The smooth luminal filling defect *(arrows)* that projects into the bladder neck is a ureterocele.

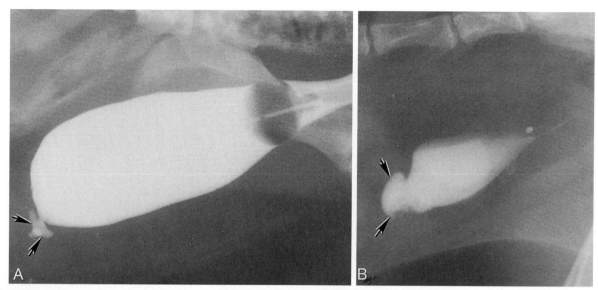

FIGURE 40–18. *A,* Positive-contrast cystogram with a small, irregular urachal diverticulum *(arrows).* The air-filled balloon on the Foley catheter causes the filling defect within the bladder neck. *B,* A traumatic bladder diverticulum is identified *(arrows).* Immediately after trauma, traumatic diverticula must be differentiated from a bladder contusion. Contusions usually heal within 48 hours, and the bladder distends symmetrically.

from the cystogram when attached filling defects are present, they may be differentiated by surgical removal or biopsy.

Contrast Extravasation Patterns From the Urinary Bladder

Retrograde positive-contrast cystography best demonstrates contrast-medium extravasation from the urinary bladder. Contrast-medium extravasation may be within the urinary tract, communicating with other visceral structures, or within the peritoneal cavity and surrounding soft tissues.

Contrast-medium extravasation from the normal bladder confined within the urinary tract may be seen with vesicoureteral reflux, urachal anomalies, and traumatic bladder diverticula (Fig. 40–18). Congenital urachal anomalies include diverticula,[38, 39] cysts, and persistent patent urachus.[40–43]

The contrast medium borders produced by extravasation within the urinary tract are usually smooth and may be identified as extensions from the urinary bladder. Contrast extravasation from the urinary bladder to adjacent visceral structures may be seen with either congenital or acquired fistulas. The organs most commonly involved are the rectum and the vagina. The communicating segment may not be outlined with contrast medium in such a way as to be detected radiographically. Such fistulas can usually be diagnosed with fluoroscopy[44] or in an indirect fashion on contrast cystograms; that is, the structure that communicates with the bladder fills simultaneously or shortly after the bladder is filled with contrast medium.

Contrast extravasation into the peritoneal cavity and surrounding soft tissues has an irregular outline and usually

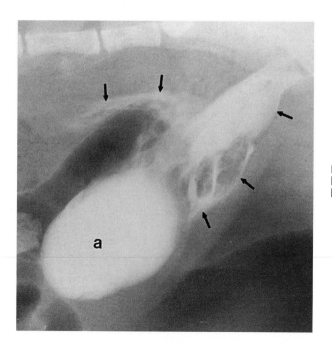

FIGURE 40–19. Positive-contrast cystogram in a cat. Contrast medium fills the urinary bladder (a) but extravasates into the peritoneal cavity *(arrows).* This complication has resulted from a tear in the bladder neck.

occurs simultaneously with injection of contrast medium into the bladder (Fig. 40–19). With small bladder neck tears, extravasation of contrast medium may be slow, with only a small volume extravasated.[6, 39] In these instances, a second radiograph may be required 5 to 10 minutes after contrast medium injection to obtain a positive diagnosis.

Pitfalls With Cystographic Interpretation

Interpretation pitfalls are changes noted on the radiograph that mimic actual pathologic changes. These changes are artifacts that are created during the cystographic procedure. Pitfalls commonly seen with contrast cystography are air bubble artifacts and pseudofilling defects.

There are three types of air bubble artifacts (Fig. 40–20): small air bubbles simulating calculi or other small luminal filling defects, a large air bubble simulating bladder wall thickening, and multiple air bubbles creating a honeycomb appearance. Air bubbles are radiolucent and have smooth distinct borders.

Pseudofilling defects may be mistaken for bladder neoplasia or other attached filling defects. These defects are created by inadequate bladder distention combined with external pressure from adjacent abdominal structures. Pseudofilling defects have a smooth surface and taper on both borders (Fig. 40–21); they can be obliterated with further bladder distention.

Ultrasound

Ultrasonographic examination of the urinary bladder, in addition to providing information for diagnosing cystic calcu-

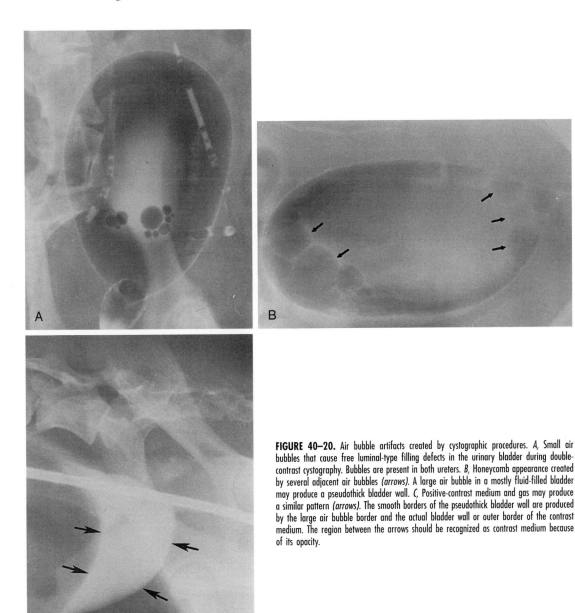

FIGURE 40–20. Air bubble artifacts created by cystographic procedures. *A,* Small air bubbles that cause free luminal-type filling defects in the urinary bladder during double-contrast cystography. Bubbles are present in both ureters. *B,* Honeycomb appearance created by several adjacent air bubbles *(arrows).* A large air bubble in a mostly fluid-filled bladder may produce a pseudothick bladder wall. *C,* Positive-contrast medium and gas may produce a similar pattern *(arrows).* The smooth borders of the pseudothick bladder wall are produced by the large air bubble border and the actual bladder wall or outer border of the contrast medium. The region between the arrows should be recognized as contrast medium because of its opacity.

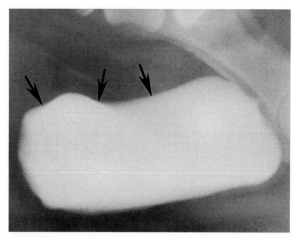

FIGURE 40–21. Lateral radiograph of a contrast medium–filled bladder during intravenous urography. Pseudofilling defects (arrows) are created by pressure on a partially distended bladder from adjacent abdominal structures.

li,[16, 17, 45] provides information for diagnosing other intraluminal and intramural diseases, including cystitis and neoplasia.[17, 46, 47] The extent and character of bladder wall disease can be determined, similarly as can be determined from a double-contrast cystogram study. Positive-contrast cystography provides information relative to bladder wall perforation and ruptures and communication with adjacent structures more readily than an ultrasound examination.

References

1. Fletcher TF: Anatomy of pelvic viscera. Vet Clin North Am 4:471, 1974.
2. International Committee on Veterinary Anatomical Nomenclature: Nomina Anatomica Veterinaria. Vienna, World Association of Veterinary Anatomists, 1973.
3. Miller ME, Christensen GC, and Evans HE: Anatomy of the Dog. Philadelphia, WB Saunders, 1964.
4. Mahaffey MB, Barsanti JA, Barber DL, et al: Pelvic bladders in dogs without urinary incontinence. J Am Vet Med Assoc 184:1477, 1984.
5. Johnston GR, Osborne CA, Jessen CR, et al: Effects of urinary bladder distension on location of the urinary bladder and urethra of healthy dogs and cats. Am J Vet Res 47:404, 1986.
6. Nickel R, Schummer A, Seiferle E, et al: The Viscera of the Domestic Mammals. Berlin, Paul Parey, 1973.
7. Park RD: Radiology of the urinary bladder and urethra. In O'Brien TR (Ed): Radiographic Diagnosis of Abdominal Disorders in the Dog and Cat. Davis, CA, Covell Park Veterinary Company, 1981, pp 543–614.
8. Adams WM, and DiBartola SP: Radiographic and clinical features of pelvic bladder in the dog. J Am Vet Med Assoc 182:1212, 1983.
9. Patnaik AK, and Greene RW: Intravenous leiomyoma of the bladder in a cat. J Am Vet Med Assoc 175:381, 1979.
10. Hansen JS: Persistent urachal ligament in the cat. Vet Med Small Anim Clin 67:1090, 1972.
11. Root CR, and Scott RC: Emphysematous cystitis and other radiographic manifestations of diabetes mellitus in dogs and cats. J Am Vet Med Assoc 158:721, 1971.
12. Ellenbogen PH, and Talner LB: Uroradiology of diabetes mellitus. Urology 8:413, 1967.
13. Middleton DJ, and Lomas GR: Emphysematous cystitis due to Clostridium perfringens in a non-diabetic dog. J Small Anim Pract 20:433, 1979.
14. Sherding RG, and Chew DJ: Nondiabetic emphysematous cystitis in two dogs. J Am Vet Med Assoc 174:1105, 1979.
15. Steyn PF, and Lowry J: Positional radiography as an aid to diagnose sand-like uroliths in the urinary bladder of feline urologic syndrome cats. Feline Pract 19:21, 1991.
16. Voros K, Waldar S, and Fenyves B: Ultrasonographic diagnosis of urinary bladder calculi in dogs. Canine Pract 19:29, 1993.
17. Prufer A: Ultrasonic diagnosis of diseases of the urinary bladder and the kidneys in dogs and cats. Kleintierpraxis 39:83, 1994.
18. Moreau PM, Lees GE, and Gross DR: Simultaneous cystometry and uroflowmetry (micturition study) for evaluation of the caudal part of the urinary tract in dogs: Studies of the technique. Am J Vet Res 44:1769, 1983.
19. Moreau PM, Lees GE, and Gross DR: Simultaneous cystometry and uroflowmetry (micturition study) for evaluation of the caudal part of the urinary tract function in dogs: Reference values for healthy animals sedated with xylazine. Am J Vet Res 44:1774, 1983.
20. Moreau PM, Lees GE, and Hobson HP: Simultaneous cystometry and uroflowmetry for evaluation of micturition in two dogs. J Am Vet Med Assoc 183:1083, 1983.
21. Rosin AE, and Barsanti JA: Diagnosis of urinary incontinence in dogs: Role of the urethral pressure profile. J Am Vet Med Assoc 178:814, 1981.
22. Oliver JE Jr, and Young WO: Air cystometry in dogs under xylazine-induced restraint. Am J Vet Res 34:1433, 1973.
23. Mooney JK Jr, Cox EC, and Heniman F: Vesical contamination from insertions of everting cot or catheter in inoculated canine urethra. Invest Urol 11:248, 1973.
24. Buchanan JW: Kinked catheter: A complication of pneumocystography. J Am Vet Radiol Soc 8:54, 1967.
25. Feeney DA, Johnston GR, Tomlinson MJ, et al: Effects of sterilized micropulverized barium sulfate suspension and meglumine iothalamate solution on the genitourinary tract of healthy male dogs after retrograde urethrocystography. Am J Vet Res 45:730, 1984.
26. Johnston GR, Stevens JB, Jessen CR, et al: Complications of retrograde contrast urethrography in dogs and cats. Am J Vet Res 44:1248, 1983.
27. Barsanti JA, Crowell W, Losonsky J, et al: Complications of bladder distention during retrograde urethrography. Am J Vet Res 42:819, 1981.
28. Farrow CS: Exercises in diagnostic radiology. Can Vet J 22:260, 1981.
29. Mahaffey MB, Barber DL, Barsanti JA, et al: Simultaneous double-contrast cystography and cystometry in dogs. Vet Radiol 25:254, 1984.
30. Ackerman N, Wingfield WE, and Corley EA: Fatal air embolism associated with pneumourethrography and pneumocystography in a dog. J Am Vet Med Assoc 160:1616, 1972.
31. Thayer GW, Carrig CB, and Evans AT: Fatal venous air embolism associated with pneumocystography in a cat. J Am Vet Med Assoc 176:643, 1980.
32. Brodeur AE, Goyer RA, and Melick W: A potential hazard of barium cystography. Radiology 85:1080, 1965.
33. Mahaffey MB, Barsanti JA, Browell WA, et al: Cystography: Effect of technique on diagnosis of cystitis in dogs. Vet Radiol 30:261, 1989.
34. Johnston GR, and Feeney DA: Radiographic evaluation of the urinary tract in dogs and cats. In Contemporary Issues in Small Animal Practice. Vol 4. Nephrology and Urology. New York, Churchill Livingstone, 1986, p 203.
35. Mostofi FK: Potentialities of bladder epithelium. J Urol 71:705, 1954.
36. Stowater JL, and Springer AL: Ureterocele in a dog: A case report. Vet Med Small Anim Clin 74:1753, 1979.
37. Archibald J: Urinary system. In Archibald J (Ed): Canine Surgery. Santa Barbara, CA, American Veterinary Publications, 1965.
38. Green RW, and Bohning RH Jr: Patent persistent urachus associated with urolithiasis in a cat. J Am Vet Med Assoc 158:489, 1971.
39. Osborne CA, Johnston GR, Kruger JM, et al: Etiopathogenesis and biological behavior of feline vesicourethral diverticula. Vet Clin North Am [Small Anim Pract] 3:697, 1987.
40. Hansen JS: Patent urachus in a cat. Vet Med Small Anim Clin 67:379, 1972.
41. Osborne CA, Rhoades JD, and Hanlon GF: Patent urachus in the dog. Anim Hosp 2:245, 1966.
42. Scherzo CS: Cystic liver and persistent urachus in a cat. J Am Vet Med Assoc 151:1329, 1967.
43. Park RD: Radiographic contrast studies of the lower urinary tract. Vet Clin North Am 4:863, 1974.
44. Osuna DJ, Stone EA, and Metcalf MR: A urethrorectal fistula with concurrent urolithiasis in a dog. J Am Anim Hosp Assoc 25:35, 1989.
45. Berry CR: Differentiating cystic calculi from colon. Vet Radiol Ultrasound 33:282, 1992.
46. Leville R, Biller DS, Partington BP, et al: Sonographic investigation of transitional cell carcinoma of the urinary bladder in small animals. Vet Radiol Ultrasound 33:103, 1992.
47. Bradley WA: Imaging technology for the delineation of a leiomyoma in the urinary bladder of a bitch. Aust Vet Pract 24:79, 1994.

STUDY QUESTIONS

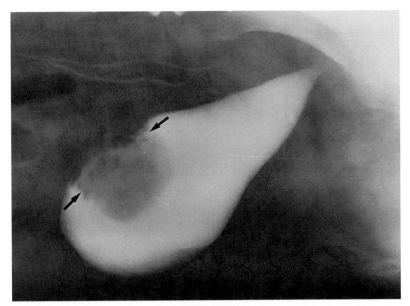

FIGURE 40–22

1. You observe the caudal aspect of the urinary bladder to be within the pelvic canal on a lateral abdominal radiograph of a dog. Is this abnormal?

2. With good serosal detail noted within the abdomen, what conditions may cause the bladder not to be visualized radiographically?

3. On a lateral survey abdominal radiograph, you observe a 1-cm round lucent area with well-defined margins in the center of the urinary bladder. What is producing this?

4. A dog is presented to you after being hit by a car. On a lateral abdominal radiograph, the serosal detail is poor, and you cannot distinctly see the urinary bladder. You suspect a ruptured urinary bladder. Which contrast examination would be most informative?

5. Why is moderate bladder distention recommended for double-contrast cystography?

6. What are the three types of artifacts that may be created by gas bubbles within the bladder?

7. How would you differentiate a pseudofilling defect from a pathologic filling defect?

8. Is visicoureteral reflux an abnormal finding when performing cystography?

9. Figure 40–22 is a lateral caudal abdominal view of a positive-contrast cystogram in a dog. What type of filling defect is present in the urinary bladder, and what is(are) the most likely diagnosis(es)?

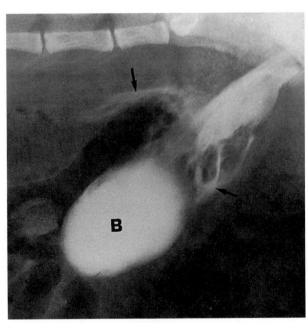

FIGURE 40–23

10. Figure 40–23 is a caudal abdominal view of a positive-contrast cystogram in a cat. What contrast pattern is present on the radiographic study, and what does it indicate?

(Answers appear on page 647.)

Chapter 41

The Urethra

Robert D. Pechman, Jr.

ANATOMY

The urethra is a sphincter and a conduit for urine from the bladder.[1] In females, the urethra is shorter and wider than in males; it terminates at the external urethral orifice on the ventral floor of the vagina. An external urethral sphincter is present in female dogs.[2]

In males, the urethra is long and thin and may be subdivided into three parts (Fig. 41–1). The prostatic urethra extends from the bladder to the caudal border of the prostate gland. The membranous urethra extends from the caudal margin of the prostate gland to the urethral bulb of the penis in dogs and to the bulbourethral glands in cats. In both species, the distal extent of the membranous urethra is approximately at the caudal margin of the ischium. The penile urethra extends from the caudal edge of the pelvis to the tip of the penis. The penile urethra is considerably smaller than the membranous urethra in cats; in dogs, it is partially surrounded dorsally by the os penis.[1, 2]

SURVEY RADIOGRAPHY

Radiographic evaluation of the urethra is performed most often in male dogs.[1] Radiographic examination of the urethra in male cats may be of value in patients with feline urologic syndrome with or without urethral obstruction.[3] Radiographic examination of the urethra is not often performed in female dogs or cats.

Survey radiographs of the urethra are rarely helpful, but they should be carefully examined for signs of urethral disease. Radiopaque urethral calculi may be seen on survey radiographs. Abnormal cranial displacement of the urinary bladder may occur secondary to urethral rupture. Pelvic fractures, particularly in male dogs, may result in urethral injury. Contrast urethrography is indicated in all instances of suspected urethral disease.[3, 4]

CONTRAST URETHROGRAPHY

Water-soluble organic iodide contrast media should be used. Oil-based contrast media, barium suspensions, and air should not be used because of the risk of urethrocavernous reflux and contrast medium embolization.[1, 4–6] Positive-contrast medium should be diluted with sterile saline or sterile water to approximately 15 percent of the original concentration.[1, 4]

A balloon-tipped catheter should be used.[4] The catheter is inserted into the urethra, and the balloon is inflated to prevent reflux of contrast medium. A 10- to 15-mL volume of contrast medium is usually used in dogs; 5 to 10 mL is adequate in cats. Radiographic exposures should be made during injection of the last 2 or 3 mL of contrast medium. A lateral view is usually adequate for diagnosis of urethral disease, but right and left ventrodorsal oblique projections are sometimes helpful. Ventrodorsal views are not often of value. In the lateral view, it is important to position the patient with the pelvic limbs pulled cranially to avoid superimposition of the femurs over the urethra.[1, 4] Distention of the urethra, particularly the prostatic urethra, and overall quality of the contrast urethrogram may be improved if the urinary bladder is fully distended with urine, contrast medium, or sterile saline during urethrography.[5] Retrograde positive-contrast urethrography should be performed with care because complications can result.[7, 8] Fortunately, most of these potential complications are transient and reversible.

Urethrography should be performed in any patient with abnormal urination or hematuria that is thought to be of

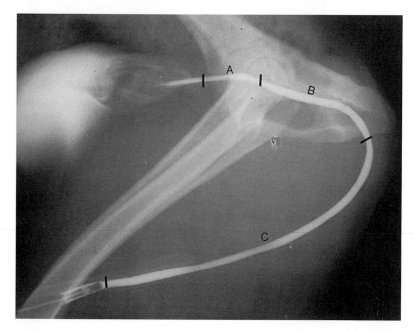

FIGURE 41–1. Normal positive-contrast retrograde urethrogram in a dog. A balloon-tipped catheter is present within the penile urethra. The urethra is divided into three segments: *A,* The prostatic urethra. *B,* The membranous urethra. *C,* The penile urethra. The urethral mucosa is smooth, and there are no filling defects in the contrast medium column.

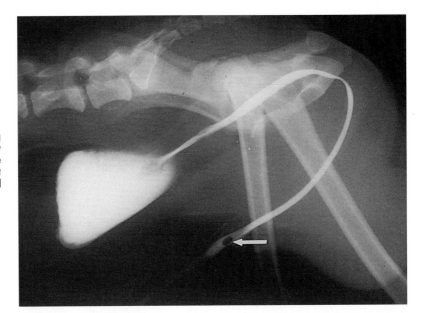

FIGURE 41–2. Positive-contrast retrograde urethrogram in a male dog with a solitary urethral calculus. In survey radiographs, a mineral-opacity calculus was seen near the proximal os penis. With urethrography, the calculus appears as a radiolucent intraluminal filling defect in the contrast medium column *(arrow)*. The margins of the calculus are smooth and sharply defined. The remainder of the urethra is normal.

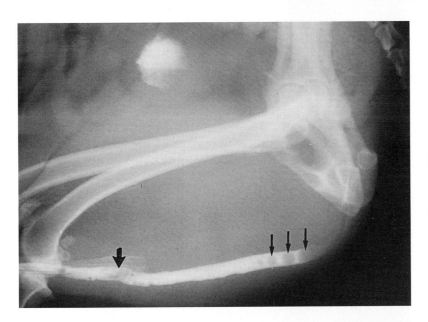

FIGURE 41–3. Retrograde positive-contrast urethrogram in a male dog with stranguria and a history of urethral calculi. There are intraluminal and intramural filling defects in the contrast medium column. Marked irregularity of the urethral mucosa is evident. An irregularly shaped intraluminal filling defect is present near the proximal os penis *(large arrow)*, and multiple smooth, ovoid intraluminal filling defects are present in the proximal penile urethra *(small arrows)*. Urethritis and a large blood clot within the urethra were found at surgery. The ovoid filling defects are intraluminal air bubbles. No urinary calculi were found.

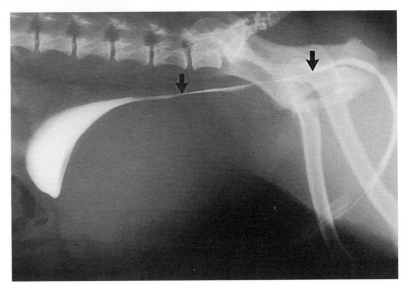

FIGURE 41–4. Retrograde positive-contrast urethrogram in a male dog with a large paraprostatic cyst. There is a long extramural filling defect (narrowing) of the urethra *(arrows)*. The margins of the filling defect are long and tapered, indicating extramural compression of the urethra. The urethra is stretched and compressed by the large prostatic mass.

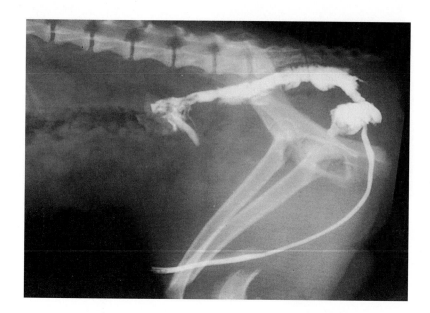

FIGURE 41–5. Positive-contrast retrograde urethrogram in a male dog with fractures of the pelvis and femur. There is extravasation of contrast medium into the perineal and pelvic soft tissues. Complete transection of the membranous urethra was found at surgery.

FIGURE 41–6. Positive-contrast urethrogram in a male dog. There is extravasation of contrast medium through a urethral laceration into the cavernous tissues of the penis. There is opacification of the dorsal vein of the penis by contrast medium *(arrows)*. The patient was examined because of stranguria. A fracture of the os penis at the site of the urethral laceration was apparent in survey radiographs. Note drainage of contrast medium into the caudal vena cava.

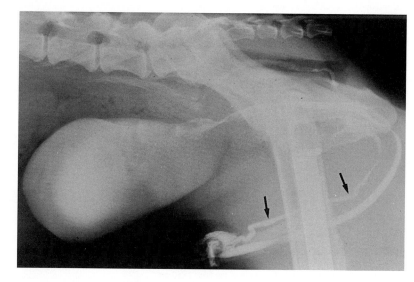

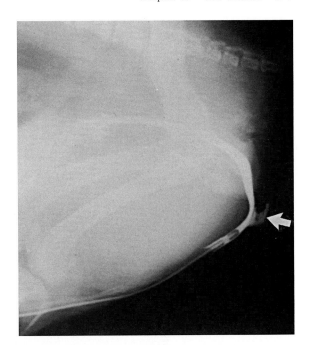

FIGURE 41–7. Iatrogenic urethral trauma. There is a small region of extravasation of contrast medium caudal to the urethra *(arrow)* near the junction of the membranous and penile portions. This urethral laceration was due to perforation of the urethra by a stiff plastic urinary catheter.

urethral origin. Pelvic fractures, especially in male dogs, are an indication for contrast urethrography if urinary tract injury is suspected.[4, 9–11]

RADIOGRAPHIC SIGNS OF URETHRAL DISEASE

Urethrographic signs of urethral disease may be classified as filling defects in the contrast medium column, extravasation of contrast medium from the urethral lumen,[1] or both.

Filling Defects

Filling defects may be intraluminal, intramural, or extramural. Intraluminal filling defects may be caused by air bubbles in the contrast medium column, mineralized or nonmineralized urethral calculi, or blood clots (Fig. 41–2). Air bubbles are round to oval and have smooth margins and a distinct, sharply defined border. Urethral calculi are variable in shape, have irregular margins, and usually are characterized by a poorly defined or blurred margin. If large enough, urethral calculi may produce widening of the urethral lumen. Blood clots are irregular in shape and have poorly defined margins.

Intramural filling defects may be due to neoplasia, inflammatory diseases, or scar tissue from previous urethral surgery, or they may result from careless instrumentation (Fig. 41–3). Intramural urethral lesions usually result in marked irregularity of the mucosal surface of the urethra and may cause widening or narrowing of the urethral lumen. The transitional zone from normal to abnormal urethra is usually abrupt and is sharply defined with intramural lesions.

Extramural filling defects result from compression by masses that surround the urethra (Fig. 41–4). Prostatic hyperplasia or neoplasia may result in extraluminal filling defects. The mucosal surface remains smooth, and the margins of the extraluminal filling defect are smooth and tapered.[1]

Extravasation of Contrast Medium

Extravasation of contrast medium indicates a disruption in the integrity of the urethra (Fig. 41–5). Contrast medium may enter the peritoneal cavity if the urethral rent is near the bladder neck. Contrast medium may also enter the systemic venous circulation if urethrocavernous reflux of contrast medium occurs (Fig. 41–6).[1, 11] Pelvic fractures or fractures of the os penis may produce urethral lacerations.[9–11] Abdominal trauma may be associated with urethral rupture at the vesicourethral junction.[10, 11] Iatrogenic urethral disruptions may result from poor catheter manipulation or as a sequela to urethral surgery (Fig. 41–7).[1]

Extravasation of urethral contrast medium may also be seen when there is communication of the urethral lumen with extraurinary organs through fistulous tracts. Urethrorectal and urethrovaginal fistulas have been reported[1, 12]; these fistulas may be congenital or acquired.[1]

References

1. Park RD: Radiology of the urinary bladder and urethra. *In* O'Brien TR (Ed): Radiographic Diagnosis of Abdominal Disorders in the Dog and Cat. Philadelphia, WB Saunders, 1978, pp 605–611.
2. Osborne CA, Low DG, and Finco DR: Canine and Feline Urology. Philadelphia, WB Saunders, 1972.
3. Johnston GR, Feeney DA, and Osborne CA: Urethrography and cystography in cats: I. Techniques, normal radiographic anatomy, and artifacts. Comp Contin Ed Vet Pract 4:823, 1982.
4. Ticer JW, Spener CP, and Ackerman N: Positive contrast retrograde urethrography: A useful procedure for evaluating urethral disorders in the dog. Vet Radiol 21:2, 1980.
5. Johnston GR, Jessen CR, and Osborne CA: Effects of bladder distention on canine and feline retrograde urethrography. Vet Radiol 24:271, 1983.
6. Ackerman N, Wingfield WE, and Corley EA: Fatal air embolism associated with pneumourethrography and pneumocystography in a dog. J Am Vet Med Assoc 160:1616, 1972.
7. Johnston GR, Stevens JB, Jessen CR, et al: Complications of retrograde contrast urethrography in dogs and cats. Am J Vet Res 44:1248, 1983.
8. Johnston GR, Feeney DA, and Osborne CA: Urethrography and cystography in cats: II. Abnormal radiographic anatomy and complications. Comp Contin Ed Vet Pract 4:931, 1982.
9. Johnston GR, Jessen CR, and Osborne CA: Lower urinary tract injuries associated with pelvic trauma. Canine Pract 1:25, 1974.
10. Kleine LJ, and Thornton GW: Radiographic diagnosis of urinary tract trauma. J Am Anim Hosp Assoc 7:318, 1971.
11. Pechman RD: Urinary trauma in dogs and cats: A review. J Am Anim Hosp Assoc 18:33, 1982.
12. Osborne CA, Engen MH, Yano BL, et al: Congenital urethrorectal fistula in two dogs. J Am Vet Med Assoc 166:999, 1975.

STUDY QUESTIONS

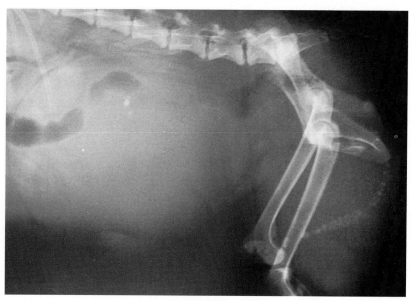

FIGURE 41-8

1. The male urethra is subdivided into three parts: the prostatic urethra, the membranous urethra, and the penile urethra. (True or False)

2. Contrast urethrography should be performed on all patients with urethral disease. (True or False)

3. What abnormal radiographic findings are present in this lateral radiograph of the caudal abdomen and perineal region of a male dog (Fig. 41–8)?

4. Positive-contrast urethrography should be performed using:
   A. Room air.
   B. 30 percent barium suspension.
   C. Oil-based contrast medium.
   D. Water-soluble organic iodide contrast medium.
   E. Carbon dioxide.

5. Urethral distention and overall quality of a urethrogram are improved if the bladder is fully distended when the examination is performed. (True or False)

6. A positive-contrast urethrogram was performed in a male dog (Fig. 41–9). What is the radiographic diagnosis?

7. Intraluminal filling defects in a positive-contrast urethrogram can be caused by air bubbles, calculi, and prostatic hyperplasia. (True or False)

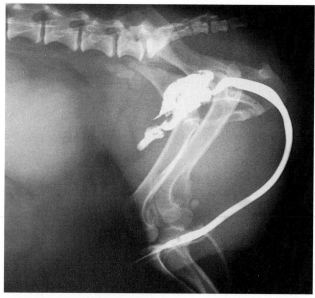

FIGURE 41-9

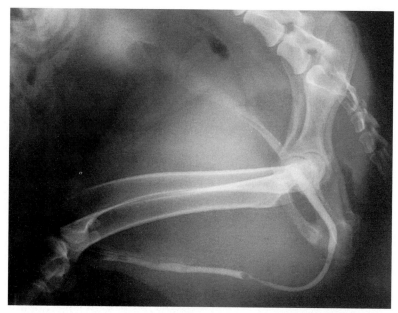

FIGURE 41–10

8. List three possible causes of intramural filling defects in a positive-contrast urethrogram.

9. This is a lateral view of a positive-contrast urethrogram (Fig. 41–10). What is the radiographic diagnosis?

10. Extravasation of contrast medium in a positive-contrast urethrogram indicates disruption of the integrity of the urethra. (True or False)

(Answers appear on page 647.)

Chapter 42

The Prostate Gland

Jimmy C. Lattimer

NORMAL ANATOMY

The prostate is a small, ovoid exocrine and endocrine accessory sex gland located just caudal to the urinary bladder.[1, 2] The urethra passes through the prostate gland slightly dorsal to center. The prostatic urethra is slightly dilated within the gland and is slightly narrowed at the caudal margin. A small papilla in the dorsal wall of the midprostatic urethra, the colliculus seminalis, marks the entry point of the vas deferens. Multiple pairs of prostatic ducts enter the urethra dorsal, lateral, ventral, and caudal to the seminal hillock, providing drainage of the prostate.[3]

The prostate is located immediately ventral to the rectum and dorsal to the pubis. The relationship of the prostate to the rectum and pubis is highly dependent on the position of the urinary bladder. If the bladder is displaced, the prostate may also be displaced.[3, 4]

After rupture of the urachal remnant at about 2 months of age, the prostate usually lies completely within the pelvic canal. As the animal matures, the prostate enlarges in response to the increase in androgen levels.[5, 6] By the time the animal is 3 or 4 years old, the gland has usually migrated cranially so that it is mostly, if not completely, within the peritoneal cavity.[7]

As the dog ages, the size of the normal prostate remains relatively constant until 10 or 11 years; at this age, the gland usually undergoes some degree of shrinkage owing to atrophy.[8] The prostate may then again become intrapelvic, although this occurrence is not constant and usually does not happen if there is pathologic enlargement of the prostate.

Position and form of the prostate in the adult male cat are much the same as in the dog. The gland is much smaller than in the dog, however, and rarely, if ever, is seen on a radiograph. Reports of abnormalities of the feline prostate are rare.[7]

Although all mammals have prostate glands, prostatic disease is rare in all except dogs and humans. Because the dog is the only domestic animal in which the prostate is visible on radiographs, the remainder of this discussion is limited to the dog.

Just as there is no average-sized dog, there is no average-sized prostate gland. The great variation in canine body size makes any statement regarding average absolute prostate size meaningless. It has been reported, however, that the relative weight of the prostate, defined as prostatic weight in grams

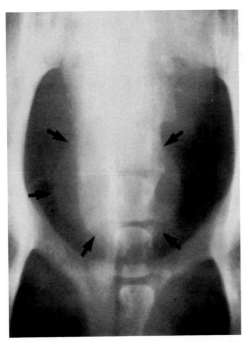

FIGURE 42–1. Ventrodorsal view of the pelvis in which a normal prostate gland *(arrows)* is visible. Note that the total diameter of the prostate gland is approximately one half to two thirds that of the pelvic canal.

divided by body weight in kilograms, is the same for all dogs except the Scottish terrier, in which it has been reported to be larger by a factor of four.[8] This author,[8] however, considered benign hyperplasia to be a normal finding, and the histologic description of the prostates from the Scottish terriers was not given. Thus, the data cannot be considered definitive evidence to support the conclusion that the prostate of the Scottish terrier is normally larger than that of other breeds because the experimental group may have had prostatic hyperplasia. Prostatomegaly, however, is observed frequently in Scottish terriers.

A number of technical and anatomic conditions make it difficult, if not impossible, to determine the absolute size of the prostate radiographically. In fact, it has been shown that estimates of prostatic weight based on radiographic measurement are consistently low.[9] The relative anatomic size of the prostate is the key indication. The normal prostate is seldom greater in diameter than two thirds of the width of the pelvic inlet as seen on the ventrodorsal radiograph. Although the central portion of the prostate is usually obscured by the sacrum and caudal vertebrae, its lateral margins are often visible (Fig. 42–1). This is often true even when the gland is completely obscured on the lateral view. Another criterion that has been described is that no dimension of the prostate should exceed 70 percent of the distance from the pubic rim to the sacral promontory.[10]

The shape of the prostate varies from almost spherical to an oval or a flattened ellipse, in which the length is approximately 1.5 times the width of the gland. The normal prostate is bilobate and bilaterally symmetric on gross examination.[2, 11] It is generally not possible to differentiate lobar borders on survey radiographs.

The prostate is of soft-tissue opacity; therefore, visualization is dependent on differential contrast with surrounding pelvic fat. If the dog is emaciated or if there is fluid in the abdomen, the prostate is obscured. When surrounded by pelvic fat, the prostate has a smooth, well-margined contour that may be seen on both the lateral and the ventrodorsal projections. On the lateral view, the cranial and ventral borders are clearly seen where a triangular area of fat separates the prostate from the bladder and the ventral abdominal wall (Fig. 42–2).[7, 12]

Because the prostate is usually in direct contact with the rectum, the dorsal border is often difficult to see, especially if the rectum contains feces. A full rectum may also completely obscure the prostate on the ventrodorsal radiograph.

The normal prostate is recognizable by its shape and opacity and the relationship of the gland to the organs around it. If the shape or position of the gland is altered, the gland may not be recognizable other than as a nondescript opacity between the bladder, rectum, and pelvis.[13]

Because the prostate enlarges in response to androgens, the removal of those hormones by castration results in atrophy of the gland. Alternatively, if the animal is neutered at an early age, the prostate remains small. Shrinkage of the prostate almost invariably follows castration, unless pre-existing disease is present.[8, 13–15] A similar effect is obtained by estrogen administration, even in an intact animal.[13] Administration of estrogen in combination with castration usually results in rapid shrinkage of the prostate, even if the diseased gland is

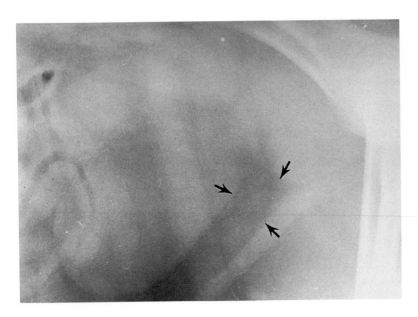

FIGURE 42–2. Lateral view of the caudal abdomen. The position and size of the prostate is apparent. The *arrows* indicate the fat triangle that marks the division between the prostate gland and the bladder.

only partially hormone responsive. After castration or estrogen therapy, a prostate tumor may exhibit rapid initial shrinkage followed by tumor regrowth.[16]

In instances in which a male dog has been castrated or was given estrogen, the prostate may be so small that it is not visible radiographically. Evidence of an enlarged prostate in such animals is often a poor prognostic sign in that it indicates a disease not responsive to normal homeostatic mechanisms.[14]

DISEASES OF THE PROSTATE

Intrinsic disease of the prostate usually results in prostatic enlargement. Enlargement may also occur in response to extraprostatic diseases, such as an androgen-producing testicular tumor and orchitis.[8] Because of the close functional association of the prostate and testes, any animal with prostatic disease should also be examined (preferably ultrasonographically) for testicular disease.

The most common prostatic abnormality is benign prostatic hypertrophy, in which instance the prostate enlarges owing to an increase in the volume of the intercellular and ductal space rather than to an increase in intracellular volume or cell numbers. Thus, once the disease reaches a certain point, the development of dilated cystic spaces and ducts is inevitable. Solid and cystic hypertrophy are therefore different stages of the same disease, with the latter being the advanced form.[8, 17] A cystic prostate usually has cysts of many different sizes. Size of the cystic spaces varies from microscopic to large; they may become so large that they distort the shape of the entire gland. The larger cysts are also prone to infection.

Another common cause of prostatic enlargement is prostatitis, which is usually bacterial.[18] The infection may arise within the prostate or may extend from other sources, such as the bladder and testicles.[19] Because many antibiotics do not readily penetrate the prostate, the gland may also be a reservoir for reinfection or primary extension to other organs.[6, 20] The degree of inflammation depends on the type of organism present and the condition of the prostate before infection. A normal prostate is more resistant to infection than is a hypertrophied gland with many secretion-filled cystic spaces. The inflammation may vary in severity from a mild transient process that causes minimal or no clinical disease to a fulminating hemorrhagic process that rapidly destroys the entire gland.[3] The latter may result in rupture of the capsule with extension of infection to the peritoneal cavity, resulting in peritonitis.[20]

Chronic, recurrent prostatitis may result in a scarred, fibrotic prostate that is smaller than normal. A prostate such as this may not be recognized radiographically unless a urethrogram is performed. Chronic scarring may result in stricture of the urethra.[16]

Prostatic abscesses may form as a result of prostatitis. As with cyst formation, abscesses may be small or large. Large abscesses distort the shape of the gland and may eventually rupture, causing peritonitis. Abscess formation may be primary or secondary to cyst infection. As previously stated, cysts form in advanced benign hypertrophy and are usually contained within the gland. Occasionally, cysts become so large that the shape of the gland is distorted, and the predominant opacity seen on the radiograph is due to the large cyst. Such large cysts are also referred to as *paraprostatic cysts* because they are no longer confined within the gland. These cysts are usually sterile but may become infected and abscessed.[21]

Occasionally, abscesses or cysts result from neoplasia.[11] Formation of functional neoplastic secretory cells without an accompanying ductal system results in a cystic structure lined with neoplastic epithelium. Osteocollagenous retention cysts are rare and of unknown origin, but they do not appear to be the direct result of cystic hypertrophy.[22]

A rare form of cyst, which is truly paraprostatic, is cystic enlargement of the wolffian ducts, termed *uterus masculinus*.[23] Enlargement of the wolffian ducts results in a bilateral tubular mass that resembles uterine enlargement. The prostate itself may or may not be enlarged and is usually not distinguishable as a separate opacity.[16]

Prostatic adenocarcinoma is relatively uncommon.[24, 25] When it occurs, this tumor is often advanced at presentation, with metastasis to regional lymph nodes, the pelvis, and distant sites such as the liver and lungs.[14, 26, 27] In some dogs, the prostate is massively enlarged by the tumor, and in others the degree of enlargement is minimal. Small in situ prostatic carcinomas are unusual, but they do occur; they are usually discovered as a result of metastasis rather than local effects. Prostatic neoplasms are often secondarily infected or necrotic, and affected dogs may therefore have clinical signs of prostatitis. These patients are difficult to diagnose because of the tendency of prostatitis to overshadow neoplasia, unless signs of metastasis are present.[28–30]

Clinical Signs

The clinical signs of prostate disease are usually referable to either urinary or rectal problems. Strangury, hematuria, and pyuria are commonly seen.[3, 19, 21, 23] Complete urethral obstruction is unusual.[17, 31] Another common complaint with prostatic disease is dyschezia, with small or ribbon-like stools.[3, 31] As the enlarging prostate displaces the colon dorsally, it compresses it against the sacrum and pelvis, resulting in a decrease in stool diameter (Fig. 42–3). Extreme straining to defecate may result in small amounts of fresh blood in the stool. Severe rectal compression by the prostate may cause clinical and radiographic signs of constipation or obstipation. Such patients may not strain or even attempt to defecate. The problem is then critical and immediate, and definitive treatment must be instituted.

Another less common but important complaint is a pelvic limb gait abnormality. The animal may refuse to climb stairs and jump. Owners often believe the animal has developed degenerative joint disease in the hips. Such animals may have severe, active septic prostatitis.[3, 19] The pain caused by the prostatic infection is markedly exacerbated by walking, climbing, and jumping. Both pelvic limbs are usually affected uniformly because the pain is central. These animals are also usually sensitive to palpation of the caudal abdomen. There may also be some erythema of the skin because of inflammation in this area. Gait abnormalities are seen rarely in uncomplicated benign prostatic hypertrophy.

Radiographic Changes

Although ultrasonography has improved the ability to diagnose prostatic abnormalities, radiography is still the first imaging procedure that should be performed in patients with suspected prostatic disease. Because of its intimate relationship to the urinary bladder, prostatomegaly displaces the bladder cranially (Fig. 42–4). If prostatomegaly is uniform, bladder displacement is cranial along the floor of the abdomen. If prostatomegaly is eccentric, as often occurs with cysts and abscesses, the direction of bladder displacement may be different. Dorsal prostatomegaly by a cyst or abscess may extend dorsal to the bladder, compressing it against the floor

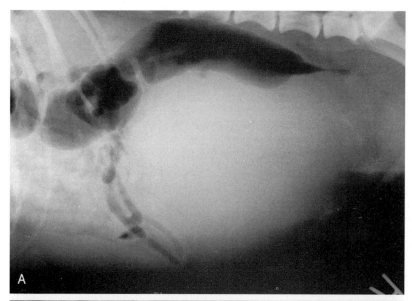

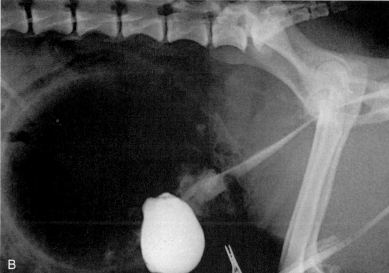

FIGURE 42–3. Prostatic enlargement and probable cyst or abscess formation. *A,* There is apparent cranial displacement of the bladder and marked dorsal displacement and compression of the descending colon. Because of the marked enlargement and inflammation present in the caudal abdomen, the normal division between the bladder and prostate gland is obscured. Without cystography or sonography, correct identification of an enlarged prostate is difficult. *B,* Same animal following a double-contrast cystogram. The huge air-filled structure is a prostatic cyst or abscess. The positive-contrast portion of the study delineates the course of the urethra, which leads to the bladder. If only the negative-contrast portion of the study had been performed, some confusion may have remained about the location and size of the bladder.

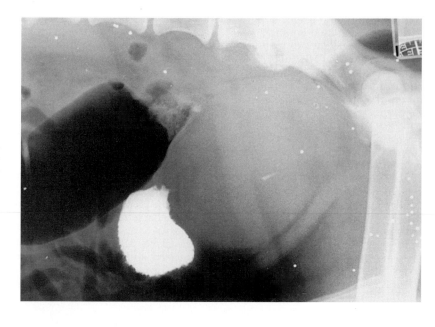

FIGURE 42–4. Marked enlargement of the prostate gland has displaced the urinary bladder cranial to its normal location. The enlargement is so extreme that the partially full urinary bladder does not contact the abdominal wall.

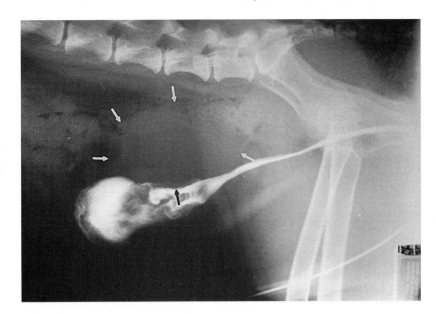

FIGURE 42–5. Urethrogram, lateral view. A large paraprostatic cyst *(arrows)* located dorsal to the neck of the urinary bladder is compressing the bladder. The bladder is also displaced cranially by the combination of the enlarged prostate gland and the cyst.

of the abdomen (Fig. 42–5). Alternatively, with ventral prostatomegaly, the bladder may be elevated (Fig. 42–6). A large prostatic cyst or abscess may extend ventral to the bladder, also resulting in craniodorsal displacement of the bladder. This latter appearance of elevation of the bladder may also be seen with severe benign prostatic hypertrophy (Fig. 42–7).

The other major radiographic sign of prostatomegaly is dorsal displacement of the colon (see Figs. 42–3 through 42–5). The colon normally lies in contact with the dorsal or dorsolateral surface of the bladder. As prostatomegaly displaces the colon dorsally, contact with the bladder is lost. Radiographically, there is separation of the ventral border of the colon and the dorsal border of the bladder. In a male dog, such a finding is virtually confirmatory of prostatomegaly.[19]

Prostatic enlargement may cause narrowing of the colon lumen. Radiographically, this compression may be visible, or the colon may simply become confluent with the prostate mass at the pelvic inlet. The latter appearance does not usually occur unless highly aggressive disease is present. The colon is often displaced laterally within the pelvic canal by a prostatic mass (Fig. 42–8). Colon contents, especially gas, often improve identification of the prostate. Air can be intro-

duced into the colon to provide a contrasting opacity in the colon. This more clearly delineates the degree of colonic compression by an enlarged prostate or other mass.

The urethra, although not really displaced relative to the prostate, may be elevated from the pelvic floor or displaced laterally by an enlarged prostate. Urethral displacement is most often seen with asymmetric prostatic disease, such as tumor and abscess. The urethra is also often elongated by its passage through an enlarged prostate. The position of the urethra is impossible to ascertain unless contrast medium is used to outline it (see Fig. 42–5).

A tremendously enlarged prostate displaces other abdominal organs cranially. Huge prostatic lesions usually lie on the floor of the abdomen, so there is some dorsal displacement of the remainder of the abdominal contents. Prostatic and paraprostatic cysts may become so large that they reach almost to the costal arch.[23] With masses of this magnitude, organ displacement is so severe that the actual source of the mass may be difficult to determine without the use of special radiographic procedures or sonography.

All common prostate diseases cause enlargement. As is the instance with most organs, the enlargement may be symmet-

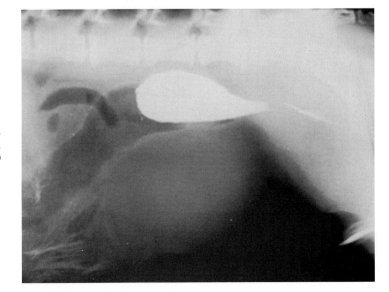

FIGURE 42–6. Marked dorsal displacement of the bladder (filled with positive-contrast medium) by a large paraprostatic cyst (soft-tissue mass ventral to bladder). Note that in contrast to the cyst in Figure 42–15B, this cyst does not appear to communicate with the urethra.

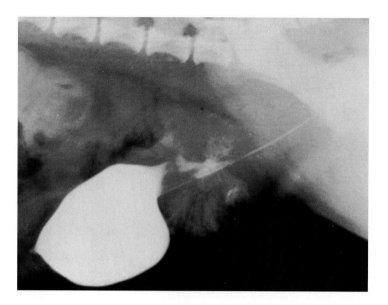

FIGURE 42–7. Positive-contrast cystogram. There is marked prostatic hypertrophy, and the bladder is displaced cranially. Note that if the bladder were less distended, it would not touch the abdominal wall. There is reflux of contrast medium into the parenchyma of the prostate gland outlining the dilated ducts.

ric (diffuse in origin), asymmetric (focal in origin), or a combination of the two. Hypertrophy and prostatitis are examples of symmetric enlargement, whereas neoplasia and cysts are examples of asymmetric enlargement. Large prostatic and paraprostatic cysts and abscesses are generally combination lesions that involve the entire prostate, but a single lobe predominates as the source of the radiographic lesion.[3] Because it is difficult to define the shape of the normal prostate precisely, it may be difficult to determine whether the enlarged prostate is symmetric or asymmetric when enlargement is mild. If the enlarged prostate is relatively symmetric in its relationship to the bladder, the enlargement is probably symmetric (Fig. 42–9); if not, the enlargement is asymmetric (Fig. 42–10).

It has been stated that, in general, prostatic size that exceeds 90 percent of the distance from the pubis to the sacral promontory is suggestive of a mass lesion (cyst, abscess, or neoplasm).[10] The actual degree of prostatic enlargement varies tremendously, however. For instance, prostatic size may vary from slight enlargement to 10 times normal size for benign prostatic hypertrophy, and the prostate may actually decrease in size in chronic prostatitis. If prostatic cysts or abscesses are present, the prostate may be as great as 20 or more times normal size, or the degree of enlargement may be minimal. Acute prostatitis and neoplasia do not usually cause huge enlargement, as seen with hypertrophy and cyst formation. Some small in situ prostatic tumors are not recognized until the animal is examined for another problem, such as cough and lameness caused by metastasis, or as an incidental finding at post mortem.

It is important where possible to evaluate the margination of the prostate. The presence of adequate amounts of abdominal fat is essential to visualize the prostatic margin. In the presence of emaciation, normally thin animals, or abdominal effusion, the prostatic margin and even the entire prostate itself may be indistinctly seen. If the prostate has a smooth margin that is easily seen, the disease involving the gland is likely to be benign or slowly progressing (see Fig. 42–2). A rough or indistinct margin in the presence of adequate abdominal fat is more likely to be due to an acute or aggressive process, such as neoplasia and prostatitis (Fig. 42–11).[12, 29, 32] Paraprostatic cysts and abscesses usually have well-defined margins that are easily seen (see Fig. 42–6). An occasional abscess is poorly marginated because of local peritonitis, although this occurrence is the exception rather than the rule. Occasionally a cyst or abscess may form in the pelvic canal; such lesions may not be readily visible on survey radiographs or produce the usual displacement of the bladder.[33] These lesions do, however, produce marked displacement and compression of the rectum and are therefore recognized as an intrapelvic mass. The lack of regional peritonitis associated with the large abscess may be due in part to the thickness of the capsule and to the organism being of a low virulence. It is seldom possible to distinguish a cyst from an abscess on the basis of radiographic examination alone.

Any change in the opacity of the prostate from its normal soft-tissue opacity indicates severe disease. Areas of calcification within the gland are a sign of either long-standing prostatitis or of neoplasia (Fig. 42–12).[10, 23, 30] Most prostate calcification is a result of neoplasia. Therefore, calcification should be considered a serious finding that warrants biopsy.[4, 12]

The presence of gas within the prostate is also an important sign. The prostate may contain air because of reflux from

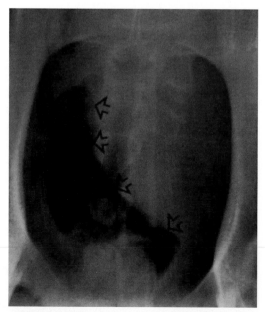

FIGURE 42–8. Ventrodorsal radiograph of the pelvic canal. *Arrows* indicate concave indentation of the colon on the left side by an enlarged prostate.

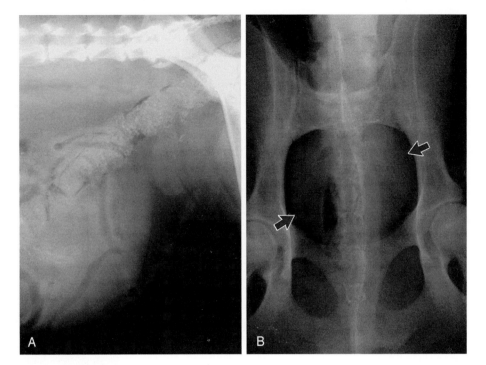

FIGURE 42–9. *A* and *B,* Moderate symmetric enlargement of the prostate gland owing to hypertrophy. The margins of the gland are smooth, and the fat triangle between the bladder and the prostate is clearly visible. Note that the dorsal portion of the prostate is superimposed on the feces-filled colon. The opacities superimposed over the prostate are artifacts.

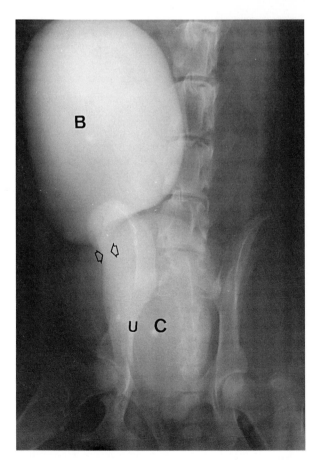

FIGURE 42–10. Positive-contrast retrograde urethrogram. There is an asymmetric prostatic mass. This large prostatic cyst (C) markedly displaces the urethra (U) to the right side of the pelvic canal. *Arrows* indicate the point at which the urethra enters the bladder; such displacement of the urethra is typical of large cystic lesions of the prostate gland. Some contrast medium is present in the prostatic cyst. B, bladder.

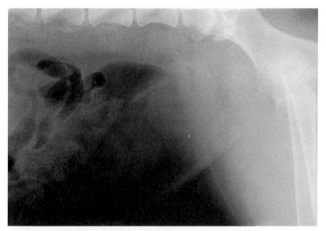

FIGURE 42–11. Prostatic adenocarcinoma. The large, irregularly shaped prostate displaces the bladder cranially. The colon is displaced dorsally, and the bladder is dorsal to the abdominal wall. Although the tumor has not yet broken through the capsule of the gland, it distorts the outline, making its shape irregular.

the bladder during a negative-contrast or double-contrast cystogram (Fig. 42–13). A small amount of reflux into prostatic ducts is a normal but not consistent occurrence. Simple filling of the ducts with air does not necessarily indicate prostatic disease. Filling of air in pockets within the prostate is abnormal, however, and is most commonly associated with cyst formation secondary to benign hypertrophy. The presence of gas within the prostate may indicate infection with a

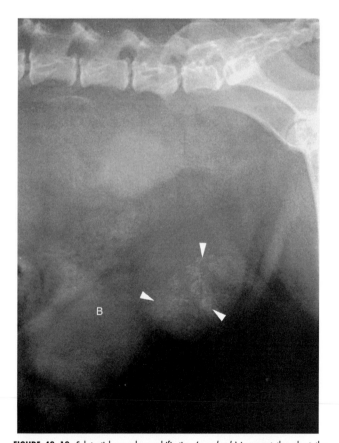

FIGURE 42–12. Substantial amorphous calcification *(arrowheads)* is present throughout the parenchyma of this enlarged prostate gland. Calcification in association with the enlarged gland is strongly suggestive of neoplasia. There is also extensive external iliac lymphadenopathy. The histologic diagnosis is carcinoma of the prostate. B, urinary bladder.

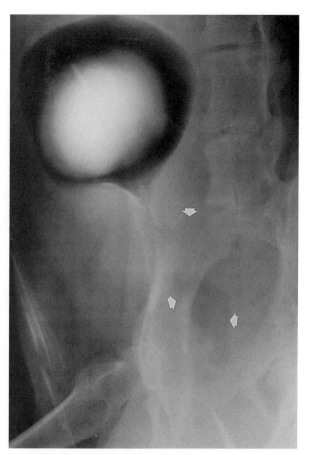

FIGURE 42–13. Oblique view of a double-contrast cystogram. There is marked enlargement of the prostate. Note that air has refluxed into the gland *(arrows)*. The cavities are irregular, suggestive of multiple abscesses or neoplasia.

gas-forming organism. Coliform or clostridial prostatitis results in severe hemorrhagic necrosis of the gland. These infections rapidly destroy the gland and extend to the abdomen, resulting in a generalized peritonitis. Because of the rapidly fatal course of these infections, identification of noniatrogenic gas within the prostate should be viewed as an unfavorable prognostic sign.

Palisade-type periosteal proliferation is sometimes seen on the ventral aspect of the caudal lumbar vertebrae and pelvis (Fig. 42–14). Such proliferation is suggestive of regional metastasis from prostatic neoplasia.[2, 4, 10, 29–31, 34]

Special Radiographic Procedures

Few special radiographic procedures are used in the diagnosis of prostatic disease. The only technique that has been found to be uniformly useful in the evaluation of the prostate is the positive-contrast retrograde urethrogram. This procedure allows evaluation of the position of the urethra in relation to a suspected prostatic mass. Asymmetric positioning of the urethra indicates the enlargement is either extrinsic to the prostate or is occurring asymmetrically within the prostate (Fig. 42–15), the latter being more common.[10] Urethrography also allows evaluation of the urethra itself. Invasion or stricture of the urethra in association with a prostatic mass is a poor prognostic finding not only because of the danger that a urinary obstruction might occur, but also because it is a sign that aggressive disease is present.[10] Evidence of either prostatic asymmetric enlargement or urethral abnormalities

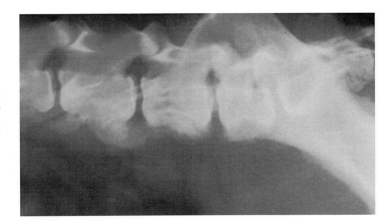

FIGURE 42–14. Palisade-type periosteal reaction along the ventral aspect of L5 through L7 and the sacrum. This lesion is not a constant feature with all prostate tumors, but when evident, it is suggestive of a prostatic or bladder-urethra carcinoma, even if there is no gross enlargement of the prostate gland. (Courtesy of Dr. L. Konde.)

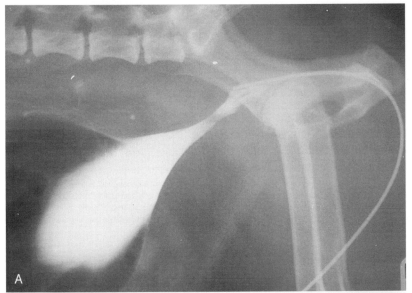

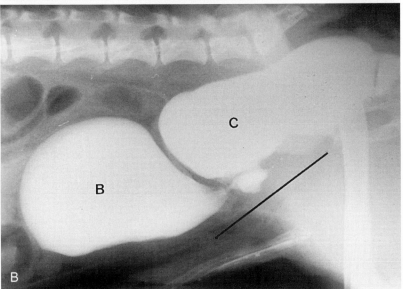

FIGURE 42–15. *A,* Double-contrast cystogram. The prostate is moderately enlarged. In the urethrogram, the position of the urethra indicates that the ventral portion of the gland is more enlarged than the dorsal portion. The off-center position of the urethra suggests the enlargement is at least in part due to either a cystic-type or neoplastic lesion. *B,* Positive-contrast cystogram. There is a large, dorsally located paraprostatic cyst (C) filled with contrast medium. Thus, the cyst communicates with the urethra. The bladder neck is displaced cranially and ventrally. Note the relatively small size of the remainder of the prostate, as indicated by the space between the cyst and the ventral abdominal wall *(line)* caudal to the bladder (B).

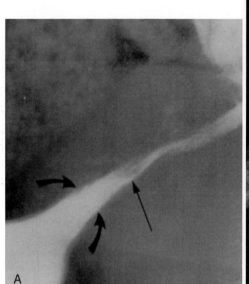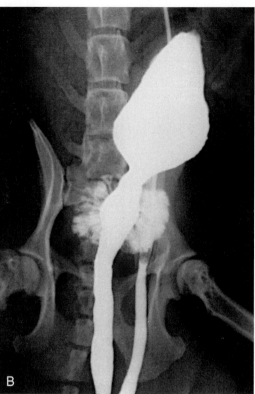

FIGURE 42–16. *A*, In this close-up view of the prostate, the normal appearance of the urethra when distended during positive-contrast retrograde urethrography can be seen. The small amount of contrast medium reflux into the gland is insignificant. The small filling defect *(straight arrow)* indicates the position of the colliculus seminalis and is a normal finding. If the prostatic urethra is not distended when radiographed, the colliculus will probably not be evident. Note that the level of the urethral sphincter *(curved arrows)* is well within the prostatic silhouette. *B*, In a ventrodorsal view of a prostatic urethrogram, there is substantial filling of the prostatic ducts with contrast medium but no filling cavities within the gland. Interpretation was normal prostatic urethrogram.

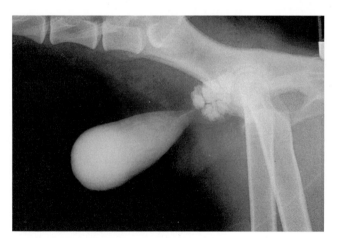

FIGURE 42–17. Prostatic cavitation without enlargement. A positive-contrast urethrogram was performed in a dog with persistent hematuria and pyuria. There are multiple cavities within the prostate that communicate with the urethra. Although this is an unusual occurrence, it illustrates that significant prostatic pathology can be present in a radiographically normal prostate gland and the utility of the urethrogram in establishing a correct diagnosis.

is a positive indication for prostatic biopsy. Such a finding also points out the difficulties likely to be encountered if resection of the disease is attempted.

A secondary benefit of the urethrogram is that it identifies the true location of the urinary bladder. In some instances, abdominal masses, such as an omental tumor and enlarged retained testicle, lie just cranial to the bladder. This positioning closely mimics the appearance of an enlarged prostate that is displacing the bladder cranially. Such tumors obviously present different clinical and diagnostic problems and should be handled accordingly.

Positive identification of the bladder and its position relative to the prostate also has definite benefits when the disease process does involve the prostate. It is not always obvious from survey radiographs or palpation what is prostate and what is bladder (see Fig. 42–4). This identification is necessary if a blind percutaneous aspirate or biopsy of the mass is to be attempted rather than a biopsy via laparotomy or with ultrasound guidance. By identifying the position of the bladder and urethra with a urethrogram, the chances of injury to the urinary tract during biopsy procedures are lessened.

Urethrography is easily performed in the male dog, and there are several methods that may be used (see Chapter 41).[35, 36] Urethrography often provides only indirect evidence of prostatic disease. If the urethra is deviated around a large

mass or does not pass directly through the center of the prostate, the disease within the prostate is asymmetric, such as a cyst. If the urethra passes directly through the middle of an enlarged prostate, the disease process is more likely to be diffuse throughout the gland, such as hypertrophy or prostatitis.

Direct signs of urethral disease of prostatic origin are urethral stricture, ulceration of the mucosa, and filling defects within the urethra. Ulceration or stricture of the prostatic urethra should be regarded as highly suggestive of neoplasia of the prostate.[6, 10]

Extravasation of contrast medium into the prostate should not be interpreted as abnormal as long as only the prostatic ducts fill with contrast medium (Fig. 42–16). This appearance is often seen in animals with a normal prostate.[37] Only if definite pooling of contrast medium within the prostate is seen should extravasation be considered abnormal (Fig. 42–17). Large, irregularly shaped cavities with rough walls that communicate with the urethra or cavitated smooth-walled lesions containing intraluminal masses are often associated with neoplasia; biopsy is then indicated (Fig. 42–18).[25, 33] Conversely, if extravasation does not occur, the prostate is not necessarily normal or solid. Many times, large cavitary lesions, such as cysts and abscesses, attain their size because they do not communicate with the urethra.[21, 23, 31] If these

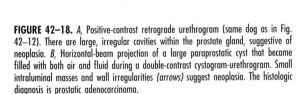

FIGURE 42–18. *A*, Positive-contrast retrograde urethrogram (same dog as in Fig. 42–12). There are large, irregular cavities within the prostate gland, suggestive of neoplasia. *B*, Horizontal-beam projection of a large paraprostatic cyst that became filled with both air and fluid during a double-contrast cystogram-urethrogram. Small intraluminal masses and wall irregularities *(arrows)* suggest neoplasia. The histologic diagnosis is prostatic adenocarcinoma.

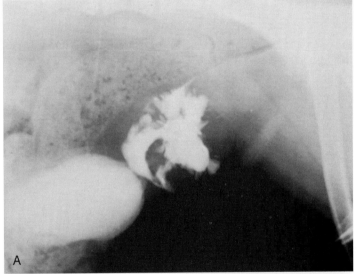

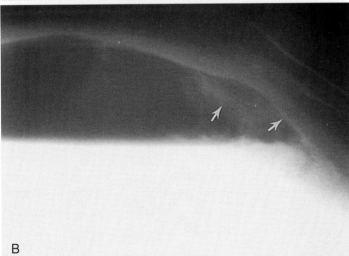

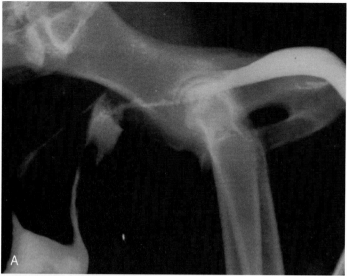

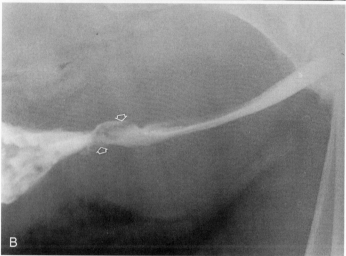

FIGURE 42–19. *A,* Positive-contrast urethrogram. There is marked irregularity of the prostatic urethral mucosa and vesicourethral junction. Such lesions may not be visible on a double-contrast cystogram, or the true extent of the lesion may be underestimated. Diagnosis was transitional cell carcinoma. *B,* Invasion of the urethra at the junction of the prostatic urethra and the urinary bladder by a prostatic carcinoma. Note the irregular filling defect within the urethra *(arrows)* delineated by the contrast medium. Such a lesion is not detectable on a routine double-contrast cystogram.

cavities do fill with contrast medium, they are usually ovoid, with smooth walls. The normal prostatic urethra as seen on the urethrogram has a smooth mucosal border. It is common to see a small filling defect in the dorsal wall of the urethra near the center of the prostate. This defect represents the colliculus seminalis and is a normal finding (see Fig. 42–16). In some dogs, there may also be a normal groove in the colliculus.

The point at which the prostatic urethra joins the trigone of the bladder should be carefully evaluated. It is possible to detect small filling defects or mucosal ulcers that may be early lesions of transitional cell carcinoma (Fig. 42–19). These small lesions may not be detected on a cystogram because they are obscured by the internal urethral sphincter, which is actually encircled by the prostate.[2]

References

1. Aumuller G, Stofft E, and Tunn U: Fine structure of the canine prostatic complex. Anat Embryol *160*:327, 1980.
2. Christensen GC: The reproductive organs. *In* Evans HE, Christensen GC (Eds): Miller's Anatomy of the Dog. Philadelphia, WB Saunders, 1979, pp 565–566.
3. Barsanti JA, and Finco DR: Canine bacterial prostatitis. Vet Clin North Am [Small Anim Pract] *9*:679, 1979.
4. Weaver AD: Prostatic disease in the dog. Vet Annu *20*:82, 1980.
5. James RW, and Heywood R: Age-related variations in the testes and prostate of Beagle dogs. Toxicology *12*:273, 1979.
6. Rogers KS, Wantschek L, and Lees GE: Diagnostic evaluation of the canine prostate. Comp Small Anim *8*:799, 1986.
7. O'Brien T: Normal radiographic anatomy of the abdomen. *In* Diagnosis of Abdominal Disorders in the Dog and Cat: Radiographic Interpretation, Clinical Signs, Pathophysiology. Philadelphia, WB Saunders, 1978, pp 9–47.
8. O'Shea JD: Studies on the canine prostate gland: I. Factors influencing its size and weight. J Comp Pathol *73*:321, 1962.
9. Juniewicz PE, Ewing LL, Dahnert WF, et al: Determination of canine prostatic size in situ: Comparison of direct caliper measurements with radiologic and transrectal ultrasonographic measurements. Prostate *14*:55, 1989.
10. Feeney DA, Johnston GR, Klausner JS, et al: Canine prostatic disease: Comparison of radiographic appearance with morphologic and microbiologic findings—30 cases (1981–1985). J Am Vet Med Assoc *190*:1018, 1987.
11. Price D: Comparative aspects of development and structure in the prostate. Natl Cancer Inst Monogr *12*:1, 1962.
12. Zontine WJ: Radiographic interpretation: The prostate gland. Mod Vet Pract *56*:341, 1975.
13. Finco DR: Diseases of the prostate gland of the dog. *In* Morrow DA (Ed): Current Therapy in Theriogenology. Philadelphia, WB Saunders, 1980, pp 654–661.
14. Gill CW: Prostatic adenocarcinoma with concurrent Sertoli tumor in a dog. Can Vet J *22*:230, 1981.
15. Klausner JS: Management of canine bacterial prostatitis. J Am Vet Med Assoc *182*:292, 1983.
16. Kornegay J: Canine prostatic disease. Southwestern Veterinarian *26*:257, 1973.
17. Metten S: A morphologic study of benign prostatic hypertrophy in the

dog. Doctoral dissertation. Fort Collins, CO, Department of Anatomy, Colorado State University, 1978.
18. Barsanti JA, Shotts EB Jr, Prasse K, et al: Evaluation of diagnostic techniques for canine prostate disease. J Am Vet Med Assoc 177:160, 1980.
19. Griener TP, and Johnson RG: Diseases of the prostate gland. In Ettinger SJ (Ed): Textbook of Veterinary Internal Medicine: Diseases of the Dog and Cat, 2nd Ed. Philadelphia, WB Saunders, 1983, pp 1459–1492.
20. Zolton GM, and Griener TP: Prostatic abscess: Surgical approach. J Am Anim Hosp Assoc 14:698, 1978.
21. Zolton GM: Surgical techniques for the prostate. Vet Clin North Am [Small Anim Pract] 9:349, 1979.
22. Rife J, and Thornburg LP: Osteocollagenous prostatic retention cyst in the canine. Canine Pract 7:44, 1980.
23. Weaver AD: Discrete prostatic (paraprostatic) cysts in the dog. Vet Rec 102:435, 1978.
24. O'Shea JD: Studies on the canine prostate gland: II. Prostatic neoplasms. J Comp Pathol 73:244, 1963.
25. Weaver AD: Fifteen cases of prostatic carcinoma in the dog. Vet Rec 109:71, 1981.
26. Grant CA: Carcinoma of the canine prostate. Acta Pathol Scand 40:197, 1957.
27. Rabut SM, and Kelch WJ: Undifferentiated carcinoma in the canine prostate. Mod Vet Pract 60:401, 1979.
28. Jameson RM: Prostatic abscess and carcinoma of the prostate. Br J Urol 40:288, 1968.
29. Leav I, and Ling GV: Adenocarcinoma of the canine prostate. Cancer 22:1329, 1968.
30. Rendano VT Jr, and Slauson DO: Hypertrophic osteopathy in a dog with prostate adenocarcinoma and without thoracic metastasis. J Am Anim Hosp Assoc 18:905, 1982.
31. Bortwiek R, and Mackenzie CP: The signs and results of treatment of prostatic disease in dogs. Vet Rec 89:374, 1971.
32. O'Brien T: Abdominal masses. In Diagnosis of Abdominal Disorders in the Dog and Cat: Radiographic Interpretation, Clinical Signs, Pathophysiology. Philadelphia, WB Saunders, 1978, pp 85–109.
33. McClain DL: Surgical treatment of perineal prostatic abscesses. J Am Anim Hosp Assoc 18:794, 1982.
34. Franks LM: The spread of prostatic carcinoma to the bones. J Pathol 66:91, 1953.
35. Root CA: Urethrography. In Ticer JW (Ed): Radiographic Techniques in Veterinary Practice, 2nd Ed. Philadelphia, WB Saunders, 1984, pp 387–394.
36. Johnston GR, Feeney DA, Osborne CA, et al: Effects of intravesical hydrostatic pressure and volume on the distensibility of the canine prostatic portion of the urethra. Am J Vet Res 46:748, 1985.
37. Ackerman N: Prostatic reflux during positive contrast retrograde urethrography in the dog. Vet Radiol 24:251, 1983.

STUDY QUESTIONS

1. Does the prostate become more or less prominent radiographically with age?

2. Enlargement of the prostate owing to benign prostatic hypertrophy usually results in cranial displacement of the bladder. What is the usual displacement seen with paraprostatic cysts?

3. Acute prostatitis classically results in a loss of distinction of the prostate silhouette. Why?

4. How can the route that the urethra takes passing through the prostate help in establishing the most likely diagnosis?

5. In Figure 42–3B, the appearance of a large air-filled cystic structure is suggestive of an abscess as a complicating factor to a prostatic cyst or neoplasm. Why?

6. See Figure 42–13. In addition to the cavitated areas in the prostate, there is another radiographic finding that is suggestive of neoplasia. What is it?

7. How does the periosteal reaction seen on the ventral aspect of the lumbar vertebrae in Figure 42–14 differ from spondylosis deformans?

8. What is the significance of fine linear air lucencies in the prostate when a double-contrast cystogram is performed?

9. What is the significance of a stricture of the prostatic urethra?

(Answers appear on pages 647 to 648.)

Chapter 43

The Uterus, Ovaries, and Testes

Daniel A. Feeney • Gary R. Johnston

IMAGING PROCEDURES

Uterus

The indications and limitations of abdominal radiography as they apply to specific uterine conditions have been described.[1–5] The major applications of survey radiographs to diseases of the uterus lie in confirming that a palpable abdominal mass is consistent with an enlarged uterus or in identifying an enlarged uterus in a bitch that is difficult to palpate. Other uses for survey radiographs include assessment for the purposes of determining (1) fetal skeletons (i.e., number, degree of mineralization); (2) progress in variations of uterine size both during pregnancy and in disease states such as pyometra; and (3) to a limited degree, fetal viability, based principally on the absence of findings consistent with fetal demise.

Adequate attention must be paid to technical procedures to ensure maximal radiographic contrast because the uterus in disease states and without the presence of skeletal structures must be differentiated from the bladder, bowel, and other nonspecific abdominal masses. Unless the patient is critically ill, ideal preparation includes withholding food for 24 hours and the administration of enemas to evacuate the colon at least 2 hours before radiography.[6] Radiographic technique is also important when the early mineralization of fetal skeletons is assessed because in the presence of a large uterus, early fetal mineralization may be masked by poor technique.

Abdominal compression has been suggested as a possible means by which the colon, uterus, and bladder may be differentiated radiographically.[6] The usefulness of this technique is basically limited to patients in which the uterus is not massively enlarged and can be aligned between the colon and urinary bladder by using a compression device—either a plastic paddle or a wooden kitchen spoon. An example of the type of separation that can be achieved is shown in Figure 43–1.

Ultrasonography is useful for the diagnosis of pregnancy in the bitch as well as for confirmation of fetal viability.[1, 5] It is also valuable in assessing a mildly enlarged uterus to determine whether the contents are fluid, as in pyometra; gestational sacs, indicative of pregnancy; or a mass, suggestive of neoplasia. Interested readers are directed to available literature on obstetric and gynecologic application of ultrasonography in small animals.[1, 2, 5, 7]

Ovary

Survey radiographs have limited applicability to the ovaries. Because these organs are the basis of reproduction, exposure to ionizing radiation should be minimized. The indications for radiographic examination of the ovaries have been defined elsewhere.[1, 2] The major application of survey radiographs to the ovary is that of identifying a mass not palpable at physical examination or further localizing an abdominal mass to the ovary. On the basis of location, displacement of adjacent organs, and radiographic opacity, the organ of origin of the mass may be determined.[6] Survey radiographs are of considerable value in differentiating ovarian, splenic, and renal masses. The limitations are that normal ovaries cannot be visualized and the internal architecture of ovarian masses cannot be assessed by radiography unless mineralization is present; such mineralization is uncommon.

Excretory urography may be of assistance in assessing ovarian masses by assisting in the identification of and distinction from the ipsilateral kidney. It may also be helpful to determine the degree of renal displacement and to separate renal parenchyma from that of the ovary if the mass has not resulted in ventral migration of the ovary into the conglomerate of small bowel away from the kidney.

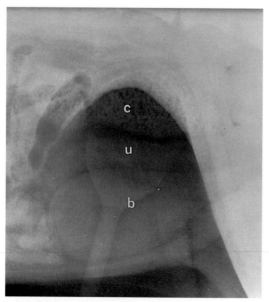

FIGURE 43–1. Lateral view of the caudal abdomen. Local compression was applied by using a wooden spoon during radiography. Note the separation of the colon (c), uterus (u), and urinary bladder (b).

Another technique that is extremely valuable in assessing intra-abdominal masses, including ovarian masses, is that of ultrasonography.[5, 7] Ultrasonographic techniques are useful in assessing general and follicular ovarian architecture that facilitates determining ovarian activity and staging of ovarian masses. Interested readers are directed to available literature on obstetric and gynecologic applications of ultrasonography in small animals.[1, 5, 7]

Testicle

Survey radiographs have limited applicability to the intrascrotal testes. Radiographs are, however, of value in the assessment of abdominal masses, which include neoplastic transformation of an intra-abdominal testicle. In addition, testicular exposure to the mutagenic effects of ionizing radiation should be limited. An additional method that does provide information on the intrascrotal and intra-abdominal testicular architecture is ultrasonography.[8] This technique is applicable to reproductive organs because as yet no major reproductive or genetic consequences have resulted from the use of the diagnostic technique. For a more extensive discussion of the role of ultrasonography in the diagnosis of testicular disease, the reader is referred to references 8 through 10.

NORMAL RADIOGRAPHIC FINDINGS

Uterus

Nonpregnant Animal

The normal uterus has a body and two horns and usually cannot be seen in the normal dog or cat unless it is enlarged by a pathologic process or pregnancy.[3] The normal uterus is tubular, about 1 cm in diameter, and located in the mid and caudal abdomen, with the uterine body between the colon and the bladder.[3] The radiopacity of the uterus is that of soft tissue, and it usually cannot be differentiated from small intestine on survey radiographs.

Pregnant Animal

The size, shape, and opacity of the canine uterus during pregnancy varies with the breed, the number of fetuses, and the stage of gestation. The fetal development and radiographic appearance of the uterus during gestation have been described in detail elsewhere,[4, 11, 12] but a brief summary follows. In general, uterine enlargement is detectable radiographically at approximately 30 days after ovulation.[4] The circumference of the uterine horns is then reported to be about 10 or 11 cm.[12] Spheric enlargements at the location of the gestational sacs are identifiable in the uterus between 30 and 40 days after ovulation.[4] The circumference at the spheric enlargement is then approximately 10 to 15 cm.[12] The uterus subsequently becomes smoothly tubular and has been described as sausage shaped at about 38 to 45 days after ovulation[4]; the circumference of the uterine horns is then approximately 12 to 17 cm.[12] Early fetal mineralization is identifiable by survey radiographs at or beyond 45 days after ovulation.[4] A near-term pregnancy in a normal bitch is shown radiographically in Figure 43–2.

The size, shape, and opacity of the feline uterus are similar to those of the dog. The feline uterus during gestation is described in considerable detail elsewhere,[13] but a brief summary follows. In the pregnant cat, radiographically detectable uterine enlargement occurs at approximately 25 to 35 days

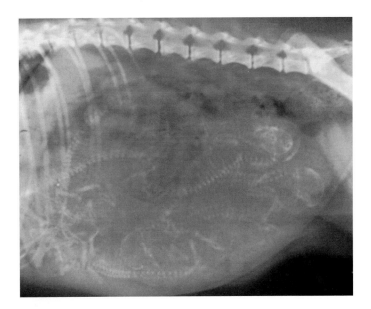

FIGURE 43–2. A normal pregnancy, near term, in a bitch (lateral view). Note the mineralization and alignment of the skull bones as well as the arrangement of the cervical through lumbar vertebrae and the pelvis with the appendages.

of gestation. Fetal mineralization is identified at approximately 36 to 45 days of gestation and progresses beyond this time.

The location of the pregnant uterus in both the dog and the cat is in the mid to caudal ventral abdomen at mid to late gestation. The enlargement of the uterus at this site causes cranial and somewhat dorsal displacement of the small intestine, with dorsal and lateral displacement of the descending colon and some degree of ventral compression of the urinary bladder.[6]

Ovary

The normal ovaries, located just caudal to the kidneys, are not seen radiographically.[5, 6] The ovaries are not, however, functionally retroperitoneal as are the kidneys, and ovarian masses gravitate ventrally without extensive ventral displacement of other abdominal viscera, such as that caused by a renal mass.[14]

Testes

Because the testicles, epididymis, and scrotum are all soft-tissue structures, radiography is of minimal value in the evaluation of these organs in small animals. The accessibility of the scrotum to visual and digital inspection further minimizes the usefulness of radiography. Radiography may occasionally provide some information on the opacity (such as mineral and air) of an abnormality detected by palpation. Ultrasonography is of assistance in noninvasively assessing the internal architecture of the testicle and epididymis as well as the nature of scrotal enlargement.[8–10]

ABNORMAL RADIOGRAPHIC FINDINGS

Uterus

Number

Absence of one of the horns in a normally bicornuate uterus has been reported,[15] but this is rare.

Size

Generalized uterine enlargement in the absence of fetal mineralization may be suggestive of a number of diseases in addition to the early phases of normal pregnancy before fetal mineralization. Differential diagnoses that should be considered under these circumstances include early pregnancy and possibly pseudopregnancy[3–6, 14, 16]; pyometra, hydrometra, and mucometra[3–6, 14, 16, 17]; uterine torsion[18, 19]; and uterine adenomyosis.[20] Representative examples of diffuse uterine enlargement are shown in Figure 43–3.

Generalized uterine enlargement in the presence of fetal mineralization is suggestive of pregnancy, but the possibility of torsion of the pregnant uterus should not be excluded. Clinical signs and history must then be used to differentiate these possibilities.

Localized uterine enlargement may be suggestive of a number of diseases, including neoplasia[3, 21]; cystic endometrial hyperplasia[2, 21]; localized or loculated pyometra, hydrometra, or mucometra[17]; uterine stump granuloma or abscess[5, 22]; cystic uterine remnant[23]; and uterine adenomyosis.[20] Focal uterine body enlargement confirmed as a uterine stump granuloma with urinary bladder invasion and a fistulous tract draining into the flank are shown in Figure 43–4.

Location

The normal location of the uterus in the caudal ventral midabdomen has been discussed, and its detection as well as location and effect on adjacent organs is highly dependent on its size.[3, 6] Herniation of the uterus through discontinuities in the abdominal wall, including the inguinal ring, may occur and may be congenital or acquired.[3, 5] It is also possible that these herniations may occur during pregnancy. An example of uterine herniation into the subcutaneous tissues via the inguinal canal is shown in Figure 43–5. This uterus was in the stages of gestation before fetal mineralization.

Radiopacity

The normal nonpregnant and early pregnant uterus are of soft-tissue or fluid radiopacity.[3–6, 11–13] Other uterine conditions that also have soft-tissue radiographic characteristics are pyometra, hydrometra, mucometra, and uterine torsion.[3–6, 14, 16–19] As previously mentioned, history and clinical signs are

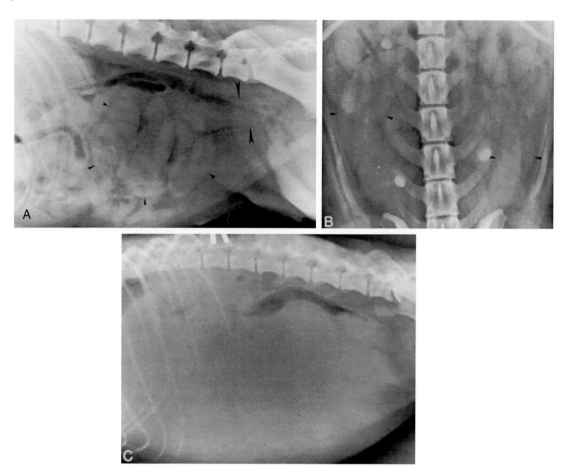

FIGURE 43–3. Lateral *(A)* and ventrodorsal *(B)* radiographs of a patient with a tubular, coiled, soft-tissue structure in the caudal abdomen that extends into the pelvis *(arrowheads)*. This structure is a moderately distended uterus, as found in pyometra. *C,* Lateral view of a patient with a caudoventral abdominal mass that occupies about 60 percent of the abdominal cavity. Displacement of the viscera is consistent with uterine enlargement.

necessary to differentiate these possibilities. Gas within the uterus is generally indicative of either fetal death[3, 5] or ischemia owing to uterine torsion.[18, 19] In both instances, the gas is due to devitalization and breakdown of the tissues. An example of an emphysematous fetus is shown in Figure 43–6. The clinician should be careful that there have been no traumatic attempts at catheterization of the cervix wherein gas could have artifactually been introduced and overinterpreted as evidence of intrauterine disease. The other possibility is that a gas-forming organism within an abscess of the

uterine stump in the neutered patient may cause focal accumulation of air, but this is highly unlikely.[6, 22]

Mineralization within the uterus is usually indicative of fetal skeletons, but it is imperative that the alignment of the structures, such as vertebrae, ribs, and limbs, and the shape and alignment of skull bones be assessed to differentiate a radiographically viable fetus, a dead fetus, and a mummified fetus.[3, 4] In general, radiographic evidence of axial or appendicular skeletal malalignment or collapse of the skull bones is suggestive of fetal death. Overlap and apparent compres-

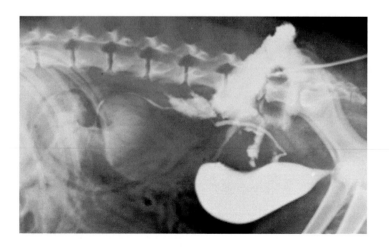

FIGURE 43–4. Lateral view after excretory urography and left flank fistulography. A draining tract in the left flank injected with contrast medium leads to a soft-tissue mass, which displaces the urinary bladder ventrally and indents it dorsally. Only the right kidney and ureter may be identified. Radiologic diagnosis was probable uterine stump granuloma with chronic obstruction of the left ureter. The diagnosis was confirmed at laparotomy.

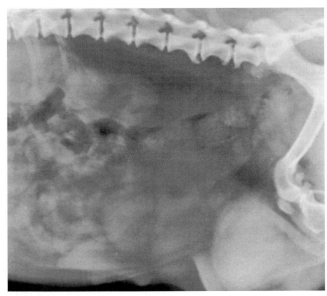

FIGURE 43–5. Lateral view of a bitch in midterm pregnancy with an inguinal mass. The tubular soft-tissue opacity representing the uterus extends into the subcutaneous peri-inguinal tissues. Radiologic diagnosis was inguinal hernia containing a portion of dilated uterus, probably secondary to pregnancy.

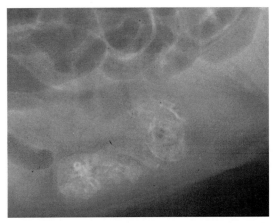

FIGURE 43–7. Lateral view of a previously pregnant bitch. An irregularly mineralized mass with some evidence of skull and tubular bones may be identified and is located outside the intestinal tract and in a region consistent with that of the uterus. Radiologic diagnosis was mummified fetus. The diagnosis was confirmed at surgery.

sion of the structures into a smaller than expected space is more suggestive of mummification than a recent history of fetal death. An example of a mummified fetus is shown in Figure 43–7.

If the fetal skeleton appears to be tightly curled, more obvious than expected than when surrounded by the uterus, or not associated with a tubular uterine radiopacity or its expected location, the possibility of ectopic pregnancy should be considered.[24–26] Peritoneal effusion may complicate the assessment of the uterine boundaries in these patients and may further confuse the diagnosis with the possibility of acute uterine rupture rather than ectopic pregnancy.[24–26] Ultrasonography is of value in this situation.[1, 5, 7]

Function

Dystocia may be due to both maternal and fetal factors.[27] Radiographs are of minimal value in determining the maternal factors, such as uterine contractility, other than assessment of the size relationship between the fetus and the maternal pelvic canal. Radiography may be helpful in assessing one of the fetal factors, positioning relative to the maternal pelvic canal, thus providing additional evidence for the necessity of cesarean section (Fig. 43–8). If there is no fetus lodged in the birth canal, another consideration is uterine inertia. Survey radiographs may also be of value in the postpartum bitch to determine the possibility of a retained fetus, but routine follow-up radiography of every pregnancy is not indicated.

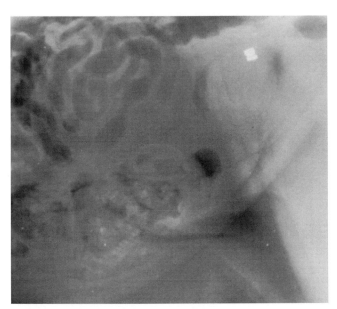

FIGURE 43–6. Close-up lateral view of the ventral abdomen. There is a moderately mineralized fetus within the soft-tissue uterine shadow. Gas, however, surrounds the fetus. Radiologic diagnosis was emphysematous fetus.

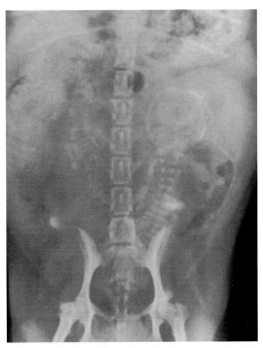

FIGURE 43–8. Ventrodorsal view of a small-breed bitch in dystocia. Note the transverse presentation of the enlarged, but as determined radiographically, viable fetus. Surgical diagnosis was viable single fetus, which subsequently died.

Ovary

Number

Usually only one, but occasionally both, ovaries may be radiographically abnormal. In the authors' opinion, the ovary must increase in size to at least the diameter of two bowel loops to be identifiable on survey radiographs. The shape of the abnormal ovary may be variable, but ovarian masses are usually well circumscribed.[6, 14] If the ovarian mass is neoplastic, peritoneal fluid may also be present.

Size

A radiographically detectable mass in the appropriate anatomic region for the ovary, which is usually caudal to the respective kidney and originating from the dorsal abdominal wall, should have certain differential considerations: follicular cyst,[28] luteal cyst,[28] tumors of gonadostromal origin,[28, 29] tumors of epithelial origin,[28, 29] germ cell tumors (see section on radiopacity),[29, 30] tumors of mesodermal origin,[29, 30] and hydrovarium.[31] An example of a well-circumscribed ovarian mass is shown in Figure 43–9.

Location

The normal ovaries lie caudal to their respective kidneys. As ovaries enlarge, they may displace the ipsilateral kidney cranially or laterally and may pull it ventrally. The degree and direction of adjacent organ displacement and the extent of ovarian mass migration depend on ovarian size and the position of the patient during radiography. Abdominal viscera other than those described specifically in the previous section may be displaced. For a more extensive discussion of the evaluation of ovarian masses, the reader is directed to the article by Root.[14]

Radiopacity

Ovarian cysts and most ovarian neoplasms are of soft-tissue opacity.[5, 28, 33] Occasionally, ovarian neoplasms may contain mineralized areas, including those with the opacity of bone or tooth enamel. Such masses are usually benign teratomas (dermoid cyst),[28, 29] but malignant teratocarcinomas have also been reported to contain mineralization.[32] On the basis of this assessment and the vast difference in prognosis for these two types of tumors, it is ill advised to base prognosis on the presence of mineralization.

Consideration

It is important to be aware of the possibility of intersex conditions, including the true hermaphrodite and pseudohermaphrodite.[34, 35] Complex anomalies encompassing the entire genital tract and involving the urinary tract should be considered in patients with other intra-abdominal abnormalities or combined urinary and reproductive signs. Although contrast radiographic procedures and ultrasonographic evaluation may be of assistance in analyzing the anomaly, it is often necessary to remove the anomalous tissue and then to evaluate it by dissection and histologic examination.[5, 7]

Testicle

Detailed discussion of the embryogenesis of the testes, gubernaculum, and scrotum is beyond the scope of this book; for further details, the reader should consult references 36 and 37. As with ovarian diseases, intersex anomalies must be considered. These anomalies may be evaluated with the use of contrast procedures of the lower and upper urinary tract as well as with ultrasonography, although the final diagnosis is usually determined surgically and microscopically.[34, 35] With

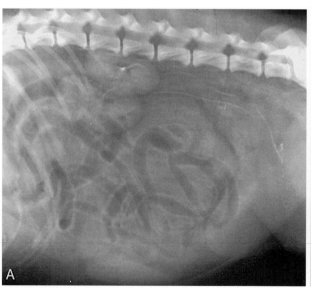
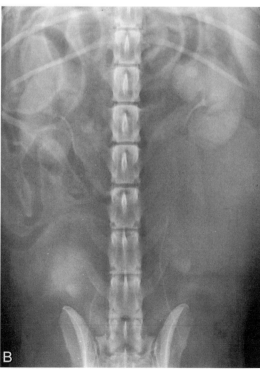

FIGURE 43–9. Lateral *(A)* and ventrodorsal *(B)* views of a patient with a soft-tissue abdominal mass approximately four times the size of the left kidney and located caudal and ventral to it. The mass is not seen clearly in the lateral view but is causing deformation of the dorsal and cranial aspects of the bladder by compression. Kidneys are opacified secondary to the injection of contrast medium. The location of the soft-tissue mass is consistent with a mass arising from the ovary. Diagnosis was ovarian cyst (at surgery).

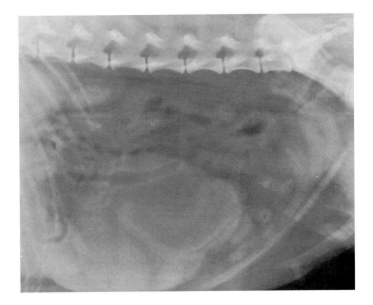

FIGURE 43–10. Lateral radiograph of a male dog with an abdominal mass and only one palpable descended testicle. The abdominal mass in the caudal midventral abdomen is approximately four to six times the size of the kidneys. Radiographic diagnosis was well-circumscribed intra-abdominal mass, probably a retained intra-abdominal testicle. The diagnosis was confirmed at laparotomy.

this preface, most of the following discussion deals with sequelae of cryptorchidism amenable to radiographic assessment.

Intra-abdominal testicles that are of normal dimension usually cannot be identified radiographically. If the intra-abdominal testicle enlarges, however, the following considerations may apply.

Size and Shape

To be detected radiographically, the enlarged intra-abdominal testicle must be two or more times the diameter of the normal small intestine. When such a structure is identified, it must also be differentiated from other soft-tissue structures in the abdomen, such as fluid-filled bowel, bladder, spleen, and possibly the prostate gland. In general, the radiologic consideration of the mass as an intra-abdominal testicle is either by knowledge that only one testicle was descended or identified at castration or by the fact that the mass cannot be associated with any other organ in a male patient. The shape of the enlarged, and probably neoplastically transformed, intra-abdominal testicle is usually fairly symmetric with varying degrees of surface irregularity.

Number and Radiopacity

Usually, only one of the testicles is responsible for the abdominal abnormalities in a given patient, even if both testicles are intra-abdominal. The radiographic opacity of intra-abdominal testicles is usually that of soft tissue, and no specificity may be assigned to the identification of calcific opacity within these masses; such an opacity is most likely to be dystrophic calcification rather than suggestive of teratoma and teratocarcinoma, as in the bitch.

Location

Intra-abdominal testicles, when identified radiographically as an abdominal mass, usually lie somewhere in a parasagittal plane between the caudal pole of the ipsilateral kidney and the inguinal canal. The authors' experience suggests these testicles usually gravitate to the ventral abdomen as they enlarge, causing dorsal and lateral displacement of the small intestine and possible indentation or caudal displacement of the urinary bladder. An example of a neoplastically trans-

formed intra-abdominal testicle is shown in Figure 43–10. Testicles may be identified in the inguinal canal or subcutaneous structures of the inguinal region. Subcutaneous soft-tissue masses in this region in a male dog may be identified radiographically, but differentiation from lymph node, subcutaneous tumor, or another nonspecific mass requires ultrasonographic assessment and probable microscopic examination of a fine-needle aspirate. An example of an enlarged, neoplastically transformed inguinal testicle is shown in Figure 43–11.

Consideration

An intra-abdominal mass identified in a male dog fitting the size, shape, and location criteria described earlier must be differentiated from other intra-abdominal organs, including

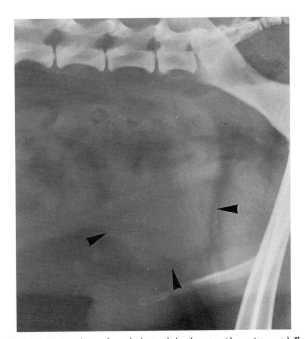

FIGURE 43–11. Lateral view of a male dog in which only one testicle was intrascrotal. There is an ovoid soft-tissue mass *(arrowheads)* in the peri-inguinal soft tissues in the region of the os penis. Surgical diagnosis was malignant transformation of an incompletely descended testicle.

the spleen, bladder, cecum, and prostate gland; a nonspecific mesenteric mass; and a mass originating within the intestinal tract. Ultrasonographic examination can be valuable in this differentiation.[10] Fine-needle aspiration biopsy and laparotomy are the alternatives worthy of consideration.

The mass, which is possibly testicle, may represent a neoplastically transformed, retained testicle[29] or torsion of an intra-abdominal testicle without neoplastic transformation.[38, 39] Differentiation between these processes is based on the history, abdominal palpation, and reproductive and cutaneous manifestations of endocrine abnormalities (i.e., feminization) associated with neoplastic testicular tissue.

Intrascrotal Testicle

Size and shape are the major features used to assess the intrascrotal testicle for potential abnormalities. Symmetric enlargement of the testicle or hemiscrotum is suggestive of orchitis,[40] hydrocele,[8, 40] intrascrotal testicular torsion,[38, 40] and nonspecific vascular abnormalities.[40] Observation of the testicular mass and spermatic cord at scrotal exploratory surgery is the most definitive means of differentiation among the scrotal contents and is not associated with the known genetic sequelae of ionizing radiation to the opposite testicle. Asymmetric enlargement of the intrascrotal testicle is suggestive of neoplasia,[29, 41, 42] varicocele,[8, 10] hematoma, abscess, and epididymitis[40]; differentiation of these possibilities may be facilitated by information from the history and fine-needle aspiration biopsy.

As mentioned previously, an additional means of assessing the internal contents of the scrotum, including the testicle, is ultrasonography.[8–10] This method permits identification of the source of scrotal enlargement as to testicle, fluid retention, associated mass, and, if the testicle is the site of enlargement, the internal architecture of the mass.

RELATED ABNORMAL INTRA-ABDOMINAL FINDINGS

Unexplained intra-abdominal calcific opacities may be related to previous uterine rupture or ectopic pregnancy and subsequent mummification of the involved fetuses. Careful radiographic scrutiny of the character of the calcified intra-abdominal masses and the possible use of serial radiographs to assess reproducibility of the location are indicated. Occasionally, ingestion of an intact body of a puppy or other small animal may complicate the differentiation of intrauterine fetal calcification or mummification and intra-abdominal ectopic pregnancy or fetal mummification from the ingested body of a fetus or other similar-sized animal.

Variations in abdominal contrast may be somewhat nonspecific in that there are numerous causes of accumulation of abdominal fluid and free intraperitoneal air. The presence of abdominal fluid, however, especially if the patient has intestinal displacement (based on intestine containing gas so it can be recognized) consistent with an enlarged uterus, may be suggestive of uterine rupture with subsequent hemorrhage, ruptured pyometra, or hemorrhage from uterine torsion. Free intraperitoneal air in such patients, especially in the presence of intrauterine (perifetal) or intrafetal air, is highly suggestive of uterine rupture and fetal death.

Peritoneal effusion, which may occur from a wide variety of causes, may result from peritoneal seeding and diffuse metastasis of malignant ovarian tumors or hemorrhage owing to rupture of an ovarian tumor.[33] Although ovarian tumors are less often the cause of malignant effusion, abdominal hemorrhage, or both, these lesions should at least be considered as differential possibilities in an intact bitch.

Medial iliac lymphadenopathy may be identified in patients with testicular disease and is most suggestive of metastasis[10, 42] or extension of an inflammatory process. Lumbar vertebral osteomyelitis and discospondylitis have been reported in patients with inflammatory diseases of the testicle, including, specifically, infection caused by *Brucella canis*.[43]

Although this chapter has emphasized survey radiographic findings, ultrasonography may play a major role as a noninvasive diagnostic technique. When access to such techniques is afforded to the clinician, the potential usefulness of this procedure should be considered.[1, 5, 7–10]

References

1. England G: Infertility in the bitch and queen. *In* Authur GH, Noakes DE, Pearson H, et al (Eds): Veterinary Reproduction and Obstetrics, 7th Ed. Philadelphia, WB Saunders, 1996, pp 516–548.
2. Morrow DA: Current Therapy in Theriogenology. Philadelphia, WB Saunders, 1986.
3. Ackerman N: Radiographic evaluation of the uterus: A review. Vet Radiol 22:252, 1981.
4. Rendano VJ: Radiographic evaluation of fetal development in the bitch and fetal death in the bitch and the queen. *In* Kirk RW (Ed): Current Veterinary Therapy VIII. Philadelphia, WB Saunders, 1983, pp 947–952.
5. Rivers B, and Johnston GR: Imaging of the reproductive organs of the bitch: Methods and limitations. Vet Clin North Am [Small Anim Pract] 21:437, 1991.
6. Root CN: Interpretation of abdominal survey radiographs. Vet Clin North Am 4:763, 1974.
7. Poffenbarger EM, and Feeney DA: Use of gray-scale ultrasonography in the diagnosis of reproductive disease in the bitch: 18 cases 1981–1984. J Am Vet Med Assoc 189:90, 1986.
8. Pugh CR, Konde LJ, and Park RD: Testicular ultrasound in the normal dog. Vet Radiol 31:195, 1990.
9. Parkinson TJ: Fertility and infertility in male animals. *In* Authur GH, Noakes DE, Pearson H, et al (Eds): Veterinary Reproduction and Obstetrics, 7th Ed. Philadelphia, WB Saunders, 1996, pp 572–633.
10. Johnston GR, Feeney DA, Rivers B, et al: Diagnostic imaging of the male canine reproductive organs: Methods and limitations. Vet Clin North Am [Small Anim Pract] 21:553, 1991.
11. Noakes DE: Pregnancy and its diagnosis. *In* Authur GH, Noakes DE, Pearson H, et al (Eds): Veterinary Reproduction and Obstetrics, 7th Ed. Philadelphia, WB Saunders, 1996, pp 63–109.
12. Tsutsui T: Process of development of uterus, fetus, and fetal appendices during pregnancy in the dog. Bull Nippon Vet Zootech Coll 30:175, 1981.
13. Boyd JS: Radiographic identification of the various stages of pregnancy in the domestic cat. J Small Anim Pract 12:501, 1971.
14. Root CR: Abdominal masses: The radiographic differential diagnosis. J Am Vet Radiol Soc 15:26, 1974.
15. Robinson GW: Uterus unicornis and unilateral renal agenesis in a cat. J Am Vet Med Assoc 147:516, 1965.
16. Stein BS: Obstetrics, surgical procedures and anesthesia. *In* Morrow DA (Ed): Current Therapy in Theriogenology. Philadelphia, WB Saunders, 1980, pp 865–869.
17. McAfee CT: Hydrouterus and hydroovarium in a Beagle bitch. Canine Pract 4:48, 1977.
18. Shull RM, Johnston SD, Johnston GR, et al: Bilateral torsion of uterine horns in a nongravid bitch. J Am Vet Med Assoc 172:601, 1978.
19. Freeman LJ: Feline uterine torsion. Comp Contin Ed Vet Pract 10:1078, 1988.
20. Pack FD: Feline uterine adenomyosis. Feline Pract 10:45, 1980.
21. Brodey RS, and Roszel JF: Neoplasms of the canine uterus, vagina, and vulva. A clinicopathologic survey. J Am Vet Med Assoc 151:1294, 1967.
22. Spackman CJA, Caywood DD, Johnston GR, et al: Granulomas of the uterine and ovarian stumps: A case report. J Am Anim Hosp Assoc 20:449, 1984.
23. Franklin RT, and Prescott JVB: Tenesmus and stranguria from a cystic uterine remnant. Vet Radiol 24:139, 1983.
24. Carrig CB, Gourley IM, and Philbrick AL: Primary abdominal pregnancy in a cat subsequent to OHE. J Am Vet Med Assoc 160:308, 1972.
25. Tomlinson J, Jackson ML, and Pharr JW: Extrauterine pregnancy in a cat. Feline Pract 10:18, 1980.
26. DeNooy PP: Extrauterine pregnancy and severe ascites in a cat. Vet Med [Small Anim Clin] 74:349, 1979.
27. Bennett D: Canine dystocia—a review of the literature. J Small Anim Pract 15:101, 1974.
28. Dow C: Ovarian abnormalities in the bitch. J Comp Pathol 70:59, 1960.
29. Barrett RE, and Theiler LH: Neoplasms of the canine and feline reproductive tracts. *In* Kirk RW (Ed): Current Veterinary Therapy VI. Philadelphia, WB Saunders, 1977, pp 1263–1267.

30. Riser WH, Marcus JF, Gaibor EC, et al: Dermoid cyst of the canine ovary. J Am Vet Med Assoc 134:27, 1959.
31. McAfee LT: Hydroureters and hydrovarium in a Beagle bitch. Canine Pract 4:48, 1977.
32. Patnaik AK, Schaer M, Parks JL, et al: Metastasizing ovarian teratocarcinoma in dogs. J Small Anim Pract 17:235, 1976.
33. Greene JA, Richardson RP, Thornhill JA, et al: Ovarian papillary cystadenoma in a bitch. J Am Anim Hosp Assoc 15:351, 1979.
34. Murti GS, Gilbert DL, and Bougmann AP: Canine intersex states. J Am Vet Med Assoc 149:1183, 1966.
35. Todoroff RJ: Canine urogenital anomalies. Comp Contin Ed Small Anim Pract 1:780, 1979.
36. Wensing CJ: Developmental anomalies, including cryptorchidism. In Morrow DA (Ed): Current Therapy in Theriogenology. Philadelphia, WB Saunders, 1980, pp 583–589.
37. Bauran V, Dijkstra F, and Wensing CJ: Testicular descent in the dog. Anat Histol Embryol 10:97, 1981.
38. Pearson A, and Relly DF: Testicular torsion in the dog: A review of 13 cases. Vet Rec 97:200, 1975.
39. Naylor RW, and Thompson SMR: Intra-abdominal testicular torsion—a report of 2 cases. J Am Anim Hosp Assoc 15:763, 1979.
40. Leio DH: Canine orchitis. In Kirk RA (Ed): Current Veterinary Therapy VI. Philadelphia, WB Saunders, 1977, pp 1255–1259.
41. McNeil PE, and Weaver AD: Massive scrotal swelling in two unusual cases of canine sertoli cell tumor. Vet Rec 106:144, 1980.
42. Simon J, and Rubin SB: Metastatic seminoma in a dog. Vet Med [Small Anim Clin] 74:941, 1979.
43. Henderson RA, Hoerline BF, Kramer TT, et al: Discospondylitis in three dogs infected with Brucella canis. J Am Vet Med Assoc 165:451, 1974.

STUDY QUESTIONS

1. The normal uterine body in a nulliparous bitch is:
   A. Easily detectable on routine survey radiographs.
   B. Is difficult or impossible to detect on routine survey radiographs.
   C. Usually lies between the distal colon and the urinary bladder near the midline.
   D. Usually lies between the urinary bladder and the rectus abdominis muscle on the midline.
   E. B and C.

2. The uterine horns in a bitch may:
   A. Be indistinguishable from the small intestine, if normal.
   B. Sometimes be distinguishable from the small intestine if only mildly enlarged, provided that the small intestine contains gas.
   C. Displace the kidneys cranially because both the uterine horns and the kidneys are retroperitoneal.
   D. A and B.
   E. A, B, and C.

3. Gas in the uterus can be the result of:
   A. Fetal demise.
   B. Uterine ischemia.
   C. Vaginitis.
   D. Intrauterine fetal growth retardation.
   E. A and B.

4. Which of the following survey radiographic findings are indications of late term fetal death?
   A. Malalignment of fetal structures.
   B. Collapse of the fetal skull.
   C. Tightly curled fetus.
   D. Emphysematous fetus.
   E. All of the above.

5. Which of the causes of dystocia listed can be diagnosed from survey radiographs?
   A. Uterine inertia.
   B. Fetus too large for maternal pelvic canal.
   C. Fetus lodged in the maternal pelvic canal.
   D. Fetus in a position such that it is blocking the entrance to (or unlikely to pass through) the maternal pelvic canal.
   E. B, C, and D.

6. An ovarian mass can:
   A. Displace the bowel, particularly the colon, ventrally as can be seen with retroperitoneal masses originating in the kidney.
   B. Migrate ventrally among the small intestinal loops, if enlarged.
   C. May induce peritoneal fluid, if malignant and there has been peritoneal seeding.
   D. A, B, and C.
   E. B and C.

7. Mineralization of an ovarian mass as detected by survey radiography:
   A. Is useful to differentiate malignant from benign masses because only benign masses undergo mineralization.
   B. Is useful to differentiate malignant from benign masses because only malignant masses undergo mineralization.
   C. Eliminates consideration of an ovarian cyst because benign ovarian cysts never undergo mineralization.
   D. A and C.
   E. None of the above.

8. Intra-abdominal testes:
   A. Are readily detected on survey radiographs, even if not enlarged.
   B. Are difficult to impossible to detect on survey radiographs, unless quite enlarged.
   C. Have a radiographically specific appearance when enlarged and can be easily differentiated from masses originating in the bowel, mesentery, or abdominal wall.
   D. A and C.
   E. B and C.

9. Acute testicular torsion:
   A. Is readily diagnosed on survey radiographs because of gas in the scrotum.
   B. Is readily diagnosed on survey radiographs because of mineralization in the scrotum.
   C. Is readily differentiated from other intrascrotal problems such as hydrocele or mass using survey radiographs.
   D. Cannot be diagnosed by survey radiographs and is best defined using a combination of acute history of pain, symmetric testicular enlargement at palpation, and, if available, Doppler ultrasonography to assess blood flow.
   E. A and C.

10. The normal ovary:
    A. Can have mineralization detectable on survey radiographs.
    B. Can be determined as to its phase in the estrous cycle using survey radiographic techniques.
    C. Can be easily identified on survey radiographs and can be readily differentiated from the small intestine.
    D. A, B, and C.
    E. None of the above.

(Answers appear on page 648.)

Chapter 44

The Stomach

Don L. Barber • Mary B. Mahaffey

ANATOMY

The stomach is a musculoglandular organ that connects the esophagus and duodenum. The cranial surface of the stomach is in close apposition to the caudal surface of the liver. In the normal dog and cat, the empty stomach usually lies cranial to the last pair of ribs,[1, 2] but it may extend slightly caudal to the costal arch. The stomach lies in a transverse plane, primarily to the left of the median plane.

The stomach is subdivided into the cardia, fundus, body, and pyloric portions (Fig. 44–1).[1] The cardia is a small area at the esophagogastric junction. The fundus is the dome or outpouching from the left dorsal aspect of the stomach. The body is the middle portion from the fundus to the pyloric portion and is the largest portion of the stomach. The distal one third of the stomach is the pyloric portion, which is further subdivided into the pyloric antrum and the pyloric canal. The pyloric antrum is the proximal two thirds of the pyloric portion and is relatively thin walled and slightly expanded. The pyloric canal, the distal one third of the pyloric portion, is more muscular and contains a double sphincter.

Additional landmarks of the stomach include the greater and lesser curvatures and the angular incisure (notch).[1] The greater curvature is the convex surface of the stomach that originates at the cardia and extends caudoventrally around to the pylorus. The lesser curvature is the concave surface that originates to the right of the cardia and extends cranioventrally to the pylorus. It is the shortest distance between the cardia and the pylorus. The angular notch is the point of acute angulation of the lesser curvature, located approximately at the junction of the body and the pyloric antrum. The mucosal surface of the stomach is characterized by numerous folds or ridges called *rugal folds* or *rugae*.

RADIOGRAPHIC EXAMINATION

Preparation

Ingesta within the stomach may obscure some lesions or simulate other lesions and thus create false-negative or false-positive results. Therefore, under ideal conditions, routine radiographic examination of the stomach should be performed on an animal that has been fasted for 12 to 24 hours.[3, 4] Nonirritating cleansing enemas may also be useful. This method of preparation allows for more accurate evaluation of the stomach and for contrast studies if needed. Fasting is not feasible in many situations, however, and the inability to fast the patient is not a contraindication for abdominal radiography. Additionally, there are exceptions to fasting because patients with emesis or anorexia may not require fasting. Also, fasting and enemas should be avoided in patients with acute abdominal disorders in which time delays are medically contraindicated or fluid and gas patterns in the bowel may be of diagnostic importance.

A consideration of medications is also important. Many drugs used for treatment of gastrointestinal disorders or for chemical restraint affect gastric motility and the radiographic appearance of the stomach, and these preparations should be avoided or discontinued for an appropriate interval before any contrast study.[5–7]

Radiographic Technique

Survey radiographs may be sufficient to diagnose some gastric abnormalities. If contrast studies are deemed necessary, survey radiography of the stomach should always precede contrast studies. Various radiographic techniques are available and include conventional barium sulfate gastrography, low-volume gastrography, double-contrast gastrography, pneumogastrography, gastrography using iodinated contrast media, and gastric emptying studies using barium-food mixtures.[2, 3, 5, 8–16]

In veterinary medicine, most radiographs are made with overhead x-ray tubes. Fluoroscopy is a valuable tool for evaluation of the stomach because it allows dynamic visualization of stomach function. Because the stomach frequently undergoes cyclic changes in appearance and anatomic changes characteristic of a particular disease may not be continuously present, fluoroscopy is a valuable tool in evaluating some diseases of the stomach.

For complete evaluation of the stomach, four conventional views may be necessary: the ventrodorsal view with the animal in dorsal recumbency, the dorsoventral view with the animal in ventral recumbency, the right recumbent lateral view, and the left recumbent lateral view. Oblique views may occasionally be of value to isolate or project certain areas of the stomach, such as the pylorus.

NORMAL RADIOGRAPHIC FINDINGS

The radiographic appearance of the normal stomach is variable and depends on many factors, such as the species, breed, degree of gastric distention, volume and type of gastric content, position of the patient during radiography, and whether contrast medium was used.

The stomach is usually easy to recognize by its location and shape and the content of gas, ingesta, or both. The entire

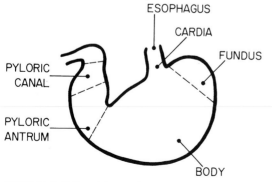

FIGURE 44–1. Divisions of the stomach.

stomach may not be discernible on survey radiographs if it is empty or if the gastric fluid content silhouettes with the liver or other abdominal structures. As a general guide, on the lateral view, the axis of the stomach from the fundus through the body and pylorus is perpendicular to the spine, parallel to the ribs, or somewhere between these angles (Fig. 44–2A). On the lateral view, the pylorus may be superimposed over the body or located slightly cranial to the body. On the ventrodorsal view of the dog, the cardia, fundus, and body of the stomach are located to the left of midline, and the pyloric portions are located to the right of midline. The pyloric sphincter is usually located in the right cranial abdominal quadrant at about the level of the 10th or 11th ribs and is usually cranial to the pyloric canal.[2] In immature dogs, the pylorus may be located closer to midline than in adults.[8]

The long axis of the stomach may be perpendicular to the spine with the stomach appearing to run transversely across the abdomen, making the angular notch difficult to identify (see Fig. 44–2B). The stomach may also have a U-shaped appearance with a more obvious angular notch and still be within its normal location (see Fig. 44–2C). On the ventrodorsal view of the cat, the stomach is more acutely angled with the pylorus located at or near the midline (see Fig. 44–2D). Variations in the appearance of the stomach in the

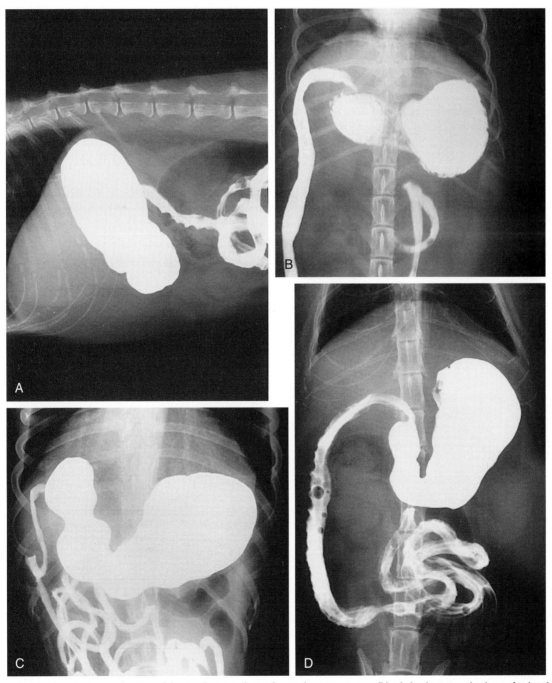

FIGURE 44–2. Gastrograms demonstrating normal positions of the stomach. *A,* Lateral view of a cat. The gastric axis is parallel with the ribs. *B,* Ventrodorsal view of a dog. The gastric axis of this dog is perpendicular to the spine. *C,* Ventrodorsal view of a dog. The stomach is U shaped, and the pyloric sphincter and fundus are normally located. *D,* Ventrodorsal view of a cat. The stomach is acutely angled, with the pylorus located at midline.

dog based on the shape of the thorax and cranial abdomen, that is, breed conformation, have been described.[2] The actual shape of the stomach also varies with the degree of gastric distention because different portions of the stomach vary in their distensibility.

One of the most important factors in the appearance of the stomach is the position of the patient during radiography.[17] The relationship between the position of the patient and the radiographic appearance of the stomach is an important concept that must be understood for interpretation of radiographs and for demonstration of some gastric lesions. Variation in appearance of the stomach with different patient positions is caused by shifts in fluid and gas distribution within the lumen of the stomach. The stomach usually contains both fluid and gas, with the fluid being either of water opacity or positive–contrast medium opacity. This fluid and gas distribution varies with the position of the patient because fluid settles dependently owing to gravity, and gas rises to the highest part of the lumen. Gas and positive-contrast medium are relatively easy to visualize on radiographs, whereas fluid within the stomach may be more difficult to see because it may silhouette with other structures of similar opacity.

To aid in understanding the radiographic appearance of the stomach, the stomach can be described as J shaped and positioned in a transverse plane in the cranial abdomen. Thus, as an example, with a patient positioned in dorsal recumbency for a ventrodorsal view, fluid within the lumen settles dependently to the fundus and body of the stomach. If enough fluid is present, the pyloric portion of the stomach also fills. Gas rises to the uppermost portion, which is in the pyloric antrum and body near midline (Fig. 44–3). Figure 44–3 is a computed tomographic cross-sectional view of the cranial abdomen at the level of the stomach acquired with the dog in dorsal recumbency. Note the fluid opacity filling most of the stomach with the gas bubble floating near midline. With this image as an example, it is possible to predict how the fluid and gas would be distributed if the animal were rotated in 90-degree increments for a left recumbent lateral view, a dorsoventral view in sternal recumbency, a right recumbent lateral view, and back to a ventrodorsal view

in dorsal recumbency. These variations in appearance of the stomach are further altered by the volume and ratio of fluid to gas within the stomach. Examples of the appearance of the stomach with various views are illustrated in Figure 44–4, which were made with a vertically directed x-ray beam.

On the ventrodorsal view (see Fig. 44–4A), gas is located in the pyloric antrum and body near midline. Fluid settles to fill the fundus, body, and pyloric portions of the stomach. Less fluid with a larger volume of gas would fill additional areas of the stomach with gas. If completely empty, the fundus and body may appear as a soft-tissue mass on the ventrodorsal view. On a dorsoventral view (see Fig. 44–4B), gas rises to the cardia and fundus, and fluid settles dependently to fill the pyloric portions and part of the body. On the left recumbent lateral view (see Fig. 44–4C), gas rises to the pyloric portion of the stomach, which is on the patient's right side and is thus the uppermost point of the stomach. Fluid settles dependently to the fundus and body. Occasionally a gas pocket may be trapped in the fundic region. In this position, the fundus and body are well visualized with positive-contrast medium but are more difficult to visualize if filled with fluid (Fig. 44–5A). On the right recumbent lateral view (see Fig. 44–4D), gas rises to the fundus and body, which are on the patient's left side and thus are uppermost. With this view, the gas is often more spread out to fill the fundus and body (see Fig. 44–5B) and may not stand out as discretely as on the left recumbent lateral view. In addition, fluid settles dependently to fill the pyloric portions and part of the body of the stomach. In this position, the pyloric portion is well visualized with positive-contrast medium. Occasionally the pyloric antrum and distal part of the body may appear in survey radiographs as a soft-tissue mass in the right recumbent lateral view (see Fig. 44–5B).

The radiographic appearance of the normal stomach is quite variable. It is thus important to recognize variations that exist in the appearance of the normal stomach and to understand how the appearance of the stomach may be altered by factors such as the position of the patient and the volume and ratio of fluid and gas within the stomach. It is also important to be able to take advantage of fluid and gas shifts within the stomach to visualize certain portions of the stomach more clearly.

Rugal folds are not seen well on survey radiographs. With positive-contrast gastrography, rugal folds are best seen at the peripheral portions of the stomach, where they may be visualized end-on as regular, small filling defects at the mucosal surface (Fig. 44–6). If projected en face, rugal folds are not visible with positive-contrast gastrography unless the barium is well penetrated by the x-ray beam or the stomach has emptied much of the original dose. Rugal folds then appear as relatively radiolucent, linear filling defects separated by barium in the interrugal spaces (see Fig. 44–7B). Double-contrast gastrography provides the most detailed evaluation of the gastric mucosa and rugal folds.

Radiographic assessment of rugal folds is usually subjective. Rugal folds vary in size and number,[5] and the appearance of rugal folds depends on the degree of gastric distention. Rugal folds are more tortuous in the nondistended stomach and become more uniform and parallel to the gastric curvature with increasing distention.[5, 9] Rugal folds are smaller and more spiral in the pyloric antrum.[19] Rugal folds may not be visible if the stomach is overdistended.[10] Rugal folds are smaller and fewer in number in cats than in dogs.[2]

Gastric peristalsis and gastric emptying may be observed directly during fluoroscopy by using positive-contrast medium. Without fluoroscopy, gastric peristalsis cannot be evaluated. Although a peristaltic contraction may be seen on a conventional radiograph during gastrography, visualization

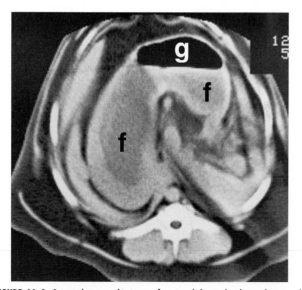

FIGURE 44–3. Computed tomographic image of a normal dog in dorsal recumbency at the level of the stomach. Fluid (f) fills most of the stomach, and the gas bubble (g) floats near the midline. (From Barber DL: Imaging: Radiography II. Vet Radiol *22*:149, 1981; with permission.)

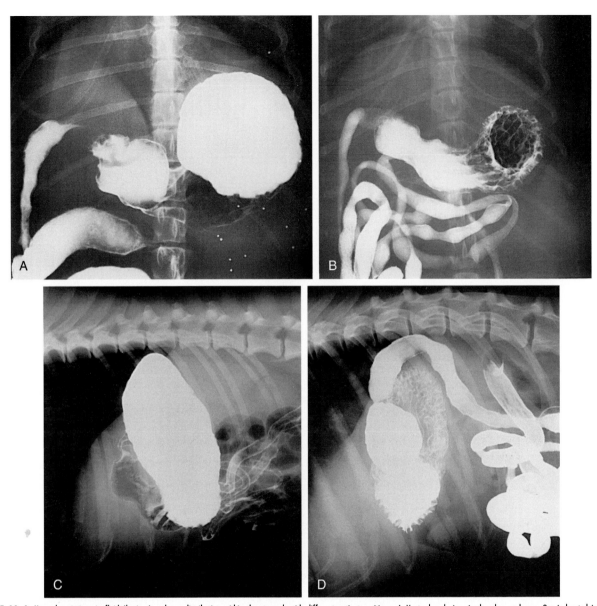

FIGURE 44-4. Normal variations in fluid (barium) and gas distribution within the stomach with different patient positions. A, Ventrodorsal view, in dorsal recumbency. Gas is located in the body and pyloric antrum. Fluid settles dependently to fill the fundus, body, and pyloric portions (compare with Fig. 44-3). B, Dorsoventral view, in ventral recumbency. Gas rises to the cardia and fundus, and fluid settles dependently to fill pyloric portions and part of the body. C, Left recumbent lateral view. Gas rises to the pyloric portion, and fluid settles dependently to fill the fundus and body. D, Right recumbent lateral view. Gas rises to the fundus and body, which are coated with barium. Fluid settles dependently to fill the pyloric portion and part of the body.

of peristalsis is a chance event dependent on when the radiograph was made during the contractile cycle of the stomach. A peristaltic contraction appears as an indentation of the wall of the stomach with slight dilation of the lumen immediately preceding the contraction. Peristaltic contractions are stronger and more obvious in the pyloric portion of the stomach.

Following administration of barium sulfate, gastric emptying should start within 15 minutes in most normal patients.[2, 20, 21] During gastrography with barium sulfate, the stomach generally empties within 1 to 4 hours in dogs.[5, 20] Minimal significance should be applied to rapid emptying of the stomach; delayed emptying is more significant.

The rate of gastric emptying is a complex phenomenon that is altered by a variety of factors, such as volume of contents, chemical and physical properties of chyme entering the duodenum, various reflex mechanisms, certain medications, and the type of contrast medium used. Thus, a standard approach must be used to evaluate the rate of gastric emptying radiographically. Because the stomach starts to empty faster with an increased intraluminal volume,[11] the dose of contrast medium should be standardized. Low doses may result in delayed gastric emptying, which, in turn, may lead to a false-positive diagnosis of pyloric obstruction. The type of contrast medium used, the volume administered, and the presence or absence of medications that affect gastric emptying are all factors that must be considered and standardized. If these factors can be excluded as a cause of delayed gastric emptying, such delays are most often caused by psychological influences or actual disease at the pylorus. Emotional stress and noise may inhibit gastric movement.[22] Anxiety, fear, rage, or pain induced by physical manipulation of the patient, gastric intubation, and physical restraint may contribute to delayed gastric emptying. Thus, patients with delayed gastric emptying must be allowed to calm down in a quiet environment before diagnostic significance is placed on delayed gas-

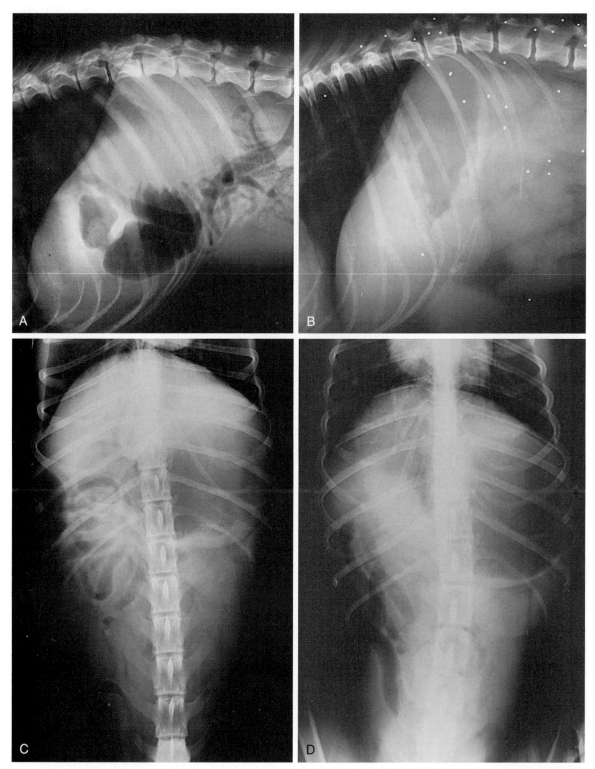

FIGURE 44–5. Normal variations in fluid and gas distribution within the stomach on survey radiographs. *A,* Left recumbent lateral view. Gas rises to the pyloric portion and part of the body, and a gas pocket remains near the cardia. Fluid settles dependently to the fundus and body, which are difficult to visualize when filled with fluid (compare to Fig. 44–4*C*). *B,* Right recumbent lateral view. Gas rises to fill the fundus and the body. Fluid settles dependently to the pyloric portion, which appears as a soft-tissue mass (compare to Fig. 44–4*D*). *C,* Ventrodorsal view made in dorsal recumbency. Gas rises across much of the stomach to outline the pylorus and body. *D,* Dorsoventral view made in ventral recumbency (same dog as in *C*). Gas rises to fill the body and fundus. Fluid settles dependently to fill the pyloric portion, which is difficult to visualize when filled with fluid (compare to Fig 44–4*B*).

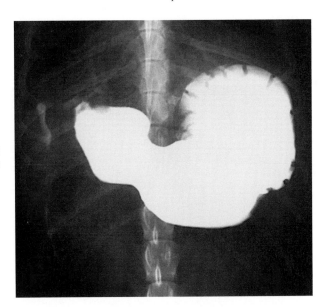

FIGURE 44–6. Dorsoventral gastrogram. Rugal folds at the periphery of the stomach are viewed end-on and create small filling defects at the mucosal surface. Radiolucent linear filling defects are due to rugal folds projected en face.

tric emptying. Also for these reasons, minimal significance is usually placed on slight or minor delays in gastric emptying if the stomach proceeds to empty in a normal manner after an initial delay.

Studies using barium-food mixtures have been performed in an attempt to evaluate gastric function further.[12, 13] Emptying times for individual dogs were repeatable; however, the range of normal gastric emptying times was so wide (7 to 15 hours) that the procedure is not useful for evaluation of gastric emptying unless gross abnormalities are present.[12]

ABNORMAL RADIOGRAPHIC FINDINGS

Displacement

The position of the stomach may be a useful indicator for recognition or localization of some extragastric abnormalities in the cranial abdomen. Some diseases of the liver, spleen, pancreas, and diaphragm may affect the stomach. The relationship between the stomach and extragastric abnormality may help define the primary organ involved or the nature of the primary lesion.

The cranial surface of the stomach is in close apposition with the caudal surface of the liver. Thus, changes in size or position of the liver may cause a change in position of the stomach. Generalized hepatomegaly often produces caudal and dorsal displacement of the stomach.[23] This displacement may be asymmetric if it is caused by a mass lesion.[2] Because the cardia of the stomach is relatively fixed in position, however, even generalized hepatomegaly produces a nonuniform displacement of the stomach. Thus, on the lateral view, generalized hepatomegaly often produces caudal and dorsal displacement of the pylorus and body of the stomach. This displacement changes the axis of the stomach so that the axis is no longer parallel with the ribs (Fig. 44–7A). On the ventrodorsal or dorsoventral views, generalized hepatomegaly often causes displacement of the body and pylorus of the stomach caudally and toward the left from normal (see Fig. 44–7B). This displacement changes the axis of the stomach so that the axis is no longer transverse.

Because there is a minimal amount of objective radiographic criteria of liver size, displacement of the stomach aids in recognition of hepatomegaly. Gastric displacement becomes especially valuable when the liver is not visible per

se because of emaciation or abdominal effusion. In such patients, air within the stomach may often be used to define the axis of the stomach. A small volume of barium may also be given to confirm the axis of the stomach.

If the diaphragm is intact, cranial displacement of the stomach relative to the diaphragm can occur only with a decrease in the size of the liver. This displacement results from cranial displacement of the pylorus and body of the stomach (Fig. 44–8). Contrast studies are often of value to confirm cranial displacement of the stomach because a patient with a small liver may also be emaciated or have abdominal effusion, making the stomach difficult to see. Cranial displacement of the stomach may also occur with rupture of the diaphragm and herniation of the liver, part of the liver, or the stomach. Thus, even though the stomach may not pass through a diaphragmatic hernia, the position of the stomach is an important consideration in patients suspected of having a diaphragmatic hernia. A cranial shift of the axis of the stomach may help define whether the liver has herniated cranially through the diaphragm. A normal axis of the stomach in such instances, however, may still not completely exclude the possibility of herniation of part of the liver.

Abdominal masses that originate caudal to the stomach do not displace the stomach cranially because of the presence of the liver. Instead, such masses may distort the shape of the stomach as they press against and indent the stomach, or they may displace the stomach to the right or left. The relationship of an abdominal mass to the stomach is often of value in helping define whether the mass originates in the liver, spleen, or pancreas (Fig. 44–9).

Gastric Foreign Bodies

Radiopaque material within the stomach is easily visualized and is commonly present on survey radiographs. These opacities are most often the result of ingested bone fragments and are present as an incidental finding with no clinical significance. More clinically significant foreign bodies, such as fishhooks and needles, are also readily visualized and present no diagnostic problem. Occasionally the stomach may contain nondescript radiopaque material that is of questionable significance. Close correlation with clinical signs is important. Another important factor is persistence of the abnor-

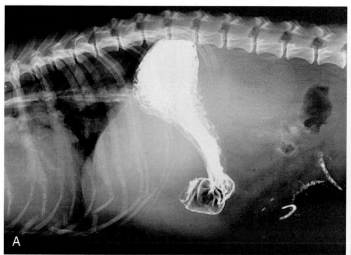

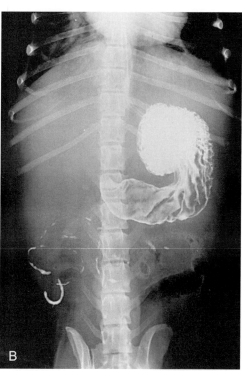

FIGURE 44–7. Gastric displacement due to hepatomegaly. *A,* Lateral view. The pylorus and body are displaced caudally. *B,* Ventrodorsal view. The pylorus and body are displaced caudally and to the left. Final diagnosis was chronic passive hepatic congestion as a result of heartworm disease.

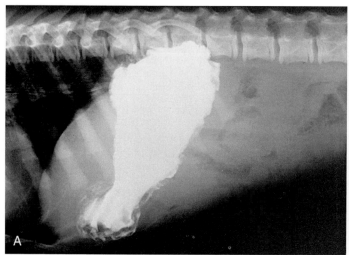

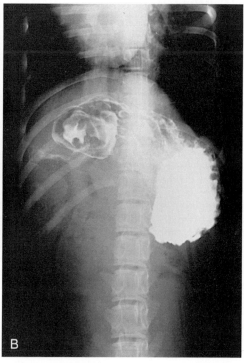

FIGURE 44–8. Gastric displacement because of a small liver. The pylorus and body are displaced cranially on lateral *(A)* and ventrodorsal *(B)* views. Final diagnosis was portosystemic shunt.

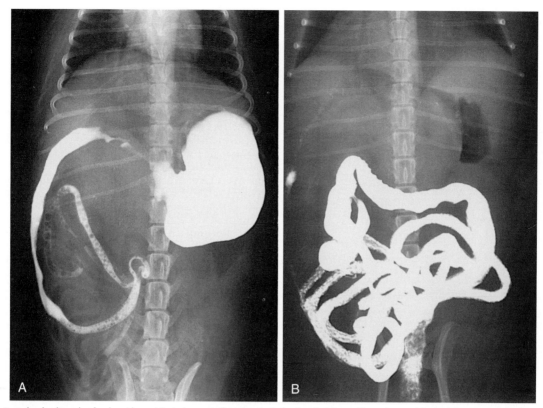

FIGURE 44–9. Ventrodorsal radiographs of a dog with an abdominal mass. *A,* The pylorus is displaced to the left; in addition, the cranial duodenal flexure and proximal part of the descending duodenum have a broad arc around the cranial surface of the mass, which itself is not visible. *B,* The transverse colon is displaced and curves caudally around the caudal surface of the mass. The mass is located between the proximal duodenum, the pylorus, and the transverse colon. Final diagnosis was pancreatic abscess.

mality. If the patient is stable, repeat radiographs made 1 to 3 days later may provide valuable information (Fig. 44–10).

A greater problem exists with radiographic diagnosis of nonopaque gastric foreign bodies. Such objects are usually difficult to see on survey radiographs. Gastric endoscopic examination is valuable if the equipment is available. Contrast studies may be necessary for diagnosis. Several solutions exist to aid in radiographic identification of nonopaque gastric foreign bodies. The simplest technique is to use different patient positions. If the foreign body does not shift dependently with gastric fluid, a different view may help to outline the foreign body with gas. This approach is most valuable if the foreign body remains in the pyloric portion of the stomach and can be outlined with gas in a left recumbent lateral view (Fig. 44–11). Giving a small amount of barium or performing a double-contrast gastrogram may make such foreign bodies easier to visualize than does a standard gastrogram using a large volume of barium because a large volume of barium may completely obscure the foreign body and thus lead to a false-negative result. Knowledge of patient positioning is again important because gas within the stomach during a contrast study may simulate a filling defect comparable with that of a foreign body.

The appearance of a foreign body on a gastrogram varies depending on the type of foreign body present. An object such as a solid ball creates a round, discrete filling defect within the barium (Fig. 44–12). If the object has a nonabsorbent surface, it may not be visible after the stomach has emptied. Conversely a rag or sock may not create an initial filling defect because the contrast medium may permeate the object. Because of absorption and retention of contrast medium, however, the foreign body may be better visualized after the stomach has emptied.

Acute Gastric Dilation and Volvulus

Acute gastric dilation and gastric volvulus produce gaseous distention of the stomach. Although both fluid and gas are present in the stomach, gaseous distention is the predominant abnormality in these conditions.

Acute gastric dilatation of the stomach may be due to a complex variety of causes. Gaseous distention of the stomach may also be caused by aerophagia that is secondary to severe dyspnea or pain. In such instances, the gastric distention is usually less severe, and other correlative findings may be present to aid in differential diagnosis. With acute gastric dilation, the stomach is enlarged and is filled primarily with gas but retains its normal position and anatomic relationships. Thus, the pylorus is still located on the right and the fundus on the left. The normal position of the stomach can usually be determined on survey radiographs by using and comparing the right recumbent and left recumbent lateral views or the ventrodorsal and dorsoventral views. Recognition of the pylorus of a distended stomach is usually easier on lateral views than on ventrodorsal or dorsoventral views. Contrast gastrography may help in this localization but is usually not necessary.

Gastric volvulus is also associated with acute gaseous distention of the stomach. Gastric volvulus is differentiated from acute gaseous dilation by the presence of stomach rotation. Different directions and degrees of rotation of the stomach may be present at the time of radiography, and the radiographic appearance of the stomach varies depending on the type and degree of rotation and the amount of distention.[24, 25] As the stomach dilates, the greater curvature rotates (clockwise when viewed from caudal to cranial) to lie along the ventral abdominal wall. The pylorus continues to shift dor-

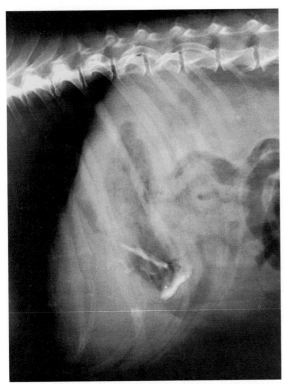

FIGURE 44–10. Persistent gastric foreign body. This radiopaque plastic material was also present on radiographs made 3 days previously; it was eventually removed by gastroscopy.

sally, cranially, and to the left, and the body of the stomach shifts toward the right.[19] Because of the gastrosplenic ligament, the spleen follows the greater curvature toward the right.

The major radiographic feature of gastric volvulus is gas and fluid distention of the stomach (more gas than fluid). Additionally the pylorus is usually displaced dorsally and to the left. Thus, radiographic determination of the location of the pylorus is the key differentiating feature between dilation and volvulus. Radiographic localization of the pylorus is best accomplished by making left and right recumbent lateral views or ventrodorsal and dorsoventral views. Lateral views are usually of most value. When filled with gas, the pyloric portion of the stomach appears more tubular and more narrow than the rest of the stomach. Although the stomach is filled primarily with gas, it usually contains enough fluid so that the pyloric portion may fill with fluid and thus not be seen. Both lateral views may be needed to be sure that the pylorus fills with gas and can thus be recognized.

With the pylorus shifted to the left and with the patient in left recumbency, fluid in the stomach fills the pylorus, and gas fills the rest of the stomach. With the patient in right recumbency, gas fills the pyloric portion and fluid shifts to the fundus or body of the stomach. Thus, the radiographic finding that the pyloric portion fills with fluid on the left recumbent lateral view and fills with gas on the right recumbent lateral view indicates that the pylorus in on the left side and that the stomach has rotated (Figs. 44–13 and 44–14). Recognition of this shift is usually more difficult on the ventrodorsal and dorsoventral views because specific recognition of the pyloric portion may be more difficult. Positive-contrast gastrography may be performed but is usually not needed. An additional variation is a volvulus of 360 degrees, in which the pylorus and fundus are on their normal sides (Fig. 44–15) and diagnosis is dependent on findings at physical examination.

Gastric volvulus may also be present without severe gastric distention. This situation may often exist for days or weeks after previous gastric decompression[24] or may be present at the time of initial presentation.[27] The aforementioned radiographic principles still apply as a means to recognize rotation of the stomach (Fig. 44–16).

Compartmentalization is a term that refers to the radiographic appearance of soft-tissue bands that project into or across the gas-filled lumen of the rotated stomach. These soft-tissue bands are due to folding of the stomach on itself as the folded wall projects into the lumen and is outlined by gas within the lumen.[2] These bands may become more obvious with greater degrees of distention. With progressive distention of the stomach, the stomach wall becomes thinner. Gas within the gastric wall has also been described but is infrequent.[2]

As the stomach enlarges, other mobile structures within the abdomen are displaced caudally. With severe gastric distention, it is often difficult to visualize other abdominal organs because of crowding. The spleen is also usually involved in gastric volvulus and may shift with the stomach. The spleen is usually enlarged owing to impaired circulation, but its location may vary. The greater the gastric distention, the less likely the spleen is visualized radiographically because of crowding of abdominal viscera. Thus, splenomegaly and splenic displacement may be more easily visualized with less severe gastric volvulus. Other changes that may be seen with volvulus include reflex paralytic ileus of the small intestine, esophageal dilation, and cardiovascular changes within the thorax associated with shock.

Chronic Pyloric Obstruction

Obstruction of gastric emptying at the pylorus may be acute or chronic. Causes of acute obstruction include gastric volvulus as well as foreign bodies. Chronic pyloric obstruction is usually the result of narrowing of the pyloric orifice secondary to diseases affecting the wall or blocking the orifice, such as hypertrophic pyloric stenosis, pylorospasm, inflammation or fibrosis, neoplasia, and mucosal antral hypertrophy. These conditions usually cause a chronic, partial obstruction at the pylorus leading to chronic retention of gastric content.

Chronic, partial obstruction of the pylorus is often manifest on survey radiographs as fluid-filled gastric distention as opposed to the acute gaseous distention of gastric volvulus (Fig. 44–17). The stomach may be quite large with chronic partial obstruction of the pylorus. The enlarged stomach, however, may be more difficult to identify on survey radiographs when it is filled with fluid than when it is filled with gas. Even when distended with fluid, the stomach still contains some gas. In these instances, however, the gas does not totally outline or fill the entire stomach. Instead the smaller amount of gas floats as a bubble on top of the fluid and should not be mistaken as the limits of the stomach (see Fig. 44–17B).

The major effect of pyloric obstructive diseases is to restrict gastric emptying. Survey radiographic findings may vary from normal gastric size to enlargement, depending on the severity and duration of the obstruction. With contrast studies, the major radiographic abnormality is delayed gastric emptying. An initial delay in gastric emptying, however, may be of no clinical significance because of the influence of various psychological factors discussed previously. This point is especially important to remember if the stomach starts to empty normally after an initial delay or after the animal is allowed to calm down. Of more significance is a pronounced delay in gastric emptying when only a small amount of contrast medium passes from the stomach in a few hours.

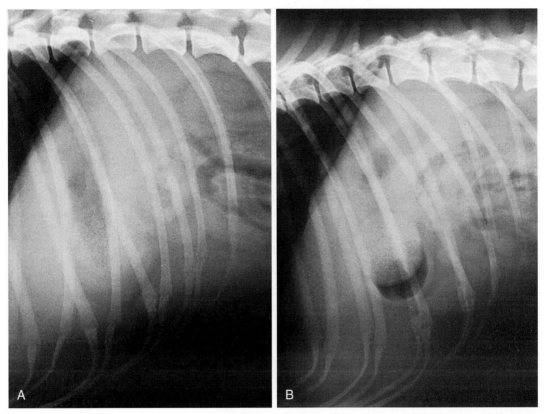

FIGURE 44–11. *A,* Gastric foreign body (ball) in the pyloric portion that is not seen well on the right recumbent lateral view because of fluid in the pylorus. *B,* In the left recumbent lateral view, gas rises to the pylorus to better outline the ball.

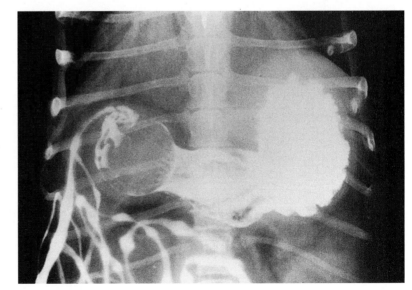

FIGURE 44–12. Gastric foreign body (ball) that creates a round intraluminal filling defect on the gastrogram.

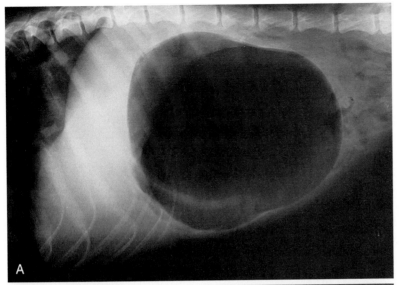

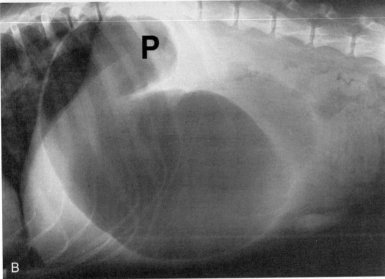

FIGURE 44–13. Gastric volvulus. *A,* Left recumbent lateral view. The stomach is greatly distended with gas in the fundus and the body. Fluid fills the pyloric portion, which is not well visualized. *B,* Right recumbent lateral view. The fluid shifts into the fundic portion, and gas outlines the pyloric portion (P). These changes indicate that the pylorus is on the left and the fundus is on the right and that there is a gastric volvulus. In this particular patient, the pylorus is directed caudally.

FIGURE 44–14. Gastric volvulus, right recumbent lateral view. The pylorus (P) is directed cranioventrally (compare with Fig. 44–13*B*). The soft-tissue mass in the ventral abdomen just caudal to the stomach is the spleen, which is displaced as a result of the gastric malpositioning. The splenic enlargement is suggestive of splenic vein compression or obstruction, and splenic torsion should be considered.

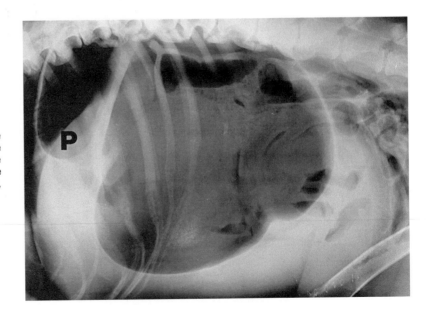

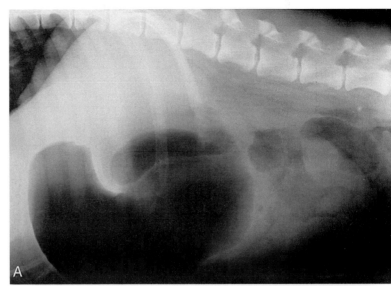

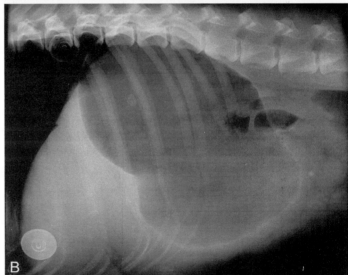

FIGURE 44–15. Left recumbent *(A)* and right recumbent *(B)* lateral views of a dog with acute gastric dilation. On the basis of these radiographic findings, the pylorus and the fundus are on normal sides of the abdomen. The esophagus was dilated, however, and a gastric tube could not be passed into the stomach. Final diagnosis was 360-degree gastric volvulus.

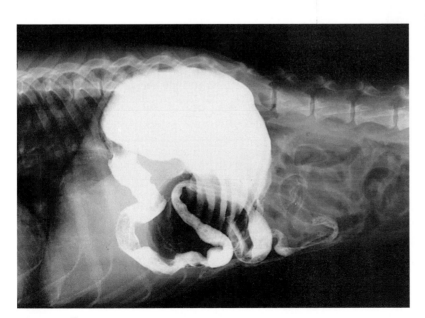

FIGURE 44–16. Left recumbent lateral view of a dog a few days after gastric decompression. Gastric volvulus is still present but without extreme dilation.

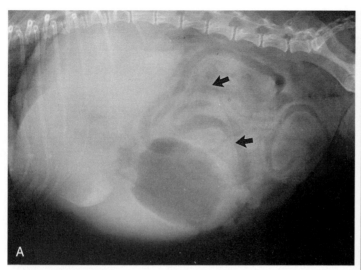

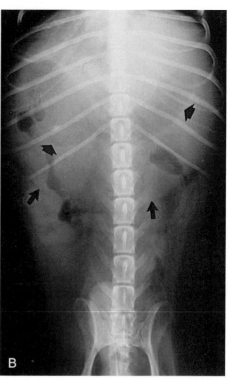

FIGURE 44–17. Lateral *(A)* and ventrodorsal *(B)* radiographs of two dogs with fluid-filled gastric distention because of chronic pyloric obstruction. The stomach is more difficult to identify when filled with fluid instead of gas. The *long arrows* in *A* and *B* indicate the caudal margin of the stomach. The smaller gastric gas pocket *(short arrows in B)* should not be mistaken for limits of the stomach. The dog shown in *A* also had hepatomegaly and cholelithiasis.

Because the normal stomach should be empty 1 to 4 hours after administration of contrast medium, retention of most of the barium within the stomach 3 or 4 hours after administration usually indicates pyloric obstructive disease (Fig. 44–18).

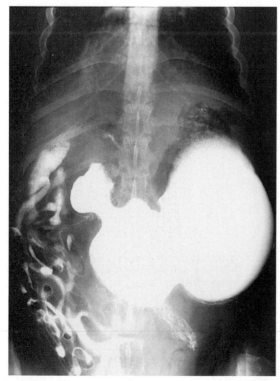

FIGURE 44–18. Dorsoventral radiograph 5 hours after barium was given. There is a pronounced delay in gastric emptying, with most of the contrast medium retained within the stomach. Note the strong peristaltic contraction of the pyloric portion.

It is often difficult to differentiate the pyloric obstructive diseases radiographically, especially without fluoroscopy. The stomach is a dynamic organ that rapidly changes appearance because of peristaltic waves, and a radiograph captures the morphology of the stomach during only a fraction of a second. Thus, the appearance of the stomach on a radiograph depends on when the exposure was made. Although some diseases may produce characteristic radiographic abnormalities, such abnormalities may be visible only during certain moments within the gastric cycle and thus are not likely to be seen on a randomly exposed radiograph. The advantage of fluoroscopy is that sequential changes of the shape of the stomach can be visualized, and thus momentary changes that may best demonstrate certain lesions of the stomach may be documented. Even with fluoroscopy, however, it is often not possible to differentiate some pyloric obstructive diseases. For example, hypertrophic pyloric stenosis, neoplasia, and mural scarring all may produce an annular type of stricture of the pylorus that prevents the pylorus from opening adequately. Thus, it may be more practical to divide obstructive pyloric diseases into those that encircle the pylorus and are thus restrictive and those that obstruct the pylorus by blocking its orifice.

Restrictive diseases of the pylorus include hypertrophic pyloric stenosis, pylorospasm, inflammation or scarring, and neoplasia. If characteristic abnormalities are present on radiographs, they are usually those of an annular type of stricture narrowing the pyloric sphincter. If barium fills only the entrance of the lumen at the pyloric sphincter, the resultant radiographic appearance is referred to as the *beak sign*.[27] If barium fills the length of the narrowed lumen through the pyloric sphincter, the resultant radiographic appearance is referred to as the *string sign*.[27] A *tit sign* has been described as a relatively sharp, pointed, outpouching of the pyloric antrum along the lesser curvature as a peristaltic wave pushes contrast medium in a peristaltic pouch up against the mass-type lesion around the pylorus.[27] Variations in severity, symmetry, and radiographic projection all contribute to create variations in the radiographic appearance of pyloric restrictive lesions (Fig. 44–19).

The second group of pyloric obstructive diseases includes gastric foreign bodies, mucosal inflammation or hypertrophy, and some mural lesions of the pyloric antrum. These types of lesions are more likely to produce filling defects within the lumen that occlude the orifice of the pyloric sphincter (Fig. 44–20). It is again emphasized that radiographic recognition of such a lesion is usually diagnostically adequate and that specific differentiation of the underlying cause may not be possible on radiographs.

Gastric Ulcers

Gastric ulcers are difficult to identify on conventional radiographs. Gastric ulcers produce craters in the wall of the stomach that appear as outpouchings from the lumen (Fig. 44–21). The radiographic appearance of a gastric ulcer may be variable, depending on whether the ulcer is projected in profile, en face, or obliquely.[28] The appearance of the ulcer may be altered further by gastric peristalsis. Manipulation of the patient during fluoroscopy allows a more complete and continuous evaluation of the margin and contour of the stomach. Double-contrast gastrography may also be of value because ulcers that are projected en face may be visualized with double-contrast studies but are obscured with positive-contrast gastrography.

Gastric ulcers may be benign or malignant. Benign gastric ulcers may result from a variety of causes.[19, 29, 30] Use of nonsteroidal anti-inflammatory drugs has become a common cause of benign gastric ulcers.[31–33] Malignant gastric ulcers occur in association with gastric neoplasia and may be caused by tumor necrosis.[30] Criteria have been established for the

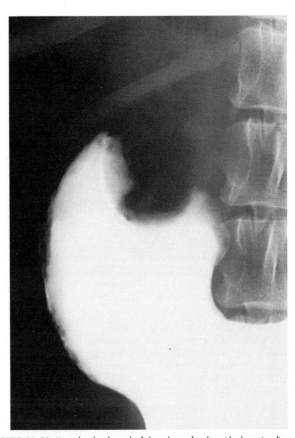

FIGURE 44–20. Ventrodorsal radiograph of the pylorus of a dog with obstructive disease of the pylorus. There is a hemispheric filling defect at the pylorus that projects into the lumen. There was pronounced delay in gastric emptying (same dog as in Fig. 44–18). The filling defect was due to mucosa that was hypertrophied in a symmetric band around the pylorus. Final diagnosis was chronic plasmocytic gastritis.

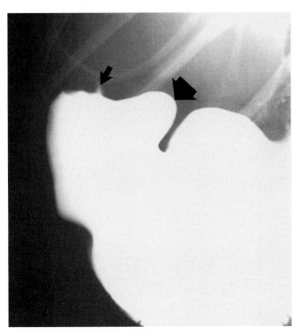

FIGURE 44–19. Ventrodorsal radiograph of the pyloric region of a dog with restrictive disease of the pylorus. The *beak sign (small arrow)* is caused by barium that fills only the entrance of the lumen of the pyloric sphincter because of an annular type of stricture. The peristaltic pouch *(large arrow)* is the outpouching of the pyloric antrum along the lesser curvature as a peristaltic wave pushes contrast medium up against the mass-type lesion encircling the pylorus. There was also a pronounced delay in gastric emptying (same dog as in Fig. 44–17*B*). Final diagnosis was pyloric stenosis owing to inflammation caused by an ulcer.

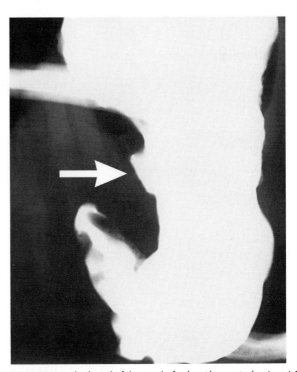

FIGURE 44–21. Lateral radiograph of the stomach of a dog with a gastric ulcer *(arrow)*. The stomach tube is still in place. Mass lesions of the stomach are not definitive, and the ulcer is the only definitive radiographic abnormality. Final diagnosis was gastric adenocarcinoma.

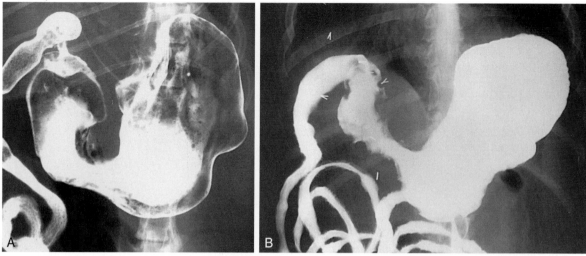

FIGURE 44–22. *A*, Dorsoventral double-contrast gastrogram of a cat. There is a nodular filling defect owing to a mass lesion along the lesser curvature. Final diagnosis was lymphosarcoma. *B*, Dorsoventral gastrogram of a dog. An annular mass encircles the pyloric portion and part of the body. This area failed to distend, even in sternal recumbency, and the abnormality persisted throughout the study. Final diagnosis was gastric adenocarcinoma.

radiographic differentiation of benign and malignant gastric ulcers in humans.[28, 34, 35] Thus, although radiography may provide an excellent method for the recognition of gastric ulcers, infrequent use of single-contrast and double-contrast gastrography, lack of fluoroscopy, and insufficient views all combine to limit the recognition of gastric ulcers in dogs and cats. In addition, experience is limited in radiographically differentiating benign and malignant gastric ulcers in dogs and cats. Ulceration is often associated with gastric carcinoma,[36, 37] and gastric ulcers in dogs that are recognized on radiographs are often the result of neoplasia.[38] Thus, the radiographic recognition of a gastric ulcer should lead to strong consideration of neoplasia and further evaluation of the stomach with endoscopic and biopsy studies or by surgical exploration.

Gastric Neoplasia

Several types of gastric neoplasms occur in the stomach, and any region of the stomach may be involved. Polyps may often be clinically silent and are most often found incidentally.[39] Adenocarcinoma is the most common malignant gastric tumor in dogs.[37, 40] This tumor may occur in any region of the stomach but appears to be found most often in the pyloric portion.[36, 41] Gastric neoplasia occurs less frequently in the cat than in the dog,[42] and lymphosarcoma is the most common type of feline gastric neoplasm.[43]

The radiographic appearance of gastric neoplasia is variable and depends primarily on the size, shape, and location of the tumor. The major radiographic feature is that of a mass lesion that projects into the gastric lumen, creating a filling defect within the contrast medium. The more nodular and pedunculated the lesion, the easier it is to recognize as a distinct mass (Fig. 44–22*A*). Smaller mass lesions may be totally obscured by a relatively large volume of barium. Oblique projections, conformation of the stomach, and peristaltic contractions all may contribute to obscure some mass lesions of the stomach.

Tumors that are more diffuse and less discrete are more difficult to identify. Diffuse, infiltrative lesions of the stomach wall may not produce distinct filling defects. Instead, they

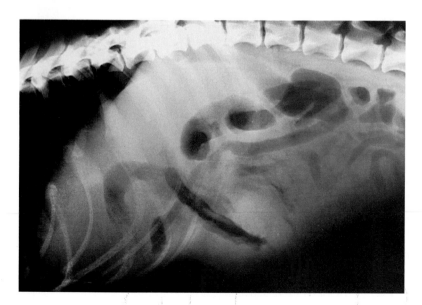

FIGURE 44–23. Lateral survey radiograph of the abdomen of a dog with a thick gastric wall. The thickened wall is best visualized in the ventral midabdomen and is associated with a narrow, tubular, gas-filled lumen. Rugal folds were enlarged on a gastrogram. Final diagnosis was chronic hypertrophic gastritis.

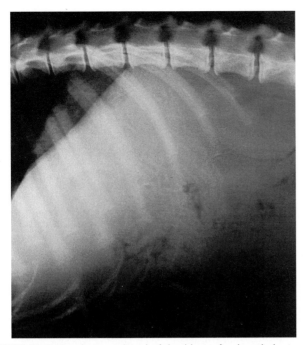

FIGURE 44–24. Lateral survey radiograph of the abdomen of a dog with chronic renal failure. Thin, linear, mineralized opacities that parallel the axis of the ribs are due to gastric calcification.

may alter the shape of the stomach and produce decreased motility of the involved area. If such diffuse lesions encircle a portion of the stomach, the radiographic appearance may be that of an annular narrowing or one in which the stomach has decreased distensibility in the affected area (see Fig. 44–22B). Because of variations in appearance of the stomach created by peristalsis, persistence of a suspected abnormality on sequential radiographs is important. The radiographic recognition of a gastric ulcer should also suggest the possibility of gastric neoplasia.

Diffuse Diseases of the Stomach

The stomach may be involved diffusely by a variety of diseases that produce inflammation, hypertrophy, atrophy, or mineralization. Acute gastritis may result from a variety of causes and is rarely associated with radiographic abnormalities. Chronic gastritis is infrequently diagnosed clinically and may also result from a variety of causes. Examples include diseases such as chronic atrophic gastritis, chronic hypertrophic gastritis, eosinophilic gastritis, and phycomycosis.[44, 45] Paucity of rugal folds, large rugal folds, nodules, or a thickened gastric wall may be seen with these diseases (Fig. 44–23).[44]

Soft-tissue calcification may occur in association with chronic renal failure.[46, 47] In such patients, mineralization of the gastric wall may be visible radiographically as thin, linear, mineralized opacities (Fig. 44–24).[46] Rugal mineralization is often more easily visualized when the stomach is empty and the mineralized mucosal fold pattern is more tightly grouped.

References

1. Evans HE, and Christensen GC: Miller's Anatomy of the Dog, 2nd Ed. Philadelphia, WB Saunders, 1979.
2. O'Brien TR: Radiographic Diagnosis of Abdominal Disorders in the Dog and Cat. Philadelphia, WB Saunders, 1978.
3. Brawner WR, and Bartels JE: Contrast radiography of the digestive tract: Indications, techniques, and complications. Vet Clin North Am 13:599, 1983.
4. Root CR: Interpretation of abdominal survey radiographs. Vet Clin North Am 4:763, 1974.
5. Gomez JA: The gastrointestinal contrast study: Methods and interpretation. Vet Clin North Am 4:805, 1974.
6. Bargai U: The effect of xylazine hydrochloride on the radiographic appearance of the stomach and intestine in the dog. Vet Radiol 23:60, 1982.
7. Hogan PM, and Aronson E: Effect of sedation on transit time of feline gastrointestinal contrast studies. Vet Radiol 29:85, 1994.
8. Miyabayashi T, and Morgan JP: Upper gastrointestinal examinations: A radiographic study of clinically normal Beagle puppies. J Small Anim Pract 32:83, 1991.
9. Evans SM, and Lauffer I: Double-contrast gastrography in the normal dog. Vet Radiol 22:2, 1981.
10. Evans SM, and Biery DN: Double-contrast gastrography in the cat: technique and normal radiographic appearance. Vet Radiol 24:3, 1983.
11. Root CR, and Morgan JP: Contrast radiography of the upper gastrointestinal tract in the dog. J Small Anim Pract 10:279, 1969.
12. Burns, J, and Fox SM: The use of a barium meal to evaluate total gastric emptying time in the dog. Vet Radiol 27:169, 1986.
13. Miyabayashi T, and Morgan JP: Gastric emptying in the normal dog: A contrast radiographic technique. Vet Radiol 25:187, 1984.
14. Allan GS, Rendano VT, Quick CB, et al: Gastrografin as a gastrointestinal contrast medium in the cat. Vet Radiol 20:110, 1979.
15. Agut A, Sanchezvalverde MA, Torrecillas FE, et al: Iohexol as a gastrointestinal contrast medium in the cat. Vet Radiol Ultrasound 35:164, 1994.
16. Williams J, Biller DS, Miyabayashi T, et al: Evaluation of iohexol as a gastrointestinal contrast medium in normal cats. Vet Radiol Ultrasound 34:310, 1993.
17. Grandage J: The radiologic appearance of stomach gas in the dog. Aust Vet J 50:529, 1974.
18. Jakovljevic S, and Gibbs C: Radiographic assessment of gastric mucosal fold thickness in dogs. Am J Vet Res 54:1827, 1993.
19. Twedt DC, and Wingfield WE: Diseases of the stomach. In Ettinger SJ (Ed): Textbook of Veterinary Internal Medicine, Vol 2, 2nd Ed. Philadelphia, WB Saunders, 1983, pp 1233–1277.
20. Funkquist B, and Garmer L: Pathogenetic and therapeutic aspects of torsion of the canine stomach. J Small Anim Pract 8:523, 1967.
21. Gibbs C, and Pearson H: The radiological diagnosis of gastrointestinal obstruction in the dog. J Small Anim Pract 14:61, 1973.
22. Gue M, Fioramonti J, Frexinos J, et al: Influence of acoustic stress by noise on gastrointestinal motility in dogs. Dig Dis Sci 32:1411, 1987.
23. Suter PF: Radiographic diagnosis of liver disease in dogs and cats. Vet Clin North Am [Small Anim Pract] 12:153, 1982.
24. Funkquist B: Gastric torsion in the dog: I. Radiological picture during nonsurgical treatment related to the pathological anatomy and to the future clinical course. J Small Anim Pract 20:73, 1979.
25. Kneller SK: Radiographic interpretation of the gastric dilation—volvulus complex in the dog. J Am Anim Hosp Assoc 12:154, 1976.
26. Frendin J, Funkquist B, and Stavenborn M: Gastric displacement in dogs without clinical signs of acute dilation. J Small Anim Pract 29:775, 1988.
27. Rhodes WH, and Brodey RS: The differential diagnosis of pyloric obstructions in the dog. J Am Vet Radiol Soc 6:65, 1965.
28. Zboralske FF: Gastric ulcer. In Margulis AR, and Burhenne HJ (Eds): Alimentary Tract Roentgenology. St. Louis, CV Mosby, 1967.
29. Howard EB, Sawa TR, Nielson SW, et al: Mastocytoma and gastroduodenal ulceration. Vet Pathol 6:146, 1969.
30. Robbins SL: Pathologic Basis of Disease. Philadelphia, WB Saunders, 1974.
31. Jones RD, Baynes RE, and Nimitz CT: Nonsteroidal anti-inflammatory drug toxicosis in dogs and cats: 240 cases (1989–1990). J Am Vet Med Assoc 201:475, 1992.
32. Stanton ME, and Bright RM: Gastroduodenal ulceration in dogs. J Vet Intern Med 3:238, 1989.
33. Wallace MS, Zawie DA, and Garvey MS: Gastric ulceration in the dog secondary to the use of nonsteroidal antiinflammatory drugs. J Am Anim Hosp Assoc 26:467, 1990.
34. Nelson SW: The discovery of gastric ulcers and the differential diagnosis between benignancy and malignancy. Radiol Clin North Am 7:5, 1969.
35. Porcher P, and Buffard P: Malignancy of the stomach. In Margulis AR, and Burhenne HJ (Eds): Alimentary Tract Roentgenology. St. Louis, CV Mosby, 1967.
36. Hayden DW, and Nelson SW: Canine alimentary neoplasia. Zentralbl Veterinarmed [A] 20:1, 1973.
37. Sautter JH, and Hanlon GF: Gastric neoplasms in the dog: A report of 20 cases. J Am Vet Med Assoc 166:691, 1975.
38. Barber DL: Radiographic aspects of gastric ulcers in dogs: A comparative review and report of 5 case histories. Vet Radiol 23:109, 1982.
39. Willard MD: Diseases of the stomach. In Ettinger SJ, Feldman EC (Eds): Textbook of Veterinary Internal Medicine, Vol 2, 4th Ed. Philadelphia, WB Saunders, 1995, pp 1143–1168.

40. Murray M, Robinson PB, McKeating FJ, et al: Primary gastric neoplasia in the dog: A clinico-pathological study. Vet Rec 91:474, 1972.
41. Patnaik AK, Hurvitz AI, and Johnson GE: Canine gastric adenocarcinoma. Vet Pathol 15:600, 1978.
42. Brodey RS: Alimentary tract neoplasms in the cat: A clinicopathologic survey of 46 cases. Am J Vet Res 27:74, 1966.
43. Tyler DE: Gastric neoplasia in the dog and cat (Abstract). Arch Am Coll Vet Surg 6:47, 1977.
44. Twedt DC, and Magne ML: Diseases of the stomach. In Ettinger SJ (Ed):

Textbook of Veterinary Internal Medicine, Vol 2, 3rd Ed. Philadelphia, WB Saunders, 1989, pp 1289–1322.
45. Miller RI: Gastrointestinal phycomycosis in 63 dogs. J Am Vet Med Assoc 165:473, 1985.
46. Barber DL, and Rowland GN: Radiographically detectable soft-tissue calcification in chronic renal failure. Vet Radiol 20:117, 1979.
47. Parfitt AM: Soft-tissue calcification in uremia. Arch Intern Med 124:544, 1969.

STUDY QUESTIONS

1. Which one of the following methods of restraint is preferable in performing a gastrogram in a dog?
   A. Psychic persuasion.
   B. Manual restraint.
   C. Chemical restraint with tranquilization.
   D. Chemical restraint with general anesthesia.

2. You wish to demonstrate radiographically a geometric abnormality of the pyloric antrum of the stomach of a dog. The stomach, however, contains a large amount of gas in addition to the barium sulfate you have administered. Which two of the following views should be used to fill best the *pyloric portion* of the stomach with barium?

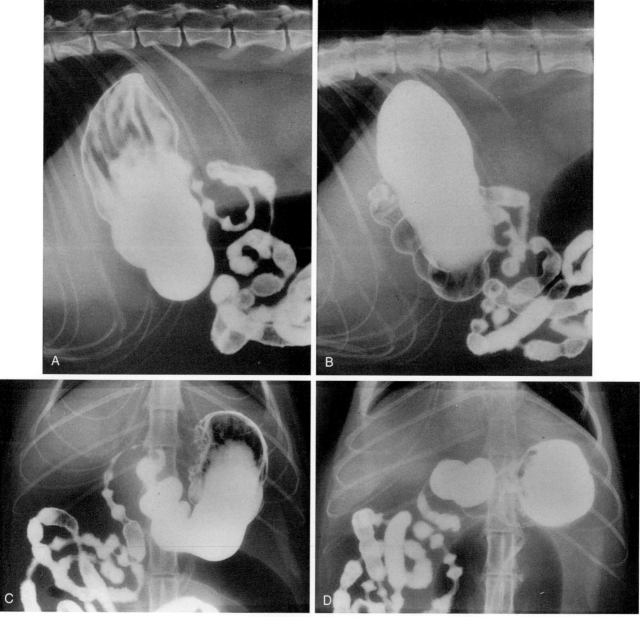

FIGURE 44–25. *A, B, C,* and *D*

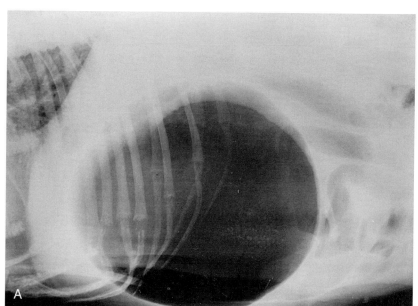

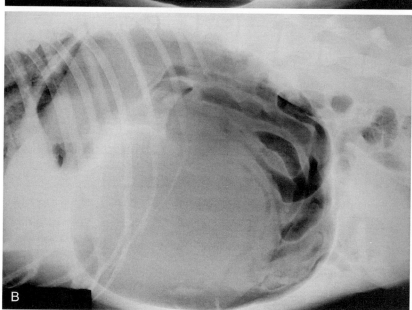

FIGURE 44–26. *A* and *B*

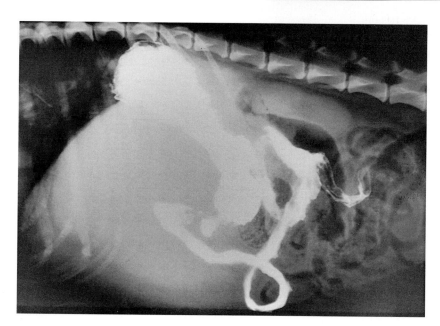

FIGURE 44–27

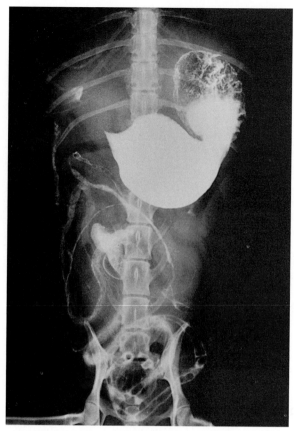

FIGURE 44–28

1. Left recumbent lateral view.
2. Right recumbent lateral view.
3. Ventrodorsal (dorsal recumbency) view.
4. Dorsoventral (ventral recumbency) view.
   A. 1 and 3.
   B. 1 and 4.
   C. 2 and 3.
   D. 2 and 4.

3. You perform a standard upper gastrointestinal series on a dog by using manual restraint, passing a stomach tube, and administering 1 ounce of liquid barium sulfate per 5 pounds of body weight. On subsequent radiographs, the following sequence is observed: 40 minutes, stomach starts to empty; 3 hours, stomach is empty. This sequence is:
   A. Rapid—definite significance.
   B. Rapid—doubtful significance.
   C. Delayed—definite significance.
   D. Delayed—doubtful significance.

4. Water-soluble, organic, iodinated contrast media formulated for the alimentary tract are the preferred media to use routinely for gastrography. (True or False)

5. Figure 44–25A to D shows close-up views of the stomach of a cat made during an upper gastrointestinal series. Which of the following sequences matches the views in the order they are projected?
   A. *A*, Left lateral; *B*, right lateral; *C*, ventrodorsal; *D*, dorsoventral.
   B. *A*, Right lateral; *B*, left lateral; *C*, ventrodorsal; *D*, dorsoventral.

C. *A*, Left lateral; *B*, right lateral; *C*, dorsoventral; *D*, ventrodorsal.
D. *A*, Right lateral; *B*, left lateral; *C*, dorsoventral; *D*, ventrodorsal.

6. These radiographs are left recumbent lateral (Fig. 44–26A) and right recumbent lateral (see Fig. 44–26B) radiographs of the abdomen of a dog with abdominal distention. Describe the radiographic abnormalities present.

7. This lateral radiograph of the abdomen of a dog (Fig. 44–27) was made 15 minutes after administration of barium sulfate. Which one of the following radiographic diagnoses is correct?
   A. Hepatomegaly.
   B. Hepatic neoplasia.
   C. Small liver.
   D. Chronic pyloric outlet obstruction.
   E. Gastric neoplasia.

8. This ventrodorsal abdominal radiograph (Fig. 44–28) was made 4.0 hours after initiation of an upper gastrointestinal series in a dog. Which one of the following *radiographic* diagnoses is correct?
   A. Hypertrophic pyloric stenosis.
   B. Pyloric neoplasia.
   C. Pylorospasm.
   D. Pyloric foreign body.
   E. Delayed gastric emptying—probable pyloric disease.

9. These lateral (Fig. 44–29A) and ventrodorsal (see Fig. 44–29B) radiographs of the abdomen of a dog were made 30 minutes after administration of barium sulfate.

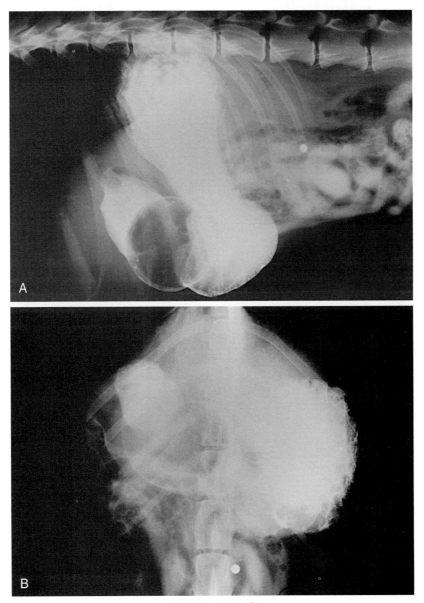

FIGURE 44–29. *A* and *B*

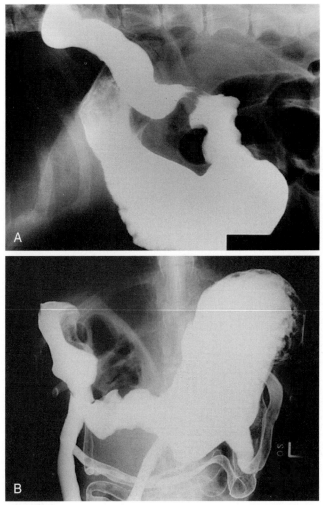

FIGURE 44–30. *A* and *B*

Describe the radiographic abnormalities present and the most likely cause.

10. These lateral (Fig. 44–30*A*) and ventrodorsal (see Fig. 44–30*B*) radiographs of the abdomen of a dog were

made 15 minutes after administration of barium sulfate. Describe the radiographic abnormalities present and the most likely cause.

(Answers on page 648.)

Chapter 45

The Small Bowel

Sandra V. McNeel • Elizabeth A. Riedesel

Vomiting, diarrhea, weight loss, abdominal pain, and palpation of a midabdominal mass are the most common clinical signs of intestinal disease in small animals. Abdominal radiographs may help make a positive diagnosis or provide information that may be helpful when deciding whether medical or surgical treatment is required. Survey radiographs and intestinal contrast examinations may be useful aids in the diagnosis of both acute and chronic intestinal disorders but

should not take precedence over a complete history, thorough physical examination, and pertinent laboratory tests. The animal that does not respond to symptomatic therapy for vomiting or diarrhea should be given a more extensive work-up, including radiographic or sonographic studies or both. The following information is provided as a guide to interpretation of radiographic changes that occur in the small intestinal tract. Although radiographic changes are not pres-

Table 45–1
ROENTGEN SIGNS IN THE SMALL INTESTINE

> Margination—serosal surface definition
> Size—diameter of lumen
> Position—Location within abdominal cavity
> Shape—contour of bowel loops
> Radiopacity—bowel wall and lumen contents
> Architecture—mucosa/bowel wall smoothness
> Motility—contrast medium transit time

ent in every intestinal disorder, many lesions are characterized by one or more of the roentgen signs discussed in the following sections.

ROENTGEN SIGNS IN THE NORMAL SMALL BOWEL

Table 45–1 is a summary of the roentgen signs that are most useful in the interpretation of intestinal radiographs. Margination, size, position, contour, and radiopacity of the bowel can often be evaluated on survey radiographs, but mucosal irregularities and abnormal peristalsis or transit time must be determined from contrast studies.

Margination

A mature dog or cat with a moderate amount of intra-abdominal fat deposition usually has good radiographic definition of intestinal serosal surfaces (Fig. 45–1). Serosal margins should be smooth and are most easily seen adjacent to the abdominal wall, where there is less superimposition of other structures. Conversely, serosal margins of normal bowel located in the midabdomen just caudal to the greater curvature of the stomach frequently appear indistinct, and this finding should not be misinterpreted as a sign of abdominal fluid. Animals younger than 6 months of age or those who are emaciated have poor serosal definition owing to lack of intra-abdominal fat.[1]

Size

Because of the great variation in canine body size, a specific measurement for normal diameter of the small bowel is difficult to establish. Several schemes for relative bowel diameter have been reported, however, using lumbar vertebral body height as the reference structure. These reports suggest that maximum normal small bowel diameter should not exceed the height of the central part of the body of a lumbar vertebra.[2] An alternate criterion states the diameter of the normal canine small intestine should not exceed twice the width of a rib.[3] Because cats tend to be similar in body size, a more specific criterion can be made: The diameter of normal feline small bowel should not exceed 12 mm,[5] or twice the height of the central portion of the L4 vertebral body (Fig. 45–2).[4] Although the duodenum may be slightly wider, the jejunum and ileum should have approximately the same luminal diameter.[6] Attempting to judge the thickness of the intestinal wall on survey radiographs is hazardous; a normal empty bowel loop with a small volume of intraluminal air may be mistaken for a pathologically thickened segment. True thickening of the intestinal wall is better judged by a contrast study, by abdominal palpation, or by ultrasound.[7]

Position

The small bowel should be uniformly distributed throughout the peritoneal cavity, occupying space not taken up by distensible organs (stomach or urinary bladder), solid organs (liver, spleen, or kidneys), or fat. Common variations in the position of the small bowel seen in normal dogs and cats include (1) a full stomach displacing the bowel caudally; (2) a distended urinary bladder displacing the bowel cranially; (3) intra-abdominal fat deposition in obese cats causing the small bowel to be located centrally and on the right side; (4) in very obese cats, fat displacing the bowel into the central region of the abdominal cavity; and (5) the bowel in obese dogs occupying the most ventral portion of the pendulous abdominal cavity.

In the dog, the cranial duodenal flexure is fixed along the caudal surface of the right side of the liver by the hepatoduodenal ligament. The descending duodenum lies along the right abdominal wall. The caudal duodenal flexure is located at midabdomen, with the ascending duodenum continuing from this point directly cranial to the caudal portion of the stomach. Distal to this point, the loops of jejunum may take any position not occupied by other organs.

In the cat, the cranial duodenal flexure usually creates a sharper angle with the pylorus than in the dog. The descend-

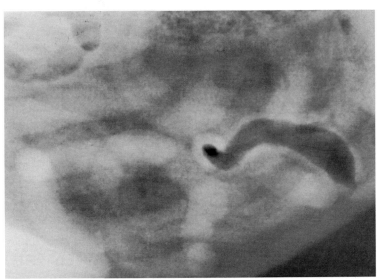

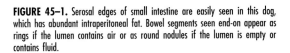
FIGURE 45–1. Serosal edges of small intestine are easily seen in this dog, which has abundant intraperitoneal fat. Bowel segments seen end-on appear as rings if the lumen contains air or as round nodules if the lumen is empty or contains fluid.

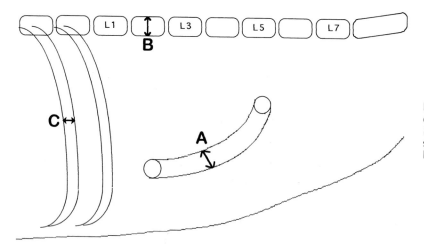

FIGURE 45–2. In the normal dog, small bowel diameter *(A)* should not exceed the height of the central portion of the body of a lumbar vertebra *(B)* or twice the width of a rib *(C)*. In the normal cat, small bowel diameter should not exceed 12 mm or twice the height of the central part of the L4 vertebral body.

ing duodenum then courses in a gently curved loop, with the caudal duodenal flexure at approximately midabdomen. As in the dog, the ascending duodenum courses in a cranial direction until it reaches the stomach; the jejunal loops are then located throughout the rest of the mesogastric area.

Shape and Contour

On survey radiographs, the small bowel may be seen as smooth, continuous, curved tubes or as solid circles or rings (especially in fat animals). These shapes are produced by the contractile activity of the smooth muscle. Segmental contractions give rise to spherical shapes, whereas peristaltic contractions cause long tubular shapes. Contrast studies are often necessary to identify abnormal shape of bowel loops.

Radiopacity

The radiopacity of the normal small intestine is variable because of differing opacities of material within the lumen. In a nonfasted animal, any of the following contents may be seen in the lumen: air; ingesta, with a grainy or mottled appearance; fluid, which is of homogeneous soft-tissue opacity; or bone. The bowel lumen of a fasted dog or cat can be a homogeneous fluid or soft-tissue radiopacity, or it may contain a small amount of ingested air. Nonintestinal conditions that cause increased aerophagia (e.g., struggling during positioning or dyspnea owing to respiratory disease) frequently result in increased numbers of air-filled bowel loops. The bowel wall should also be a uniform soft-tissue opacity. This uniformity is most easily evaluated in portions of the intestine that contain air.

Architecture of Mucosal Surface

On survey radiographs, the mucosal surface can be seen only in air-filled segments of bowel. Barium studies are the procedures of choice to evaluate the mucosa appropriately.

SURVEY RADIOGRAPHY

Technique

Patient Preparation

In the patient with acute abdominal pain, acute onset of persistent vomiting, or palpable enlarged fluid-filled or air-

filled bowel loops, no specific preparation for abdominal radiographs is necessary. In fact, it is important to assess the abdomen radiographically in such patients before gas or fluid patterns, which may be diagnostically helpful, are disturbed by an enema. For elective abdominal radiographs, withholding food for 24 hours and administering a cleansing enema 2 to 4 hours before radiographic examination produces the desired empty intestinal tract.

Radiographic Projections

Standard views to evaluate the small bowel are the right lateral recumbent and ventrodorsal views. Additional views that may be useful include left lateral recumbent, for changes in position of fluid or gas; standing lateral with horizontal x-ray beam, for gas-capped fluid levels sometimes seen with obstruction; and left lateral decubitus (or erect ventrodorsal) with horizontal x-ray beam, for free gas in the peritoneal cavity (as might result from bowel perforation).

Abnormal Roentgen Signs

Margination

See Chapter 37 for a more complete description of peritoneal disorders. Some pathologic conditions cause bowel serosal surfaces to be less or more distinct than expected. Decreased or absent definition of serosal edges is found with a lack of intra-abdominal fat (abdominal walls are tucked up in the emaciated patient) or with fluid in the peritoneal space (abdominal walls are often distended in the patient with a large volume of peritoneal fluid). The type of fluid in the peritoneal cavity cannot be determined by radiography; abdominal paracentesis with cytologic evaluation of fluid is required. Common causes of peritoneal fluid are peritonitis, trauma, right-sided heart failure, and neoplasia.

Unusually clear definition of serosal edges can be seen when air is present in the peritoneal cavity. This situation can occur following puncture of the abdominal wall or perforation of the intestine (or other hollow viscus); iatrogenic induction (recent abdominal surgery); bacterial fermentation; and fat deposition, which may be normal in obese animals.

Size (Increased Luminal Diameter)

The most common alteration in size is distention with air, fluid, or a combination of both. Failure of intestinal contents to pass through the tract is termed *ileus*. Ileus may be mechanical, caused by physical obstruction of the bowel lumen, or functional (paralytic), in which the peristaltic contractions of the bowel cease owing to vascular or neuromuscular abnormalities of the intestinal wall. In functional ileus, the bowel lumen remains patent.

Evaluation of both the approximate length of bowel affected and the degree of luminal distention may aid in establishing a list of reasonable differential diagnoses. The following guidelines are presented to assist in the evaluation of bowel distention. Pathologic conditions described here and summarized in Table 45–2 usually have the radiographic sign being discussed. These lists are not meant to be complete, however, because a single disease process may have different radiographic appearances during its clinical course.

Focal/Mild. When used in this chapter, *focal* refers to involvement of one to three small bowel loops. *Mild* distention is defined as luminal distention equal to 1.5 to 2 times the normal bowel diameter. Possible causes for focal/mild distention include regional enteritis, regional peritonitis (e.g.,

Table 45–2

PATHOLOGIC CONDITIONS BY LENGTH AND RELATIVE DISTENTION OF AFFECTED BOWEL

	Intraluminal	Intramural	Extramural
Focal/Mild Distention			
Early functional ileus		X	
Regional enteritis		X	
Regional peritonitis			X
Mechanical ileus— partial obstruction	X		
Vascular compromise		X	
Focal/Severe Distention			
Mechanical Ileus			
Foreign object	X		
Intussusception	X		
Bowel wall neoplasia		X	
Granulomatous wall infiltrate		X	
Bowel stricture		X	
Stenosis/atresia		X	
Postsurgical adhesion			X
Herniation			X
Functional ileus			
Parvoviral enteritis		X	
Generalized/Mild Distention			
Functional ileus			
Enteritis		X	
Anticholinergic drugs		X	
Partial obstruction at ileocolic junction (usually in cats)		X	
Malabsorption		X	
Electrolyte imbalance		X	
Abdominal pain		X	
Generalized/Severe Distention			
Mechanical Ileus			
Complete obstruction, distal bowel			
Bowel wall neoplasia		X	
Intussusception	X		
Foreign object	X		
Functional ileus			
Recent abdominal surgery		X	
Spinal trauma (neurologic injury)		X	
Intestinal volvulus (rare)		X	

secondary to pancreatitis), thrombosis of a segmental mesenteric artery (early, developing functional ileus), and recent or incomplete obstruction in the proximal intestinal tract (mechanical ileus).

Focal/Severe. In this category, one to three loops of small bowel are greatly distended (greater than twice the normal bowel diameter), whereas other visible portions of the small bowel may be less distended (nonuniform enlargement of luminal diameter). Complete mechanical obstruction of the mid to distal intestine (Fig. 45–3) is the most common cause of focal/severe dilation. It may be caused by intraluminal occlusion (foreign body, intussusception), intramural lesions (neoplasia, granulomatous infiltration as seen with histoplasmosis, strictures after trauma or previous surgery, congenital stenosis or atresia), or extraluminal pressure (adhesions, hernias). A less frequent cause of focal or severe bowel dilation is functional ileus caused by parvoviral enteritis. Therefore, in immature or young adult dogs with questionable parvoviral vaccination status and no palpable mass, barium studies or sonography may be required to rule out intestinal obstruction. As mechanical obstruction becomes more chronic or more complete, the bowel wall becomes atonic, and functional ileus may develop.

Severe focal bowel dilation is a significant radiographic sign of intestinal disease. Because of the potentially life-threatening lesions that may be present, rapid surgical exploration is often warranted, especially when an abdominal mass is also palpable.

Generalized/Mild. All small bowel loops appear mildly enlarged; they may be distended with variable proportions of air and fluid. Possible causes include mild functional ileus owing to bacterial or viral enteritis, malabsorption, hypokalemia, the use of anticholinergic drugs such as atropine, or abdominal pain (Fig. 45–4).

Generalized/Severe. If all bowel loops are uniformly distended, functional ileus is present. Possible causes of diffuse functional ileus are recent abdominal surgery with manipulation of bowel, neurologic injury (spinal trauma), and volvulus of the entire small bowel around the mesenteric root.

If bowel loops are not uniformly distended, mechanical ileus in the distal portion of the small bowel is likely. This appearance may be seen with foreign body obstruction, tumor, stricture, or intussusception. The high probability of obstructive ileus as the cause of severe generalized small bowel distention often allows the clinician to proceed with surgical correction without contrast radiography. Specific identification of the site and type of obstruction usually cannot be made on survey radiographs.

Position

Displacement of small bowel is usually caused by enlargement of adjacent organs, space-occupying mass lesions (see Chapter 36), or herniation. Potential sites for herniation of small bowel are illustrated in Figure 45–5. Contrast studies often help define position abnormalities, especially if there is only a small amount of air in the bowel lumen. The most common sites of small intestinal herniation are through the diaphragm, abdominal wall, inguinal canal, or pelvic diaphragm.[6]

Shape and Contour

Stacked loops is the term used to describe bowel segments (usually distended) that are layered parallel to each other. This appearance also suggests sharp hairpin turns (Fig. 45–6). Stacked loops are usually seen with mechanical ileus.

Irregular or tortuous contour of intestinal loops may be

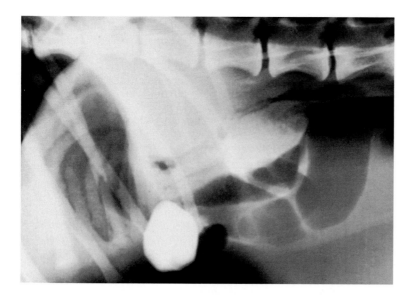

FIGURE 45–3. Mechanical ileus caused by a radiopaque foreign object (rock). Note the focal, extensive air-distended small bowel loops (approximately 2.5 times normal bowel diameter).

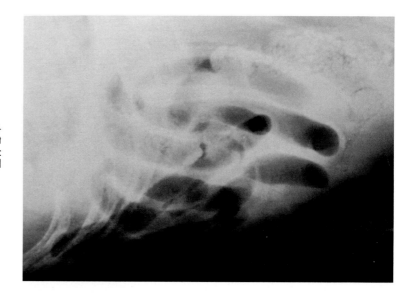

FIGURE 45–4. Mild, generalized enlargement of small bowel lumen (approximately four times the width of the adjacent rib). This appearance is consistent with mild, early functional ileus. This dog had a recently ruptured splenic hemangiosarcoma (not visible on this image) leading to abdominal pain and subsequent functional ileus.

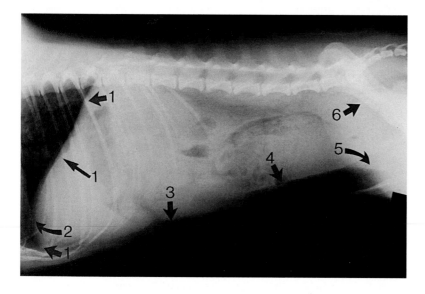

FIGURE 45–5. Potential locations for displacement of bowel in traumatic or congenital herniation. 1, diaphragmatic; 2, peritoneopericardial; 3, umbilical; 4, ventral; 5, inguinal; 6, pelvic diaphragmatic.

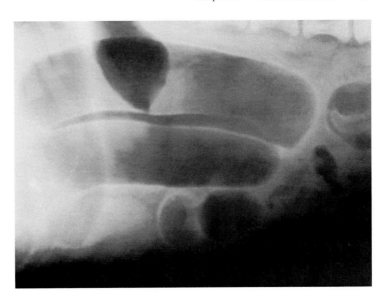

FIGURE 45–6. *Stacked loops* are greatly distended segments of small bowel that lie parallel and may be connected by sharp 180-degree hairpin turns. Stacking is usually seen with obstructive (mechanical) ileus, as in this dog with a corncob (not visible) jejunal obstruction.

due to partial obstruction by linear foreign material[8] (Fig. 45–7) or the occurrence of multiple serosal adhesions. Abnormalities in shape and contour are often easier to identify with contrast studies.

Radiopacity

Luminal Contents

Increased radiopacity occurs most commonly with radiopaque foreign objects (mineral or metallic content) (see Fig. 45–3). Small particles of radiopaque ingesta and debris may also accumulate proximal to a chronic or partial obstruction (Fig. 45–8). Identification of opaque objects small enough to pass through the normal bowel should raise the index of suspicion for a partial obstruction.

Decreased radiopacity is usually the result of ingested air (aerophagia), especially if the location of the lucency changes on serial radiographs. A persistent decreased radiopacity within the bowel lumen may be a radiolucent foreign object. Fruit pits, corncobs, and other nonopaque objects may be recognized by their geometrically shaped radiolucencies on survey radiographs (Fig. 45–9).[9] Based on clinical signs, 24-hour serial survey radiographs or a contrast study may be necessary to confirm the diagnosis of partial obstruction suggested by abnormal luminal contents.

Bowel Wall

Alterations in radiopacity of the bowel wall are unusual and may be difficult to differentiate from opacities within the lumen. Increased radiopacity occurs with dystrophic calcification within a neoplasm, granuloma, or abscess. Radiolucent defects within the intestinal wall, although rare, have been seen with intestinal necrosis secondary to infarction of mesenteric vessels or volvulus.

Architecture of Mucosal Surface

The mucosa cannot be adequately evaluated on survey radiographs. An irregularly scalloped appearance of the mucosa

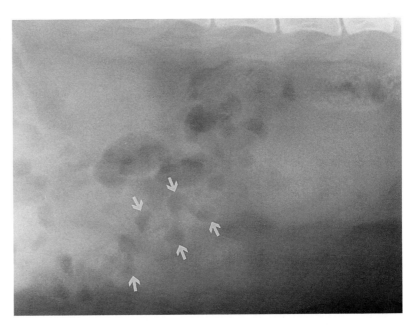

FIGURE 45–7. Plicated, zig-zag, accordion-like contour of the small intestine *(arrows)* in a cat with a linear intestinal foreign object. A string was removed at surgery.

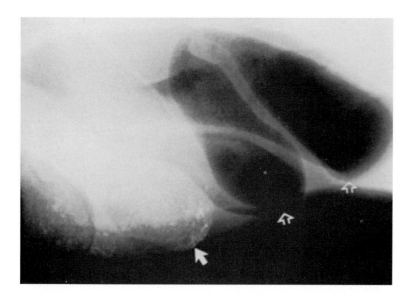

FIGURE 45–8. Mechanical ileus in a dog with an ileocolic intussusception. Although intussusception cannot be diagnosed from this image, the radiographic findings are strongly suggestive of mechanical obstruction. Air-distended stacked loops *(open arrows)* and small particles of radiopaque ingesta *(solid arrow)* are trapped proximal to the obstruction. The latter finding is commonly seen in instances of chronic or slowly developing partial obstruction.

seen in air-filled segments of bowel, however, may provide an additional indication for contrast radiography (Figs. 45–10 and 45–11).

CONTRAST RADIOGRAPHY

Indications

The information gained from a barium upper gastrointestinal tract study is often limited. This limitation is generally the result of poor patient selection and preparation or inappropriate technique. The complete radiographic evaluation of the stomach and small bowel is time-consuming for the veteri-

narian and expensive for the animal's owner. Because of the potential for a low yield of diagnostic information from this procedure, a contrast study should be reserved for the patient in which a diagnosis or approach to treatment cannot be made from clinical information and survey radiographs. In many patients, sonography is also capable of providing useful information about the small bowel, and this information often negates the need for doing an upper gastrointestinal examination.

The clinical signs that most frequently warrant an intestinal contrast study are (1) acute, persistent vomiting with no changes seen on survey radiographs; (2) recurrent vomiting (especially in those animals refractory to symptomatic therapy and without other organ involvement to explain the

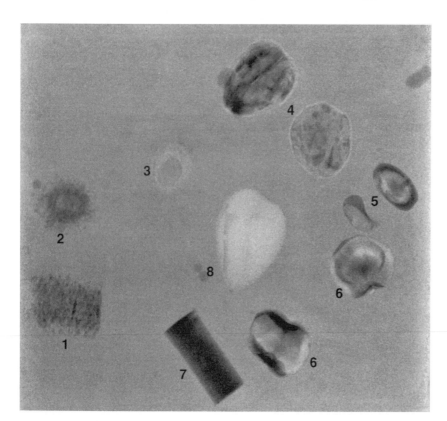

FIGURE 45–9. Various nonopaque foreign bodies radiographed in a water bath. 1, section of corncob viewed side-on; 2, section of corncob viewed end-on; 3, peach pit; 4, walnuts; 5, acorns; 6, chestnuts; 7, wine cork; 8, avocado pit. (From Lamb CR, and Hansson K: Radiological identification on nonopaque intestinal foreign bodies. Vet Radiol Ultrasound 35:87, 1994; with permission).

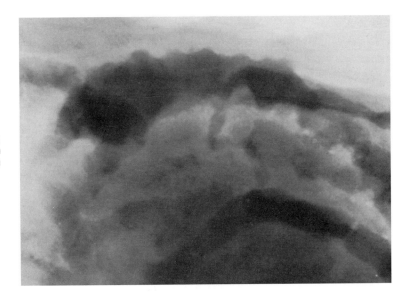

FIGURE 45–10. Survey radiograph in which focal dilation and an irregular, scalloped mucosal surface of a small bowel segment may be seen. Evaluation of the length of intestine affected and the severity of changes in the mucosa require a barium study.

vomiting); (3) palpable abdominal mass without obstruction on survey radiographs; (4) hematemesis; (5) melena; (6) acute abdominal pain with an unusual or unexplained abnormality seen on survey radiographs; and (7) weight loss with intermittent or recurrent diarrhea.[6, 10–13]

Unfortunately, contrast gastrointestinal tract studies are frequently not informative in patients with chronic diarrhea but without vomiting. Additional information that can be gained from a contrast study in these patients includes (1) more thorough evaluation of mucosal abnormalities, (2) length of intestine affected (focal, regional, or generalized), (3) thickness of bowel wall, (4) abnormalities in peristaltic activity and intestinal transit time, (5) improved determination of luminal size, (6) more complete evaluation of luminal contents, and (7) determination of patency of the lumen.

Contraindications

Contrast examination is not warranted in the patient with survey radiographic evidence of obstructive ileus and a palpable abdominal mass.[11] Minimal additional information is to be gained because contrast medium passes only slowly through the atonic bowel proximal to the obstruction, especially in the weakened or debilitated animal. If the clinical and survey radiographic findings are suggestive of mechanical obstruction, surgery is indicated. Further attempts to define the specific site and type of obstructing lesion only delay and possibly complicate surgery and cause additional patient stress. In the young dog, if parvoviral infection cannot be ruled out, contrast procedures should be delayed until parvoviral status is determined.

Technique

An empty gastrointestinal tract is preferred for obtaining optimal information from the contrast study. In patients with severe acute abdominal distress, however, no preparation is usually possible. Additionally, patients with an acute abdominal crisis may suffer additional injury from administration of laxatives or enemas.

For the elective upper gastrointestinal tract examination, a 24-hour fast is recommended before contrast medium administration. An enema should be given 2 to 4 hours before the contrast study to allow emptying of residual fluid and air.

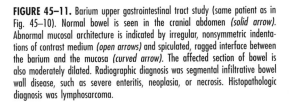
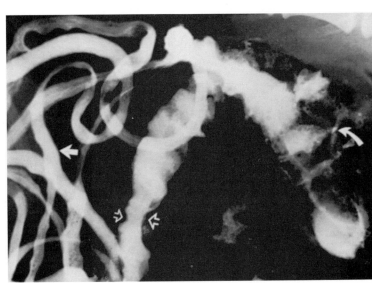

FIGURE 45–11. Barium upper gastrointestinal tract study (same patient as in Fig. 45–10). Normal bowel is seen in the cranial abdomen *(solid arrow)*. Abnormal mucosal architecture is indicated by irregular, nonsymmetric indentations of contrast medium *(open arrows)* and spiculated, ragged interface between the barium and the mucosa *(curved arrow)*. The affected section of bowel is also moderately dilated. Radiographic diagnosis was segmental infiltrative bowel wall disease, such as severe enteritis, neoplasia, or necrosis. Histopathologic diagnosis was lymphosarcoma.

Table 45-3
INTESTINAL CONTRAST AGENTS

Contrast Agent	Advantages	Disadvantages	Uses
Barium sulfate suspensions	Very radiopaque Excellent mucosal detail Remains in suspension Resists dilution Physiologically inert Low cost	May induce granulomas or adhesions if leaked into peritoneal cavity	Routine gastrointestinal tract contrast studies
Barium sulfate, USP	Inexpensive	Inadequate mucosal detail Tends to precipitate	Not recommended

Organic iodine (ionic) solutions	Rapid transient time
	Nonirritating to serosal surfaces
	Rapidly resorbed following extraluminal leakage
		May form precipitates
		May be absorbed across mucosa and excreted by urinary tract
		Hypertonicity causes:
		    Fluid flux into lumen
		    Dilution of contrast
		    Electrolyte imbalance
		    Dehydration
			Suspected intestinal perforation
			
			Young or debilitated patient

Organic iodine (nonionic) solutions	Rapid transit time Nonirritating Resorbed following extraluminal leakage Low osmolality Does not become progressively dilute	Expensive	Suspected perforation Pre-endoscopy

Because most sedative drugs affect gastrointestinal motility, their use should be avoided. General anesthetics and tranquilizers, such as promazine hydrochloride, fentanyl/droperidol, and xylazine hydrochloride, have all been shown to slow passage of barium through the intestine.[14, 15] When sedation of a cat is necessary, a ketamine/diazepam combination (2.7 mg/kg ketamine hydrochloride and 0.09 mg/kg diazepam in separate syringes given intramuscularly 20 minutes before administration of barium) has been shown to have minimal effect on motility.[16] Low-dose (0.05 mg/kg) intravenous acetylpromazine has been recommended for sedation of fractious dogs.[17] Medications that contain anticholinergic drugs should also be discontinued at least 24 hours (preferably 48 to 72 hours) before the contrast study.[10]

Ventrodorsal and right lateral recumbent positions are routinely used. Oblique views to project the pyloric sphincter or a particular abnormality may be added as needed.[18, 19]

Contrast Medium

Barium sulfate suspension is the contrast medium of choice in most situations. Micropulverized preparations are available in a dry powder form (Barosperse, Lafayette Pharmaceuticals, Lafayette, IN) or as a liquid suspension (Liquid Barosperse, Lafayette Pharmaceuticals; Novapaque, Picker International, Cleveland, OH; E-Z-Paque, E-Z Em, Inc., Westbury, NY). The advantages of barium sulfate suspension are summarized in Table 45-3.[10, 13, 20–23] If perforation of the intestinal tract is suspected, use of barium sulfate is not recommended; the combination of barium and ingesta within the peritoneal cavity may cause more severe peritonitis, foreign body granulomas, or serosal adhesions.[11, 24–26] Therefore, an organic iodine preparation designed for the gastrointestinal tract should be used (Gastrografin, meglumine diatrizoate oral solution, Bracco Diagnostics, Princeton, NJ; Oral Hypaque, sodium

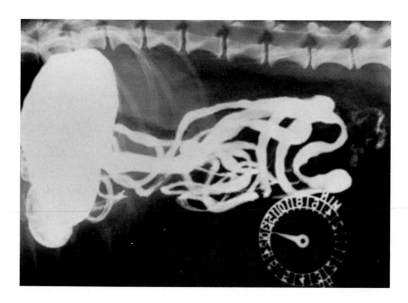

FIGURE 45-12. Normal canine barium upper gastrointestinal tract study, 30 minutes after contrast medium administration. Note the excellent radiopacity of the contrast medium and the sharp definition of the mucosal surface.

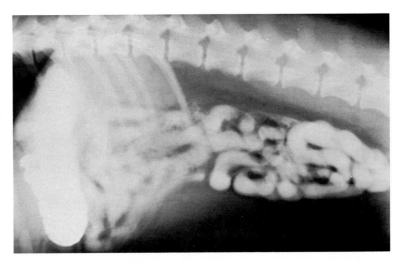

FIGURE 45–13. Normal canine iodine-preparation upper gastrointestinal tract study, 30 minutes after contrast medium administration. Whereas contrast medium opacity is good in the bowel located in the caudal abdomen, the contrast medium is diluted (decreased opacity and poor definition of mucosa) in the cranial abdomen because of fluid entering the bowel in response to the hyperosmolar nature of the contrast medium.

diatrizoate liquid, Nycomed, Princeton, NJ). Occasionally a small tear is missed because the iodine is reabsorbed rapidly by the serosa. If a tear is still suspected after an iodine study, barium may demonstrate the leak more obviously (see Fig. 45–20). Because of the rapid passage of iodine preparations through the gastrointestinal tract, these agents may also be used to determine quickly the patency of the lumen. The potentially hazardous adverse effects from the hyperosmolarity of the iodine contrast media, however, should always be kept in mind. Nonionic, water-soluble iodinated contrast media, such as iohexol, which are of low osmolality, have been used for gastrointestinal contrast studies in animals.[22, 23, 27, 30] Because they are transparent, these agents allow endoscopic evaluation to be performed immediately following completion of the imaging study. These agents cause less fluid movement into the bowel lumen but are relatively costly. Examples of the appearance of barium and iodine in normal small bowel are presented in Figures 45–12 and 45–13. The advantages and disadvantages of the water-soluble contrast media are summarized in Table 45–3.

The volume of barium present within the intestinal lumen is a critical factor. The intestine should be distended to its reasonable physiologic maximum. Failure to administer an adequate volume of contrast medium is one of the most frequent causes for nondiagnostic barium studies. The recommended doses for contrast medium are given in Table 45–4.

Complete descriptions of the procedure for performing an upper gastrointestinal tract study and excellent examples of the normal appearance of the contrast-filled small bowel are available elsewhere.[5, 10, 12, 13, 18] A summary of the organs usually seen at specific intervals after contrast medium administration is presented in Table 45–5.

Normal Roentgen Signs

Margin

The same considerations are present as described for the noncontrast bowel study.

Size

During contrast radiography, nonpersistent narrowing of the bowel lumen is caused by segmental or peristaltic contractions associated with normal bowel motility.

Position

Individual segments of the intestinal tract can be identified and their locations more specifically evaluated during contrast procedures than in survey radiographs.

Table 45–4
RECOMMENDED DOSE RATE FOR CONTRAST MEDIUM

Contrast Medium	Dog	Cat
Barium sulfate suspension*	6–12 mL/kg 20% (w/w)[25] or 6–10 mL/kg 60% (w/w)	12–16 mL/kg[5]
Organic iodine preparation (full strength)	2–3 mL/kg[6, 12, 13]	2 mL/kg[13]
Organic iodine-nonionic (240–300 mg I/mL)	10 mL/kg[22] (1 : 2 dilution)	10 mL/kg[23, 30] (1 : 2 dilution)

*A large volume of relatively dilute contrast medium is preferred by some to distend the intestinal lumen but not to obscure radiolucent luminal filling defects. The authors prefer use of full-strength barium suspension for its superior mucosal pattern definition.

Table 45–5
UPPER GASTROINTESTINAL TRACT FILM SEQUENCE

	Barium	Ionic and Nonionic Organic Iodine	Structures Usually Opacified in Normal Animals*
Dog	Immediate	Immediate	Stomach
	15 minutes		Stomach, duodenum
	30 minutes	15 minutes	Stomach, duodenum, jejunum
	1 hour		Stomach, duodenum, jejunum
	2 hours	30 minutes	Stomach, all parts of small bowel
	4 hours	1 hour	Small bowel, colon
Cat	Immediate	Immediate	Stomach
	5 minutes	5 minutes	Stomach, duodenum
	30 minutes	30 minutes	All parts of small bowel
	1 hour	1 hour	Small bowel, colon

*Owing to the extreme variability of individual transit times, this list is only an approximation of the parts of the gastrointestinal tract seen at these times.

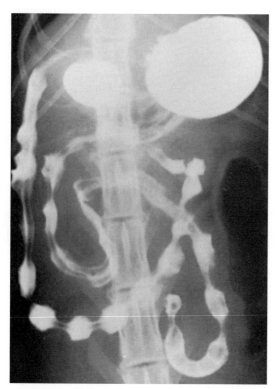

FIGURE 45–14. Normal feline barium upper gastrointestinal tract study. Prominent circular muscle contractions cause almost complete obliteration of the duodenal lumen during segmental peristalsis. This *string-of-pearls* appearance is commonly seen in feline barium studies of the small bowel. The linear filling defect is a normal variant, attributed to a longitudinal fold of mucosa in the incompletely distended intestine. This has been called a *pseudostring sign.*

Shape and Contour

In a barium study in a normal cat, distinct bead-like segments of contrast medium are frequently seen in the duodenum (Fig. 45–14). This *string-of-pearls* appearance is normal and is due to the strong circular muscle contractions that occur during segmental intestinal peristalsis in the cat.

Radiopacity

The opacity of the lumen during a contrast study depends on the volume and type of contrast medium used as well as the

volume of air present. When the bowel lumen is filled with contrast medium, it appears uniformly opaque (Fig. 45–15). Bowel loops containing contrast medium and air have bubble-like radiolucent defects or contrast medium–coated walls with air distention of the lumen (see Fig. 45–15).

Architecture of Mucosal Surface

The normal cat duodenum or jejunum may be characterized by a longitudinally oriented linear filling defect during a barium upper gastrointestinal tract study (see Fig. 45–14). Sometimes called a *pseudostring* sign, this appearance is due to an indentation of a mucosal fold into the lumen. It is usually seen in those intestinal segments that are poorly distended by contrast medium. See the description of roentgen signs of a linear foreign body to differentiate the pseudostring sign from a foreign object.

During a barium upper gastrointestinal tract study, the mucosa/barium interface of the normal dog may be smooth or finely fimbriated (Figs. 45–15 and 45–16). The degree of fimbriation (fringing at the barium/mucosa interface) in the normal dog is variable. This appearance has been attributed to barium dissecting between groups of aggregated villi.[28] Another variation in the normal appearance of the mucosa is the occurrence of pseudoulcers in the canine descending duodenum (Fig. 45–17). These distinct outpouchings are more commonly seen in younger dogs and are mucosal depressions in the antimesenteric side of the bowel wall over lymphoid follicles.[6] Their location, consistently square or conical shape without accompanying spasm, or irregularity of the opposite duodenal wall helps distinguish these normal structures from true ulcers. Cats do not have pseudoulcers.

Motility

Transit time of contrast medium through the intestinal tract and frequency of segmental peristaltic contractions may provide some gross evidence of bowel motility. There is a wide range of normal transit times in dogs, whereas cats have a more consistent, shorter small bowel transit time.[5, 18, 29] A guideline to organs that usually opacify during the upper gastrointestinal tract contrast study is given in Table 45–5. Normal peristaltic waves produce symmetric indentations along the bowel (Fig. 45–18). These indentations do not persist in the same bowel loop when serial radiographs are compared.

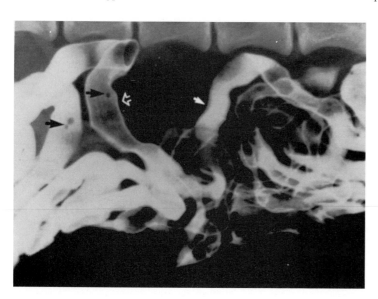

FIGURE 45–15. Normal canine barium upper gastrointestinal tract study. The bowel segments filled with barium are uniformly opaque *(solid white arrow)*. The mucosal surface/barium interface is flat and smooth. Bowel loops containing air have a double-contrast effect; barium coating the mucosa is seen as a thin opaque line, whereas intraluminal air is radiolucent *(open white arrow)*. Small intraluminal gas bubbles may be seen as sharply defined focal radiolucencies in two bowel segments *(black arrows)*.

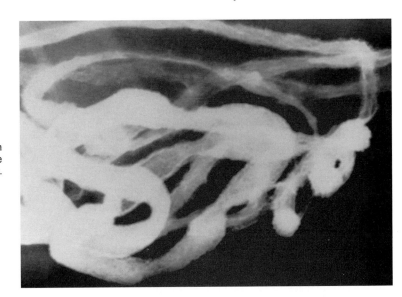

FIGURE 45–16. Normal canine barium upper gastrointestinal tract study in which a finely fimbriated mucosal surface may be seen. This appearance of the interface between the barium and the mucosa is seen in some normal animals.

Abnormal Roentgen Signs

The constant movement of the intestinal tract owing to segmental and peristaltic contractions may produce some unusual appearances of the contrast medium column. Any single radiograph is an image of what is occurring within the gastrointestinal tract during one small fraction of a second. To avoid mistaking a contraction or a peristaltic wave for a pathologic lesion, the clinician should remember that in an upper gastrointestinal tract study, the probability of a suspicious opacity being a real lesion varies directly with its frequency of occurrence; the more often the same abnormality is seen, the more likely it is to be a real lesion.

Position

Displacement of the small intestine within the confines of the peritoneal cavity is usually caused by a space-occupying mass. A complete description of the direction of displacement caused by organ enlargement is available in Chapter 36.

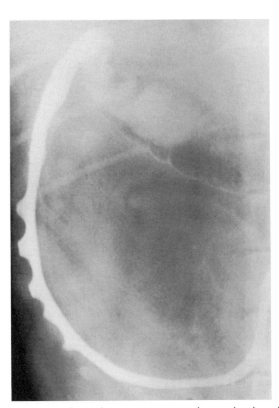

FIGURE 45–17. Normal canine barium upper gastrointestinal tract study with pseudoulcers along the descending duodenum. These indentations are normal variations in the appearance of the duodenum of young dogs and are due to depressions in the mucosa at sites of lymphoid follicles.

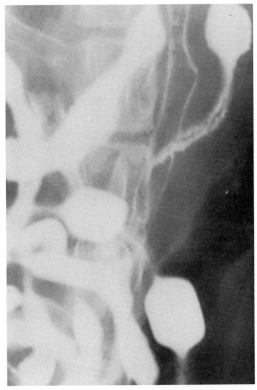

FIGURE 45–18. Normal segmental intestinal contractions during a canine upper gastrointestinal tract study are indicated by symmetric indentations of the bowel wall on each side proximal and distal to the formed bolus of contrast medium.

Pathologic gathering, or crowding, of bowel loops in the midabdomen occurs most frequently because of an ingested linear foreign object or adhesions from peritonitis owing to penetrating foreign object, pancreatitis, bite wound, or, uncommonly, as a result of organizing hemorrhage (after surgery or trauma) or bowel infarction.[31, 32]

Herniation is another common cause of bowel displacement. Most herniations are actually ruptures of one of the tissues that form the boundaries of the peritoneal cavity—diaphragm, abdominal wall, or pelvic diaphragm. Figure 45–5 is an illustration of the most common sites at which traumatic herniation occurs. Congenital hernias usually affect the diaphragm, the scrotum, and the umbilicus.[6]

Shape and Contour

Because the contour of the normal small intestinal wall is gently rounded or curved, abnormal patterns are seen as segments of bowel with persistent straight or flat walls or those that are excessively coiled or plicated. Straight wall contour is seen with infiltrative diseases (lymphosarcoma, scirrhous adenocarcinoma, and histoplasmosis). Fibrosis or adhesions as might occur after trauma or focal peritonitis may also cause loss of bowel wall pliability.

A characteristic pleated (plicated, ribbon-candy) appearance occurs commonly when linear foreign material has been ingested (Fig. 45–19); compare with the normal cat intestine in Figure 45–14.[6] Because this type of foreign material tends to cause only incomplete blockage, the luminal diameter is usually not greatly distended, especially on survey radiographs.[33] Often an increased number of bizarre-shaped (e.g., teardrop, paisley print, fleur-de-lis) gas bubbles may be the

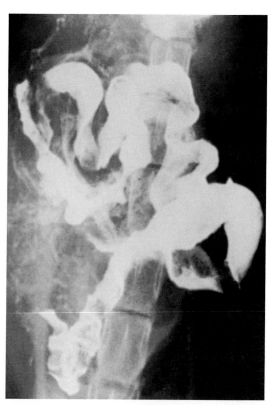

FIGURE 45–20. Leakage of contrast medium into the peritoneal cavity occurred owing to bowel wall necrosis at multiple sites. Iodine-containing, water-soluble contrast media are the agents of choice when bowel perforation is suspected. After this cat vomited iodine several times, barium was used to achieve a diagnostic study.

only change seen on the survey radiographs (see Fig. 45–7).[33] This gas pattern, in conjunction with loss of serosal detail, suggests laceration of the bowel wall with secondary peritonitis.[8] Contrast medium may leak from these lacerations (Fig. 45–20). Common linear foreign objects include string, thread, or tinsel in the cat and fabric (scarves, socks, pantyhose, carpet) or plastic (meat wrappers, trash bags) in the dog.[8]

Radiopacity

The shape of a large radiolucent filling defect within the contrast medium column may indicate not only the presence of obstruction, but also the type of lesion causing the blockage. Barium is often able to dissect between an intraluminal object and the bowel wall, allowing a more complete image of the obstruction. The following lesions may be recognized by the given shape of the intraluminal filling defect (Fig. 45–21):

1. *Spheric*—rubber ball (common), benign tumor such as a leiomyoma (rare).
2. *Elliptic*—fruit pit, nut.
3. *Straight*—plastic, leather, wood splinter.
4. *Hemispheric*—retrograde intussusception.
5. *Curved linear*—ascarid (Fig. 45–22).

Other foreign objects have distinctive shapes that allow their positive identification (Fig. 45–23). Contrast medium trapped in irregular contours or crevices of some foreign objects frequently persists after the main column of contrast medium has passed. If patient preparation is inadequate, particles of ingesta may appear as filling defects in the barium

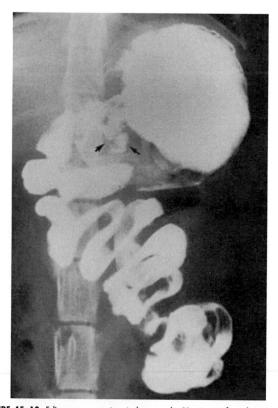

FIGURE 45–19. Feline upper gastrointestinal tract study, 20 minutes after administration of barium. The tightly pleated or ribbon candy appearance indicates the presence of linear foreign material. The proximal end of the foreign material is often wrapped around the base of the tongue or is caught in the pyloric antrum of the stomach *(arrows)*.

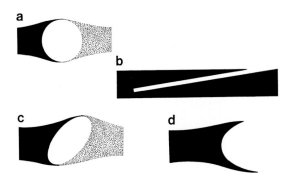

FIGURE 45–21. Shapes of contrast interface with an intraluminal object. The barium column *(black)* fills the intestine and outlines one or several surfaces of the object. Partial obstruction of the lumen allows a smaller quantity of barium *(stippling)* to pass. With complete obstruction, there is no barium in the bowel distal to it and therefore no definition of the caudal surface of the object. *A,* Rubber ball, spherical mass arising from the bowel mucosa (leiomyoma—rare). *B,* Flat, straight foreign object, such as hard plastic, leather, and wood splinter. *C,* Fruit pit or nut. *D,* Retrograde intussusception (invagination of bowel in the opposite direction of normal ingesta passage).

column (Fig. 45–24), which significantly reduces the information available from the study.

Size and Architecture

The following descriptions refer to the size of the bowel lumen, the appearance of the mucosal surface, and the extent of the small intestine that is affected. The term *focal* indicates that one to three loops of bowel are involved; *regional* is used when more than three loops but less than 50 percent of the small bowel is affected; and *generalized* applies to lesions present in more than 50 percent of the small bowel segments.

Dilated Lumen/Smooth Mucosa. This combination of roentgen signs is most frequently seen with obstruction.[34] In Figure 45–27, barium within distended bowel segments proximal to a site of mechanical obstruction can be seen.

With focal or regional involvement, this radiographic sign is usually seen with mechanical obstruction of recent onset or when the obstruction is located in the duodenum or cranial portion of the jejunum. The bowel distal to the obstruction and the unaffected bowel proximal to the obstruction are normal in size and show evidence of peristalsis. If

the obstruction of the lumen is almost complete, the small volume of barium that passes the lesion may not be sufficient to distend the lumen of the remainder of the bowel (see Fig. 45–23). This finding may lead to a false impression of narrowed bowel diameter distal to the obstruction.

Generalized involvement is indicated if all loops of bowel are distended uniformly, no peristaltic indentations are seen along the intestinal walls, and functional or paralytic ileus is present. Mechanical ileus may be generalized because of chronic obstruction in the distal small bowel or at the ileocolic junction. Generalized mechanical ileus may proceed to functional ileus as the bowel wall stretches and becomes atonic and then progressively ischemic. Other causes of functional ileus include parvovirus infection, parasympatholytic drug administration, peritoneal inflammation, spinal cord trauma, intestinal vascular injury, or thrombosis.

Dilated Lumen/Irregular Mucosa. Usually seen as focal or regional involvement, the mucosa has an irregularly scalloped or spiculated surface; this appearance often is associated with ulceration. Regional infiltration of the jejunum by lymphosarcoma is shown in Figure 45–11. Other pathologic processes that may show similar changes in the bowel include

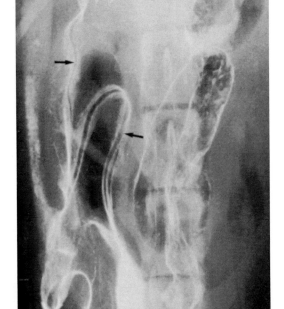

FIGURE 45–22. The thin, radiolucent filling defects are ascarids *(arrows).* Note that the defects taper at their cranial and caudal ends and that there is no evidence of abnormal size, shape, or contour of the bowel.

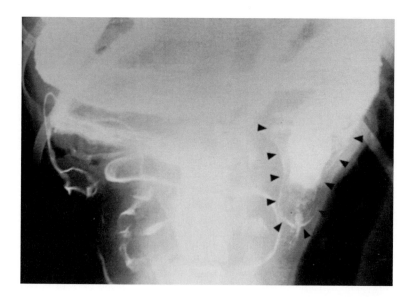

FIGURE 45–23. Mechanical obstruction of the jejunum by a foreign object (baby bottle nipple [arrows]).

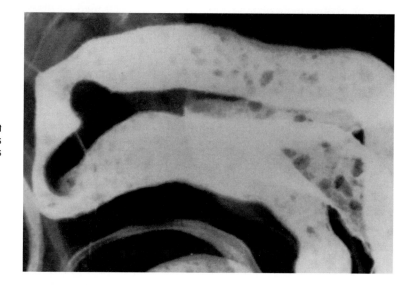

FIGURE 45–24. Food particles mixed with barium in a patient that had not been fasted before the contrast study. The food particles create filling defects that compromise the ability to define small intraluminal objects or nodules arising from the mucosa.

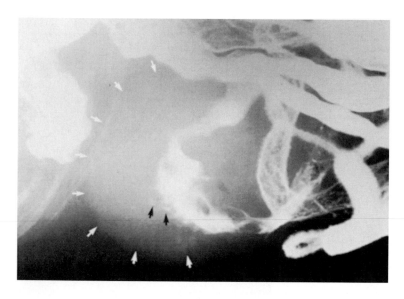

FIGURE 45–25. Adenocarcinoma of the jejunum during a barium upper gastrointestinal tract study. Roentgen signs include soft-tissue mass (white arrows), mild focal enlargement of bowel lumen, irregular contour of mucosa, and extravasation of a small amount of contrast medium into the mass (black arrows).

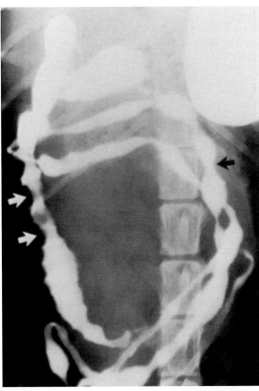

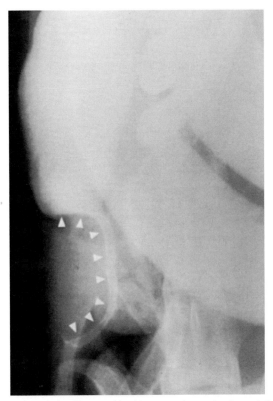

FIGURE 45–26. Irritation of duodenum and jejunum is indicated by irregular, serrated mucosal surface *(white arrows)* of duodenum and hypersegmentation *(black arrow).* The midcentral area, which is devoid of bowel loops, was caused by necrotic, hemorrhagic pancreatitis with abscess formation that resulted 10 days after a penetrating wound.

FIGURE 45–27. Eccentrically narrowed bowel lumen, smooth mucosal surface, and dilation of bowel proximal to the narrowing characterize this focal intramural obstruction *(arrowheads).* Histopathologic diagnosis was adenocarcinoma of bowel wall. Eccentric narrowing usually occurs with a mass lesion; a post-traumatic or postinflammatory stricture usually causes more symmetric narrowing.

adenocarcinoma (often produces a focal mass that is palpable; Fig. 45–25) and histoplasmosis.[35, 36]

Narrowed Lumen/Smooth Mucosa. With focal or regional involvement, localized irritation of the bowel may cause spasm of the circular muscle component of the wall and induce hyperperistalsis, leading to hypersegmentation of the barium column (Fig. 45–26). A single, persistent focus of narrowed lumen may also be seen with stricture owing to an intramural mass, such as a granuloma and an adenocarcinoma (Fig. 45–27)[37–40]; stenosis after injury of the wall; or when barium given orally reaches an intussusception that

has occurred in the direction of normal peristalsis (forward or direct intussusception). Signs of mechanical ileus may also be present in these patients.

Diffuse enteritis or peritonitis caused by a variety of bacterial organisms or chemical irritants can cause a more generalized distribution of hyperperistalsis (Fig. 45–28). An insufficient volume of barium (from either inadequate dosage or vomiting following administration) may fail to distend the bowel and may artifactually create an impression of bowel narrowing.

FIGURE 45–28. Hyperperistalsis is seen in this barium upper gastrointestinal tract study 5 minutes after contrast medium administration. Hypersegmentation causes numerous bead-like accumulations of contrast medium *(solid arrow).* Thin strands of barium that extend for several centimeters *(open arrow)* can be seen when transit time through the small bowel is faster than normal, as in this patient.

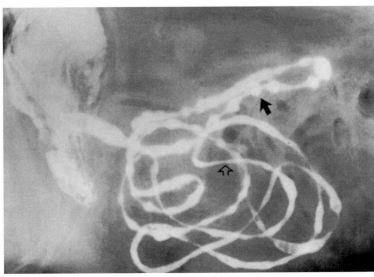

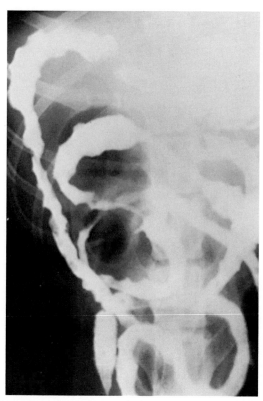

FIGURE 45–29. Numerous radiolucent mural indentations, resulting in filling defects, are seen in the duodenum and less prominently in the jejunum. These defects appear as thumbprint-like indentations of the barium column. The lumen diameter of the descending duodenum is narrowed. Possible causes include chronic severe inflammation and infiltrative neoplasia. Histopathologic diagnosis was lymphocytic-plasmacytic enteritis.

Narrowed Lumen/Irregular Mucosa/Filling Defects. When this roentgen sign is seen at a single site or within a focal region of small bowel, possible causes include ulceration, mucosal polyps, or inflammatory bowel disease. Diseases that can produce secondary ulceration, which may be detected by a contrast study, include mast cell tumors, hepatic disorders, uremia, and recurrent pancreatitis.[41–45] Ulcerated primary intestinal tumor, such as adenocarcinoma, may also have a narrowed lumen and ragged, irregular mucosa, some-

times described as *apple core* in appearance.[46, 47] Although rare, an ulcerated granuloma occurring secondary to foreign object penetration or systemic fungal spread should also be considered.

When the distribution is more regional or generalized, severe inflammatory conditions of the mucosa and bowel wall may have numerous nodular filling defects or thumbprint indentations along the mucosal surface (Figs. 45–29 and 45–30). Possible causes include inflammatory bowel disease, eosinophilic enteritis, hemorrhagic gastroenteritis, intestinal lymphosarcoma or ischemia, and necrosis.[32, 48–54] Spastic contraction of circular muscles of the intestinal wall may either mimic or contribute to the scalloped appearance of the barium column. Although the typical appearance is a narrowed lumen, identification of a widened diameter should not exclude consideration of severe infiltrative bowel disorders.

Transit Time and Peristaltic Activity

Because of the great variation in time required for barium to pass through the small bowel in the dog and the cat, only those transit times that are significantly outside the normal parameters should be considered indicative of a pathologic condition. The best methods for the evaluation of peristaltic activity are image-intensified fluoroscopy and ultrasonography. Because of the limited availability of this equipment, however, those inferences concerning bowel motility that can be made from barium studies are mentioned here.

Prolonged Transit. If barium is not cleared from the small bowel of the dog after 5 hours or after 3 hours in the cat, transit is considered abnormally slow. If luminal diameter is normal, possible causes for slow transit include anticholinergic drug administration or a volume of barium insufficient to stimulate intestinal centers of peristaltic activity.[55] If the luminal diameter is distended, atony as a result of mechanical or functional ileus is present.

Rapid Transit. When rapid opacification of small bowel loops occurs in combination with multiple, closely spaced peristaltic contractions, hypermotility is present. This finding is most commonly associated with acute enteritis or serosal irritation (peritonitis). Motility may be increased secondary to the increased volume and fluid nature of intestinal contents in the animal with profuse diarrhea.[56] If early opacification of many segments of the small bowel is seen without distinct peristaltic contractions, enteritis or one of the infil-

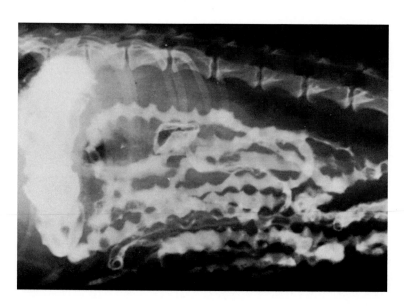

FIGURE 45–30. Generalized asymmetric thumbprint indentations throughout the small bowel. This pattern is unusual but suggests extensive infiltrative mucosal disease (such as lymphosarcoma, parvoviral enteritis, lymphocytic-plasmacytic enteritis), wall spasm, or both.

trative diseases that cause malabsorption may be reducing compliance of the intestinal wall.

References

1. Root CR: Interpretation of abdominal survey radiographs. Vet Clin North Am 4:763, 1974.
2. Jergens AE, Moore FM, Haynes JS, et al: Idiopathic inflammatory bowel disease in dogs and cats: 84 cases (1987–1990). J Am Vet Med Assoc 201:1603, 1992.
3. Owens JM: Radiographic Interpretation for the Small Animal Clinician. St. Louis, Ralston Purina, 1982.
4. Riedesel E: Unpublished data, 1996.
5. Morgan JP: The upper gastrointestinal examination in the cat: Normal radiographic appearance using positive-contrast medium. Vet Radiol 22:159, 1981.
6. O'Brien TR: Small intestine. In O'Brien TR (Ed): Radiographic Diagnosis of Abdominal Disorders in the Dog and Cat. Philadelphia, WB Saunders, 1978, pp 279–351.
7. Penninck DG, Nyland T, Fisher P, et al: Ultrasonography of normal canine gastrointestinal tract. Vet Radiol 30:272, 1989.
8. Evans KL, Smeak DD, and Biller DS: Gastrointestinal linear foreign bodies in 32 dogs: A retrospective evaluation and feline comparison. J Am Anim Hosp Assoc 30:445, 1994.
9. Lamb CR, and Hansson K: Radiological identification on nonopaque intestinal foreign bodies. Vet Radiol Ultrasound 35:87, 1994.
10. Brawner WR, and Bartels JE: Contrast radiography of the digestive tract: Indications, techniques and complications. Vet Clin North Am [Small Anim Pract] 13:599, 1983.
11. Gomez JA: The gastrointestinal contrast study. Vet Clin North Am 4:805, 1974.
12. Morgan JP, and Silverman S: Radiographic evaluation of the digestive tract. In Techniques of Veterinary Radiography, 3rd Ed. Davis, CA, Veterinary Radiology Associates, 1982.
13. Root CR: Contrast radiography of the alimentary tract. In Ticer JW (Ed): Radiographic Technique in Veterinary Practice. Philadelphia, WB Saunders, 1984.
14. Hsu WH, and McNeel SV: Effect of yohimbine on xylazine-induced prolongation of gastrointestinal transit in dogs. J Am Vet Med Assoc 183:297, 1983.
15. Zontine WJ: Effect of chemical restraint drugs on the passage of barium sulfate through the stomach and duodenum of dogs. J Am Vet Med Assoc 162:878, 1973.
16. Hogan PM, and Aronson E: Effect of sedation on transit time of feline gastrointestinal contrast studies. Vet Radiol 29:85, 1988.
17. Kerr LV, and Koblik PD: Contrast radiography. In Morgan R (Ed): Handbook of Small Animal Practice. New York, Churchill Livingstone, 1988.
18. Farrow CS, Green R, and Shively M: Radiology of the Cat. St. Louis, Mosby-Year Book, 1994.
19. Ticer JW: The abdomen. In Ticer JW (Ed): Radiographic Technique in Veterinary Practice. Philadelphia, WB Saunders, 1984.
20. Allan GS, Rendano VT, Quick CB, et al: Gastrografin as a gastrointestinal contrast medium in the cat. Vet Radiol 20:3, 1979.
21. Root CR, and Morgan JP: Contrast radiography of the upper gastrointestinal tract in the dog: A comparison of micropulverized barium sulfate and U.S.P. barium sulfate suspensions in clinically normal dogs. J Small Anim Pract 10:279, 1969.
22. Agut A, Sanchez-Valverde MA, Lasaosa JM, et al: Use of iohexol as a gastrointestinal contrast medium in the dog. Vet Radiol Ultrasound 34:71, 1993.
23. Agut A, Sanchez-Valverde ME, Torrecillas FE, et al: Iohexol as a gastrointestinal contrast medium the cat. Vet Radiol Ultrasound 35:164, 1993.
24. Foley MJ, Ghahremani GG, and Rogers LF: Reappraisal of contrast media used to detect upper gastrointestinal perforations. Radiology 144:231, 1982.
25. Ott DJ, and Gelfand DW: Gastrointestinal contrast agents: Indications, uses, and risks. JAMA 249:2380, 1983.
26. Seltzer SE, Jones B, and McLaughlin GC: Proper choice of contrast agents in emergency gastrointestinal radiology. Crit Rev Diagn Imaging 12:79, 1979.
27. Williams J, Biller DS, Myer CW, et al: Use of iohexol as a gastrointestinal contrast agent in three dogs, five cats and one bird. J Am Vet Med Assoc 202:624, 1993.
28. Thrall DE, and Leininger JR: Irregular intestinal mucosal margination in the dog: Normal or abnormal? J Small Anim Pract 17:305, 1976.
29. Miyabayashi T, Morgan JP, Atilola MAO, et al: Small intestinal emptying time in normal Beagle dogs: A contrast radiographic study. Vet Radiol 27:164, 1986.
30. Williams J, Biller DS, Miyabayashi T, et al: Evaluation of Iohexol as a gastrointestinal contrast medium in normal cats. Vet Radiol Ultrasound 34:310, 1993.
31. Suter PF, and Olsson S-E: The diagnosis of injuries to the intestines, gallbladder and bile ducts in the dog. J Small Anim Pract 11:575, 1970.
32. Vest B, and Margulis AR: Experimental infarction of small bowel in dogs. AJR 92:1080, 1964.
33. Felts JF, Fox PP, and Burk RL: Thread and sewing needles as gastrointestinal foreign bodies in the cat: A review of 64 cases. J Am Vet Med Assoc 184:56, 1984.
34. Kleine LJ: The role of radiography in the diagnosis of intestinal obstruction in dogs and cats. Comp Contin Ed Pract 1:44, 1979.
35. Brodey RS: Alimentary tract neoplasms in the cat: A clinicopathologic survey of 46 cases. Am J Vet Res 27:74, 1966.
36. Patnaik AK, Hurvitz AI, and Johnson GF: Canine gastrointestinal neoplasms. Vet Pathol 14:547, 1977.
37. Gibbs C, and Pearson H: Localized tumours of the canine small intestine: A report of twenty cases. J Small Anim Pract 27:507, 1986.
38. Patnaik AK, Liu S-K, and Johnson GF: Feline intestinal adenocarcinoma. Vet Pathol 13:1, 1976.
39. Feeney DA, Klausner JS, and Johnston GR: Chronic bowel obstruction caused by primary intestinal neoplasia: A report of five cases. J Am Anim Hosp Assoc 18:67, 1982.
40. Bruecker KA, and Withrow SJ: Intestinal leiomyosarcomas in six dogs. J Am Anim Hosp Assoc 24:281, 1988.
41. Happe RP, van der Gaag I, Lamers CBHW, et al: Zollinger-Ellison syndrome in three dogs. Vet Pathol 17:177, 1980.
42. Moreland KJ: Ulcer disease of the upper gastrointestinal tract in small animals: Pathophysiology, diagnosis, and management. Comp Contin Ed Vet Pract 10:1265, 1988.
43. Murray M, McKeating FJ, Baker GJ, et al: Peptic ulceration in the dog: A clinico-pathological study. Vet Rec 91:441, 1972.
44. Zontine WJ, Meierhenry EF, and Hicks RF: Perforated duodenal ulcer associated with mastocytoma in a dog: A case report. J Am Vet Radiol Soc 18:162, 1977.
45. Middleton DJ, Watson ADJ, and Culvenor JE: Duodenal ulceration associated with gastrin-secreting pancreatic tumor in a cat. J Am Vet Med Assoc 183:461, 1983.
46. Patnaik AK, Hurvitz AI, and Johnson GF: Canine intestinal adenocarcinoma and carcinoid. Vet Pathol 17:149, 1980.
47. Theilen GH, and Madewell BR: Tumors of the digestive tract. In Theilen GH, Madewell BR (Eds): Veterinary Cancer Medicine. Philadelphia, Lea & Febiger, 1979, pp 307–331.
48. Burrows CF: Canine hemorrhagic gastroenteritis. J Am Anim Hosp Assoc 13:451, 1977.
49. Hayden DW, and Van Kruiningen HJ: Lymphocytic-plasmacytic enteritis in German shepherd dogs. J Am Anim Hosp Assoc 18:89, 1982.
50. Smith SL, Tutton RH, and Ochsner SF: Roentgenographic aspects of intestinal ischemia. AJR 116:249, 1972.
51. Hendrick M: A spectrum of hypereosinophilic syndromes exemplified by six cats with eosinophilic enteritis. Vet Pathol 18:1888, 1981.
52. Couto CG, Rutgers HC, Sherding RG, et al: Gastrointestinal lymphoma in twenty dogs. J Vet Intern Med 3:73, 1989.
53. Tams TR: Chronic feline inflammatory bowel disorders: II. Feline eosinophilic enteritis and lymphosarcoma. Comp Contin Ed Vet Pract 8:464, 1986.
54. Weichselbaum RC, Feeney DA, and Hayden DW: Comparison of upper gastrointestinal radiographic findings to histopathologic observations: A retrospective study of 41 dogs an cats with suspected small bowel infiltrative disease. Vet Radiol Ultrasound 35:418, 1994.
55. Ehrlein H-J: A new technique for simultaneous radiography and recording of gastrointestinal motility in unanesthetized dogs. Lab Anim Sci 30:879, 1980.
56. Sherding RG: Diseases of the small bowel. In Ettinger SJ (Ed): Textbook of Veterinary Internal Medicine. Philadelphia, WB Saunders, 1983, pp 1278–1345.

STUDY QUESTIONS

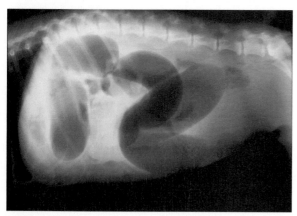

FIGURE 45–31. Right lateral view of a 14-month-old dog with intermittent vomiting for 5 days. An abdominal mass is palpable. Same dog as in Figure 45–32. See Answer Section, 45–3 for interpretation.

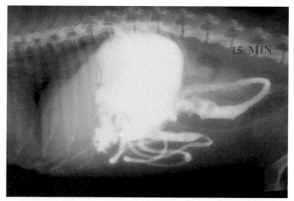

FIGURE 45–33. Right lateral view at 15 minutes after barium administration in an 11-year-old male Shih tzu with chronic anemia and melena. See Question 4 for more history and laboratory results. Same dog as in Figure 45–34 and Figure 45–35. See Answer Section, 45–4 for interpretation.

1. Serosal surfaces of the small intestines would be expected to be poorly defined in which of the following conditions? (more than one may be correct)
   A. A 9-year-old fat dog presented for acute onset of vomiting, polyuria, and polydipsia.
   B. A 14-year-old cat with anorexia and severe weight loss.
   C. A 4-month-old puppy with vomiting and palpable abdominal mass.
   D. An obese 7-year-old cat, inappetent for 3 weeks with icterus.

2. The duodenum frequently has a *string-of-pearls* shape in the normal young dog and cat, but this appearance can be seen only on a barium upper gastrointestinal contrast study. (True or False)

3. A 14-month-old male mixed-breed dog is presented for intermittent vomiting of 5 days' duration. A mass in the

abdomen and gas-filled loops of bowel can be palpated. Figures 45–31 and 45–32 are right lateral and ventrodorsal survey views. What is your interpretation of the radiographs, recommendation to the owner based on your findings, and rationale for the recommendation?

4. An 11-year-old male Shih tzu has had chronic anemia and melena for about 40 days. There is a tense abdomen; pale mucous membranes; and dark, formed feces. Urinalysis and routine blood chemistries were unremarkable (hemoglobin = 3.9 g/dL, packed cell volume = 12 percent). A barium upper gastrointestinal study was performed: Figure 45–33 is a right lateral view at 15 minutes, Figure 45–34 is a ventrodorsal view at 1 hour, and Figure 45–35 is a ventrodorsal view at 2 hours after barium administration. Describe any significant radiographic abnormality, and list differential diagnostic possibilities.

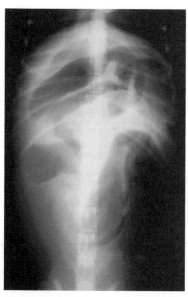

FIGURE 45–32. Ventrodorsal view of same dog as in Figure 45–31.

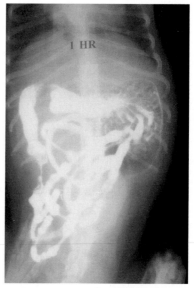

FIGURE 45–34. Ventrodorsal view at 1 hour after barium administration. Same dog as in Figures 45–33 and 45–35.

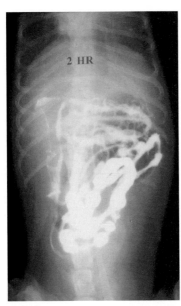

FIGURE 45–35. Ventrodorsal view at 2 hours after barium administration. Same dog as in Figures 45–33 and 45–34.

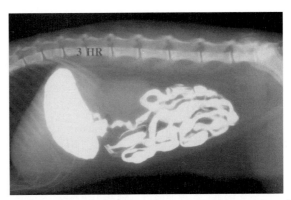

FIGURE 45–38. Right lateral view at 3 hours after barium administration in a 1-year-old cat with a 1-month history of pyrexia, weight loss, and general debilitation. See Question 6 for additional history and laboratory results. Same cat as in Figure 45–39. See Answer Section, 45–6 for interpretation.

5. Figures 45–36 and 45–37 are right lateral and ventrodorsal survey abdominal radiographs of a 15-year-old neutered male cat reported to be ill for 5 days with dark diarrhea. On physical examination, the cat is depressed and distended bowel loops are palpable. Describe the appearance of the gastrointestinal tract. What is your interpretation?

6. A 1-year-old neutered male seal-point Siamese cat had a 1-month history of pyrexia, weight loss, and general debilitation. The owner reported recent onset of diarrhea. The cat was depressed and lethargic with thickened, painful bowel on palpation. Additional tests included fecal (negative), total serum protein = 8.7 g/dL, and negative serology for feline leukemia virus and toxoplasmosis. Figures 45–38 and 45–39 are right lateral and ventrodorsal views made 3 hours after barium administration. Describe any radiographic abnormalities demonstrated by the barium study. List possible explanations for observed abnormalities.

7. What is one of the most common causes of technically inadequate barium upper gastrointestinal studies?

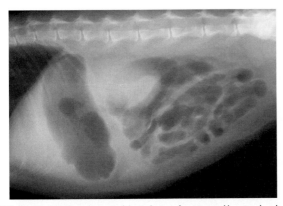

FIGURE 45–36. Right lateral survey abdominal view of a 15-year-old neutered male cat ill for 5 days with dark diarrhea. Distended bowel loops are palpable. For interpretation see Answer Section, 45–5. Same cat as in Figure 45–37.

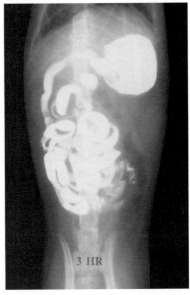

FIGURE 45–39. Ventrodorsal view at 3 hours after barium administration. Same cat as in Figure 45–38.

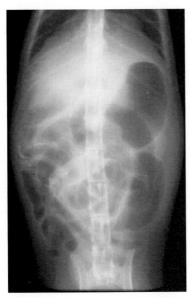

FIGURE 45–37. Ventrodorsal survey abdominal view of same cat as in Figure 45–36.

8. List the reason why there may be no abnormalities from an intestinal obstruction on survey abdominal radiographs.

9. Filling defects in the barium-filled small bowel lumen may or may not be pathologic. What roentgen signs could be used to determine whether filling defects are pathologically significant?

10. Small bowel wall thickening is more reliably determined by palpation than by survey radiography. (True or False)

(Answers appear on pages 648 to 649.)

Chapter 46

The Large Bowel

Darryl N. Biery

IMAGING OPTIONS FOR LARGE BOWEL DISEASES

Survey and contrast radiographic studies are diagnostic procedures that frequently enable recognition of large bowel disease.[1-3] After a survey radiographic examination, however, endoscopy (colonoscopy) now has largely replaced the radiographic contrast studies of the colon. More than 80 percent of colonic diseases now are reported to be diagnosed using endoscopy, especially when a flexible endoscope enables visualization of the transverse colon, ascending colon, and cecum.[4-6]

Ultrasound is also becoming more important for examination of the large bowel by providing additional and complementary information to the clinical, endoscopic, and survey radiographic findings. Although air and feces in the bowel are a limiting factor for ultrasound studies, an ultrasound examination can assess near-field bowel wall thickness and symmetry, mural and extramural bowel masses, the regional lymph nodes, and other abdominal viscera. On ultrasound, an intussusception can be readily identified. Needle aspiration and biopsy specimens of the colon can also be obtained using ultrasound-guided techniques.[7, 8]

Other much less commonly used imaging techniques for colonic diseases include rectocolonic lymphangiography, mesenteric angiography, and colonic transit scintigraphy. These techniques enable assessment of anatomic or functional abnormalities and require specialized equipment and expertise.[9-11]

NORMAL RADIOGRAPHIC ANATOMY

The large bowel of the dog and cat is composed of the cecum, colon, rectum, and anal canal (Fig. 46–1). The cecum, a

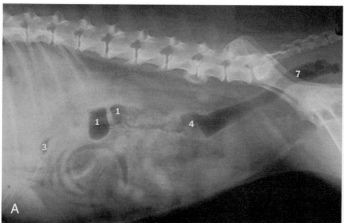
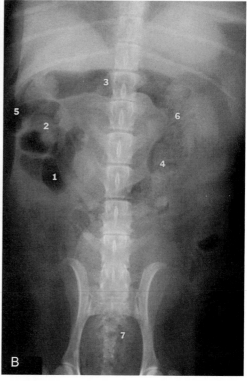

FIGURE 46–1. Survey lateral *(A)* and ventrodorsal *(B)* radiographs of a normal canine abdomen. The large bowel is divided into the cecum (1), ascending colon (2), transverse colon (3), descending colon (4), hepatic flexure (5), splenic flexure (6), rectum (7), and anal canal. Note the admixture of gas and feces present in the cecum, colon, and rectum. In *B*, the descending colon is displaced toward the right by a normally distended urinary bladder.

diverticulum of the proximal colon, has different anatomic and radiographic appearances in the dog and the cat (Fig. 46–2).[1] The canine cecum is semicircular (corkscrew or C shaped) and compartmentalized with a cecocolic junction and normally contains some intraluminal gas. The intraluminal gas and characteristic shape enable easy recognition of the cecum in the right midabdomen on most survey radiographs. The feline cecum, however, is usually not visible on survey radiographs. It is a short, cone-like diverticulum of the colon with no distinct cecocolic junction and no compartmentalization; it rarely contains gas.

The colon of the dog and the cat, the longest segment of the large bowel, is a thin-walled distensible tube that is divided into ascending, transverse, and descending parts. These divisions are easily recognized on survey abdominal radiographs based on their shape, size, and location. The distal ileum enters the ascending colon from a medial direction via the ileocecal sphincter. This circular sphincter is usually not visible on survey radiographs, but it is usually easy to identify with a barium enema. The colon has a shape similar to that of a question mark or shepherd's crook (see Fig. 46–1). The junction between the ascending and transverse colon is called the *hepatic* or *right colic flexure*, and the junction between the transverse and descending colon is called the *splenic* or *left colic flexure*. The ascending colon and hepatic flexure are located to the right of midline. The transverse colon, which passes from right to left, lies cranial to the root of the mesentery. The splenic flexure and proximal descending colon are located to the left of midline. The distal descending colon courses to the midline and enters the pelvic canal to become the rectum. The rectum is the terminal portion of the colon, beginning at the pelvic inlet and ending at the anal canal.

The anatomic relation of the large bowel to other viscera is extremely important for the radiographic recognition of diseases of the large bowel and adjacent organs (Fig. 46–3). The ascending colon lies adjacent to the descending duodenum, right limb of the pancreas, right kidney, mesentery, and small bowel. The transverse colon lies adjacent to the greater curvature of the stomach, left limb of the pancreas, liver, small intestine, and root of the mesentery. The proximal descending colon lies in close proximity to the left kidney and ureter, spleen, and small bowel. The midportion of the descending colon lies adjacent to the small bowel, urinary bladder, and uterus. Because it is less fixed, the midportion of the descending colon has a variety of normal positions in the caudal left abdomen. Normal variations are caused by various amounts of ingesta within the bowel, degree of urinary bladder distention, and amount of intra-abdominal fat. Some dogs appear to have an excess of length of colon. Termed *redundant colon*, this finding is considered a variant of normal and is not clinically significant.[1, 12]

Frequently the distended urinary bladder displaces the descending colon toward the midline or to the right of midline (see Fig. 46–1). The distal portions of the descending colon and rectum are also closely associated with the urethra, the medial iliac and sacral lymph nodes, the prostate or uterus and vagina, and the pelvic diaphragm.

RADIOGRAPHIC TECHNIQUES OF LARGE BOWEL EVALUATION

Because feces and gas produce contrasting radiographic opacities and are usually present in the large bowel, a part or all of the large bowel is identifiable on survey radiographs of the abdomen. The different body positions used for survey radiography distribute intraluminal gas to different parts of the large bowel, largely because of gravity. Thus, gas is usually present in the more nondependent portions of the colon. When present, foreign bodies (i.e. pieces of bone, safety pin, wire) are easily recognized on survey radiographs. The colonic mucosal pattern cannot be evaluated from survey radiographs.

When the large bowel is evaluated radiographically, it is essential that the entire abdomen and pelvic area be included on two orthogonal radiographic views and that the radiographs be of diagnostic quality. The urinary bladder should be empty. Rectal examination, vigorous abdominal palpation,

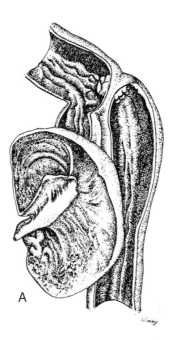
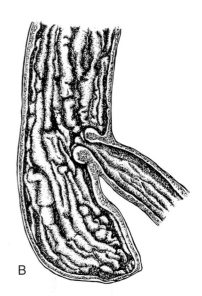

FIGURE 46–2. The cecum of the dog *(A)* and of the cat *(B)* are anatomically and radiographically different. The canine cecum is semicircular and compartmentalized and normally contains some gas. The feline cecum, however, is a short, cone-like structure with no compartmentalization; it rarely contains gas. (From O'Brien TR: Radiographic Diagnosis of Abdominal Disorders in the Dog and Cat. Davis, CA, Covell Park Veterinary, 1981; with permission.)

A

B

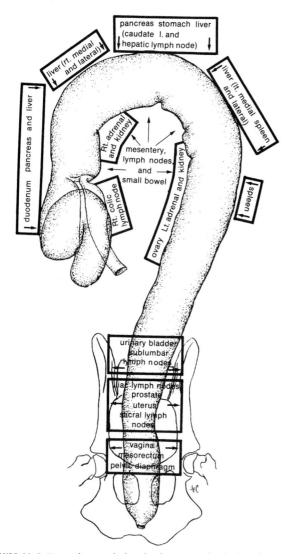

FIGURE 46–3. Viscera adjacent to the large bowel, on a ventrodorsal radiographic view, may cause anatomic-radiographic variations that may be alterations indicative of disease or variants of normal. *Arrows* indicate usual direction of large bowel position displacement when an organ enlarges (see Fig. 46–9). (From O'Brien TR: Radiographic Diagnosis of Abdominal Disorders in the Dog and Cat. Davis, CA, Covell Park Veterinary, 1981; with permission.)

aerophagia from restraint and struggling, and enemas before survey radiography may increase the amount of gas or fluid present within the colon and other parts of the gastrointestinal tract. Although an abnormality in position, size, or shape of the large bowel may be seen on survey radiographs, it may not be a significant finding, and a diagnosis may not be possible.

Compression radiography of the abdomen is a simple technique that may aid in further delineating the presence of a lesion. When the colon is compressed with a wooden or plastic spoon or paddle, adjacent bowel or masses are displaced or compressed, which enhances radiographic detail (Fig. 46–4). More definitive radiographic evaluation of the large bowel usually requires a contrast study using barium sulfate suspension (barium enema), air (pneumocolon), or a combination of barium sulfate suspension and air (double-contrast study).

After survey radiographs, the barium enema is the most commonly used radiographic study for the examination of the large bowel. Currently a barium enema is most indicated when (1) lumen narrowing prevents passage of an endoscope, (2) endoscope limitations prevent examination of all of the colon and cecum, and (3) a mural or extramural lesion is suspected and the mucosa was found to be normal on endoscopic examination.[4] Survey radiographs should not only be made as a first diagnostic step, but also before the contrast study to determine correct radiographic exposure techniques and to ascertain adequate patient preparation for the contrast study. For a high-quality diagnostic study, the colon should be thoroughly cleansed before the contrast study. This is best done by withholding food for 24 to 36 hours and cleansing the colon with both an orally administered cathartic and warm water enemas. The colonic mucosa and lumen should be free of fecal material with a clear effluent visible on an enema immediately before the study. Generally the radiographic technique should be increased 6 to 8 kVp over the survey technique when barium is used. Although the techniques of doing a contrast study may vary, barium at room temperature is administered through an inflatable cuffed catheter placed in the distal rectum to prevent the barium from leaking from the colon and to obtain adequate distention of the colon.[1, 12, 14] General anesthesia is almost always necessary. Micropulverized barium suspension is the contrast medium of choice for obtaining a smooth coating of the mucosal surface. The colon should be slowly filled with barium using a gravity system and preferably with fluoroscopic observation. Because fluoroscopic equipment may not be available and the volume of barium needed to fill the colon is extremely variable, the contrast medium should be given in several small increments until the desired effect is seen radiographically. Usually the barium dose is 7 to 15 mL of barium per kilogram body weight. Multiple radiographic views (i.e., left lateral, ventrodorsal, and ventral right–dorsal left and ventral left–dorsal right obliques) should be made when the colon is distended with barium and again after evacuation of the barium from the colon. The detection of subtle mucosal lesions may be enhanced by a double-contrast study. In most instances, this is done by removing as much of the barium as possible and inflating the colon with room air through the catheter.

When distended with barium, the normal colon has a smooth contrast medium/mucosa interface and uniform diameter. After evacuation of the barium, longitudinal mucosal folds are visible. If air is then infused, a double-contrast study is obtained, which provides the most detailed visualization of the mucosal surface.

A variety of radiographic appearances result from barium adhering to mucus, clumping and flocculation of barium, and filling defects of feces within the lumen or adhered to the wall. The colon of the dog and cecum and colon of the cat have lymph follicles in the mucosa, which appear as spicules on a barium enema study or as pinpoint radiopacities when visualized en face with a double-contrast study. These normal follicles must be differentiated from small ulcers.

The large bowel cannot be properly evaluated following oral administration of contrast medium because there is usually inadequate large bowel luminal distention as well as intraluminal filling defects owing to feces.

Complete large bowel contrast studies are time-consuming and must be done meticulously to assess the mucosa, wall, lumen, and adjacent viscera as well as to avoid artifacts, complications, and messes, such as contrast medium on the veterinarian, equipment, and patient. Partial large bowel contrast studies, which are less thorough, quicker, and easier, may be performed with the introduction of small amounts of air or barium into the rectum via dose syringe. These studies

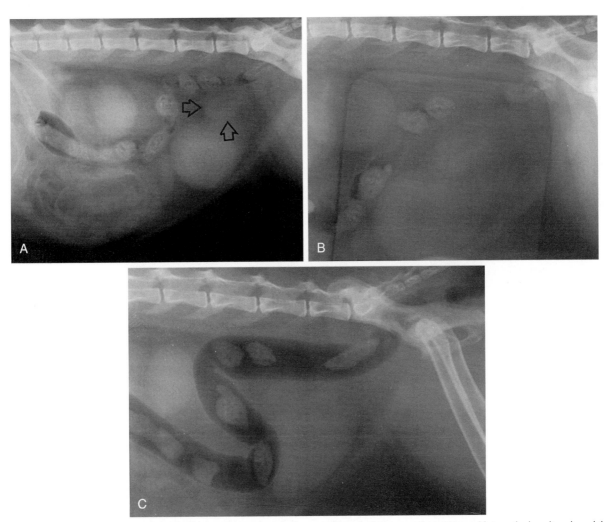

FIGURE 46–4. A 5-year-old neutered domestic shorthair female cat. *A,* Survey radiograph. There is an abnormal soft-tissue mass *(arrows)* interposed between the descending colon and the urinary bladder. At surgery, the mass was a uterine stump pyometra. *B,* Survey lateral recumbent radiograph of the abdomen with a compression paddle applied. The mass appears fixed and separate from the descending colon and urinary bladder. *C,* Survey lateral radiograph of the abdomen after a partial pneumocolon study via retrograde introduction of gas. The soft-tissue mass (uterine stump pyometra) is visualized as an extramural mass. Feces were not removed before the contrast study was conducted.

do not allow visualization of the entire large bowel or small lesions, such as mucosal irregularities; however, they may enable visualization of large intraluminal lesions and differentiation of the colon from adjacent organs and masses (see Fig. 46–4C).

Complications related to contrast studies of the colon may occur. The most serious complication is perforation and subsequent peritonitis (Fig. 46–5). Rupture can occur from a cleansing enema, improper selection or use of a barium enema catheter, and overdistention of weakened or diseased bowel or after a biopsy.[15–17] If colonic perforation is suspected, a 15 to 20 percent concentration of nonionic aqueous iodine contrast media can be substituted for the barium, but mucosal detail will be significantly diminished.[13] A common complication that is inconsequential is retrograde filling of the distal small bowel; such reflux may obscure visualization of the colon. This complication has been reported in about one third of dogs and may occur without overdistention of the colon.[12] Spasm, which is usually transient, may also occur when the contrast medium is cold, when narcotic premedications are used, or the wall is irritated by the catheter (Fig. 46–6).

RADIOGRAPHIC FINDINGS IN LARGE BOWEL DISEASE

Disease involving or adjacent to the large bowel may produce radiographic alterations in size, shape, location, and radiopacity.[1–4] Although function cannot be evaluated radiographically, the quantity or location of feces may suggest impaired motility. Most radiographic findings in large bowel diseases are not pathognomonic. Many different diseases have similar radiographic findings, and any particular disease may have a spectrum of different appearances. In addition, parasitic, dietary, and other inflammatory causes of large bowel disease commonly have no visible radiographic abnormality.

In the normal large bowel, the colon contains most of the feces, with small amounts or no feces in the rectum (see Fig. 46–1). The diameter of the normal colon varies with the amount of feces present and defecation habits. As a rule of thumb, the diameter of the normal colon should be less than the length of L7.[1]

Colonic impaction is characterized radiographically by accumulation of feces that is more radiopaque than normal as a consequence of constipation, obstipation, or megacolon.

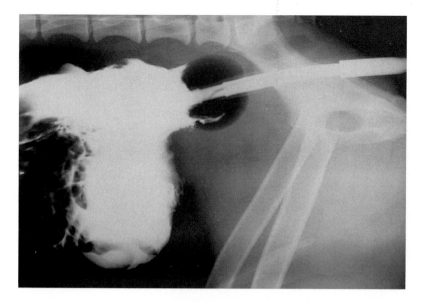

FIGURE 46–5. Lateral radiograph of a 5-year-old male Irish setter in which perforation of the colon occurred during a barium enema study. This complication may occur secondary to improper type and use of a catheter or to disease of the colon. The dog had a 4-month history of weight loss and straining to defecate. At necropsy, chronic prostatitis with adhesions to the colon and a localized peritonitis were evident.

Chronic impaction can also result in generalized enlargement of the colon.

Localized dilation of the colon is usually related to impaction or localized diseases such as mechanical obstructions owing to ileocolic intussusception, cecocolic intussusception, narrowed pelvic canal from fracture, intramural or extramural colonic tumor (Fig. 46–7), stricture, and foreign body.

Abnormal generalized enlargement of the colon is commonly referred to as megacolon, a condition caused by mechanical or functional obstruction and characterized by diffuse colonic dilation with ineffective motility. Megacolon may be idiopathic or associated with numerous underlying causes, such as (1) chronic constipation and obstipation, (2) feline idiopathic megacolon, (3) spinal anomalies (i.e., cauda equina syndrome, sacrococcygeal agenesis in Manx cats), (4) neuromuscular disorders (i.e., feline dysautonomia, aganglionosis, or Hirschsprung's disease [Fig. 46–8]), (5) metabolic disorders (i.e., hypokalemia, hypothyroidism), (6) surgical ureterocolic diversion techniques, and (7) anorectal congenital anomalies.[1, 10, 11]

Congenital anomalies of the colon are rare in the dog and the cat.[1, 3, 18–20] Anomalies reported include imperforate anus; rectal atresia; colonic atresia; fistulization; diverticuli; duplication of the large bowel and rectum; and a short, straight colon with the cecum in the left hemiabdomen.

The size and shape of the colon may also be altered by numerous chronic inflammatory diseases of the large bowel and adjacent viscera. These inflammatory changes may result in localized or generalized irregularity and ulceration of the mucosa with diverticuli, adhesions, or shortening of the colon.

Abnormal location of the large bowel is a common radiographic alteration seen with large bowel disease in the dog and cat. Although there is some normal variability in the location of the large bowel, mass lesions, particularly those of organs adjacent to the colon, cause displacement of the cecum, colon, or rectum (Fig. 46–9; see also Fig. 46–3 and Chapter 36). Masses or enlargement of the uterus, prostate, and lymph nodes (mesenteric, para-aortic, and iliac) commonly alter the position and shape of the large bowel.

It is important to recognize the radiographic differences in appearance for lesions of the large bowel that are intraluminal, intramural, and extramural. These classifications as to site or origin allow differentiation of conditions such as foreign bodies, intussusception, inflammation, and benign or malignant tumors (see Chapter 45). For example, a lesion that is plaque-like is intramural and arises from the mucosal or submucosal tissues. An extramural mass usually causes extrinsic narrowing of the lumen, displacement of the bowel and adjacent viscera, or both.

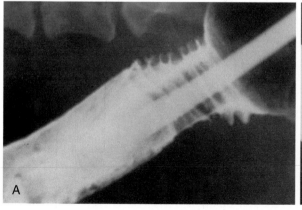
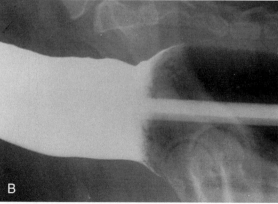

FIGURE 46–6. Narrowing and irregularity of the descending colon are present immediately cranial to the air-inflated catheter cuff. This was a spasm (A) and was transient based on a subsequent radiograph (B) made several minutes later.

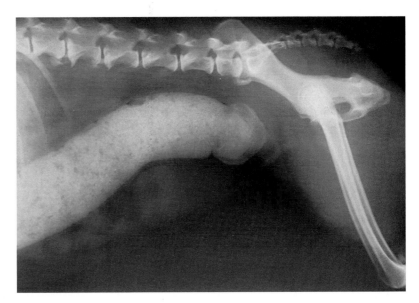

FIGURE 46–7. Survey lateral recumbent radiograph of the abdomen of a 9-year-old female, neutered mixed-breed dog with 5 months of progressive difficulty urinating and straining to defecate. The stools were flattened, and a rectal mass was palpable. The mass within the pelvis was a fibroleiomyoma causing partial colonic obstruction and megacolon. Unrelated L7–S1 spondylosis deformans is present.

Many large bowel diseases exhibit radiographic changes in the colon that are similar to those often present in other parts of the gastrointestinal tract. These conditions include (1) foreign bodies; (2) obstruction, including ileocolic (Fig. 46–10) and cecocolic intussusception (Fig. 46–11)[21, 22]; (3) inflammation (Fig. 46–12); (4) stricture (Fig. 46–13); (5) neoplasms (Fig. 46–14); (6) perforation; (7) adhesions; and (8) diverticula or hernia (Fig. 46–15). Most of the radiographic findings of these diseases have been discussed elsewhere in this text (Chapters 25, 36, 44, and 45) or are described in other textbooks.[1–4]

In most diseases of the large bowel, particularly those that are not extramural, a contrast study is required for detection and for decision making as to the most probable diagnosis (Fig. 46–16). The radiographic findings (barium enema or double-contrast study) in large bowel disease include (1) irregularity of the barium/mucosa interface, (2) spasm of the bowel lumen, (3) partial or complete occlusion of the bowel lumen, (4) outpouching of the bowel wall owing to a hernia or diverticulum, (5) displacement of bowel, and (6) perforation with peritonitis.

As with the alterations seen on survey radiographs, the contrast study findings are also usually nonspecific. Although spasm and mucosal irregularity are commonly associated with severe local inflammation, other causes include toxicity, reflex mechanism, and idiopathic factors. Bowel inflammation (typhlitis and colitis) may have generalized or regional areas of bowel wall thickening owing to edema and small ulcerations. Frequently the acute stages of bowel inflammation have no abnormal radiographic findings. A severe form of inflammatory disease in the dog, known as *ulcerative colitis,* has a spectrum of radiographic findings that consist of mucosal and submucosal ulcers, spasticity, rigidity, and shortening of the colon (see Fig. 46–12).

Narrowing of the large bowel lumen results from spasm or constriction caused by neoplasia, scar tissue, or direct trauma to the bowel wall. In contrast to constriction, spasm is transient and frequently is secondary to the barium enema technique (see Fig. 46–6). When evaluating a constriction with the use of a barium enema examination, the base and length of the defect, the mucosal surface, and the mural involvement should be assessed (see Fig. 46–13). Most constrictions of the large bowel are produced by neoplasms (usually carcinoma and lymphosarcoma), but benign disease, such as ade-

Text continued on page 570

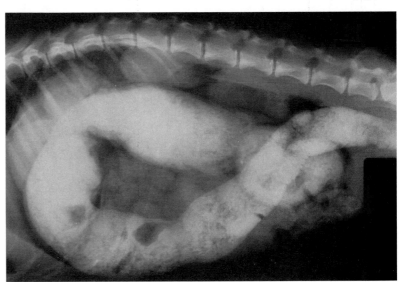

FIGURE 46–8. Generalized megacolon is present. This 5-month-old female mixed-breed dog had functional and histologic evidence of Hirschsprung's disease.

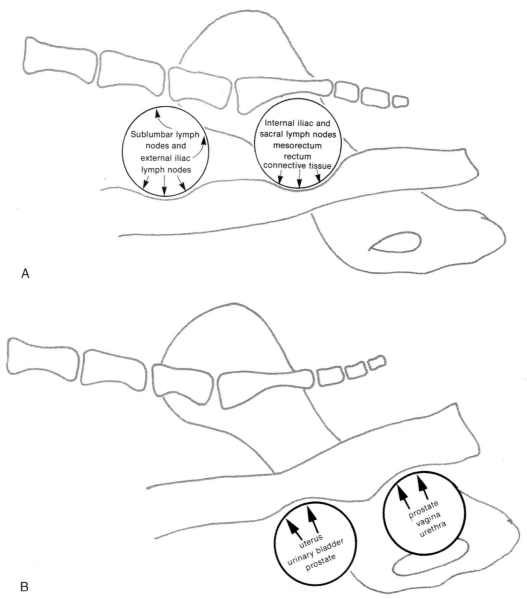

FIGURE 46–9. Terminal colon and rectal displacement by adjacent organ enlargement. *A*, Ventral displacement of the terminal colon and rectum commonly results from medial iliac (previously termed *sublumbar* or *external iliac lymph nodes*) and sacral lymph node enlargement. Although less common, a hematoma, abscess, or tumor may produce similar displacement alterations. *B*, Dorsal displacement of the rectum commonly results from enlargement of the prostate, uterus, vagina, or intrapelvic urinary bladder. (From O'Brien TR: Radiographic Diagnosis of Abdominal Disorders in the Dog and Cat. Davis, CA, Covell Park Veterinary, 1981; with permission.)

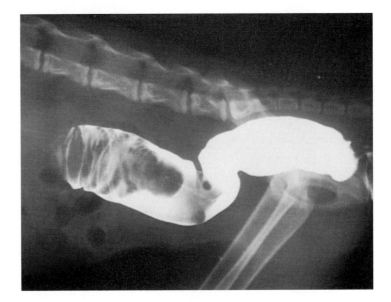

FIGURE 46–10. A 4.5-month-old male Siamese cat with ileocolic intussusception. Note the radiolucent filling defect and the coiled-spring appearance created by the intussusceptum being outlined by barium.

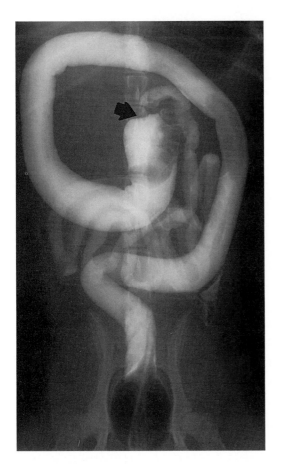

FIGURE 46–11. A 14-month-old male Beagle had intermittent diarrhea with shreds of mucosa and blood in the stool for 5 months. On the ventrodorsal view during a barium enema examination, a cecocolic intussusception is visible as a radiolucent filling defect. Note that the remainder of the large bowel, ileocolic junction *(arrow)*, and distal ileum are normal. The cecocolic intussusception had not been visible on two previous barium upper gastrointestinal tract studies.

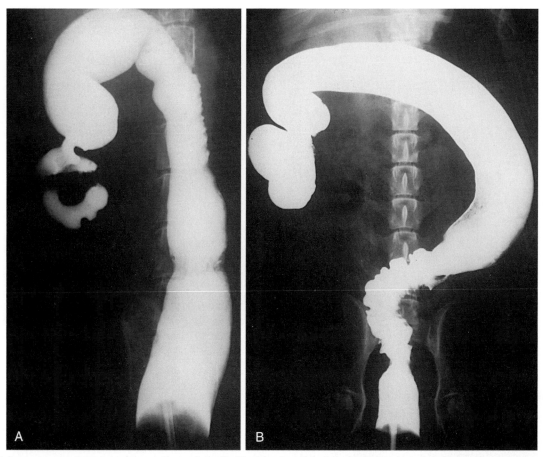

FIGURE 46–12. Barium enema examination in two dogs, one with generalized colitis *(A)* and the other with localized colitis *(B)*. Note the nondistensible descending colon and cecum and shortening of the colon in the more advanced and generalized disease. The localized colitis is characterized by nondistensibility and mucosal irregularity of the distal portion of the descending colon.

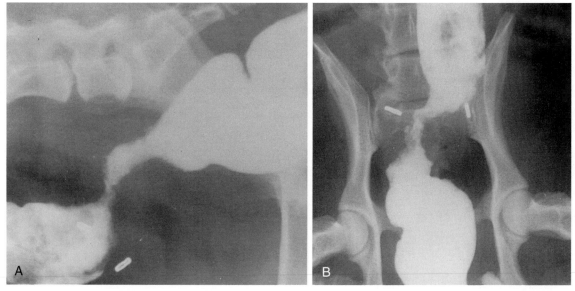

FIGURE 46–13. An 11-year-old female, neutered miniature Schnauzer had a 3-year history of straining to defecate with occasional soft and bloody stools. Lateral *(A)* and ventrodorsal *(B)* views of the barium enema examination demonstrate an irregular and circumferential narrowing at the junction of the descending colon and rectum. At surgery and biopsy, this narrowing was a benign stricture, presumed secondary to previous ovariohysterectomy (note surgical clips).

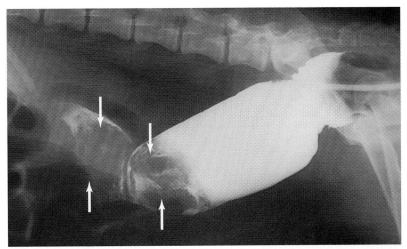

FIGURE 46–14. A barium enema study in a 6-year-old female German shepherd. An intraluminal mass *(arrows)* is seen as a polypoid filling defect in the midportion of the descending colon. The mass was lymphoma of the colon.

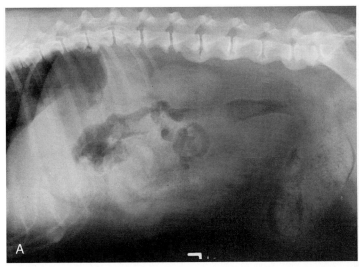

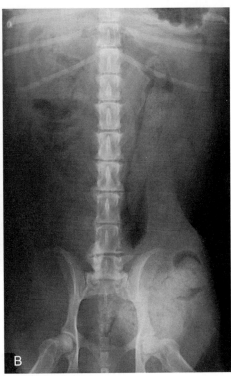

FIGURE 46–15. A 17-month-old female, neutered mixed-breed dog had a painful abdomen and lethargy after fighting with a larger dog. In survey lateral *(A)* and ventrodorsal *(B)* radiographs, a localized and dilated feces-filled segment of the descending colon was seen. This represents a partial obstruction, within a left inguinal hernia.

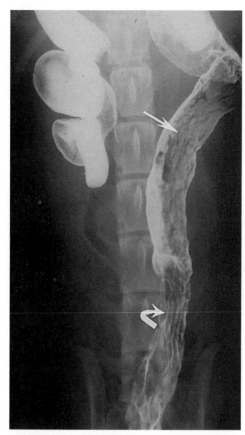

FIGURE 46–16. Postevacuation ventrodorsal radiograph of a barium enema. Normal longitudinal mucosal folds of the colon *(curved arrow)* and an abnormal mucosal pattern *(straight arrow)* are visualized. The abnormal area was localized colitis and was not visible on other radiographs obtained with the colon distended with barium.

References

1. O'Brien TR: Radiographic Diagnosis of Abdominal Disorders in the Dog and Cat. Davis, CA, Covell Park Veterinary, 1981.
2. Farrow CS, Green R, and Shiveley M: Radiology of the Cat. St. Louis, Mosby, 1995.
3. Kealy KJ: Diagnostic Radiology of the Dog and Cat, 2nd Ed. Philadelphia, WB Saunders, 1987.
4. Leib M, and Matz M: Diseases of the Large Intestine. *In* Ettinger SJ, Feldman EC (Eds): Textbook of Veterinary Internal Medicine: Diseases of the Dog and Cat, 4th Ed. Philadelphia, WB Saunders, 1995, pp 1232–1260.
5. Richter K: Diseases of the large bowel. *In* Ettinger SJ (Ed): Textbook of Veterinary Internal Medicine: Diseases of the Dog and Cat, 3rd Ed. Philadelphia, WB Saunders, 1989, pp 1397–1420.
6. Washabau RJ: Personal communication, 1995.
7. Homco LD: Gastrointestinal lract. *In* Green R (Ed): Small Animal Ultrasound. Philadelphia, Lippincott-Raven, 1996.
8. Penninck DG: Ultrasonography of the gastrointestinal tract. *In* Nyland T Mattoon J (Eds): Veterinary Diagnostic Ultrasound. Philadelphia, WB Saunders, 1995.
9. Becker M, Adler L, and Parish JF: Rectal lymphangiography in dogs. Radiology *91*:1037, 1968.
10. Gomez JA, Korobkin M, Lawson TL, et al: Selective abdominal angiography in the dog. J Am Vet Radiol Soc *14*:72, 1973.
11. Krevsky B, Somers MB, Mauere AH, et al: Quantitative measurement of feline colonic transit. Am J Physiol *255*:G529, 1988.
12. Ticer JW: Radiographic Technique in Veterinary Practice, 2nd Ed. Philadelphia, WB Saunders, 1984.
13. Kleine LJ, and Lamb CR: Comparative organ imaging: The gastrointestinal tract. Vet Radiol *30*:133, 1989.
14. Brawner WB, and Bartels JE: Contrast radiography of the digestive tract: Indications, techniques, and complications. Vet Clin North Am *13*:599, 1983.
15. Seaman WB, and Walls J: Complications of the barium enema. Gastroenterology *48*:728, 1965.
16. Toombs JP, Caywood DD, Lipowitz AJ, et al: Colonic perforation following neurosurgical procedures and corticosteroid therapy in four dogs. J Am Vet Med Assoc *177*:68, 1980.
17. Toombs JP, Collins LG, Graves GM, et al: Colonic perforation in corticosteroid-treated dog. J Am Vet Med Assoc *188*:145, 1986.
18. Rawlings CA, and Capps WF: Rectovaginal fistula and imperforate anus in a dog. J Am Vet Med Assoc *159*:320, 1971.
19. Fluke MH, Hawkins EC, Elliott GS, et al: Short colon in two cats and a dog. J Am Vet Med Assoc *195*:87, 1989.
20. Jakowski RM: Duplication of colon in a Labrador retriever with abnormal spinal column. Vet Pathol *14*:256, 1977.
21. Guffy MM, Wallace L, and Anderson NV: Inversion of the cecum into the colon of a dog. J Am Vet Med Assoc *156*:183, 1970.
22. Kolata RJ, and Wright JH: Inflammation and inversion of the cecum in a cat. J Am Vet Med Assoc *162*:958, 1976.

noma, scar tissue, eosinophilic colitis, and ulcerative colitis, may mimic the radiographic findings of a malignant lesion.

STUDY QUESTIONS

1. If inflammatory disease of the large bowel is suspected clinically, which one of the following examinations would usually be indicated after survey radiographs?
   A. pneumocolonography
   B. barium enema
   C. ultrasonography
   D. endoscopy
   E. mesenteric arteriography

2. The cecum of the dog and cat have a similar anatomical and radiographic appearance. (True or False)

3. Which one of the following is not recommended prior to a barium enema radiographic study?
   A. withhold water for 8–12 hours
   B. withhold food for 24–36 hours
   C. empty the urinary bladder
   D. administer gastric lavage solutions
   E. administer warm water cleansing enemas

4. The large bowel cannot be fully evaluated radiographically with an upper gastrointestinal barium study. (True or False)

5. Ulcerative mucosal lesions of the colon are best visualized radiographically with which one of the following techniques?
   A. survey radiographs
   B. pneumocolon
   C. barium enema
   D. double contrast study
   E. survey radiographs made with compression

6. In dogs and cats, the most common reason for displacement of the descending colon is due to:
   A. distended urinary bladder (full bladder)
   B. enlarged right kidney
   C. enlarged prostate
   D. pancreatitis
   E. congenital anomaly

7. Most constrictive and infiltrative lesions of the colon are caused by which one of the following?

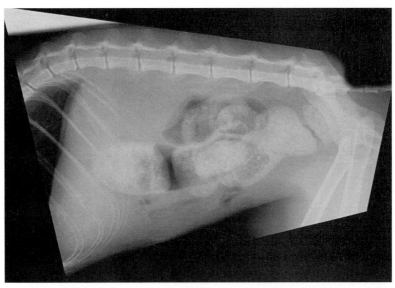

FIGURE 46–17

A. tumor
B. colitis
C. trauma from previous enemas
D. perineal hernia
E. prostatic infection

8. Since being adopted as a stray several weeks earlier, a female domestic short hair cat has had recurrent episodes of constipation. On two survey radiographs of the abdominal and pelvic regions (Figs. 46–17 and 46–18), what is your radiographic diagnosis for the most likely cause of the constipation?

A. foreign body of the descending colon
B. intraluminal mass in the descending colon
C. old pelvic fractures with malunion and secondary narrowing of the descending colon
D. perineal and abdominal hernia
E. idiopathic megacolon

9. In the same cat (refer to question 8 and Figs. 46–19 to 46–22), a barium enema and double contrast barium enema were done. Based on the contrast studies, which one of the following conditions is present? Note: the intraluminal filling defects are due to feces.

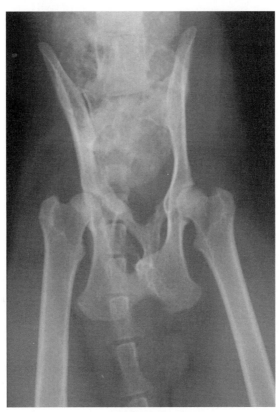

FIGURE 46–18

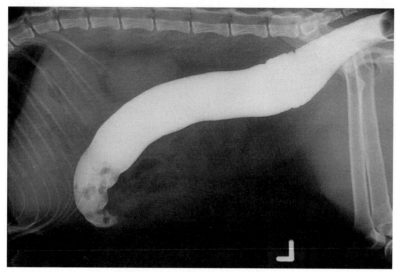

FIGURE 46–19

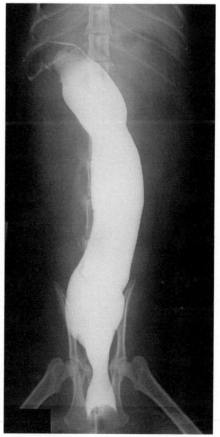

FIGURE 46–20

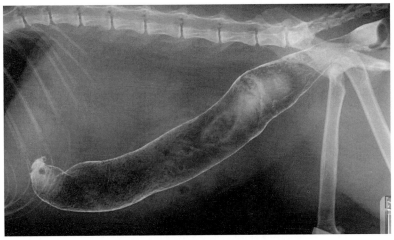

FIGURE 46–21

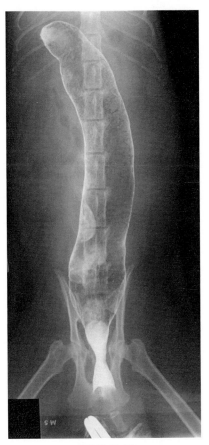

FIGURE 46–22

A. normal feline cecum and colon
B. intraluminal mass in descending colon, probably tumor
C. partial obstruction of descending colon secondary to previous trauma
D. perineal hernia with partial obstruction of the descending colon
E. colitis

10. In the same cat (refer to questions 8 and 9 and Figs. 46–19, 46–20, 46–21, and 46–22), what is your radio-

graphic interpretation for the cecum and ascending portion of the colon? Note: the intraluminal filling defects are due to feces.
A. normal feline cecum and ascending colon
B. cecocolic inversion
C. cecal aplasia
D. redundant colon
E. colitis

(Answers appear on page 649.)

RADIOGRAPHIC ANATOMY

Chapter 47

Radiographic Anatomy of the Dog and Horse

James E. Smallwood • Kathy A. Spaulding

To use the roentgen-sign method of recognizing abnormal radiographic findings effectively, one must first have an understanding of normal radiographic anatomy for the specific area of interest. This chapter provides the veterinary student and practitioner with a limited reference for the anatomy of the more frequently radiographed regions in the dog and horse.

By inclusion of labeled radiographs of selected areas of clinically normal animals (Figs. 47–1 through 47–85), basic resource information for veterinarians is provided in support of their more effective utilization of the roentgen-sign method of radiographic interpretation. For more detailed information, readers are referred to comprehensive textbooks on radiographic anatomy.[1, 2]

The radiographic nomenclature used in this chapter is that approved by the American College of Veterinary Radiology in 1983.[3] The xeroradiographs of the equine limbs presented in this chapter (Figs. 47–51 through 47–71) have been taken from previous publications[4–6] and are reproduced here with permission of the journals and author. Figures 47–72 through 47–85, which are radiographs of the equine shoulder, elbow, stifle, pelvis, cervical vertebrae, and head, have been added to the third edition of this book.

Text continued on page 630

RADIOGRAPHIC ANATOMY OF THE DOG

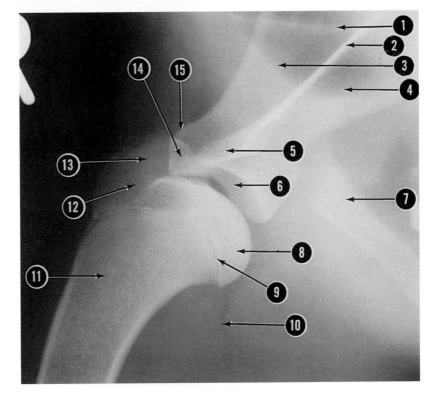

FIGURE 47–1. Mediolateral Radiograph of Canine Shoulder Joint.

1. Tracheal cartilages
2. Spine of scapula
3. Supraspinous fossa of scapula
4. Infraspinous fossa of scapula
5. Acromion of scapula
6. Glenoid cavity of scapula
7. Manubrium of sternum
8. Head of humerus
9. Proximal physis of humerus
10. Radiolucent area created by concentration of fat, caudal to shoulder joint capsule
11. Diaphysis of humerus
12. Intertubercular groove of humerus
13. Greater tubercle of humerus
14. Coracoid process of scapula
15. Supraglenoid tubercle of scapula

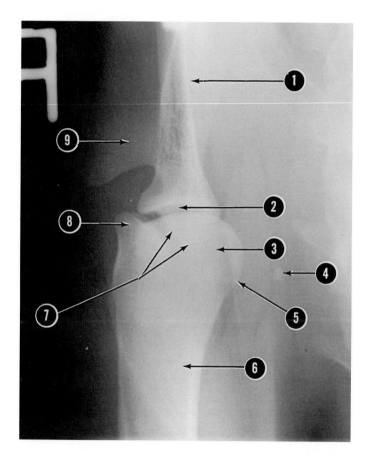

FIGURE 47–2. Caudocranial Radiograph of Canine Shoulder Joint.

1. Body of scapula
2. Glenoid cavity of scapula
3. Head of humerus
4. Clavicle
5. Lesser tubercle of humerus
6. Body of humerus
7. Supraglenoid tubercle of scapula
8. Greater tubercle of humerus
9. Spine of scapula

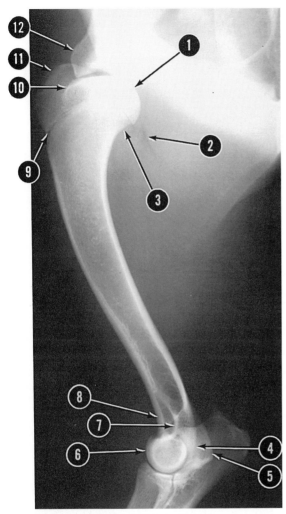

FIGURE 47–3. Mediolateral Radiograph of Canine Humerus.

1. Head of humerus
2. Radiolucent area created by concentration of fat, caudal to shoulder joint capsule
3. Neck of humerus
4. Caudal border of lateral epicondyle of humerus
5. Caudal border of medial epicondyle of humerus
6. Condyle of humerus
7. Cranial border of lateral epicondyle of humerus
8. Cranial border of medial epicondyle of humerus
9. Proximal physis of humerus
10. Cranial border of lesser tubercle of humerus
11. Cranial border of greater tubercle of humerus
12. Supraglenoid tubercle of scapula

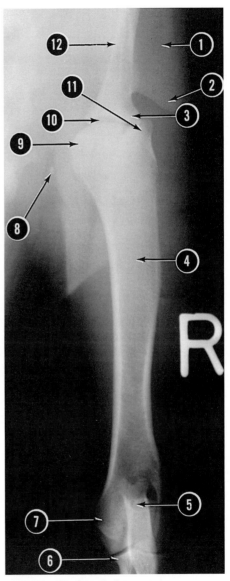

FIGURE 47–4. Caudocranial Radiograph of Canine Humerus.

1. Spine of scapula
2. Acromion of scapula
3. Ventral (glenoid) angle of scapula
4. Body of humerus
5. Tuber olecrani of ulna
6. Medial coronoid process of ulna
7. Medial epicondyle of humerus
8. Clavicle
9. Lesser tubercle of humerus
10. Shoulder (humeral) joint
11. Greater tubercle of humerus
12. Body of scapula

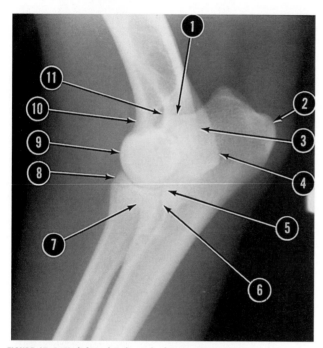

FIGURE 47–5. Mediolateral Radiograph of Canine Elbow Joint.

1. Anconeal process of ulna
2. Tuber olecrani of ulna
3. Caudal border of lateral epicondyle of humerus
4. Caudal border of medial epicondyle of humerus
5. Lateral coronoid process of ulna
6. Proximal radioulnar joint
7. Medial coronoid process of ulna
8. Head of radius
9. Condyle of humerus
10. Cranial border of medial epicondyle of humerus
11. Cranial border of lateral epicondyle of humerus

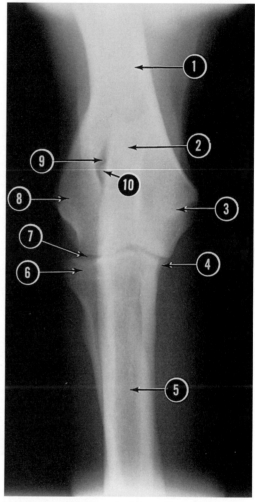

FIGURE 47–6. Craniocaudal Radiograph of Canine Elbow Joint.

1. Body of humerus
2. Tuber olecrani of ulna
3. Medial epicondyle of humerus
4. Medial coronoid process of ulna
5. Superimposed bodies of radius and ulna
6. Head of radius
7. Elbow (cubital) joint
8. Lateral epicondyle of humerus
9. Supratrochlear foramen of humerus
10. Anconeal process of ulna

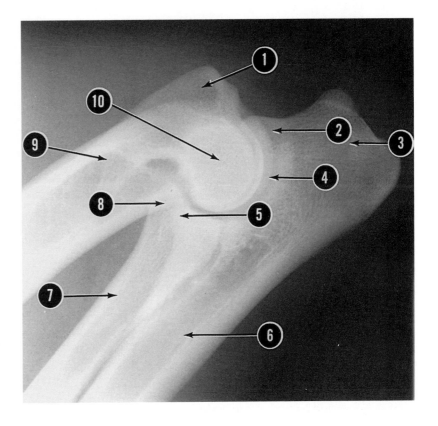

FIGURE 47–7. Mediolateral Radiograph of Flexed Canine Elbow Joint.

1. Medial epicondyle of humerus
2. Anconeal process of ulna
3. Olecranon of ulna
4. Medial border of humeral condyle
5. Medial coronoid process of ulna
6. Body of ulna
7. Body of radius
8. Head of the radius
9. Body of humerus
10. Condyle of humerus

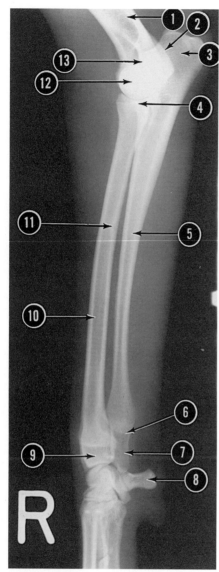

FIGURE 47–8. Mediolateral Radiograph of Canine Antebrachium.

1. Body of humerus
2. Caudal border of medial epicondyle of humerus
3. Olecranon of ulna
4. Medial coronoid process of ulna
5. Body of ulna
6. Distal physis of ulna
7. Styloid process (distal epiphysis) of ulna
8. Accessory carpal bone
9. Distal epiphysis of radius
10. Body of radius
11. Nutrient foramen of radius
12. Condyle of humerus
13. Anconeal process of ulna

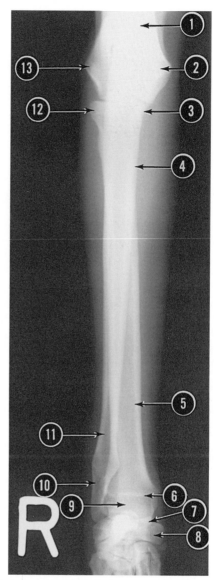

FIGURE 47–9. Craniocaudal Radiograph of Canine Antebrachium.

1. Body of humerus
2. Medial epicondyle of humerus
3. Medial coronoid process of ulna
4. Body of ulna
5. Body of radius
6. Distal physis of radius
7. Medial styloid process of radius
8. Intermedioradial carpal bone
9. Distal epiphysis of radius
10. Styloid process (distal epiphysis) of ulna
11. Body of ulna
12. Head of radius
13. Lateral epicondyle of humerus

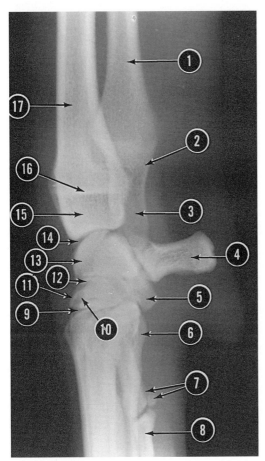

FIGURE 47–10. Mediolateral Radiograph of Canine Carpus.

1. Body of ulna
2. Distal physis of ulna
3. Styloid process (distal epiphysis) of ulna
4. Accessory carpal bone
5. Ulnar carpal bone
6. Metacarpal bone 5
7. Metacarpal bone 1 and proximal sesamoid bone of digit 1
8. Proximal phalanx of digit 1
9. Carpometacarpal joints
10. Distal border of second carpal bone
11. Third carpal bone
12. Middle carpal joint
13. Intermedioradial carpal bone
14. Antebrachiocarpal joint
15. Distal epiphysis of radius
16. Distal physis of radius
17. Body of radius

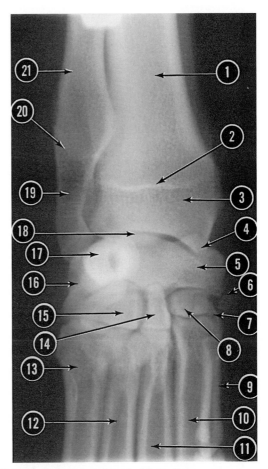

FIGURE 47–11. Dorsopalmar Radiograph of Canine Carpus.

1. Body of radius
2. Distal physis of radius
3. Distal epiphysis of radius
4. Medial styloid process of radius
5. Intermedioradial carpal bone
6. Sesamoid bone of abductor pollicis longus muscle
7. First carpal bone
8. Second carpal bone
9. Metacarpal bone 1
10. Metacarpal bone 2
11. Metacarpal bone 3
12. Metacarpal bone 4
13. Metacarpal bone 5
14. Third carpal bone
15. Fourth carpal bone
16. Ulnar carpal bone
17. Accessory carpal bone
18. Antebrachiocarpal joint
19. Styloid process of ulna
20. Distal physis of ulna
21. Body of ulna

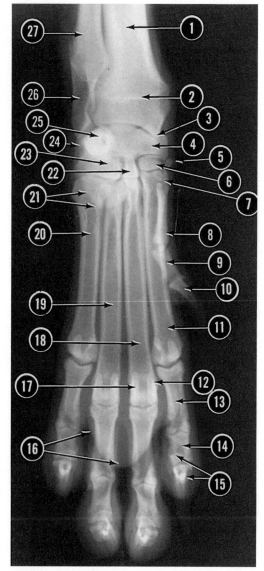

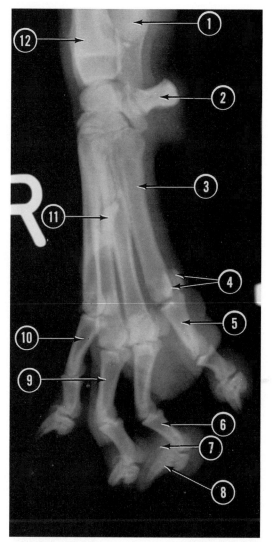

FIGURE 47–12. Dorsopalmar Radiograph of Canine Manus.

1. Body of radius
2. Distal physis of radius
3. Medial styloid process of radius
4. Intermedioradial carpal bone
5. Sesamoid bone of abductor pollicis longus muscle
6. Second carpal bone
7. First carpal bone
8. Metacarpal bone 1
9. Proximal phalanx of digit 1
10. Distal phalanx of digit 1
11. Metacarpal bone 2
12. Abaxial proximal sesamoid bone of digit 3
13. Proximal phalanx of digit 2
14. Middle phalanx of digit 2
15. Distal phalanx of digit 2
16. Metacarpal pad
17. Axial proximal sesamoid bone of digit 3
18. Metacarpal bone 3
19. Metacarpal bone 4
20. Metacarpal bone 5
21. Carpal pad
22. Carpal bone 3
23. Carpal bone 4
24. Ulnar carpal bone
25. Accessory carpal bone
26. Styloid process of ulna
27. Body of ulna

FIGURE 47–13. Palmaromedial-Dorsolateral Oblique Radiograph of Canine Manus.

1. Ulna
2. Accessory carpal bone
3. Metacarpal bone 5
4. Proximal sesamoid bones of digit 5
5. Proximal phalanx of digit 5
6. Middle phalanx of digit 4
7. Unguicular crest of distal phalanx of digit 4
8. Unguicular process of distal phalanx of digit 4
9. Proximal phalanx of digit 3
10. Proximal phalanx of digit 2
11. Proximal phalanx of digit 1
12. Radius

FIGURE 47–14. Right-Left Lateral Radiograph of Canine Pelvis.

1. Caudal vertebra 1
2. Sacrum
3. Right hip (coxal) joint
4. Superimposed tubera ischiadica
5. Superimposed obturator foramina
6. Superimposed rami of ischia
7. Body of right femur
8. Body of left femur
9. Iliopubic eminence
10. Head of left femur
11. Intervertebral disc space between L7 and S1
12. Vertebral canal at level of L7
13. Caudal extremity (fossa) of body of L5

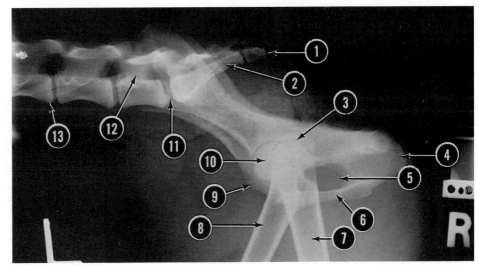

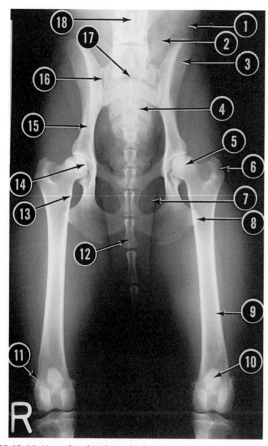

FIGURE 47–15. Ventrodorsal Radiograph of Canine Pelvis.

1. Feces in descending colon
2. Left transverse process of L7
3. Wing of left ilium
4. Sacrum
5. Dorsal border of left acetabulum superimposed on femoral head
6. Greater trochanter of left femur
7. Left obturator foramen
8. Left tuber ischiadicum superimposed on femur
9. Body of left femur
10. Left patella
11. Lateral sesamoid bone of right gastrocnemius muscle
12. Caudal vertebra 5
13. Lesser trochanter of right femur
14. Fovea capitis of right femoral head
15. Body of right ilium
16. Right sacroiliac joint
17. Intervertebral disc space between L7 and S1
18. Spinous process of L6

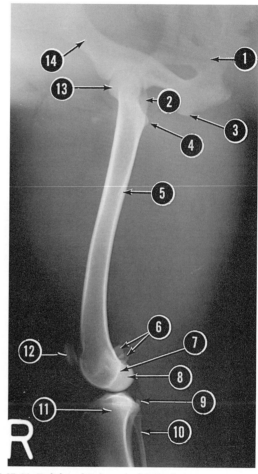

FIGURE 47–16. Mediolateral Radiograph of Canine Femur.

1. Pelvic symphysis
2. Intertrochanteric crest
3. Tuber ischiadicum
4. Lesser trochanter of femur
5. Body of femur
6. Medial and lateral sesamoid bones of gastrocnemius muscle
7. Wall of intercondylar fossa of femur
8. Superimposed medial and lateral condyles of femur
9. Sesamoid bone of popliteus muscle
10. Fibula
11. Tibia
12. Patella
13. Head of femur
14. Body of ilium

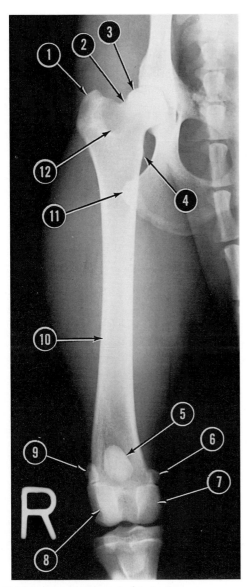

FIGURE 47–17. Craniocaudal Radiograph of Canine Femur.

1. Greater trochanter of femur
2. Neck of femur
3. Head of femur
4. Lesser trochanter of femur
5. Patella
6. Medial sesamoid bone of gastrocnemius muscle
7. Medial condyle of femur
8. Lateral condyle of femur
9. Lateral sesamoid bone of gastrocnemius muscle
10. Body of femur
11. Lateral border of tuber ischiadicum
12. Trochanteric fossa and intertrochanteric crest

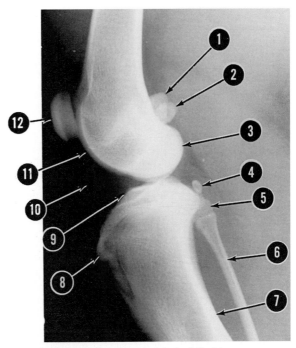

FIGURE 47–18. Mediolateral Radiograph of Canine Stifle Joint.

1. Lateral sesamoid bone of gastrocnemius muscle
2. Medial sesamoid bone of gastrocnemius muscle
3. Superimposed medial and lateral condyles of femur
4. Sesamoid bone of popliteus muscle
5. Head of fibula
6. Body of fibula
7. Body of tibia
8. Tibial tuberosity; incompletely fused to body of tibia
9. Cranial intercondylar area of tibia
10. Infrapatellar fat body
11. Trochlea of femur
12. Patella

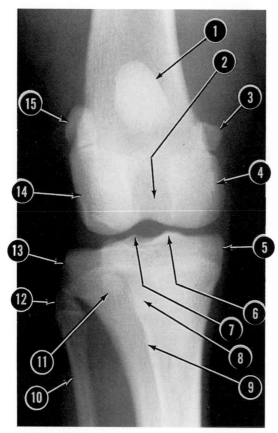

FIGURE 47–19. Craniocaudal Radiograph of Canine Stifle Joint.

1. Patella
2. Intercondylar fossa of femur
3. Medial sesamoid bone of gastrocnemius muscle
4. Medial condyle of femur
5. Medial condyle of tibia
6. Medial intercondylar tubercle of tibia
7. Lateral intercondylar tubercle of tibia
8. Tibial tuberosity
9. Cranial border of tibia
10. Body of fibula
11. Sesamoid bone of popliteus muscle
12. Head of fibula
13. Lateral condyle of tibia
14. Lateral condyle of femur
15. Lateral sesamoid bone of gastrocnemius muscle

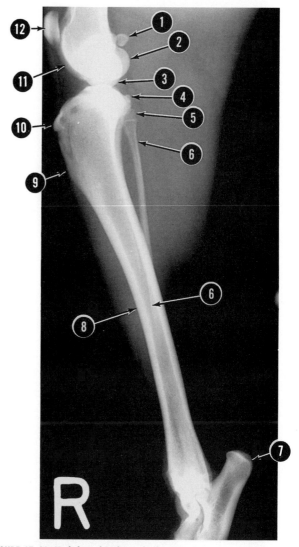

FIGURE 47–20. Mediolateral Radiograph of Canine Crus.

1. Medial sesamoid bone of gastrocnemius muscle
2. Medial condyle of femur
3. Lateral condyle of femur
4. Sesamoid bone of popliteus muscle
5. Head of fibula
6. Body of fibula
7. Tuber calcanei
8. Body of tibia
9. Cranial border of tibia
10. Tibial tuberosity
11. Trochlea of femur
12. Patella

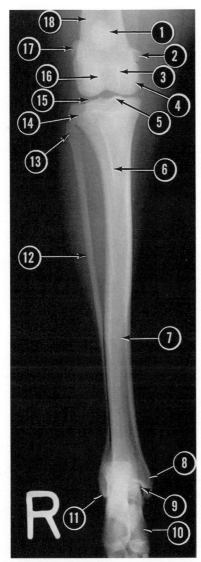

FIGURE 47–21. Craniocaudal Radiograph of Canine Crus.

1. Patella
2. Medial sesamoid bone of gastrocnemius muscle
3. Medial wall of intercondylar fossa of femur
4. Medial condyle of femur
5. Medial intercondylar tubercle of tibia
6. Cranial border of tibia
7. Body of tibia
8. Medial malleolus of tibia
9. Tarsocrural joint
10. Talus
11. Lateral maleollus of fibula
12. Body of fibula
13. Head of fibula
14. Lateral condyle of tibia
15. Stifle (genual) joint
16. Lateral wall of intercondylar fossa of femur
17. Lateral sesamoid bone of gastrocnemius muscle
18. Body of femur

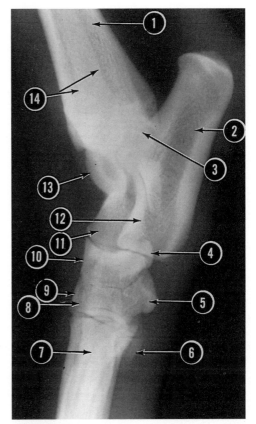

FIGURE 47–22. Mediolateral Radiograph of Canine Tarsus.

1. Body of tibia
2. Calcaneus
3. Tarsocrural joint
4. Plantar process of central tarsal bone
5. Fourth tarsal bone
6. Metatarsal bone 1
7. Superimposed metatarsal bones 2 through 5
8. Superimposed dorsal borders of second and fourth tarsal bones
9. Dorsal border of third tarsal bone
10. Dorsal border of central tarsal bone
11. Head of talus
12. Superimposed talus and calcaneus
13. Trochlea of talus
14. Body of fibula

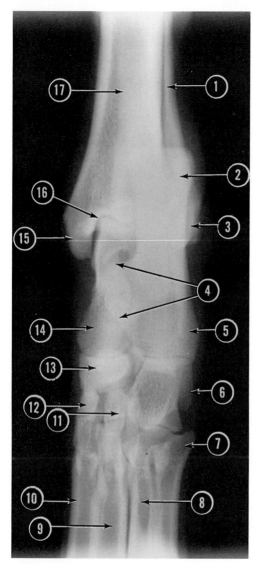

FIGURE 47–23. Dorsoplantar Radiograph of Canine Tarsus.

1. Body of fibula
2. Tuber calcanei
3. Lateral malleolus of fibula
4. Sustentaculum tali of calcaneus
5. Calcaneus
6. Fourth tarsal bone
7. Base of metatarsal bone 5
8. Metatarsal bone 4
9. Metatarsal bone 3
10. Metatarsal bone 2
11. Third tarsal bone
12. Superimposed first and second tarsal bones
13. Central tarsal bone
14. Talus
15. Medial malleolus of tibia
16. Tarsocrural joint
17. Common calcanean tendon superimposed on tibia

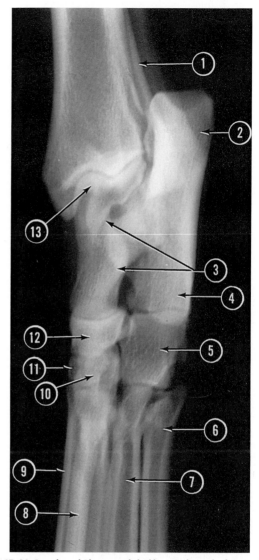

FIGURE 47–24. Dorsolateral-Plantaromedial Oblique Radiograph of Canine Tarsus.

1. Fibula
2. Tuber calcanei
3. Sustentaculum tali superimposed on talus
4. Calcaneus
5. Fourth tarsal bone
6. Fifth metatarsal bone
7. Fourth metatarsal bone
8. Superimposed third and second metatarsal bones
9. Second metatarsal bone
10. First tarsal bone superimposed on third tarsal bone
11. Superimposed dorsomedial aspects of second and third tarsal bones
12. Central tarsal bone
13. Medial ridge of trochlea tali

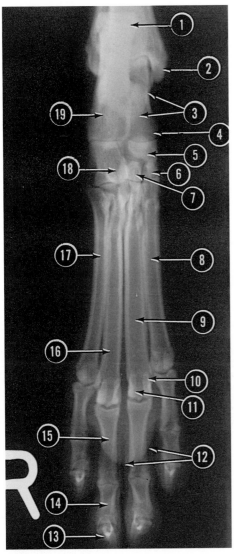

FIGURE 47–25. Dorsoplantar Radiograph of Canine Pes.

1. Tuber calcanei
2. Medial malleolus of tibia
3. Sustentaculum tali of calcaneus
4. Head of talus
5. Central tarsal bone
6. Superimposed first and second tarsal bones
7. Third tarsal bone
8. Metatarsal bone 2
9. Metatarsal bone 3
10. Abaxial proximal sesamoid bone of digit 3
11. Axial proximal sesamoid bone of digit 3
12. Metatarsal pad
13. Distal phalanx of digit 4
14. Middle phalanx of digit 4
15. Proximal phalanx of digit 4
16. Metatarsal bone 4
17. Metatarsal bone 5
18. Fourth tarsal bone
19. Calcaneus

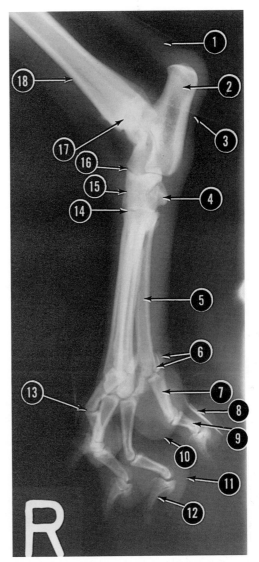

FIGURE 47–26. Mediolateral Radiograph of Canine Pes With Digits Spread.

1. Common calcanean tendon
2. Calcaneus
3. Tape used in positioning
4. Fourth tarsal bone
5. Metatarsal bone 5
6. Proximal sesamoid bones of digit 5
7. Proximal phalanx of digit 5
8. Tape used in positioning
9. Middle phalanx of digit 5
10. Metatarsal pad
11. Digital pad of digit 4
12. Unguicular process of distal phalanx of digit 4
13. Proximal interphalangeal joint of digit 2
14. Tarsometatarsal joints
15. Distal intertarsal (centrodistal) joint
16. Proximal intertarsal (talocalcaneocentral) joint
17. Tarsocrural joint
18. Body of tibia

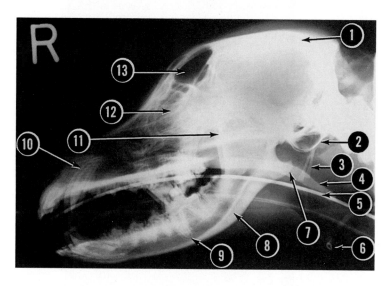

FIGURE 47–27. Left-Right Lateral Radiograph of Canine Head.

1. Calvaria
2. Tympanic bullae
3. Stylohyoid bones
4. Soft palate
5. Endotracheal tube
6. Basihyoid bone
7. Angular processes of mandibles
8. Bodies of mandibles
9. Mandibular canals
10. Roots of superior canine teeth
11. Coronoid processes of mandibles
12. Ethmoidal conchae
13. Frontal sinuses

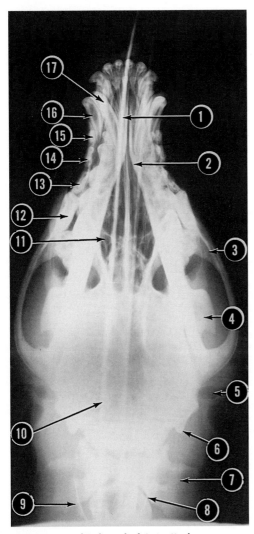

FIGURE 47–28. Dorsoventral Radiograph of Canine Head.

1. Endotracheal tube
2. Medial surface of left mandible
3. Temporal process of left zygomatic bone
4. Coronoid process of left mandible
5. Air within left external acoustic meatus
6. Left paracondylar process of occipital bone
7. Left wing of atlas
8. Atlantoaxial joint
9. Thyroid cartilage of larynx
10. Endotracheal tube
11. Ethmoidal conchae
12. Right superior premolar 4
13. Right superior premolar 3
14. Right superior premolar 2
15. Right superior premolar 1
16. Right superior canine tooth
17. Right inferior canine tooth

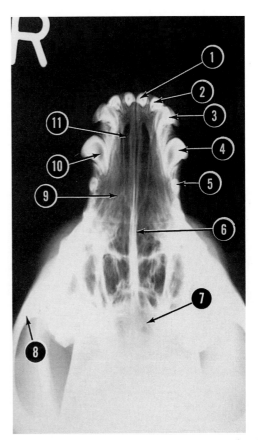

FIGURE 47–29. Open-Mouth Ventrodorsal Radiograph of Canine Nasal Cavity.

1. Left superior incisor 1
2. Left superior incisor 2
3. Left superior incisor 3
4. Left superior canine tooth
5. Left superior premolar 1
6. Nasal septum
7. Left ethmoidal conchae
8. Temporal process of right zygomatic bone
9. Superimposed right dorsal and right ventral nasal conchae
10. Dental cavity of right superior canine tooth
11. Right palatine fissure

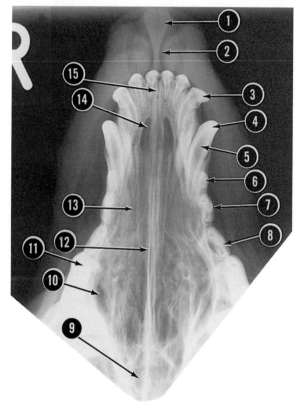

FIGURE 47–30. Intraoral Dorsoventral Radiograph of Canine Nasal Cavity.

1. Cartilaginous nasal septum
2. Left nostril
3. Left superior incisor 3
4. Left superior canine tooth
5. Dental cavity of left superior canine tooth
6. Left superior premolar 1
7. Left superior premolar 2
8. Left superior premolar 3
9. Right ethmoidal conchae
10. Right maxillary recess
11. Right superior premolar 4
12. Nasal septum
13. Superimposed right dorsal and right ventral nasal conchae
14. Right palatine fissure
15. Interincisive suture

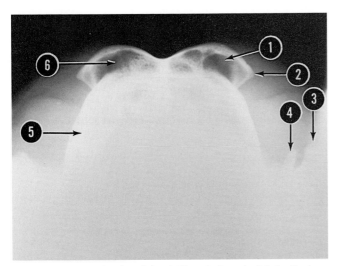

FIGURE 47–31. Rostrodorsal-Caudodorsal Oblique Radiograph of Canine Head.

1. Left lateral frontal sinus
2. Zygomatic process of left frontal bone
3. Left zygomatic arch
4. Coronoid process of left mandible
5. Calvaria
6. Right lateral frontal sinus

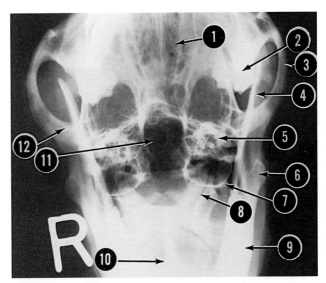

FIGURE 47–32. Rostroventral-Caudodorsal Oblique Radiograph of Canine Tympanic Bullae.

1. Left half of nasal cavity
2. Left superior cheek teeth
3. Left zygomatic arch
4. Coronoid process of left mandible
5. Left petrous temporal bone
6. Angular process of left mandible
7. Left tympanic bulla
8. Atlanto-occipital joint
9. Body of left mandible
10. Axis
11. Nasopharynx
12. Right zygomatic arch

FIGURE 47–33. Left Caudal–Right Rostral Oblique Radiograph of Canine Tympanic Bullae and Left Temporomandibular Joint.

1. Left paracondylar process
2. Right stylohyoid bone
3. Air within nasopharynx
4. Soft palate lying over endotracheal tube
5. Right epihyoid bone
6. Left tympanic bulla
7. Right tympanic bulla
8. Left retroarticular process
9. Left temporomandibular joint
10. Left tympanohyoid cartilage

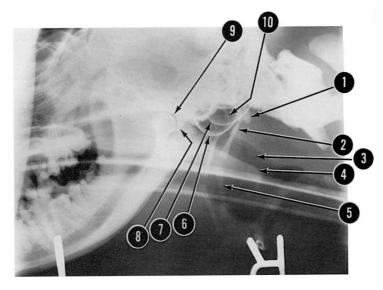

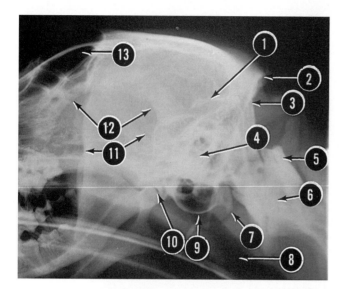

FIGURE 47-34. Left Dorsal–Right Ventral Oblique Radiograph of Left Canine Tympanic Bulla and Temporomandibular Joint.

1. Tentorium cerebelli osseum
2. External occipital protuberance
3. Occipital bone
4. Right tympanic bulla superimposed on left petrous temporal bone
5. Dorsal arch of atlas
6. Dens of axis
7. Left paracondylar process
8. Junction of oropharynx, nasopharynx, and laryngopharynx
9. Left tympanic bulla
10. Left temporomandibular joint
11. Coronoid process of right mandible
12. Right zygomatic arch
13. Frontal sinuses

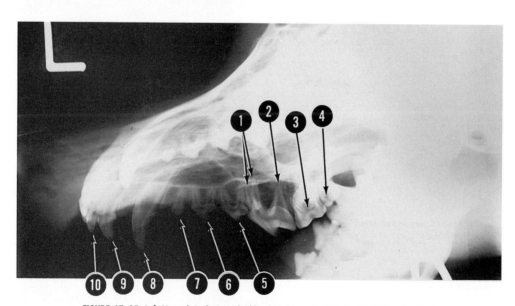

FIGURE 47-35. Left Ventral–Right Dorsal Oblique Radiograph of Canine Right Superior Teeth.

1. Rostral roots of right superior premolar 4
2. Caudal root of right superior premolar 4
3. Right superior molar 1
4. Right superior molar 2
5. Right superior premolar 3

6. Right superior premolar 2
7. Right superior premolar 1
8. Right superior canine tooth
9. Right superior incisor 3
10. Right superior incisor 2

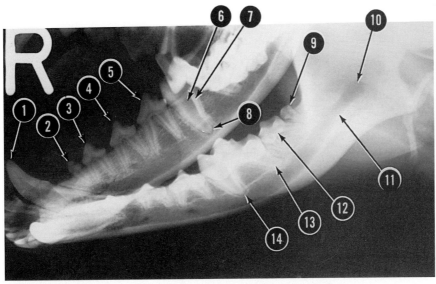

FIGURE 47–36. Left Dorsal–Right Ventral Oblique Radiograph of Canine Inferior Teeth.

1. Right inferior canine tooth
2. Right inferior premolar 1
3. Right inferior premolar 2
4. Right inferior premolar 3
5. Right inferior premolar 4
6. Dental cavity of right inferior molar 1
7. Dentin of rostral root of right inferior molar 1

8. Peridontal ligament (membrane[7])
9. Left inferior molar 3
10. Left mandibular foramen
11. Left mandibular canal
12. Left inferior molar 2
13. Caudal root of left inferior molar 1
14. Cortical bone forming wall of alveolus (lamina dura)

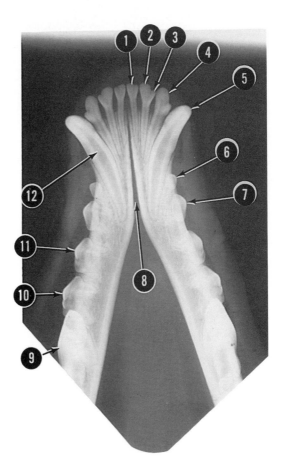

FIGURE 47–37. Ventrodorsal Intraoral Radiograph of Canine Inferior Teeth.

1. Left inferior incisor 1
2. Major tubercle of left inferior incisor 2
3. Minor tubercle of left inferior incisor 2
4. Left inferior incisor 3
5. Left inferior canine tooth
6. Left inferior premolar 1
7. Left inferior premolar 2
8. Intermandibular joint
9. Right inferior molar 1
10. Right inferior premolar 4
11. Right inferior premolar 3
12. Dental cavity of right inferior canine tooth

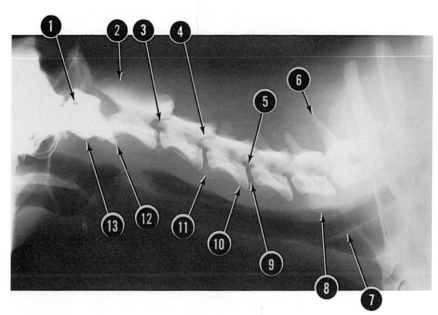

FIGURE 47–38. Left-Right Lateral Radiograph of Canine Cervical Spine.

1. Lateral vertebral foramina of atlas
2. Spinous process of axis
3. Cranial articular processes of C3
4. Caudal articular processes of C3
5. Intervertebral foramina between C4 and C5
6. Spinous process of C7
7. Trachea

8. Expanded transverse processes of C6
9. Intervertebral disc space between C4 and C5
10. Caudal physis of C4
11. Transverse processes of C4
12. Transverse processes (wings) of atlas
13. Ventral tubercle of atlas

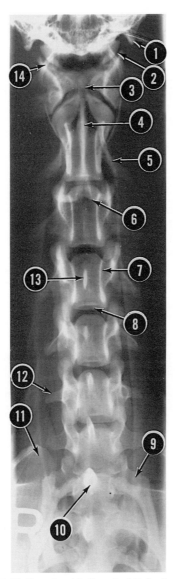

FIGURE 47–39. Ventrodorsal Radiograph of Canine Cervical Spine.

1. Left paracondylar process of occipital bone
2. Atlanto-occipital joint
3. Dens of axis
4. Spinous process of axis
5. Left transverse process of axis
6. Left caudal articular process of axis
7. Left pedicle of C4
8. Intervertebral disc space between C4 and C5
9. Tubercle of left rib 1
10. Spinous process of T1
11. Right scapula
12. Right transverse process of C6
13. Spinous process of C4
14. Right thyrohyoid bone superimposed on cranial articular fovea of atlas

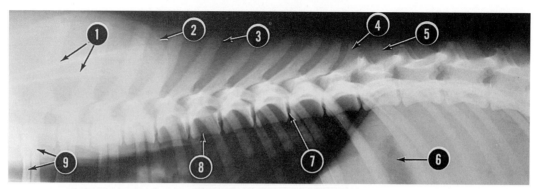

FIGURE 47–40. Left-Right Lateral Radiograph of Canine Thoracic Spine.

1. Spines of scapulae
2. Dorsal border of scapula
3. Spinous process of T5
4. Spinous process of T10 (caudally inclined)
5. Spinous process of T11 (anticlinal vertebra)
6. Gas within stomach
7. Intervertebral disc space between T8 and T9
8. Vertebral body of T6
9. First pair of ribs

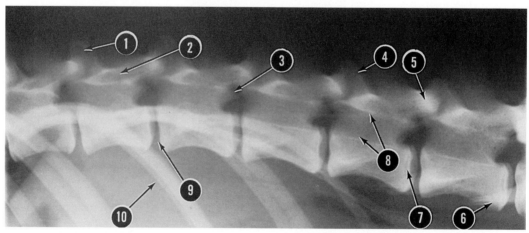

FIGURE 47–41. Left-Right Lateral Radiograph of Canine Thoracolumbar Spine.

1. Cranial articular processes of T12
2. Laminae of T12
3. Accessory processes of T13
4. Cranial articular processes of L2
5. Caudal articular processes of L2
6. Transverse processes of L4 superimposed on body of L3
7. Caudal extremity (fossa) of L2
8. Dorsal and ventral walls of vertebral canal
9. Intervertebral disc space between T12 and T13
10. Eleventh pair of ribs

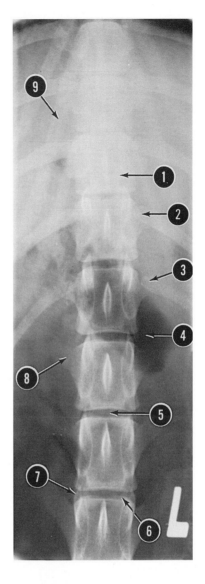

FIGURE 47–42. Ventrodorsal Radiograph of Canine Thoracolumbar Spine.

1. Body of T11
2. Head of left rib 12
3. Tubercle of left rib 13
4. Gas within colon
5. Intervertebral disc space between L1 and L2
6. Left caudal articular process of L2
7. Right cranial articular process of L3
8. Right transverse process of L1
9. Costal cartilage of right rib 9

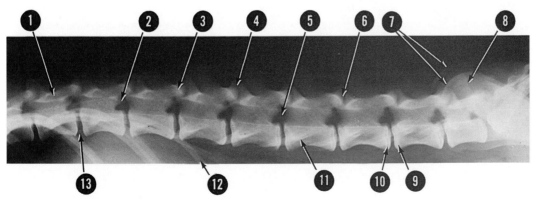

FIGURE 47–43. Left-Right Lateral Radiograph of Canine Lumbar Spine.

1. Laminae of T12
2. Accessory processes of T13
3. Caudal articular processes of L1
4. Cranial articular processes of L3
5. Intervertebral foramina between L3 and L4
6. Synovial joints between L4 and L5
7. Crests of ilia
8. Spinous process of L7
9. Cranial extremity (head) of L6
10. Caudal extremity (fossa) of L5
11. Transverse processes of L4
12. Thirteenth pair of ribs
13. Intervertebral disc space between T12 and T13

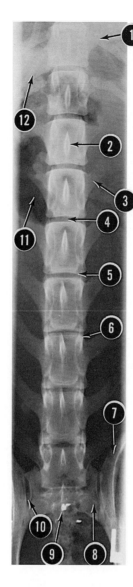

FIGURE 47–44. Ventrodorsal Radiograph of Canine Lumbar Spine.

1. Left rib 12
2. Spinous process of L1
3. Left transverse process of L2
4. Intervertebral disc space between L2 and L3
5. Left caudal articular process of L3
6. Left cranial articular process of L5
7. Wing of left ilium
8. Left wing of sacrum
9. Metallic foreign body within descending colon
10. Right sacroiliac joint
11. Gas within colon
12. Costal cartilage of right rib 10

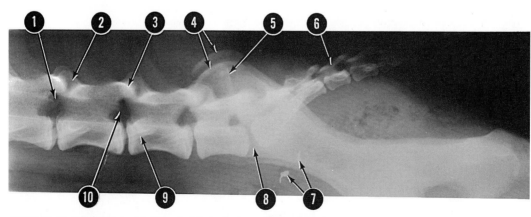

FIGURE 47–45. Left-Right Lateral Radiograph of Canine Lumbosacral Spine.

1. Accessory processes of L4
2. Cranial articular processes of L5
3. Caudal articular processes of L5
4. Crests of ilia
5. Spinous process of L7

6. Caudal vertebra 1
7. Metallic foreign bodies within descending colon
8. Intervertebral disc space between L7 and S1
9. Transverse processes of L6
10. Intervertebral foramina between L5 and L6

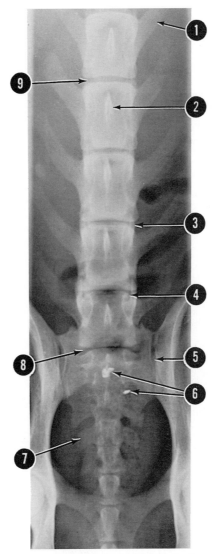

FIGURE 47–46. Ventrodorsal Radiograph of Canine Lumbosacral Spine.

1. Left transverse process of L3
2. Spinous process of L4
3. Left cranial articular process of L6
4. Left caudal articular process of L6
5. Left sacroiliac joint
6. Metallic foreign bodies within descending colon
7. Caudal vertebra 1
8. Intervertebral disc space between L7 and S1
9. Intervertebral disc space between L3 and L4

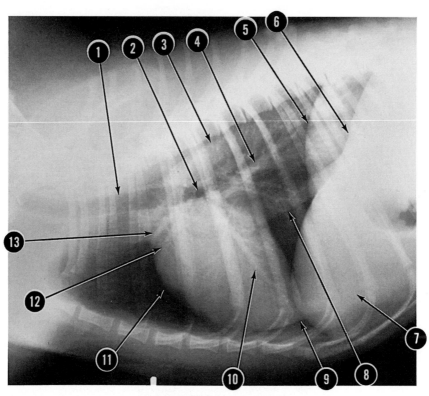

FIGURE 47–47. Right-Left Lateral Radiograph of Canine Thorax.

1. Trachea
2. Right cranial lobar bronchus[8]
3. Descending aorta
4. Superimposed caudal lobar branches of pulmonary arteries and veins
5. Left crus of diaphragm; typically extends cranial to right crus in left lateral recumbency[9]
6. Right crus of diaphragm
7. Liver

8. Caudal vena cava
9. Apex of cardiac silhouette; falls away from sternum in left lateral recumbency
10. Middle lobar branch of right pulmonary artery
11. Right ventricular wall
12. Right cranial lobar pulmonary vein
13. Cranial lobar branch of right pulmonary artery; the right cranial lobar bronchus is located between 12 and 13.[10]

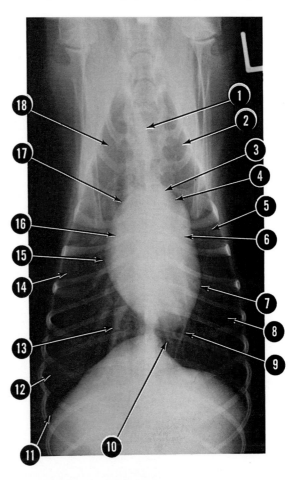

FIGURE 47–48. Ventrodorsal Radiograph of Canine Thorax.

1. Cranial mediastinum
2. Cranial part of cranial lobe of left lung
3. Aortic arch
4. Pulmonary trunk
5. Caudal part of cranial lobe of left lung
6. Left auricle of heart
7. Left ventricle of heart
8. Caudal lobe of left lung
9. Caudoventral mediastinum
10. Accessory lobe of right lung
11. Right costodiaphragmatic recess
12. Caudal lobe of right lung
13. Caudal lobar branch of right pulmonary vein superimposed on caudal vena cava
14. Middle lobe of right lung
15. Right ventricle of heart
16. Right atrium of heart
17. Right auricle of heart
18. Cranial lobe of right lung

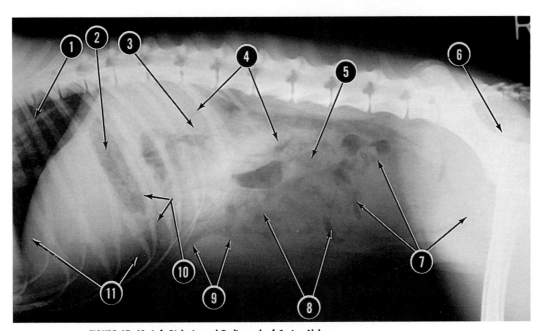

FIGURE 47–49. Left-Right Lateral Radiograph of Canine Abdomen.

1. Caudal lobar branches of pulmonary vessels
2. Gas within body of stomach; surrounding gastric folds
3. Ventral border of right kidney; contrasted by perirenal fat
4. Cranial and caudal borders of left kidney; cranial extremity of left kidney superimposed on right kidney
5. Gas and feces within descending colon
6. Feces within rectum
7. Borders of urinary bladder
8. Loops of small intestine (jejunum)
9. Ventral extremity of spleen
10. Greater curvature of stomach
11. Liver

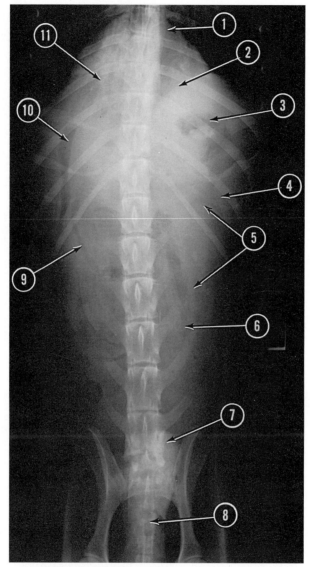

FIGURE 47–50. Ventrodorsal Radiograph of Canine Abdomen.

1. Cupula of diaphragm
2. Left crus of diaphragm
3. Gas within stomach
4. Body of spleen
5. Cranial and caudal borders of left kidney
6. Gas within descending colon
7. Prepuce superimposed over L7 and sacrum
8. Os penis
9. Gas within loop of jejunum
10. Gas within descending duodenum
11. Caudal lobar branches of pulmonary vessels superimposed on liver

RADIOGRAPHIC ANATOMY OF THE HORSE

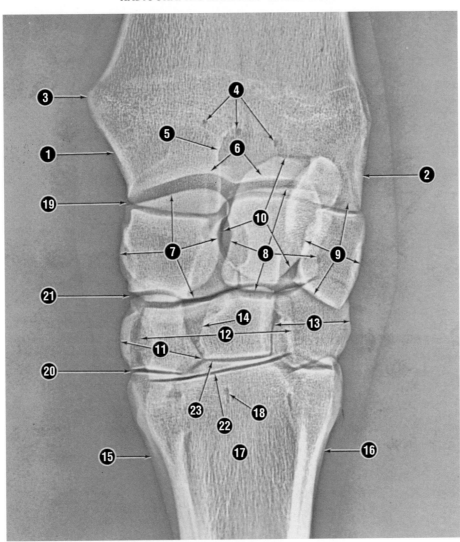

FIGURE 47–51. Dorsopalmar (DPa) Xeroradiograph of Left Equine Carpus.

1. Medial styloid process
2. Lateral styloid process
3. Projection at proximomedial aspect of 1
4. Vascular channels
5. Caudolateral border of 1
6. Junction of carpal articular surface with cranial surface of radius
7. Radial carpal bone (Cr)
8. Intermediate carpal bone (Ci)
9. Ulnar carpal bone (Cu)
10. Accessory carpal bone (Ca)
11. Second carpal bone (C2)
12. Third carpal bone (C3)
13. Fourth carpal bone (C4)
14. Medial border of palmar process of C3
15. Second metacarpal bone
16. Fourth metacarpal bone
17. Third metacarpal bone
18. Vascular channel
19. Antebrachiocarpal joint
20. Carpometacarpal joints
21. Middle carpal joint
22. Shadow cast by dorsal aspects of carpometacarpal joints
23. Shadow cast by palmar aspects of carpometacarpal joints

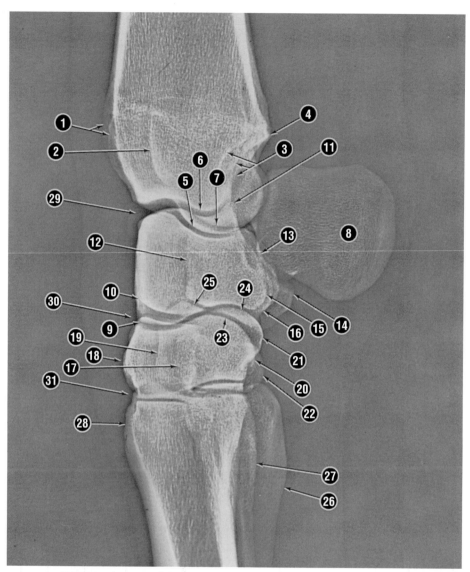

FIGURE 47–52. Lateromedial (LM) Xeroradiograph of Left Equine Carpus.

1. Ridges on cranial surface of radius
2. Ridge adjacent to lateral border of common digital extensor tendon
3. Caudal border of radial trochlea
4. Transverse crest of radius
5. Medial part of carpal articular surface
6. Intermediate part of carpal articular surface
7. Lateral part of carpal articular surface
8. Accessory carpal bone
9. Dorsodistal border of radial carpal bone
10. Dorsodistal border of intermediate carpal bone
11. Proximal process of Ci
12. Dorsal surface of ulnar carpal bone
13. Articulation of Ca with Cu
14. Palmar border of Cu
15. Palmar border of Ci

16. Palmar border of Cr
17. Dorsal border of C2
18. Dorsal border of C3
19. Dorsal border of C4
20. Palmar border of C2
21. Palmar border of C3
22. Palmar border of C4
23. Proximal border of C2
24. Proximal border of C3
25. Proximal border of C4
26. Fourth metacarpal bone
27. Second metacarpal bone
28. Metacarpal tuberosity
29. Antebrachiocarpal joint
30. Middle carpal joint
31. Carpometacarpal joints

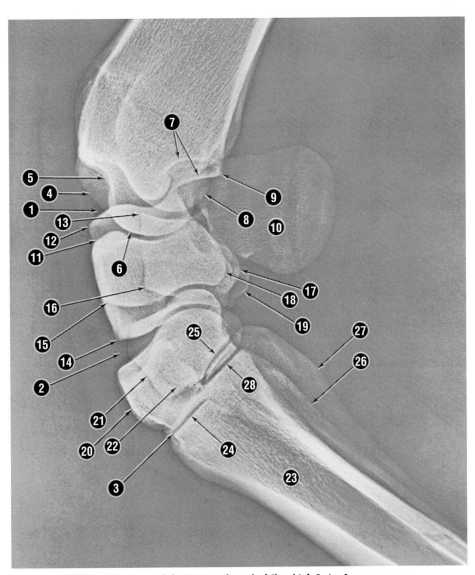

FIGURE 47–53. Lateromedial (LM) Xeroradiograph of Flexed Left Equine Carpus.

1. Antebrachiocarpal joint
2. Middle carpal joint
3. Carpometacarpal joints
4. Medial border of medial part of carpal articular surface
5. Lateral border of medial part of carpal articular surface
6. Medial styloid process
7. Shadows from caudal aspect of intermediate part of radial trochlea
8. Lateral styloid process
9. Transverse crest of radius
10. Accessory carpal bone
11. Dorsoproximal border of Cr
12. Dorsoproximal border of Ci
13. Dorsoproximal border of Cu
14. Dorsodistal border of Cr (isolated)

15. Dorsodistal border of Ci
16. Dorsodistal border of Cu
17. Palmar border of Cr
18. Palmar border of Ci
19. Palmar border of Cu
20. Dorsal border of C3
21. Dorsal border of C4
22. Dorsal border of C2
23. Third metacarpal bone
24. Third carpometacarpal joint
25. Second carpometacarpal joint
26. Second metacarpal bone
27. Fourth metacarpal bone
28. Fourth carpometacarpal joint

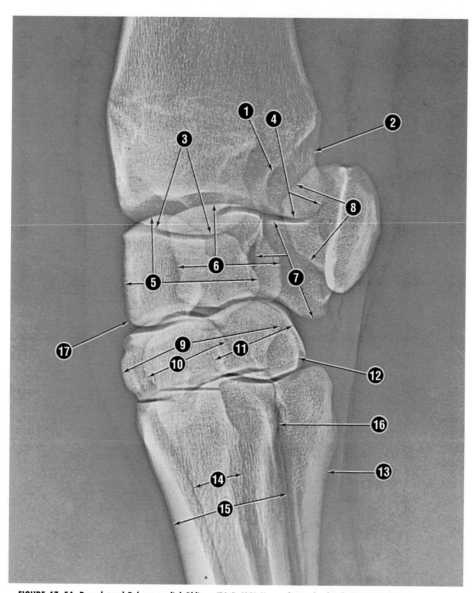

FIGURE 47–54. Dorsolateral-Palmaromedial Oblique (DL-PaMO) Xeroradiograph of Left Equine Carpus.

1. Radiolucent area at line of fusion between lateral styloid process and radius
2. Lateral styloid process
3. Medial part of radial trochlea
4. Lateral styloid process
5. Radial carpal bone
6. Intermediate carpal bone
7. Ulnar carpal bone
8. Articulations of accessory carpal bone with 2 and 7

9. Third carpal bone
10. Second carpal bone
11. Fourth carpal bone
12. Palmar projection of C4
13. Fourth metacarpal bone
14. Second metacarpal bone
15. Third metacarpal bone
16. Location of metacarpal interosseous ligaments
17. Distal aspect of dorsomedial border of Cr (isolated)

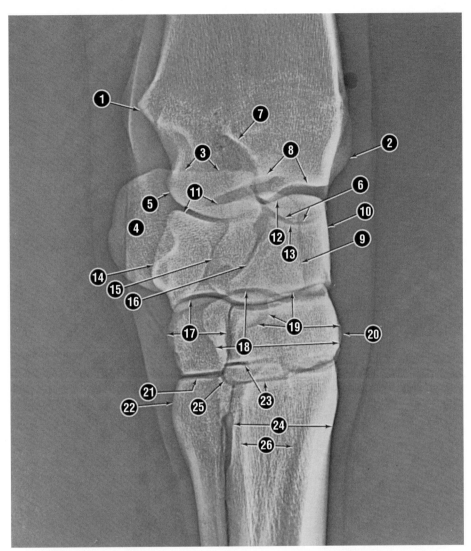

FIGURE 47–55. Dorsomedial-Palmarolateral Oblique (DM-PaLO) Xeroradiograph of Left Equine Carpus.*

1. Projection of radius for attachment of medial collateral ligament
2. Ridge that forms lateral border of groove for common digital extensor tendon
3. Proximal border of accessory carpal bone
4. Accessory carpal bone
5. Medial styloid process of radius
6. Lateral styloid process
7. Ridge on caudal aspect of radius
8. Ridge at junction of cranial surface of radius with carpal articular surface
9. Dorsolateral border of Cr
10. Dorsolateral borders of Cu and Ci
11. Proximal surface of Cr
12. Proximal surface of Ci
13. Proximal surface of Cu

14. Palmaromedial border of Cr
15. Palmaromedial border of Ci
16. Palmaromedial border of Cu
17. Second carpal bone
18. Third carpal bone
19. Fourth carpal bone
20. Dorsolateral borders of C3 and C4
21. Articulation between C2 and MC 2
22. Second metacarpal bone
23. Articulation between C3 and MC 3
24. Third metacarpal bone
25. Inconstant articulation between C3 and MC 2
26. Fourth metacarpal bone

*Xeroradiographs are not translucent. Therefore, it is impossible to orient all xeroradiographs in the conventional manner with cranial (dorsal) to the left.

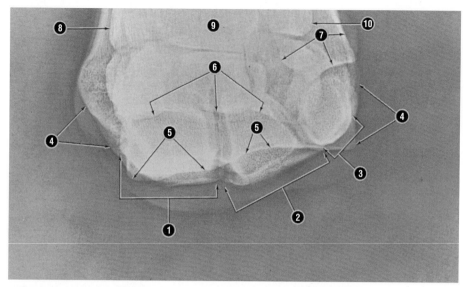

FIGURE 47–56. Dorsoproximal-Dorsodistal Oblique (DPr-DDiO) Xeroradiograph of Proximal Row of Equine Carpal Bones.

1. Dorsal surface of radial carpal bone
2. Dorsal surface of intermediate carpal bone
3. Dorsal surface of ulnar carpal bone
4. Radius
5. Carpal articular surface of radial trochlea
6. Dorsal surfaces of distal carpal bones
7. Accessory carpal bone
8. Second metacarpal bone
9. Third metacarpal bone
10. Fourth metacarpal bone

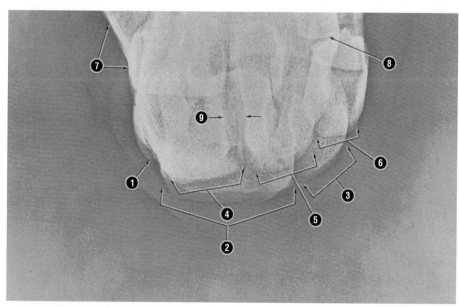

FIGURE 47–57. Dorsoproximal-Dorsodistal Oblique (DPr-DDiO) Xeroradiograph of Distal Row of Equine Carpal Bones.

1. Dorsal surface of second carpal bone
2. Dorsal surface of third carpal bone
3. Dorsal surface of fourth carpal bone
4. Dorsal surface of radial carpal bone
5. Dorsal surface of intermediate carpal bone
6. Dorsal surface of ulnar carpal bone
7. Radius
8. Accessory carpal bone
9. Interosseous space between Cr and Ci

FIGURE 47–58. Lateromedial (LM) Xeroradiograph of Left Equine Foredigit.

1. Proximal interphalangeal joint (DIJ)
2. Extensor process of distal phalanx (Pd)
3. Distal interphalangeal joint
4. Part of DIJ that extends between Pd and the distal sesamoid (navicular) bone
5. Proximal extent of tubular horn forming stratum medium of hoof wall
6. Junction of stratum medium and laminar horn of stratum internum
7. Transverse part of sole canal of Pd; accommodates terminal arch of digital vessels
8. Sole border of Pd
9. Planum cuneatum (sole surface) of Pd
10. Vascular channels extending from sole canal to sole border of Pd
11. Flexor surface of Pd
12. Flexor surface of navicular bone
13. Superimposed medial and lateral palmar processes of Pd
14. Radiolucent areas created by fat within synovial folds
15. Borders of DDF tendon; defined by fat within synovial folds of digital sheath

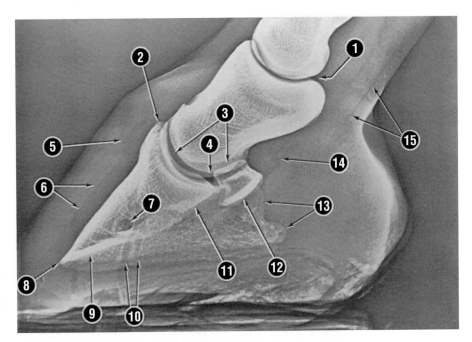

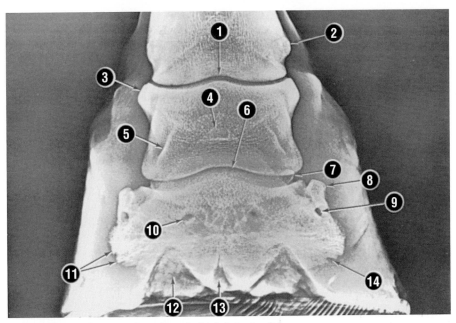

FIGURE 47–59. Dorsopalmar (DPa) Xeroradiograph of Left Equine Foredigit.

1. Proximal interphalangeal joint
2. Lateral distal collateral tubercle of proximal phalanx (Pp)
3. Medial proximal collateral tubercle of middle phalanx (Pm)
4. Extensor process of Pd
5. Wall of depression in Pm for attachment of medial collateral ligament of DIJ
6. Distal interphalangeal joint
7. Lateral extremity of navicular bone
8. Lateral palmar process of Pd
9. Foramen in lateral palmar process of Pd that accommodates dorsal branches of digital vessels
10. Medial sole foramen of Pd; receives digital vessels as they enter sole canal
11. Sole border of Pd; typically irregular because of notches for vascular channels
12. Medial collateral groove of frog
13. Central groove of frog
14. Notch in sole border associated with vascular channel from sole canal of Pd

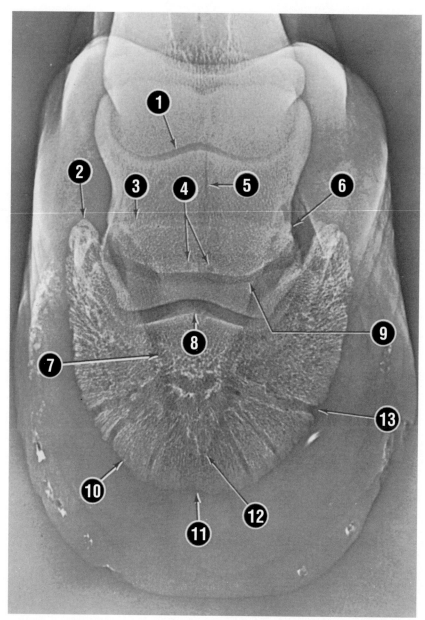

FIGURE 47–60. Dorsal 65-Degree Proximal-Palmarodistal Oblique (D65Pr-PaDiO) Xeroradiograph of Left Equine Foredigit.

1. Proximal interphalangeal joint
2. Medial palmar process of Pd
3. Proximal border of navicular bone
4. Vascular foramina and synovial fossae along distal border of navicular bone
5. Air within central groove of frog
6. Lateral extremity of navicular bone
7. Sole canal of Pd
8. Distal interphalangeal joint
9. Articulation of Pd with navicular bone; part of DIJ
10. Sole border of Pd
11. Crena marginis solearis
12. Apex of frog
13. Vascular channel from sole canal to sole border of Pd

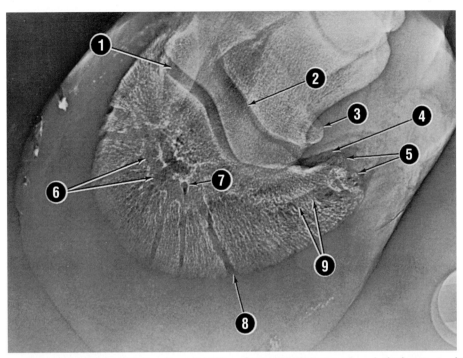

FIGURE 47–61. Dorsoproximolateral-Palmarodistomedial Oblique (D65Pr45L-PaDiMO) Xeroradiograph of Left Equine Foredigit.

1. Distal interphalangeal joint
2. Articulation of Pd with navicular bone; part of DIJ
3. Lateral extremity of navicular bone
4. Air within lateral collateral groove of frog
5. Lateral palmar process of Pd
6. Sole canal of Pd

7. End-on perspective of vascular channel from sole canal to parietal surface of Pd
8. Vascular channel from sole canal to sole border of Pd
9. Lateral parietal groove of Pd; accommodates dorsal branches of digital vessels.

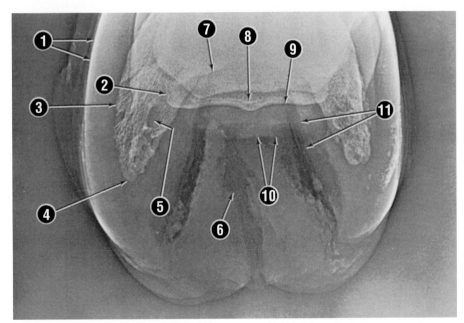

FIGURE 47–62. Palmaroproximal-Palmarodistal Oblique (PaPr-PaDiO) Xeroradiograph of Left Equine Foredigit.

1. Proximal border of hoof wall
2. Lateral extremity of navicular bone
3. Sole border of Pd
4. Lateral palmar process of Pd
5. Foramen of lateral palmar process
6. Air within central groove of frog

7. Articulation of Pm with navicular bone; part of DIJ
8. Sagittal ridge of navicular bone
9. Flexor surface of navicular bone
10. DDF tendon
11. Air within medial collateral groove of frog

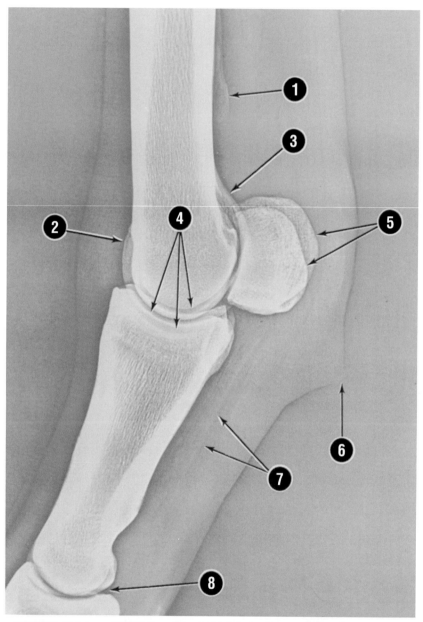

FIGURE 47–63. Lateromedial (LM) Xeroradiograph of Left Equine Metacarpophalangeal Joint (McPJ).

1. Distal end (head) of small metacarpal bone
2. Dorsal part of sagittal ridge of MC 3
3. Palmar part of sagittal ridge of MC 3
4. Metacarpophalangeal joint

5. Proximal sesamoid bones
6. Ergot
7. Straight sesamoid ligament
8. Proximal interphalangeal joint

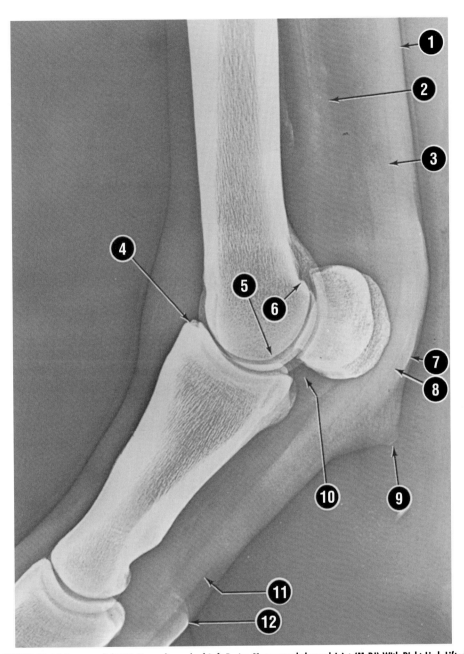

FIGURE 47–64. Lateromedial (LM) Xeroradiograph of Left Equine Metacarpophalangeal Joint (McPJ) With Right Limb Lifted to Increase Weight on Left Limb.

1. Superficial digital flexor (SDF) tendon
2. Interosseus
3. Deep digital flexor (DDF) tendon
4. Dorsoproximal aspect of Pp
5. Subtle transverse ridge on head of MC 3
6. Distinct transverse ridge at palmar edge of articular surface
7. Palmar annular ligament of metacarpophalangeal joint

8. SDF tendon
9. Ergot
10. Increased distance between proximal sesamoid bones and Pp (see Fig. 47–63)
11. DDF tendon
12. Distal digital annular ligament

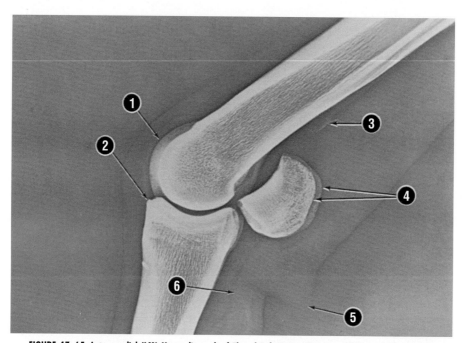

FIGURE 47–65. Lateromedial (LM) Xeroradiograph of Flexed Left Equine Metacarpophalangeal Joint (McPJ).

1. Sagittal ridge on head of MC 3
2. Dorsoproximal aspect of Pp
3. Distal end of small metacarpal bone

4. Proximal sesamoid bones
5. Ergot
6. DDF tendon

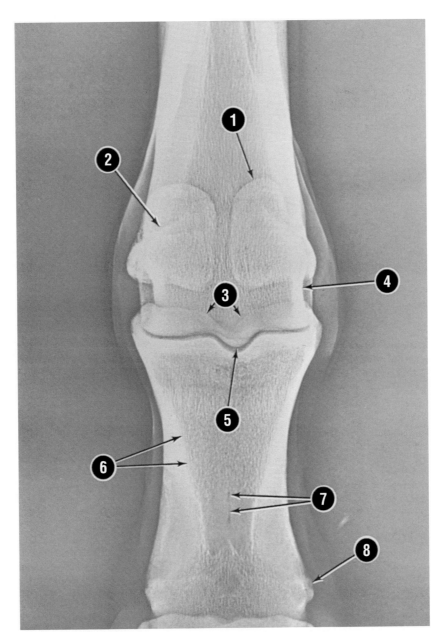

FIGURE 47–66. Dorsoproximal-Palmarodistal Oblique (DPr-PaDiO) Xeroradiograph of Left Equine Metacarpophalangeal Joint (McPJ).

1. Lateral proximal sesamoid bone
2. Depression in interosseus (abaxial) surface of medial proximal sesamoid bone for attachment of interosseus tendon
3. Palmaroproximal edge of Pp
4. Depression in MC 3 for attachment of lateral collateral ligament of McPJ
5. Sagittal ridge on head of MC 3
6. Area of oblique ridge on palmar surface of Pp for attachment of medial oblique sesamoid ligament
7. Nutrient canal through dorsal cortex of Pp
8. Lateral distal collateral tubercle of Pp

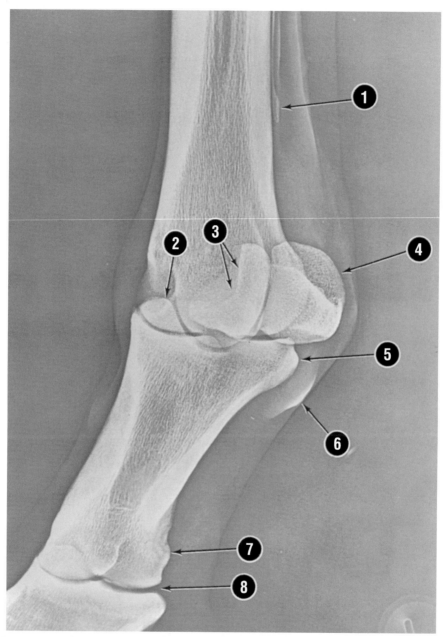

FIGURE 47–67. Dorsolateral-Palmaromedial Oblique (D45L-PaMO) Xeroradiograph of Left Equine Metacarpophalangeal Joint (McPJ).

1. Distal end of MC 4
2. Dorsoproximal aspect of Pp
3. Depression in interosseus surface of medial proximal sesamoid bone for attachment of interosseus tendon
4. Palmaroabaxial border of lateral proximal sesamoid bone
5. Lateral proximal collateral tubercle of Pp
6. Ergot
7. Lateral distal collateral tubercle of Pp
8. Proximal interphalangeal joint

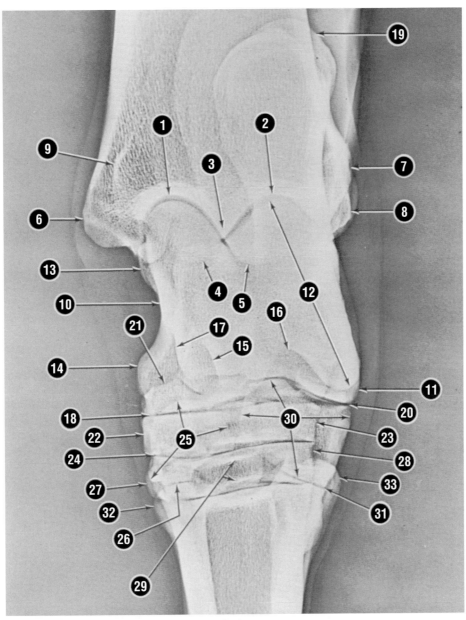

FIGURE 47–68. Dorsoplantar (DPl) Xeroradiograph of Left Equine Tarsus.

1. Medial groove of tibial cochlea
2. Lateral groove of tibial cochlea
3. Oblique ridge separating 1 and 2
4. Pointed caudal end of 3
5. Rounded cranial end of 3
6. Medial malleolus
7. Caudal part of lateral malleolus
8. Cranial part of lateral malleolus
9. Radiopaque shadow
10. Talus
11. Calcaneus
12. Lateral ridge of trochlea tali
13. Proximal tubercle of talus
14. Distal tubercle of talus
15. Medial ridge of trochlea tali
16. Groove between 12 and 15
17. Medial edge of sustentaculum tali

18. Proximal intertarsal (talocalcaneocentral) joint
19. Tuber calcanei
20. Calcaneoquartal joint
21. Proximoplantar aspect of central tarsus bone (Tc)
22. Medial aspect of Tc
23. Lateral aspect of Tc
24. Distal (centrodistal intertarsal) joint
25. Fused first and second tarsal bones (T1 + T2)
26. Articulation between 25 and MT 2
27. Medial aspect of third tarsal bone (T3)
28. Lateral aspect of T3
29. Radiopaque lines produced by walls of nonarticular depressions on T3
30. Fourth tarsal bone
31. Tarsometatarsal joints (also, 26)
32. Base of second metatarsal bone
33. Base of fourth metatarsal bone

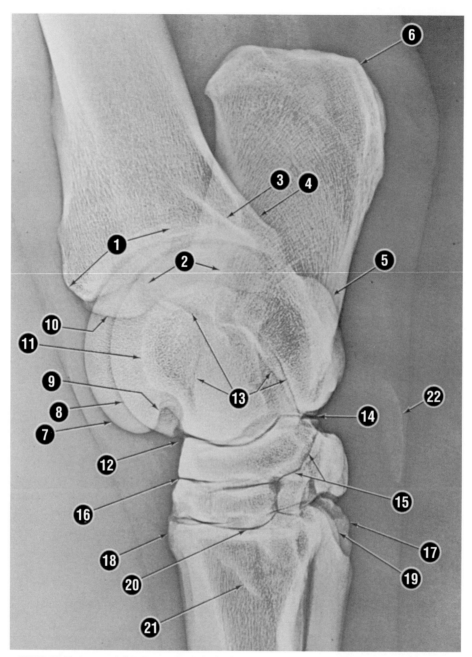

FIGURE 47–69. Lateromedial (LM) Xeroradiograph of Left Equine Tarsus.

1. Lateral malleolus
2. Medial malleolus
3. Radiopaque line produced by ridge on caudal surface of tibia
4. Medial part of caudal surface of tibia
5. Sustentaculum tali
6. Tuber calcanei
7. Lateral ridge of trochlea tali
8. Medial ridge of trochlea tali
9. Larger notch associated with lateral ridge of trochlea tali
10. Intermediate part of tibial cochlea
11. Groove of trochlea tali—defined by radiopaque line

12. Proximal intertarsal joint
13. Articular facets between talus and calcaneus
14. Plantar aspect of proximal intertarsal joint
15. Articulation between Tc and T1 + T2
16. Distal intertarsal joint
17. Base of MT 2
18. Base of MT 3
19. Base of MT 4
20. Tarsometatarsal joint
21. Groove on proximolateral aspect of MT 3 for dorsal metatarsal artery 3
22. Chestnut (torus tarseus)

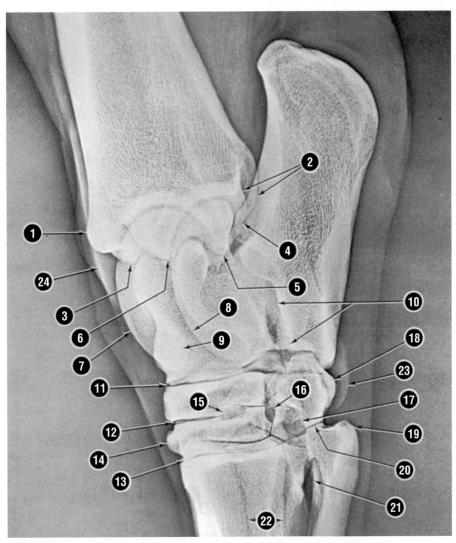

FIGURE 47–70. Dorsolateral-Plantaromedial Oblique (DL-PlMO) Xeroradiograph of Left Equine Tarsus.

1. Cranial aspect of medial malleolus
2. Shadows produced by borders of groove in lateral malleolus
3. Distal projection of medial malleolus
4. Distal projection of lateral malleolus
5. Caudal aspect of intermediate ridge of tibial cochlea
6. Cranial aspect of intermediate ridge of tibial cochlea
7. Medial ridge of trochlea tali
8. Lateral ridge of trochlea tali
9. Radiopaque area produced by distal tubercle of talus
10. Sinus tarsi
11. Dorsomedial aspect of proximal intertarsal joint
12. Dorsomedial aspect of distal intertarsal joint
13. Dorsomedial aspect of third tarsometatarsal joint
14. Ridge on dorsomedial aspect of T3
15. Nonarticular area between Tc and T3
16. Dorsal opening of tarsal canal
17. Plantar opening of tarsal canal
18. Plantar tuberosity on T4
19. Base of MT 4
20. Articulation between T4 and MT 4
21. Interosseous space between MT 3 and MT 4
22. Second metatarsal bone
23. Chestnut
24. Tendons crossing flexor surface of tarsus

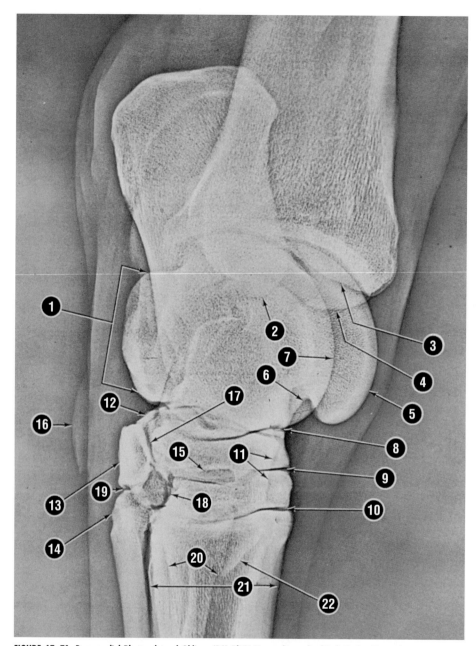

FIGURE 47–71. Dorsomedial-Plantarolateral Oblique (DM-PlLO) Xeroradiograph of Left Equine Tarsus.*

1. Sustentaculum tali
2. Distal extremity of medial malleolus
3. Distal extremity of lateral malleolus
4. Intermediate ridge of tibial cochlea
5. Lateral ridge of trochlea tali
6. Notch distal to 5.
7. Medial ridge of trochlea tali
8. Dorsolateral aspect of proximal intertarsal joint
9. Dorsolateral aspect of distal intertarsal joint
10. Dorsolateral aspect of third tarsometatarsal joint
11. Dorsal aspect of T4
12. Plantaromedial aspect of Tc

13. Plantaromedial aspect of T1 + T2
14. Plantaromedial aspect of MT 2
15. Nonarticular depression between Tc and T3
16. Chestnut
17. Articulation between T1 + T2 and Tc
18. Articulation between T1 + T2 and T3
19. Articulation between T1 + T2 and MT 2
20. Fourth metatarsal bone
21. Third metatarsal bone
22. Radiopaque line produced by border of groove for dorsal metatarsal artery 3

*Xeroradiographs are not translucent. Therefore, it is impossible to orient all xeroradiographs in the conventional manner with cranial (dorsal) to the left.

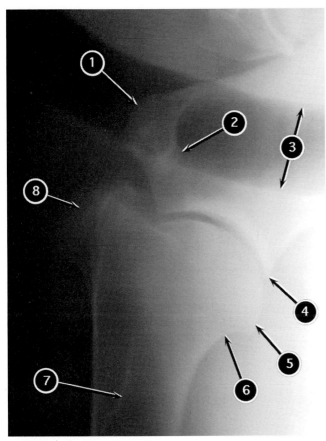

FIGURE 47–72. Mediolateral (ML) Radiograph of Equine Shoulder Joint.

1. Supraglenoid tubercle of scapula
2. Coracoid process of scapula
3. Air in trachea
4. Caudal border of glenoid cavity of scapula
5. Head of humerus
6. Neck of humerus
7. Deltoid tuberosity of humerus
8. Superimposed greater, lesser, and intermediate tubercles of humerus

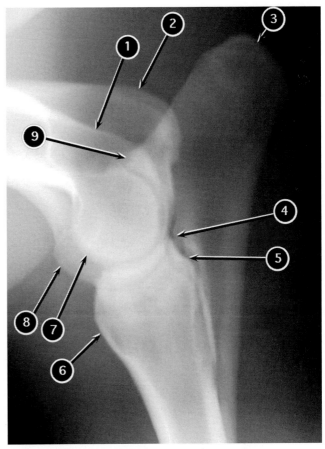

FIGURE 47–73. Mediolateral (ML) Radiograph of Equine Elbow Joint.

1. Caudal border of lateral epicondyle of humerus
2. Caudal border of medial epicondyle of humerus
3. Tuber olecrani of ulna
4. Lateral coronoid process of ulna
5. Proximal radioulnar joint
6. Radial tuberosity
7. Capitulum of humeral condyle
8. Trochlea of humeral condyle
9. Anconeal process of ulna

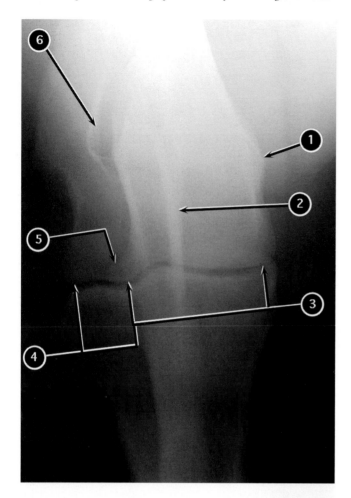

FIGURE 47–74. Craniocaudal (Cr-Cd) Radiograph of Equine Elbow Joint.

1. Medial epicondyle of humerus
2. Olecranon of ulna
3. Trochlea of humeral condyle
4. Capitulum of humeral condyle
5. Lateral coronoid process of ulna
6. Lateral border of olecranon fossa of humerus

FIGURE 47–75. Lateromedial (LM) Radiograph of Equine Stifle Joint.

1. Base of patella
2. Gliding part of articular surface of patella
3. Locking (resting) part of articular surface of patella
4. Lateral ridge of femoral trochlea
5. Extensor fossa of femur
6. Fibula
7. Tibial tuberosity
8. Intercondylar eminence of tibia
9. Apex of patella
10. Medial ridge of femoral trochlea

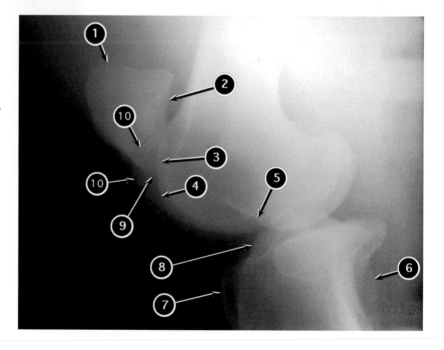

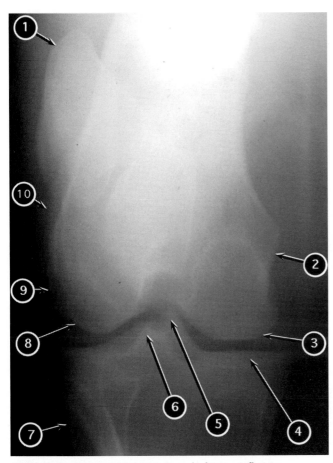

FIGURE 47–76. Caudocranial (Cd-Cr) Radiograph of Equine Stifle Joint.

1. Base of patella
2. Medial epicondyle of femur
3. Medial condyle of femur
4. Medial condyle of tibia
5. Medial tubercle of intercondylar eminence of tibia
6. Lateral tubercle of intercondylar eminence of tibia
7. Fibula
8. Lateral condyle of femur
9. Lateral epicondyle of femur
10. Lateral ridge of femoral trochlea

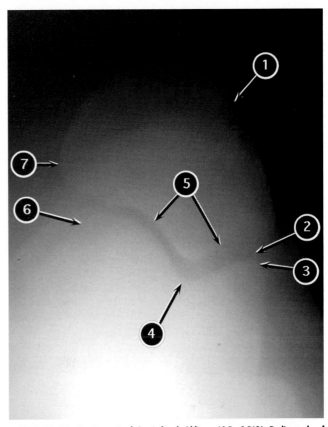

FIGURE 47–77. Cranioproximal-Craniodistal Oblique (CrPr-CrDiO) Radiograph of Equine Stifle Joint.

1. Cranial surface of patella
2. Femoropatellar joint
3. Lateral ridge of femoral trochlea
4. Groove of femoral trochlea
5. Articular surface of patella
6. Medial ridge of femoral trochlea
7. Osseous part of cartilaginous process of patella

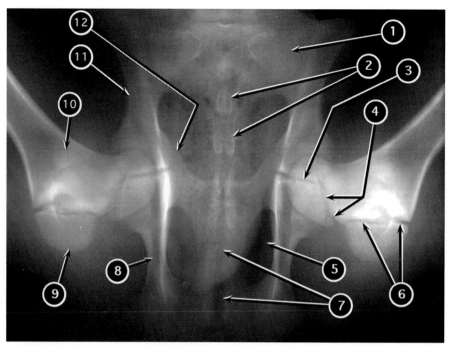

FIGURE 47–78. Ventrodorsal (VD) Radiograph of Foal Pelvis.

1. Wing of sacrum
2. Spinous processes of sacral vertebrae
3. Cartilaginous junction between ilium and ischium
4. Proximal physis (epiphyseal cartilage) of femur
5. Obturator foramen
6. Cartilaginous junction between greater trochanter and femoral body

7. Cartilaginous pelvic symphysis
8. Body of ischium
9. Greater trochanter of femur
10. Lesser trochanter of femur
11. Body of ilium
12. Cranial ramus of pubis near iliopubic eminence

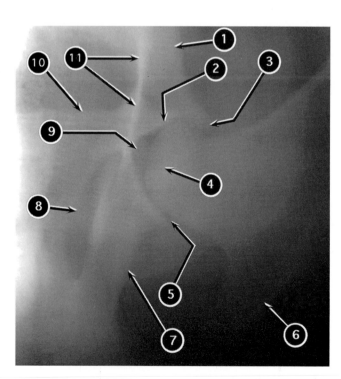

FIGURE 47–79. Ventrodorsal (VD) Radiograph of Equine Hip Joint.

1. Body of ilium
2. Cranial border of acetabulum
3. Craniodorsal border of acetabulum
4. Fovea of femoral head for attachment of round and accessory ligaments
5. Hip (coxal) joint
6. Greater trochanter of femur, caudal part
7. Body of ischium
8. Obturator foramen
9. Acetabular fossa and notch
10. Pecten (cranial border) of pubis
11. Ischiatic spine

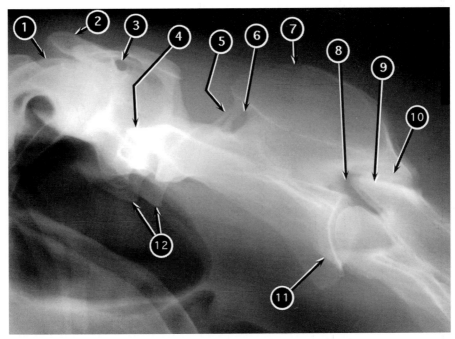

FIGURE 47–80. Left-Right Lateral Radiograph of Equine Atlas and Axis.

1. Occipital condyles
2. Cranial articular fovea of atlas
3. Lateral vertebral foramen of atlas for passage of cervical nerve 1
4. Dens of axis
5. Ossified ligaments forming cranial borders of 6; not ossified in young horses
6. Lateral vertebral foramina of axis for passage of cervical nerve 2
7. Spinous process of axis
8. Intervertebral foramina between C2 and C3 for passage of cervical nerve 3
9. Cranial articular processes of C3
10. Caudal articular processes of C2 (axis)
11. Ventral tubercles of transverse processes of C3
12. Wings of atlas

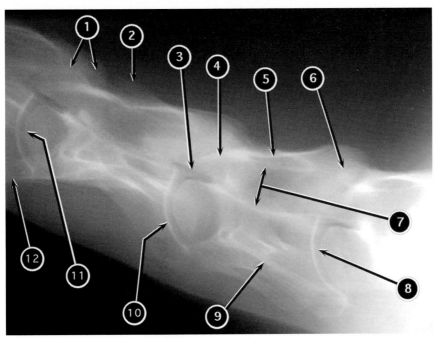

FIGURE 47–81. Left-Right Lateral Radiograph of Equine C4 and C5.

1. Caudal articular processes of C3
2. Spinous process of C4
3. Intervertebral foramina between C4 and C5 for passage of cervical nerve 5
4. Cranial articular processes of C5
5. Laminae of C5
6. Caudal articular processes of C5
7. Vertebral foramen of C5
8. Intervertebral disc space between C5 and C6
9. Dorsal tubercles of transverse processes of C5
10. Caudal extremity (fossa) of C4
11. Cranial extremity (head) of C4
12. Ventral tubercles of transverse processes of C4

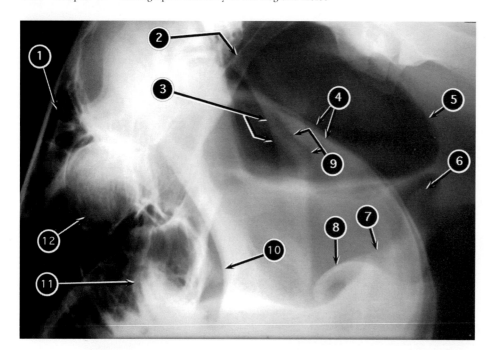

FIGURE 47–82. Left-Right Lateral Radiograph of Equine Guttural Pouch Region.

1. Superimposed conchofrontal sinuses (frontal parts)
2. Basilar part of occipital bone
3. Rostral borders of stylohyoid bones dividing compartments of guttural pouches
4. Caudal borders of mandibles
5. Caudal extent of medial compartments of guttural pouches
6. Corniculate processes of arytenoid cartilages of larynx
7. Aryepiglottic folds connecting arytenoid and epiglottic cartilages of larynx
8. Epiglottis (formed by epiglottic cartilage of larynx)
9. Caudal extent of lateral compartments of guttural pouches
10. Rostral borders of mandibles
11. Embedded part of superior molars 3
12. Ethmoidal conchae

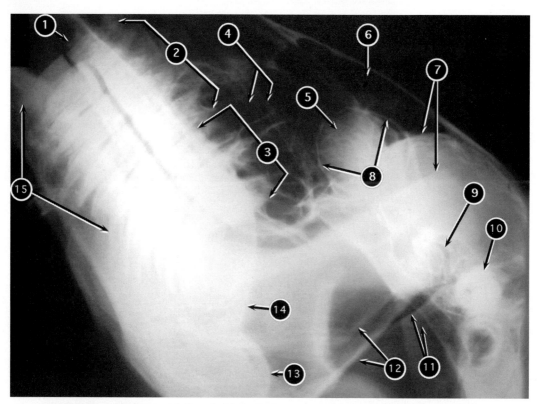

FIGURE 47–83. Left-Right Lateral Radiograph of Equine Head.

1. Wolf tooth (superior premolar 1)
2. Superior premolars 2–4
3. Superior molars 1–3
4. Infraorbital canals
5. Ethmoidal conchae
6. Superimposed conchofrontal sinuses
7. Rostral borders of coronoid processes of mandibles
8. Edges of orbits
9. Temporomandibular joint
10. Petrous temporal bone
11. Rostral borders of stylohyoid bones dividing compartments of guttural pouches
12. Caudal borders of mandibles
13. Caudal surface of epiglottis (formed by epiglottic cartilage of larynx)
14. Dorsal surface of soft palate overlying root of tongue
15. Inferior premolars 2–4

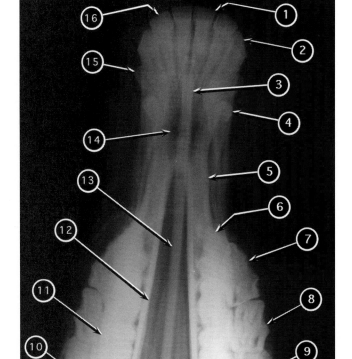

FIGURE 47–84. Ventrodorsal (VD) Radiograph of Rostral Part of Equine Head.

1. Left central incisors (I1)
2. Left corner incisors (I3)
3. Rostral part of nasal septum superimposed on palatine processes of incisive bones
4. Left superior canine tooth
5. Buccal (lateral) surface of body of mandible
6. Left inferior premolar 2
7. Left superior premolar 2
8. Left superior premolar 3
9. Left superior premolar 4
10. Right inferior molar 1
11. Right inferior premolar 4
12. Lingual (medial) surface of body of mandible
13. Nasal septum superimposed on vomer
14. Right palatine fissure
15. Right inferior canine tooth
16. Right intermediate incisors (I2)

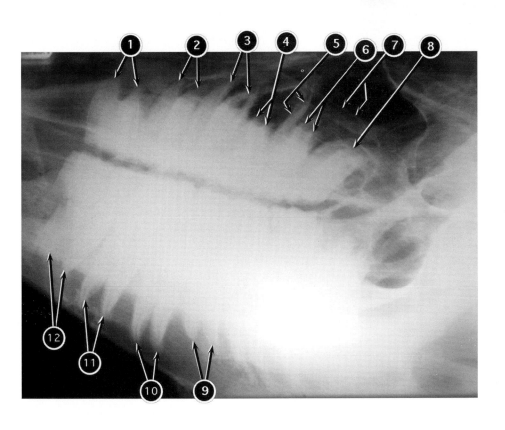

FIGURE 47–85. Left Ventral–Right Dorsal Oblique Radiograph of Equine Head.

1. Roots of left superior premolar 2
2. Roots of left superior premolar 3
3. Roots of left superior premolar 4
4. Roots of left superior molar 1
5. Maxillary septum between left rostral and caudal maxillary sinuses
6. Roots of left superior molar 2
7. Left infraorbital canal
8. Roots of left superior molar 3
9. Roots of right inferior molar 1
10. Roots of right inferior premolar 4
11. Roots of right inferior premolar 3
12. Roots of right inferior premolar 2

References

1. Schebitz H, and Wilkens H: Atlas of Radiographic Anatomy of the Dog and Cat, 4th Ed. Philadelphia, WB Saunders, 1986.
2. Schebitz H, and Wilkens H: Atlas of Radiographic Anatomy of the Horse, 3rd Ed. Philadelphia, WB Saunders, 1978.
3. Smallwood JE, Shively MJ, Rendano VT, et al: A standardized nomenclature for radiographic projections used in veterinary medicine. Vet Radiol 26:2–9, 1985.
4. Smallwood JE, and Shively MJ: Radiographic and xeroradiographic anatomy of the equine carpus. Equine Pract 1:22–38, 1979.
5. Smallwood JE, and Holladay SD: Xeroradiographic anatomy of the equine digit and metacarpophalangeal region. Vet Radiol 28:166–173, 1987.
6. Shively MJ, and Smallwood JE: Radiographic and xeroradiographic anatomy of the equine tarsus. Equine Pract 2:19–35, 1980.
7. Zontine WJ: Canine dental radiology: Radiographic technic, development, and anatomy of the teeth. J Am Vet Radiol Soc 16:75, 1975.
8. Burk RL, Corwin LA, Bahr RJ, et al: The right cranial lung lobe bronchus of the dog: Its identification in a lateral chest radiograph. J Am Vet Radiol Soc 19:210, 1978.
9. Spencer CP, Ackerman N, and Burt JK: The canine lateral thoracic radiograph. Vet Radiol 22:262, 1981.
10. Thrall DE, and Losonsky JM: A method of evaluating canine pulmonary circulatory dynamics from survey radiographs. J Am Anim Hosp Assoc 12:457, 1976.

Answers

SECTION I • PRINCIPLES OF INTERPRETATION

Chapter 1 • Radiation Physics, Radiation Protection, and Darkroom Theory

1. (C) X-rays are produced in atomic shells by electron interactions, and gamma rays originate from unstable atomic nuclei.

2. (C) X-rays have no charge. See Table 1–2.

3. (B) Protective aprons and gloves are not designed to protect against the primary beam; they have insufficient absorption capability to do so.

4. (A) X-rays are produced primarily by radiative interactions.

5. (B) The anode is angled to improve image quality by reducing the effective size of the focal spot.

6.

Criterion	Absorption Process
Independent of atomic number	Compton
Results in most exposure to radiographers	Compton
Desirable process for diagnostic radiology	Photoelectric
Provides for differential absorption of x-rays by tissue	Photoelectric

7.

$$\frac{mAs_1}{mAs_2} = \frac{(d_1)^2}{(d_2)^2}$$

$$\frac{10}{mAs_2} = \frac{(40)^2}{(60)^2};$$

$$\frac{10}{mAs_2} = \frac{1600}{3600};$$

$$\frac{10}{mAs_2} = 0.44;$$

$$mAs_2 = \frac{10}{0.44};$$

$$mAs_2 = 22.7 \, mAs.$$

8.

Best detail	No screen
Poorest detail	High-speed screen
Most film blackness	High-speed screen
Least film blackness	No screen

9. A. It was overexposed/<u>underexposed</u>.
   B. A grid <u>was</u>/was not used.
   C. The grid was/<u>was not</u> aligned.
   D. The developer temperature was too <u>low</u>/high.
   E. The developer was new/<u>exhausted</u>.
   F. The film was in the developer too long/<u>not long enough</u>.
   G. The film was <u>fresh</u>/old.
   H. The screens had <u>high</u>/low resolution.
   I. The film was first placed in the developer/<u>fixer</u>.

10. The black crescent mark was caused by the film being mishandled before processing. The mishandling could have occurred when the film was placed into the cassette or when it was processed. The mishandling resulted in a crimp, the pressure of which resulted in exposure of the silver halide film crystals in the area. Crimping results when film, particularly large format sheets such as 14 inch × 17 inch, is handled with only one hand and the film drapes over the fingers.

11. The black arborizing artifacts resulted from static electricity. Static electricity is likely to be produced when film is slid along another surface, such as when it is removed from a cassette. Rapid movements of the film should be avoided.

12. Gloved hands are in the primary x-ray beam. Lead gloves and aprons are designed to prevent exposure associated with scattered x-rays. Lead gloves and aprons do not protect the wearer against the primary x-ray beam, and body parts must never be placed in the primary beam.

13. The most likely cause for this artifact is a piece of hair in the cassette. The hair prevents light produced by the intensifying screen from reaching the film. Another cause might be scratching of the emulsion off the film. These two causes could be differentiated by looking closely at the film. The emulsion scratch would produce a physical defect on the surface of the film, whereas hair in the cassette would not.

14. This artifact was caused by a focused grid being positioned in the x-ray beam upside down. This results in a malalignment between the diverging x-ray beam and the spaces between the lead strips in the grid (see Fig. 1–28). A similar-appearing artifact could result from a focused grid being used at the incorrect focal spot–film distance, but the extent of grid cutoff would not be as severe.

Chapter 2 • Introduction to Radiographic Interpretation

1. When the thickness of the substance with the greater effective atomic number or physical density (or both) is much greater than the other substance.

2. Air (gas), fat, water (soft tissue), bone, metal.

3. Size, shape, number, location, margination, opacity.

4. (B) The silhouette sign.

5. The small radiopacity cannot be a tracheal foreign body because its margin extends beyond the wall of the trachea. The opacity cannot be a tracheal wall mass because the wall of the trachea can be clearly seen through the mass. This opacity was created by an engorged tick present on the side of the dog's neck. It appears so intensely opaque because of the principle described in Figure 2–15. The gas superimposed on the dorsal aspect of the opacity is gas in the cervical esophagus, a normal finding. The small opacity slightly dorsocaudal to the larger opacity is a film artifact created by dirt in the cassette.

6. No, the dorsal (cranial) aspect of the subject should be facing to the left, not to the right.

7. A dorsoplantar view. Distal to the antebrachiocarpal (tarsocrural) joint, the front surface of the limb is termed the *dorsal surface*; the back surface of the forelimb is the *palmar surface,* and the back surface of the hindlimb is the *plantar surface.*

8. (A) The left coronary artery would not be visible because it silhouettes with the myocardium. The other

three structures are surrounded by air-containing lung and will be clearly visible.

9. (A) Intrapericardial lipoma is least likely because the fat-containing tumor would be visible as a mass of decreased opacity in the cardiac silhouette. The other conditions would result in a homogeneously opaque, enlarged cardiac silhouette.

10. True. For easily accessible parts, such as the canine elbow, reversing the position of the x-ray tube and cassette results in minimal differences in the appearance of the radiograph.

Chapter 3 • Visual Perception and Radiographic Interpretation

1. Shadows.
2. Contours.
3. Percepts.
4. Masses, kidneys, pulmonary cavitary lesions, pulmonary nodules.
5. Plurality (or multistability) of perception.
6. Exposure (or assimilation of the concept).
7. Dime.
8. 30.
9. Fills in.
10. Sensory detection and perception.

Chapter 4 • Aggressive Versus Nonaggressive Bone Lesions

1. Possible differential diagnoses for focal lytic and proliferative lesions at multiple skeletal sites include metastatic neoplasia, hematogenous osteomyelitis, and fungal osteomyelitis.

2. There are two options. You could biopsy the lesion, or you could reradiograph the area in 2 to 4 weeks to determine if there is progression of bone lysis or evidence of fracture healing. Because this is a fibular fracture, surgical fixation would not be necessary, so placing the dog in a splint or other external support and waiting to reradiograph would be a reasonable option.

3. The three patterns of bone destruction are geographic (less aggressive), moth-eaten (moderately aggressive), and permeative (highly aggressive).

4. Differential diagnoses for geographic bone lysis include cyst, abscess, and benign bone neoplasia.

5. False. The margins are more indicative of how aggressive a lesion is than the length of the transition zone between normal and abnormal bone. Smooth margins indicate a more benign process, whereas irregular or moth-eaten margins indicate a more aggressive process.

6. True. Interrupted periosteal new bone formation is consistent with an aggressive lesion. It can have smooth margins and still appear nonhomogeneous, disorganized, or irregular.

7. True. Many skeletal diseases have tendencies to affect certain areas of bone. For example, osteosarcoma is more often seen in metaphyseal areas, panosteitis is usually diaphyseal, osteochondrosis affects subchondral bone of

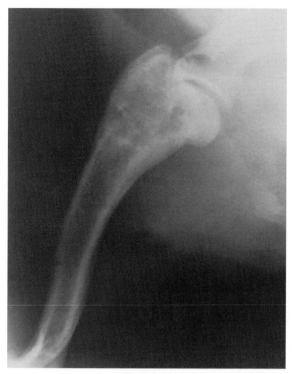

FIGURE 4–14

specific joints, and nutritional secondary hyperparathyroidism diffusely affects all bones.

8. The pattern of bone destruction is moth-eaten. There is interrupted periosteal new bone formation seen on the cranial and caudal aspect of the humeral metaphysis and epiphysis. The periosteal bone on the caudal aspect is somewhat lamellated with a mixed smooth and irregular margin. The edge margin is moth-eaten and indistinct with a short transition zone. The radiographic changes indicate a moderately aggressive bone lesion. Neoplasia and osteomyelitis are possible differential diagnoses. Bone biopsy indicated a pyogranulomatous osteomyelitis. A lateral radiograph obtained 6 months later (Fig. 4–14) after treatment shows a smooth, continuous periosteal reaction, more sharply marginated zone between normal and abnormal bone, and some normal bone production intermixed with residual moth-eaten bone lysis. There is no progression of the lysis, and changes seen suggest healing.

9. The lysis in the proximal tibia is moth-eaten with an irregular, indistinct edge margin. There is cortical bone destruction. Nonhomogeneous, interrupted periosteal new bone formation is seen on the caudal, medial, and lateral areas around the lesion. Changes indicate a moderately aggressive bone lesion. Neoplasia and osteomyelitis are possible differential diagnoses. Final diagnosis was osteosarcoma.

10. The lysis is primarily geographic with a few moth-eaten areas. The edge margin is irregular. There is sharp demarcation between normal and abnormal bone. There is no periosteal new bone formation present. The changes suggest an aggressive lesion owing to the irregular margins and the subtle moth-eaten appearance but perhaps a slower-growing lesion. Differential diagnoses include neoplasia, bone abscess, and bone cyst. Final diagnosis was lymphosarcoma.

SECTION II • AXIAL SKELETON—COMPANION ANIMALS

Chapter 5 • Cranial Vault and Associated Structures

1. Common radiographic features of hydrocephalus include doming and cortical thinning of the calvaria, decreased prominence of the normal calvarial convolutional markings, persistent fontanelles, and a homogeneous appearance to the brain. Commonly affected breeds include the Chihuahua, Yorkshire terrier, and many other miniature and toy breeds.

2. Common fractures that occur with high-rise syndrome include mandibular and maxillary symphyseal separation with splitting of the hard palate and associated carpal dislocations, crushing injuries to the carpi, and forelimb and femoral fractures.

3. The primary radiographic feature of hyperparathyroidism is a general loss of bone opacity with loss of the lamina dura of the dental alveolus and cortical thinning of all bones. Hyperostotic fibrous osteodystrophy (excessive replacement of bone with fibrous tissue) may occur, especially in exotic animals and primates.

4. Benign tumors tend to appear much less aggressive than malignant tumors and often result in focal areas of bone proliferation with little or no evidence of bone lysis. Malignant neoplasms tend to appear less contained and to be characterized by progressive and unrestrained bone lysis with varying amounts of proliferation.

5. Clinical features of nasopharyngeal polyps are age (affected animals are generally young) and the presence of respiratory signs, including nasal discharge, sneezing, and stridor. Radiographically a focal soft-tissue mass may be visible within the nasal pharynx on the lateral skull radiograph; however, the most obvious radiographic signs involve the tympanic bullae. One or both bullae may be severely thickened and contain a diffuse soft-tissue opacity suggestive of otitis media.

6. Radiographic signs of otitis media depend on the duration and severity of the disease and vary from mild to severe thickening of the affected tympanic bulla, which also appears mildly to severely increased in radiopacity. Otitis externa is common and may result in thickening or mineralization of the external ear canal, which therefore appears less well aerated than normal. Radiographic evaluation is not complete without the inclusion of both oblique views, a dorsoventral or ventrodorsal view, and a rostral-caudal open-mouth projection of the bulla. This allows evaluation with a minimum of superimposed bone and soft tissue and optimizes comparison of the two bullae.

7. Radiographic signs of periapical infection include widening of the periodontal space surrounding the apex, bone lysis or sclerosis adjacent to the apex, resorption of the tooth root, and osteomyelitis of the adjacent bone.

8. The three types of epuli are fibromatous, ossifying, and acanthomatous. The acanthomatous epulis is considered to be the most aggressive because of its potential to infiltrate into adjacent bone.

9. On the radiograph, there is complete lack of aeration of the right external ear canal with severe bone lysis of the caudal aspect of the right zygomatic arch and destruction of the right temporomandibular joint. The right tympanic bulla appears thickened, which could be confirmed by obtaining oblique and open-mouth views of the region. Although the history is one of chronic infection, the extensive bone lysis indicates a much more aggressive process, and neoplasia of the external ear canal or of the zygomatic arch must be high on the list of differential diagnoses. A biopsy of the area is indicated and in this case confirmed the presence of a cerruminous gland adenocarcinoma of the ear canal.

10. There is extensive lysis of bone around the base of the fourth maxillary premolar and first maxillary molar with apparent displacement of these teeth. Notice also that the roots of the fourth maxillary premolar tooth are narrow and pointed, suggesting lysis of these roots as well as of the adjacent bone. Extension of this process into the adjacent nasal passage is also likely due to the increased soft-tissue opacity above the tooth. Although the clinical signs suggest a carnassial tooth abscess, the severity of the bone and tooth root lysis is more consistent with a much more aggressive lesion, and a tumor of soft-tissue origin must be highly considered. Additional radiographs of the nasal passages should be obtained to allow better assessment of the suspected extension of this process. A biopsy of the mass is also indicated, and in this dog the diagnosis was an acanthomatous epulis. The dog was treated aggressively with a partial maxillectomy followed by radiation therapy.

Chapter 6 • Nasal Cavity and Paranasal Sinuses

1. Radiographic evaluation should include lateral and open-mouth or occlusal views of the nasal passages as well as a rostrocaudal view of the frontal sinuses. Oblique views of the maxilla may also prove helpful.

2. Fractures generally appear as straight or curved radiolucent lines with malalignment and discontinuity of the adjacent maxillary cortex. Fractures are often multiple, and subcutaneous hemorrhage and air accumulation are common. Hemorrhage into the nasal passages, which appears as an ill-defined area of increased soft-tissue opacity superimposed over normal or disrupted conchae, is also common.

3. Nasal conchae appear as fine, semiparallel radiopaque lines that extend caudally from the level of the canine teeth to the third premolars. The midline is marked by the sagittal groove of the vomer bone, and the ethmoidal turbinates appear as a fine fan-like bone pattern between the conchae and the cribriform plate. The presence of fine, bony scrolls covered by nasal mucosa and surrounded by air accounts for the radiographic appearance of the normal nasal passages.

4. Four common causes of acute rhinitis are allergy, foreign bodies, bacterial infections, and viral infections. In many animals with acute rhinitis, radiographs of the nasal passages may appear normal. Unilateral or bilateral increase in soft-tissue opacity in the nasal passages and frontal sinuses may be seen. Focal increases in opacity may be seen around a soft-tissue foreign body, or the foreign body may be visible itself if it is radiopaque.

5. Chronic rhinitis generally results in focal-to-diffuse areas of increased soft-tissue opacity superimposed over the normal conchal structures. This may be unilateral or bilateral, and there may be secondary involvement of the frontal sinuses as well, especially in the cat.

6. The most common causative agent of destructive rhinitis is *Aspergillus*, especially *Aspergillus fumigatus*. Rhinitis secondary to these agents is more aggressive in radiographic

appearance than that caused by bacterial agents. Therefore, conchal destruction is generally present—this may vary from small, punctate areas of lucency to larger, more ill-defined areas of conchal destruction.

7. The most common type of tumor is the carcinoma with adenocarcinomas predominating.

8. Factors that affect the radiographic appearance of an animal with a nasal tumor include the type and duration of the tumor as well as any previous surgical or medical therapy.

9. There is a diffuse increase in opacity of the middle and caudal portions of the right nasal passage with decreased conchal definition. Because of the blood-tinged discharge, the differential diagnosis should include erosive rhinitis and neoplasia. The caudal and unilateral location of the lesion as well as the advanced age of the dog makes neoplasia the most likely possibility; therefore, a biopsy is recommended, and nasal endoscopy should be performed. An *Aspergillus* titer could also be obtained. In this particular animal, the *Aspergillus* titer was negative, and an undifferentiated adenocarcinoma was diagnosed on the biopsy.

10. The short white arrow indicates an area of periosteal new bone formation. There is a diffuse increase in soft-tissue opacity of the caudal nasal passages primarily on the right side with large areas of conchal destruction and erosion of the vomer. The frontal sinuses are also opacified. These changes indicate an aggressive, destructive process originating in the right caudal nasal passage with extension through the maxilla and frontal bones and either extension of this process into the frontal sinuses or occlusion of sinus drainage with mucus accumulation. The most likely cause for this appearance is a malignant neoplasm, and a biopsy or fine-needle aspirate is recommended. A poorly differentiated adenocarcinoma was diagnosed.

Chapter 7 • Anatomic and Physiologic Imaging of the Canine and Feline Brain

1. (A) Falx cerebri shift.

2. (D) Planar scintigraphy.

3. (D) All of the above.

4. (C) Inherent attenuation differences of the objects located within the volumetric slice being imaged.

5. (A) Oligodendroglioma.

6. (C) Excite the net magnetization moments.

7. (A) Hypointense.

8. (D) Meningioma.

9. (B) ^{99m}Tc-glucoheptate.

10. (D) Ventricular dilation and asymmetry.

Chapter 8 • The Vertebrae

1. Possible explanations include (A) the anomalous presence of an extra lumbar vertebra, (B) agenesis or partial formation of the 13th pair of ribs, or (C) incomplete fusion of the first sacral vertebra to the sacrum.

2. True.

3. (A) Agenesis, (B) fracture, or (C) fusion failure of the

odontoid process or (D) rupture of the stabilizing ligaments between C1 and C2.

4. C4–C5, C5–C6, and C6–C7 are the most frequently affected sites.

5. (A) Sacrum subluxates ventral to L7, (B) lumbosacral stenosis, (C) collapse of the lumbosacral disc space, (D) narrowing of the sacral vertebral canal or neural foramina, and (E) protruding degenerative disc.

6. Discospondylitis is sepsis of the intervertebral disc space and adjacent ends of the adjoining vertebral bodies. Spondylosis deformans is a noninflammatory vertebral body remodeling that may vary in extent from formation of small spurs to complete bridging of adjacent vertebrae.

7. Neoplasia does not routinely result in end plate lysis occurring simultaneously cranial and caudal to an intervertebral disc.

8. Most primary vertebral neoplasms are osteosarcomas and reside within one vertebra. Most secondary vertebral neoplasms are carcinomas and may reside in one or more vertebrae.

9. Discospondylitis at L4–L5 and probably at L7–S1; probable lumbosacral instability with spondylosis deformans.

10. The column of contrast medium from the epidurogram is displaced dorsally by the protruding disc at L7–S1. There is slight spondylosis ventral to S1. The dog has cauda equina syndrome from a herniating disc at L7–S1, possibly owing to lumbosacral instability.

Chapter 9 • Intervertebral Disc Disease and Myelography

1. (B) Fibroid degeneration.

2. (C) The pia is the thinnest meningeal layer and covers the spinal cord.

3. (F) All of the above.

4. Multipoint centering, use of detail film-screen combinations, and paying strict attention to patient positioning.

5. Narrowed intervertebral articular process joint space, narrowed intervertebral disc space, cloudy intervertebral foramen, small intervertebral foramen, and presence of extruded, mineralized disc material within the vertebral canal.

6. (B) Disc mineralization is a dystrophic change.

7. (F) None of the above.

8. Intradural extramedullary.

9. Slight epidural leakage of contrast medium around the needle.

10. Extradural.

SECTION III • AXIAL SKELETON—EQUIDAE

Chapter 10 • The Equine Skull

1. The mandible is sclerotic in the region of the roots of the first mandibular cheek tooth (second mandibular premolar). There are small focal radiolucent areas immediately adjacent to the rostral and caudal roots of this tooth. These signs are consistent with a tooth root ab-

scess and associated osteomyelitis (e.g., mandibular periostitis).

2. There is diffuse thickening of the proximal portion of the left stylohyoid bone. This is probably the result of trauma. Involvement of the adjacent temporal bone is presumed.

3. There is retropharyngeal soft-tissue swelling, which is compressing the dorsal aspect of the nasopharynx. There is a displaced bone fragment superimposed over the medial guttural pouch compartments. This was the tip of one paracondylar process. The basisphenoid and basioccipital bones appear intact. The appearance of the fracture is also consistent with an avulsion fracture associated with tearing of the insertion of the longus capitis muscle.

4. (D) All of the above.

5. True.

6. False.

7. (A) May result from infection of the middle ear or guttural pouch.

8. (C) Temporal bone.

9. False.

10. Retained deciduous premolars.

Chapter 11 • Equine Nasal Passages and Sinuses

1. Immediately dorsal to the fourth premolar. This represents an oblique laminar bony line as seen on lateral and some oblique radiographs.

2. The maxillary sinus surrounds the alveolar recess of these tooth roots. As the horse ages, the roots of the premolars and molars impinge less and less on the maxillary sinuses. Thus these sinuses actually become larger as the animal ages.

3. Multiple views are required to rule out the possibility of depressed fractures of the maxilla where there are fragments displaced into the nasal passages or a sinus. Such depressed fragments may not be visible on routine lateral and ventrodorsal radiographs, and the physical deformity in the bone may be masked by soft-tissue swelling.

4. Increased soft-tissue opacity to the caudal part of the nasal cavity and fluid lines in the frontal and caudal maxillary sinuses. Note that there is no fluid in the rostral maxillary sinus.

5. The ventrodorsal view. Lesions of the septum are poorly seen at best on any other view.

6. Although the mandible and teeth overlie the medial side of the maxilla and may obscure lesions in these areas, it is the masseter muscles that overlie the lateral part of the caudal maxillary sinus. On straight ventrodorsal views of the maxilla, these muscles impart a fluid-like opacity to the sinus, which could be mistaken for fluid in the sinus.

7. It is unlikely that any lesion other than neoplasia would result in fragmentation and displacement of a piece of cortical bone or a tooth. Expansion and displacement of cortical bone may occur with cystic lesions, but fragmentation and lysis of that bone is not a feature of these diseases.

8. The bony infraorbital canal. This structure becomes more visible as the animal ages owing to the progressive downward movement of the tooth roots.

Chapter 12 • The Equine Vertebral Column

1. (E) All of the above.

2. Caudal.

3. 2, 5.

4. Iopamidol.

5. True.

6. (A) Arabians.

7. (D) *Brucella.*

8. (A) C3–C4, C6–C7, C5–C6, and C4–C5.

9. The contrast myelogram is normal. The narrowing of the ventral contrast medium column on this flexion study is a normal finding. Notice that the dorsal contrast medium column remains normally wide.

10. In this extended view, there is compression of the ventral and dorsal contrast medium columns at C5–C6 and C6–C7. The vertebra labeled with the arrow is the sixth cervical vertebra and is identifiable in the vast majority of horses because of the large lateral process with the separate center of ossification at the caudal aspect.

SECTION IV • APPENDICULAR SKELETON—COMPANION ANIMALS

Chapter 13 • Diseases of the Immature Skeleton

1. True. Although vacuum phenomenon has been associated with shoulder joint osteochondrosis, it is also seen in normal shoulder joints and joints with degenerative arthritis, so it is not specific to osteochondrosis. The joint should be scrutinized carefully, however, for the presence of osteochondrosis if vacuum phenomenon is observed.

2. True. As a general rule, larger osteochondrosis lesions are more likely to have cartilaginous flaps and more likely to have clinical signs of pain and lameness.

3. The anconeus should fuse to the ulna by 4 to 5 months, so an ununited anconeus is diagnosed after 5 months of age.

4. False. A medial coronoid fragment is often not radiographically visible because it is frequently composed of cartilage and therefore not radiopaque.

5. Hypertrophic osteodystrophy is the most likely diagnosis. The radiographic changes and clinical signs described are characteristic of hypertrophic osteodystrophy. Hematogenous osteomyelitis could also be considered.

6. Panosteitis is typically located in the diaphysis, near nutrient foramina. Medullary sclerosis with or without continuous periosteal new bone formation is a classic change associated with this disease.

7. Malignant neoplastic transformation is a potential sequela of multiple cartilaginous exostoses. Any rapid growth of previously inert lesions should be radiographed and biopsied.

8. There is increased medullary opacity in the distal humeral diaphysis (compare the humeral medullary opacity with the relatively lucent proximal radial diaphysis). Radioulnar joint incongruity is present with a small stairstep at the articular junction of the radius and ulna. Subtle enthesophyte bone production is present on the anconeal process. The area of the coronoid is not well

defined. Mild bone sclerosis is present along the sub-trochlear bone and adjacent to the lateral coronoid process. Changes are consistent with panosteitis in the distal humerus, elbow dysplasia (joint incongruity), minor degenerative joint disease, and possible fragmented medial coronoid process. Additional views of the medial coronoid process are recommended. The panosteitis is probably responsible for a major portion of the lameness, but the joint incongruity, minor arthritis, and possible fragmented medial coronoid process could also cause the lameness to persist after resolution of the panosteitis.

9. There is cranial and medial bowing of the radius. There is a retained cartilaginous core in the distal ulna. The radial and ulnar physes appear normal and open. There is mild humeral-ulnar joint subluxation seen on the craniocaudal view. The caudal radial cortex is thickened, probably secondary to abnormal weight bearing. The angular limb deformity is probably secondary to growth interruption of the distal ulnar physis by the retained cartilaginous core. Ulnar ostectomy is the recommended surgical procedure.

10. There is subchondral bone flattening and lucency in the medial humeral condyle. Bone sclerosis is seen adjacent to the lucency. Minor enthesophyte formation is present on the medial aspect of the medial condyle. Radiographic diagnosis is osteochondrosis of the medial humeral condyle with mild degenerative joint disease.

Chapter 14 • Fracture Healing and Complications

1. C   2. E   3. C   4. C   5. D   6. D   7. C
8. B   9. D   10. A

Chapter 15 • Bone Tumors Versus Bone Infections

1. (C) The zone of hypertrophied chondrocytes.
2. (E) Rigid fracture fixation.
3. (C) Retains sharp margins radiographically.
4. (C) Periosteal vessels, metaphyseal vessels, and nutrient vessels.
5. (E) None of the above.
6. (D) Sclerotic fragment ends and a closed marrow cavity.
7. (C) Healing fracture but fragments malaligned.
8. (B) Osteomyelitis is highly likely.
9. (D) Healed fracture with disuse osteoporosis.
10. (A) Fragment distraction with probable low-grade osteomyelitis.

Chapter 16 • Radiographic Signs of Joint Disease

1. Traction, rotation, wedge, compression, shear.
2. Coxofemoral joint subluxation, seen as an increase in the radiolucent joint space.
3. 100 mg I/mL.
4. Radiographic signs of joint disease are (1) synovial effusion, (2) altered subchondral bone opacity, (3) osteophyte/enthesophyte proliferation, (4) soft-tissue mineralization, (5) intra-articular calcification, (6) bone cyst formation, (7) subchondral bone erosion, (8) joint mal-formation, (9) joint displacement, (10) altered joint space thickness.

5. (1) Immune mediated (e.g., rheumatoid arthritis), (2) infectious arthritis, (3) chronic hemarthrosis.

6. Synovial sarcoma.

7. (1) Osteochondritis dissecans, (2) avulsion of the origin of the long digital extensor tendon, (3) avulsion of the tendon of origin of the popliteal muscle, (4) avulsion of the origin or insertion of a cruciate ligament, (5) meniscal calcification, (6) synovial osteochondroma formation, (7) degenerative joint disease, (8) septic arthritis.

8. There is a triangular radiolucent region in the subchondral region of the distal radius. Stress radiography was done. Look at Figure 16–26B. There is an articular fracture and a large bone fragment.

9. Slight unilateral joint laxity (right) was evident in Figure 16–27A, but when a distraction (PennHip) view (Fig. 16–27B) is made, it is evident that joint laxity was not disclosed by the extended view. Diagnosis was hip dysplasia.

10. Most of the changes seen in Figure 16–28A and B appear benign and consist of new bone formation around the elbow. Some condylar erosion and soft-tissue mineralization are also evident, consistent with degenerative joint disease. Periosteal new bone proliferation on the caudal surface of the ulna is not, however, consistent with the presence of degenerative joint disease. Figure 16–28C is a microradiograph of a transverse slab of bone taken through the distal humerus at necropsy. It reveals extensive bone destruction. Histologic diagnosis was degenerative joint disease and synovial sarcoma.

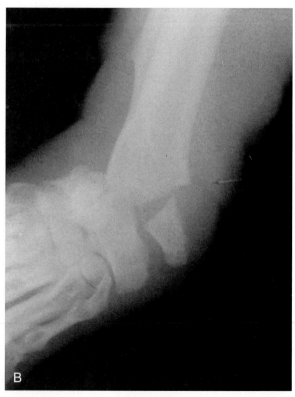

FIGURE 16–26. *B*

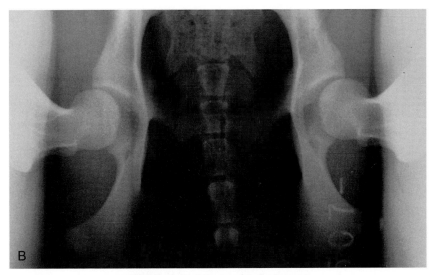

FIGURE 16–27. *B* (Courtesy of Dr. Ray Ferguson.)

SECTION V • APPENDICULAR SKELETON—EQUIDAE

Chapter 17 • Physeal Disorders of the Immature Horse

1. (D) All of the above.
2. (B) Distal femur.
3. (C) Epiphysis.
4. (A) Infectious physitis.
5. (C) Physeal dysplasia of the distal tibia.

Chapter 18 • The Stifle and Tarsus

1. (A) Medial femoral condyle.
2. (C) 40%.
3. (D) Secondary to umbilical infection.

4. (D) Failure of the lateral malleolus to unite with the tibia.
5. (C) Dorsolateral-plantaromedial.
6. (A) Calcaneus.
7. False.
8. False.

Chapter 19 • The Carpus

1. Five. These include the dorsopalmar, lateromedial, flexed lateromedial, dorsal–60-degree lateral-palmaromedial oblique and dorsal–60-degree medial-palmarolateral oblique. Dorsoproximal-dorsodistal oblique views are special views.

2. (A) Intracapsular soft-tissue swelling. (B) The radiographic findings seen in the five standard projections do not correlate with the clinical signs or joint capsule distention.

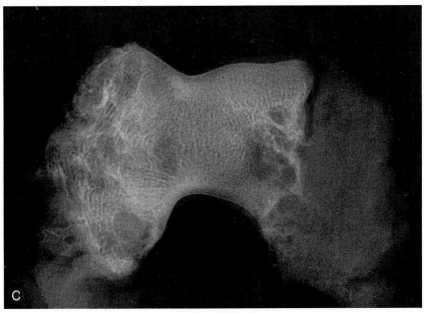

FIGURE 16–28. *C*

3. By the location of the intracapsular soft-tissue swelling (i.e., distention of the middle carpal joint indicates the need for a distal row examination, and distention of the antebrachiocarpal indicates a need for the distal radius).

4. Closer to the dorsopalmar projection. The angle being described is relative to the dorsal surface of the carpus.

5. Chip, corner, and slab fractures.

6. Radial carpal bone.

7. (A) Determine the origin of the deviation (i.e., growth plate of distal radius, abnormal carpal bone development, or joint capsule laxity). (B) Determine the extent of the bony changes. (C) Provide a basis to evaluate treatment success.

8. Treatment may correct growth imbalances associated with the carpus as the foal develops. A growth imbalance resulting in bone and joint changes at the metacarpophalangeal joint cannot be corrected if the physes have closed or have limited growth potential remaining. Radiographic closure of the physis of the distal radius is approximately 30 months, and for the distal third metacarpus and proximal aspect of the proximal phalanx, it is approximately 6 to 8 months.

9. A more complete radiographic examination consisting of 5 routine views and a dorsoproximal-dorsodistal oblique view are needed to determine (1) change in the slab fracture (i.e., displacement or comminution), (2) presence of additional fractures, (3) size and thickness of the slab using the dorsoproximal-dorsodistal view, (4) the degree to which the fracture reduces on the flexed lateromedial view, (5) evidence of secondary joint disease in the carpus.

10. The intermediate carpal bone is more proximal than the radial carpal bone. Therefore, the dorsoproximal intermediate and the dorsodistal radial carpal bones are seen without being overshadowed.

Chapter 20 • The Metacarpus and Metatarsus

1. False.
2. True.
3. False.
4. True.
5. True.
6. True.
7. Distal condyle (sagittal), dorsal-distal cortex (saucer), palmar/plantar proximal cortex.
8. Mach bands.
9. Nutrient foramen.
10. Suspensory ligament (branches).

Chapter 21 • The Metacarpophalangeal (Metatarsophalangeal) Articulation

1. (D) Should be made prior to making special projections or contrast studies of the joint.

2. (C) The result of repetitive or single event trauma.

3. There is flattening and excavation of subchondral bone at the palmar articular radius of the third metacarpus with sclerosis and compression of trabecular bone deep to the area of flattening. Findings are consistent with osteochondrosis. Additional radiographic examination should include dorsopalmar and oblique projections. Radiography of the contralateral limb is advised.

4. (B) May involve any of the bony components of the fetlock joint.

5. (A) Similar to villonodular synovitis except that it occurs at the plantar (palmar) surface of the bone.

6. There is extensive soft-tissue swelling around the joint; the axis of the metacarpophalangeal joint is straight, and the cartilage space of the entire joint is wide. There is lysis and destruction of subchondral bone of the distal third metacarpus and the epiphysis of the proximal phalanx. Linear opacities with sharp, distinct margins are present at the joint surfaces. Findings are an indication of advanced septic arthritis with multiple sequestra.

7. (C) Is a nonspecific term for progressive deterioration of all tissue components of the joint.

8. (C) Is often diagnosed in Standardbreds at the proximal palmar (plantar) margin of the proximal phalanx.

9. There is a smooth osseous fragment of bone along the plantar margin of the proximal phalanx, medial to the sagittal groove, and there has been remodeling and separation of bone of the medial plantar eminence. These findings are reported as fractures or osteochondrosis and given the respective classification of type I and type II fragments.

10. (B) Is often associated with changes in the suspensory ligament and tissues removed from the fetlock joint.

Chapter 22 • The Phalanges

1. The correct choice is (A), severe chronic degenerative joint disease. The high-load/low-motion character of the proximal interphalangeal joint makes it prone to degenerative joint disease, in which subchondral bone resorption is a common feature identified by radiography. Selection (B), osteochondrosis, is incorrect because although one form of equine osteochondrosis is typified by subchondral bone lucency in the distal end of the proximal phalanx, it is uncommon to have more than one subchondral defect. Joint space narrowing and osteophytes, however, can be a sequela of osteochondrosis. Selection (C) acute, active septic osteoarthritis, is incorrect because the initial radiographic appearance of this condition is most often unremarkable except for soft-tissue swelling associated with joint capsule distention. Untreated, septic arthritis progresses to the appearance of joint space widening owing to cartilage loss and subchondral bone lysis. As illustrated in Figure 22–24*E*, chronic low-grade septic osteoarthritis could appear as described for this patient.

2. A dorsopalmar view (using a horizontal beam) or a dorsal–45-degree proximal-palmarodistal oblique view would be the best. Calcification in the collateral cartilages would be easily seen and appear within the soft tissues medial and lateral to the distal interphalangeal joint. If the calcification was within the deep digital flexor tendon, it would be superimposed by the bone opacity of the middle and distal phalanges and would not be readily visible on the dorsopalmar view.

3. Common radiographic signs seen with chronic laminitis include

(A) Palmar rotation/deviation of the distal phalanx.
(B) Gas dissection between the laminae.

(C) Increased number of circular vascular channel lucencies in the midbody of the distal phalanx on the dorsal–65-degree proximal-palmarodistal oblique view.

(D) Fractures along the solar margin of the distal phalanx, especially at the toe region.

(E) Long hoof wall at the toe.

(F) Domed dorsal margin of the distal phalanx (lateral view).

4. The opacity of the periosteal reaction should be carefully compared to the opacity of the underlying cortex. If similar, the opacity (along with the smooth surface margin) would suggest that this reaction is considerably older than 10 days and is unlikely to be associated with the current cause of lameness. Another consideration is whether any soft-tissue attachments occur in the area of the periosteal reaction. If yes, the periosteal reaction may indicate a previous strain injury, with a recent reinjury to the tendon, ligament, or joint capsule superimposed on the older osseous response.

5. The linear radiolucency may be a fracture line, or it may be a vascular channel in the distal phalanx. The most useful additional radiographic projection would be a dorsal–65-degree proximal–45-degree lateral-palmarodistomedial oblique view. If the lucency is a fracture, the primary beam will pass straight through the fracture plane on the oblique view and enhance its visualization. If it is a fracture that extends into the distal interphalangeal joint, displacement of the subchondral bone margin will be visible on the oblique view. A hoof tester should also be used to determine if there is focal sensitivity to pressure in the suspect area.

6. The most important preparations involve removing any extraneous material from the patient's foot, including bandages, shoes, pads, and medications. The sulci of the frog should be thoroughly cleaned with a narrow-bladed hoof pick to ensure that no small bits of gravel remain in the deepest crevices of the frog. The sulci should then be packed with a material that has the same radiopacity as soft tissue.

7. Abnormal radiographic signs on the lateral view include moderate palmar rotation of the distal phalanx, gas dissection between the hoof wall and underlying lamina, and a faint bone opacity at the tip of the toe of the distal phalanx. The dorsal–65-degree proximal-palmarodistal oblique view exposed to show the entire distal phalanx shows no changes in the body and the distal interphalangeal joint. On the dorsal–65-degree proximal-palmarodistal oblique exposed to optimize evaluation of the toe, there is a fracture along the solar margin of the distal phalanx from the toe through the lateral quarter. Radiographic diagnosis was chronic laminitis with type VI distal phalanx fractures.

8. Three variable length radiolucent lines are seen within the middle phalanx on the lateral view; two enter the middle region of the proximal interphalangeal joint resulting in mild distraction at the joint surface. The longer line involves the distal interphalangeal joint at the palmar condylar surface just dorsal to the distal border of the navicular bone, without significant distraction. The fracture is not visible on the dorsopalmar view. A slight step effect is evident, however, in the lateral half of the proximal subchondral bone of the middle phalanx, which indicates the fracture location at this articulation. An additional finding is a fracture through the lateral aspect of the navicular bone seen as an oblique linear lucency through the lateral part of the bone on the dorsopalmar view. This fracture accounts for the unusual shape of the proximal margin of the navicular bone in the lateral view, as the lateral fragment is distracted proximally. Radiographic diagnosis was biarticular middle phalanx fracture with minimal distraction. Navicular bone fracture. *Comment:* Fracture visibility on any one view depends on the completeness of the fracture and the distracting forces on the fragments. When the fragments are minimally displaced, the fracture plane may be optimally visualized only on one view. In this horse, oblique views may have increased the visibility of the fracture plane. *Follow-up:* The distal limb was placed in a cast. Three months later, the middle phalanx fracture was radiographically healed. Osteoarthritis of the proximal interphalangeal joint (but not the distal interphalangeal joint) was evident radiographically. There was no osseous union of the navicular fracture. At that time, the horse was not lame when allowed free movement in the pasture.

9. The area of sole debridement is seen at the toe. A focal area of osteolysis in the toe of the distal phalanx, just medial to the midsagittal plane, is seen in all views. On the dorsal–65-degree proximal-palmarodistal oblique view, the osteolysis is seen as a larger defect in the bone, and a bone opacity is separated from the toe. The line drawing of the dorsal–65-degree proximal-palmarodistal oblique view (Fig. 22–37) can be correlated with the radiograph. Radiographic diagnosis was septic pedal osteitis with bone fragment consistent with sequestrum formation. Treatment was deeper curettage of the abscess and removal of the bone fragment. *Comments:* Debridement of the sole can create a defect that is not often amenable to successful packing with soft-tissue equivalent material, especially in the field. The artifacts created by the nonuniformity of the sole make interpretation of the toe region of the distal phalanx difficult on the dorsal–65-degree proximal-palmarodistal oblique view. When this situation is encountered, the dorsopalmar view using a horizontally directed beam direction should also be used.

10. Osseous abnormalities include malalignment of the proximal interphalangeal joint (flexural deformity) as seen on the lateral view and extensive periosteal proliferation around the distal third of the proximal phalanx. The density of the bony proliferation indicates that the peri-

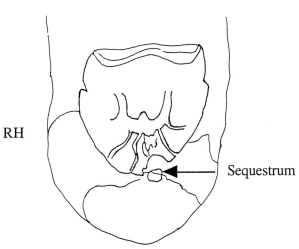

FIGURE 22–37

osteal stimulus is chronic, whereas the irregular surface margin suggests an active process. Soft-tissue thickening is also identifiable, especially along the lateral and medial sides of the proximal interphalangeal joint. Radiographic diagnosis was chronic flexural deformity of the proximal interphalangeal joint with severe secondary osteoarthritis. *Comments:* The flexural deformity could not be reduced by manipulation of the joint or by having the foal place full weight on the leg. Surgical arthrodesis was recommended because of the extent of the deformity and progression of secondary joint disease.

Chapter 23 • The Navicular Bone

1. (C) Proximal border and extremities.
2. (B) 65-degree dorsoproximal-palmarodistal.
3. (D) Cortical erosion of the flexor surface.
4. (A) Most prominent in the distal border.
   (C) Increased size but triangular shape suggests age/work changes.
   (D) Lollipop shape is abnormal.
5. True.
6. (E) All of the above.
7. False.
8. (1) Constant fragment motion. (2) Poor osteoprogenitor cell availability. (3) Influx of synovial fluid hampers healing.
9. (A) Within 3 to 12 weeks.
10. (B) Progressive navicular bursitis.
    (C) Degenerative arthrosis.
    (E) Ischemic necrosis.

SECTION VI • NECK AND THORAX—COMPANION ANIMALS

Chapter 24 • The Larynx, Pharynx, and Trachea

1. (D) All of the above.
2. False.
3. False.
4. True.
5. True.
6. False.
7. False.
8. True.
9. True.
10. True.

Chapter 25 • The Esophagus

1. (C) Foreign body and dystrophic mineralization.
2. False.
3. (D) All of the above.
4. Radiographic findings:

   Zone of reduced radiopacity dorsal to and superimposed on the cervical trachea.

Distinct hypaxial soft-tissue interface in cranial thorax.

Ventral displacement of trachea.

Paired soft-tissue stripes in caudal thorax between aorta and caudal vena cava on lateral view and on either side of spine converging at the hiatus of the diaphragm on the dorsoventral view.

Gas-distended stomach.

Reduced airway through larynx with change in shape of hyoid apparatus.

Radiographic conclusions:

Megaesophagus.

Gastric dilation.

Soft-tissue swelling of larynx.

Cause: Acute laryngeal edema with secondary aerophagia causing megaesophagus and gastric distention. A generalized neuropathy or toxicity could also result in these findings, but weakness or other signs of toxicosis were not reported.

5. (C) Rightward and ventral displacement of the intrathoracic trachea.
6. (E) All of the above.
7. (B) Barium sulfate paste.
8. (D) Aorta and azygous vein.
9. (A) Periesophageal hiatal hernia. (B) Esophageal diverticulum.
10. They provide selection of a suitable radiographic technique, and they allow assessment of the esophagus, surrounding tissue, and lung to determine coexisting disease and rule in or out the need for contrast examination.

Chapter 26 • The Thoracic Wall

1. (A) Lower the kVp and compensatorily raise the mAs. Presuming satisfactory radiographic visualization of thoracic visceral structures (because they are usually well contrasted by pulmonary air) using relatively high kVp and relatively low mAs on initial radiographs (to attempt to reduce the stark contrast between fluid opacity structures and ribs), lowering kVp and raising mAs will produce better distinction among the components of the chest wall (ribs, intercostal muscles, subcutaneous muscles, subcutaneous fat, and intrafascial fat).

2. Fistulography of the thoracic wall

   Indications:
   A. Chronic draining tract involving the thoracic wall (or any other site) that has failed to respond to therapy.
   B. Draining lesion of the thoracic wall (or any other site) that has recurred after having been treated either medically or surgically.

   Contraindications:
   A. Regional infection, especially if not confined.
   B. Suspected communication with a body cavity.
   C. Multiple interconnected tracts through the skin.
   D. Large tract that cannot be sealed well enough to be back-filled with contrast material.

   Patient preparation:
   A. General anesthesia.
   B. Clip, clean, and surgical scrub of the area of the lesion.

   Supplies:
   A. Sterile syringes.
   B. Organic iodide contrast material.

C. Pediatric Foley catheter.
D. Catheter adapters.

Procedure:
A. Load the syringe and Foley catheter (or catheter adapter) with contrast material diluted to 5 to 10 percent (w/v).
B. Cannulate the tract with the Foley catheter, and inflate the cuff to seat the catheter against the inside of the tract *or* wedge a catheter adapter into the skin lesion.
C. Fill the tract with diluted contrast material, taking care to prevent significant leakage onto the skin.
D. Radiograph the lesion in conventional projections and with supplemental tangential and oblique views.

Complications:
A. Loss of contrast material around the catheter or catheter adapter.
B. Obliteration of small or faintly radiopaque filling defects by insufficiently diluted contrast material.
C. Spread of infection into adjacent body cavities.

Potential radiographic signs:
A. Communication of contrast material with underlying body cavities, underlying skeletal structures, or distant subcutaneous tracts.
B. Demonstration of filling defects (sequestered soft tissue, foreign bodies).

3. Wet hair, dirty hair (cutaneous debris).

4. Subcutaneous lipoma differs from other focal lucency in that the former is generally better circumscribed and usually slightly more opaque than cutaneous gas from lacerations or puncture wounds.

Subcutaneous lipoma differs from a benign subcutaneous neoplasm in that the former is less opaque than the latter, even though both are usually fairly well circumscribed.

Subcutaneous lipoma differs from a subcutaneous injection in that the latter is a focal (but poorly circumscribed) fluid opacity with small gas bubbles, whereas the former is well circumscribed and has opacity that is midway between gas and fluid.

Subcutaneous lipoma differs from obesity in that the former is focal and usually well circumscribed, whereas the latter is widespread. Opacity of both is the same or similar (but is thickness dependent).

Subcutaneous lipoma differs from hypodermoclysis fluid in that the latter is diffuse and is a fluid opacity; the former is neither.

Subcutaneous lipoma differs from a subcutaneous or intrafascial abscess in that the latter is a fluid opacity and may have associated gas pockets, whereas the former is a fat opacity. Either is usually well circumscribed and focal.

Subcutaneous lipoma differs from subcutaneous emphysema in that the latter is a gas lucency and is often diffuse, whereas the former is a fat opacity and is usually localized and well circumscribed.

5. (A, C, F) Intercostal masses and expansile rib lesions may enlarge to the point that cranially and caudally adjacent ribs are displaced. Fractured ribs may be displaced but usually do not cause adjacent ribs to change position. Laceration or tearing of intercostal muscles allows adjacent ribs to separate to varying degrees depending on various factors, including fractures of nearby ribs and intrathoracic trauma (see Figs. 26–4 and 26–9).

6. (A, B, C, D) Each may produce the *extrapleural sign* by displacement of the parietal pleura medially. Soft-tissue swelling (hemorrhage, edema) associated with fractured ribs is less dramatic and usually must be radiographed tangentially to be appreciated.

7. False. Stippled mineralization of costal cartilages is a normal aging change, is quite often seen, and usually proceeds from caudal to cranial as the animal matures.

8. Pectus excavatum and peritoneopericardial diaphragmatic hernia may be seen concomitantly, with or without reduction in the normal number (eight) of sternebrae, because formation of the caudal sternum, the diaphragmaticopericardial ligament, the ventral diaphragm, the pericardial sac, the pleural cavity, and the peritoneal cavity are all developing simultaneously in the fetus.

9. Image interpretation: Left lateral thoracic radiograph of a dog with draining soft-tissue swelling at the ventral aspect of the midportion of the sternum. The major radiographic signs include sclerosis (increased radiopacity), periosteal reaction, and end plate lysis involving the fourth and fifth sternebrae. There is also a mild associated extrapleural sign dorsal to the affected sternebrae. The final diagnosis was osteomyelitis of the sternum.

Chapter 27 • The Diaphragm

1. (A) The position of the x-ray tube (i.e., over the thorax or abdomen). (B) Position of the animal (i.e., ventral or dorsal recumbency).

2. The diaphragmatic crus closest to the table is displaced cranially.

3. Any substance of soft-tissue opacity adjacent to the thoracic surface of the diaphragm obliterates the outline.

4. (A) Cranial displacement of abdominal organs, particularly the liver, stomach, and spleen. (B) Cranial or lateral displacement of thoracic structures by a soft-tissue structure or structures.

5. The dorsal peritoneopericardial mesothelial remnant.

6. (A) Cranial displacement of the gastric cardia. (B) A soft-tissue mass in the thorax adjacent to the diaphragm in the area of the caudal esophagus.

7. A scalloped ventral diaphragmatic margin noted on the lateral thoracic radiograph.

8. Radiographic signs lateral view:
A. The cranial diaphragmatic border is not visible.
B. The caudal cardiac border is not visible.
C. Focal gas opacities in the caudal ventral thorax, suspect small bowel loops.

Radiographic signs ventrodorsal view:
A. The mediastinum *(solid arrow)* and heart are displaced to the left of midline.
B. There is a soft-tissue opacity in the caudal right thorax.
C. Focal gas opacities in the caudal right thorax, suspect small bowel loops *(open arrows)*.

Specific or differential diagnosis:
A. Traumatic diaphragmatic hernia with abdominal organs in the caudal right thorax.
B. Loculated pleural fluid or soft-tissue mass in the caudal right thorax.
C. Possible lung mass in the caudal right lung lobe.

9. 1. Right and left lateral decubitus views to see if the diaphragmatic border can be visualized.
2. Filling the stomach and small bowel with contrast material (barium upper gastrointestinal study).

3. Positive-contrast peritoneography.

4. Ultrasound.

10. 1. On the right lateral decubitus view, left side up (see Fig. 27–22A), the thoracic border of the diaphragm is visualized (arrows), and air-filled lung is in the caudal left thorax.

2. On the left lateral decubitus view, right side up (see Fig. 27–22B), the thoracic border of the diaphragm is not visualized, and there are soft-tissue and gas opacities in the caudal right thorax.

3. On the ventrodorsal view made after contrast material administration (see Fig. 27–23), the pyloric antrum and small bowel filled with barium are visualized in the right caudal thorax.

Chapter 28 • The Mediastinum

1. (A) The mediastinum is not a closed space. It communicates with fascial planes of the neck and the retroperitoneal space.

2. The cranioventral and caudoventral mediastinal reflections are commonly visualized.

3. Because the mediastinum is essentially a midline structure, it is much easier to assess it in ventrodorsal or dorsoventral views. In lateral radiographs, the mediastinum is viewed en face, and it is not possible to tell if a mass is within or superimposed on the mediastinum.

4. The following radiographic signs indicate that the opacity seen cranial to the heart is in the mediastinum.
   A. Compression of the trachea on the lateral view.
   B. Mass is on the midline on the ventrodorsal view.
   C. The trachea is displaced to the left on the ventrodorsal view.

5. Pneumomediastinum. There is visualization of the adventitial surface of the trachea and esophagus and cranial mediastinal vessels. These signs are consistent with pneumomediastinum.

6. Peritoneal lymphatics drain into the sternal lymph node. In this dog, barium might have become trapped in the sternal lymph node, thereby increasing its radiographic opacity.

7. A horizontal-beam ventrodorsal thoracic radiograph or mediastinal sonography.

8. An intrapulmonary laceration with retrograde dissection of air along peribronchial and perivascular spaces into the mediastinum.

9. False. Pneumothorax does not progress to pneumomediastinum, but the opposite is true.

10. True. There may be elevation, depression, or no change in the position of the tracheal bifurcation in dogs with tracheobronchial lymphadenopathy.

Chapter 29 • The Pleural Space

1. (A) The x-ray beam must strike the fluid-containing fissure tangentially.

2. False. In ventrodorsal radiographs, the fluid has more opportunity to enter an interlobar fissure and be struck tangentially by the x-ray beam. In dorsoventral radiographs, the fluid collects just dorsal to the sternum.

3. False. A straight fluid line will only be seen when a horizontal-beam x-ray beam is used and there is a free gas–free fluid interface.

4. (A) Retraction of lung margins from the thoracic wall with soft-tissue opacity between lung and thoracic wall.
   (B) Visualization of interlobar fissures of a soft-tissue opacity.
   (C) Silhouetting of the diaphragm by an intrathoracic soft-tissue opacity.

5. The dog was in dorsal recumbency. If the dog had been in sternal recumbency, the heart would not be visible because of the effusion collected around it.

6. (C) The finding of simultaneous peritoneal and pleural effusion is typically associated with a poor prognosis.

7. True. Visualization of interlobar fissures is more common with pleural effusion. With pneumothorax, the pulmonary collapse prevents gas from entering the pleural space.

8. Three radiographic signs of a tension pneumothorax are
   A. A contralateral mediastinal shift.
   B. Caudal displacement of the diaphragm, possibly with visualization of the costal attachments of the diaphragm.
   C. Complete collapse of the lung against the hilum.

9. Two things that can be confused with pneumothorax are
   A. A skin fold.
   B. The thoracic wall conformation of chondrodystrophoid breeds.

10. The concave aspect of costal is cranial, whereas the concave aspect of interlobar fissures is caudal.

Chapter 30 • The Heart and Great Vessels

1. The range of normal patient sizes is large, various breeds have markedly different thoracic anatomic conformations, and it is difficult (if not impossible) to correlate routinely precise patient positioning, maximum thoracic inflation, and cardiac cycle with radiographic exposure.

2. Dorsal displacement of the left main stem bronchus in the lateral projection (A) and divergence of the left and right main stem bronchi in the ventrodorsal or dorsoventral projection (C) are reliable radiographic signs of left atrial enlargement, provided that the patient was positioned without obliquity. Further, loss of the left atrioventricular "waist" is often seen radiographically with left atrial enlargement in the lateral projection.

3. Decrease in the tracheovertebral angle in the lateral projection is not a reliable indication of left atrial enlargement when there is a large volume of free pleural fluid.

4. With right ventricular dilation, there is increased cardiosternal contact, whereas right ventricular hypertrophy (in the lateral projection) may cause elevation of the apex of the cardiac silhouette without effecting increased contact between the heart and the sternum.

5. Dorsal deviation of the left main stem bronchus (B), alveolar pulmonary infiltrate (E), and elevation of the trachea (G) are commonly seen in left-sided heart failure. However, (B) and (G), without (E), are also commonly seen in dogs with compensated left heart enlargement (i.e., no left-sided heart failure), whereas alveolar pulmonary infiltrate caused by cardiogenic pulmonary edema is a reliable sign of left-sided heart failure.

6. Increased cardiosternal contact (A), hepatomegaly (C),

ascites (D), and free pleural fluid (H) are often seen in right-sided congestive heart failure.

7. Survey radiographic signs associated with PDA include

Segmental enlargement of the distal aortic arch (distinct bulge along the left cranial portion of the heart), *pulmonary knob sign* owing to enlargement of the main pulmonary artery segment (pulmonary trunk), left atrial enlargement with at least "loss of the caudal waist," elongation of the left ventricle, and enhancement of the pulmonary vascular pattern owing to overcirculation.

Survey radiographic signs associated with aortic stenosis include

Widening of the caudal aspect of the cranial mediastinum (owing to poststenotic dilation of the aortic arch) and elongation of the left ventricle in the dorsoventral view and distortion of the junction between the heart and cranial vena cava in the lateral view ("loss of the cranial waist") owing to poststenotic dilation of the ascending aorta and aortic arch.

Survey radiographic signs associated with pulmonic stenosis include

Dilation of the main pulmonary artery (pulmonary knob), right ventricular enlargement, and possible hypovascular pulmonary parenchyma.

8. Survey radiographic signs associated with heartworm disease include

Dilation of the main pulmonary artery (pulmonary knob), right ventricular enlargement, dilation of the right and left pulmonary arteries with truncation ("pruning") and possible arterial tortuosity, and possible signs of right-sided heart failure (ascites, hydrothorax).

Survey radiographic signs associated with mitral insufficiency include

Elevation of the left main stem bronchus and loss of the caudal "waist" (enlarged left atrium), decrease in the tracheovertebral angle (enlarged left ventricle), possible caudodorsal unstructured interstitial or alveolar pulmonary infiltrate (pulmonary edema), and possible dilation of the pulmonary veins.

9. Radiographic interpretation (Fig. 30–24): The major radiographic sign is globoid enlargement of the cardiac silhouette. Necropsy revealed the presence of a large amount of hemorrhagic fluid in the pericardial sac because of a mass involving the wall of the right atrium (histopathologic diagnosis was hemangiosarcoma).

10. Radiographic interpretation (Fig. 30–25): The major radiographic sign is generalized cardiomegaly. Sonographically, there was poor cardiac contractility and severely dilated cardiac ventricles consistent with dilatory cardiomyopathy.

Chapter 31 • The Pulmonary Vasculature

1. (A) On the left lateral recumbent thoracic view, there is right cranial lobar pulmonary arterial enlargement because the artery is larger than its counterpart vein. On the dorsoventral view, both caudal lobar pulmonary arteries are larger than the ninth rib at their intersection. The right caudal lobar pulmonary artery is more enlarged than the left. There is also main pulmonary artery enlargement and right heart enlargement. The diagnosis is heartworm disease.

2. (B) Mitral insufficiency was documented on two-dimen-

sional echocardiography, and a mitral murmur was heard on auscultation.

3. (C) Both caudal pulmonary arteries and veins where they intersect with the ninth rib are larger in diameter than the rib width. A ventricular septal defect was apparent when the heart was examined with two-dimensional echocardiography. The pulmonary arteries and veins are enlarged because of volume overload associated with the left-to-right shunt.

4. (C) Heartworm disease.

5. (B) Severe blood loss (hypovolemia).

6. (A) On the lateral thoracic view, the large left pulmonary artery is dorsal to the trachea.

7. (A) Pulmonary arteries are lateral to pulmonary veins.

8. (B) Dorsoventral view.

9. (A) Left lateral recumbency.

10. (C) Mitral insufficiency.

Chapter 32 • The Canine Lung

1. (A) False. (B) False. (C) False. Localized pulmonary lesions, including nodules, are normally most visible radiographically when the patient is radiographed with the affected side uppermost (i.e., when the lesion is in the nondependent lung). If the patient is large, some magnification of lesions in the nondependent lung may be apparent owing to geometric distortion.

2. Obesity (reduces radiographic contrast by increasing scattered radiation; tends to reduce visibility of intrathoracic structures, such as the cranial lung lobes; necessitates higher radiographic exposures, which may lead to underexposure or excessively long exposure times).

Brachycephalic conformation (often associated with obesity; poor conformation of the upper airway in many brachycephalic dogs may contribute to underinflation of the lung).

Prolonged recumbency (may result in collapse of the dependent lung, which can obscure lesions).

Movement (owing to rapid breathing, panting, coughing, or voluntary patient movement may result in motion blur, which obliterates fine detail on radiographs; hence small lesions may become invisible).

3. There is a rounded soft-tissue mass (or large nodule) in the right lung, probably in the caudal lobe; the borders of the mass are distinct, indicating a sharp demarcation between the lesion and adjacent aerated lung; the mass is located in the periphery of the lobe, but no lesions are apparent in the adjacent ribs.

Differential diagnoses for a solitary pulmonary mass should include

Primary lung neoplasm.

Pulmonary metastasis.

Granuloma.

Fluid-filled bulla.

Hematoma.

Abscess.

Cyst (see Table 32–2).

The right caudal lobe was removed surgically. The histologic diagnosis was bronchoalveolar carcinoma.

4. Opacity of the lung is greater at peak expiration than

inspiration because air (the lucent component) is expelled. An expiratory thoracic radiograph may be useful when a small-volume pneumothorax is suspected because this maximizes contrast between the lung and air-filled pleural space.

5. Pulmonary vessels seen end-on

   Are smaller than the nearest side-on vessel.

   Are smaller in the periphery of the lung.

   Are less numerous in the periphery of the lung.

   Pulmonary nodules

   May be larger than adjacent vessels.

   May be large in the periphery of the lung.

   Can occur anywhere in the lung.

6. If the appearance of the lesion changes markedly within 24 hours, it is more likely to be the result of fluid in the lung (e.g., edema, hemorrhage) than of cellular infiltrates.

   An increase (or decrease) in size indicates that the disease is progressing (or resolving) rapidly.

7. True. Aspiration bronchopneumonia frequently affects the ventral parts of the lung (see Fig. 32–27); lesions in the ventral part of the lung are often most visible on a ventrodorsal radiograph because of the combined effects of optimal aeration of the nondependent lung and geometric distortion (see Fig. 32–3).

8. The pulmonary pattern is mixed: The left cranial lobe is uniformly opacified compatible with an alveolar pattern; the left caudal lobe has a diffuse interstitial infiltrate that obscures the vessels and cardiac border; nodules are visible in the left lateral radiograph, presumably in the *right* cranial lobe. Note that the consolidated left cranial lobe is not visible on the left lateral radiograph.

   The other relevant radiographic sign is mediastinal shift to the right; this indicates that the left-sided lesion is expansile.

   This dog died. The pathologic diagnosis was primary carcinoma in the left cranial lobe with intrapulmonary metastasis.

9. (A) 4. (B) 3. (C) 2. (D) 1.

10. Differential diagnoses for pulmonary calcification include

    Bronchial calcification.

    Heterotopic bone.

    Calcified mass (e.g., granuloma, primary neoplasm, metastasis).

    Diffuse interstitial calcification (e.g., associated with hyperadrenocorticism, hyperparathyroidism, chronic uremia).

    Idiopathic (see Table 32–6).

SECTION VII • NECK AND THORAX—EQUIDAE

Chapter 33 • Larynx, Pharynx, and Proximal Airway

1. During extension, the pharynx is drawn rostrally causing it to appear dorsally compressed, as if by an overlying mass.

   During flexion, the pharynx becomes foreshortened, resembling encroachment by a rostrally located mass.

Dark pharyngeal radiographs are characterized by decreased image contrast, often concealing abnormal tissue margins and low-opacity lesions.

2. By employing *laryngography,* contrast medium is administered orally, the horse allowed to swallow, and images of the pharynx and proximal airway are made. If contrast medium is present in the larynx or trachea, the epiglottis is functionally—and often anatomically—abnormal. The absence of upper airway opacification, however, does not exclude the possibility of laryngeal dysfunction because the epiglottis may be abnormal but still prevent opaques from entering the larynx.

3. (G) Pharyngitis produces no radiographically visible alterations in the pharynx and thus is typically associated with a *normal* radiograph.

4. Epiglottitis is typically an acute inflammation of the epiglottis, often infectious, which may cause proximal airway obstruction, especially in foals.

   Radiographic recognition of epiglottitis is entirely dependent on the amount of resultant epiglottic enlargement. Accordingly, severe inflammation is most apt to be detected radiographically, whereas mild inflammation is likely to go unobserved.

5. The most common cause of laryngeal calcification is age-related metaplasia, which does not affect laryngeal function. Dystrophic calcification typically occurs following tissue injury, and is more likely to be relevant.

6. Superimposition. Lateral imaging of the guttural pouches results in additive subject opacities. This means that an air-distended pouch makes the adjacent normal pouch appear darker, whereas a partially fluid-filled pouch makes the nearby normal pouch appear lighter. Thus, there is often uncertainty as to which pouch is diseased unless there is external swelling.

Chapter 34 • The Pleural Space

1. (A) Is composed of two potential spaces, each lined by visceral, parietal, diaphragmatic, and costal pleura, separated by the mediastinum.

2. (C) May require three or four projections in both left and right lateral, horizontal-beam configurations.

3. The descending aorta can be seen with improved detail, the dorsal margin of one lung border is retracted ventrally, and a lung margin is displaced from the diaphragm. Free air is present in the left pleural space, but no cause is apparent. Trauma resulting in spontaneous pneumothorax was suspected.

4. (D) May require a fluid or air volume in excess of 2 L for detection by radiography of the thorax.

5. (D) Clear definition of the dorsal lung margins and aorta.

6. A fluid line (fluid-air interface) is superimposed over the trachea, and there is loss of detail of heart and vessels ventral to the fluid line. The cranial dorsal margin of the aorta has improved detail owing to free air in the cranial dorsal pleural space. Pleural effusion and pneumothorax are present.

7. (B) Results in progressive obscuration of the margins of the heart, diaphragm, and vena cava on radiographic images.

8. (A) When the disease is in the mediastinum or deep to lung tissue.

9. The diaphragm is concave and displaced caudally by lung with increased air volume and detail. Caudal to the heart, there is a thick tissue opacity extending to the diaphragm and outlining the irregular margin of an air-filled compartment. These findings are the result of cavitary disease suspected to be contained in the pleural space owing to the absence of obvious pulmonary disease. Findings and assessment were documented using ultrasound and pleuroscopy.

10. (C) By radiography of the thorax.

Chapter 35 • The Equine Lung

1. Pleuropneumonia is a combined infection of the lungs and pleura. It is generally believed that pleuropneumonia begins in the lungs and subsequently extends to the pleura.

   Pleuropneumonia is obviously worse than pneumonia because of its pleural component. Pleurisy (infection of the pleura) directly affects the lungs' ability to expand and indirectly impedes inflation through fluid buildup in the pleural space.

   Where large volumes of pleural fluid are present, radiographic evaluation of the lung may not be possible. In such instances—and assuming there is consolidation of portions of the lung surface—sonography can be used to confirm lung involvement, although it is not always possible to differentiate consolidation from atelectasis.

2. The visible blood vessels of the lung are useful indicators of both the general and regional circulation. For example, if the lung vessels are small and few in number, and the heart is also small, the cause may be a smaller than normal blood volume (e.g., shock). If the vessels are large and more numerous than normal and accompanied by cardiomegaly, the blood volume may be increased (e.g., heart failure).

   Pneumonia often results in a regional pulmonary hyperemia.

   Emphysema is usually associated with a generalized pulmonary oligemia.

   The absence of major arteries, implying thrombosis, is extremely difficult to determine using only lateral radiographs.

   The assessment of vessel size and number is best done subjectively using two or more normal comparison films of comparably sized individuals. The measurement of individual blood vessels is unreliable.

3. Lung abscess.

4. The large size of the subject and the inability to obtain a ventrodorsal projection of the thorax.

5. True.

6. Because of the inability to obtain ventrodorsal or dorsoventral projections of the thorax.

7. Dorsocaudal lung field.

8. Ventral lung field.

9. By obtaining radiographs with the left and right side of the thorax adjacent to the cassette and determining in which radiograph the lesion margins are most distinct.

SECTION VIII • ABDOMEN—COMPANION ANIMALS

Chapter 36 • Abdominal Masses

1. Structures that are nearly always seen in abdominal radiographs include the stomach, the liver, the urinary bladder, the small bowel, and the colon.

   Structures that are often only partially seen are the spleen, the kidneys (especially the right kidney in dogs), and the prostate gland.

   Structures that are seldom seen unless they are abnormal include the pancreas, the adrenal glands, the ovaries, and the mesenteric lymph nodes.

2. The head of the spleen is attached to the stomach by the gastrosplenic ligament. The rest of the spleen is free to move around in the abdomen, between the body wall and the rest of the viscera. Therefore, the spleen is better seen (radiographically) with the patient in right lateral recumbency because this position allows the body and tail of the spleen to swing across the ventral midline, where it is seen caudoventral to the body of the stomach and cranioventral to the urinary bladder. With the patient in left lateral recumbency, the spleen slips between the bowel and the dependent body wall, where it seems disappear because none of its edges are presented tangent to the x-ray beam.

3. (B) Positional radiography. This should be considered before any of the other choices because it is both cheaper and quicker and because it may provide displacement information that is significant in differential diagnosis.

4. An upper gastrointestinal series (C), pneumoperitoneography (D), and celiography (E) all may provide significant information in differential diagnostic assessment of a right cranioventral abdominal mass. Neither excretory urography nor cystography is helpful in assessment of such a lesion.

5. The stomach, the urinary bladder, and the uterus all undergo considerable normal variation in size.

6. (A) Right lateral lobe of the liver. None of the other choices should be expected to create the described displacement of adjacent structures. Pancreatic masses should displace the descending duodenum *laterally* and should pull it ventrally. Masses of the right kidney should displace the descending duodenum ventrally. Colic lymphadenopathy should pull the transverse and ascending portions of the colon ventrally. Masses in the root of the mesentery should displace the small bowel peripherally.

7. (D) All of the above. Masses originating from the left kidney, the left 13th rib, and the left sublumbar muscles all should be expected to produce the described visceral displacements. Make sure to try to find the kidney; if you cannot, a left kidney mass is the most likely choice for the described displacement.

8. (Fig. 36–24) The radiographic signs include mild ventral displacement of the descending duodenum and caudal and left displacement of the jejunum. Histopathologic diagnosis was severe suppurative subacute pancreatic necrosis, obstructing the common bile duct. Bowel displacement in this case is typical of pancreatic masses.

9. (Fig. 36–25) The radiographic signs include poor serosal detail and the suggestion of mass effects in the caudal and lateral aspects of the abdomen. Surgical exploration revealed torsion and hemorrhagic distention of both

horns of the uterus. The patient made a complete recovery after ovariohysterectomy.

10. (Fig. 36–26) The radiographic signs include multiple small soft-tissue metallic opacities (shotgun pellets—probably an incidental finding of no current clinical significance) and a large dorsal left fluid opacity mass displacing the descending colon and small intestine ventrally and medially. Histopathologic diagnosis was renal carcinoma.

Chapter 37 • The Peritoneal Space

1. Abdominal effusion. There is increased fluid opacity within the abdomen causing severe loss of serosal surface visualization. Also, the abdomen is pendulous. The final diagnosis was hepatic atrophy, portal fibrosis, and intrahepatic and extrahepatic portocaval shunts. The peritoneal fluid was caused by portal hypertension.

2. Sublumbar lymphadenopathy and small liver. There is a soft-tissue mass in the retroperitoneal space ventral to the caudal lumbar vertebra and dorsal to the colon, which is displaced ventrally. The stomach and small intestine are located more cranially than usual indicating decreased liver size. Final diagnosis was lymphosarcoma. The cause of the small liver was not determined, but the primary rule-out was fibrosis.

3. (B) Lateral view, patient in dorsal recumbency.

4. (C) Abdominal mass.

5. Blood, urine, inflammation (abscessation).

6. (A) Mediastinum.
   (B) Pelvic canal.

7. (A) Adrenal glands.
   (B) Sublumbar lymph nodes.

8. There is loss of serosal surface visualization in the midventral abdomen. Gas is seen in the craniodorsal abdomen outlining the liver lobes (Fig. 37–25C). Free gas is also seen as thin radiolucent lines between the stomach, liver, and diaphragm on both views. Radiographic diagnosis was free peritoneal gas and focal peritoneal fluid/peritonitis compatible with intestinal rupture.

A horizontal-beam radiograph (see Fig. 37–12A) was made to confirm the presence of free gas. At surgery, a string foreign body extending from the duodenum to the cecum was found. It had eroded through the mesenteric surface at multiple sites.

9. This is usually an incidental finding with no clinical significance.

10. Less sensitive.

Chapter 38 • The Liver and Spleen

1. True.

2. (B) The liver margin extends well beyond the costal arch, and there is dramatic elevation of the pyloric region of the stomach. The caudal liver edge is rounded. Masses are not seen.

3. (D) With extrahepatic shunts, more common in small breeds, there are reduced levels of hepatic growth factors delivered to the liver resulting in microhepatica.

4. False. Only mineralization causes an increase in radiopacity of the liver.

5. (A) Operative portography does not require sophisticated imaging equipment and can be performed in most small animal practices.

6. (B) The stomach is caudally displaced and appears to wrap around a round mass cranial to it, a liver mass.

7. True.

8. False. The opposite circumstance is correct.

9. (D) A large midabdominal mass is caudal to the stomach. A splenic mass is the most common cause of a midventral abdominal mass.

10. False. The precise cause of a mass in the spleen cannot be determined from a radiograph. The mass could be a hematoma.

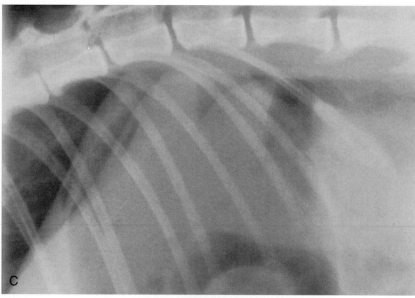

FIGURE 37–25. C

Chapter 39 • The Kidneys and Ureters

1. (B) Intravenous urography.
2. (E) Is there adequate urine production, and is the patient adequately hydrated?
3. (E) All of the above.
4. (E) Retroperitoneal fluid, lack of retroperitoneal fat, and infiltrative retroperitoneal mass.
5. (E) Multifocal metastatic cancer and polycystic renal disease.
6. (D) Ureteral obstruction.
7. (B) Hydronephrosis.
8. (D) Acute extrarenal obstruction.
9. (E) Hydronephrosis, infiltrative renal disease, and compensatory hypertrophy.
10. (E) Ectopic ureter, urinary bladder mass causing obstruction of one ureter at the trigone and ascending pyelonephritis.

Chapter 40 • The Urinary Bladder

1. No. There is no clinical correlation with abnormal clinical signs when the urinary bladder of a dog is located partially within the pelvic canal.
2. (A) Displacement of the bladder caudally or ventrally from the normal location.

   (B) No urine within the bladder; postvoiding.
3. The lucent area is gas within the urinary bladder. It is in the center of the bladder because with a lateral recumbent position the highest part of the bladder is the center on the up side. Calculi are either more opaque or the same opacity as urine; therefore, this could not represent a calculus.
4. Positive-contrast cystogram.
5. Complete distention of the bladder may obliterate mucosal and bladder wall lesions.
6. (A) Small air bubbles that may be mistaken for calculi.

   (B) A large air bubble that may be mistaken for bladder wall thickening.

   (C) Multiple adjacent bubbles producing a honeycomb pattern.
7. A pseudofilling defect has a smooth mucosal surface, and the borders of the filling defect taper gradually.
8. No.
9. (A) The filling defect in the dorsal bladder is an attached filling defect extending into the lumen from the dorsal bladder wall. The filling defect has a sharply angled border with the bladder wall on the cranial and caudal margins *(arrows)* indicating an intramural origin.

   (B) The most likely diagnosis would be neoplasia, and a transitional cell carcinoma would be the common type of neoplasia with these radiographic signs. A hematoma within the bladder wall can also produce such radiographic changes but is an uncommon lesion.
10. (A) The contrast pattern is an extravasation pattern. Contrast medium is leaking into the peritoneal cavity (arrows) from the urinary bladder (B).

    (B) This indicates the bladder is ruptured or perforated.

Chapter 41 • The Urethra

1. True.
2. False. See Figure 41–8. No urethrogram is necessary in this patient.
3. The radiographic diagnosis is multiple, variably sized, radiopaque urethral calculi and a greatly distended bladder that is likely due to urethral obstruction. Calculi are also present in the bladder, and the prostate gland is enlarged.
4. (D) Barium and oil-based contrast media should not be used for urethrography. Room air and carbon dioxide are negative contrast agents.
5. True. Distention of the prostatic urethra is especially improved if the bladder is fully distended when the urethrogram is performed.
6. There are pelvic fractures and extravasation of contrast medium into the soft tissues of the pelvic canal indicating urethral rupture, most likely traumatic in origin.
7. False. Prostatic hyperplasia would cause extramural compression of the urethra, not an intraluminal filling defect.
8. Neoplasia, inflammatory diseases, or scar tissue from prior urethral surgery.
9. There is an intraluminal filling defect just proximal to the os penis that represents a urethral calculus. Small filling defects at the level of the ischium could be additional calculi or air bubbles.
10. True. See Figure 41–9.

Chapter 42 • The Prostate Gland

1. Generally the prostate enlarges slowly throughout life in the male dog.
2. Displacement with paraprostatic cysts is quite variable, and no set rules can be established. Generally the displacement is cranial, but there is tremendous variation in individual patients.
3. Loss of a distinct margin of the prostate in patients with acute prostatitis is due to a low-grade regional peritonitis secondary to the inflammation in the prostate. It is usually not septic but may be so in some patients.
4. Asymmetric placement of the urethra within the prostate is a sign of a mass lesion, such as a cyst, abscess, or tumor. It is not seen with benign prostatic hypertrophy. Conversely a centrally placed prostate is unusual with prostatic mass lesions.
5. This cystic structure is thick walled and has an indistinct margin, especially at the caudal end. These are typical findings with abscesses and cystic neoplasms.
6. There is asymmetric impingement of the prostate on the neck of the urinary bladder. As with the urethra, asymmetry in impingement on the neck of the bladder is a sign of a mass lesion.
7. Spondylosis deformans is composed of compact bone, and the ventral margin of it is generally quite smooth. It also arises from the end plate of the vertebrae and subsequently involves the body of the vertebrae. This reaction is not arising directly from the end plate but rather from the adjacent body.
8. This is a normal finding.
9. A stricture of the prostatic urethra is a poor prognostic

sign. Because of the central placement of the urethra in the prostate, it is generally not constricted in benign disease. A stricture may result from scarring but is difficult to treat in many cases. Typically, it is a finding associated with neoplasia.

Chapter 43 • The Uterus, Ovaries, and Testes

1. (E) Is difficult or impossible to detect on routine survey radiographs and usually lies between the distal colon and urinary bladder near the midline.

2. (D) May be indistinguishable from the small intestine, if normal, and sometimes may be indistinguishable from the small intestine if only mildly enlarged, provided that the small intestine contains gas.

3. (E) Fetal demise and uterine ischemia.

4. (E) All of the above.

5. (E) Fetus too large for maternal pelvic canal, fetus lodged in maternal pelvic canal, and fetus in a position so that it is blocking the entrance to (or is unlikely to pass through) the maternal pelvic canal.

6. (E) Migrate ventrally among the small intestinal loops, if enlarged, and may induce peritoneal fluid if malignant and there has been peritoneal seeding.

7. (E) None of the above.

8. (B) Are difficult or impossible to detect on survey radiographs, unless quite enlarged.

9. (D) Cannot be diagnosed on survey radiographs and is best defined using a combination of history of acute pain, symmetric testicular enlargement at palpation, and, if available, Doppler ultrasonography to assess blood flow.

10. (E) None of the above.

Chapter 44 • The Stomach

1. (B) Manual restraint is preferred if possible for routine gastrography to avoid effects on the stomach induced by chemical restraint drugs.

2. (D) The right lateral recumbent view and the dorsoventral view made in ventral recumbency both place the pyloric portion of the stomach in a dependent position and thus best allow filling of the pyloric antrum with liquid contrast medium.

3. (D) Although at 40 minutes there is a slight delay in initiation of gastric emptying, the stomach then proceeds to empty in a normal manner. The technical procedure used in initiating the study most likely accounts for the initial delay through psychic factors. Thus, the initial delay is of doubtful significance.

4. (B) Routine gastrography is preferably performed with liquid barium sulfate. Most water-soluble, organic, iodinated contrast media formulated for the alimentary tract can induce adverse physiologic effects. Newer iodinated contrast media of lower osmolality are expensive for routine gastrography.

5. (D) The sequence is as follows: right lateral, left lateral, dorsoventral, and ventrodorsal. In right lateral recumbency, the liquid barium sulfate fills the dependent pyloric portion of the stomach, and gas rises to the fundus. In left lateral recumbency, the liquid barium sulfate fills the dependent fundus and body, and gas rises to the pyloric portion of the stomach. In the dorsoventral view in ventral recumbency, the liquid barium sulfate fills the dependent pyloric portion of the stomach, and gas rises to the fundus. In the ventrodorsal view in dorsal recumbency, the liquid barium fills the dependent fundic and pyloric portions of the stomach, and gas rises across the body of the stomach.

6. The stomach is greatly distended with gas and some fluid. In left recumbency (A), the gas outlines a round portion of the stomach representing the fundus and body of the stomach, but the pyloric portion of the stomach is not identified because it is filled with fluid. In right recumbency (B), gas rises to outline the pyloric portion of the stomach, which indicates that the pyloric portion of the stomach is located on the left side. Fluid shifts to more uniform distribution throughout the body and fundus of the stomach. The pylorus is displaced dorsally and to the left, and the fundus and body are displaced ventrally and to the right. Changes indicate gastric volvulus.

7. (A) The stomach is shifted in position such that the body and pylorus of the stomach are displaced caudally. This pattern of displacement is characteristic of hepatomegaly. The specific cause of the hepatomegaly is not identified.

8. (E) In this dog, the stomach has emptied little after 4.0 hours. A little of the contrast medium has exited the stomach, but the bulk of the contrast medium is retained in the stomach. Thus, gastric emptying is significantly delayed. There appears to be an annular restriction around the pyloric sphincter, but this is not confirmed on this one image. In this dog, changes were due to restrictive disease of the pyloric sphincter that was identified fluoroscopically and at surgery.

9. There is a large, round, sharply marginated filling defect within the pyloric antrum. At surgery, a large, round rubber ball was removed from the stomach.

10. There is an annular mural filling defect encircling the pyloric antrum. There is also an outpouching of luminal barium sulfate on the cranial surface of the annular filling defect. This outpouching is an ulcer that is located in the middle of the annular mass. The duodenum is located more dorsally than usual, but no significance was attached. Endoscopic evaluation of the stomach confirmed the ulcer, and surgery was performed. Final diagnosis was gastric adenocarcinoma with ulceration.

Chapter 45 • The Small Bowel

1. (B and C) Fat is essential for the contrast that allows visualization of intestinal serosal surfaces. Anything that severely reduces the amount of intraperitoneal fat (such as animals under 6 months of age and animals with severe weight loss) causes the bowel surfaces to be poorly defined. Additionally, peritoneal effusions and crowding of the bowel loops by space-occupying masses reduce bowel serosal delineation.

2. False. The string-of-pearls appearance of the duodenum is seen only in the normal cat, not the normal dog.

3. There is extensive dilation of the lumen of a focal portion of the intestinal tract. The diameter of the intestinal lumen is 4.5 to 6 times larger than the height of the central part of a lumbar vertebral body. These radiographic signs in a young dog with an acute history of vomiting and a palpable abdominal mass are most consistent with bowel obstruction (mechanical ileus). *Recom-*

mendation: Exploratory laparotomy. *Rationale:* Although the source and location of the obstructive disease cannot be determined with the available information, once the diagnosis of obstructive bowel disease has been made, the treatment is the same—surgical intervention. An intussusception was found at surgery.

4. Abnormal radiographic signs include focal site of irregular, thumbprint mucosa/barium interface with narrowed bowel lumen in the midportion of the descending duodenum. The remainder of the small intestine as seen on these images is unremarkable. The apple-core appearance of the duodenal lesion is seen most frequently with abnormalities that originate in the bowel wall and produce ulceration of the mucosa. Possible causes include primary intestinal neoplasia; bowel ulceration secondary to mast cell tumors, uremia, hepatic disorders, or recurrent pancreatitis; or granuloma. The diagnosis was bowel carcinoma.

5. There is a generalized, mild distention of the stomach and small intestinal tract with air. Portions of the colon are also air filled. This appearance is most consistent with functional ileus, which may be caused by bacterial or viral enteritis, abdominal pain, use of anticholinergic drugs, or malabsorption. Further work-up indicated recent seroconversion to feline immunodeficiency virus–positive status. Presumptive diagnosis was bacterial or viral enteritis secondary to immune suppression associated with feline immunodeficiency virus.

6. Passage of barium through the stomach and small intestinal segments is abnormally slow. In a normal cat, the stomach should be empty of barium by 1 hour postadministration. By 3 hours, the stomach and small bowel should both be empty, with the remaining barium located in the colon. Delayed contrast passage could be due to recent administration of parasympathomimetic drugs, inadequate volume of barium (either through underdosing or patient vomiting), or functional ileus. In this cat, barium volume was adequate, and no inhibitory drugs had been given. Radiographic diagnosis was functional ileus. The cat was euthanized; necropsy diagnosis was granulomatous (noneffusive) feline infectious peritonitis.

7. Administration of an inadequate volume of barium at the beginning of the study. If the patient vomits the contrast medium, redosing can often be accomplished without subsequent bouts of vomiting.

8. Mechanical obstruction of the intestine could show no radiographic signs on survey radiographs if (A) the obstruction is only partial; (B) the obstructing object is radiolucent and located in the proximal duodenum. Any air or fluid accumulating proximal to this site will be evacuated by vomiting.

9. Radiographic signs:
   A. Shape of the filling defects—if round, likely to be air bubbles; if elliptical, likely to be ingesta such as rice.
   B. Other abnormal radiographic signs increase the possibility that the filling defects are pathologic (i.e., lumen distention, irregular mucosa, or abnormal location of the affected bowel segment).

10. True. Either palpation or ultrasonography would be more accurate to determine bowel wall thickness than survey abdominal radiographs.

Chapter 46 • The Large Bowel

1. (D) Mesenteric arteriography.
2. False.
3. (A) Withhold water for 8 to 12 hours.
4. True.
5. (D) Double contrast study.
6. (A) Distended urinary bladder.
7. (A) Tumor.
8. (C) Old pelvic fractures with malunion and secondary narrowing of the descending colon.
9. (C) Partial obstruction of the descending colon secondary to previous trauma.
10. (A) Normal feline cecum and ascending colon.

Index

Note: Page numbers in *italics* refer to illustrations; page numbers followed by t refer to tables.